AACN Essentials of Progressive Care Nursing
Fourth Edition

Suzanne M. Burns, MSN, ACNP-BC, CCRN, RRT, FAAN, FCCM, FAANP
Professor Emerita, School of Nursing
University of Virginia
Charlottesville, Virginia

Sarah A. Delgado, MSN, RN, ACNP-BC
Clinical Practice Specialist
American Association of Critical-Care Nurses
Aliso Viejo, California

Mc
Graw
Hill
Education

New York   Chicago   San Francisco   Athens   London   Madrid   Mexico City
Milan   New Delhi   Singapore   Sydney   Toronto

1 2 3 4 5 6 7 8 9   LWI   23 22 21 20 19 18

ISBN 978-1-260-11673-1
MHID 1-260-11673-5

NOTICE

Medicine is an ever-changing science. As new research and clinical experience broaden our knowledge, changes in treatment and drug therapy are required. The authors and the publisher of this work have checked with sources believed to be reliable in their efforts to provide information that is complete and generally in accord with the standards accepted at the time of publication. However, in view of the possibility of human error or changes in medical sciences, neither the authors nor the publisher nor any other party who has been involved in the preparation or publication of this work warrants that the information contained herein is in every respect accurate or complete, and they disclaim all responsibility for any errors or omissions or for the results obtained from use of the information contained in this work. Readers are encouraged to confirm the information contained herein with other sources. For example and in particular, readers are advised to check the product information sheet included in the package of each drug they plan to administer to be certain that the information contained in this work is accurate and that changes have not been made in the recommended dose or in the contraindications for administration. This recommendation is of particular importance in connection with new or infrequently used drugs.

This book was set in Minion Pro by Cenveo® Publisher Services.
The editors were Susan Barnes and Christina M. Thomas.
The production supervisor was Richard Ruzycka.
Project management was provided by Surbhi Mittal, Cenveo Publisher Services.
The cover designer was W2 Design.

This book is printed on acid-free paper.

Library of Congress Cataloging-in-Publication Data

Names: Burns, Suzanne M., author. | Delgado, Sarah A., author.
Title: AACN essentials of progressive care nursing / Suzanne M. Burns, Sarah
  Delgado.
Other titles: Essentials of progressive care nursing
Description: Fourth edition. | New York : McGraw-Hill, [2018] | Includes
  bibliographical references and index.
Identifiers: LCCN 2018040692| ISBN 9781260116731 (paperback) | ISBN
  1260116735 (paperback)
Subjects: LCSH: Progressive patient care. | Nursing. | BISAC: MEDICAL /
  Nursing / Psychiatric.
Classification: LCC RT120.I5 A167 2018 | DDC 610.73—dc23

*To our progressive care nursing colleagues around the world
whose wonderful work and efforts ensure the safe passage of patients
through the progressive care environment. Your knowledge, skills, and care are what make
a positive difference in the outcomes of our patients and families. We humbly and sincerely
thank you for your commitment to providing excellent patient care.*

Suzi Burns and Sarah Delgado

Contents

Contents in Detail

Contributors

Earnest Alexander, PharmD, FCCM
Assistant Director, Clinical Pharmacy Services
Program Director, PGY2 Critical Care Residency
Department of Pharmacy Services
Tampa General Hospital
Tampa, Florida
Chapter 7: Pharmacology
Chapter 22: Pharmacology Tables

Suzanne M. Burns, MSN, ACNP-BC, CCRN, RRT, FAAN, FCCM, FAANP
Professor Emerita, School of Nursing
University of Virginia
Charlottesville, Virginia
Chapter 21: Normal Laboratory Reference Values

Jie Chen, MSN, RN, ACNP-BC, CMSRN
Advanced Practice Nurse
Abdominal Solid Organ Transplant Program
University of Virginia Health System
Charlottesville, Virginia
Chapter 15: Renal System

Yvonne D'Arcy, MS, CRNP, CNS, FAANP
Pain Management and Palliative Care Nurse Practitioner
Consultant: Pain management and education
Ponte Vedra Beach, Florida
Chapter 6: Pain and Sedation Management

Sarah A. Delgado, MSN, RN, ACNP-BC
Clinical Practice Specialist
American Association of Critical-Care Nurses
Aliso Viejo, California
Chapter 8: Ethical and Legal Considerations
Chapter 21: Normal Laboratory Reference Values

Diane K. Dressler, MSN, RN, CCRN
Clinical Assistant Professor
College of Nursing
Marquette University
Milwaukee, Wisconsin
Chapter 13: Hematologic and Immune Systems

Julie Grishaw, MSN, RN, CCRN, ACNP-C
Acute Care Nurse Practitioner-MICU
University of Virginia
Charlottesville, Virginia
Chapter 11: Multisystem Problems

Benjamin W. Hughes, RN, MSN, MS
Director of Clinical Operations
Neurology
University of Louisville
School of Medicine
Louisville, Kentucky
Chapter 17: Trauma

Carol Jacobson, MN, RN
Partner, Cardiovascular Nursing Education Associates
Burien, Washington
Chapter 3: Interpretation and Management of Basic Cardiac Rhythms
Chapter 18: Advanced ECG Concepts
Chapter 23: Cardiac Rhythms, ECG Characteristics, and Treatment Guide

Robert E. St. John, MSN, RN, RRT
Clinical Director—US Patient Monitoring and Recovery
Medtronic
Nellcor, Microstream, BIS, INVOS
Ballwin, Missouri
Chapter 5: Airway and Ventilatory Management

Sara Knippa, MS, RN, ACCNS-AG, CCRN, PCCN
Clinical Nurse Specialist/Educator, Cardiac ICU and ICU
   Educator Supervisor
Professional Development
University of Colorado Hospital
Aurora, Colorado
Chapter 6: Pain and Sedation Management

Barbara Leeper, MN, RN-BC, CNS M-S, CCRN, FAHA
Clinical Nurse Specialist
Cardiovascular Services
Baylor University Medical Center at Dallas
Dallas, Texas
Chapter 9: Cardiovascular System
Chapter 19: Advanced Cardiovascular Concepts

Mary E. Lough, PhD RN, CCNS, FCCM
Nurse Scientist; Clinical Nurse Specialist
Office of Patient Care Research
Stanford Health Care
Stanford, California
Chapter 16: Endocrine System

**Leanna R. Miller, MN, RN, CCRN-CMC, PCCN-CSC,
   CEN, CNRN, NP**
Instructor of Nursing
Western Kentucky University
Bowling Green, Kentucky
Chapter 4: Hemodynamic Monitoring

DaiWai M. Olson, PhD, RN, CCRN FNCS
Associate Professor
Department of Neurology and Neurotherapeutics
University of Texas Southwestern
Dallas, Texas
Chapter 12: Neurological System
Chapter 20: Advanced Neurologic Concepts

Beth Quatrara, DNP, RN, CMSRN, ACNS-BC
Advanced Practice Nurse 3-Clinical Nurse Specialist
Director of Nursing Research and Clinical Assistant
   Professor
University of Virginia Health System
Charlottesville, Virginia
Chapter 14: Gastrointestinal System

**Maureen A. Seckel, MSN, APRN, ACNS-BC, CCNS,
   CCRN, FCCM**
Lead Critical Care Clinical Nurse Specialist and
   Sepsis Leader
Medical Intensive Care Unit and Department of Medicine
Christiana Care Health Services,
Newark, Delaware
Chapter 5: Airway and Ventilatory Management
Chapter 10: Respiratory System

Kathrina Siaron, BSN-RN
Staff RN- Neurosurgical ICU
UT Southwestern Medical Center, Zale Lipshy
   University Hospital
Dallas, Texas
Chapter 12: Neurological System
Chapter 20: Advanced Neurologic Concepts

Mary Fran Tracy, PhD, RN, APRN, CNS, FAAN
Associate Professor, University of Minnesota School
   of Nursing
Nurse Scientist, University of Minnesota Medical Center
Minneapolis, Minnesota
*Chapter 1: Assessment of Progressive Care Patients and
   Their Families*
*Chapter 2: Planning Care for Progressive Care Patients and
   Their Families*

**Allen C. Wolfe Jr., MSN, CNS, APRN, CFRN, CCRN,
   CTRN, CMTE**
Director of Clinical Education/Critical Care
   Clinical Specialist
Clinical Education
Air Methods
Aurora, Colorado
Chapter 17: Trauma

Reviewers

Thomas Ahrens, DNS, RN, CCNS, FAAN
Chief Learning Officer
NovEX, Novice to Expert
St Louis, Missouri

Staccie Anne Allen, DNP, MSN, BSBA, ARNP, EMT-P,
A-G ACNP, PM-FNP, CFRN
Flight Nurse Practitioner/Paramedic
Emergency Nurse Practitioner
Department of Emergency Medicine
University of Florida Health Shands Hospital
Gainesville, Florida

Richard Arbour, MSN, RN, CCRN, CNRN, CCNS, CCTC,
FAAN, FCCM
Neuroscience/Critical Care Clinical Nurse Specialist
Lancaster General Health/Penn Medicine
Lancaster, Pennsylvania

Kwame Asante Akuamoah-Boateng, MSN, RN, ACNP-BC
Lead APP Acute Care Surgical Services Division
Virginia Commonwealth University Health-Surgical
Trauma Intensive Care
Richmond, Virginia

Pamela S. Anderson, MS, ANP-BC, RN, CCRN
Adult NP-Vascular Surgery St. Vincent Medical Group
Staff Nurse, ICU
Tipton Hospital
Tipton, Indiana

Carla Aresco, MSN, RN, CRNP
Senior Lead Nurse Practitioner
University of Maryland R Adams Cowley Shock Trauma
Center, Trauma Neurosurgery, APMS, Multitrauma
Critical Care and Critical Care Resuscitation Unit
Baltimore, Maryland

Deborah Becker, PhD, ACNP, BC, CHSE, FAAN
Practice Professor of Nursing
Director, Adult Gerontology ACNP, Streamlined Post MSN
Adult Gero NP
Adult Gerontology CNS and Adult Oncology
Minor Programs
Director, Helene Fuld Pavilion for Innovative Learning
and Simulation
University of Pennsylvania, School of Nursing
Philadelphia, Pennsylvania

Elida Benitez, DNP, AG-ACNP
Advance Practice Provider
UF Health, Department of Surgery, Surgical, Trauma,
and Cardiothoracic ICUs
Gainesville, Florida

Nancy P. Blumenthal, DNP, ACNP-BC, CCTC
Director of Clinical Practice & Senior Nurse Practitioner
Lung Transplant Program
Hospital of the University of Pennsylvania
Philadelphia, Pennsylvania

Steven W. Branham, PhD, ACNP-BC, FNP-BC, FAANP,
CCRN
Associate Professor of Nursing
Texas Tech Health Sciences Center School of Nursing
Lubbock, Texas

Elizabeth Bridges, PhD, RN, CCNS, FCCM, FAAN
Professor-University of Washington School of Nursing,
Seattle, Washington
Clinical Nurse Researcher
University of Washington Medical Center
Seattle, Washington

Beth Epstein, PhD, RN, FAAN
Associate Professor & Chair
Department of Acute and Specialty Care
University of Virginia School of Nursing and
    Associate Professor
Center for Biomedical Ethics and Humanities
University of Virginia School of Nursing
Charlottesville, Virginia

Charles A. Fisher, MSN, RN, ACNP-BC
APN 1 Medical ICU and Medical units
University of Virginia Health System
Charlottesville, Virginia

Elizabeth Good, MSN, RN, ACNS-BC, ACNP-BC
Nurse Practitioner - Surgical Oncology
University of Virginia Health System
Emily Couric Clinical Cancer Center
Charlottesville, Virginia

Vicki S. Good, DNP RN CPHQ CPPS
Vice President of Quality/Safety
Mercy Hospital
Springfield, Missouri

Tonja Hartjes, DNP, ACNP/FNP-BC, CCRN-CSC, FAANP
Clinical Associate Professor, Adult-Gerontology Acute
    Care DNP Track Coordinator
University of Florida
Gainesville, Florida

Shannon Hilton, DNP, ANP-BC, ACNS-BC
Adult Nurse Practitioner, Adult Clinical Nurse Specialist
The Alaska Hospitalist Group, Intensive Care Unit
Anchorage, Alaska

**Randall Steven Hudspeth, PhD, MBA, MS, APRN-CNP/
    CNS, FRE, FAANP**
Clinical Practice Consultant, Pain Management and
    Substance Use Disorder
Retired: Saint Alphonsus Health System, Program Director
    Pain Management/Palliative Care
Boise, Idaho

Deborah Kiley, DNP, NP-C, FNP-BC, FAANP, FNAP
Nurse Practitioner
Alaska Center for Pain Management and Fearless
    Wellness LLC
Anchorage, Alaska

**Deborah Klein, MSN, APRN, ACNS-BC, CCRN,
    CHFN, FAHA**
Clinical Nurse Specialist
Cleveland Clinic
Coronary ICU, Heart Failure ICU, Cardiac Short Stay/
    PACU/CARU
Cleveland, Ohio

JoAnne Konick-McMahan, MSN, RN, PCCN
Certification Practice Specialist
AACN Certification Corporation
Aliso Viejo, California
Staff Nurse, Intermediate and Respiratory Care Unit
UPMC Pinnacle Health System
Harrisburg, Pennsylvania

Donna Lester, DNP, MS, ACNP-BC, CC-CNS
Clinical Assistant Professor at the University of Florida
Adjunct Faculty at Georgetown University
Acute Care Nurse Practitioner: Cardiothoracic and
    Vascular Surgery
Lakeland Regional Health
Lakeland, Florida

Donna W. Markey, MSN, RN, ACNP-BC
Nurse Practitioner, Hematology/Oncology
Augusta Health Cancer Center
Fishersville, Virginia

Matthew Morrisette, PharmD
Critical Care Pharmacy Specialist
Thoracic and Cardiovascular Surgical Intensive Care Unit
University of Virginia Health System
Charlottesville, Virginia

Wendy Phillips, MS, RD, CNSC, CLE, FAND
Division Director of Clinical Nutrition
Morrison Healthcare
St. George, Utah

Karah Cripe Sickler, DNP, AGACNP-BC
Adult Gerontology Acute Care Nurse Practitioner
UF Health, Surgical Critical Care
Gainesville, Florida

Chrissie Shirley, PharmD, MPH
Clinical Pharmacist, Critical Care
University of Virginia Health System
Charlottesville, Virginia

Mary A. Stahl, MSN, RN, CCNS, CCRN-K
Clinical Practice Specialist
American Association of Critical Care Nurses, Practice
    Excellence
Aliso Viejo, California

**Terri Townsend, MA, RN, CCRN-CMC, CVRN-BC,
    CMSRN**
Clinical Educator
Cardiovascular and Outpatient Services
Community Hospital Anderson
Anderson, Indiana

Maxine V. Wanzer, MSN, AGACNP-BC, CCRN
Advanced Practice Provider
Ohio Health, MICU
Columbus, Ohio

Preface

Progressive care nursing is a complex, challenging area of nursing practice where clinical expertise is developed over time by integrating progressive care knowledge, clinical skills, and caring practices. This textbook, the first to specifically address the educational needs of the progressive care nurse, succinctly presents essential information about how best to safely and competently care for acutely ill patients and their families.

As it has since the first edition, the American Association of Critical-Care Nurses reaffirms this book's value to the AACN community and especially to clinicians at the point of care. The title continues to carry AACN's name, as it has since the first edition.

AACN Essentials of Progressive Care Nursing provides essential information on the care of adult acutely ill patients and families. The book recognizes the learner's need to assimilate foundational knowledge before attempting to master more complex progressive care nursing concepts. Written by nationally acknowledged clinical experts in critical and progressive care nursing, this textbook sets the standard for progressive care nursing education.

AACN Essentials of Progressive Care Nursing:

- Succinctly presents essential information for the safe and competent care of progressive care patients and their families, building on the clinician's significant medical-surgical nursing knowledge base, avoiding repetition of previously acquired information
- Stages the introduction of advanced concepts in progressive care nursing after essential concepts have been mastered
- Provides clinicians with clinically relevant tools and guides to use as they care for progressive care patients and families
- Includes principles of management to summarize key concepts and case studies to demonstrate their application

The AACN Essentials of Progressive Care Nursing is divided into four parts:

- **Part I: The Essentials** presents essential information that clinicians must understand to provide safe, competent nursing care to the majority of progressive care patients, regardless of their underlying medical diagnoses. This part includes content on assessment, diagnosis, planning, and interventions common to progressive care patients and families; interpretation and management of cardiac rhythms; hemodynamic monitoring; airway and ventilatory management; pain and sedation management; pharmacology; and ethical and legal considerations. Chapters in Part I present content in enough depth to ensure that essential information is available for the new progressive care clinician to develop competence, while sequencing pathological conditions in Part II and advanced content in a later part of the book (Part III).
- **Part II: Pathologic Conditions** covers pathologic conditions and management strategies commonly encountered in progressive care, closely paralleling the blueprint for the PCCN certification examination. Chapters in this part are organized by body systems and selected progressive care conditions (cardiovascular, respiratory, multisystem, neurologic, hematologic and immune, gastrointestinal, renal, endocrine, and trauma).
- **Part III: Advanced Concepts** presents advanced progressive care concepts or pathologic conditions that are more complex and represent expert level information. Specific advanced chapter content includes ECG, cardiovascular, and neurologic concepts.
- **Part IV: Key Reference Information** contains selected reference information that clinicians will find helpful in the clinical area (normal laboratory and diagnostic values; cardiac rhythms, ECG characteristics and

treatment guide and summary tables of progressive care medications). Content in part IV is presented primarily in table format for quick reference.

Each chapter in Part I, II, and III, begins with "Knowledge Competencies" that can be used to guide informal or formal teaching and to gauge the learner's progress. In addition, each of the chapters provide "Essential Content Case" studies that focus on key information presented in the chapters in order to assist clinicians in understanding the chapter content and how to best assess and manage conditions and problems encountered in progressive care. The case studies also are designed to enhance the learners understanding of the magnitude of the pathologic problems/conditions and their impact on patients and families. Questions and answers are provided for each case so learners may test their knowledge of the essential content.

We believe that there is no greater way to protect our patients than to ensure that an educated clinician cares for them. Competent, skilled, knowledgeable, and caring clinicians ensure safe passage in progressive care. We sincerely believe that this textbook will help you make it so! Thank you!

Suzi Burns and Sarah Delgado

ACKNOWLEDGMENTS

Special thanks to those who made contributions to the previous editions of both the *Essentials of Critical Care Nursing* and the *Essentials of Progressive Care Nursing*.

To Cathie Guzzetta, PhD, RN, FAAN and Barbara Dossey, MS, RN, FAAN for their early work in creating the *Handbook of Critical Care Nursing* which preceded the *Essentials of Critical Care Nursing* and the *Essentials of Progressive Care Nursing* books.

To Marianne Chulay, PhD, RN, FAAN, for her many contributions and mentoring during the development of the first two editions of the *Essentials of Critical Care Nursing* and the *Essentials of Progressive Care Nursing* books.

Thank you to the many authors for their past contributions:

Tom Ahrens, DNS, RN, CCNS, FAAN (Chapter 4 and key reference materials)
Sue Simmons-Alling, MSN, RN (Chapter 2)
Deborah A. Andris, MSN, APNP (Chapter 14)
Suzanne M. Burns, MSN, RN, RRT, ACNP, CCRN, FAAN, FCCM, FAANP (Chapters 4, 5, 6, 10, 11, 22)
Deb Byram, MS, RN (Chapter 1)
Karen Carlson, MN, RN (Chapter 15)
Joan Michiko Ching, MN, RN, CPHQ (Chapter 6)
Marianne Chulay, PhD, RN, FAAN (Chapter 10, and the key reference materials)
Maria Connolly, DNSc, RN (Chapters 5, 10)

Dorrie Fontaine, DNSc, RN, FAAN (Chapter 17)
Bradi Granger, PhD, RN (Chapter 9)
Anne Marie Gregoire, MSN, RN, CRNP (Chapter 19)
Carol Hinkle, MSN, RN (Chapter 15)
Christine Kessler, MN, RN, CNS, ANP-BC, ADM-BC (Chapter 16)
Ruth Kleinpell, PhD, RN, ACNP, FAAN, FCCM, FAANP (Chapter 11)
Joe Krenitsky, MS, RD (Chapter 14)
Joanne Krumberger, MSN, RN, CHE, FAAN (Chapters 14, 16)
Elizabeth Krzywda, MSN, RN, APNP (Chapter 14)
Dea Mahanes, MSN, RN, CCRN, CNRN, CCNS (12, 20)
Sally Miller, PhD, RN, APN, FAANP (Chapter 14)
Carol Rees Parrish, MS, RD (Chapter 14)
Carol A. Rauen, MS, RN, CCNS, CCRN, PCCN (Chapter 17)
Juanita Reigle, MSN, RN, ACNP (Chapter 8)
Anita Sherer, MSN, RN (Chapter 2)
Jamie Sinks, MS, RN (Chapter 17)
Greg Susla, PharmD, FCCM (Chapters 7 and key reference materials)
Debbie Tribett, MS, RN, CS, LNP (Chapter 13)
Debra Lynn-McHale Wiegand, PhD, RN, CS (Chapter 19)
Lorie Wild, PhD, RN (Chapter 6)
Susan Woods, PhD, RN (Chapters 3, 18)
Marlene Yate, MSN, RN (Chapter 2)

THE ESSENTIALS

I

Assessment of Progressive Care Patients and Their Families

1

Mary Fran Tracy

KNOWLEDGE COMPETENCIES

1. Discuss the importance of a consistent and systematic approach to assessment of progressive care patients and their families.
2. Identify the assessment priorities for different stages of an acute illness:
   • Prearrival assessment
   • Arrival quick check

• Comprehensive initial assessment
• Ongoing assessment
3. Describe how the assessment is altered based on the patient's clinical status.

The assessment of acutely ill patients and their families is an essential competency for progressive care nurses. Information obtained from an assessment identifies the immediate and future needs of the patient and family so a plan of care can be initiated to address or resolve these needs.

Traditional approaches to patient assessment include a complete evaluation of the patient's history and a comprehensive physical examination of all body systems. This approach is ideal, though progressive care clinicians must balance the need to gather data while simultaneously prioritizing and providing care to acutely ill patients. Traditional approaches and techniques for assessment are modified in progressive care to balance the need for information, while considering the acute nature of the patient and family's situation.

This chapter outlines an assessment approach that recognizes the dynamic nature of an acute illness. This approach emphasizes the collection of assessment data in a phased or staged manner consistent with patient care priorities. The components of the assessment can be used as a generic template for assessing most progressive care patients and families. The assessment can then be individualized based on the patient's diagnosis. These specific components of the assessment are identified in subsequent chapters.

Crucial to developing competence in assessing progressive care patients and their families is a consistent and systematic approach. Without this approach, it would be easy to miss subtle signs or details that may identify an actual or potential problem and also indicate a patient's changing status. Assessments focus first on the patient, then on the technology. The patient is the focal point of the progressive care practitioner's attention, with technology augmenting the information obtained from the direct assessment.

There are two standard approaches to assessing patients—the head-to-toe approach and the body systems approach. Most progressive care nurses use a combination—a systems approach applied in a top-to-bottom manner. The admission and ongoing assessment sections of this chapter are presented with this combined approach in mind.

ASSESSMENT FRAMEWORK

Assessing the progressive care patient and family begins from the moment the nurse is aware of the pending admission or transfer and continues until transitioning to the next phase of care. The assessment process can be viewed as four distinct stages: (1) prearrival, (2) arrival quick check ("just the basics"), (3) comprehensive initial assessment, and (4) ongoing assessment.

Prearrival Assessment

Patients admitted to a progressive care unit may be transitioning from a more intensive level of care, as they become more stable and improve in condition. Conversely, they may be transferred from a less acute level of care, because their physiologic status may be deteriorating. In either case, the progressive care patient has the potential to have a rapid change in status. A prearrival assessment begins the moment the information is received about the upcoming admission of the patient to the progressive care unit. This notification comes from the initial healthcare team contact. The contact may be a transfer from another facility or a transfer from other areas within the hospital such as the emergency room, operating room, the intensive care unit (ICU), or medical/surgical nursing unit. The prearrival assessment paints the initial picture of the patient and allows the progressive care nurse to begin anticipating the patient's physiologic and psychological needs. This assessment also allows the progressive care nurse to determine the appropriate resources that are needed to care for the patient. The information received in the prearrival phase is crucial because it allows the progressive care nurse to adequately prepare the environment to meet the specialized needs of the patient and family.

Arrival Quick Check

An arrival quick check assessment is obtained immediately upon arrival and is based on assessing the parameters represented by the ABCDE acronym (Table 1-1). The arrival quick check assessment is a quick overview of the adequacy of ventilation and perfusion to ensure early intervention for any life-threatening situations. This assessment is a high-level view of the patient but is essential because it validates that basic cardiac and respiratory function is sufficient, and it can be used as a baseline for potential future changes in a condition.

Comprehensive Initial Assessment

A comprehensive assessment is performed as soon as possible, with the timing dictated by the degree of physiologic stability and emergent treatment needs of the patient. If the patient is being admitted directly to the progressive care unit from outside the hospital, the comprehensive assessment is an in-depth assessment of the past medical and social history and

TABLE 1-1. ABCDE ACRONYM

*A*irway
*B*reathing
*C*irculation, *C*erebral perfusion, and *C*hief complaint
*D*rugs and *D*iagnostic tests
*E*quipment

a complete physical examination of each body system. If the patient is being transferred to the progressive care unit from another area in the hospital, the comprehensive assessment includes a review of the admission assessment data and comparison to the current assessment of the patient. The comprehensive assessment is vital to successful outcomes because it provides insight into which proactive interventions are needed.

Ongoing Assessment

After the baseline comprehensive assessment is completed, ongoing assessments—an abbreviated version of the comprehensive assessment—are performed at varying intervals. The assessment parameters outlined in this section are usually completed for all patients, in addition to other ongoing assessment requirements related to the patient's specific condition, treatments, and response to therapy.

Patient Safety Considerations in Admission Assessments

Admission of an acutely ill patient can be a chaotic event with multiple disciplines involved in many activities. It is at this time, however, that healthcare providers are particularly cognizant of accurate assessments and data gathering to ensure the patient is cared for safely with appropriate interventions. Obtaining inaccurate information on admission can lead to ongoing errors that may not be easily rectified or discovered and lead to poor patient outcomes.

Obtaining information from an acutely ill patient may be difficult, if possible at all. If the patient is unable to supply information, other sources are utilized such as family members, electronic health records (EHRs), past medical records, transport records, or information from the patient's belongings. Of particular importance at admission is obtaining accurate patient identification, as well as past medical history and any known allergies. Obtaining current medication regimens as soon as possible is essential, as they can provide clues to the patient's medical condition and any potential contributing factors to the current condition, and ensures medication reconciliation to continue appropriate medications and avoid medication interactions. With the use of EHRs, there are opportunities for timely access to past and current medical history information of patients. Healthcare providers may have access to both inpatient and outpatient records within the same healthcare system, assisting them to quickly identify the patient's most recent medication regimen and laboratory and diagnostic results. In addition, healthcare systems within the same geographic locations may offer intersystem access to the medical records of patients treated at multiple healthcare institutions. This is particularly beneficial when patients are unable to articulate essential medical information including advance directives, allergies, and next of kin.

Careful physical assessment on admission to the progressive care unit is pivotal for the prevention and/or early treatment for complications associated with the illness. Of particular importance is the assessment of risk for pressure injury, alteration in mental status, infection, and/or falls. Risks associated with accurate patient identification never lessen, particularly as these relate to interventions such as performing invasive procedures, medication administration, blood administration, and obtaining laboratory tests. Nurses need to be cognizant of safety issues as treatment begins as well; for example, accurate programming of pumps infusing high-risk medications is essential. It is imperative that nurses use all safety equipment available to them such as pre-programmed drug libraries in infusion pumps and bar-coding technology. Healthcare providers also ensure the safety of invasive procedures that may be performed emergently.

PREARRIVAL ASSESSMENT: BEFORE THE ACTION BEGINS

A prearrival assessment begins when information is received about the pending arrival of the patient. The prearrival report, although abbreviated, provides key information about the chief complaint, diagnosis, or reason for admission, pertinent history details, and physiologic stability of the patient (Table 1-2). It also contains the gender and age of the patient and information on the presence of invasive tubes and lines, medications

TABLE 1-2. SUMMARY OF PREARRIVAL AND ARRIVAL QUICK CHECK ASSESSMENTS

Prearrival Assessment
- Abbreviated report on patient (age, gender, chief complaint, diagnosis, allergies pertinent history, physiologic status, invasive devices, equipment, and status of laboratory/diagnostic tests)
- Complete room setup, including verification of proper equipment functioning
- Do Not Resuscitate (DNR) status
- Isolation status

Admission Quick Check Assessment
- General appearance (consciousness)
- *Airway*:
  Patency
  Position of artificial airway (if present) such as tracheostomy
- *Breathing*:
  Quantity and quality of respirations (rate, depth, pattern, symmetry, effort—use of accessory muscles)
  Breath sounds
  Presence of spontaneous breathing
- *Circulation and Cerebral Perfusion*:
  Electrocardiogram (ECG) (rate, rhythm, and presence of ectopy)
  Blood pressure
  Peripheral pulses
  Capillary refill
  Skin color, temperature, moisture
  Presence of bleeding
  Level of consciousness, responsiveness
- *Chief Complaint*:
  Primary body system
  Associated symptoms
- *Drugs and Diagnostic Tests*:
  Drugs prior to admission (prescribed, over-the-counter, illicit)
  Current medications
  Review diagnostic test results
- *Equipment*:
  Patency of vascular and drainage systems
  Appropriate functioning and labeling of all equipment connected to patient

TABLE 1-3. EQUIPMENT FOR STANDARD ROOM SETUP

- Bedside ECG or telemetry monitoring and invasive pressure monitor with appropriate cables
- ECG electrodes
- Blood pressure cuff
- Pulse oximetry
- End-tidal CO_2
- Thermometer
- Suction gauges and canister setup
- Suction catheters
- Bag valve mask device
- Oxygen flow meter, appropriate tubing, and appropriate oxygen delivery device
- IV poles and infusion pumps
- Bedside supplies to include alcohol swabs, non-sterile gloves, syringes, bed pads, and dressing supplies
- Admission kit that usually contains bath basin and general hygiene supplies (if direct admission)
- Bedside computer and/or paper admission documentation forms

being administered, other ongoing treatments, and pending or completed laboratory or diagnostic tests. This basic information may indicate a need to consider whether the patient will need a specialty bed such as a bariatric bed or a bed to optimize skin integrity. Determining this in advance is helpful as it may take time to acquire a specialty bed. It is also important to consider the potential isolation requirements for the patient, including neutropenic precautions, contact precautions, or special respiratory isolation. Being prepared for isolation needs prevents potentially serious exposures to the patient, roommates, or the healthcare providers. This information assists the clinician in anticipating the patient's physiologic and emotional needs prior to admission or transfer and in ensuring that the bedside environment is set up to provide all monitoring, supply, and equipment needs prior to the patient's arrival.

Many progressive care units have a standard room setup, guided by the major diagnosis-related groups of patients each unit receives. The standard monitoring and equipment list for each unit varies; however, there are certain common requirements (Table 1-3). The standard room setup is modified for each admission to accommodate patient-specific needs (eg, additional equipment, intravenous [IV] fluids, medications). Proper functioning of all bedside equipment is verified prior to the patient's arrival.

It is also important to prepare the medical record forms, which usually consist of a computerized data entry system or paper flow sheets to record vital signs, intake and output, medication administration, patient care activities, and patient assessment. The prearrival report may suggest pending procedures, necessitating the organization of appropriate supplies at the bedside. Having the room prepared and all equipment available facilitates a rapid, smooth, and safe admission of the patient.

ADMISSION QUICK CHECK ASSESSMENT

From the moment the patient arrives in the progressive care unit setting, his or her general appearance is immediately observed and assessment of ABCDEs is quickly performed (see Table 1-1). The condition of the patient is determined so any urgent needs can be addressed first. The patient is connected to the appropriate monitoring and support equipment, medications being administered are verified, and essential laboratory and diagnostic tests are ordered. Simultaneously with the ABCDE assessment, the patient's nurse validates that the patient is appropriately identified through a hospital wristband, personal identification documents, or family identification. In addition, the patient's allergy status is verified, including the type of reaction that occurs and what, if any, treatment is used to alleviate the allergic response.

ESSENTIAL CONTENT CASE

Prearrival Assessment

The charge nurse notifies Sue that she will be receiving a 26-year-old man from the ICU who was involved in a serious car accident 14 days ago. The ICU nurse caring for the patient has called to give Sue a report following the hospital's standardized report format.

Case Question 1: What basic information will Sue want to know from the prearrival communication with the ICU nurse?

Case Question 2: What patient issues are likely to need immediate assessment and/or intervention on arrival to the progressive care unit in order to ensure the appropriate equipment is set up in the room?

Case Question 3: What information should be included in the more formal handoff between the ICU nurse and Sue after the patient is settled in his room in the progressive care unit?

Answers

1. Patient name/age, type and date of accident, extent of accident injuries, pertinent medical history, allergies, vital signs, placement of lines and tubes, medications being administered, significant laboratory results, anticipated plan for care and discharge plan, presence of family, and any other special instructions.

    The patient suffered a closed head injury and chest trauma with collapsed left lung. The patient had been intubated and placed on a mechanical ventilator. The patient had developed pneumonia when in the ICU, and though he now exhibited stable oxygenation, a tracheostomy was required to manage copious secretions. He had now been weaned off the ventilator and was requiring 30% Fio_2. A central line with a central venous pressure (CVP) setup and a left chest tube to water seal were in place. Sue questions the critical care nurse regarding whether the patient has been agitated, his level of consciousness (LOC) and neuro deficits, if a Foley catheter or nasogastric (NG) tube is present, and whether the family has been notified of the transfer to the progressive care unit.

2. Vital signs, neurologic status, the tracheostomy and oxygen requirements of the patient, medications are appropriately infusing, and whether the patient is agitated or experiencing extensive pain.

    Sue goes to check the patient's room prior to admission and begins to do a mental check of what will be needed. "The patient has a tracheostomy so I'll connect the AMBU bag to the oxygen source, check for suction catheters, and make sure the suction systems are working. The pulse oximeter is ready to use. I'll also ensure the telemetry pack has fully charged batteries and have the ECG electrodes ready to apply. The CVP line flush system and transducer are also ready to be connected. The IV infusion devices are set up. This patient has an altered LOC, which means frequent neuro checks. I have my penlight handy. The computer in the room is on and ready for me to begin documentation. I think I'm ready."

3. Using an SBAR (**S**ituation, **B**ackground, **A**ssessment, and **R**ecommendations) format, the ICU nurse can give more detailed information about the injuries from the car accident, the patient's complete medical history as known, reiteration of known allergies, a system by system assessment review, significant diagnostic test results, confirmation of all invasive lines and equipment settings, the anticipated plan for ongoing assessments, interventions, and discharge planning, and any pertinent family information. Sue can also clarify any remaining questions she might have.

There may be other healthcare professionals present to receive the patient and assist with arrival tasks. The progressive care nurse, however, is the leader of the receiving team. While assuming the primary responsibility for assessing the ABCDEs, the progressive care nurse directs the team in completing delegated tasks, such as changing over to the unit equipment or attaching monitoring cables. Without a leader, care can be fragmented and vital assessment clues overlooked.

The progressive care nurse rapidly assesses the ABCDEs in the sequence outlined in this section. If any aspect of this preliminary assessment deviates from normal, interventions are immediately initiated to address the problem before continuing with the arrival quick check assessment. Additionally, regardless of whether the patient appears to be conscious or not, it is important to talk to him or her throughout this admission process regarding what is occurring with each interaction and intervention.

Airway and Breathing

Patency of the patient's airway is verified by having the patient speak, watching the patient's chest rise or fall, or both. If the airway is compromised, verify that the head has been positioned properly to prevent the tongue from occluding the airway. Inspect the upper airway for the presence of blood, vomitus, and foreign objects before inserting an oral airway if indicated. If the patient already has an artificial airway, such as a cricothyrotomy or tracheostomy, ensure that the airway is secured properly. Note the position of the tracheostomy and size of the airway. Suctioning of the upper airway, either through the oral cavity or artificial airway, may be required to ensure that the airway is free from secretions. Note the amount, color, and consistency of secretions that are removed.

Assessment of the patient's breathing also includes observation of the rate, depth, pattern, and symmetry of breathing; the effort of breathing; the use of accessory muscles; and, if mechanically ventilated, whether breathing is in synchrony with the ventilator. Do not overlook nonverbal signs of respiratory distress including restlessness, anxiety, or change in mental status. Auscultate the chest for presence of bilateral breath sounds, quality of breath sounds, and bilateral chest expansion. Optimally, both anterior and posterior breath sounds are auscultated, but during this arrival quick check assessment, time generally dictates that just the anterior chest is assessed. If noninvasive oxygen saturation monitoring is available, observe and quickly analyze the values.

If chest tubes are present, note whether they are pleural or mediastinal chest tubes. Ensure that they are connected to suction, if appropriate, and are not clamped or kinked. In addition, assess whether the chest tubes are functioning properly (eg, air leak, fluid fluctuation with respirations) and the amount and character of the drainage.

Circulation and Cerebral Perfusion

The arrival quick check assessment of circulation includes quickly palpating a pulse and viewing the ECG monitor for the heart rate, rhythm, and presence of ectopy if ECG monitoring is ordered. Obtain blood pressure and temperature. Assess peripheral perfusion by evaluating the color, temperature, and moisture of the skin along with capillary refill. Based on the prearrival report and reason for admission, there may be a need to inspect the body for any signs of blood loss and determine if active bleeding is occurring.

Evaluating cerebral perfusion in the arrival quick check assessment is focused on determining the functional integrity of the brain as a whole, which is done by rapidly evaluating the gross LOC. Assess whether the patient is alert and oriented, aware of his or her surroundings, or whether a verbal or painful stimulus is required to obtain a response, or whether the patient is unresponsive. Observing the response of the patient during movement from the stretcher to the progressive care unit bed can supply additional information about the LOC. Note whether the patient's eyes are open and watching the events around him or her; for example, does the patient follow simple commands such as "Place your hands on your chest" or "Slide your hips over?" If the patient is unable to talk because of trauma or the presence of an artificial airway, note whether they nod appropriately to questions.

Chief Complaint

Optimally, the description of the chief complaint is obtained from the patient, but this may not be realistic. The patient may be unable to respond or may face a language barrier. Data may need to be gathered from family, friends, or bystanders, or from the completed admission database if the patient has been transferred from another area in the hospital. For patients who face a language barrier, an approved hospital translator or phone translating service can assist with the interview and subsequent evaluations and communication. Avoid asking family and friends to translate for the patient to protect the patient's privacy, avoid errors due to family not understanding appropriate medical terminology for translation, and to eliminate well-intentioned but potential bias in translating for the patient. In the absence of a history source, practitioners need to depend on the physical findings (eg, presence of medication patches, permanent pacemaker, or old surgery scars), knowledge of pathophysiology, access to prior electronic medical records (EMRs), and transport records to identify the potential causes of the admission.

Assessment of the chief complaint focuses on determining the body systems involved and the extent of associated symptoms. Additional questions explore the time of onset, precipitating factors, and severity. Although the arrival quick check phase is focused on obtaining a quick overview of the key life-sustaining systems, a more in-depth assessment of a particular system may need to be done at this time; for example, in the prearrival case study scenario presented, completion of the ABCDEs is followed quickly by more extensive assessment of both the nervous and respiratory systems.

Drugs and Diagnostic Tests

Information about infusing medications and diagnostic tests is integrated into the priority of the arrival quick check. If IV access is not already present, it is immediately obtained and intake and output records started. If IV medications are infusing, check the medication and verify the concentration and correct infusion of the desired dosage and rate.

Determine the latest results of any diagnostic tests already performed. Augment basic screening tests (Table 1-4) with additional tests appropriate to the underlying diagnosis, chief complaint, transfer status, and recent procedures. Review available laboratory or diagnostic data for abnormalities or indications of potential problems that may develop. The abnormal laboratory and diagnostic data for specific pathologic conditions will be covered in subsequent chapters.

TABLE 1-4. COMMON DIAGNOSTIC TESTS OBTAINED DURING ARRIVAL QUICK CHECK ASSESSMENT

Serum electrolytes
Glucose
Complete blood count with platelets
Coagulation studies
Chest x-ray
ECG

Equipment

The last phase of the arrival quick check is an assessment of the equipment in use. Quickly evaluate all vascular, feeding and drainage tubes for location and patency, and connect them to appropriate monitoring or suction devices. Note the amount, color, consistency, and odor of drainage secretions. Verify the appropriate functioning of all equipment attached to the patient and label as required. While connecting the monitoring and care equipment, it is important for the nurse to continue assessing the patient's respiratory and cardiovascular status until it is clear that all equipment is functioning appropriately and can be relied on to transmit accurate patient data.

The arrival quick check assessment is accomplished in a matter of a few minutes. After completion of the ABCDE assessment, the comprehensive assessment begins. If at any phase during the arrival quick check a component of the ABCDEs has not been stabilized and controlled, energy is focused first on resolving the abnormality before proceeding to the comprehensive admission assessment.

After the arrival quick check assessment is complete, and if the patient requires no urgent intervention, there may now be time for a more thorough report from the healthcare providers transferring the patient to the progressive care unit. Handoffs with transitions of care are intervals when safety gaps may occur. Omission of pertinent information or miscommunication at this critical juncture can result in patient care errors. Use of a standardized handoff format—such as the "SBAR" format, which includes communication of the **S**ituation, **B**ackground, **A**ssessment, and **R**ecommendations—can minimize the potential for miscommunication. Use the handoff as an opportunity to confirm observations such as dosage of infusing medications, abnormalities found on the quick check assessment, and any potential inconsistencies noted between the arrival quick check assessment and the prearrival report. It is easier to clarify questions while the transporters are still present, if possible.

This may also be an opportunity for introductory interactions with the patient's family members or friends, if present. The relationship between the family and the healthcare team begins with a professional introduction, reassurance, and confirmation of the intent to give the patient the best care possible (Table 1-5). If feasible, allow the family to stay with the patient in the room during the arrival process. If this is not possible, give them an approximate time frame when they can expect to receive an update on the patient's condition. Another member of the healthcare team can assist by escorting them to the appropriate waiting area.

COMPREHENSIVE INITIAL ASSESSMENT

Comprehensive assessments determine the physiologic and psychosocial baseline to which future changes are compared to determine whether the status is improving or deteriorating. The comprehensive assessment also defines the patient's

TABLE 1-5. EVIDENCE-BASED PRACTICE: FAMILY NEEDS ASSESSMENT

Quick Assessment
- Offer realistic hope
- Give honest answers and information
- Give reassurance

Comprehensive Assessment
- Use open-ended communication and assess their communication style
- Assess family members' level of anxiety
- Assess perceptions of the situation (knowledge, comprehension, expectations of staff, expected outcome)
- Assess family roles and dynamics (cultural and religious practices, values, spokesperson)
- Assess coping mechanisms and resources (what do they use, social network, and support)
- Assess knowledge and capacity for providing support after discharge

pre-event health status, determining problems or limitations that may impact patient status during this admission as well as potential issues for future transitioning of care. The content presented in this section is a template to screen for abnormalities or determine the extent of injury or disease. Any abnormal findings or changes from baseline warrant a more in-depth evaluation of the pertinent system.

The comprehensive assessment includes the patient's medical and social history, and physical examination of each body system. The comprehensive assessment of the progressive care patient is similar to admission assessments for medical-surgical patients. This section describes only those aspects of the assessment that are unique to progressive care patients or require more extensive information than is obtained from a medical-surgical patient. The entire assessment process is summarized in Tables 1-6 and 1-7.

An increasing proportion of patients in progressive care units are older adults, requiring assessments that incorporate the effects of aging. Although assessment of the aging adult does not differ significantly from the younger adult, understanding how aging alters the physiologic and psychological status of the patient is important. Key physiologic changes pertinent to the progressive care older adult are summarized in Table 1-8. Additional emphasis is also placed on the past medical history because the older adult frequently has multiple coexisting chronic illnesses and is taking several prescriptive and over-the-counter medications. Social history addresses issues related to home environment, support systems, and self-care abilities. The interpretation of clinical findings in the older adult also takes into consideration the fact that the coexistence of several disease processes and the diminished reserves of most body systems often result in more rapid physiologic deterioration than in younger adults.

Past Medical History

If the patient is being directly admitted to the progressive care unit, it is important to determine prior medical and surgical conditions, hospitalizations, medications, and symptoms besides the primary event that brought the patient to the hospital (see Table 1-7). A thorough review of medications

TABLE 1-6. SUMMARY OF COMPREHENSIVE INITIAL ASSESSMENT REQUIREMENTS

Past Medical History
- Medical conditions, surgical procedures
- Psychiatric/emotional problems
- Hospitalizations
- Medications (prescription, over-the-counter, illicit drugs) and time of last medication dose
- Allergies
- Review of body systems (see Table 1-7)

Social History
- Age, gender, self-identified gender
- Ethnic origin
- Height, weight
- Highest educational level completed
- Preferred language
- Occupation
- Marital status
- Primary family members/significant others/decision makers
- Religious affiliation
- Advance Directive and Durable Power of Attorney for Health Care, Medical Orders for Life-Sustaining Treatment (MOLST)
- Substance use/abuse (alcohol, illicit drugs or prescription medications, caffeine, tobacco)
- Domestic abuse or vulnerable adult screen
- Dependence on others—family members or paid caregivers—for assistance with activities of daily living

Psychosocial Assessment
- General communication
- Coping styles
- Anxiety and stress[a]
- Expectations of progressive care unit
- Current stresses
- Family needs

Spirituality
- Faith/spiritual preference
- Healing practices

Physical Assessment
- Nervous system
- Cardiovascular system
- Respiratory system
- Renal system
- Gastrointestinal system
- Endocrine, hematologic, and immune systems
- Integumentary system

[a]*Pain may need to be assessed in each body system rather than as a stand-alone assessment—see Table 1-9.*

TABLE 1-7. SUGGESTED QUESTIONS FOR REVIEW OF PAST HISTORY CATEGORIZED BY BODY SYSTEM

Body System	History Questions
Nervous	• Have you ever had a seizure? • Have you ever had a stroke? • Have you ever fainted, blacked out, or had delirium tremens (DTs)? • Do you ever have numbness, tingling, or weakness in any part of your body? • Do you have any difficulty with your hearing, vision, or speech? • Has your daily activity level changed due to your present condition? • Do you require any assistive devices such as canes? • Have you fallen in the past 6 months?
Cardiovascular	• Have you experienced any heart problems or disease such as heart attacks or heart failure? • Do you have any problems with extreme fatigue? • Do you have an irregular heart rhythm? • Do you have high blood pressure? • Do you have a pacemaker or an implanted defibrillator?
Respiratory	• Do you ever experience shortness of breath? • Do you have any pain associated with breathing? • Do you have a persistent cough? Is it productive? • Have you had any exposure to environmental agents that might affect the lungs? • Do you have sleep apnea?
Renal	• Have you had any change in frequency of urination? • Do you have any burning, pain, discharge, or difficulty when you urinate? • Have you had blood in your urine?
Gastrointestinal	• Has there been any recent weight loss or gain? • Have you had any change in appetite? • Do you have any problems with nausea or vomiting? • Do you have any difficulty swallowing? • How often do you have a bowel movement and has there been a change in the normal pattern? Do you have blood in your stools? • Do you have dentures? • Do you have any food allergies?
Integumentary	• Do you have any problems with your skin?
Endocrine	• Do you have any problems with bleeding?
Hematologic	• Do you have problems with chronic infections?
Immunologic	• Have you recently been exposed to a contagious illness? • Have you recently traveled outside the country?
Psychosocial	• Do you have any physical conditions, which make communication difficult (hearing loss, visual disturbances, language barriers, etc)? • How do you best learn? Do you need information repeated several times and/or require information in advance of teaching sessions? • What are the ways you cope with stress, crises, or pain? • Who are the important people in your family or network? • Who do you want to make decisions with you, or for you? • Have you had any previous experiences with acute illness? • Have you ever been hurt, or been threatened verbally, with physical harm? • Do you feel safe at home? • Have you ever been abused? • Have you ever experienced trouble with anxiety, irritability, being confused, mood swings, or suicidal thoughts or attempts? • What are the cultural practices, religious influences, and values that are important to you or your family? • What are family members' perceptions and expectations of the progressive care staff and the setting?
Spiritual	• What is your faith or spiritual preference? • What practices help you heal or deal with stress? • Would you like to see a chaplain, priest, or other spiritual guide?

includes the use of over-the-counter medication use as well as any herbal or alternative supplements. For every positive symptom response, additional questions should be asked to explore the characteristics of that symptom (Table 1-9). If the patient is a transfer from another area in the hospital, review the admission assessment information, and clarify as needed with the patient and family. Be aware of opportunities for health teaching and transition planning needs for discharge to home or to a rehabilitation facility.

Social History

The social history includes asking about the use and abuse of caffeine, alcohol, tobacco, and other substances such as illicit drugs or prescription medications. Because the use of these agents can have major implications for the progressive care

TABLE 1-8. PHYSIOLOGIC EFFECTS OF AGING

Body System	Effects
Nervous	Diminished hearing and vision, short-term memory loss, altered motor coordination, decreased muscle tone and strength, slower response to verbal and motor stimuli, decreased ability to synthesize new information, increased sensitivity to altered temperature states, increased sensitivity to sedation (confusion or agitation), decreased alertness levels
Cardiovascular	Increased effects of atherosclerosis of vessels and heart valves, decreased stroke volume with resulting decreased cardiac output, decreased myocardial compliance, increased workload of heart, diminished peripheral pulses
Respiratory	Decreased compliance and elasticity, decreased vital capacity, increased residual volume, less effective cough, decreased response to hypercapnia
Renal	Decreased glomerular filtration rate, increased risk of fluid and electrolyte imbalances
Gastrointestinal	Increased presence of dentition problems, decreased intestinal mobility, decreased hepatic metabolism, increased risk of altered nutritional states
Endocrine, hematologic, and immunologic	Increased incidence of diabetes, thyroid disorders, and anemia; decreased antibody response and cellular immunity
Integumentary	Decreased skin turgor, increased capillary fragility and bruising, decreased elasticity
Miscellaneous	Altered pharmacokinetics and pharmacodynamics, decreased range of motion of joints and extremities
Psychosocial	Difficulty falling asleep and fragmented sleep patterns, increased incidence of depression and anxiety, cognitive impairment disorders, difficulty with change

patient, questions are aimed at determining the frequency, amount, and duration of use. Honest information regarding alcohol and substance abuse, however, may not be always forthcoming. Alcohol use is common in all age groups. Phrasing questions about alcohol use by acknowledging this fact may be helpful in obtaining an accurate answer (eg, "How much alcohol do you drink?" vs "Do you drink alcohol and how much?"). Family or friends might provide additional information that could assist in assessing these parameters. The information revealed during the social history can often be verified during the physical assessment through the presence of signs such as needle track marks, nicotine stains on teeth and fingers, or the smell of alcohol on the breath.

Patients are also asked about physical and emotional safety in their home environment in order to uncover potential domestic or elder abuse. It is best if patients can be assessed for vulnerability when they are alone to prevent placing them in a position of answering in front of family members or friends who may be abusive. Questions such as "Is anyone hurting you?" or "Do you feel safe at home?" are included in a non-threatening manner. Any suspicion of abuse or vulnerability warrants a consultation with social work to determine additional assessments.

Physical Assessment by Body System

The physical assessment section is presented in the sequence in which the combined system, head-to-toe approach, is followed. Although content is presented as separate components, generally the history questions are integrated into the physical assessment. The physical assessment section uses the techniques of inspection, auscultation, and palpation. Although percussion is a common technique in physical examinations, it is infrequently used in progressive care patients.

Pain assessment is generally linked to each body system rather than considered as a separate system category; for example, if the patient has chest pain, assessment and documentation of that pain is incorporated into the cardiovascular assessment. Rather than have general pain assessment questions repeated under each system assessment, they are presented here.

Pain and discomfort are clues that alert both the patient and the progressive care nurse that something is wrong and needs prompt attention. Pain assessment includes differentiating acute and chronic pain, determining related physiologic symptoms, and investigating the patient's perceptions and emotional reactions to the pain. The qualities and characteristics of pain are listed in Table 1-9. Pain is a subjective assessment, and progressive care practitioners sometimes struggle with applying their own values when attempting to evaluate the patient's pain. To resolve this dilemma, use the patient's own words and descriptions of the pain whenever possible and use a patient-preferred pain scale (see Chapter 6, Pain and Sedation Management) to evaluate pain levels objectively and consistently.

TABLE 1-9. IDENTIFICATION OF SYMPTOM CHARACTERISTICS

Characteristic	Sample Questions
Onset	How and under what circumstances did it begin? Was the onset sudden or gradual? Did it progress?
Location	Where is it? Does it stay in the same place or does it radiate or move around?
Frequency	How often does it occur?
Quality	Is it dull, sharp, burning, throbbing, and so on?
Intensity	Rank pain on a scale (numeric, word description, FACES, FLACC)
Quantity	How long does it last?
Setting	What are you doing when it happens?
Associated findings	Are there other signs and symptoms that occur when this happens?
Aggravating and alleviating factors	What things make it worse? What things make it better?

Nervous System

The nervous system is the master computer of all systems and is divided into the central and peripheral nervous systems. With the exception of the peripheral nervous system's cranial nerves, almost all attention in the acutely ill patient is focused on evaluating the central nervous system (CNS). The physiologic and psychological impact of an acute illness, in addition to pharmacologic interventions, frequently alters CNS functioning. The single most important indicator of cerebral functioning is the LOC. The LOC is assessed using the Glasgow Coma Scale (GCS).

Additional neurological assessment includes evaluating the patient's pupils for size, shape, symmetry, and reactivity to direct light. Certain medications such as atropine, morphine, or illicit drugs may affect pupil size. Baseline pupil assessment is important even in patients without a neurologic diagnosis because some individuals have unequal or unreactive pupils normally. If pupils are not checked as a baseline, a later check of pupils during an acute event could inappropriately attribute pupil abnormalities to a pathophysiologic event.

LOC and pupil assessment are followed by motor function assessment of the upper and lower extremities for symmetry and quality of strength. Traditional motor strength exercises include having the patient squeeze the nurse's hands and plantar flexing and dorsiflexing of the patient's feet. If the patient cannot follow commands, an estimate of strength and quality of movements can be inferred by observing activities such as pulling on side rails or thrashing around. If the patient has no voluntary movement or is unresponsive, check the gag reflex.

If head trauma is involved or suspected, check for evidence of fluid leakage around the nose or ears, differentiating between cerebral spinal fluid and blood (see Chapter 12, Neurological System). Complete cranial nerve assessment is rarely warranted, with specific cranial nerve evaluation based on the injury or diagnosis; for example, extraocular movements are routinely assessed in patients with facial trauma. Sensory testing is a baseline standard for spinal cord injuries, extremity trauma, and epidural analgesia.

Now, it is a good time to assess mental status if the patient is responsive. Assess orientation to person, place, and time. Ask the patient to state their understanding of what is happening. As they answer questions, observe for eye contact, pressured or muted speech, and rate of speech. Rate of speech is usually consistent with the patient's psychomotor status. Underlying cognitive impairments such as dementia and developmental delays are typically exacerbated during an acute illness due to physiologic changes, medications, and environmental changes. Many hospitals routinely perform baseline and ongoing assessments for delirium in patients by using tools such as the Confusion Assessment Method (CAM). The family may be able to provide information about the patient's baseline level of functioning.

It is also important to assess patients for the risk of a fall. Progressive care patients often have increased mobility as a goal so it is imperative that the nurse understand the fall risk for each individual patient and implement interventions to minimize the potential for a fall. The patient's physical strength, memory and ability to follow instructions to wait for assistance before getting up all contribute to the risk for falling. Verify and document settings for any electronic devices (eg, bed or chair alarms) that are being used to prevent falls.

Laboratory data pertinent to the nervous system include serum electrolytes and urine electrolytes, osmolarity, and specific gravity. Drug toxicology and alcohol levels may be evaluated to rule out potential sources of altered LOC.

Cardiovascular System

The cardiovascular system assessment is directed at evaluating central and peripheral perfusion. Revalidate your admission quick check assessment of the blood pressure, heart rate, and rhythm. If the patient is being monitored, assess the ECG for T-wave abnormalities and ST-segment changes and determine the PR, QRS, and QT intervals and the QTc measurements. Note any abnormalities or indications of myocardial damage, electrical conduction problems, and electrolyte imbalances. Note the pulse pressure. If treatment decisions will be based on the cuff pressure, blood pressure is taken in both arms to determine if they are the same. If different, a decision is made about which will be used. If an arterial pressure line is in place, use a fast flush test to assess the dynamic response and accuracy. Determine which pressure is the most accurate and will be followed for future treatment decisions. Switching between methods may lead the healthcare team to inappropriately attribute fluctuations in blood pressure to physiologic changes rather than anatomic differences.

Note the color and temperature of the skin, with particular emphasis on lips, mucous membranes, and distal extremities. Also evaluate nail color and capillary refill. Inspect for the presence of edema, particularly in the dependent parts of the body such as feet, ankles, and sacrum. Measurement scales to quantify the severity of peripheral edema vary between sources and institutions. Nurses are encouraged to check nursing manuals and electronic skill programs or institutional skill sources, as appropriate, to ensure consistency.

Auscultation of heart sounds includes assessment of S_1 and S_2 quality, intensity, and pitch, and for the presence of extra heart sounds, murmurs, clicks, or rubs. Listen to one sound at a time, consistently progressing through the key anatomic landmarks of the heart each time. Note whether there are any changes with respiration or patient position.

Palpate the peripheral pulses for amplitude and quality, using the 0 to +4 scale (Table 1-10). Check bilateral pulses simultaneously, except the carotid, comparing each pulse to its partner. If the pulse is difficult to palpate, an ultrasound (Doppler) device is used. To facilitate finding a weak pulse for subsequent assessments, mark the location of the pulse with an indelible pen. It is also helpful to compare quality of the pulses to the ECG to evaluate the perfusion of heartbeats.

TABLE 1-10. PERIPHERAL PULSE RATING SCALE

- 0 Absent pulse
- +1 Palpable but thready; easily obliterated with light pressure
- +2 Normal; cannot obliterate with light pressure
- +3 Full
- +4 Full and bounding

Electrolyte levels, complete blood counts (CBCs), coagulation studies, and lipid profiles are common laboratory tests evaluated for abnormalities of the cardiovascular system. Cardiac biomarkers (troponin, creatine kinase MB, β-natriuretic peptide) are obtained for any complaint of chest pain or suspected chest trauma or a concern for heart failure. Drug levels of commonly used cardiovascular medications, such as digoxin, may be warranted for certain types of arrhythmias. A 12-lead ECG may be evaluated, either due to the chief reason for admission (eg, with complaints of chest pain, irregular rhythms, or suspected myocardial bruising from trauma) or as a baseline for future comparison if needed.

Note the type, size, and location of IV catheters, and verify their patency. If continuous infusions of medications such as antiarrhythmics are being administered, ensure that they are being infused into an appropriately sized vessel and are compatible with any piggybacked IV solution.

Verify that all monitoring system alarm parameters are active with appropriate limits set. Note the size and location of invasive monitoring lines such as arterial and central venous catheters. Confirm that the appropriate flush solution is hanging with the correct amount of pressure applied. Level the invasive line to the appropriate anatomic landmark and zero the monitor as needed. Interpret hemodynamic pressure readings against normal value ranges and with respect to the patient's underlying pathophysiology. Assess waveforms to determine the quality of the waveform (eg, dampened or hyperresonant) and whether the waveform appropriately matches the expected characteristics for the anatomic placement of the invasive catheter (see Chapter 4, Hemodynamic Monitoring); for example, a right ventricular waveform for a CVP line indicates a problem with the position of the central venous line that needs to be corrected. Evaluate all cardiovascular devices that are in place as feasible, such as a pacemaker, or any ventricular assist device. Verify and document equipment settings, appropriate function of the device, and the patient response to that device function.

Respiratory System

Oxygenation and ventilation are the focus of respiratory assessment parameters. Reassess the rate and rhythm of respirations and the symmetry of chest wall movement. If the patient has a productive cough or secretions are suctioned from an artificial airway, note the color, consistency, and amount of secretions. Evaluate whether the trachea is midline or shifted. Inspect the thoracic cavity for shape, anterior-posterior diameter, and structural deformities (eg, kyphosis or scoliosis). Palpate for equal chest excursion, presence of crepitus, and any areas of tenderness or fractures. If the patient is receiving supplemental oxygen, verify the mode of delivery and percentage of oxygen against provider orders.

Auscultate all lobes anteriorly and posteriorly for bilateral breath sounds to determine the presence of air movement and the presence of adventitious sounds such as crackles or wheezes. Note the quality and depth of respirations, and the length and pitch of the inspiratory and expiratory phases. Ask the patient to report their level of comfort with breathing.

Arterial blood gases (ABGs) may be used to assess oxygenation, ventilatory status, and acid-base balance. Hemoglobin and hematocrit values are interpreted for their impact on oxygenation and fluid balance. If the patient's condition warrants, the oxygen saturation values may be continuously monitored or periodically assessed via a noninvasive oxygen saturation monitor.

If the patient is connected to a mechanical ventilator, verify the ventilatory mode, tidal volume, respiratory rate, positive end expiratory pressure, and percentage of oxygen against prescribed settings. Observe whether the patient has spontaneous breaths, noting both the rate and the average tidal volume of each breath. Note the amount of pressure required to ventilate the patient for later comparisons to determine changes in pulmonary compliance. If the patient has a tracheostomy, note the size and type of tube in place and the location to assist future comparisons for proper placement. If the patient is on biphasic positive airway pressure (BiPAP), note and verify the pressure settings against ordered parameters. Also assess the patient's tolerance to the full face or nasal mask. Patients frequently exhibit anxiety with BiPAP and have difficulty tolerating the feeling of the mask.

If chest tubes are present, palpate the area around the insertion site for crepitus. Note the amount and color of drainage and whether an air leak is present. Verify whether the chest tube drainage system is a water seal or is connected to suction.

Renal System

Urinary characteristics and electrolyte status are the major parameters used to evaluate the kidney function. In conjunction with the cardiovascular system, the renal system's impact on fluid volume status is also assessed.

Some progressive care patients have an indwelling urinary catheter or a urinary collection device in place to evaluate urine output. Note the amount, clarity, and color of the urine and, if warranted, obtain a sample to assess for the abnormal presence of glucose, protein, and blood. Inspect the external genitalia for inflammation, swelling, ulcers, and drainage. If suprapubic tubes or a ureterostomy are present, note the position as well as the amount and characteristics of the drainage. Observe whether any drainage is leaking around the drainage tube or device. For those with indwelling catheters, evaluate whether the patient meets the criteria for continuation of urinary catheter use and consider switching to a less invasive method of measuring output.

In addition to the urinalysis, urine electrolytes, serum electrolyte levels, blood urea nitrogen, creatinine, and urinary and serum osmolarity are common diagnostic tests used to evaluate kidney function.

Gastrointestinal System

The key factors when reviewing the gastrointestinal system are the nutritional and fluid status. Inspect the abdomen for overall symmetry, noting whether the contour is flat, round, protuberant, or distended. Note the presence of discoloration or striae. Nutritional status is evaluated by looking at the patient's weight and muscle tone, the condition of the oral mucosa, and laboratory values such as serum albumin and transferrin. If there are any indications of swallowing difficulty, either patient reported or observed, follow hospital protocol to perform a swallow screen and/or request a formal swallow evaluation by speech pathology.

Auscultation of bowel sounds is performed in all four quadrants in a clockwise order, noting the frequency and presence or absence of sounds. Bowel sounds are usually rated as absent, hypoactive, normal, or hyperactive. Before noting absent bowel sounds, a quadrant is listened to for at least 60 to 90 seconds. Characteristics and frequency of the sounds are noted. After listening for the presence of normal sounds, determine whether any adventitious bowel sounds such as friction rubs, bruits, or hums are present.

Light palpation of the abdomen identifies areas of fluid, rigidity, tenderness, pain, and guarding or rebound tenderness. Remember to auscultate before palpating because palpation may change the frequency and character of the patient's peristaltic sounds.

Assess the location and function of any drainage tubes, and note the characteristics of any drainage. Validate the proper placement and patency of NG tube or percutaneously placed gastric tubes. Check placement and assess for any drainage or leaking around the tubes. Check emesis and stool for occult blood as appropriate. Evaluate ostomies for location, color of the stoma, and color and consistency of their output.

Endocrine, Hematologic, and Immune Systems

The endocrine, hematologic, and immune systems often are overlooked when assessing progressive care patients. The assessment parameters used to evaluate these systems are included under other system assessments, but consciously considering these systems when reviewing these parameters is essential. Assessing the endocrine, hematologic, and immune systems is based on a thorough understanding of the primary function of each of the hormones, blood cells, or immune components of each of the respective systems.

Assessment of the endocrine system is challenging because symptoms of changes in hormone secretion are the same as symptoms that occur due to disorders in the other systems. The patient's history may help differentiate the source, but any abnormal assessment findings detected with regard to fluid balance, metabolic rate, altered LOC, color and temperature of the skin, electrolytes, glucose, and acid-base balance require the progressive care nurse to consider the potential involvement of the endocrine system. For example, are the signs and symptoms of hypervolemia related to cardiac insufficiency or excessive amounts of antidiuretic hormone? Serum blood tests for specific hormone levels may be required to rule out involvement of the endocrine system.

Assessment parameters specific to the hematologic system include laboratory evaluation of the red blood cells (RBCs) and coagulation studies. Diminished RBCs may affect the oxygen-carrying capacity of the blood which is evidenced by pallor, cyanosis, light-headedness, tachypnea, and tachycardia. Check the patient for bruising, oozing of blood from puncture sites or mucous membranes, or overt bleeding, which may indicate low platelet count, or deficiency in clotting factors. See Chapter 13 (Hematologic and Immune Systems) for additional discussion of the hematologic and immunologic assessment.

The immune system's primary function of fighting infection is assessed by evaluating the white cell and differential counts from the CBC, and assessing puncture sites and mucous membranes for drainage, inflammation, and redness. Spiking or persistent low-grade temperatures often are indicative of underlying infections. The absence of these symptoms, however, may not indicate the absence of infection. Many progressive care patients have impaired immune systems and the normal response to infection, such as white pus around an insertion site or elevated temperature and WBC, may not be evident. If an infection is suspected, consider potential sources that can be readily addressed such as an invasive line or urinary catheter.

Integumentary System

The skin is the first line of defense against infection so assessment parameters are focused on evaluating the intactness of the skin. Skin assessment can be undertaken while performing other system assessments; for example, while listening to breath sounds or bowel sounds, the condition of the thoracic cavity or abdominal skin can be observed, respectively. It is important that a thorough head-to-toe, anterior, posterior, and between skin folds assessment is performed and documented on admission to the progressive care unit to identify any preexisting skin integrity concerns that need to be immediately addressed and to establish a baseline for comparison with future assessments.

Inspect the skin for overall integrity, color, temperature, and turgor. Note the presence of rashes, striae, discoloration, scars, or lesions. For any abrasions, lesions, pressure injuries, or wounds, note the size, depth, and presence or absence of drainage. Consider use of a skin integrity risk assessment tool to determine immediate interventions that may be needed to prevent development or progression of pressure injury.

Psychosocial Assessment

The rapid physiologic and psychological changes associated with acute illnesses, coupled with pharmacologic and biological treatments, can profoundly affect behavior. Patients may suffer from illnesses that lead to predictable psychological responses, and, if untreated, may threaten recovery or life. To avoid making assumptions about how a patient feels about his or her care, there is no substitute for asking the patient directly or asking a collateral informant, such as the family or significant other.

General Communication

Factors that affect communication include culture, developmental stage, physical condition, stress, perception, neurocognitive deficits, emotional state, and language skills. The nature of an acute illness coupled with pharmacologic and airway technologies can interfere with patients' usual methods of communication. It is essential to determine pre-illness communication abilities and identify methods and styles to ensure optimal communication with the progressive care patient and family. The inability of some progressive care patients to communicate verbally necessitates that progressive care practitioners become expert at assessing nonverbal clues to determine important information and needs of patients. Important assessment data include body gestures, facial expressions, eye movements, involuntary movements, and changes in physiologic parameters, particularly heart rate, blood pressure, and respiratory rate. Often, nonverbal data may be more reflective of patients' actual feelings, particularly if they are denying symptoms and attempting to be the "good patient" by not complaining.

Anxiety and Stress

Anxiety is both psychologically and physiologically exhausting. Being in a prolonged state of arousal is hard work and uses adaptive reserves needed for recovery. The progressive care environment can be stressful, full of constant auditory, visual, and tactile stimuli, and may contribute to a patient's anxiety level. The progressive care setting may force isolation from social supports, dependency, loss of control, trust in unknown care providers, helplessness, and an inability to solve problems. Restlessness, distractibility, hyperventilation, and unrealistic demands for attention are warning signs of escalating anxiety.

Medications such as interferon, corticosteroids, angiotensin-converting enzyme inhibitors, and vasopressors can induce anxiety. Abrupt withdrawal from benzodiazepines, caffeine, nicotine, and narcotics as well as akathisia from phenothiazines may mimic anxiety. Additional etiologic variables associated with anxiety include pain, sleep loss, delirium, hypoxia, ventilator synchronization or weaning, fear of death, loss of control, high-technology equipment, and a dehumanizing setting. Admission to or repeated transfers may also induce anxiety.

Coping Styles

Individuals cope with an acute illness in different ways and understanding their pre-illness coping style, personality traits, or temperament allows the nurse to anticipate coping styles in the progressive care setting. Include the patient's family when assessing previous resources, coping skills, or defense mechanisms that strengthen adaptation or problem-solving resolution. For instance, some patients want to be informed of everything that is happening with them in the progressive care unit. Providing information reduces their anxiety and gives them a sense of control. Other patients prefer to have others receive information about them and make decisions for them. Giving them detailed information only exacerbates their level of anxiety and diminishes their ability to cope. Understanding the meaning that the patient and family assign to this illness event is crucial to evaluating their ability to cope. Does the coping resource fit with the event and meet the patient's and family's need?

This may also be the time to conduct a brief assessment of the spiritual beliefs and needs of the patient and family as this may be a powerful tool to assist them in their coping. Minimally, patients are asked if they have a faith or spiritual preference and offered the support of a chaplain, priest, or other spiritual guide. In addition, patients are also asked about spiritual and cultural healing practices that are important to them to determine whether those can be continued during their progressive care unit stay.

Patients express their coping styles in a variety of ways. Persons who are stoic by personality or culture usually present as the good patient. Such patients may be wary of "bothering" the busy staff and may not admit they have pain because family or others are nearby. Other patients express their anxiety and stress through manipulative behavior. Patients' and families use different modes of interacting and coping to feel safe. Impulsive behaviors, deception, low tolerance for frustration, unreliability, superficial charm, splitting among the healthcare team, and general avoidance of rules or limits may be modes of interacting and coping and attempts to feel safe. Still other patients may withdraw and actually request use of sedatives and sleeping medications to blunt the stimuli and stress of the environment.

Fear has an identifiable source and plays an important role in the ability of the patient to cope. Treatments, procedures, pain, and separation are common objects of fear. The dying process elicits specific fears, such as fear of the unknown, loneliness, loss of body, loss of self-control, suffering, pain, loss of identity, and loss of everyone loved by the patient. The family, as well as the patient, experiences the grieving process, which includes the phases of denial, shock, anger, bargaining, depression, and acceptance.

Family Needs

The concept of family is not limited to the nuclear family but includes any loving, supportive person regardless of social and legal boundaries. Ideally the patient is asked to identify their family and to select who should receive information about them, and who is the decision maker if they become unable to make decisions on their own. This may also be an opportune time to ask whether they have an advance directive or a Medical Order for Life-Sustaining Treatment (MOLST) on file, or if they have discussed their wishes with any family members or friends. Progressive care practitioners need to be flexible around traditional legal requirements of "next of kin" as well as patient wishes surrounding "next of kin" so that communication is extended to, and sought from, surrogate decision makers and whomever the patient designates.

Families can have a positive impact on the patient's ability to cope with and recover from an acute illness. The family's access to the patient is crucial and open visitation, with policies and protections in place to prevent violence and incivility, is encouraged. Each family system is unique and varies by culture, values, religion, previous experience with crisis, socioeconomic status, psychological integrity, role expectations, communication patterns, health beliefs, and ages. It is important to assess the family's needs and resources to develop interventions that will optimize family impact on the patient and support family collaboration with the healthcare team. Areas for family needs assessments are outlined in Table 1-5.

Unit Orientation

The progressive care nurse takes the time to educate the patient (if alert) and family about the specialized progressive care unit environment. Provide simple explanations of the equipment being used, the visitation policies, the routines of the unit, and how the patient can communicate needs to the unit staff. Give the family the unit telephone number and the names of the nurse manager as well as the nurse caring for the patient in case problems or concerns arise during the progressive care unit stay. Explain to the patient and family how they will be involved in receiving updates and given opportunities to ask questions.

Referrals

After completing the comprehensive assessment, the progressive care nurse analyzes the information gathered and determines the need to make referrals to other healthcare providers and resources (Table 1-11). To ensure appropriate and timely discharge and appropriate resource management, referrals are initiated as soon as possible to maintain continuity of care and avoid worsening decline of status. If any ancillary service referrals have already been initiated in the ICU or medical-surgical unit, those services are notified regarding the transfer in order to avoid any gaps in coverage.

Transition/Discharge Planning

It is important that transition and/or discharge planning starts on arrival of the patient to the progressive care unit. Lengths of stay continue to decrease for patients in progressive care, creating a challenge for progressive care nurses to assess the appropriate transition location for the progressive care patient adequately. Educational and logistical processes need to be put into place in a timely manner so as to avoid

TABLE 1-11. EXAMPLES OF POTENTIAL REFERRALS NEEDED FOR PROGRESSIVE CARE PATIENTS

Referral	Resources Needed
Social work	• Financial needs/resources for patient and/or family • Coping resources for patient and/or family • Resources to assist with transition planning
Nutrition	• Nutritional status at risk and in need of in-depth nutritional assessment • Altered nutritional status on admission • Education to patient/family about nutrition and diet after discharge
Therapies	• Physical therapy for maintaining or improving physical flexibility and strength • Occupational therapy for assistive devices • Speech therapy for assessment of ability to swallow or communication needs • All above three therapies for input on the appropriate discharge plan
Pastoral care	• Spiritual guidance for patient and/or family • Coping resources for patient and/or family
Enterostomal nursing	• Stoma assessment and needs • In-depth skin integrity needs • Teaching for patient/family how to care for new stoma
Ethics committee	• Decisions involving significant ethical complexity • Decisions involving disagreements over care between care providers or between care providers and patient/family
Care coordinator	• Anticipate transition needs throughout and post hospitalization
Palliative care	• Additional support, symptom management, goals of care conversations

any delays in patient progress and recovery. This necessitates early and active involvement by all appropriate healthcare team members to ensure smooth transitioning.

ONGOING ASSESSMENT

After the arrival quick check and comprehensive assessments are completed, all subsequent assessments are used to determine trends, evaluate response to therapy, and identify new potential problems or changes from the comprehensive baseline assessment. Ongoing assessments become more focused, and the frequency is driven by the stability of the patient; however, routine periodic assessments are the norm. Stable patients are assessed according to unit protocol, but an increased level of frequency is required for patients who are exhibiting changes in physiological status. Additional assessments are done when any of the following situations occur:

- Caregivers change
- Before and after any major procedural intervention, such as chest tube insertion
- Before and after transport out of the progressive care unit for diagnostic procedures or other events
- Deterioration in physiologic or mental status
- Initiation of any new therapy

TABLE 1-12. ONGOING ASSESSMENT TEMPLATE

Body System	Assessment Parameters
Nervous	• LOC • Pupils • Motor strength of extremities
Cardiovascular	• Blood pressure • Heart rate and rhythm • Heart sounds • Capillary refill • Peripheral pulses • Patency of IVs • Verification of IV solutions and medications • Hemodynamic pressures and waveforms
Respiratory	• Respiratory rate and rhythm • Breath sounds • Color and amount of secretions • Noninvasive technology information (eg, pulse oximetry) • Mechanical ventilatory parameters • Location, patency, and function of chest tubes • Arterial and venous blood gases
Renal	• Intake and output • Color, clarity, and amount of urinary output • Blood urea nitrogen (BUN)/creatinine values
Gastrointestinal	• Bowel sounds • Contour of abdomen • Position and patency of drainage tubes • Position of feeding tube • Color and amount of secretions • Bilirubin and albumin values
Endocrine, hematologic, and immunologic	• Fluid balance • Electrolyte and glucose values • CBC and coagulation values • Temperature • WBC with differential count
Integumentary	• Color and temperature of skin • Skin integrity • Areas of redness
Pain/discomfort	• Assessed in each system • Response to interventions
Psychosocial	• Mental status and behavioral responses • Reaction to acute illness experience (eg, stress, anxiety, coping, mood) • Presence of cognitive impairments (dementia, delirium), depression, or demoralization • Family functioning and needs • Ability to communicate needs and participate in care • Sleep patterns • Preparation for transition to the next level of care

As with the arrival quick check, the ongoing assessment section is offered as a generic template that can be used as a basis for all patients (Table 1-12). More in-depth and system-specific assessment parameters are added based on the patient's diagnosis and pathophysiologic problems.

PRINCIPLES OF MANAGEMENT

- There are four distinct components in the assessment of a patient admitted to progressive care: (1) the pre-arrival assessment, (2) the admission quick check, (3) the comprehensive initial assessment, and (4) ongoing assessment.
- The admission quick check is systematic so as not to miss subtle signs or cues. It is also used to ensure that patients' urgent needs are met. For instance, the patient's mental status can be observed during transfer from stretcher to hospital bed and addressed quickly.
- A common standard assessment approach is a combination of a body systems approach and a head-to-toe approach. A consistent process is applied to ensure complete information is gathered, while additional attention is given to certain systems according to the patient's presenting pathology.
- Assessment focuses first on the patient and then on the technology.
- Planning for the transition of the patient out of progressive care begins at the time of admission.

SELECTED BIBLIOGRAPHY

Progressive Care Assessment

American Association of Critical-Care Nurses. *Practice Alert: Assessment and Management of Delirium across the Lifespan.* Aliso Viejo, CA: AACN; 2016. https://www.aacn.org/clinical-resources/practice-alerts/assessment-and-management-of-delirium-across-the-life-span.

American Association of Critical-Care Nurses. *Practice Alert: Ensuring Accurate ST Monitoring.* Aliso Viejo, CA: AACN; 2016. https://www.aacn.org/clinical-resources/practice-alerts/st-segment-monitoring.

American Association of Critical-Care Nurses. *Practice Alert: Obtaining Accurate Non-Invasive Blood Pressure Measurements in Adults.* Aliso Viejo, CA: AACN; 2016. https://www.aacn.org/clinical-resources/practice-alerts/obtaining-accurate-noninvasive-blood-pressure-measurements-in-adults.

Bickley LS. *Bates' Guide to Physical Examination and History Taking.* 12th ed. Philadelphia, PA: Lippincott Williams & Wilkins; 2016.

Hartjes TM. *AACN Core Curriculum for High Acuity, Progressive and Critical Care.* 7th ed. St. Louis, MO: Elsevier; 2018.

Prin M, Wunsch H. The role of stepdown beds in hospital care. *Am J Respir Crit Care Med.* 2014;190(11):1210-1216.

Stacy KM. Progressive care units: different but the same. *Crit Care Nurs.* 2011;31(3):77-83.

Weigand DLM. *AACN Procedure Manual for High Acuity, Progressive and Critical Care.* 7th ed. St. Louis, MO: Elsevier; 2017.

Evidence-Based Practice

Davidson JE, Harvey MA. Patient and family post intensive care syndrome. *AACN Adv Crit Care.* 2016;27(2):184-186.

Gephart SM. The art of effective handoffs. What is the evidence? *Adv Neonatal Care.* 2012;12(1):37-39.

Hilligoss B, Cohen MD. The unappreciated challenges of between-unit handoffs: negotiating and coordinating across boundaries. *Ann Emerg Med.* 2013;61(1):15-160.

Maxwell KE, Stuenkel D, Saylor C. Needs of family members of critically ill patients: a comparison of nurse and family perceptions. *Heart Lung.* 2007;36(5):367-376.

Murphy TH, Labonte P, Klock M, Houser L. Falls prevention for elders in acute care: an evidence-based nursing practice initiative. *Crit Care Nurs Q.* 2008;31(1):33-39.

Sendelbach S, Guthrie PF, Schoenfelder DP. Acute confusion/delirium. Identification, assessment, treatment, and prevention. *J Gerontol Nurs.* 2009;35(11):11-18. doi: 10.3928/00989134-20090930-01.

Stafos A, Stark S, Barbay K, et al. Identifying hospital patients at risk for harm: a comparison of nurse perceptions vs. electronic risk assessment tool scores. *Am J Nurs.* 2017;117(4):26-31.

Staggers N, Blaz JW. Research on nursing handoffs for medical and surgical settings: an integrative review. *J Adv Nurs.* 2013;69(2):247-262.

Tescher AN, Branda ME, OByrne TJ, Naessens JM. All at-risk patients are not created equal. Analysis of Braden pressure ulcer risk scores to identify specific risks. *J Wound Ostomy Continence Nurs.* 2012;39(3):282-291.

Verhaeghe S, Defloor T, Van Zuuren F, Duijnstee M, Grypdonck M. The needs and experiences of family members of adult patients in an intensive care unit: a review of the literature. *J Clin Nurs.* 2005;14:501-509.

Planning Care for Progressive Care Patients and Their Families

Mary Fran Tracy

2

KNOWLEDGE COMPETENCIES

1. Discuss the importance of an interprofessional plan of care for optimizing clinical outcomes.

2. Describe interventions for prevention of common complications in progressive care patients:
   - Venous thromboembolism
   - Infection
   - Sleep pattern disturbances
   - Fall
   - Skin breakdown
   - Delirium

3. Discuss interventions to maintain psychosocial integrity and minimize anxiety for the progressive care patient and family members.

4. Describe interventions to promote family-centered care, and patient and family education.

5. Identify necessary equipment and personnel required to safely transport the progressive care patient within the hospital.

6. Describe transfer-related complications and preventive measures to be taken before and during patient transport.

It is important to be mindful of the unique needs of patients and their families as they transition from the intensive care or medical-surgical environment to a progressive care environment. Since lengths of stay in progressive care are typically short, preparation for the next anticipated level of care is initiated on arrival to the progressive care unit. Patient and family education is key to preparing for care transitions or potential discharge to home. It is also important to recognize anxiety that the patient may experience during transitions of care. If the patient is transferring from critical care to progressive care, the patient and family may feel nervous at the perceived decrease in level of nursing vigilance and technology. This can create questions on the part of the patient and family as to whether staff will be available to respond quickly to patient needs and changes in condition. Conversely, if a patient is transferred to the progressive care unit from a medical-surgical area because of declining physiologic status, anxiety on the part of the patient and family is related to the uncertainty of the patient condition. In either case, it is important to reassure the patient and family that the progressive care nurses have the skills and equipment needed to monitor and meet the needs of the patient.

The achievement of optimal clinical outcomes in the progressive care patient requires a coordinated approach to care delivery by interprofessional team members. Experts in nutrition, respiratory therapy, progressive care nursing and medicine, psychiatry, and social work, as well as other disciplines, work collaboratively to effectively and efficiently provide optimal care.

An interprofessional plan of care is a useful approach to facilitate the coordination of a patient's care by the interprofessional team and optimize clinical outcomes. These interprofessional plans of care are increasingly being used to replace individual, discipline-specific plans of care. Each clinical condition presented in this text discusses the management of patient needs or problems with an integrated, interprofessional approach.

The following section provides an overview of interprofessional plans of care and their benefits. In addition, this chapter discusses patient management approaches to needs or problems during acute illnesses that are not diagnosis specific, but common to a majority of progressive care patients, such as sleep deprivation, pressure injury, and patient and family education. Additional discussion of these needs or problems is also presented in other chapters related to specific disease management.

INTERPROFESSIONAL PLAN OF CARE

An *interprofessional plan of care* is a set of expectations for the major components of care a patient receives during the hospitalization to manage a specific medical or surgical problem. Other types of plans include *clinical pathways*, *protocols*, and *care maps*. The interprofessional plan of care expands the concept of a medical or nursing care plan and provides a multidisciplinary, comprehensive blueprint for patient care. The result is a diagnosis-specific plan of care that focuses the entire care team on expected patient outcomes.

The interprofessional plan of care outlines the tests, medications, care, and treatments needed to discharge the patient in a timely manner with all patient outcomes met. These plans have a variety of benefits to both patients and the hospital system:

- Improved patient outcomes (eg, survival rates, morbidity)
- Increased quality and continuity of care
- Improved communication and collaboration
- Identification of hospital system problems
- Coordination of necessary services and reduced duplication
- Prioritization of activities
- Reduced length of stay (LOS) and healthcare costs

Teams of individuals who closely interact with a specific patient population develop interprofessional plans of care. It is this process of multiple disciplines communicating and collaborating around the needs of the patient that creates benefits for the patients. Representatives of disciplines commonly involved in developing plans of care include providers, nurses, respiratory therapists, physical therapists, social workers, and dieticians. The format for the interprofessional plans of care typically includes the following categories:

- Discharge outcomes
- Patient goals (eg, pain control, activity level, absence of complications)
- Assessment and evaluation
- Consultations
- Tests
- Medications
- Nutrition
- Activity
- Education
- Discharge planning

The suggested activities within each of these categories may be divided into daily activities or grouped into phases of the hospitalization (eg, preoperative, intraoperative, and postoperative phases). All staff members who use the plan of care require education as to its specifics. This team approach in development and utilization optimizes communication, collaboration, coordination, and commitment in using the plan to achieve patient outcomes.

Interprofessional plans of care are evolving into many different forms and the documentation varies widely across institutions. Some electronic formats mimic the paper version. Other institutions may incorporate pieces of the plan of care into varied electronic flow sheets (eg, orders, assessments, interventions, education, outcomes, specific plans of care). Regardless of the specific format, a wide range of disciplines use interprofessional plans of care. Each individual who assesses progress toward patient goals and implements various aspects of the interprofessional plan of care is accountable for documenting on the care plan in the approved format. Specific patient goals on the plan of care can then be evaluated and tracked to determine if they are met, not met, or are not applicable. Goals on the plan of care that are not completed typically are termed *variances*, which are deviations from the expected activities or goals outlined. Goal outcomes on the plan of care that occur early are termed *positive variances*. *Negative variances* are those planned outcomes that are not accomplished on time. Negative variances typically include goals not completed or achieved due to the patient's condition, hospital system challenges (diagnostic studies or therapeutic interventions not completed within the optimal time frame), or lack of orders. Assessing patient progression on the plan of care helps caregivers to have an overall picture of patient recovery as compared to the goals and can be helpful in early recognition and resolution of problems. It is important to remember that individual discipline documentation on the plan of care does not preclude the need for ongoing, direct communication and collaboration between disciplines in order to facilitate optimal patient care and achievement of goals.

PLANNING CARE THROUGH STAFFING CONSIDERATIONS

Planning care for individual acutely ill patients begins with ensuring each nurse caring for a patient has the corresponding competencies and skills to meet the patient's needs. The American Association of Critical-Care Nurses has developed the AACN Synergy Model for Patient Care to delineate core patient characteristics and needs that drive the core competencies of nurses required to care for patients and families (Table 2-1). All eight competencies identified in the Synergy Model are essential for the progressive care nurse's practice, though the extent to which any particular competency is needed on a daily basis depends on the patient's needs at that point in time. When making patient staffing assignments, the charge nurse or nurse manager assesses the priority needs of the patient and assigns a nurse who has the proficiencies to meet those patient needs. By matching the competencies

TABLE 2-1. CORE PATIENT CHARACTERISTICS AND NURSE COMPETENCIES AS DEFINED IN THE SYNERGY MODEL

Patient Characteristics	Description
Resiliency	The capacity to return to a restorative level of functioning using compensatory/coping mechanisms
Vulnerability	Susceptibility to actual or potential stressors that may adversely affect patient outcomes
Stability	The ability to maintain a steady-state equilibrium
Complexity	The intricate entanglement of two or more systems
Resource availability	Extent of resources (technical, fiscal, personal, psychological, and social) the patient/family bring to the situation
Participation in care	Extent to which patient/family engages in aspects of care
Participation in decision making	Extent to which patient/family engages in decision making
Predictability	Characteristic that allows one to expect a certain course of events or course of illness

Nurse Competencies	Description
Clinical judgment	Clinical reasoning (clinical decision making, critical thinking, and global understanding of situation) coupled with nursing skills (formal and informal experiential knowledge and evidence-based practice)
Advocacy and moral agency	Working on another's behalf and representing concerns of patients/families and nursing staff
Caring practices	Activities that create a compassionate, supportive, and therapeutic environment
Collaboration	Working with others in a way that promotes each person's contributions toward achieving optimal patient/family goals
Systems thinking	Body of knowledge that allows the nurse to manage environment and system resources for patients, families, and staff
Response to diversity	Sensitivity to recognize, appreciate, and incorporate differences into provision of care
Facilitation of learning	Ability to facilitate learning for patients, families, and staff
Clinical inquiry	Ongoing process of questioning and evaluating practice and providing informed practice

Data from American Association of Critical-Care Nurses. The AACN Synergy Model for Patient Care. Aliso Viejo, CA: AACN. Available at: http://www.aacn.org/WD/Certifications/Content/synmodel.content?menu=Certification.

of the nurse with the needs of the patient, synergy occurs resulting in optimal patient outcomes.

PATIENT SAFETY CONSIDERATIONS IN PLANNING CARE

Progressive care units are high-technology, high-intervention environments with multiple disciplines caring for the patient. Progressive care nurses need to be especially thoughtful of minimizing the safety risks inherent in such an environment. Progressive care units are constantly working to improve ways to optimize care and minimize risks to patients.

As the nurse develops an ongoing plan of care, safety considerations are also incorporated. Conditions of acutely ill patients can change quickly, so ongoing awareness and vigilance is the key even when the patient appears to be stable or improving. The progressive care unit environment itself can contain safety issues. Inappropriate use of medical gas equipment or ventilator settings, electrical equipment with invasive lines, certain types of restraints, bedside rails, and cords and tubing lying on the floor may all be hazardous to the acutely ill patient. In addition, with so many healthcare disciplines involved in the care of each patient, it is imperative that communication remain accurate and timely. Use of a standardized handoff communication tool (eg, SBAR; see Chapter 1, Assessment of Progressive Care Patients and Their Families) is a fundamental step in preventing errors related to poor communication among healthcare providers.

Finally, as described in more detail later, many common complications can be prevented by patient safety initiatives that reduce the risk of ventilator-acquired pneumonia, central line-associated bloodstream infections, catheter-associated

---

ESSENTIAL CONTENT CASE

Synergy between Patient Characteristics and Nurse Competencies

MG is an 83-year-old woman with a history of coronary heart disease and metastatic breast cancer who is transferred to the progressive care unit with shortness of breath. Her respiratory status is continuing to worsen and CPAP is initiated though the physician is evaluating MG for potential intubation and sedation. In addition, MG is experiencing episodes of tachycardia. It has been determined the shortness of breath is due to a large, pleural effusion. MG is widowed with three children who are very supportive but all live at least 5 hours away and are unclear about their mother's wishes regarding medical treatment or her goals of care.

Case Question 1: Based on the Synergy Model (see Table 2-1), what four priority patient characteristics would the charge nurse consider in making a nurse assignment for MG?

Case Question 2: The charge nurse assigns Rebecca to care for MG. What particular skills will Rebecca use in caring for MG during the upcoming shift?

Answers
1. MG's priority characteristics include instability, minimally resilient, vulnerable, and currently unable to fully participate in decision making.
2. Clinical judgment, advocacy and moral agency, and caring practices.

urinary tract infections, and *Clostridium difficile* and multidrug resistant organisms (MDROs). Initiatives that promote hand hygiene, meticulous care of patients, and attention to the environment including cleaning of reusable equipment can prevent transmission of pathogens from one patient to another. Another approach is incorporating daily discussions with the healthcare team about the use of invasive lines and catheters. Removing invasive equipment as soon as clinically appropriate can prevent pathogen exposure from becoming an infection.

PREVENTION OF COMMON COMPLICATIONS

The development of an acute illness, regardless of its cause, predisposes the patient to a number of physiologic and psychological complications. A major focus when providing care to progressive care patients is the prevention of complications associated with acute illness. The following content describes some of the most common complications.

Physiologic Instability

Ongoing assessments and monitoring of progressive care patients (see Table 1-13) are key to early identification of physiologic changes and to ensuring that the patient is progressing to the identified transition goals. It is important for the nurse to use critical thinking skills throughout the provision of care to accurately analyze patient changes.

After each assessment, the data obtained are looked at in totality as they relate to the status of the patient. When an assessment changes in one body system, rarely does it remain an isolated issue, but rather it frequently either impacts or is a result of changes in other systems. Only by analyzing the entire patient assessment can the nurse see what is truly happening with the patient and anticipate interventions and responses.

When assuming care of the patient, define patient goals to achieve by the end of the shift, either as identified by the plan of care or by the patient assessment. This provides opportunities to evaluate care over a period of time. It prevents a narrow focus on the completion of individual tasks and interventions and encourages a broader consideration of the overall progression of the patient toward various goals. In addition, this broader view allows the nurse to anticipate the potential patient responses to interventions. For instance, the nurse notices that a patient requires an increase in the insulin infusion in response to higher glucose levels every morning around 10 AM. When looking at the whole picture, the nurse realizes that the patient is receiving several medications in the early morning that are mixed in a dextrose diluent. Recognition of this pattern helps the nurse to stabilize swings in blood glucose.

Venous Thromboembolism

Progressive care patients are at increased risk of venous thromboembolism (VTE) due to their underlying condition and immobility. Routine interventions can prevent this potentially devastating complication from occurring. There is increasing evidence to support early and progressive mobility of patients to decrease the risk of VTEs in addition to improving respiratory function and muscle strength. It takes a team effort to fully implement early mobility protocols, including nurses, physical therapists, respiratory therapists, and providers. Increased mobility is emphasized as soon as the patient is stable. Even transferring the patient from the bed to the chair changes positioning of extremities and improves circulation. Additionally, use of sequential compression devices assists in enhancing lower extremity circulation. Avoid placing intravenous (IV) access in the groin site or lower limbs as this impedes mobility and potentially impedes blood flow and can thus increase VTE risk. Ensure adequate hydration. Many patients may also be placed on low-dose heparin or enoxaparin protocols as a preventative measure.

Hospital-Acquired Infections

Acutely ill patients are vulnerable to infection during their stay in the progressive care unit. It is estimated that 20% to 60% of progressive care patients acquire some type of infection. In general, the risk of hospital-acquired infections is due to the use of multiple invasive devices and the frequent presence of debilitating underlying diseases. Hospital-acquired infections increase the patient's LOS and hospitalization costs, and can markedly increase mortality rates depending on the type and severity of the infection and the underlying disease. Although urinary tract infections are the most common hospital-acquired infections in the progressive care setting, hospital-acquired pneumonias are the second most common infection and the most common cause of mortality from infections. Details of specific risk factors and control measures for the prevention of hospital-acquired pneumonias are presented in Chapter 10 (Respiratory System). Other frequent infections include bloodstream and surgical site infections. In addition, *C. difficile* and MDRO infections have been steadily increasing in incidence over the past decades. This is particularly concerning as there are very limited options for treating these MDROs. It is imperative for progressive care practitioners to understand the processes that contribute to these potentially lethal infections and their roles in preventing them.

Prevention

Standard precautions, sometimes referred to as *universal precautions* or *body substance isolation*, refer to the basic precautions that are to be used on all patients, regardless of their diagnosis. The general premise of standard precautions is that all body fluids have the potential to transmit any number of infectious diseases, both bacterial and viral. Certain basic principles are followed to prevent direct and indirect transmission of these organisms. Nonsterile examination gloves are worn when performing venipuncture, touching

TABLE 2-2.   ISOLATION CATEGORIES AND RELATED INFECTION EXAMPLES

Isolation Categories	Infection Examples When Used
Standard precautions	Used with care of all patients
Airborne precautions	Tuberculosis, measles (rubeola), varicella
Droplet precautions	*Neisseria meningitidis, Haemophilus influenzae,* pertussis, mumps, whooping cough
Contact precautions	Vancomycin-resistant enterococcus (VRE), methicillin-resistant *Staphylococcus aureus* (MRSA), *Clostridium difficile,* scabies, impetigo, varicella, respiratory syncytial virus

nonintact skin or mucous membranes of the patient or for touching any moist body fluid. This includes urine, stool, saliva, emesis, sputum, blood, and any type of drainage. Other personal protective equipment, such as face shields and protective gowns, is worn whenever there is a risk of splashing body fluids into the face or onto clothing. This protects not only the healthcare worker, but also prevents any contamination that may be transmitted between patients via the caregiver. Specific control measures are aimed at specific routes of transmission. See Table 2-2 for examples of isolation precaution categories and the types of infections for which they are instituted.

Other interventions to prevent nosocomial infections are similar regardless of the site. Maintaining glycemic control in both diabetic and nondiabetic patients may decrease the patient's risk for developing an infection. Invasive lines or tubes never remain in place longer than absolutely necessary and never for staff convenience or patient preference. Use closed drainage systems whenever possible and avoid breaks in systems such as urinary drainage systems, IV lines, and ventilator tubing. Use of aseptic technique is essential if breaks into these systems are necessary. Hand hygiene before and after any manipulation of invasive lines is essential.

The current recommendation from the United States Centers for Disease Control and Prevention (CDC) is that peripheral IV lines remain in place no longer than 72 to 96 hours. There is no standard recommendation for routine removal of central venous catheters when required for prolonged periods. If the patient begins to show signs of sepsis that could be catheter-related, these catheters are removed. More important than the length of time the catheter is in place is how carefully the catheter was inserted and cared for while in place. All catheters placed in an emergency situation are replaced as soon as possible or within 48 hours. Dressings are kept dry and intact and changed at the first signs of becoming damp, soiled, or loosened. IV tubing is changed no more frequently than every 72 hours, with the exception of tubing for blood, blood products, or lipid-based products, each of which has specific criteria for how often the tubing is changed.

Strategies to prevent aspiration, a risk factor for hospital-acquired pneumonia include the following: maintain the head of the bed at greater than or equal to 30°, assess tolerance to enteral feeding and adjust feeding rates accordingly,

and wash hands before and after contact with patient secretions or respiratory equipment (refer to Chapters 5 and 14 for specific content related to these recommendations). Consider performing a swallow screen with patient reports of swallowing difficulties or with observed difficulty swallowing such as coughing or choking with oral intake. Performing routine oral care will also decrease the risk of microaspiration of oral bacteria.

Hand hygiene is one of the most important defenses to preventing infection. Hand hygiene is defined by the CDC as using either hand washing (soap and water), antiseptic hand wash, antiseptic hand rub (alcohol-based hand sanitizer including foam or gel), or surgical hand antisepsis. It has been estimated that healthcare workers cleanse their hands as much as 50% fewer times than necessary. It is important to involve all disciplines in encouraging and reminding each other to perform hand hygiene when it has been overlooked. Some institutions also encourage patients and families to be partners in hand hygiene efforts by asking care providers if they have cleansed their hands prior to patient contact.

Hand washing is defined by the CDC as vigorous rubbing together of lathered hands with soap and water for 15 seconds followed by a thorough rinsing under a stream of running water. Particular attention is paid around rings and under fingernails. It is best to keep natural fingernails well trimmed and unpolished. Cracked nail polish is a good place for microorganisms to hide.

Artificial fingernails are not worn in any healthcare setting because they are virtually impossible to clean without a nailbrush and vigorous scrubbing. Hand washing with soap and water is performed when hands are visibly soiled, after exposure to known or suspected *C. difficile,* after known or suspected exposure to infectious diarrhea during norovirus outbreak, before eating, and after using restroom. Use of alcohol-based waterless cleansers is convenient and effective when no visible soiling or contamination has occurred and after all other activities. Hand hygiene is performed prior to donning examination gloves to carry out patient-care activities and after removing examination gloves.

Dry, cracked skin, a long-standing problem associated with hand washing, has new significance with the emergence of blood-borne pathogens. Frequent hand washing, especially with antimicrobial soap, can lead to extremely dry skin. The frequent use of latex examination gloves has been associated with increased sensitivities and allergies, causing even more skin breakdown. Breaks in skin integrity can put the healthcare provider at risk for blood-borne pathogen transmission, as well as for colonization or infection with bacteria. Attention to skin care is extremely important for the progressive care practitioner who is using antimicrobial soap and latex gloves frequently. Lotions and emollients are used to prevent dryness and reduce the risk of cracking. If skin breakdown does occur, the employee health nurse is consulted for possible treatment or work restriction until the condition resolves.

Pressure Injury

Pressure injury is a major risk with progressive care patients due to immobility, poor nutrition, invasive lines, surgical sites, poor circulation, edema, and incontinence issues. Skin can become fragile and easily tear. Pressure injury can start to occur in as little as 2 hours in an immobile patient. Healthy people constantly reposition themselves, even in their sleep, to relieve areas of pressure. Progressive care patients who cannot reposition themselves rely on caregivers to assist them. Pay particular attention to pressure points that are most prone to injury, namely, heels, elbows, coccyx, and occiput. When receiving progressive care patients following prolonged surgical procedures, ask the perioperative providers about the patient's positioning during the procedure. This will help determine the need for close monitoring of the related pressure points for early indication of deep tissue injury. Also be cognizant of equipment that may contribute to pressure injury, such as drainage tubes and even bed rails, if patients are positioned in constant contact with them. As the patient's condition changes, so does the risk of developing a pressure injury. Routine use of a risk assessment tool alerts the caregiver to increasing or decreasing risk of pressure injury and the need for changes in interventions.

There are many simple interventions to maintain skin integrity: (1) reposition the patient minimally every 2 hours, particularly if they are not spontaneously moving; (2) use pressure-reduction mattresses for patients at high risk of injury; (3) elevate heels off the bed using pillows placed under the calves or heel protectors; (4) consider elbow pads; (5) avoid long periods of sitting in a chair without repositioning; (6) inflatable cushions (donuts) are never used for either the sacrum or the head because they can actually cause increases in pressure on surrounding skin surfaces; and (7) use a skin care protocol with ointment barriers for patients experiencing incontinence to prevent skin irritation and tissue breakdown. There is also emerging evidence for use of polyurethane foam dressings prophylactically over bony prominences that are exposed to shear and friction, though this intervention needs to be carefully considered based on individual patients and their conditions.

Sleep Pattern Disturbance

Progressive care patients are at risk for altered sleep patterns. Sleep is a problem for patients for many reasons, not the least of which are the pain and anxiety of an acute illness within an environment that is inundated with the multiple activities of healthcare providers. Table 2-3 identifies the many reasons for patients to experience sleep deprivation. The priority of sleep in the hierarchy of patient needs is often perceived to be low by clinicians. This contradicts patients' own statements about the progressive care experience. Patients complain about lack of sleep as a major stressor along with the discomfort of unrelieved pain. The vicious cycle of undertreated pain, anxiety, and sleeplessness continues unless clinicians

TABLE 2-3. FACTORS CONTRIBUTING TO SLEEP DISTURBANCES IN PROGRESSIVE CARE

Illness
- Metabolic changes
- Underlying diseases (eg, cardiovascular disease, chronic obstructive pulmonary disease [COPD], dementia)
- Pain
- Anxiety, fear
- Delirium

Medications
- Analgesics
- Antidepressants
- Beta-blockers
- Bronchodilators
- Benzodiazepines
- Corticosteroids

Environment
- Noise
- Roommate or other patients
- Staff conversations
- Television/radio
- Equipment alarms
- Frequent care interruptions
- Lighting
- Lack of usual bedtime routine
- Room temperature
- Uncomfortable sleep surface

intervene to break the cycle with simple but essential interventions individualized to each patient.

Noise from patient-care activities, monitor alarms, lights, and frequent patient interruptions are common in many progressive care settings, with staff able to tune out the disturbances after they have worked in the setting for even a short period of time. Subjecting patients to these environmental stimuli and interruptions to rest/sleep can quickly lead to sleep deprivation. Psychological changes in sleep deprivation include confusion, irritability, and agitation. Physiologic changes include depressed immune and respiratory systems and a decreased pain threshold. Patients may already be sleep-deprived when they are admitted to the progressive care setting. The progressive care unit routine can help start to reestablish a healing sleep pattern.

Enhancing patients' sleep potential in the progressive care setting involves knowledge of how the environment affects the patient and where to target interventions to best promote sleep and rest. A nighttime sleep protocol where patients are closely monitored but untouched from 1 to 5 AM is an excellent example of eliminating the hourly disturbances that may have been occurring in the ICU. Encouraging blocks of time for sleep and careful assessment of the quantity and quality of sleep are important to patient well-being. The middle-of-the-night bath is not a standard of care for any patient. Table 2-4 details basic recommendations for sleep assessment, protecting or shielding the patient from the environment, and modifying the internal and external environments of the patient. When these activities are incorporated into standard practice routines, progressive care patients receive optimal opportunity to achieve sleep.

TABLE 2-4. EVIDENCE-BASED PRACTICE: SLEEP PROMOTION IN PROGRESSIVE CARE

- Assess patient's usual sleep patterns
- Minimize effects of underlying disease process as much as possible (eg, reduce fever, control pain, minimize metabolic disturbances)
- Avoid medications that disturb sleep patterns
- Consult with providers to continue behavioral medications during hospital stay
- Mimic patients' usual bedtime routine as much as possible
- Minimize environmental impact on sleep as much as possible
- Utilize complementary therapies to promote sleep as appropriate

Falls

Progressive care patients are encouraged to increase mobility following a prolonged critical illness, or they may be fairly mobile at baseline and require progressive care for an acute illness. While patients who are mobile face a lower risk of complications such as pressure injury and VTE, this increase in activity does introduce a concern for falls, particularly when physical mobility is coupled with impaired cognitive function. Planning the care of patients at risk for falls includes consideration of side rail position, bed height, frequency of patient observation, and consistent simple instructions to the patient and family.

Many hospitals have specific programs for assessing all patients for the risk of falls and interventions to implement based on the individual risk for each patient. For example, patients who are at high risk of falling may be better served when placed in rooms where they can be easily observed. Keeping items of importance, such as the television remote, the urinal, and the call light within easy reach may also prevent a fall. Patients who recurrently attempt to get out of bed independently may be safer if they are assisted to a chair, if they have family present, or if staffing permits, with ongoing observation by a staff member.

A vulnerable time for a potential fall is when patients need to urgently use the restroom or after being assisted to the restroom, they believe they can return to bed unassisted. Interventions to address this risk are routine rounding on patients to address their hygiene and other essential needs proactively as well as staying near or in the bathroom with the patient who is at a high risk for falls and who may be reluctant to ask for help returning to bed. Collaboration with other professionals such as physical therapy and occupational therapy may be instrumental in identifying additional interventions to prevent falls. Delirium in a mobile patient may present a particularly high risk for falls, and in these cases, interventions to address the delirium, as described later, take on added importance.

Psychosocial Impact

Basic Tenets

Healthcare providers are becoming increasingly aware that time spent in the intensive care unit (ICU) can have long-term physical, mental, and cognitive changes, impacting patients and families for years following the illness. This Post-Intensive Care Syndrome (PICS) can result in survivors and their family members exhibiting signs of posttraumatic stress disorder (PTSD). The progressive care nurse may see evidence of this in patients and families in the progressive care unit. While evidence is still emerging on strategies to prevent and treat PICS, there are basic interventions that can be done on the progressive care unit. Keys to maintaining psychological integrity during and after an acute illness include (1) keeping stressors at a minimum; (2) encouraging family participation in care; (3) promoting a proper sleep-wake cycle; (4) encouraging communication, questions, and honest and positive feedback; (5) empowering the patient to participate in decisions as appropriate; (6) providing patient and family education about unit expectations and rules, procedures, medications, and the patient's physical condition; (7) ensuring pain relief and comfort; and (8) providing continuity of care providers. It is also important to have the patient's usual sensory and physical aids available, such as glasses, hearing aids, and dentures, as they may help prevent confusion. Encourage the family to bring something familiar or personal from home, such as a family or pet picture.

Delirium

Delirium is evidenced by disorientation, confusion, perceptual disturbances, restlessness, distractibility, and sleep-wake cycle disturbances. Any prior LOS in an ICU may have already resulted in, or put a patient at risk for, development of confusion. Causes of confusion are usually multifactorial and include metabolic disturbances, polypharmacy, immobility, infections (particularly urinary tract and respiratory infections), dehydration, electrolyte imbalances, sensory impairment, and environmental challenges. Treatment of delirium is a challenge and therefore prevention is ideal.

Delirium occurs most often in postsurgical and elderly patients and is the most common cause of disruptive behavior in progressive care. It is not unusual for providers to suspect delirium when acutely ill patients are confused and restless; however, in reality there are several different subtypes of delirium: hyperactive (restlessness, agitation, irritability, aggression); hypoactive (slow response to verbal stimuli, psychomotor slowing); and mixed delirium (both hyperactive and hypoactive behaviors). Assessment of delirium should be routine in the progressive care unit, and there are several valid and reliable tools that can be used to identify delirium.

Often mislabeled as psychosis, delirium is not psychosis. Sensory overload is a common risk factor that contributes to delirium in the acutely ill. Medications that may also play a role in instigating delirium include prochlorperazine, diphenhydramine, famotidine, benzodiazepines, opioids, and antiarrhythmic medications.

After recognizing the risk for delirium, nurses can take action to prevent it. The best approaches are multimodal, employing a variety of interventions simultaneously, often referred to as a "bundle" of care. A typical bundle to prevent delirium might include addressing pain, implementing early mobility, ensuring adequate sleep, providing assistive devices such as glasses and hearing aids to address sensory deficits and minimizing the use of medications that contribute to delirium. Family involvement in reorienting the patient and providing familiar faces and voices is also helpful in preventing delirium.

Once delirium develops, the first priority is to identify the cause. Is there a physiologic change such as an electrolyte abnormality, hypoxemia, or an adverse reaction to a medication? Are the patient's underlying health problems, such as heart failure, poorly controlled? Could the patient have a new infection? Is the patient in pain? Once a cause is identified, collaborate with providers in the selection of an appropriate treatment plan. Medication for managing delirium is best reserved for those cases in which behavioral interventions have failed. Restraints are discouraged because they tend to increase agitation.

If the patient demonstrates a paranoid element in his or her delirium, avoid confrontation and remain at a safe distance. Accept bizarre statements calmly, without agreement. Explain to the family that the behaviors are symptoms that will most likely resolve with time, resumption of normal sleep patterns, and medication. Delirious patients usually remember the events, thoughts, conversations, and provider responses that occur during delirium. The recovered patients may be embarrassed and feel guilty if they were combative during their illness.

Depression

Depression occurring with a medical illness affects long-term recovery by lengthening the course of the illness, and increasing morbidity and mortality. Risk factors that predispose for depression with medical disorders include social isolation, recent loss, pessimism, financial pressures, history of mood disorder, alcohol or substance abuse/withdrawal, previous suicide attempts, and pain. Many patients arrive in the hospital with a history of treatment for depression that can be exacerbated by an acute illness crisis. It is important that healthcare providers maintain the patient's psychiatric medication regimen if at all possible in order to avoid worsening of the patient's psychological status.

Educating the patient and family about the temporary nature of most depressions during acute illness assists in providing reassurance that this is not an unusual phenomenon. Severe depressive symptoms often respond to pharmacologic intervention, so a psychiatric consultation may be warranted. Keep in mind that it may take several weeks for antidepressants to reach their full effectiveness. The best way to assess for depression is to ask directly. Allow the patient to direct the conversation. If negative distortions about illness and treatment are communicated, it is appropriate to correct, clarify, and reassure with realistic information to promote a more hopeful outcome. Consistency in care providers promotes trust in an ongoing relationship and enhances recovery.

A patient who has attempted suicide or is suicidal can be frightening to hospital staff. Staff members are often uncertain of what to say when the patient says, "I want to kill myself … my life no longer has meaning." Ask the patient if they are feeling suicidal; such questions do not promote suicidal thoughts. Many times the communication of feeling suicidal is a cover for wanting to discuss fear, pain, or loneliness. A psychiatric referral is recommended in these situations for further evaluation and intervention. Patients who are suicidal with an active plan are monitored for safety to prevent self-harm, based on the facility's policy and on psychiatry recommendations.

Anxiety

Medical disorders can cause anxiety and panic-like symptoms, which are distressing to the patient and family and may exacerbate the medical condition. Treatment of the underlying medical condition may decrease the concomitant anxiety. Both pharmacologic and nonpharmacologic interventions can be helpful in managing anxiety during acute illness. Pharmacologic agents for anxiety are discussed in Chapter 6 (Pain and Sedation Management) and Chapter 7 (Pharmacology). Goals of pharmacologic therapy are to titrate the drug dose so that the patient can remain cognizant and interactive with staff, family, and environment; to complement pain control; and to assist in promoting sleep. There are also a variety of nonpharmacologic interventions to decrease or control anxiety:

- *Breathing techniques:* These techniques target somatic symptoms and include deep and slow abdominal breathing patterns. It is important to demonstrate and do the breathing with patients, as their heightened anxiety decreases their attention span. Practicing this technique may decrease anxiety and assist the patient through difficult procedures.
- *Muscle relaxation:* Reduce psychomotor tension with muscle relaxation. Again, the patient will most likely be unable to cue himself or herself, so this is an excellent opportunity for the family to participate as the cuing partner. Cuing might be, "The mattress under your head, elbow, heel, and back feels heavy against your body, press harder, and then try to drift away from the mattress as you relax." Mobile applications and websites with commercial relaxation techniques are available but are not as useful as the cuing by a familiar voice.
- *Imagery:* Interventions targeting cognition, such as imagery techniques, depend on the patient's capacity for attention, memory, and processing. Visualization imagery involves recalling a pleasurable, relaxing situation; for example, a hot bath, lying on a warm beach, listening to waves, or hearing birds sing. Guided imagery and hypnosis are additional therapies, but require some competency to be effective; thus, a referral is suggested. Patients who practice meditation as an alternative for stress control are encouraged to continue, but the environment may need modification to optimize the effects.

- *Preparatory information:* Providing the patient and family with preparatory information is extremely helpful in controlling anxiety. Allowing the patient and family to control some aspects of the treatment process, even if only minor aspects of care, can be anxiolytic.
- *Distraction techniques:* Distraction techniques can also interrupt the anxiety cycle. Methods for distracting can be listening to familiar music, watching videos, or counting backward from 200 by 2 rapidly.
- *Use of previous coping methods:* Identify how the patient and family have dealt with stress and anxiety in the past and suggest that approach if feasible. Supporting previous coping techniques may well be adaptive.

PATIENT AND FAMILY EDUCATION

Patient and family education in the progressive care environment is essential to providing information regarding diagnosis, prognosis, treatments, and procedures. In addition, education provides patients and family members a mechanism by which fears and concerns can be put in perspective and confronted so that they can become active members in the decisions made about care.

Providing patient and family education in acute care is challenging; multiple barriers (eg, environmental factors, patient stability, patient and family anxiety) are overcome or adapted to provide this essential intervention. The importance of education, coupled with the barriers common in progressive care, necessitates that education be a continuous ongoing process engaged in by all members of the team.

Education in the progressive care setting is most often done informally, though some patients may be able to tolerate limited sessions in a classroom setting. Education of the patient and family can often be subtle, occurring with each interaction between the patient, family, and members of the healthcare team. Education may also be more direct, particularly in relation to self-care or managing equipment at home. Use of a family member or friend who is a learning partner during patient education provides for the most effective learning process and outcomes.

Assessment of Learning Readiness

Assessment of the patient's and family's learning needs focuses primarily on learning readiness. *Learning readiness* refers to that moment in time when the learner is able to comprehend and synthesize the shared information. Without learning readiness, teaching may not be useful. Questions to assess learning readiness are listed in Table 2-5.

Strategies to Address Patient and Family Education

Prior to teaching, the information gathered in the assessment is prioritized and organized into a format that is meaningful

TABLE 2-5. ASSESSMENT OF LEARNING READINESS

General Principles
• Do the patient and the family have questions about the diagnosis, prognosis, treatments, or procedures?
• What do the patient and the family desire to learn about?
• What is the knowledge level of the individuals being taught? What do they already know about the issues that will be taught?
• What is their current situation (condition and environment) and have they had any prior experience in a similar situation?
• Do the patient or the family have any communication barriers (eg, language, illiteracy, culture, listening/comprehension deficits)?
• What is patient's or family members' preferred method of learning?

Special Considerations in Progressive Care
• Does the patient's condition allow you to assess this information from them (eg, physiologic/psychological stability)?
• Is the patient's support system/family/significant other available or ready to receive this information?
• What environmental factors (including time) present as barriers in the progressive care unit?
• Are there other members of the healthcare team who may possess vital assessment information?

to the learner (Table 2-6). Next, the outcome of the teaching is established along with appropriate content, and then a decision is made about how to share the information. The next step is to teach the patient, family, and significant others (Table 2-7). Although this phase often appears to be the easiest, it is actually the most difficult. It is crucial during the communication of the content, regardless of the type of communication vehicle used (video, pamphlet, discussion), to listen carefully to the needs expressed by the learner and to provide clear and precise responses to those needs. Use of teach-back is a simple method to ensure the patient and family members comprehend the information provided. Teach-back involves asking the patient or family member to relay back, in their own words, what they need to do or know.

TABLE 2-6. PRINCIPLES FOR TEACHING PLANS

General Principles
• Establish the outcome of the teaching.
• Determine what content needs to be taught, given the assessment.
• Identify what support systems are in place to support your educational efforts (eg, unit leadership, education department, standardized teaching plans, teaching materials such as pamphlets, brochures, videos).
• Familiarize yourself with the content and teaching materials.
• Contact resources to clarify and provide consistency in information and to also provide additional educational support and follow-up.
• Determine the most appropriate teaching strategy (video, CDs, computer, written materials, discussion) and to whom (patient or family) it should be directed.

Special Considerations in Progressive Care
• Plan the teaching strategy *carefully*. Patients and families in the progressive care environment are stressed and an overload of information adds to their stress.
• When planning education, consider content and amount based on the assessment of the patient, nature, and severity of the patient's illness, availability of significant others, and existing environmental barriers.

TABLE 2-7. PRINCIPLES FOR EDUCATIONAL SESSIONS

General Principles
• Consider the time needed to convey the information and the support system availability.
• Consider the situation the patient is currently experiencing. Postpone the session or adjust the goal as needed.
• Be aware of the amount of content and the patient's and the family's ability to process the information.
• Be sensitive in the delivery of the information. Make sure it is conveyed at a level that the patient and the family can understand.
• Refer to and involve resources as appropriate.
• Convey accurate and precise information. Make sure this information is consistent with previous information given to the patient.
• Listen carefully and solicit feedback during the session to guide the discussion.
• Use teach-back to ensure the patient and family understood and comprehend the information provided. Re-explain and clarify any potential misinterpretations.

Special Considerations in Progressive Care
• Keep the time frame of educational sessions short to optimize learning. Education must be episodic due to the nature of the patient's condition and the environment.
• Provide repetition of the information. Stress and the progressive care environment can alter comprehension; for this reason repetition is necessary.
• More details will need to be given as the patient's condition improves and transitioning to the next level of care occurs.
• Return demonstrations may be required for self-care activities.
• Share the information given with other nurses and members of the team, including with patient transitions, so they can reinforce during their time with the patient and family.

This allows the healthcare provider to clarify or re-explain the content if learners have misunderstood or not comprehended the information relayed.

Outcome Measurement

Following educational interventions, it is essential to determine if the educational outcomes have been achieved (Table 2-8). Even if the outcome appears to have been achieved, it is not unusual that the learners may not retain all the information. Patients and families experience a great deal of stress while in the progressive care environment; reinforcement is often necessary and is anticipated.

TABLE 2-8. PRINCIPLES FOR EDUCATIONAL OUTCOME MONITORING

General Principles
• Measure the outcome. Was the outcome met? Was the outcome unmet?
• Communicate the outcome verbally and in a written format to other members of the healthcare team.
• Provide necessary follow-up and reinforcement of the teaching.
• Make referrals that may have been identified in or as a result of patient and family education.
• Evaluate the teaching process for barriers or problems, and then address those areas and be aware of these for future interactions.

Special Considerations in Progressive Care
• Recognize that repetition of information is the rule, not the exception. Be prepared to repeat information previously given, many times if necessary.

FAMILY-CENTERED CARE

There is a strong evidence base to support that family presence and involvement in the progressive care unit aids in patient recovery. Family members can help patients cope, reduce anxiety, and provide a resource for the patient. Families, however, also need support in maintaining their strength and having needs met to be able to function as a positive influence for the patient rather than having a negative impact.

Developing a partnership and a trusting relationship with the family is in everyone's best interest so that optimal functioning can occur. Research shows that there can frequently be disagreement between the nurse and family about the type or priorities of family needs. Therefore, it is important to discuss family needs and perceptions directly with each family and tailor interventions based on that assessment (Table 2-9).

Research has consistently identified five major areas of family needs (receiving assurance, remaining near the patient, receiving information, being comfortable, and having support available). These and the importance of unrestricted family visitation are addressed next.

Receiving Assurance

Family members need reassurance that the best possible care is being given to the patient. This instills confidence and a sense of security. It can also assist in either maintaining hope or can be helpful in redefining hope to a more realistic image when appropriate.

Remaining Near the Patient

Family members need to have consistent access to their loved one. Of primary importance to the family is the unit visiting policy. Specifics to be discussed include the number of

TABLE 2-9. EVIDENCE-BASED PRACTICE: FAMILY INTERVENTIONS

Planning
• Determine what the family sees as priority needs.

Interventions
• Determine spokesperson and contact person.
• Establish optimum methods to contact and communicate with family and make communication routine.
• Make referrals for support services as appropriate (eg, palliative care, social work, spiritual support).
• Provide information according to family needs.
• Include family in direct care and decision making as appropriate.
• Provide a comfortable environment.
• Consider development of a program for families to keep a "diary" of events and emotions.
• Encourage family presence and active participation during team rounds.

Evaluation
• Evaluate achievement of meeting family needs through multiple methods (eg, feedback, satisfaction surveys, care conferences, follow-up after discharge).

Data from Leske JS. Interventions to decrease family anxiety. Crit Care Nurse. 2002 Dec;22(6): 61-65 and Coombs M, Puntillo KA, Franck LS, et al. Implementing the SCCM Family-Centered Care Guidelines in Critical Care Nursing Practice. AACN Adv Crit Care. 2017 Summer;28(2):138-147.

TABLE 2-10. EVIDENCE-BASED PRACTICE: FAMILY VISITATION IN PROGRESSIVE CARE

- Establish ways for families to have access to the patient (eg, open visitation, contract visitation, unit phone numbers).
- Ask patients their preferences related to visiting.
- Promote access to patients with consistent unit policies and procedures with options for individualization, including policies to address incivility or violence from visitors.
- Prepare families for visit.
- Model interaction with patient.
- Give information about the patient's condition, equipment, and technology being used.
- Monitor the response of the patient and family to visitation.

visitors allowed at one time, age restrictions, visiting times if not flexible or open, and how to gain access to the unit (Table 2-10). There is increasing evidence to support the presence of a family member with the patient during invasive procedures, as well as during cardiopulmonary resuscitation (CPR). Although this practice may still be controversial, family members have reported a sense of relief and gratitude at being able to remain close to the patient. It is recommended that written policies be developed through an interprofessional approach prior to implementing family presence at CPR or procedures.

Receiving Information

Communication with the patient and family should be open and honest. Keep promises (be thoughtful before making promises), describe expectations, apologize for inconveniences and mistakes, and maintain confidentiality. Avoid contracting for secrets or accommodating requests for preferred care providers. Use concise, simplistic explanations without medical jargon or alphabet shorthand to facilitate understanding. Contact interpreters, as appropriate, when language barriers exist.

Evaluate the effectiveness of communication by asking the patient and family for their understanding of the message, its content and intent. When conflict occurs, find a private place for discussion. Avoid taking the confrontation personally. Consider what the issue is and what needs to occur to reach resolution. If too much emotion is present, agree to address the issue at a later time, if possible.

It is helpful to establish a communication tree by designating one family member to be called if there are changes in the patient's condition. Establish a time for that person to call the unit for updates. Reassure the family by being present or offering to refer them to other system supports. Unit expectations and rules can be conveyed in a pamphlet for the family to refer to over time. Content that is helpful includes orientation about the philosophy of care; routines such as shift changes and provider rounds; the varied roles of personnel who work with patients; and information to address the family's needs such as food services, bathrooms, waiting areas, chapel services, transportation, and lodging. Clarify what they see and hear. Mobilize resources and include them in patient care and problem solving, as appropriate.

Some progressive care units invite family members to interprofessional rounds for the discussion of their loved ones. Adequate communication can decrease anxiety, increase a sense of control, and assist in improving decision making by families.

Being Comfortable

Ensure that space in or near the progressive care unit to meet comfort needs of the family is available. This space may include comfortable furniture, access to phones and restrooms, and assistance with finding overnight accommodations. Encourage the family to admit when they are overwhelmed, take breaks, go to meals, rest, sleep, take care of themselves, and not to abandon members at home. Helping the family with basic comfort needs helps decrease their distress and maintain their reserves and coping mechanisms. This improves their ability to be a valuable resource for the patient.

Having Support Available

Utilize all potential resources in meeting family needs. Relying on nurses to fulfill all family needs while they are also trying to care for progressive care patients can create tension and frustration. Assess the family for their own resources that can be maximized. Utilize hospital referrals that can assist in family support such as chaplains, social workers, palliative care, and child-family life departments.

Family Visitation

There is an abundance of evidence demonstrating that unrestricted access of the patient's support network (family, significant others, trusted friends) benefits the patient by providing emotional and social support; improving the healthcare team's understanding of the patient's goals of care; increasing communication, and increasing patient and family satisfaction. However, many hospitals continue to have policies that restrict visitation. There are certainly individual circumstances where open visiting can be ill-advised due to medical, therapeutic, or safety considerations (eg, disruptive behavior, infectious disease concerns, patient privacy, or per patient request). On admission to the progressive care unit, ask the patient to identify the people who comprise their "family" and to state their visiting preferences. Collaborate with the interprofessional team and the patient and family to accommodate those preferences while meeting safety, privacy, and decision-making needs.

For the family, the progressive care setting symbolizes a variety of hopes, fears, and beliefs that range from hope of a cure to end-of-life care. A family-centered approach can promote coping and cohesion among family members and minimize the isolation and anxiety for patients. Anticipating family needs, focusing on the present, fostering open communication, and providing information are vital to promoting psychological integrity for families. By using the event of hospitalization as a point of access, progressive care clinicians assume a major role in primary prevention and assisting families to cope positively with crisis and grow from the experience.

TRANSPORTING THE PROGRESSIVE CARE PATIENT

Preventing common complications and maintaining physiologic and psychosocial stability is a challenge even when in the controlled environment of the progressive care unit. It is even more challenging when transporting the progressive care patient to other areas of the hospital for diagnostic and therapeutic purposes. The decision to transport the progressive care patient out of the well-controlled environment of the progressive care unit elicits a variety of responses from clinicians. It is not uncommon to hear phrases like these: "What if something happens en route?" "Who will take care of my other patients while I'm gone?" Responses like these underscore the clinician's understanding of the risks involved in transporting progressive care patients.

Transporting a progressive care patient involves more than putting the patient on a stretcher and rolling him or her down the hall. Safe patient transport requires thoughtful planning, organization, and interprofessional communication and cooperation. The goal during transport is to maintain the same level of care, regardless of the location in the hospital. The transfer of progressive care patients always involves some degree of risk to the patient. The decision to transfer, therefore, is based on an assessment of the potential benefits of transfer weighed against the potential risks.

The reason for moving a progressive care patient is typically the need for care, technology, or specialists not available in the progressive care unit. Whenever feasible, diagnostic testing or simple procedures are performed at the patient's bedside within the progressive care unit. If the diagnostic test or procedural intervention under consideration is unlikely to alter management or outcome of the patient, then the risk of transfer may outweigh the benefit. It is imperative that every member of the healthcare team assists in clarifying what, if any, benefit may be derived from transport.

Assessment of Risk for Complications

Prior to initiating transport, a patient's risk for development of complications during transport is systematically assessed. The switching of technologies in the progressive care unit to portable devices may lead to undesired physiologic changes. In addition, complications may arise from environmental conditions outside the progressive care unit that are difficult to control, such as body temperature fluctuations or inadvertent movement of invasive devices (eg, tracheostomies, chest tubes, IV devices). Common complications associated with transportation are summarized in Table 2-11.

Pulmonary Complications
Maintaining adequate ventilation and oxygenation during transport is a challenge. Patients who are not intubated prior to their transfer are at risk for developing airway

TABLE 2-11. POTENTIAL COMPLICATIONS DURING TRANSPORT

Pulmonary
- Hyperventilation
- Hypoventilation
- Airway obstruction
- Aspiration
- Recurrent pneumothorax
- Arterial blood gas changes

Cardiovascular
- Hypotension
- Hypertension
- Arrhythmias
- Decreased tissue perfusion
- Cardiac ischemia
- Peripheral ischemia

Neurologic
- Increased intracranial pressure
- Cerebral hypoxia
- Cerebral hypercarbia
- Paralysis

Gastrointestinal
- Nausea
- Vomiting

Pain

compromise. This is particularly a problem in patients with decreased levels of consciousness. Continuous monitoring of airway patency is critical to ensure rapid implementation of airway strategies, if necessary.

Hypoventilation or hyperventilation can result in pH changes, which may lead to deficits in tissue perfusion and oxygenation. Therefore, respiratory and nursing personnel who are properly trained in the mechanisms of manual ventilation need to provide ventilation during transport, if portable ventilators are not available or are not tolerated by the patient. Patients requiring continuous bilevel positive airway pressure (BiPAP) or high-flow oxygen may experience changes in respiratory status during transport. The percentage of inspired oxygen (FiO_2) may need to be increased during transport. Increasing the FiO_2 for any patient requiring transfer may help avoid other complications from hypoxia. Ensuring the appropriate portable equipment to maintain adequate oxygenation may be complex but imperative. The patient's special respiratory equipment may also be transported to the destination so that he or she can be placed back on the equipment during the procedure.

Cardiovascular Complications
Whether related to their underlying disease processes or the anxiety of being taken out of a controlled environment, the potential for cardiovascular complications exists in all patients being transported. These complications include hypotension, hypertension, arrhythmias, tachycardia, ischemia, and acute pulmonary edema. Many of these complications can be avoided by adequate patient preparation with pharmacologic agents to maintain hemodynamic stability and manage pain and anxiety. Continuous infusions are

carefully maintained during transport, with special attention given to IV lines during movement of the patient from one surface to another. Additional emergency equipment may need to be taken on the transport such as hand pumps for patients on ventricular assist devices.

Neurologic Complications

The potential for respiratory and cardiovascular changes during transport increases the risk for cerebral hypoxia, hypercarbia, and intracranial pressure (ICP) changes. Patients with high baseline ICP may require additional interventions to stabilize cerebral perfusion and oxygenation prior to transport (eg, hyperventilation, increased partial pressure of oxygen in arterial blood [Pao_2], blood pressure control). In addition, patients with suspected cranial or vertebral fractures are at high risk for neurologic damage during repositioning from bed to transport stretchers or diagnostic tables. Proper immobilization of the spine is imperative in these situations, as is the avoidance of unnecessary repositioning of the patient. Positioning the head in the midline position with the head of the bed elevated, when not contraindicated, may decrease the risk of increases in ICP.

Gastrointestinal Complications

Gastrointestinal (GI) complications may include nausea or vomiting, which can threaten the patient's airway, as well as cause discomfort. Premedicating patients at risk for GI upset with an H_2-blocker, proton pump inhibitor, or an antiemetic as appropriate may be helpful. For patients with large volume nasogastric (NG) drainage, preparations to continue NG drainage during transportation or in the destination location may be necessary.

Pain and Anxiety

The level of pain experienced by the patient is likely to be increased during transport. Many of the diagnostic tests and therapeutic interventions in other hospital departments are uncomfortable or painful. Anxiety associated with transport may also increase the level of pain. Additional analgesic or anxiolytic agents, or both may be required to ensure adequate pain and anxiety management during the transport process. Keeping the patient and family members well informed is also helpful in decreasing anxiety levels.

Level of Care Required During Transport

During transport, there should be no interruption in the monitoring or maintenance of the patient's vital functions. The equipment used during transport as well as the skill level of accompanying personnel is to be equivalent with the interventions required or anticipated for the patient while in the progressive care unit (Table 2-12). Intermittent and continuous monitoring of physiologic status (eg, cardiac rhythm, blood pressure, oxygenation, ventilation) continue during transport and while the patient is away from the progressive care unit (Table 2-13).

TABLE 2-12. TRANSPORT PERSONNEL AND EQUIPMENT REQUIREMENTS

Personnel
- Patients whose conditions are unstable, or are at risk for instability, or who require a specific type of monitoring should be accompanied by staff competent in managing the instability and in interpreting and intervening appropriately, based on the monitoring data.
- Additional personnel may include a respiratory therapist, registered nurse, transport aide, or provider.

Equipment
The following minimal equipment should be available:
- Cardiac monitor/defibrillator
- Airway management equipment and resuscitation bag of proper size and fit for the patient.
- Oxygen source of ample volume to support the patient's needs for the projected time out of the progressive care unit, with an additional 30-minute reserve.
- Standard resuscitation drugs: epinephrine, atropine, amiodarone.
- Blood pressure cuff (sphygmomanometer) and stethoscope.
- Ample supply of the IV fluids and continuous infusion medications (regulated by battery-operated infusion pumps) being administered to the patient.
- Additional medications to provide the patient's scheduled intermittent medication doses and to meet anticipated needs (eg, sedation) with appropriate orders to allow their administration if a provider is not present.
- Resuscitation cart and suction equipment need not accompany each patient being transferred, but such equipment should be stationed in areas used by acutely ill patients and be readily available (within 4 minutes) by a predetermined mechanism for emergencies that may occur en route.

Data from Day D. Keeping patients safe during intrahospital transport. Crit Care Nurse. 2010 Aug;30(4):18-32.

Questions that need to be answered to prepare for transfer include the following:

- What is the current level of care (equipment, personnel)?
- What will be needed during the transfer or at the destination to maintain that level of care?
- What additional therapeutic interventions may be required before or during transport (eg, pain and sedation medications or titration of infusions)?
- Do I have all the necessary equipment needed in the event of an emergency during the transport?

To confirm what capabilities exist at the destination, call the receiving area in advance to ask about their resources; for example, are there adequate outlets to plug in electrical equipment rather than continuing to use battery power,

TABLE 2-13. MONITORING DURING TRANSFER

- If technologically possible, patients being transferred should receive the same physiologic monitoring (eg, ECG, BP, SPo_2, vital signs; continuous or intermittent) during transfer that they were receiving in the progressive care unit.
- In addition, selected patients, based on clinical status, may benefit from continuous measurement of blood pressure and intermittent measurement of CVP.

Data from: Day D. Keeping patients safe during intrahospital transport. Crit Care Nurse. 2010 Aug;30(4):18-32.

do they have capability for high levels of suction pressure if needed, or what specialty instructions need to be followed in magnetic resonance imaging? Will they be ready to take the patient immediately into the procedure with no waiting? Are they aware of and can accommodate required isolation precautions?

Preparation

Before transfer, the plan of care for the patient during and after transfer is coordinated to ensure continuity of care and availability of appropriate resources (Table 2-14). The receiving units are contacted to confirm that all preparations for the patient's arrival have been completed. Communication, both written and verbal, between team members delineates the current status of the patient, management priorities, and the process to follow in the event of untoward events (eg, unexpected hemodynamic instability or airway problems).

After assessing the patient's risk for transport complications, prepare the patient for transfer, both physically and mentally. While organizing the equipment and monitors, explain the transfer process to the patient and family. The explanation includes a description of the sensations the

TABLE 2-14. PRETRANSFER COORDINATION AND COMMUNICATION

- Provider-to-provider and/or nurse-to-nurse communication regarding the patient's condition and treatment preceding and following the transfer should be documented in the medical record when the management of the patient will be assumed by a different team while the patient is away from the progressive care unit.
- The area to which the patient is being transferred (x-ray, operating room, nuclear medicine, etc) must confirm that it is ready to receive the patient and immediately begin the procedure or test for which the patient is being transferred.
- Ancillary services (eg, security, respiratory therapy, escort) must be notified as to the timing of the transfer and the equipment and support needed.
- Documentation in the medical record must include the indication for transfer, the patient's status during transfer and whether the patient is expected to return to the progressive care unit.

Data from: Day D. Keeping patients safe during intrahospital transport. Crit Care Nurse. 2010 Aug;30(4):18-32.

patient may expect, an estimate of the procedure's length, and the role of individual members of the transport team. It is important to allay any patient or family anxiety by identifying current caregivers who will accompany the patient during transport. The availability of emergency equipment and medications and how communication is handled during

---

ESSENTIAL CONTENT CASE

Risk Factors During Transport

Mr. W, a 45-year-old man, was involved in a motor vehicle accident when he fell asleep on his way home from work. He was not wearing a seat belt, and there were no air bags in the car. His injuries included chest contusions and broken ribs from the steering wheel and lacerations of his scalp from the windshield. He was in the ICU for 7 days with the insertion of a chest tube to relieve his left pneumothorax and on mechanical ventilation for 6 days. Twenty-four hours ago, he was transferred to the progressive care unit. Mr. W is assigned to a progressive care nurse, Nancy, who has three other patients. One of these patients is recovering from repair of an abdominal aortic aneurysm 2 days ago, the second patient is recovering from a large anterior myocardial infarction suffered after a total hip replacement, and the third patient will be discharged to home today after a 3-day stay for an exacerbation of heart failure. Mr. W is now complaining of a new onset of shortness of breath and requires 50% Fio_2 per face mask for slowly falling oxygen saturations. A chest computed tomography (CT) had been ordered for him.

Case Question 1: Which of Mr. W's physiologic systems or clinical states are at particular risk of compromise during the transport for his CT scan?

Case Question 2: Why is Nancy concerned about the possibility of Mr. W experiencing pain and anxiety during the transport?

Answers
1. Respiratory, cardiovascular, pain, anxiety. Nancy was aware of the possible complications he might experience during transport—respiratory, cardiovascular, or safety

compromises. Possible respiratory complications included upper airway obstruction, respiratory depression, hypoxia, or hypercarbia, especially in a patient who has head and chest trauma and whose oxygenation is already compromised. Cardiovascular risks included hypotension, tachycardia due to cardiac tamponade, and decreased tissue perfusion because of decreased cardiac output and increased tissue oxygen demand during the transfer. Acute pain may occur or be exacerbated as a result of increased anxiety, patient movement and positioning, and hard surfaces during transport as well as potential manipulation/movement of invasive devices such as chest tubes. Nancy noted that anxiety from both the activity of transfer and from the uncertainty of Mr. W's future could certainly result in adverse physiologic changes during transport.

2. In addition to Nancy's goal to keep Mr. W comfortable while under her care, she also recognizes that increasing pain and anxiety can result in an increasing respiratory rate, heart rate, and blood pressure. All of these physiologic changes can exacerbate his worsening respiratory status and increased oxygen demands. It is important that the potential for these complications be minimized, particularly when Mr. W is being transported for the CT scan where addressing any physiologic decompensation or emergency situations is more challenging.

Anticipating complications, Nancy planned ahead. She asked the respiratory therapist to gather the appropriate oxygen equipment and accompany Nancy on the transport. With his respiratory status stable for the time being, Mr. W could be safely medicated with small dosages for pain and anxiety, ultimately decreasing his oxygen demand.

transportation also may be information that will reassure the patient and family.

Transport

Once preparations are complete, the actual transfer can begin. Ensure that the portable equipment has adequate battery life to last well beyond the anticipated transfer time in case of unanticipated delays. Connect each of the portable monitoring devices prior to disconnection from the bedside equipment, if possible. This enables a comparison of vital sign values with the portable equipment.

Once vital sign measurement equipment and noninvasive oxygenation monitors are in place and values verified, disconnect the patient from the bedside oxygen source and begin portable oxygenation. Assess for clinical signs and symptoms of respiratory distress and changes in ventilation and oxygenation. It may be easier to transfer the patient on the bed if it will fit in elevators and spaces in the receiving area. Check IV lines, pressure lines, monitor cables, NG tubes, chest tubes, urinary catheters, or drains of any sort to ensure proper placement during transport and to guard against accidental removal during transport.

During transport, the progressive care nurse is responsible for continuous assessment of cardiopulmonary status (ie, electrocardiograph, blood pressures, respiration, oxygenation) and interventions as required to ensure stability.

Throughout the time away from the progressive care environment, vigilant monitoring to evaluate the patient's response to the transport, and to the procedure or therapeutic intervention is imperative. Alterations in medication administration, particularly analgesics, sedatives, and vasoactive agents, are frequently needed during the time away from the progressive care unit to maintain physiologic stability. Documentation of assessment findings, interventions, and the patient's responses continue throughout the transport process.

Following return to the progressive care unit, monitoring systems and interventions are reestablished and the patient is completely reassessed. Often, some adjustment in pharmacologic therapy or oxygen support is required following transport. Allowing for some uninterrupted time for the family to be at the patient's bedside and for patient rest is another important priority following return to the unit. Documentation of the patient's overall response to the transport situation is included in the medical record.

Interfacility Transfers

Interfacility patient transfers, although similar to transfers within a hospital, can be more challenging. The biggest differences between the two are the isolation of the patient in the transfer vehicle, limited equipment and personnel, and a high complication rate due to longer transport periods and inability to control environmental conditions (eg,

---

ESSENTIAL CONTENT CASE

Preparing for Transport

Having recognized and addressed Mr. W's risk factors, his nurse, Nancy, organizes the team for the transport of Mr. W to CT scan, making sure another nurse is able to care for her other patients while she was off the unit. Recognizing Mr. W's risk for respiratory compromise, Nancy requests a respiratory therapist for the transport. Other members of the transport team include two transporters to help manage the equipment, open doors, and hold elevators.

Case Question 1: Nancy decided to contact the Imaging Department prior to transporting Mr. W. What types of questions should Nancy ask of the radiology nurse?

Case Question 2: What information could Nancy provide to Mr. W and his wife to allay some of their concerns?

Answers

1. Examples of questions that Nancy asked for clarification: Is there a nurse in the CT suite who can care for Mr. W once he arrives there? How long should she expect him to be gone from the progressive care unit? Are there electrical outlets for all the equipment in CT? Is there oxygen available in CT? Is there suction equipment in the CT suite? When will they be ready to receive Mr. W?

    Nancy gathered the portable equipment and connected it to Mr. W. This included a cardiac monitor, a blood pressure monitor, and a pulse oximeter. IV lines were organized so that only essential infusions were transported with Mr. W.

Other concerns that Nancy considered included: How long will the equipment batteries last? Will the water seal for the chest tube hang on the bed? Will he need suctioning? What medications does Mr. W need while he is off the progressive care unit? Does he need something for pain or his next dose of antibiotic? Will he need new IV fluids while he is gone? If he is able, does he understand the procedure that he's going to have? Where is his family? Do they know what is going on?

Fortunately for Nancy, one battery-operated machine was able to monitor pressures, cardiac rhythm, and pulse oximetry. The respiratory therapist brought high-flow oxygen equipment on the transport in case it was needed during the CT scan. The chest tube drain fit over the rail around the bed, maintaining the water seal without suction. The urinary catheter also had a special hook allowing it to hang safely on the side of the bed.

2. Mr. W was understandably anxious about what was going on, as was his wife. Nancy talked to both of them about what to expect during the transport, as well as in the CT suite. She explained how long the procedure would last, and where Mr. W's wife could wait while the procedure was in progress. She reassured them that a nurse would be with Mr. W throughout the procedure and that any pain or discomfort would be adequately treated. She allowed Mr. W's wife to stay with her husband as long as possible during the transfer.

temperature, atmospheric pressure, sudden movements), which may cause physiologic instability.

The primary consideration in interfacility transfer is maintaining the same level of care provided in the progressive care unit. Accordingly, the mode of transfer is selected with this in mind. The resources available in the sending facility are made as portable as possible and accompany the patient; for example, ventricular assist devices are continued without interruption. This requirement often challenges progressive care practitioners' skills and abilities, as well as the equipment resources necessary to ensure a safe transport.

TRANSITIONING TO THE NEXT STAGE OF CARE

Planning the transition of the patient to the next stage of care (eg, transfer from progressive care to rehabilitation, skilled nursing facility or to home) begins soon after the patient is admitted to the progressive care unit. It involves assessing minimally where and with whom the patient lives, what external resources were being used prior to admission, and what resources are anticipated to be required on transfer out of the progressive care unit. Complex patients require extensive preplanning to achieve a successful transition. As the patient stabilizes and improves, the thought of leaving the progressive care unit can be frightening as it is perceived as moving to a level of care where there are fewer staff to monitor the patient. Reinforce the positive aspect of planning for the transition in that it is a sign that the patient is improving and making progress.

If the patient is transferring to another institution, such as an acute or subacute rehabilitation facility, suggest that the family visit the facility prior to transfer. This gives them an opportunity to meet the new caregivers, ask any questions they may have, and alleviate the patient's anxiety about the transfer. If the transfer is internal to another patient-care unit and the patient's care is complex, consider working with the receiving unit staff in advance to inform them of the anticipated plan of care and any patient preferences. Identify a primary nurse in advance from the receiving unit, if possible, who may be able to take the time to meet the patient before the transfer. Clinical nurse specialists or nurse managers may also be able to meet the patient and family, describe the receiving unit, and act as a resource after the transfer, again giving a sense of control to the patient and family.

SUPPORTING PATIENTS AND THEIR FAMILIES DURING THE DYING PROCESS

Transitioning of care also includes planning care for the patient who is dying. Caring for the dying patient and his or her family can be the most rewarding challenge. The use of advance directives and Orders for Life Sustaining Treatment provides a means for the acutely ill patient to communicate wishes regarding end-of-life care. A dialogue with the patient about end-of-life care is an appropriate avenue for discussing values and beliefs associated with dying and living and understanding their goals of care. Hopefully, discussions prior to a traumatic event or progressive care admission have occurred so the patient is empowered to institute stopping or continuing life-support measures and has designated a surrogate decision maker. If advance directives are in place, then advocating for those wishes and promoting comfort are primary responsibilities of clinicians. If previous discussions have not taken place, as with an unexpected traumatic accident, then requesting system resources such as palliative care to assist the family is appropriate. Providing for clergy to assist with spiritual needs and rituals also can help the family to cope with the crisis.

An awareness of personal feelings about death is essential when caring for dying persons. Be genuine in providing care, touch, and presence, and do not feel compelled to talk. Take cues from the patient. Crying or laughing with the patient and family is an acknowledgment of humanness—an existential relationship and a rare gift in a unique encounter.

PRINCIPLES OF MANAGEMENT

1. Use of interprofessional plans of care improves communication and collaboration in achieving optimal patient outcomes.
2. Optimal care of acutely ill patients includes preventing complications common in the progressive care unit setting such VTEs, hospital-acquired infections, pressure injury, falls and sleep disturbances.
3. Prevention and prompt treatment of delirium, depression, and anxiety may prevent or ameliorate the negative long-term consequences of progressive care stays for both patients and families.
4. Meeting patient and family needs through patient and family-centered care and education includes providing vital information regarding the patient's condition and care to allay their fears and concerns.
5. Careful planning and organization can minimize risks of intrafacility transport of acutely ill patients.
6. Planning for the transition of patients out of progressive care begins on admission.

SELECTED BIBLIOGRAPHY

Patient and Family Needs

American Association of Critical-Care Nurses. AACN Practice Alert. Family visitation in the adult intensive care unit. 2016. https://www.aacn.org/~/media/aacn-website/clincial-resources/practice-alerts/famvisitpafeb2016ccnpages.pdf. Accessed June 15, 2017.

Chapman DK, Collingridge DS, Mitchell LA, et al. Satisfaction with elimination of all visitation restrictions in a mixed-profile intensive care unit. *Am J Crit Care.* 2016;25(1):46-50.

Coombs M, Puntillo KA, Franck LS, et al. Implementing the SCCM family-centered guidelines in critical care nursing practice. *AACN Adv Crit Care.* 2017;28(2):138-147.

DeCourcey M, Russell AC, Keister KJ. Animal-assisted therapy: evaluation and implementation of a complementary therapy to improve the psychological and physiological health of critically ill patients. *Dimens Crit Care Nurs.* 2010;29(5):211-214.

Hardin SR, Kaplow R. *Synergy for Clinical Excellence: The AACN Synergy Model for Patient Care.* 2nd ed. Burlington, MA: Jones & Bartlett; 2017.

Høghaug G, Fagermoen MS. Lerdal A. The visitor's regard of their need for support, comfort, information, proximity, and assurance in the intensive care unit. *Intensiv Crit Care Nurs.* 2012;28(5):263-268.

Jacob M, Horton C, Rance-Ashley S, et al. Needs of patients' family members in an intensive care unit with continuous visitation. *Am J Crit Care.* 2016;25(2):118-125.

Kozub E, Scheler S, Necoechea G, O'Byrne N. Improving nurse satisfaction with open visitation in an adult intensive care unit. *Crit Care Nurs Q.* 2017;40(2):144-154.

Obringer K, Hilgenberg C, Booker K. Needs of adult family members of intensive care unit patients. *J Clin Nurs.* 2012;21(11-12):1651-1658.

Infection Control

Centers for Disease Control and Prevention. Surveillance for bloodstream infections, 2017. https://www.cdc.gov/nhsn/acute-care-hospital/clabsi/index.html. Accessed June 13, 2017.

Centers for Disease Control and Prevention. Surveillance for *C. difficile*, MRSA and other drug-resistant organisms, 2017. https://www.cdc.gov/nhsn/acute-care-hospital/cdiff-mrsa/index.html. Accessed June 13, 2017.

Centers for Disease Control and Prevention. Surveillance for urinary tract infections, 2017. https://www.cdc.gov/nhsn/acute-care-hospital/cauti/index.html. Accessed June 13, 2017.

Centers for Disease Control and Prevention. Surveillance for ventilator-associated events, 2017. https://www.cdc.gov/nhsn/acute-care-hospital/vae/index.html. Accessed June 13, 2017.

Patient and Family Education

Always Use Teach-Back! Welcome to the Always Use Teach-Back! training toolkit, 2017. www.teachbacktraining.org. Accessed June 15, 2017.

Centrella-Nigro AM, Alexander C. Using the teach-back method in patient education to improve patient satisfaction. *J Contin Educ Nurs.* 2017;48(1):47-52.

Gillam SW, Gillam AR, Casler TL, Curcio K. Education for medications and side effects: a two part mechanism for improving the patient experience. *Appl Nurs Res.* 2016;31:72-78.

Psychological Problems

Davidson JE, Harvey MA. Patient and family post-intensive care syndrome. *AACN Adv Crit Care.* 2016;27(2):184-186.

Garrett KM. Best practices for managing pain, sedation, and delirium in the mechanically ventilated patient. *Crit Care Nurs Clin North Am.* 2016;28(4):437-450.

ICU Delirium and Cognitive Impairment Study Group. Vanderbilt University; 2013. http://www.icudelirium.org/. Accessed June 13, 2017.

Selim AA, Ely EW. Delirium the under-recognised syndrome: survey of healthcare professionals' awareness and practice in the intensive care units. *J Clin Nurs.* 2017;26(5-6):813-824.

Slooter AJ, Van de Leur RR, Zaal IJ. Delirium in critically ill patients. *Handb Clin Neurol.* 2017;141:449-466.

Sleep Deprivation

Blissitt PA. Sleep and mechanical ventilation. *Crit Care Nurs Clin North Am.* 2016;28:195-203.

Engwall M, Fridh I, Johansson L, Bergbom I, Lindahl B. Lighting, sleep and circadian rhythm: an intervention study in the intensive care unit. *Intensive Crit Care Nurs.* 2015;31(6):325-335.

Hopper K, Fried TR, Pisani MA. Health care worker attitudes and identified barriers to patient sleep in the medical intensive care unit. *Heart Lung.* 2015;44(2):95-99.

Kaplow R. Sleep disturbances and critical illness. *Crit Care Nurs Clin North Am.* 2016;28:169-182.

Owens RL, Huynh TG, Netzer G. Sleep in the intensive care unit in a model of family-centered care. *AACN Adv Crit Care.* 2017;28(2):171-178.

Shaw R. Using music to promote sleep for hospitalized adults. *Am J Crit Care.* 2018;25(2):181-184.

Transport of Critically Ill Patients

Comeau OY, Armendariz-Batiste J, Woodby SA. Safety first! Using a checklist for intrafacility transport of adult intensive care patients. *Crit Care Nurse.* 2015;35(5):16-25.

Day D. Keeping patients safe during intrahospital transport. *Crit Care Nurse.* 2010;30(4):18-32.

Warren J, Fromm RE, Orr RA, et al. Guidelines for the inter- and intrahospital transport of critically ill patients. *Crit Care Med.* 2004;32:256-262.

Evidence-Based Practice

Agency for Healthcare Research and Quality. Preventing pressure ulcers in hospitals: a toolkit for improving quality of care, 2014. www.ahrq.gov/professionals/systems/hospital/pressureulcertoolkit/index.html. Accessed June 15, 2017.

American Association of Critical-Care Nurses. AACN Practice Alert. Assessment and management of delirium across the life span. *Crit Care Nurse.* 2016;36(5):e14-e19.

American Association of Critical-Care Nurses. AACN Practice Alert. Family presence during resuscitation and invasive procedures. *Crit Care Nurse.* 2016;36(2):e11-e14.

American Association of Critical-Care Nurses. AACN Practice Alert. Oral care for acutely and critically ill patients. *Crit Care Nurse.* 2017;37(3):e19-e21.

American Association of Critical-Care Nurses. AACN Practice Alert. Prevention of aspiration in adults. *Crit Care Nurse.* 2016;36(1):e20-e24.

American Association of Critical-Care Nurses. AACN Practice Alert. Prevention of catheter-associated urinary tract infections in adults. *Crit Care Nurse.* 2017;37(3):e1-e3. Accessed at www.ccnonline.org

American Association of Critical-Care Nurses. AACN Practice Alert. Preventing venous thromboembolism in adults. *Crit Care Nurse*. 2016;36(5):e20-e23.

American Association of Critical-Care Nurses. AACN Practice Alert. Prevention of ventilator-associated pneumonia in adults. *Crit Care Nurse*. 2017;37(3):e22-e25.

Barr J, Fraser GL, Puntillo K, et al. Clinical practice guidelines for the management of pain, agitation, and delirium in the intensive care unit. *Crit Care Med*. 2013;41(1):263-306.

Centers for Disease Control and Prevention. Hand hygiene in healthcare settings. Show me the science, 2016. https://www.cdc.gov/handhygiene/science/index.html. Accessed June 15, 2017.

Flynn F, Evanish JQ, Fernald JM, Hutchinson DE, Lefaiver C. Progressive care nurses improving patient safety in limiting interruptions during medication administration. *Crit Care Nurse*. 2016;36(4):19-35.

Geerts WH, Bergqvist D, Pineo GF, et al. Prevention of venous thromboembolism: American College of Chest Physicians Evidence-Based Clinical Practice Guidelines (8th Edition). *Chest*. 2008;133(6 Suppl):381S-453S.

National Pressure Ulcer Advisory Panel, European Pressure Ulcer Advisory Panel, Pan Pacific Pressure Ulcer Injury Alliance. Prevention and Treatment of Pressure Ulcers: Quick Reference Guide, 2014. Haesler, E. (Ed.). Osborne Park, Western Australia: Cambridge Media. Available at https://www.npuap.org/wp-content/uploads/2014/08/updated-10-16-14-Quick-Reference-Guide-DIGITAL-NPUAP-EPUAP-PPPIA-16Oct2014.pdf. Accessed June 15, 2017.

Reames CO, Price DM, King EA, Dickinson S. Mobilizing patients along the continuum of critical care. *Dimens Crit Care Nurs*. 2016;35(1):10-15.

Sedwick MB, Lance-Smith M, Reeder SJ, Nardi J. Using evidence-based practice to prevent ventilator-associated pneumonia. *Crit Care Nurse*. 2012;32(4):41-50.

Williams T, King MW, Thompson JA, Champagne MT. Implementing evidence-based medication safety interventions on a progressive care unit. *Am J Nurs*. 2014;114(11):53-62.

INTERPRETATION AND MANAGEMENT OF BASIC CARDIAC RHYTHMS

3

Carol Jacobson

KNOWLEDGE COMPETENCIES

1. Correctly identify key elements of electrocardiogram (ECG) waveforms, complexes, and intervals:
   • P wave
   • QRS complex
   • T wave
   • ST segment
   • PR interval
   • QT interval
   • RR interval
   • Rate (atrial and ventricular)

2. Compare and contrast the etiology, ECG characteristics, and management of common cardiac rhythms and conduction abnormalities:
   • Sinus node rhythms
   • Atrial rhythms
   • Junctional rhythms
   • Ventricular rhythms
   • AV blocks

3. Describe the indications for, and use of, temporary pacemakers, defibrillation, and cardioversion for the treatment of serious cardiac dysrhythmias.*

*While different professional organizations may prefer the use of the term arrhythmia versus dysrhythmia, they are synonymous. This chapter uses dysrhythmia, the exception being the use of arrhythmia in selected professional statements, protocols, and practice statements.

Continuous monitoring of cardiac rhythm in the critically or acutely ill patient is an important aspect of cardiovascular assessment. Frequent analysis of electrocardiogram (ECG) rate and rhythm provides for early identification and treatment of alterations in cardiac rhythm, as well as abnormal conditions in other body systems. This chapter presents a review of basic cardiac electrophysiology and information essential to the identification and treatment of common cardiac dysrhythmias. Advanced cardiac dysrhythmias, and 12-lead ECG interpretation, are described in Chapter 18, Advanced ECG Concepts.

BASIC ELECTROPHYSIOLOGY

The electrical impulse of the heart is the stimulus for cardiac contraction. The cardiac conduction system is responsible for the initiation of the electrical impulse and its sequential spread through the atria, atrioventricular (AV) junction, and ventricles. The conduction system of the heart consists of the following structures (Figure 3-1):

Sinus node: The sinus node is a small group of cells in the upper right atrium that functions as the normal pacemaker of the heart because it has the highest rate of automaticity of all potential pacemaker sites. The sinus node normally depolarizes at a regular rate of 60 to 100 times/min.

AV node: The AV node is a small group of cells in the low right atrium near the tricuspid valve. The AV node has three main functions:

1. Its major job is to slow conduction of the impulse from the atria to the ventricles to allow time for the atria to contract and empty their blood into the ventricles.

2. Its rate of automaticity is 40 to 60 beats/min and can function as a backup pacemaker if the sinus node fails.

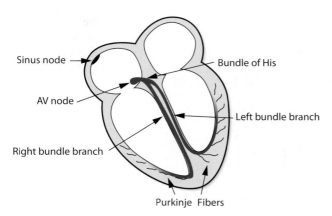

Figure 3-1. The conduction system of the heart.

3. It screens out rapid atrial impulses to protect the ventricles from dangerously fast rates when the atrial rate is very rapid.

Bundle of His: The bundle of His is a short bundle of fibers at the bottom of the AV node leading to the bundle branches. Conduction velocity accelerates in the bundle of His and the impulse is transmitted to both bundle branches.

Bundle branches: The bundle branches are bundles of fibers that rapidly conduct the impulse into the right and left ventricles. The *right bundle branch* travels along the right side of the interventricular septum and carries the impulse into

the right ventricle. The *left bundle branch* has two main divisions: the anterior fascicle and the posterior fascicle, which carry the impulse into the left ventricle.

Purkinje fibers: The Purkinje fibers are hairlike fibers that spread out from the bundle branches along the endocardial surface of both ventricles and rapidly conduct the impulse to the ventricular muscle cells. Cells in the Purkinje system have automaticity at a rate of 20 to 40 beats/min and can function as a backup pacemaker if all other pacemakers fail.

The electrical impulse normally begins in the sinus node and spreads through both atria in an inferior and leftward direction, resulting in depolarization of the atrial muscle. When the impulse reaches the AV node, its conduction velocity is slowed before it continues into the ventricles. When the impulse emerges from the AV node, it travels rapidly through the bundle of His and down the right and left bundle branches into the Purkinje network of both ventricles, and results in depolarization of the ventricular muscle. The spread of this wave of depolarization through the heart produces the classic surface ECG, which can be recorded by an electrocardiograph (ECG machine) or monitored continuously on a bedside cardiac monitor.

ECG WAVEFORMS, COMPLEXES, AND INTERVALS

The ECG waveforms, complexes, and intervals are illustrated in Figure 3-2.

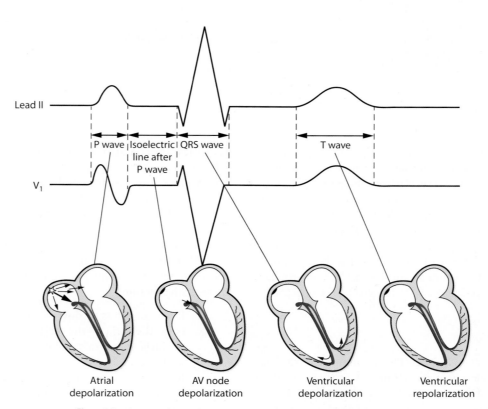

Figure 3-2. Electrocardiographic waves, complexes, and intervals in leads II and V_1.

P Wave

The P wave represents atrial muscle depolarization. It is normally 2.5 mm or less in height and 0.11 second or less in duration. P waves can be upright, inverted, or biphasic depending on how the electrical impulse conducts through the atria and on which lead it is being recorded.

QRS Complex

The QRS complex represents ventricular muscle depolarization. A Q wave is an initial negative deflection from baseline. An R wave is the first positive deflection from baseline. An S wave is a negative deflection that follows an R wave. The shape of the QRS complex depends on the lead being recorded and the ventricular activation sequence; not all leads record all waves of the QRS complex. Regardless of the shape of the complex, ventricular depolarization waves are called QRS complexes (Figure 3-3). The width of the QRS complex represents intraventricular conduction time and is measured from the point at which it first leaves the baseline to the point at which the last wave ends. Normal QRS width is 0.04 to 0.10 second in an adult. When describing the shape of the QRS complex in writing, a capital letter is used when the voltage of a wave is 5 mm or more, and a lower case letter is used for smaller waves, as in Figure 3-3.

T Wave

The T wave represents ventricular muscle repolarization. It follows the QRS complex and is normally in the same direction as the QRS complex. T waves can be upright, flat, or inverted depending on many things, including the presence of myocardial ischemia (MI), electrolyte levels, drug effect, myocardial disease, and the lead being recorded.

U Wave

The U wave is a small, rounded wave that sometimes follows the T wave and is thought to be due to repolarization of the M-cells (mid-myocardial cells) in the ventricles. U waves should be positive, especially when the T wave is positive. Large U waves can be seen when repolarization is abnormally prolonged; with electrolyte imbalances such as hypokalemia, hypocalcemia, hypomagnesemia; increased intracranial pressure; left ventricular hypertrophy; or with certain medications.

PR Interval

The PR interval is measured from the beginning of the P wave to the beginning of the QRS complex and represents the time required for the impulse to travel through the atria, AV junction, and to the Purkinje system. The normal PR interval in adults is 0.12 to 0.20 second. The PR segment extends from the end of the P wave to the beginning of the QRS complex.

ST Segment

The ST segment represents early ventricular repolarization. It begins at the end of the QRS complex (J point) and extends to the beginning of the T wave. The J point is where the QRS complex ends and the ST segment begins. The ST segment should be at the isoelectric line.

QT Interval

The QT interval measures the duration of ventricular depolarization and repolarization and varies with age, gender, and heart rate. The QT interval is measured from the beginning of the QRS complex to the end of the T wave. Because heart rate greatly affects the length of the QT interval, the QT interval must be corrected to a heart rate of 60 beats/min (corrected QT interval [QTc]). This correction is usually done using the Bazett formula:

QTc = measured QT interval divided by the square root of the RR interval (all measurements in seconds)

The QTc should not exceed 0.45 second in men and 0.46 second in women.

BASIC ELECTROCARDIOGRAPHY

The ECG is a graphic record of the electrical activity of the heart. The spread of the electrical impulse through the heart produces weak electrical currents that can be detected and amplified by the ECG machine and recorded on calibrated graph paper. These amplified signals form the ECG tracing which consists of the previously described waveforms and intervals inscribed onto grid paper. The grid on the paper consists of a series of small and large boxes, both horizontal and vertical; horizontal boxes measure time and vertical boxes measure voltage (Figure 3-4). On the horizontal axis, each small box is equal to 0.04 second, and each large box is equal to 0.20 second. On the vertical axis, each small box measures 1 mm and is equal to 0.1 mV; each large box measures 5 mm and is equal to 0.5 mV. In addition to the grid,

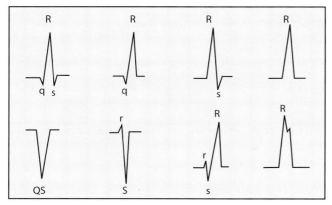

Figure 3-3. Examples of different configurations of QRS complexes. (*Reproduced with permission from Jacobson C, Marzlin K, Webner C. Cardiovascular Nursing Practice: A Comprehensive Resource Manual and Study Guide for Clinical Nurses. Burien, WA: Cardiovascular Nursing Education Associates; 2014.*)

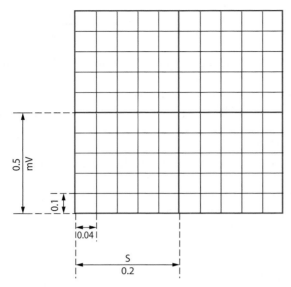

Figure 3-4. Time and voltage lines on ECG paper at standard paper speed of 25 mm/s. Horizontal axis measures time: each small box = 0.04 second, one large box = 0.20 second. Vertical axis measures voltage and also represents mm of ST segment deviation: each small box = 0.1 mV or 1 mm, one large box = 0.5 mV or 5 mm. (*Reproduced with permission from Woods SL, Froelicher ES, Motzer SU. Cardiac Nursing, 3rd ed. Philadelphia, PA: JB Lippincott; 1995.*)

TABLE 3-1. EVIDENCE-BASED PRACTICE: BEDSIDE CARDIAC MONITORING FOR DYSRHYTHMIA DETECTION

Electrode Application
• Make sure skin is clean and dry before applying monitoring electrodes. • Place arm electrodes on shoulder (front, top, or back) as close as possible to where arm joins torso. • Place leg electrodes below the rib cage or on hips. • Place V_1 electrode at the fourth intercostal space at right sternal border. • Place V_6 electrode at the left midaxillary line at the V_4 level. • Replace electrodes daily. • Mark electrode position with indelible ink to ensure consistent lead placement.
Lead Selection
• Use lead V_1 as the primary dysrhythmia monitoring lead whenever possible. • Use lead V_6 if lead V_1 is not available. • Display at least 2 leads whenever possible. • Use lead II to identify atrial activity if unclear in other leads and for R wave visualization during synchronized cardioversion. • If using a 3-wire system, use MCL_1 as the primary lead and MCL_6 as the second choice lead.
Alarm Limits
• Set heart rate alarms as appropriate for patient's current heart rate and clinical condition. • Never turn heart rate alarms off while patient's rhythm is being monitored. • Set alarm limits on other parameters based on goals of patient care if using a computerized dysrhythmia monitoring system.
Documentation and Reporting

• Document the monitoring lead on every rhythm strip.
• Document heart rate, PR interval, QRS width, QT interval every shift and with any significant rhythm change.
• Document rhythm strip with every significant rhythm change:
  – Onset and termination of tachycardias.
  – Symptomatic bradycardias or tachycardias.
  – Conversion into or out of atrial flutter or atrial fibrillation.
  – All rhythms requiring immediate treatment.
• Place rhythm strips flat on page (avoid folding or winding strips into chart).
• Report episodes of atrial fibrillation if no documented history of atrial fibrillation.
• Report rhythms with a short PR interval of < 0.12 seconds (may indicate presence of accessory pathway)
• Report episodes of life-threatening dysrhythmias and rhythms requiring treatment

Transporting Monitored Patients
• Continue cardiac monitoring using a portable, battery-operated monitor-defibrillator if patient is required to leave a monitored unit for diagnostic or therapeutic procedures. • Monitored patients must be accompanied by a healthcare provider skilled in ECG interpretation and defibrillation during transport. • Do not transport patients off the unit who have a corrected QT interval (QTc) of 0.50 seconds or greater until the prolonged QTc has been addressed.

Data from Drew, Califf, Funk, et al. 2004 and the American Association of Critical Care Nurses, 2016.

most ECG papers place a vertical line in the top margin at 3-second intervals or place a mark at 1-second intervals.

CARDIAC MONITORING

Cardiac monitoring provides continuous observation of the patient's heart rate and rhythm and is a routine nursing procedure in all types of acute and critical care units as well as in emergency departments, postanesthesia recovery units, and many operating rooms. Cardiac monitoring has also become common in areas where patients receive treatments or procedures requiring moderate sedation or where the administration of certain medications could result in cardiac dysrhythmias. The goals of cardiac monitoring can range from simple heart rate and basic rhythm monitoring to sophisticated dysrhythmia diagnosis and ST-segment monitoring to detect cardiac ischemia. Cardiac monitoring can be done using a 3-wire, 5-wire, or 10-wire cable, which connects the patient to the cardiac monitor or portable telemetry box.

The choice of monitoring lead is based on the goals of monitoring in a particular patient population and by the patient's clinical situation. Because dysrhythmias are the most common complication of ischemic heart disease and myocardial infarction (MI), monitoring for dysrhythmia diagnosis is a priority in these patients. Although many dysrhythmias can be recognized in any lead, research consistently shows that leads V_1 and V_6, or their bipolar substitutes MCL_1 and MCL_6, are the best leads for differentiating wide QRS rhythms (Table 3-1). The QRS morphologies displayed

in these leads are useful in differentiating ventricular tachycardia (VT) from supraventricular tachycardia (SVT) with aberrant intraventricular conduction and for recognizing right and left bundle branch block (see Chapter 18, Advanced ECG Concepts).

TABLE 3-2. ADVANTAGES OF COMMON MONITORING LEADS

Lead	Advantages
Preferred Monitoring Leads	
V_1 and V_6 (or MCL_1 and MCL_6 if using a 3-wire system)	Differentiate between right and left bundle branch block
	Morphology clues to differentiate between ventricular beats and supraventricular beats with aberrant conduction
	Differentiate between right and left ventricular ectopy
	Differentiate between right and left ventricular pacing
	Usually shows well-formed P waves
	Placement of electrodes keeps apex clear for auscultation or defibrillation
Other Monitoring Leads	
Lead II	Usually shows well-formed P waves
	Often best lead for identification of atrial flutter waves
	Usually has tall, upright QRS complex on which to synchronize machine for cardioversion
	Allows identification of retrograde P waves
Lead III or aVF	Assists in diagnosis of hemiblock
	Allows identification of retrograde P waves
	Allows identification of atrial flutter waves
	Best limb leads for ST-segment monitoring when 12-lead ECG showing ischemic fingerprint not available
Lewis lead (negative electrode at second right intercostal space, positive electrode at fourth right intercostal space)	Good lead to identify atrial activity when unclear in other leads
Atrial electrogram (recorded from atrial epicardial pacing wire)	Good lead to identify atrial activity when unclear in other leads

Correct placement of monitoring electrodes is critical to obtaining accurate information from any monitoring lead. Most currently available bedside monitors utilize either a 3-wire or a 5-wire monitoring cable. A 5-wire system offers several advantages over the 3-wire system (Table 3-2). With a 5-wire system, it is possible to monitor more than one lead at a time and it is possible to monitor a true unipolar V_1 lead, which is superior to its bipolar substitute MCL_1 in differentiating wide QRS rhythms. With a 5-wire system, all 12 standard ECG leads can be obtained by selecting the desired lead on the bedside monitor and moving the one chest lead to the appropriate spot on the thorax to record the precordial leads V_1 through V_6 (see Chapter 18, Advanced ECG Concepts). Figure 3-5 illustrates correct lead placement for a 5-wire system. Arm electrodes are placed on the shoulders as close as possible to where the arms join the torso. Placing the arm electrodes on the posterior shoulder keeps the anterior chest area clear for defibrillation paddles if needed and avoid irritating the skin in the subclavicular area where an intravenous (IV) catheter might need to be placed. Leg electrodes are placed at the level of the lowest ribs on the thorax or on the hips. Placing the chest electrode at the appropriate location on the chest and selecting "V" on the bedside monitor obtains the desired V or precordial lead. To monitor in V_1, place the chest electrode in the fourth intercostal space at the right sternal border. To monitor in V_6, place the chest electrode at the left midaxillary line at the V_4 level (V_4 level is fifth intercostal space, midclavicular line).

When using a 3-wire monitoring system with electrodes placed in their conventional locations on the right and left shoulders and on the left hip or low thorax, leads I, II, or III can be monitored by selecting the desired lead on the bedside monitor. It is not possible to obtain a true unipolar V_1 or V_6 lead with a 3-wire system. In this case, the bipolar substitutes MCL_1 and MCL_6 can be used but to obtain them requires placing electrodes in unconventional sites. Figure 3-5 shows electrode placement for a 3-wire system that allows the user to monitor either MCL_1 or MCL_6. Place the right arm electrode on the left shoulder, the left arm electrode at the V_1 position (fourth intercostal space at the right sternal border), and the left leg electrode in the V_6 position (fifth intercostal space at the left midaxillary line). With electrodes in this position, select "lead I" on the monitor to obtain MCL_1 and switch to lead II on the monitor to record MCL_6.

The electrode sites on the skin should be clean, dry, and relatively flat. Remove excess hair, if present, and clean the skin with alcohol to remove any oils. Mildly abrade the skin with a gauze or abrading pad supplied on electrode packaging to improve transmission of the ECG signal. Apply the pregelled electrodes to the chest in the appropriate locations. Set the heart rate alarm limits based on the patient's clinical situation and current heart rate. Bedside monitoring systems have default alarms that adjust the high- and low-rate limits based on the learned heart rate. Electrodes are changed daily to prevent pressure injury and provide artifact-free tracings.

DETERMINATION OF THE HEART RATE

Heart rate can be obtained from the ECG strip by several methods. The first, and most accurate if the rhythm is regular, is to count the number of small boxes (one small box = 0.04 second) between two R waves, and then divide that number into 1500. There are 1500 boxes of 0.04-second interval in a 1-minute strip (Figure 3-6A). Another method is to count

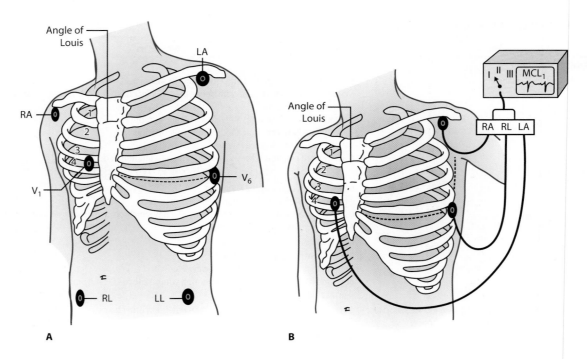

Figure 3-5. **(A)** Correct electrode placement for using a 5-wire monitoring cable. Right and left arm electrodes are placed on the shoulders and right and left leg electrodes are placed low on the thorax or on the hips. With the arm and leg electrodes placed as illustrated, leads I, II, III, aVR, aVL, and aVF can be obtained by selecting the desired lead on the bedside monitor. To obtain lead V$_1$, place the chest lead in the fourth intercostal space at the right sternal border and select "V" on the bedside monitor. To obtain lead V$_6$, place the chest lead at the level of V$_4$ in the left midaxillary line and select "V" on the bedside monitor. **(B)** Correct lead placement for obtaining MCL$_1$ and MCL$_6$ using a 3-wire lead system. Place the right arm electrode on the left shoulder; the left arm electrode in the fourth intercostal space at the right sternal border; and the left leg electrode at the level of V$_4$ in the left midaxillary line. To monitor in MCL$_1$, select lead I on the bedside monitor. To monitor in MCL$_6$, select lead II on the bedside monitor. (*Adapted with permission from Drew BJ. Bedside electrocardiogram monitoring.* AACN Clin Issues Crit Care Nurs. *1993;Feb;4(1):25-33.*)

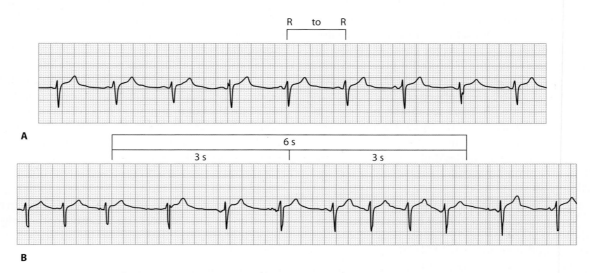

Figure 3-6. **(A)** Heart rate determination for a regular rhythm using little boxes between two R waves. One RR interval is marked at the top of the ECG paper. There are 25 little boxes between these two R waves. There are 1500 little boxes in a 60-second strip. By dividing 1500 by 25, one calculates a heart rate of 60 beats/min. Heart rate can also be determined for a regular rhythm counting large boxes between R waves. There are five large boxes between R waves. There are 300 large boxes in a 60-second strip. By dividing 300 by 5, one calculates a heart rate of 60 beats/min. **(B)** Heart rate determination for a regular or irregular rhythm using the number of RR intervals in a 6-second strip and multiplying by 10. There are seven RR intervals in this example. Multiplying by 10 gives a heart rate of 70 beats/min. (*Reproduced with permission from Woods SL, Froelicher ES, Motzer SU.* Cardiac Nursing, *3rd ed. Philadelphia, PA: JB Lippincott; 1995.*)

TABLE 3-3. HEART RATE DETERMINATION USING THE ELECTROCARDIOGRAM LARGE BOXES

Number of Large Boxes Between R Waves	Heart Rate (beats/min)
1	300
2	150
3	100
4	75
5	60
6	50
7	43
8	38
9	33
10	30

the number of large boxes (one large box = 0.20 second) between two R waves, and then divide that number into 300 or use a standardized table (Table 3-3).

The third method for computing heart rate, especially useful when the rhythm is irregular, is to count the number of RR intervals in 6 seconds and multiply that number by 10. The ECG paper is usually marked at 3-second intervals (15 large boxes horizontally) by a vertical line at the top of the paper (Figure 3-6B). The RR intervals are counted, not the QRS complexes, to avoid overestimating the heart rate.

The atrial rate can be calculated by using any of these three methods with P waves instead of R waves.

DETERMINATION OF CARDIAC RHYTHM

Correct determination of the cardiac rhythm requires a systematic evaluation of the ECG. The following steps are used to determine the cardiac rhythm:

1. Calculate the atrial (P wave) rate.
2. Calculate the ventricular (QRS complex) rate.
3. Determine the regularity and shape of the P waves.
4. Determine the regularity, shape, and width of the QRS complexes.
5. Measure the PR interval.
6. Interpret the dysrhythmia as described later.

COMMON DYSRHYTHMIAS

A *dysrhythmia* is any cardiac rhythm that is not normal sinus rhythm. The term dysrhythmia is synonymous with the term arrhythmia. A dysrhythmia may result from altered impulse formation or altered impulse conduction. The term *ectopic* refers to any beat or rhythm that arises from a location other than the sinus node. Ectopic beats can arise in the atria, AV junction, or ventricles. Dysrhythmias are named by the place where they originate and by their rate. Dysrhythmias are grouped as rhythms originating:

1. in the sinus node.
2. in the atria.
3. in the AV junction.
4. in the ventricle.
5. AV blocks

The etiology, ECG characteristics, and treatment of the basic cardiac dysrhythmias are presented here and summarized in Chapter 23, Cardiac Rhythms, ECG Characteristics, and Treatment Guide.

RHYTHMS ORIGINATING IN THE SINUS NODE

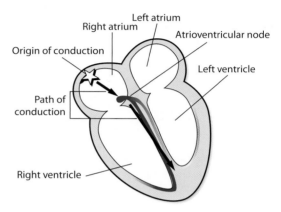

Figure 3-7. Rhythms originating in the sinus node.

Normal Sinus Rhythm

ECG Characteristics

- *Rate:* 60 to 100 beats/min.
- *Rhythm:* Regular.
- *P waves:* Precede every QRS complex; consistent in shape.
- *PR interval:* 0.12 to 0.20 second.
- *QRS complex:* 0.04 to 0.10 second.
- *Conduction:* Normal through atria, AV node, bundle branches, and ventricles.
- *Example of normal sinus rhythm:* Figure 3-8.

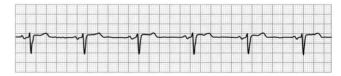

Figure 3-8. Normal sinus rhythm.

Sinus Bradycardia

All aspects of sinus bradycardia are the same as normal sinus rhythm except the rate is slower. It can be a normal finding in athletes and during sleep. Sinus bradycardia may be a response to vagal stimulation, such as carotid sinus massage, ocular pressure, or vomiting. Other causes of sinus bradycardia include inferior MI, obstructive sleep apnea, increased intracranial pressure and other central nervous system conditions (eg, stroke), anorexia nervosa, hypothyroidism, hypothermia, and some infectious diseases. Sinus bradycardia can be a response to several medications, including digitalis, beta-blockers, some calcium channel blockers, ivabradine, antiarrhythmics, and others.

ECG Characteristics

- *Rate:* Less than 60 beats/min.
- *Rhythm:* Regular.
- *P waves:* Precede every QRS; consistent in shape.
- *PR interval:* Usually normal (0.12-0.20 second).
- *QRS complex:* Usually normal (0.04-0.10 second).
- *Conduction:* Normal through atria, AV node, bundle branches, and ventricles.
- *Example of sinus bradycardia:* Figure 3-9.

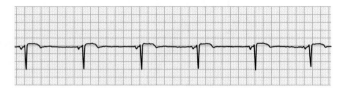

Figure 3-9. Sinus bradycardia.

Treatment

Treatment of sinus bradycardia is not required unless the patient is symptomatic. If the dysrhythmia is accompanied by hypotension, confusion, diaphoresis, chest pain, or other signs of hemodynamic compromise or by ventricular ectopy, 0.5 mg of atropine IV is the treatment of choice. Attempts are made to decrease vagal stimulation. If the dysrhythmia is due to medications, they are held until their need has been reevaluated. Temporary or permanent pacing may be necessary.

Sinus Tachycardia

Sinus tachycardia is a sinus rhythm at a rate greater than 100 beats/min. Sinus tachycardia is a normal response to exercise and emotion. Sinus tachycardia that persists at rest usually indicates some underlying problem, such as fever, acute blood loss, shock, pain, anxiety, heart failure (HF), hypermetabolic states, pulmonary disease, or anemia. Sinus tachycardia is a normal physiologic response to a decrease in cardiac output; cardiac output is the product of heart rate and stroke volume. The following medications also cause sinus tachycardia: atropine, isoproterenol, epinephrine, dopamine, dobutamine, norepinephrine, nitroprusside, and caffeine.

ECG Characteristics

- *Rate:* Greater than 100 beats/min.
- *Rhythm:* Regular.
- *P waves:* Precede every QRS; consistent in shape; may be buried in the preceding T wave.
- *PR interval:* Usually normal; may be difficult to measure if P waves are buried in T waves.

- *QRS complex:* Usually normal.
- *Conduction:* Normal through atria, AV node, bundle branches, and ventricles.
- *Example of sinus tachycardia:* Figure 3-10.

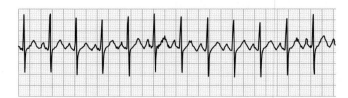

Figure 3-10. Sinus tachycardia.

Treatment

Treatment of sinus tachycardia is directed at the underlying cause. This dysrhythmia is a physiologic response to a decrease in cardiac output, and it should never be ignored, especially in the cardiac patient. Because the ventricles fill with blood and the coronary arteries perfuse during diastole, persistent tachycardia can cause decreased stroke volume, decreased cardiac output, and decreased coronary perfusion secondary to the decreased diastolic time that occurs with rapid heart rates. Carotid sinus pressure may slow the heart rate temporarily and thereby help in ruling out other dysrhythmias.

Sinus Dysrhythmia

Sinus dysrhythmia occurs when the sinus node discharges irregularly. It occurs frequently as a normal phenomenon, especially in younger people, and is commonly associated with the phases of respiration. During inspiration, the sinus node fires faster; during expiration, it slows. Digitalis toxicity may also cause this dysrhythmia. Sinus dysrhythmia looks like normal sinus rhythm except for the irregularity.

ECG Characteristics

- *Rate:* 60 to 100 beats/min.
- *Rhythm:* Irregular; phasic increase and decrease in rate, which may or may not be related to respiration.
- *P waves:* Precede every QRS complex; consistent in shape.
- *PR interval:* Usually normal.
- *QRS complex:* Usually normal.
- *Conduction:* Normal through atria, AV node, bundle branches, and ventricles.
- *Example of sinus dysrhythmia:* Figure 3-11.

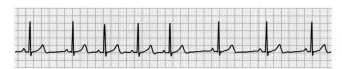

Figure 3-11. Sinus dysrhythmia.

Treatment

Treatment of sinus dysrhythmia usually is not necessary. If the dysrhythmia is thought to be because of digitalis toxicity, then digitalis is held. Atropine increases the rate and eliminates the irregularity.

Sinus Arrest

Sinus arrest occurs when sinus node firing is depressed and impulses are not formed when expected. The result is an absent P wave at the expected time. The QRS complex is also missing, unless there is escape of a junctional or ventricular impulse. If only one sinus impulse fails to form, this is usually called a *sinus pause*. If more than one sinus impulse in a row fails to form, this is termed a *sinus arrest*. Because the sinus node is not forming impulses regularly as expected, the PP interval in sinus arrest is not an exact multiple of the sinus cycle. Causes of sinus arrest include vagal stimulation, carotid sinus sensitivity, and MI interrupting the blood supply to the sinus node. Medications such as digitalis, beta-blockers, and calcium channel blockers can also cause sinus arrest.

ECG Characteristics

- *Rate:* Usually within normal range but may be in the bradycardia range.
- *Rhythm:* Irregular due to absence of sinus node discharge.
- *P waves:* Present when sinus node is firing and absent during periods of sinus arrest. When present, they precede every QRS complex and are consistent in shape.
- *PR interval:* Usually normal when P waves are present.
- *QRS complex:* Usually normal when sinus node is functioning and absent during periods of sinus arrest, unless escape beats occur.
- *Conduction:* Normal through atria, AV node, bundle branches, and ventricles when sinus node is firing. When the sinus node fails to form impulses, there is no conduction through the atria.
- *Example of sinus arrest:* Figure 3-12.

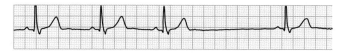

Figure 3-12. Sinus arrest.

Treatment

Treatment of sinus arrest is aimed at the underlying cause. Medications that are thought to be responsible are discontinued and vagal stimulation is minimized. If periods of sinus arrest are frequent and cause hemodynamic compromise, 0.5 mg of atropine IV may increase the rate. Pacemaker therapy may be necessary if other forms of management fail to increase the rate to acceptable levels.

DYSRHYTHMIAS ORIGINATING IN THE ATRIA

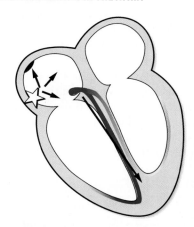

Figure 3-13. Dysrhythmias originating in the atria.

Premature Atrial Complexes

A premature atrial complex (PAC) occurs when an irritable focus in the atria fires before the next sinus node impulse is due to fire. PACs can be caused by caffeine, alcohol, nicotine, heart failure (HF), pulmonary disease, interruptions in atrial blood supply by myocardial ischemia or infarction, anxiety, and hypermetabolic states. PACs can also occur in normal hearts.

ECG Characteristics

- *Rate:* Usually within normal range.
- *Rhythm:* Usually regular except when PACs occur, resulting in early beats. PACs usually have a noncompensatory pause (interval between the complex preceding and that following the PAC is less than two normal RR intervals) because premature depolarization of the atria by the PAC usually causes premature depolarization of the sinus node as well, thus causing the sinus node to "reset" itself.
- *P waves:* Precede every QRS complex. The configuration of the premature P wave differs from that of the sinus P waves because the premature impulse originates in a different part of the atria, with atrial depolarization occurring in a different pattern. Very early P waves may be buried in the preceding T wave.
- *PR interval:* May be normal or long depending on the prematurity of the beat; very early PACs may find the AV junction still partially refractory and unable to conduct at a normal rate, resulting in a prolonged PR interval.
- *QRS complex:* May be normal, aberrant (wide), or absent, depending on the prematurity of the beat. If the ventricles have repolarized completely, they will be able to conduct the early impulse normally, resulting in a normal QRS. If the PAC occurs during the relative refractory period of the AV node, bundle branches, or ventricles, the impulse will

conduct aberrantly and the QRS will be wide. If the
PAC occurs very early during the complete refractory period of the AV node, bundle branches, or ventricles, the impulse will not conduct to the ventricles
and the QRS will be absent.
- *Conduction:* PACs travel through the atria differently
  from sinus impulses because they originate from a
  different spot; conduction through the AV node, bundle branches, and ventricles is usually normal unless
  the PAC is very early.
- *Example of PAC:* Figure 3-14A, B.

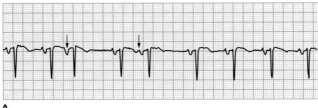

A

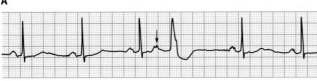

B

Figure 3-14. **(A)** PAC conducted normally in the ventricle. **(B)** PAC conducted
aberrantly in the ventricle.

Treatment

Treatment of PACs usually is not necessary because they do
not cause hemodynamic compromise. Patients with frequent
or bothersome PACs are usually counseled to avoid smoking,
alcohol, and caffeine. Frequent PACs may precede more serious dysrhythmias such as atrial fibrillation (AF). Treatment
is directed at the cause. Medications such as beta-blockers,
disopyramide, flecainide, and propafenone can be used to
suppress atrial activity, but this is rarely necessary.

Wandering Atrial Pacemaker and Multifocal Atrial Tachycardia

Wandering atrial pacemaker (WAP) refers to rhythms that
exhibit varying P-wave morphology as the site of impulse
formation shifts from the sinus node to various sites in the
atria or into the AV junction. This occurs when two (usually
sinus and junctional) or more supraventricular pacemakers
compete with each other for control of the heart. Because the
rates of these competing pacemakers are almost identical, it is
common to have atrial fusion occur as the atria are activated

by more than one wave of depolarization at a time, resulting
in varying P-wave morphology. WAP can be due to increased
vagal tone that slows the sinus pacemaker or to enhanced
automaticity in atrial or junctional pacemaker cells, causing
them to compete with the sinus node for control. The term
multifocal atrial tachycardia (MAT) is used when the rate
is faster than 100 beats/min. MAT is commonly associated
with chronic obstructive pulmonary disease (COPD) and
other pulmonary diseases such as pneumonia and pulmonary embolism. It is also seen in heart failure and coronary,
valvular, or hypertensive heart disease.

ECG Characteristics

- *Rate:* 60 to 100 beats/min. If the rate is faster than
  100 beats/min, it is called MAT.
- *Rhythm:* May be slightly irregular.
- *P waves:* Varying shapes (upright, flat, inverted,
  notched) as impulses originate in different parts of
  the atria or junction. At least three different P-wave
  shapes should be seen.
- *PR interval:* May vary depending on proximity of the
  pacemaker to the AV node.
- *QRS complex:* Usually normal.
- *Conduction:* Conduction through the atria varies as
  they are depolarized from different spots. Conduction through the bundle branches and ventricles is
  usually normal.
- *Example of WAP:* Figure 3-15. *Example of MAT:*
  Figure 3-16

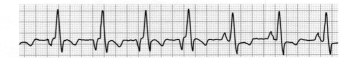

Figure 3-15. Wandering atrial pacemaker.

Treatment

Treatment of WAP usually is not necessary. If slow heart rates
lead to symptoms, atropine can be given. Treatment of MAT
is directed toward eliminating the cause, including hypoxia
and electrolyte imbalances. Intravenous beta-blockers (eg,
metoprolol) or verapamil are useful for acute ventricular rate
control. IV verapamil is sometimes effective in suppressing
atrial foci. Oral beta-blockers, verapamil, or diltiazem can be
used for management of recurrent MAT. Maintaining normal magnesium and potassium levels is important in managing MAT.

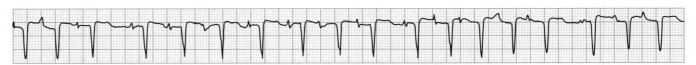

Figure 3-16. Multifocal atrial tachycardia.

Atrial Tachycardia

Atrial tachycardia (AT) is a rapid atrial rhythm occurring at a rate of 120 to 250 beats/min and can be due to abnormal automaticity or to reentry within the atrium (Figure 3-17). When the dysrhythmia abruptly starts and terminates, it is called *paroxysmal atrial tachycardia*. Rapid atrial rate can be caused by emotions, caffeine, tobacco, alcohol, fatigue, or sympathomimetic drugs. Whenever the atrial rate is rapid, the AV node begins to block some of the impulses attempting to travel through it to protect the ventricles from excessively rapid rates. In normal healthy hearts, the AV node can usually conduct each atrial impulse up to rates of about 180 to 200 beats/min. In patients with cardiac disease or who are on AV nodal blocking drugs such as digitalis, beta-blockers, or calcium channel blockers, the AV node may not be able to conduct each impulse and AT with block occurs. AT with block may indicate digitalis toxicity.

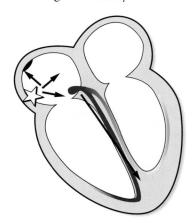

Figure 3-17. Atrial tachycardia.

ECG Characteristics

- *Rate:* Atrial rate is 120 to 250 beats/min.
- *Rhythm:* Regular unless there is variable block at the AV node.
- *P waves:* Differ in shape from sinus P waves because they are ectopic. Precede each QRS complex but may be hidden in preceding T wave. When block is present, more than one P wave will appear before each QRS complex.
- *PR interval:* May be shorter than normal but often difficult to measure because of hidden P waves.
- *QRS complex:* Usually normal but may be wide if aberrant conduction is present.

- *Conduction:* Usually normal through the AV node and into the ventricles. In AT with block, some atrial impulses do not conduct into the ventricles. Aberrant ventricular conduction may occur if atrial impulses are conducted into the ventricles while the bundle branches or ventricles are still partially refractory.
- *Example of AT:* Figure 3-18.

Treatment

Treatment of AT is directed at eliminating the cause, if possible, controlling the ventricular rate, and reestablishing sinus rhythm. If the patient is hemodynamically unstable due to a rapid AT, cardioversion can be attempted, although automatic ATs usually do not respond to cardioversion. Some ATs may terminate with IV adenosine, but more often IV verapamil or diltiazem, or an IV beta-blocker, is used for acute therapy to slow the ventricular rate, and they may occasionally terminate the AT. Other medications that can be used for management of recurrent AT are flecainide, propafenone, amiodarone, or sotalol. Catheter ablation is a class I recommendation for preventing recurrent AT. See Table 3-4 for recommendations for management of AT.

Atrial Flutter

In atrial flutter (Figure 3-19), the atria are depolarized at rates of 250 to 350 times/min. Classic or typical atrial flutter is due to a fixed reentry circuit in the right atrium around which the impulse circulates in a counterclockwise direction, resulting in negative flutter waves in leads II and III and an atrial rate between 250 and 350 beats/min (most commonly 300 beats/min). At such rapid atrial rates, the AV node usually blocks at least half of the impulses to protect the

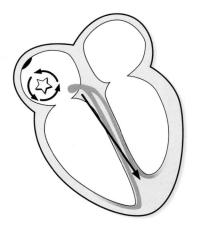

Figure 3-19. Atrial flutter.

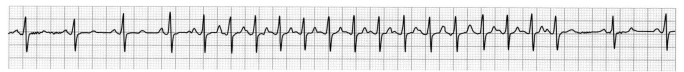

Figure 3-18. Atrial tachycardia.

TABLE 3-4. GUIDELINES FOR MANAGEMENT OF SUPRAVENTRICULAR ARRHYTHMIAS (CLASS OF RECOMMENDATION AND LEVEL OF EVIDENCE INDICATED (COR; LOE) FOR EACH RECOMMENDATION)

Treatment of SVT of Unknown Mechanism

Acute Treatment

1. Vagal maneuvers (Valsalva, CSM) for regular SVT (1, B-R)
2. Adenosine for regular SVT (1, B-R)
3. Synchronized cardioversion if hemodynamically unstable and vagal maneuvers or adenosine ineffective or not feasible (1, B-NR)
4. Synchronized cardioversion if hemodynamically stable and drug therapy ineffective or contraindicated (1, B-NR)
5. IV verapamil or diltiazem for acute treatment if hemodynamically stable (1Ia; B-R)
6. IV beta-blockers for acute treatment if hemodynamically stable (IIa; C-LD)

Ongoing Management

1. Oral beta-blockers, diltiazem, or verapamil if no pre-excitation (1; B-R)
2. EP study with option for ablation (I; B-NR)
3. Flecainide or propafenone if no structural heart disease or ischemic heart disease if ablation not an option (IIa; B-R)
4. Sotolol or dofetilide if ablation not an option and other drugs not effective (IIb; B-R)
5. Amiodarone or digoxin can be considered if ablation not an option and other drugs not effective (IIb; C-LD)

Treatment of Suspected Focal Atrial Tachycardia

Acute Treatment

1. IV beta-blockers, diltiazem, or verapamil if hemodynamically stable (I; C-LD)
2. Synchronized cardioversion if hemodynamically unstable (I; C-LD)
3. Adenosine to restore sinus rhythm or diagnose tachycardia (IIa; B-NR)
4. IV amiodarone or ibutilide if hemodynamically stable (IIb; C-LD)

Ongoing Management

1. Catheter ablation as alternative to drug therapy (I, B-NR)
2. Oral beta-blockers, diltiazem, or verapamil (IIa; C-LD)
3. Flecainide or propafenone if no structural or ischemic heart disease (IIa; C-LD)
4. Sotalol or amiodarone (IIb; C-LD)

Treatment of AVNRT

Acute Treatment

1. Vagal maneuvers or adenosine (I; B-R)
2. Synchronized cardioversion for stable or unstable AVNRT when vagal maneuvers and adenosine ineffective (I, B-NR)
3. IV beta-blockers, diltiazem, or verapamil if hemodynamically stable (IIa; B-R)
4. Oral beta-blockers, diltiazem, or verapamil if hemodynamically stable (IIb; C-LD)
5. IV amiodarone if hemodynamically stable and other drugs ineffective (IIb; C-LD)

Ongoing Management

1. Catheter ablation (I; B-NR)—considered first-line therapy
2. Oral beta-blockers, verapamil, or diltiazem if ablation not an option (I; B-R)
3. Flecainide or propafenone if ablation not an option and other drugs ineffective and no structural or ischemic heart disease (IIa; B-R)
4. Clinical follow-up without other therapy reasonable if minimally symptomatic (IIa; B-NR)
5. Oral sotalol, dofetilide, digoxin, or amiodarone if ablation not an option (IIb; B-R)
6. Pill-in-the-pocket (verapamil, diltiazem, beta-blockers) if infrequent stable episodes (IIb; C-LD)

Treatment of Orthodromic AVRT (or CMT)

Acute Treatment

1. Vagal maneuvers or adenosine (I; B-R)
2. Synchronized cardioversion for stable or unstable AVRT when vagal maneuvers and adenosine ineffective (I, B-NR)
3. Synchronized cardioversion should be performed for hemodynamically unstable pre-excited AF (I, B-NR)
4. Ibutilide or IV procainamide beneficial for pre-excited AF if hemodynamically stable (I; C-LD)
5. IV diltiazem or verapamil (IIa; B-R) or beta-blockers (IIa; C-LD) if no pre-excitation during sinus rhythm
6. IV beta-blockers, diltiazem, or verapamil might be considered in patients who have pre-excitation during sinus rhythm but have not responded to other therapies (IIb; B-R)
7. **IV digoxin, IV amiodarone, IV or oral beta-blockers, diltiazem, and verapamil are potentially harmful and contraindicated with pre-excited AF** (III harm; C-LD)

Ongoing Management

1. Catheter ablation of accessory pathway for AVRT or pre-excited AF (I; B-NR)
2. Oral beta-blockers, verapamil, diltiazem if no pre-excitation on resting ECG (I; C-LD)
3. Oral flecainide or propafenone if no structural or ischemic heart disease for AVRT or pre-excited AF if ablation not an option (IIa; B-R)
4. Oral dofetilide or sotalol for AVRT or pre-excited AF if ablation not an option (IIb; B-R)
5. Oral beta-blockers, diltiazem, or verapamil in patients with pre-excitation on resting ECG and ablation not an option (IIb, C-LD)
6. Oral amiodarone for AVRT or pre-excited AF if ablation not an option and other drugs are ineffective (IIb; C-LD)
7. Oral digoxin if no pre-excitation on resting ECG and ablation not an option (IIb; C-LD)
8. Oral digoxin potentially harmful if AF with pre-excitation on resting ECG (III harm, C-LD)

Treatment of Atrial Flutter

Acute Treatment
1. Oral dofetilide or IV ibutilide for pharmacological cardioversion (I; A)
2. IV or oral beta-blockers, diltiazem, or verapamil for rate control if hemodynamically stable (I, B-R)
3. Synchronized cardioversion if hemodynamically unstable and drugs ineffective (I; B-NR)
4. Elective synchronized cardioversion if hemodynamically stable and rhythm control is goal (I; B-NR)
5. Rapid atrial pacing for conversion of atrial flutter if atrial pacing wires in place (I; C-LD)
6. Acute antithrombotic therapy same as for AF (Table 3-5) (I; B-NR)
7. IV amiodarone for rate control (if no pre-excitation) if systolic heart failure when beta-blockers contraindicated or ineffective (IIa; B-R)

Ongoing Management
1. Catheter ablation if symptomatic or refractory to rate control drugs (I; B-R)
2. Beta-blockers, diltiazem, or verapamil for rate control if hemodynamically stable (I; C-LD)
3. Catheter ablation for "atypical" flutter after failure of at least one antiarrhythmic drug (I; C-LD)
4. Ongoing antithrombotic therapy same as for AF (see Table 3-5) (I; B-R)
5. Amiodarone, dofetilide, or sotalol useful to maintain sinus rhythm with recurrent atrial flutter (IIa; B-R)
6. There are several COR IIa recommendations for catheter ablation of atrial flutter in various situations. See source below for more information.
7. Flecainide or propafenone to maintain sinus rhythm if no structural or ischemic heart disease (IIb; B-R)
8. Catheter ablation may be reasonable for asymptomatic patients with recurrent atrial flutter (IIb; C-LD)

Treatment of Junctional Tachycardia

There are no Class I recommendations for treatment of junctional tachycardia.
Acute Treatment
1. IV beta-blockers, diltiazem, procainamide, or verapamil (IIa; C-LD)

Ongoing Management
1. Oral beta-blockers, diltiazem, or verapamil (IIa; C-LD)
2. Flecainide or propafenone if no structural or ischemic heart disease (IIb; C-LD)
3. Catheter ablation when medical therapy ineffective or contraindicated (IIb; C-LD)

Class of Recommendation (COR)
Class I: Strong; benefit >>> risk
Class IIa: Moderate; benefit >> risk
Class IIb: Weak; benefit > risk
Class III no benefit: benefit = risk, not indicated, useful, or effective
Class III harm: risk > benefit; potentially harmful, contraindicated

Level of Evidence (LOE) Definitions
Level A: High-quality evidence from multiple randomized clinical trials (RCTs) or meta-analyses of high-quality RCTs.
Level B-R (randomized): Moderate-quality evidence from one or more RCTs or meta-analysis of moderate-quality RCTs.
Level B-NR (nonrandomized): Moderate-quality evidence from one or more nonrandomized studies, observational studies, or registry studies or meta-analyses of such studies.
Level C-LD (limited data): Randomized or nonrandomized observational or registry studies with limitations of design or execution; meta-analyses of such studies.
Level C-EO (expert opinion): Consensus of expert opinion based on clinical experience.

Abbreviations: AF: atrial fibrillation; AT: atrial tachycardia; AVNRT: atrioventricular nodal reentry tachycardia; BBB: bundle branch block; CMT: circus movement tachycardia; COR: class of recommendation; CSM: carotid sinus massage; EP: electrophysiology; LOE: level of evidence; LV: left ventricular; SVT: supraventricular tachycardia.
Data from Page RL, Joglar JA, Caldwell MA, et al. 2015 ACC/AHA/HRS Guideline for the Management of Adult Patients With Supraventricular Tachycardia: A Report of the American College of Cardiology/American Heart Association Task Force on Clinical Practice Guidelines and the Heart Rhythm Society. Circulation. 2016 Apr 5;133(14):e506-e574.

ventricles from excessive rates. Causes of atrial flutter include rheumatic heart disease, atherosclerotic heart disease, thyrotoxicosis, heart failure, and myocardial ischemia or infarction. Because the ventricular rate in atrial flutter can be quite fast, symptoms associated with decreased cardiac output can occur. Mural thrombi may form in the atria due to the fact that there is no strong atrial contraction, and blood stasis occurs, leading to a risk of systemic or pulmonary emboli.

ECG Characteristics
- *Rate:* Atrial rate varies between 250 and 350 beats/min, most commonly 300. Ventricular rate varies depending on the amount of block at the AV node. New onset atrial flutter usually has a ventricular rate around 150 beats/min, and rarely 300 beats/min if 1:1 conduction occurs to the ventricles. With

medications that block AV node conduction, the ventricular rate is usually in the normal range, commonly around 75 beats/min.
- *Rhythm:* Atrial rhythm is regular. Ventricular rhythm may be regular or irregular because of varying AV block.
- *F waves:* F waves (flutter waves) are seen, characterized by a very regular, "sawtooth" pattern. One F wave is usually hidden in the QRS complex, and when 2:1 conduction occurs, F waves may not be readily apparent.
- *FR interval (flutter wave to the beginning of the QRS complex):* May be consistent or may vary.
- *QRS complex:* Usually normal; aberration can occur.
- *Conduction:* Usually normal through the AV node and ventricles.
- *Example of atrial flutter:* Figure 3-20A, B.

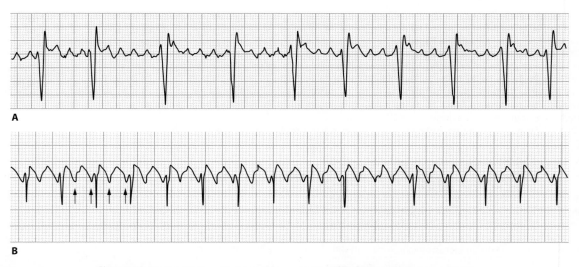

Figure 3-20. **(A)** Atrial flutter with 4:1 and 5:1 conduction. **(B)** Atrial flutter with 2:1 conduction.

Treatment

The immediate goal of treatment depends on the hemodynamic consequences of the dysrhythmia. Ventricular rate control is the priority if cardiac output is markedly compromised due to rapid ventricular rates. Electrical (direct current) cardioversion may be necessary as an immediate treatment, especially if 1:1 conduction occurs. IV calcium channel blockers (verapamil or diltiazem) or beta-blockers can be used for acute ventricular rate control. Conversion to sinus rhythm can be accomplished by electrical cardioversion, drug therapy, or overdrive atrial pacing. Oral dofetilide or IV ibutilide are useful for pharmacological cardioversion.

Medications that slow the atrial rate, like flecainide or propafenone, should not be used unless the ventricular rate has been controlled with an AV nodal blocking agent (a calcium channel blocker, beta-blocker, or digitalis). The danger of giving these medications alone is that the atrial rate may decrease from 300 beats/min to a slower rate, making it possible for the AV node to conduct each impulse and resulting in even faster ventricular rates. See Table 3-4 for treatment of atrial flutter.

Atrial Fibrillation

Atrial fibrillation (AF) is an extremely rapid and disorganized pattern of depolarization in the atria, and is the most common dysrhythmia seen in clinical practice (Figure 3-21). Atrial fibrillation commonly occurs in the presence of atherosclerotic or rheumatic heart disease, thyroid disease, HF, cardiomyopathy, valve disease, pulmonary disease, MI, congenital heart disease, and after cardiac surgery. The following classification system is used when defining AF: *paroxysmal*, episodes that terminate spontaneously or with intervention within 7 days of onset; *persistent*, episodes that last more than 7 days; *long-standing persistent*, continuous AF lasting more than 12 months; and *permanent*, continuous AF lasting more than 12 months and decision

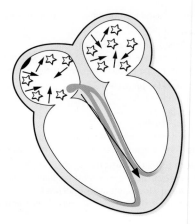

Figure 3-21. Atrial fibrillation.

has been made to stop attempts to restore and/or maintain sinus rhythm. The term *recurrent* is used when the patient has two or more episodes of AF, and the term *lone AF* is used when AF occurs in the absence of cardiac disease or any other known cause (usually in people < 60 years of age). Nonvalvular AF occurs in patients without mitral valve disease, prosthetic valve, or history of valve surgery.

Atrial fibrillation has several adverse consequences that require prompt recognition and treatment in order to prevent complications:

1. Decreased cardiac output due to loss of atrial kick, rapid ventricular rate, and irregular ventricular rhythm. Cardiac output is dependent on adequate ventricular filling, and the loss of atrial contraction and the rapid ventricular rate that commonly occurs in AF contribute to reduced ventricular filling.
2. Tachycardia-induced cardiomyopathy can occur whenever the ventricular rate is rapid for a prolonged period of time. This is more common in asymptomatic patients who are unaware that they are in AF.

3. Thromboembolism because of formation of clots in the fibrillating atria, usually in the left atrial appendage. Stroke is the most common and potentially devastating embolic event, but pulmonary embolus and embolization to any other part of the body can also occur.

ECG Characteristics

- *Rate:* Atrial rate is 400 to 600 beats/min or faster. Ventricular rate varies depending on the amount of block at the AV node. In new AF, the ventricular response is usually quite rapid, 160 to 200 beats/min; in treated atrial fibrillation, the ventricular rate is controlled in the normal range of 60 to 100 beats/min.
- *Rhythm:* Irregular; one of the distinguishing features of AF is the marked irregularity of the ventricular response.
- *F waves:* Not present; atrial activity is chaotic with no formed atrial impulses visible; irregular F waves are often seen, and vary in size from coarse to very fine.
- *PR interval:* Not measurable; there are no P waves.
- *QRS complex:* Usually normal; aberration is common.
- *Conduction:* Conduction within the atria is disorganized and follows a very irregular pattern. Most of the atrial impulses are blocked within the AV junction. Those impulses that are conducted through the AV junction are usually conducted normally through the ventricles. If an atrial impulse reaches the bundle branch system during its refractory period, aberrant intraventricular conduction can occur.
- *Example of atrial fibrillation:* Figure 3-22A, B.

Pharmacological Treatment of Atrial Fibrillation

Treatment of AF is directed toward eliminating the cause, controlling ventricular rate, restoring and maintaining sinus rhythm, and preventing thromboembolism. The American College of Cardiology, American Heart Association, and the Heart Rhythm Society have collaborated to publish guidelines for the management of AF. See Table 3-5 for the guidelines for management of AF.

Ventricular rate control is aimed at improving hemodynamics and relieving symptoms. New onset AF often results in a very rapid ventricular rate that can be mildly to moderately symptomatic or cause extreme hemodynamic instability. Patients with Wolff-Parkinson-White (WPW) syndrome have an accessory pathway that can conduct atrial fibrillation impulses directly into the ventricle via the accessory pathway, resulting in an extremely rapid ventricular rate that can cause ventricular fibrillation (VF) and sudden cardiac death (see Chapter 18, Advanced ECG Concepts). In the unstable patient, ventricular rate control is a priority, and electrical cardioversion may be necessary if the patient is hemodynamically unstable because of rapid ventricular rate. Intravenous calcium channel blockers (eg, diltiazem, verapamil) and beta-blockers are commonly used in the acute situation for ventricular rate control but should be used with caution in the presence of heart failure or hypotension and are contraindicated if WPW is present. Beta-blockers, calcium channel blockers, and digitalis can be used orally for long-term rate control.

Rhythm control is restoration of sinus rhythm using pharmacologic or electrical cardioversion, and maintenance of sinus rhythm using antiarrhythmic medications. Antiarrhythmic medications with a class I recommendation for pharmacological cardioversion of AF are flecainide, dofetilide, propafenone, and ibutilide; amiodarone is a class IIa recommendation. Medications are most effective in restoring sinus rhythm when started within 7 days of AF onset. Several antiarrhythmics can be effective in maintaining sinus rhythm after conversion, including amiodarone, dofetilide, dronedarone, flecainide, propafenone, and sotalol. Oral beta-blockers or amiodarone are often used to try to prevent postoperative AF in patients undergoing cardiac surgery. Refer to specific drug guidelines for patient selection criteria.

Preventing thromboembolism is a goal in all patients with AF regardless of rhythm or rate control strategy. Antithrombotic therapy is recommended for all patients with AF based on stroke risk. The risk of stroke must be weighed

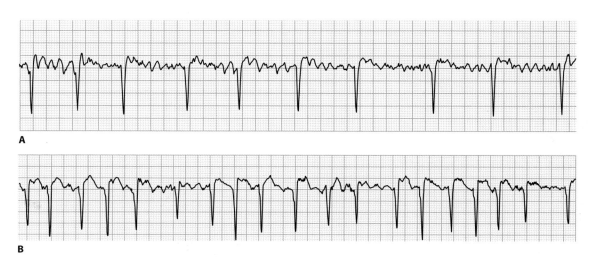

Figure 3-22. **(A)** Atrial fibrillation with a controlled ventricular response. **(B)** Atrial fibrillation with an uncontrolled ventricular response.

TABLE 3-5. GUIDELINES FOR MANAGEMENT OF ATRIAL FIBRILLATION (CLASS OF RECOMMENDATION AND LEVEL OF EVIDENCE (COR; LOE) INDICATED FOR EACH RECOMMENDATION)

Rate Control (see source for complete guidelines and more detailed information)

1. Beta-blocker, diltiazem, or verapamil for paroxysmal, persistent, or permanent AF (I; B)
2. IV beta-blocker, diltiazem, or verapamil for acute rate control if no pre-excitation (I; B)
3. Synchronized cardioversion recommended if hemodynamically unstable (I; B)
4. A resting heart rate <80 is reasonable for symptomatic AF (IIa; B)
5. IV amiodarone in critically ill patients without pre-excitation (IIa; B)
6. AV node ablation with permanent ventricular pacemaker when drug therapy ineffective (IIa; B)
7. A resting heart rate <110 is reasonable if asymptomatic and LV systolic function preserved (IIb; B)
8. Oral amiodarone if other measures ineffective (IIb; C)

Preventing Thromboembolism (see source for complete guidelines and more detailed information)

1. Selection of antithrombotic therapy based on CHA_2DS_2VASc score for assessment of stroke risk (I, B)
2. Warfarin recommended for mechanical heart valves; target INR based on type and location of valve (I; B)
3. With prior stroke, TIA, or CHA_2DS_2VASc score ≥2, oral anticoagulants with warfarin (I; A) or dabigatran, rivaroxaban, or apixaban (I, B)
4. With nonvalvular AF and CHA_2DS_2VASc score of 0, it is reasonable to omit antithrombotic therapy (IIa; B)
5. With nonvalvular AF and CHA_2DS_2VASc score of 1, no antithrombotic therapy or oral anticoagulant or aspirin may be considered (IIb; C)

Antithrombotic therapy with cardioversion (AF and atrial flutter)

1. If AF or flutter present >48 h or unknown duration, warfarin for at least 3 weeks before and 4 weeks after cardioversion (I, B); if immediate cardioversion required, anticoagulated as soon as possible and continue for at least 4 weeks (I; C)
2. If AF or flutter present <48 h and high stroke risk, IV heparin or LMWH, or factor Xa inhibitor, or direct thrombin inhibitor before or immediately after cardioversion followed by long-term anticoagulation (I; C)
3. Following cardioversion, long-term anticoagulation is based on stroke risk (I; C)
4. With AF or flutter ≥48 h or unknown duration, anticoagulation with dabigatran, rivaroxaban, or apixaban is reasonable for ≥3 weeks before and 4 weeks after cardioversion (IIa; C)
5. With AF or flutter <48 h and low stroke risk, IV heparin, LMWH, a new oral anticoagulant, or no antithrombotic therapy can be considered (IIb; C)

Cardioversion of Atrial Fibrillation and Atrial Flutter

Direct-current cardioversion

1. Cardioversion is recommended to restore sinus rhythm. If unsuccessful, attempts can be repeated. (I, B)
2. Cardioversion recommended for AF or flutter with rapid ventricular rate that does not respond to drugs (I; C)
3. Cardioversion recommended for AF or flutter with pre-excitation and hemodynamic instability (I; C)
4. It is reasonable to repeat cardioversion in persistent AF when sinus rhythm can be maintained for a clinically meaningful time period between procedures. IIb; C)

Pharmacological cardioversion

1. Flecainide, dofetilide, propafenone, and IV ibutilide in absence of contraindications (I; A)
2. Amiodarone is reasonable (IIa; A)
3. Propafenone or flecainide ("pill-in-the-pocket") to terminate AF out of hospital is reasonable once observed to be safe in a monitored setting (IIa; B)
4. Dofetilide should not be initiated out of hospital (III, B)

Maintenance of Sinus Rhythm

1. Amiodarone, dofetilide, dronedarone, flecainide, propafenone, or sotalol are recommended depending on underlying heart disease and comorbidities (I; A)
2. The risks of antiarrhythmic drugs should be considered before initiation (I; C)
3. Amiodarone should only be used after other agents have failed or are contraindicated (I; C)
4. A rhythm-control strategy with drug therapy can be useful for treatment of tachycardia induced cardiomyopathy (IIa; C)
5. It may be reasonable to continue antiarrhythmic drug therapy in the setting of infrequent, well-tolerated recurrences of AF when the drug has reduced the frequency or symptoms (IIb; C)
6. Antiarrhythmic drugs should not be continued when AF becomes permanent and dronedarone should not be used for treatment of AF in patients with NYHA class III or IV heart failure or who have had decompensated heart failure in the past 4 weeks (III, B)

Class of Recommendation (COR)

Class I: Strong; benefit >>> risk
Class IIa: Moderate; benefit >> risk
Class IIb: Weak; benefit > risk
Class III no benefit or may cause harm

Level of Evidence (LOE)

Level A: Data derived from multiple RCTs or meta-analyses.
Level B: Data derived from a single randomized trial or nonrandomized studies.
Level C: Only consensus opinion of experts, case studies, or standard-of-care.

Abbreviations: AF: atrial fibrillation; INR: international normalized ratio; LMWH: low-molecular-weight heparin; LV: left ventricular; MI: myocardial infarction; TIA: transient ischemic attack.
Data from January CT, Wann LS, Alpert JS. 2014 AHA/ACC/HRS guideline for the management of patients with atrial fibrillation: a report of the American College of Cardiology/American Heart Association Task Force on practice guidelines and the Heart Rhythm Society. Circulation. 2014 Dec 2;130(23):e199-e267.

against the risk of bleeding when considering anticoagulation for thromboembolism prevention. The CHA_2DS_2VASc score is used to assess stroke risk in AF patients and assigns 1 point for each item unless otherwise indicated: C = congestive heart failure, H = hypertension, A_2 = age > 75 years (2 points), D = diabetes, and S_2 = history of stroke, TIA, or thromboembolism (2 points), V = vascular disease (prior MI, peripheral artery disease, or aortic plaque), A = age 65-74, Sc = sex category female. Oral anticoagulation with warfarin to maintain INR between 2.0 and 3.0 (target INR = 2.5) is the usual recommendation for patients with nonvalvular AF and a CHA_2DS_2VASc score of 2 or higher and for all patients with prosthetic valves. New oral anticoagulants dabigatran, rivaroxaban, or apixaban are alternatives for patients who cannot take warfarin. For patients with a CHA_2DS_2VASc score of 1, no antithrombotic therapy or oral anticoagulant or aspirin may be considered, and for those with a score of 0, antithrombotic therapy can be omitted. See Table 3-5 for recommendations for thromboembolism prevention in patients with AF.

Nonpharmacological Management of Atrial Fibrillation

Radiofrequency (RF) catheter ablation and surgical management of AF include AV node ablation, pulmonary vein ablation, surgical or ablation Maze procedures, and occlusion or surgical removal of the left atrial appendage. These procedures are briefly described here.

ESSENTIAL CONTENT CASE

Atrial Dysrhythmia and Cardioversion

You are caring for a patient who was admitted for an elective cardioversion. She was seen in her physician's office this morning for complaints of SOB and palpitations that started around 7 AM. She has a history of hypertension and diabetes but no previous cardiac history. In the office, her ECG showed atrial fibrillation with a ventricular response between 120 and 130 beats/min. Previous ECGs had all shown normal sinus rhythm, and since her symptoms were new and time of onset was just a few hours ago, her physician elected to treat her with cardioversion. Her BP is 136/74 and she is breathing comfortably at this time. You place her on the bedside cardiac monitor in lead V_1.

Case Question 1. What are the diagnostic features of AF that you expect to see on the monitor?
Figure 3-23A shows her rhythm strip:

Case Question 2. Is her admitting diagnosis of AF correct?

Case Question 3. What other treatments besides electrical cardioversion would be appropriate for managing this rhythm?
You gather the equipment and supplies needed for the cardioversion. The cardiologist arrives and an anesthesiologist is present to sedate the patient. The cardiologist asks you to deliver a 100 joule shock after the patient is asleep.

Case Question 4. What safety considerations are necessary before delivering the cardioversion shock?
The shock is delivered and Figure 3-23B shows the post-shock rhythm.

Case Question 5. What is the rhythm?

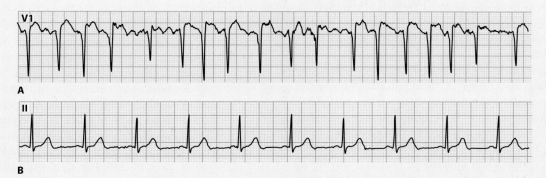

Figure 3-23. **(A)** Rhythm strip when monitoring is initiated. **(B)** Post-shock rhythm strip.

Answers
1. Atrial fibrillation is characterized by the presence of "fibrillation" waves instead of organized P waves, and an irregularly irregular ventricular response.
2. Yes. This is a typical example of AF.
3. The first goal of treatment for AF is ventricular rate control. AV nodal blocking agents such as a beta-blocker or calcium channel blocker (ie, verapamil or diltiazem) are used for rate control. Antiarrhythmics such as flecainide, dofetilide, propafenone, ibutilide, or amiodarone can be used for pharmacological conversion of atrial fibrillation to sinus rhythm. Patients with persistent AF are on chronic therapy with a rate control drug and oral anticoagulation.
4. Every member of the team participating in the procedure should be involved in assuring patient safety. The patient should be monitored with noninvasive BP monitoring and pulse oximetry. Airway management supplies, emergency drugs, and sedation reversal agents should be present at the bedside. The patient should be adequately sedated prior to shock delivery. The defibrillator must be synchronized on the QRS complex to avoid delivering the shock on the T wave, which could cause ventricular fibrillation. Prior to shock delivery, the operator should ensure that no one is touching the patient or the bed.
5. This is normal sinus rhythm, indicating a successful cardioversion.

Radiofrequency AV node ablation is the most common nonpharmacologic method of rate control in AF and is usually done only when drug therapy for rate control is ineffective or not tolerated. RF energy is directed at the AV node to heat the tissue and destroy its ability to conduct impulses to the ventricle. This procedure results in complete AV block and requires a ventricular pacemaker implant to maintain an adequate ventricular rate. AV node ablation does not stop atrial fibrillation; therefore, patients must be chronically anticoagulated to prevent stroke.

Radiofrequency ablation of AF trigger sites in the pulmonary veins or atria is the mainstay of ablation therapy for AF. The most common site of AF triggers is the first 2 to 4 cm inside the pulmonary veins leading into the left atrium, although triggers can be present in multiple sites within both atria. The most successful procedures are segmental ostial pulmonary vein isolation (PVI) and circumferential PVI. In segmental ostial PVI, specific sites of electrical conduction in the ostia of the pulmonary veins are ablated. In circumferential PVI, continuous ablation lesions encircle the ostia of all four pulmonary veins, usually in two pairs (ie, one circle of lesions around the left pulmonary veins and another circle around the right pulmonary veins). These ablation lesions completely isolate the pulmonary veins from the atrial myocardium and prevent conduction from trigger sites in to the atria.

The Cox-Maze III procedure involves creation of multiple incisions within both atria using the "cut and sew" technique during cardiac surgery. The incisions create scars in the atria that direct the impulse from the sinus node to the AV node through both atria in an orderly fashion and prevent reentry of impulses that could lead to AF. Similar scars can be created using bipolar RF ablation clamps (Cox-Maze IV procedure), which can be performed less invasively through a thoracotomy. Catheter-based RF ablation procedures create the lesions from the endocardial approach and are done percutaneously in the electrophysiology laboratory rather than requiring surgery. Hybrid procedures using ablation catheters and the surgical approach are also available.

Left atrial appendage (LAA) amputation is done along with surgical Cox-Maze procedures as well as with mitral valve procedures to reduce the likelihood of thromboembolism, since most clots develop in the LAA during AF. LAA occlusion devices can be inserted via the right femoral vein and into the LAA through a trans-septal approach and expanded within the LAA to seal it from the rest of the atrium, thus trapping clots and preventing them from embolizing.

Supraventricular Tachycardia (SVT)

A supraventricular tachycardia (SVT) by definition is any rhythm at a rate faster than 100 beats/min, which originates above the ventricle or utilizes the atria or AV junction as part of the circuit that maintains the tachycardia. Technically, SVT can include sinus tachycardia, AT, atrial flutter, atrial fibrillation, and junctional tachycardia. However, the term SVT is meant to be used to describe a regular, narrow QRS tachycardia in which the exact mechanism cannot be determined from the surface ECG. If P waves or atrial activity such a fibrillation or flutter waves can be clearly seen, then the mechanism can usually be identified. Occasionally in AT the P waves are hidden in preceding T waves and in that case use of the term SVT is appropriate.

The two most common dysrhythmias for which the term SVT is appropriate are AV nodal reentry tachycardia (AVNRT) and circus movement tachycardia (CMT) that occurs when an accessory pathway is present, such as in WPW. Another term used to describe CMT is AV reentry tachycardia (AVRT) but CMT is used here to prevent confusion between these two common dysrhythmias. The mechanisms of these SVTs are described in detail in Chapter 18, Advanced ECG Concepts. ECG characteristics of both SVTs are very similar and described here.

ECG Characteristics

- *Rate:* 140-250 beats/min.
- *Rhythm:* Regular.
- *P waves:* Usually not visible. In AVNRT, the P wave is hidden in the QRS or barely peeking out at the end of the QRS. In CMT, the P wave is usually present in the ST segment, but is often not visible.
- *PR interval:* Not measurable, since P waves are usually not visible.
- *QRS complex:* Usually normal.
- *Conduction:* In AVNRT, the impulse travels in a small circuit that includes the AV node as one limb of the circuit and a slower conducting pathway just outside the AV node as the second limb of the circuit. The impulse depolarizes the atria in a retrograde direction at the same time as it depolarizes the ventricles through the normal His-Purkinje system, resulting in a regular narrow QRS tachycardia. In CMT, the impulse follows a reentry circuit that includes the atria, AV node, ventricles, and accessory pathway. The most common type of CMT is called orthodromic CMT, in which the impulse travels from atria to ventricles through the normal AV node and His-Purkinje system, then back to the atria from the ventricles through the accessory pathway. This results in a regular, narrow QRS tachycardia because the ventricles are depolarized via the normal conduction system. If the circuit reverses direction and the ventricles depolarize through conduction down the accessory pathway, this is called antidromic CMT, and the resulting tachycardia has a wide QRS complex.
- *Example of SVT:* See Figure 3-24A, B.

Treatment

These SVTs are usually well tolerated and often paroxysmal in nature. If the ventricular rate is very rapid and sustained, symptoms such as palpitations, dizziness, or syncope can occur.

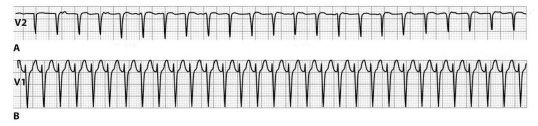

Figure 3-24. **(A)** SVT at a rate of 190 beats/min found to be AVNRT at electrophysiology study. **(B)** SVT at a rate of 214 found to be CMT at electrophysiology study.

Vagal maneuvers such as carotid sinus massage, Valsalva's maneuver, gagging or coughing, drinking ice water, or putting the face in ice water may be effective in terminating the tachycardia. Adenosine (6 mg given rapidly IV, may repeat with 12 mg if necessary) is the most effective drug to terminate the tachycardia. Drugs that slow AV conduction, like calcium channel blockers (diltiazem, verapamil) or beta-blockers, can terminate tachycardia and can be used long term to prevent recurrences. Synchronized cardioversion can be used if drugs are contraindicated or fail to terminate tachycardia. Radiofrequency ablation offers a cure for AVNRT and CMT. See Table 3-4 for recommendations for management of supraventricular tachycardias.

DYSRHYTHMIAS ORIGINATING IN THE ATRIOVENTRICULAR JUNCTION

Cells surrounding the AV node in the AV junction are capable of initiating impulses and controlling the heart rhythm (Figure 3-25). Junctional beats and junctional rhythms can appear in any of three ways on the ECG depending on the location of the junctional pacemaker and the speed of conduction of the impulse into the atria and ventricles:

- When a junctional focus fires, the wave of depolarization spreads backward (retrograde) into the atria as well as forward (antegrade) into the ventricles. If the impulse arrives in the atria before it arrives in the ventricles, the ECG shows a P wave (usually inverted because the atria are depolarizing from bottom to

top) followed immediately by a QRS complex as the impulse reaches the ventricles. In this case, the PR interval is very short, usually 0.10 second or less.
- If the junctional impulse reaches both the atria and the ventricles at the same time, only a QRS is seen on the ECG because the ventricles are much larger than the atria and only ventricular depolarization will be seen, even though the atria are also depolarizing.
- If the junctional impulse reaches the ventricles before it reaches the atria, the QRS precedes the P wave on the ECG. Again, the P wave is usually inverted because of retrograde atrial depolarization, and the RP interval (distance from the beginning of the QRS to the beginning of the following P wave) is short.

Premature Junctional Complexes

Premature junctional complexes (PJCs) are due to an irritable focus in the AV junction. Irritability can be because of coronary heart disease or MI disrupting blood flow to the AV junction, nicotine, caffeine, emotions, or medications such as digitalis.

ECG Characteristics
- *Rate:* 60 to 100 beats/min or whatever the rate of the basic rhythm.
- *Rhythm:* Regular except for occurrence of premature beats.
- *P waves:* May occur before, during, or after the QRS complex of the premature beat and are usually inverted.
- *PR interval:* Short, usually 0.10 second or less when P waves precede the QRS.
- *QRS complex:* Usually normal but may be aberrant if the PJC occurs very early and conducts into the ventricles during the refractory period of a bundle branch.
- *Conduction:* Retrograde through the atria; usually normal through the ventricles.
- *Example of a PJC:* Figure 3-26.

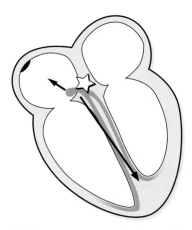

Figure 3-25. Dysrhythmias originating in the AV junction.

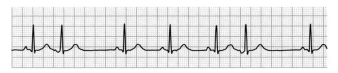

Figure 3-26. Premature junctional complexes.

Treatment
Treatment is not necessary for PJCs.

Junctional Rhythm, Accelerated Junctional Rhythm, and Junctional Tachycardia

Junctional rhythms can occur if the sinus node rate falls below the rate of the AV junctional pacemakers or when atrial conduction through the AV junction has been disrupted. Junctional rhythms commonly occur from digitalis toxicity or following inferior MI owing to disruption of blood supply to the sinus node and the AV junction. These rhythms are classified according to their rate. Junctional rhythm usually occurs at a rate of 40 to 60 beats/min, accelerated junctional rhythm occurs at a rate of 60 to 100 beats/min, and junctional tachycardia occurs at a rate of 100 to 250 beats/min.

ECG Characteristics

- *Rate:* Junctional rhythm, 40 to 60 beats/min; accelerated junctional rhythm, 60 to 100 beats/min; junctional tachycardia, 100 to 250 beats/min.
- *Rhythm:* Regular.
- *P waves:* May precede or follow QRS.
- *PR interval:* Short, 0.10 second or less.
- *QRS complex:* Usually normal.
- *Conduction:* Retrograde through the atria; normal through the ventricles.
- *Example of junctional rhythm and accelerated junctional rhythm:* Figure 3-27A, B.

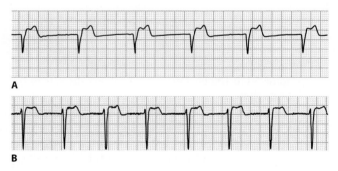

Figure 3-27. **(A)** Junctional rhythm. **(B)** Accelerated junctional rhythm.

Treatment
Treatment of junctional rhythm rarely is required unless the rate is too slow or too fast to maintain adequate cardiac output. If the rate is slow, atropine is given to increase the sinus rate and override the junctional focus or to increase the rate of firing of the junctional pacemaker. If the rate is fast, medications such as verapamil, propranolol, or beta-blockers may be effective in slowing the rate or terminating the dysrhythmia. Because digitalis toxicity is a common cause of junctional rhythms, and so is held or avoided in patients with this dysrhythmia.

DYSRHYTHMIAS ORIGINATING IN THE VENTRICLES

Ventricular dysrhythmias originate in the ventricular muscle or Purkinje system and are considered to be more dangerous

than other dysrhythmias because of their potential to initiate VT and severely decrease cardiac output (Figure 3-28). However, as with any dysrhythmia, ventricular rate is a key determinant of how well a patient can tolerate a ventricular rhythm. Ventricular rhythms can range in severity from mild, well-tolerated rhythms to pulseless rhythms leading to sudden cardiac death.

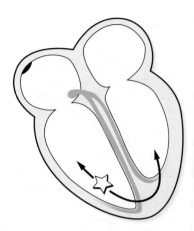

Figure 3-28. Dysrhythmias originating in the ventricles.

Premature Ventricular Complexes

Premature ventricular complexes (PVCs) are caused by premature depolarization of cells in the ventricular myocardium or Purkinje system or to reentry in the ventricles. PVCs can be caused by hypoxia, myocardial ischemia, hypokalemia, acidosis, exercise, increased levels of circulating catecholamines, digitalis toxicity, caffeine, and alcohol, among other causes. PVCs increase with aging and are more common in people with coronary disease, valve disease, hypertension, cardiomyopathy, and other forms of heart disease. PVCs are not dangerous in people with normal hearts but are associated with higher mortality rates in patients with structural heart disease or acute MI, especially if left ventricular function is reduced. PVCs are considered potentially malignant when they occur more frequently than 10 per hour or are repetitive (occur in pairs, triplets, or more than three in a row) in patients with coronary disease, previous MI, cardiomyopathy, and reduced ejection fraction.

ECG Characteristics

- *Rate:* 60 to 100 beats/min or the rate of the basic rhythm.
- *Rhythm:* Irregular because of the early beats.
- *P waves:* Not related to the PVCs. Sinus rhythm is usually not interrupted by the premature beats, so sinus P waves can often be seen occurring regularly throughout the rhythm. P waves may occasionally follow PVCs due to retrograde conduction from the ventricle backward through the atria. These P waves are inverted.

- *PR interval:* Not present before most PVCs. If a P wave happens, by coincidence, to precede a PVC, the PR interval is short.
- *QRS complex:* Wide and bizarre; greater than 0.10 second in duration. These may vary in morphology (size, shape), if they originate from more than one focus in the ventricles (multifocal PVCs).
- *Conduction:* Impulses originating in the ventricles conduct through the ventricles from muscle cell to muscle cell rather than through Purkinje fibers, resulting in wide QRS complexes. Some PVCs may conduct retrograde into the atria, resulting in inverted P waves following the PVC. When the sinus rhythm is undisturbed by PVCs, the atria depolarize normally.
- *Example of PVCs:* Figure 3-29A, B.

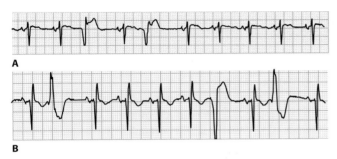

Figure 3-29. Premature ventricular complexes.

Treatment

The significance of PVCs depends on the clinical setting in which they occur. Many people have chronic PVCs that do not need to be treated, and most of these people are asymptomatic. There is no evidence that suppression of PVCs reduces mortality, especially in patients with no structural heart disease. If PVCs cause bothersome palpitations, patients are told to avoid caffeine, tobacco, other stimulants, and try stress reduction techniques. Low-dose beta-blockers may reduce PVC frequency and the perception of palpitations and can be used for symptom relief.

In the setting of an acute MI, PVCs may be precursors of more dangerous ventricular dysrhythmias, especially when they occur near the apex of the T wave (R on T PVCs). Unless PVCs result in hemodynamic instability or symptomatic VT, treatment is not recommended. Beta-blockers are often effective in suppressing repetitive PVCs and have become the drugs of choice for treating post-MI PVCs that are symptomatic. Several antiarrhythmic medications are effective in reducing the frequency of PVCs but are not recommended due to the risk of prodysrhythmia and their association with sudden cardiac death in patients with structural heart disease. Amiodarone and sotalol can be used for PVC suppression in symptomatic patients but they do not improve mortality. Catheter ablation is an option in patients with left ventricular dysfunction associated with PVCs.

Idioventricular Rhythm and Accelerated Idioventricular Rhythm (AIVR)

Idioventricular rhythm occurs when an ectopic focus in the ventricle fires at a rate less than 50 beats/min. This rhythm occurs as an escape rhythm when the sinus node and junctional tissue fail to fire or fail to conduct their impulses to the ventricle. Accelerated idioventricular rhythm (AIVR) occurs when an ectopic focus in the ventricles fires at a rate of 50 to 100 beats/min. AIVR commonly occurs in patients with acute MI, especially inferior wall MI, and is a common dysrhythmia after thrombolytic therapy, when reperfusion of the damaged myocardium occurs. However, AIVR is not a sensitive or specific marker for successful reperfusion.

ECG Characteristics

- *Rate:* Less than 50 beats/min for ventricular rhythm and 50 to 100 beats/min for accelerated ventricular rhythm.
- *Rhythm:* Usually regular.
- *P waves:* May be seen but at a slower rate than the ventricular focus, with dissociation from the QRS complex.
- *PR interval:* Not measured.
- *QRS complex:* Wide and bizarre.
- *Conduction:* If sinus rhythm is the basic rhythm, atrial conduction is normal. Impulses originating in the ventricles conduct via muscle cell-to-cell conduction, resulting in the wide QRS complex.
- *Example of escape ventricular rhythm and accelerated ventricular rhythm:* Figure 3-30A, B.

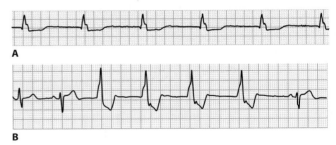

Figure 3-30. (A) Escape ventricular rhythm. **(B)** Accelerated ventricular rhythm.

Treatment

The treatment of AIVR depends on its cause and how well the patient is able to tolerate it. This dysrhythmia is usually transient and not harmful because the ventricular rate is within normal limits. Suppressive therapy is not indicated because abolishing the ventricular rhythm may leave an even less desirable heart rate. If the patient is symptomatic because of the loss of atrial kick, atropine can be used to increase the rate of the sinus node and overdrive the ventricular rhythm. If the ventricular rhythm is an escape rhythm, then treatment is directed toward increasing the rate of the escape rhythm or pacing the heart temporarily. Usually, accelerated ventricular rhythm is transient and benign and does not require treatment.

Ventricular Tachycardia

Ventricular tachycardia (VT) is a rapid ventricular rhythm at a rate greater than 100 beats/min. VT can be classified according to: (1) duration, *nonsustained* (lasts less than 30 seconds), *sustained* (lasts longer than 30 seconds), or *incessant* (VT present most of the time); and (2) morphology (ECG appearance of QRS complexes), *monomorphic* (QRS complexes have the same shape during tachycardia), *polymorphic* (QRS complexes vary randomly in shape), or *bidirectional* (alternating upright and negative QRS complexes during tachycardia). Polymorphic VT that occurs in the presence of a long QT interval is called *torsades de pointes* (meaning "twisting of the points"). The most common cause of VT is coronary artery disease, including acute ischemia, acute MI, and prior MI. Other causes include heart failure, cardiomyopathy, valvular heart disease, congenital heart disease, arrhythmogenic right ventricular dysplasia, cardiac tumors, cardiac surgery, and the proarrhythmic effects of many drugs. See Chapter 18 (Advanced ECG Concepts) for more information on VTs and the differential diagnosis of wide QRS tachycardias.

ECG Characteristics

- *Rate:* Ventricular rate is faster than 100 beats/min.
- *Rhythm:* Monomorphic VT is usually regular; polymorphic VT can be irregular.
- *P waves:* Dissociated from QRS complexes. If sinus rhythm is the underlying basic rhythm, they are regular. P waves may be seen but are not related to QRS complexes. P waves are often buried within QRS complexes.
- *PR interval:* Not measurable because of dissociation of P waves from QRS complexes.
- *QRS complex:* Usually 0.12 second or more in duration.
- *Conduction:* Impulse originates in one ventricle and spreads via muscle cell-to-cell conduction through both ventricles. There may be retrograde conduction through the atria, but more often the sinus node continues to fire regularly and depolarize the atria normally.
- *Example of VT:* Figure 3-31.

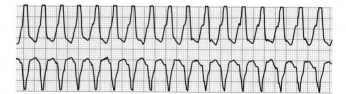

Figure 3-31. Monomorphic ventricular tachycardia.

Treatment

Immediate treatment of VT depends on how well the rhythm is tolerated by the patient. The two main determinants of patient tolerance of any tachycardia are ventricular rate and underlying left ventricular function. VT can be an emergency if cardiac output is severely decreased because of a very rapid rate or poor left ventricular function.

Hemodynamically unstable VT is treated with synchronized cardioversion. If VT is pulseless then immediate defibrillation is required. VT that is hemodynamically stable can be treated with pharmacologic therapy. Amiodarone is often the drug of choice but lidocaine or procainamide can also be used. Medications used to treat VT on a long-term basis include amiodarone, sotalol, and beta-blockers. Some VTs can be treated with radiofrequency catheter ablation to abolish the ectopic focus. The implantable cardioverter defibrillator (ICD) is frequently used for recurrent VT in patients with reduced ejection fractions or drug refractory VT. See Table 3-6 for recommendations for management of ventricular dysrhythmias based on guidelines released in 2006. At the time of this writing, more recent guidelines were underway but not yet published. Please check the American College of Cardiology and the American Heart Association websites to determine if revised guidelines are available.

Ventricular Fibrillation

Ventricular fibrillation (VF) is rapid, ineffective quivering of the ventricles and is fatal without immediate treatment (Figure 3-32). Electrical activity originates in the ventricles and spreads in a chaotic, irregular pattern throughout both ventricles. There is no cardiac output or palpable pulse with VF.

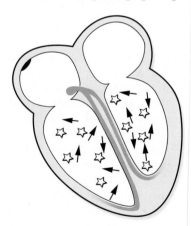

Figure 3-32. Ventricular fibrillation.

ECG Characteristics

- *Rate:* Rapid, uncoordinated, ineffective.
- *Rhythm:* Chaotic, irregular.
- *P waves:* None seen.
- *PR interval:* None.
- *QRS complex:* No formed QRS complexes seen; rapid, irregular undulations without any specific pattern.
- *Conduction:* Multiple ectopic foci firing simultaneously in ventricles and depolarizing them irregularly and without any organized pattern. Ventricles are not contracting.
- *Example of ventricular fibrillation:* Figure 3-33.

TABLE 3-6. TREATMENT OF VENTRICULAR ARRHYTHMIAS

Ventricular Tachycardia

Acute Treatment
1. Patients with a wide-QRS tachycardia should be presumed to have VT if the diagnosis is unclear. (Class I, LOE C-EO)
2. Patients presenting with ventricular arrhythmias (VA) with hemodynamic instability should undergo direct current cardioversion. (Class I, LOE A)
3. In patients with hemodynamically stable VT, administration of intravenous procainamide can be useful to attempt to terminate VT. (Class IIa, LOE A)
4. In patients with hemodynamically stable VT, administration of intravenous amiodarone or sotalol may be considered to attempt to terminate VT. (Class IIb, LOE B-R)
5. In patients with a recent MI who have VT/VF that repeatedly recurs despite direct current cardioversion and antiarrhythmic medications (VT/VF storm), an intravenous beta-blocker can be useful. (Class IIa, LOE B-NR)
6. In patients with suspected AMI, prophylactic administration of lidocaine or high-dose amiodarone for the prevention of VT is potentially harmful. (Class III, LOE B-R)
7. In patients with a wide QRS complex tachycardia of unknown origin, calcium channel blockers (eg, verapamil and diltiazem) are potentially harmful. (Class III, LOE C-LD)

Ongoing Management
1. In patients with ischemic heart disease, who either survive sudden cardiac arrest due to VT/VF or experience hemodynamically unstable VT (LOE B-R) or stable VT (LOE B-NR) not due to reversible causes, an ICD is recommended if meaningful survival greater than 1 year is expected. (Class I)
2. In patients with ischemic heart disease and unexplained syncope who have inducible sustained monomorphic VT on electrophysiological study, an ICD is recommended if meaningful survival of greater than 1 year is expected. (Class I, LOE B-NR)
3. In patients with ischemic heart disease and recurrent VA, with significant symptoms or ICD shocks despite optimal device programming and ongoing treatment with a beta-blocker, amiodarone or sotalol is useful to suppress recurrent VA. (Class I, LOE B-R)
4. In patients with prior MI and recurrent episodes of symptomatic sustained VT, or who present with VT or VF storm and have failed or are intolerant of amiodarone (LOE B-R) or other antiarrhythmic medications (LOE B-NR), catheter ablation is recommended. (Class I)
5. In patients with ischemic heart disease and ICD shocks for sustained monomorphic VT or symptomatic sustained monomorphic VT that is recurrent, or hemodynamically tolerated, catheter ablation as first-line therapy may be considered to reduce recurrent VA. (Class IIb, LOE C-LD)
6. In patients with prior MI, class IC antiarrhythmic medications (eg, flecainide and propafenone) should not be used. (Class III, LOE B-R)
7. In patients with ischemic heart disease and sustained monomorphic VT, coronary revascularization alone is an ineffective therapy to prevent recurrent VT. (Class III, LOE C-LD)
8. In patients with incessant VT or VF, an ICD should not be implanted until sufficient control of the arrhythmia is achieved to prevent repeated ICD shocks. (Class III, LOEC-LD)

Polymorphic Ventricular Tachycardia

Acute Treatment
1. In patients with polymorphic VT or VF with ST-elevation MI, angiography with emergency revascularization is recommended. (Class I, LOE B-NR)
2. In patients with polymorphic VT due to myocardial ischemia, intravenous beta-blockers can be useful. (Class IIa, LOE B-R)

Torsades de Pointes

Acute Treatment
1. For patients with QT prolongation due to a medication, hypokalemia, hypomagnesemia, or other acquired factor and recurrent torsades de pointes, administration of intravenous magnesium sulfate is recommended to suppress the arrhythmia. (Class I, LOE C-LD)
2. In patients with recurrent torsades de pointes associated with acquired QT prolongation and bradycardia that cannot be suppressed with intravenous magnesium administration, increasing the heart rate with atrial or ventricular pacing or isoproterenol are recommended to suppress the arrhythmia. (Class I, LOE B-NR)
3. For patients with torsades de pointes associated with acquired QT prolongation, potassium repletion to 4.0 mmol/L or more and magnesium repletion to normal values are beneficial. (Class I, LOE C-LD)
4. In patients with congenital or acquired long QT syndrome, QT-prolonging medications are potentially harmful. (Class III, LOE B-NR)

Class of Recommendation (COR)
Class I: Strong; benefit >>> risk
Class IIa: Moderate; benefit >> risk
Class IIb: Weak; benefit > risk
Class III: No benefit or may cause harm

Level of Evidence (LOE)
A: High quality evidence from > 1 randomized clinical trial (RTC), meta analyses of high quality RCTs.
B-R (randomized): Moderate quality evidence from 1 or more RCTs, meta analyses of moderate quality RCTs.
B-NR (nonrandomized): Moderate quality evidence from 1 or more well-designed nonrandomized studies, observational studies, or registry studies.
C-LD (limited data): Randomized or nonrandomized observational or registry studies with limitations of design or execution, meta analyses of such studies.
C-EO (expert opinion): Consensus of expert opinion based on clinical experience.

Data from Al-Khatib SM, Stevenson WG, Ackerman MJ, et al: 2017 AHA/ACC/HRS Guideline for Management of Patients With Ventricular Arrhythmias and the Prevention of Sudden Cardiac Death: A Report of the American College of Cardiology/American Heart Association Task Force on Clinical Practice Guidelines and the Heart Rhythm Society. Circulation. 2017 Oct 30.

Treatment

VF requires immediate defibrillation. Synchronized cardioversion is not possible because there are no formed QRS complexes on which to synchronize the shock. Cardiopulmonary resuscitation (CPR) must be performed until a defibrillator is available, and then defibrillation at 200 J (biphasic defibrillation) or 360 J (monophasic defibrillation) is recommended followed by CPR and pharmacologic therapy. IV amiodarone is the recommended antiarrhythmic during the resuscitation effort and as maintenance therapy for 24 to 48 hours following return of spontaneous circulation.

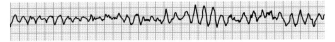

Figure 3-33. Ventricular fibrillation.

Beta-blockers, amiodarone, and sotalol are most often used for long-term drug therapy. The ICD has become the standard of care for survivors of VF that occurs in the absence of acute ischemia.

Ventricular Asystole

Ventricular asystole is the absence of any ventricular rhythm: no QRS complex, no pulse, and no cardiac output (Figure 3-34). Ventricular asystole is always fatal unless the cause can be identified and treated immediately. If atrial activity is still present, the term "ventricular standstill" is used.

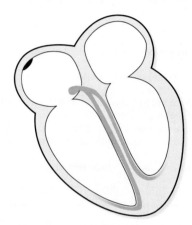

Figure 3-34. Ventricular asystole.

ECG Characteristics
- *Rate:* None.
- *Rhythm:* None.
- *P waves:* May be present if the sinus node is functioning.
- *PR interval:* None.
- *QRS complex:* None.
- *Conduction:* Atrial conduction may be normal, if the sinus node is functioning. There is no conduction into the ventricles.
- *Example of ventricular asystole:* Figure 3-35.

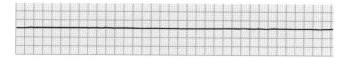

Figure 3-35. Ventricular asystole.

Treatment
CPR must be initiated immediately if the patient is to survive. IV epinephrine is the only drug currently recommended for treating asystole. The cause of asystole should be determined and treated as rapidly as possible to improve the chance of survival. Asystole has a very poor prognosis despite the best resuscitation efforts because it usually represents extensive myocardial ischemia or severe underlying metabolic problems. Pacing and atropine are no longer recommended for treatment for asystole.

ATRIOVENTRICULAR BLOCKS

The term *atrioventricular block* is used to describe dysrhythmias in which there is delayed or failed conduction of supraventricular impulses into the ventricles. AV blocks have been classified according to location of the block and severity of the conduction abnormality.

First-Degree Atrioventricular Block

First-degree AV block is defined as prolonged AV conduction time of supraventricular impulses into the ventricles (Figure 3-36). This delay usually occurs in the AV node, and all impulses are conducted to the ventricles, but with delayed conduction times. First-degree AV block can be due to coronary heart disease, rheumatic heart disease, or administration of digitalis, beta-blockers, or calcium channel blockers. First-degree AV block can be normal in people with slow heart rates or high vagal tone.

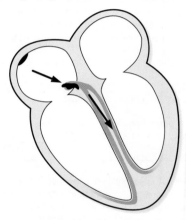

Figure 3-36. First-degree AV block.

ECG Characteristics
- *Rate:* Can occur at any sinus rate, usually 60 to 100 beats/min.
- *Rhythm:* Regular.
- *P waves:* Normal; precede every QRS complex.
- *PR interval:* Prolonged above 0.20 second.
- *QRS complex:* Usually normal.
- *Conduction:* Normal through the atria, delayed through the AV node, and normal through the ventricles.
- *Example of first-degree AV block:* Figure 3-37.

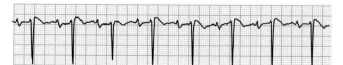

Figure 3-37. First-degree AV block.

Treatment
Treatment of first-degree AV block is usually not required, but the rhythm should be observed for progression to more severe block.

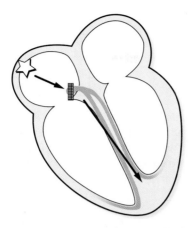

Figure 3-38. Type I second-degree AV block.

Second-Degree Atrioventricular Block

Second-degree AV block occurs when one atrial impulse at a time fails to be conducted to the ventricles. Second-degree AV block can be divided into two distinct categories: type I block, occurring in the AV node, and type II block, occurring below the AV node in the bundle of His or bundle-branch system (Figure 3-38).

Type I Second-Degree Atrioventricular Block

Type I second-degree AV block, often referred to as *Wenckebach block,* is a progressive increase in conduction times of consecutive atrial impulses into the ventricles until one impulse fails to conduct, or is "dropped." The PR intervals gradually lengthen until one P wave fails to conduct and is not followed by a QRS complex, resulting in a pause, after which the cycle repeats itself. This type of block is commonly associated with inferior MI, coronary heart disease, aortic valve disease, mitral valve prolapse, atrial septal defects, and administration of digitalis, beta-blockers, or calcium channel blockers.

ECG Characteristics

- *Rate:* Can occur at any sinus or atrial rate.
- *Rhythm:* Irregular. Overall appearance of the rhythm demonstrates "group beating."
- *P waves:* Normal. Some P waves are not conducted to the ventricles, but only one at a time fails to conduct to the ventricle.
- *PR interval:* Gradually lengthens on consecutive beats. The PR interval preceding the pause is longer than that following the pause (unless 2:1 conduction is present).
- *QRS complex:* Usually normal unless there is associated bundle branch block.
- *Conduction:* Normal through the atria; progressively delayed through the AV node until an impulse fails to conduct. Ventricular conduction is normal. Conduction ratios can vary, with ratios as low as 2:1 (every other P wave is blocked) up to high ratios such as 15:14 (every 15th P wave is blocked).
- *Example of second-degree AV block type I:* Figure 3-39.

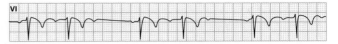

Figure 3-39. Second-degree AV block, type I.

Treatment

Treatment of type I second-degree AV block depends on the conduction ratio, the resulting ventricular rate, and the patient's tolerance for the rhythm. If ventricular rates are slow enough to decrease cardiac output, the treatment is atropine to increase the sinus rate and speed conduction through the AV node. At higher conduction ratios where the ventricular rate is within a normal range, no treatment is necessary. If the block is due to digitalis, calcium channel blockers, or beta-blockers, those medications are held. This type of block is usually temporary and benign, and seldom requires pacing, although temporary pacing may be needed when the ventricular rate is slow.

Type II Second-Degree Atrioventricular Block

Type II second-degree AV block is sudden failure of conduction of an atrial impulse to the ventricles without progressive increases in conduction time of consecutive P waves (Figure 3-40). Type II block occurs below the AV node and is usually associated with bundle branch block; therefore, the dropped beats are usually a manifestation of bilateral bundle branch block. This form of block appears on the ECG much the same as type I block except that there is no progressive increase in PR intervals before the blocked beats and the QRS is almost always wide. Type II block is less common than type I block, but is a more serious form of block. It occurs in rheumatic heart disease, coronary heart disease, primary disease of the conduction system, and in the presence of acute anterior MI. Type II block is more dangerous than type I because of a higher incidence of associated symptoms and progression to complete AV block.

ECG Characteristics

- *Rate:* Can occur at any basic rate.
- *Rhythm:* Irregular due to blocked beats.

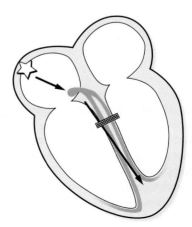

Figure 3-40. Type II second-degree AV block.

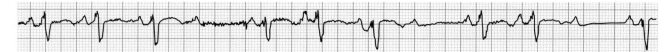

Figure 3-41. Second-degree AV block, type II.

- *P waves:* Usually regular and precede each QRS. Periodically a P wave is not followed by a QRS complex.
- *PR interval:* Constant before conducted beats. The PR interval preceding the pause is the same as that following the pause.
- *QRS complex:* Usually wide because of associated bundle branch block.
- *Conduction:* Normal through the atria and through the AV node but intermittently blocked in the bundle branch system and fails to reach the ventricles. Conduction through the ventricles is abnormally slow due to associated bundle branch block. Conduction ratios can vary from 2:1 to only occasional blocked beats.
- *Example of second-degree AV block type II:* Figure 3-41.

Treatment

Treatment usually includes pacemaker therapy because this type of block is often permanent and progresses to complete block. External pacing can be used for treatment of symptomatic type II block until transvenous pacing can be initiated. Atropine is not recommended because increasing the number of impulses conducting through the AV node may bombard the diseased bundles with more impulses than they can handle, resulting in further conduction failure and a slower ventricular rate.

High-Grade Atrioventricular Block

High-grade (or advanced) AV block is present when two or more consecutive atrial impulses are blocked when the atrial rate is reasonable (<135 beats/min) and conduction fails because of the block itself and not because of interference from an escape pacemaker. High-grade AV block may be type I, occurring in the AV node, or type II, occurring below the AV node. The importance of high-grade block depends on the conduction ratio and the resulting ventricular rate. Because ventricular rates tend to be slow, this dysrhythmia is frequently symptomatic and requires treatment.

ECG Characteristics
- *Rate:* Atrial rate less than 135 beats/min.
- *Rhythm:* Regular or irregular, depending on conduction pattern.
- *P waves:* Normal. Present before every conducted QRS, but several P waves appear without subsequent QRS complexes.
- *PR interval:* Constant before conducted beats. May be normal or prolonged.
- *QRS complex:* Usually normal in type I block and wide in type II block.

- *Conduction:* Normal through the atria. Two or more consecutive atrial impulses fail to conduct to the ventricles. Ventricular conduction is normal in type I block and abnormally slow in type II block.
- *Example of high-grade AV block:* Figure 3-42.

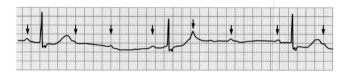

Figure 3-42. High-grade AV block.

Treatment

Treatment of high-grade block is necessary, if the patient is symptomatic. Atropine can be given and is generally more effective in type I block. An external pacemaker may be required until transvenous pacing can be initiated, and permanent pacing is often necessary in type II high-grade block.

Third-Degree Atrioventricular Block (Complete Block)

Third-degree AV block is complete failure of conduction of all atrial impulses to the ventricles (Figure 3-43A, B). In third-degree AV block, there is complete AV dissociation; the atria are usually under the control of the sinus node, although complete block can occur with any atrial dysrhythmia; and either a junctional or ventricular pacemaker controls the ventricles. The ventricular rate is usually less than 45 beats/min; a faster rate could indicate an accelerated junctional or ventricular rhythm that interferes with conduction from the atria into the ventricles by causing physiologic refractoriness in the conduction system, thus causing a physiologic failure of conduction that must be differentiated from the abnormal conduction system function of complete AV block. Causes of complete AV block include coronary heart disease, MI, Lev disease, Lenègre disease, cardiac surgery, congenital heart disease, and medications that slow AV conduction such as digitalis, beta-blockers, and calcium channel blockers.

ECG Characteristics
- *Rate:* Atrial rate is usually normal. Ventricular rate is less than 45 beats/min.
- *Rhythm:* Regular.
- *P waves:* Normal but dissociated from QRS complexes.
- *PR interval:* No consistent PR intervals because there is no relationship between P waves and QRS complexes.
- *QRS complex:* Normal if ventricles are controlled by a junctional pacemaker. Wide if controlled by a ventricular pacemaker.

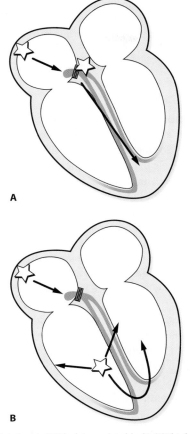

A

B

Figure 3-43. Third-degree AV block (complete block). **(A)** Third-degree AV block with junctional escape pacemaker. **(B)** Third-degree AV block with ventricular escape pacemaker. (*Reproduced with permission from Woods SL, Froelicher ES, Motzer SU.* Cardiac Nursing, *3rd ed. Philadelphia, PA: JB Lippincott; 1995.*)

- *Conduction:* Normal through the atria. All impulses are blocked at the AV node or in the bundle branches, so there is no conduction to the ventricles. Conduction through the ventricles is normal if a junctional escape rhythm occurs, and abnormally slow if a ventricular escape rhythm occurs.
- *Examples of third-degree AV block:* Figure 3-44A, B.

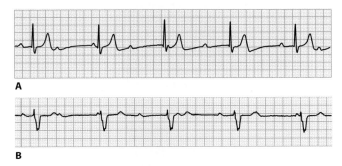

A

B

Figure 3-44. **(A)** Third-degree AV block with a junctional escape pacemaker at a rate of about 36 beats/min. **(B)** Third-degree AV block with a ventricular escape pacemaker at a rate of about 40 beats/min.

Treatment

Third-degree AV block can occur without significant symptoms if it occurs gradually and the heart has time to compensate for the slow ventricular rate. If it occurs suddenly in the presence of acute MI, its significance depends on the resulting ventricular rate and the patient's tolerance. Treatment of complete heart block with symptoms of decreased cardiac output includes external pacing until transvenous pacing can be initiated. Atropine can be given but is not usually effective in restoring conduction.

TEMPORARY PACING

Indications

If the heart fails to generate or conduct impulses to the ventricle, the myocardium can be electrically stimulated using a cardiac pacemaker. A cardiac pacemaker has two components: a pulse generator and a pacing electrode or lead. Temporary cardiac pacing is indicated in any situation in which bradycardia results in symptoms of decreased cerebral perfusion or hemodynamic compromise and does not respond to pharmacologic therapy. Signs and symptoms of hemodynamic instability are hypotension, change in mental status, angina, or pulmonary edema. Temporary pacing is also used to terminate some rapid reentrant tachycardias by briefly pacing the heart at a faster rate than the existing rate. When pacing is stopped, the sinus node may resume control of the rhythm if the tachycardia has been terminated. This type of pacing is termed *overdrive pacing* to distinguish it from pacing for bradycardic conditions.

Temporary cardiac pacing is accomplished by transvenous, epicardial, or external pacing methods. If continued cardiac pacing is required, insertion of permanent pacemakers is done electively. The following section presents an overview of temporary ventricular pacing principles. A more detailed explanation of pacemaker functions is covered in Chapter 18, Advanced ECG Concepts.

Transvenous Pacing

Transvenous pacing is usually done by percutaneous puncture of the internal jugular, subclavian, antecubital, or femoral vein and advancing a pacing lead into the apex of the right ventricle so that the tip of the pacing lead contacts the wall of the ventricle (Figure 3-45A). The transvenous pacing lead is attached to an external pulse generator that is kept either on the patient or at the bedside. Transvenous pacing is usually necessary only for a few days until the rhythm returns to normal or a permanent pacemaker is inserted.

Epicardial Pacing

Epicardial pacing is done through electrodes placed on the atria or ventricles during cardiac surgery. The pacing electrode end of the lead is looped through or loosely sutured to the epicardial surface of the atria or ventricles and the other

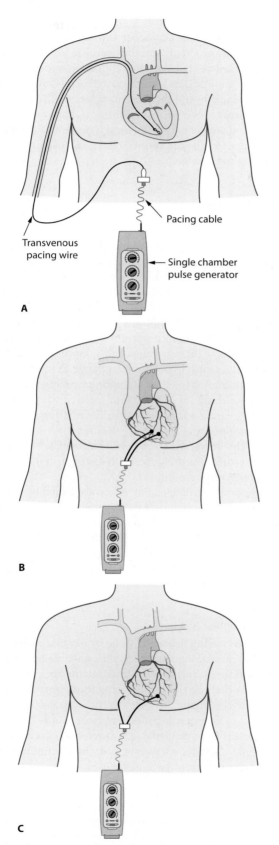

A

B

C

Figure 3-45. Temporary single chamber ventricular pacing. **(A)** Transvenous pacing with pacing lead in apex of right ventricle. **(B)** Bipolar epicardial pacing with two epicardial wires on ventricle. **(C)** Unipolar epicardial pacing with one wire on ventricle and one ground wire in mediastinum.

end is pulled through the chest wall, sutured to the skin, and attached to an external pulse generator (Figure 3-45B, C). A ground wire is often placed subcutaneously in the chest wall and pulled through with the other leads. The number and placement of leads varies with the surgeon.

Components of a Pacing System

The basic components of a cardiac pacing system are the pulse generator and the pacing lead. The *pulse generator* contains the power source (battery) and all of the electronic circuitry that controls pacemaker function. A temporary pulse generator is a box that is kept at the bedside and is usually powered by a regular 9-V battery. It has controls on the front that allow the operator to set pacing rate, strength of the pacing stimulus (output), and sensitivity settings (Figure 3-46).

The *pacing lead* is an insulated wire used to transmit the electrical current from the pulse generator to the myocardium. A unipolar lead contains a single wire and a bipolar lead contains two wires that are insulated from each other. In a unipolar lead, the electrode is an exposed metal tip at the end of the lead that contacts the myocardium and serves as the negative pole of the pacing circuit. In a bipolar lead, the end of the lead is a metal tip that contacts myocardium and serves as the negative pole, and the positive pole is an exposed metal ring located a few millimeters proximal to the distal tip.

Basics of Pacemaker Operation

Electrical current flows in a closed-loop circuit between two pieces of metal (poles). For current to flow, there must be conductive material (ie, a lead, muscle, or conductive solution) between the two poles. In the heart, the pacing lead, cardiac muscle, and body tissues serve as conducting

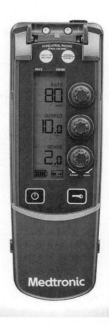

Figure 3-46. Temporary pacemaker pulse generator. (*Reproduced with permission of Medtronic, Inc.*)

material for the flow of electrical current in the pacing system. The pacing circuit consists of the pacemaker pulse generator (the power source), the conducting lead (pacing lead), and the myocardium. The electrical stimulus travels from the pulse generator through the pacing lead to the myocardium, through the myocardium, and back to the pulse generator, thus completing the circuit.

Temporary transvenous pacing is done using a bipolar pacing lead with its tip in the apex of the RV (see Figure 3-45A). Epicardial pacing can be done with either bipolar or unipolar leads. The term *bipolar* means that both of the poles in the pacing system are in or on the heart (see Figure 3-45A, B). In a bipolar system, the pulse generator initiates the electrical impulse and delivers it out the negative terminal of the pacemaker to the pacing lead. The impulse travels down the lead to the distal electrode (negative pole or cathode) that is in contact with myocardium. As the impulse reaches the tip, it travels through the myocardium and returns to the positive pole (or anode) of the system, completing the circuit. In a transvenous bipolar system, the positive pole is the proximal ring located a few millimeters proximal to the distal tip. The circuit over which the electrical impulse travels in a bipolar system is small because the two poles are located close together on the lead. This results in a small pacing spike on the ECG as the pacing stimulus travels between the two poles. If the stimulus is strong enough to depolarize the myocardium, the pacing spike is immediately followed by a P wave if the lead is in the atrium or a wide QRS complex if the lead is in the ventricle.

A unipolar system has only one of the two poles in or on the heart (see Figure 3-45C). In a temporary unipolar epicardial pacing system, a ground lead placed in the subcutaneous tissue in the mediastinum serves as the second pole. Unipolar pacemakers work the same way as bipolar systems, but the circuit over which the impulse travels is larger because of the greater distance between the two poles. This results in a large pacing spike on the ECG as the impulse travels between the two poles.

Capture and Sensing

The two main functions of a pacing system are capture and sensing. *Capture* means that a pacing stimulus results in depolarization of the chamber being paced (Figure 3-47A). Capture is determined by the strength of the stimulus, which is measured in milliamperes (mA), the amount of time the stimulus is applied to the heart (pulse width), and by contact of the pacing electrode with the myocardium. Capture cannot occur unless the distal tip of the pacing lead is in contact with healthy myocardium that is capable of responding to the stimulus. Pacing in infarcted tissue usually prevents capture. Similarly, if the catheter is floating in the cavity of the ventricle and not in direct contact with myocardium, capture will not occur. In temporary pacing, the output dial on the face of the pulse generator controls stimulus strength, and can be set and changed easily by the operator. Temporary pulse generators usually are capable of delivering a stimulus of 0.1 to 20 mA.

Sensing means that the pacemaker is able to detect the presence of intrinsic cardiac activity (Figure 3-47B). The sensing circuit controls how sensitive the pacemaker is to intrinsic cardiac depolarizations. Intrinsic activity is measured in millivolts (mV), and the higher the number, the larger the intrinsic signal; for example, a 10-mV QRS complex is larger than a 2-mV QRS. When pacemaker sensitivity needs to be increased to make the pacemaker "see" smaller signals, the sensitivity number must be decreased; for example, a sensitivity of 2 mV is more sensitive than one of 5 mV.

A fence analogy may help to explain sensitivity. Think of sensitivity as a fence standing between the pacemaker and what it wants to see, the ventricle; for example, if there is a 10-ft-high fence (or a 10-mV sensitivity) between the two, the pacemaker may not see what the ventricle is doing. To make the pacemaker able to see, the fence needs to be

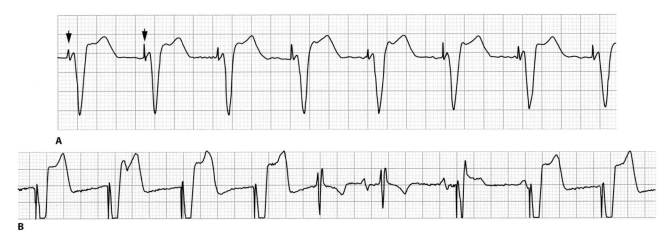

Figure 3-47. (A) Ventricular pacing with 100% capture. Arrows show pacing spikes, each one followed by a wide QRS complex indicating ventricular capture. **(B)** Rhythm strip of a ventricular pacemaker in the demand mode. There is appropriate sensing of intrinsic QRS complexes and appropriate pacing with ventricular capture when the intrinsic QRS complexes fall below the preset rate of the pacemaker. The seventh beat is fusion between the intrinsic QRS and the paced beat, a normal phenomenon in ventricular pacing.

lowered. Lowering the fence to 2 ft would probably enable the pacemaker to see the ventricle. Changing the sensitivity from 10 to 2 mV is like lowering the fence—the pacemaker becomes more sensitive and is able to "see" intrinsic activity more easily. Thus, to increase the sensitivity of a pacemaker, the millivolt number (fence) must be decreased.

Asynchronous (Fixed-Rate) Pacing Mode

A pacemaker programmed to an asynchronous mode paces at the programmed rate regardless of intrinsic cardiac activity. This can result in competition between the pacemaker and the heart's own electrical activity. Asynchronous pacing in the ventricle is unsafe because of the potential for pacing stimuli to fall in the vulnerable period of repolarization and cause VF.

Demand Mode

The term *demand* means that the pacemaker paces only when the heart fails to depolarize on its own, that is, the pacemaker fires only "on demand." In demand mode, the pacemaker's sensing circuit is capable of sensing intrinsic cardiac activity and inhibiting pacer output when intrinsic activity is present. Sensing takes place between the two poles of the pacemaker. A bipolar system senses over a small area because the poles are close together, and this can result in "undersensing" of intrinsic signals. A unipolar system senses over a large area because the poles are far apart, and this can result in "oversensing." A unipolar system is more likely to sense myopotentials caused by muscle movement and inappropriately inhibit pacemaker output, potentially resulting in periods of asystole if the patient has no underlying cardiac rhythm. The demand mode should always be used for ventricular pacing to avoid the possibility of VF.

A paced ventricular beat begins with a pacing spike, which indicates that the pacemaker released an electrical stimulus (Figure 3-48). If the pacing stimulus is strong enough to depolarize the ventricle, the spike is followed by a wide QRS complex and a T wave that is oriented in the opposite direction of the QRS complex. Figure 3-47A illustrates ventricular pacing with consistent capture.

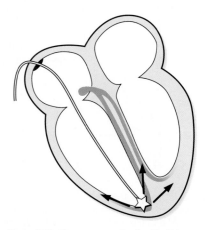

Figure 3-48. Temporary pacing lead in RV apex.

Figure 3-47B is the ECG of a ventricular pacemaker that is functioning correctly in the demand mode. The pacemaker generates an impulse when it senses that the heart rate has decreased below the set pacing rate. Therefore, the pacemaker senses the intrinsic cardiac rhythm of the patient and only generates an impulse when the rate falls below the preset pacing rate. Refer to Chapter 18, Advanced ECG Concepts, for more detailed information on single and dual chamber pacing.

Initiating Transvenous Ventricular Pacing

Temporary transvenous pacing leads are bipolar and have two tails, one marked "positive" or "proximal" and the other marked "negative" or "distal," which are connected to the pulse generator. To initiate ventricular pacing using a transvenous lead (see Figure 3-45A):

1. Connect the negative terminal of the pulse generator to the distal end of the pacing lead.
2. Connect the positive terminal of the pulse generator to the proximal end of the pacing lead.
3. Set the rate at 70 to 80 beats/min or as ordered by physician.
4. Set the output at 5 mA, then determine stimulation threshold and set two to three times higher.
5. Set the sensitivity at 2 mV and adjust according to sensitivity threshold.

Initiating Epicardial Pacing

To initiate bipolar ventricular pacing (two leads on the ventricle; see Figure 3-45B):

1. Connect the negative terminal of the pulse generator to one of the ventricular leads.
2. Connect the positive terminal of the pulse generator to the other ventricular lead.
3. Set the rate at 70 to 80 beats/min or as ordered.
4. Set the output at 5 mA, then determine stimulation threshold and set two to three times higher.
5. Set the sensitivity at 2 mV and adjust according to sensitivity threshold.

To initiate unipolar ventricular pacing (one lead on the ventricle; see Figure 3-45C):

1. Connect the negative terminal of the pulse generator to the ventricular lead.
2. Connect the positive terminal of the pulse generator to the ground lead.
3. Set the rate at 70 to 80 beats/min or as ordered by physician.
4. Set the output at 5 mA, then determine stimulation threshold and set two to three times higher.
5. Set the sensitivity at 2 mV and adjust according to sensitivity threshold. See Chapter 18, Advanced ECG Concepts, for information on how to obtain capture and sensing thresholds.

External (Transcutaneous) Pacemakers

The emergent nature of many bradycardic rhythms requires immediate temporary pacing. Because transvenous catheter placement is difficult to accomplish quickly, external pacing is the preferred method for rapid, easy initiation of cardiac pacing in emergent situations until a transvenous pacemaker can be inserted. External pacing is done through large-surface adhesive electrodes attached to the anterior and posterior chest wall and connected to an external pacing unit (Figure 3-49). The pacing current passes through skin and chest wall structures to reach the heart; therefore, large energies are required to achieve capture. Sedation and analgesia are usually needed to minimize the discomfort felt by the patient during pacing. Transcutaneous pacing spikes are usually very large, often distorting the QRS complex. The presence of a pulse with every pacing spike confirms ventricular capture.

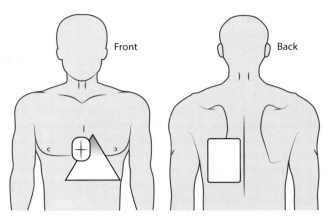

Figure 3-49. External pacemaker with pacing electrode pads on anterior and posterior chest and back.

ESSENTIAL CONTENT CASE

Heart Block and Epicardial Pacemaker

A patient underwent an aortic valve replacement yesterday. He has been extubated, he has a mediastinal chest tube, and two ventricular epicardial pacing leads are in place and coiled under a dressing. He is in sinus rhythm at a rate in the 80s, BP is 146/80, RR is 16, and he is breathing comfortably. The monitor alarm sounds and when you enter the room he is pale and complaining of dizziness but no chest pain. The monitor shows the following rhythm:

Figure 3-50A

Case Question 1. What is his rhythm?
He is dizzy and his BP is 92/60.

Case Question 2. What can you do to treat this dysrhythmia?

Case Question 3. Describe how to initiate epicardial ventricular pacing.
You connect the pacing leads to a temporary pulse generator and set the rate at 70 beats/min.
This is the rhythm:

Figure 3-50B

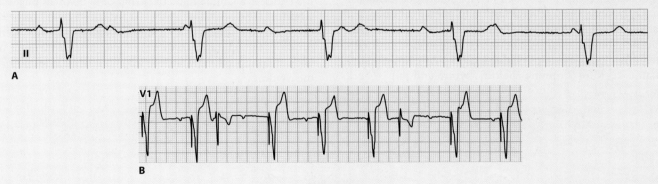

Figure 3-50.

Case Question 4. What is this rhythm?

Case Question 5. Evaluate pacemaker function in terms of ventricular capture and ventricular sensing.

Answers
1. This rhythm is third-degree AV block with a ventricular pacemaker at a rate of about 40 beats/min.
2. Third-degree AV block is best treated with pacing. Atropine may speed up the rate of the sinus rhythm but it does not improve conduction in complete heart block. Since this patient has ventricular epicardial pacing leads in place, the best treatment is to initiate temporary ventricular pacing.
3. To initiate ventricular epicardial pacing with two ventricular leads present, connect one epicardial lead to the negative terminal of the temporary pacemaker pulse generator and connect the other lead to the positive terminal of the pacemaker. Set the desired rate, output, and sensitivity and turn the pacemaker on.
4. Ventricular paced rhythm at a rate of 70 beats/min. Sinus P waves are present and two of them are conducted to the ventricles.
5. Capture is good: every ventricular pacing spike is followed by a wide QRS complex. Sensing is also good: the two conducted beats are sensed and the pacemaker inhibits its output appropriately.

DEFIBRILLATION AND CARDIOVERSION

Defibrillation

Defibrillation is the therapeutic delivery of electrical energy to the myocardium to terminate life-threatening ventricular dysrhythmias (VF and pulseless VT). The defibrillating shock depolarizes all cells in the heart simultaneously, stopping all electrical activity and allowing the sinus node to resume its function as the normal pacemaker of the heart. Early defibrillation is the only treatment for VF or pulseless VT and should not be delayed for any reason when a defibrillator is available. If a defibrillator is not immediately available, CPR should be started until a defibrillator arrives.

Defibrillation is done externally using two paddles or adhesive pads applied to the skin in the anterolateral position (Figure 3-51A). One paddle or pad is placed under the right clavicle to the right of the sternum and the other paddle or pad is placed to the left of the cardiac apex. If paddles are used, place conductive gel pads on the patient's skin, then place paddles on the gel pads using 25 lb of pressure to decrease transthoracic impedance and protect the skin from burns. Avoid placing paddles over medication patches or over pacemaker or ICD pulse generators.

Advanced Cardiac Life Support (ACLS) guidelines recommend an initial energy of 360 J with a monophasic defibrillator and the manufacturer's recommended energy level for biphasic defibrillators. If the manufacturer's suggested energy level is not known, a 200-J shock is recommended. Make sure no one is touching the patient, the bed, or anything attached to the patient when the shock is delivered; call "all clear" and visually verify before delivering the shock. Depress the discharge button to release the energy. If using paddles, depress both discharge buttons (one on each paddle) simultaneously. The shock is delivered immediately when buttons are pushed (Figure 3-52A). Immediately resume CPR for 2 minutes before rhythm and pulse check

(this may be modified in a monitored situation where ECG and hemodynamic monitoring is available).

Automatic External Defibrillators

An automatic external defibrillator (AED) is a device that incorporates a rhythm-analysis system and a shock advisory system for use by trained laypeople or medical personnel in treating victims of sudden cardiac death. The American Heart Association recommends that AEDs should be available in selected areas where large gatherings of people occur and where immediate access to emergency care may be limited, such as on airplanes, in airports, sports stadiums, health and fitness facilities, and so on. It is well known that early defibrillation is the key to survival in patients experiencing VF or pulseless VT. Any delay in the delivery of the first shock, including delays related to waiting for the arrival of trained medical personnel and equipment, can decrease the chance of survival. The availability of an AED in public areas can prevent unnecessary delays in treatment and improve survival in victims of sudden cardiac death.

Operation of an AED is quite simple and can be performed by laypeople. Instructions for use are printed on the machines and voice commands also guide the operator in using the AED. Adhesive pads are placed in the standard defibrillation position on the chest (see Figure 3-51A), the machine is turned on, and the rhythm analysis system analyzes the patient's rhythm. If the rhythm analysis system detects a shockable rhythm, such as VF or rapid VT, a voice advises the operator to shock the patient. Delivery of the shock is a simple maneuver that only involves pushing a button. The operator is advised to "stand clear" prior to delivering the shock. After a shock is delivered, the system prompts the operator to resume CPR. After 2 minutes of CPR, it prompts the operator to stop CPR while it reanalyzes the rhythm.

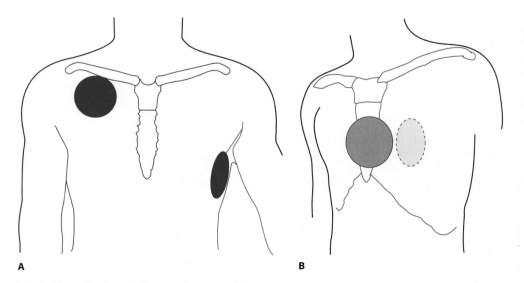

Figure 3-51. Paddle or adhesive pad placement for external defibrillation via **(A)** anterolateral position and **(B)** anteroposterior position.

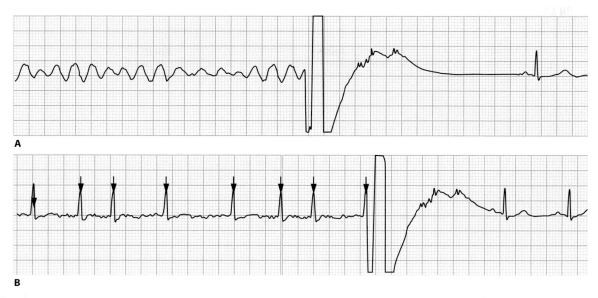

Figure 3-52. **(A)** Defibrillation of VF to sinus rhythm. **(B)** Cardioversion of atrial fibrillation to sinus rhythm. Note the synchronization mark on the QRS.

Cardioversion

Cardioversion is the delivery of electrical energy that is synchronized to the QRS complex so that the energy is delivered during ventricular depolarization in order to avoid the T wave and the vulnerable period of ventricular repolarization. The delivery of electrical energy near the T wave can lead to ventricular fibrillation. Synchronized cardioversion is used to terminate both SVT and VTs and is usually an elective procedure, although it should be performed urgently if the patient is hemodynamically unstable. Cardioversion can be performed via anterolateral electrode placement (see Figure 3-51A) or via anteroposterior (AP) electrode placement (see Figure 3-51B). Anteroposterior placement is preferred because less energy is required and the success rate is higher when energy travels through the short axis of the chest. Either paddles or hands-free adhesive pads can be used.

Sedation is required for cardioversion since the patient is usually awake and alert and able to feel the pain caused by the procedure. The selection of medications to accomplish sedation depends on physician discretion and hospital policy, or an anesthesiologist may be called to place the patient under deep sedation. Because sedation is used, an emergency cart equipped with emergency medications (lidocaine, epinephrine, amiodarone, atropine), sedation-reversal agents, O_2-delivery equipment, and suction equipment should be immediately available. The patient's blood pressure and oxygen saturation are continuously monitored during the procedure until the patient is completely awake and recovered.

Initial energy level for cardioversion is typically 50 to 100 J and varies with different dysrhythmias. If the first shock is unsuccessful, energy level is increased for subsequent shocks. The machine must be synchronized to the QRS complex for cardioversion. Most machines put a bright dot or similar marker on the QRS complex when in the "synch" mode (Figure 3-52B). The machine will not discharge its energy until it sees the synch marker. Make sure to visually verify that the synch marker is actually on the QRS complex and not on a tall T wave. When delivering energy during cardioversion, push and hold the discharge button until the energy is delivered; the synchronized machine will not discharge until it sees a QRS complex. When the energy is released, the machine automatically returns to the asynchronous mode, so if subsequent shocks are needed the machine must be resynchronized.

SELECTED BIBLIOGRAPHY

Badhwar N. Ventricular tachycardia. In: Crawford MH, eds. *CURRENT Diagnosis & Treatment: Cardiology.* 5th ed. New York, NY: McGraw-Hill; 2014. http://accessmedicine.mhmedical.com.offcampus.lib.washington.edu/content.aspx?bookid=2040&sectionid=152994681. Accessed April 19, 2017.

Hongo RH, Goldschlager F. Conduction disorders & cardiac pacing. In: Crawford MH, eds. *CURRENT Diagnosis & Treatment: Cardiology.* 5th ed. New York, NY: McGraw-Hill; 2014. http://accessmedicine.mhmedical.com.offcampus.lib.washington.edu/content.aspx?bookid=2040&sectionid=152994803. Accessed April 19, 2017.

Hsu J, Scheinman MM. Atrial fibrillation. In: Crawford MH, eds. *CURRENT Diagnosis & Treatment: Cardiology.* 5th ed. New York, NY: McGraw-Hill; 2014. http://accessmedicine.mhmedical.com.offcampus.lib.washington.edu/content.aspx?bookid=2040&sectionid=152994617. Accessed April 19, 2017.

Jacobson C, Marzlin K, Webner C. *Cardiovascular Nursing Practice: A Comprehensive Resource Manual and Study Guide for Clinical Nurses.* 2nd ed. Burien, WA: Cardiovascular Nursing Education Associates; 2014.

Lee BK. Supraventricular tachycardias. In: Crawford MH, eds. *CURRENT Diagnosis & Treatment: Cardiology.* 5th ed. New York, NY: McGraw-Hill; 2014. http://accessmedicine.mhmedical.com.offcampus.lib.washington.edu/content.aspx?bookid=2040&sectionid=152994423. Accessed April 19, 2017.

Link MS, Atkins DL, Passman RS, et al. Electrical therapies: automated external defibrillators, defibrillation, cardioversion, and pacing: 2010 American Heart Association Guidelines for Cardiopulmonary Resuscitation and Emergency Cardiovascular Care. *Circulation*. 2010:122(suppl 3), Part 6, S706-S719.

Evidence-Based Practice

AACN Practice Alert: Accurate dysrhythmia monitoring in adults. *Crit Care Nurs*. 2016;36(6):e26-e34.

Drew BJ, Califf RM, Funk M, et al. Practice standards for electrocardiographic monitoring in hospital settings. *Circulation*. 2004:110;2721-2746.

Furie KL, Goldstein LB, Albers GW, et al. Oral antithrombotic agents for the prevention of stroke in nonvalvular atrial fibrillation: a science advisory for healthcare professionals from the American Heart Association/American Stroke Association. *Stroke*. 2012:43;3442-3453.

January CT, Wann LS, Alpert JS, et al. 2014 AHA/ACC/HRS guideline for the management of patients with atrial fibrillation: a report of the American College of Cardiology/American Heart Association Task Force on Practice Guidelines and the Heart Rhythm Society. *Circulation*. 2014;130:e199-e267.

Link MS, Berkow LC, Kudenchuk PJ, et al. Part 7: adult advanced cardiovascular life support: 2015 American Heart Association guidelines update for cardiopulmonary resuscitation and emergency cardiovascular care. *Circulation*. 2015;132:S444.

Page RL, Joglar JA, Caldwell MA, et al. ACC/AHA/HRS guideline for the management of adult patients with supraventricular tachycardia: a report of the American College of Cardiology/American Heart Association Task Force on Practice Guidelines and the Heart Rhythm Society. *Circulation*. 2016;133:e506-e574.

Pedersen CT, Kay GN, Kalman J, et al. EHRA/HRS/APHRS expert consensus on ventricular arrhythmias. *Europace*. 2014;16:1257-1283.

Priori SG, Blomstrom-Lundqvist C, Mazzanti A, et al. 2015 ESC guidelines for the management of patients with ventricular arrhythmias and the prevention of sudden cardiac death. *Eur Heart J*. 2015;36:2793-2867.

Sandau K, Funk M, Auerbach A, et al. Update to practice standards for electrocardiographic monitoring in hospital settings: a scientific statement from the American Heart Association. *Circulation*. 2017;136:e273-e344. https://doi.org/10.1161/CIR.0000000000000527

Zipes D, Camm A, Borggrefe M, et al. ACC/AHA/ESC 2006 guidelines for management of patients with ventricular arrhythmias and the prevention of sudden cardiac death: a report of the American College of Cardiology/American Heart Association Task Force and the European Society of Cardiology Committee for Practice Guidelines. *Circulation*. 2006:114;e385-e484.

HEMODYNAMIC MONITORING

4

Leanna R. Miller

KNOWLEDGE COMPETENCIES

1. Identify the characteristics of normal and abnormal waveform pressures for the following hemodynamic monitoring parameters:
   - Central venous pressure
   - Arterial blood pressure
2. Describe the basic elements of arterial and venous pressure-monitoring equipment and methods used to ensure accurate pressure measurements.
3. Discuss the indications, contraindications, and general management principles for the

following common hemodynamic monitoring parameters:
   - Central venous pressure
   - Arterial blood pressure
4. Describe the clinical application of $Svo_2/Scvo_2$ monitoring.
5. Discuss the potential use of bioimpedance/bioreactance monitoring and the use of functional hemodynamics for fluid resuscitation in a progressive care population.

The term *hemodynamics* refers to the interrelationship of blood pressure (BP), blood flow, vascular volumes, heart rate (HR), ventricular function, and the physical properties of the blood. A working knowledge of how to obtain accurate information about a patient's hemodynamic state, including their responsiveness to fluid resuscitation is a key element of progressive care nursing.

Clinical examination findings such as mental status, urine output, edema, capillary refill, and jugular venous distension provide some data about a patient's fluid balance, oxygenation, and blood flow. Additional data can be obtained through invasive hemodynamic monitoring and through functional hemodynamic assessment. Parameters such as arterial BP, cardiac output (CO), pulmonary arterial pressure (PAP), and intracardiac pressures can be directly measured and monitored with special indwelling catheters. Noninvasive evaluations including the passive leg raise (PLR) test, cardiovascular ultrasound, and analysis of changes in the arterial waveforms in patients on positive pressure mechanical ventilation can also provide information about the patient's fluid balance that guides management.

This chapter includes a description of hemodynamic parameters obtained from a pulmonary artery (PA) catheter. While these catheters are seldom used except in intensive care units, the concepts are helpful to understand pathologic conditions such as heart failure and sepsis and the different causes of shock. More extensive discussion of other hemodynamic monitoring systems such as the PA catheter is found in the *AACN Essentials of Critical Care Nursing*.

HEMODYNAMIC PARAMETERS

A description of the various parameters derived from the PA catheter follows and reference values may be found in Table 4-1.

Cardiac Output

Cardiac output is the amount of blood pumped by the ventricles each minute. It is the product of the HR and the stroke volume (SV), which is the amount of blood ejected by the ventricle with each contraction; Figure 4-1. This is evaluated

TABLE 4-1. NORMAL HEMODYNAMIC AND BLOOD FLOW PARAMETERS

Parameter	Abbreviation	Formula	Normal Range
Cardiac output	CO	Stroke volume (SV) × heart rate (HR)	4-8 L/min
Cardiac index	CI	CO/BSA ÷ 1000	2.5-4.3 L/min/m^2
Mean arterial pressure	MAP	2(DBP) + SBP ÷ 3	70-105 mm Hg
Right atrial pressure	RAP	cm H$_2$O = mm Hg × 1.34	2-8 mm Hg
Pulmonary artery wedge pressure	PAOP		8-12 mm Hg
Pulmonary artery systolic	PAS		15-35 mm Hg
Pulmonary artery diastolic	PAD		10-15 mm Hg
Pulmonary vascular resistance	PVR	PAM – PAOP × 80 ÷ CO	100-250 dynes/s/cm^{-5}
Pulmonary vascular resistance index	PVRI	PAM – PAOP × 80 ÷ CI	255-285 dynes/s/cm^{-5}/m^2
Pulmonary artery mean	PAM		15-20 mm Hg
Systemic vascular resistance	SVR	MAP – RAP × 80 ÷ CO	800-1200 dynes/s/cm^{-5}
Systemic vascular resistance index	SVRI	MAP – RAP × 80 ÷ CI	1970-2390 dynes/s/cm^{-5}/m^2
Right ventricular stroke work index	RVSWI	(PAM – RAP) SVI × 0.0138	7-12 g/m/m^2/beat
Left ventricular stroke work index	LVSWI	(MAP – PAOP) SVI × 0.0138	35-85 g/m/m^2/beat
Oxygen delivery	DO$_2$	CaO$_2$ × CO × 10	900-1100 mL/min
Oxygen delivery index	DO$_2$I	CaO$_2$ × CI × 10	360-600 mL/min/m^2
Oxygen consumption	VO$_2$	C(a – v)O$_2$ × CO × 10	200-250 mL/min
Oxygen consumption index	VO$_2$I	C(a – v)O$_2$ × CI × 10	108-165 mL/min/m^2
Stroke volume	SV	CO/HR × 1000	60-100 mL/beat
Stroke volume index	SVI	CI/HR × 1000	33-47 mL/beat/m^2
Ejection fraction	EF		> 60%
Right ventricular end-diastolic volume	RVEDV	SV/EF	100-160 mL
Right ventricular end-diastolic volume index	RVEDVI	EDV/BSA	600-100 mL/m^2
Right ventricular end-systolic volume	RVESV	EDV – SV	50-100 mL
Right ventricular end-systolic volume index	RVESVI	ESV/BSA	30-60 mL/m^2
Right ventricular ejection fraction	RVEF	SV/EDV	40%-60%
Mixed venous saturation	Svo$_2$		60%-80%
Oxygen extraction ratio	O$_2$ER	(Cao$_2$ – Cvo$_2$)/Cao$_2$ × 100	22%-30%
Oxygen extraction index	O$_2$EI	Sao$_2$ – Svo$_2$/Sao$_2$ × 100	22%-30%

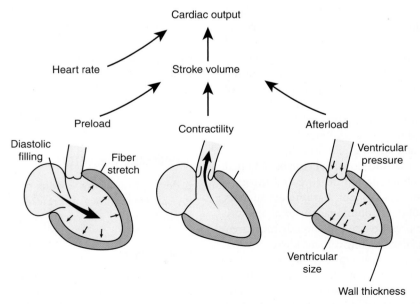

Figure 4-1. Factors affecting CO. (*Reproduced with permission from Price S, Wilson L.* Pathophysiology: Clinical Concepts of Disease Processes. *Philadelphia, PA: Mosby; 1992.*)

with a PA catheter and some noninvasive monitoring technologies such as Doppler echocardiography and bioimpedance/bioreactance systems.

$$CO = HR \times SV$$

The normal value of CO is 4.0 to 8.0 L/min. It is important to note that these values are relative to size. Values within the normal range for a person 5 ft tall weighing 100 lb may be totally inadequate for a 6-ft, 200-lb individual. Cardiac index (CI) is the CO that has been adjusted to individual body size. It is determined by dividing the CO by the individual's body surface area (BSA), which may be obtained from the DuBois BSA chart. The conversion to CI has been automated within current monitors. The normal value for CI is 2.5 to 4.3 L/min/m^2 (see Table 4-1).

$$CI = CO/BSA$$

Cardiac output measurements are used to assess the patient's perfusion status, response to therapy, and as a rapid means to evaluate the patient's hemodynamic status. As mentioned, CO is composed of HR and SV, or the amount of blood ejected with each contraction of the ventricle. Normal SV range is 60 to 100 mL/beat. SV depends on preload, afterload, and contractility. Therefore, CO is determined by:

1. HR (and rhythm)
2. Preload
3. Afterload
4. Contractility

Low-Cardiac Output/Cardiac Index

As the SV of the left ventricle is a component used in the determination of CO, any condition or disease process which impairs the pumping (ejection) or filling of the ventricle may contribute to a decreased CO. Alterations that lead to diminished CO can be divided into two general categories: inadequate ventricular filling and inadequate ventricular emptying.

Inadequate Ventricular Filling

Factors that lead to inadequate ventricular filling include arrhythmias, hypovolemia, cardiac tamponade, mitral or tricuspid stenosis, constrictive pericarditis, and restrictive cardiomyopathy. Each of these abnormalities leads to a decrease in preload (the amount of volume in the ventricle at end diastole), which results in a decrease in SV and CO.

Inadequate Ventricular Ejection

Factors that lead to inadequate ventricular emptying include mitral/tricuspid insufficiency, myocardial infarction, increased afterload (hypertension, aortic/pulmonic stenosis), myocardial diseases (myocarditis, cardiomyopathy), metabolic disorders (hypoglycemia, hypoxia, severe acidosis), and use of negative inotropic drugs (beta-blockers, calcium channel blockers).

High-Cardiac Output/Index

In theory, in the normal, healthy individual, any factor that increases HR and contractility and decreases afterload can contribute to an increase in CO. Hyperdynamic states, such as sepsis, anemia, pregnancy, and hyperthyroid crisis, may cause CO values to increase. Increased HR is a major component in hyperdynamic states; however, in sepsis a profound decrease in afterload also contributes to an increased CO.

Components of Cardiac Output/Cardiac Index

Heart Rate and Rhythm

Rate

Normal HR is 60 to 100 beats/min. In a normal, healthy individual, an increase in HR can lead to an increase in CO. In a person with cardiac dysfunction, increases in HR can lead to a decreased CO and often myocardial ischemia. An increase in HR to 130 beats/min or greater decreases the ventricular filling time causing a drop in preload and SV and a subsequent decrease in CO. An increase in HR also decreases diastolic time, which results in a decrease in coronary artery perfusion. A lower HR does not necessarily result in a decrease in CO. Decreased HRs with normal COs are often found in athletes. Their training and conditioning strengthens the myocardium such that each cardiac contraction produces an increased SV. In individuals with left ventricular (LV) dysfunction, a slow HR can produce a decrease in CO. This is caused by decreased contractility, as well as fewer cardiac contractions each minute.

Because CO is a product of SV times HR, any change in SV normally produces a change in the HR. Bradycardias and tachycardias are potentially dangerous because they may result in a decrease in CO if adequate SV is not maintained. Bradycardias that develop suddenly are almost always associated with a falling CO. The cause of tachycardia, on the other hand, must be determined because it may not reflect a low-output state but rather a normal physiologic response (eg, tachycardia secondary to fever). HR varies between individuals and is related to many factors. Some are described here.

DECREASED HEART RATE

- Parasympathetic stimulation (vagus nerve stimulation) is a common occurrence in the acute care setting. It can occur with Valsalva maneuvers such as excessive bearing down during a bowel movement, vomiting, coughing, and suctioning.
- Conduction abnormalities, especially second- and third-degree blocks, are often seen in patients with cardiovascular diseases. Many medications used in the progressive care setting may lead to a decreased HR, including digitalis, beta-blockers, calcium channel blockers, and phenylephrine (neosynephrine).
- Athletes often have resting HRs below 60 beats/min without compromising CO.
- The actual HR is not as important as the systemic effect of the HR. If the patient's HR leads to diminished perfusion (manifested by decreased level of consciousness, decreased urinary output, hypotension, prolonged capillary refill, new-onset chest pain, and the like), treatment is initiated to increase the HR.

INCREASED HEART RATE

- Stress, anxiety, pain, and conditions resulting in compensatory release of endogenous catecholamines such as hypovolemia, fever, anemia, and hypotension may all produce tachycardia.
- Medications with a direct positive chronotropic effect include epinephrine and dopamine.

Tachycardia is very common in acutely ill patients. Causes include pain, fever, anxiety, medication side effect, and a compensatory response to anemia or to a drop in SV. The two most common reasons for a low SV are hypovolemia and LV dysfunction. Both causes of low SV can produce an increased HR if no abnormality exists in regulation of the HR (such as autonomic nervous system dysfunction or use of medications that interfere with the sympathetic or parasympathetic nervous system such as beta-blockers).

An increased HR can compensate for a decrease in SV, although this compensation is limited. The faster the HR, the less time exists for ventricular filling. As an increased HR reduces diastolic filling time, the potential exists to eventually reduce the SV. There is no specific HR where diastolic filling is reduced so severely that SV decreases. However, as the HR increases, it is important to remember that SV may be negatively affected.

Increased HR also has the potential to increase myocardial oxygen consumption (MVO_2). The higher the HR, the more likely it is that the heart consumes more oxygen. Some patients are more sensitive to elevated MVO_2 than others; for example, a young person may tolerate a sinus tachycardia as high as 160 beats/min for several days, whereas a patient with coronary artery disease may decompensate and develop pulmonary edema with a HR in the 130s. Keeping HRs low—particularly in patients with altered myocardial blood flow—is one way of protecting myocardial function.

Heart Rhythm

Many of us have observed the deleterious effects produced by a supraventricular tachycardia, or a change from normal sinus rhythm to atrial fibrillation or flutter. Loss of "atrial kick" may contribute to decreased SV and therefore to a decrease in CO. Normally, atrial contraction contributes 20% to 40% of the ventricular filling volume. With tachycardia, that atrial contribution to SV may diminish significantly. Although those with normal cardiac function are unlikely to experience compromise, it is more likely in those with impaired cardiac function.

Stroke Volume and Stroke Volume Index

Stroke volume is the amount of blood ejected from each ventricle with each heartbeat. The right and left ventricles eject nearly the same amount, which normally is from 50 to 100 mL per heartbeat.

$$SV = CO/HR \times 1000$$

Stroke volume indexed to the patient's BSA is stroke volume index (SVI). Indexing helps compare values regardless of the patient's size. Normal SVI is 33 to 47 mL/beat/m^2. Common causes of decreased stroke volume/stroke volume index (SV/SVI) are inadequate blood volume (preload), impaired ventricular contractility (strength), increased systemic vascular resistance (SVR; afterload), and cardiac valve dysfunction. High SV/SVI occurs when the vascular resistance is low (sepsis, use of vasodilators, neurogenic shock, and anaphylaxis).

Ejection Fraction

The ejection fraction (EF) is defined as how much blood is pumped with each contraction in relation to the volume of available blood; for example, assume the LV end-diastolic volume (LVEDV, the amount of blood left in the heart just before contraction) is 100 mL. If the SV is 80 mL, the EF is 80%; 80 mL of the possible 100 mL in the ventricle were ejected. Right ventricular volumes are roughly equal to those of the left ventricle (RVEF) (see Table 4-1). A normal EF is usually over 60%. This is evaluated with a PA catheter or with noninvasive methods such as the echocardiogram.

The EF may change before the SV in certain conditions, such as LV failure and sepsis; for example, the left ventricle may dilate in response to LV dysfunction from coronary artery disease, and LVEDV increases. Although the increase in LVEDV may prevent a drop in SV, EF may not be preserved. Thus, EF and LVEDV are early indicators of ventricular dysfunction and are ideal monitoring parameters. It is important to remember that approximately 50% of the patients with heart failure have a normal EF which will influence monitoring and volume resuscitation. Unfortunately, EF and LVEDV are not routinely available. SV and SVI, then, are the best available measures to assess left and right ventricular dysfunction.

Factors Affecting Stroke Volume/Stroke Volume Index
Preload

Preload is the volume of blood that exerts a force or pressure (stretch) on the ventricles during diastole. It may also be described as the filling pressure of the ventricles at the end of diastole or the amount of blood that fills the ventricles during diastole.

According to the Frank-Starling law of the heart, the force of contraction is related to myocardial fiber stretch prior to contraction. As the fibers are stretched, the contractile force increases up to a certain point. Beyond this point, the contractile force decreases and is referred to as ventricular failure (Figure 4-2). With increased preload there is an increase in the volume of blood delivered to the ventricle, the myocardium is stretched, and a more forceful ventricular contraction is produced. This forceful ventricular contraction yields an increase in SV, and therefore, CO. Too much preload causes the ventricular contraction to be less effective. A commonly referred to analogy uses the properties of a rubber band. The more a rubber band is stretched, the greater "snap" is produced when released. The rubber band may be

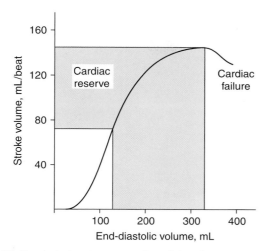

Figure 4-2. Ventricular function curve. As the end-diastolic volume increases, so does the force of ventricular contraction. The SV becomes greater up to a critical point after which SV decreases (cardiac failure). (*Reproduced with permission from Langley LF. Review of Physiology, 3rd ed. New York, NY: McGraw-Hill; 1971.*)

stretched further and further, until it reaches a point where it loses its tautness and fails to recoil. Preload is measured with a CVP catheter and/or a PA catheter.

Passive Leg Raise Maneuver

A noninvasive method for assessing preload and volume responsiveness in acutely ill patients is the passive leg raising (PLR) maneuver. It is a transient, reversible autotransfusion that temporarily increases preload (approximately 300 mL). Place the patient in a semirecumbent position and perform a baseline measurement (BP, CI, SVI, etc). Lay the patient flat and lift both legs above a 45° angle (Figure 4-3). The peak effects of PLR occur within 30 to 60 seconds, so perform the new measurement (BP, CI, SVI, etc) within this period. Using SVI as the hemodynamic measurement, a positive PLR would be an increase in SVI by greater than 10% of the baseline. This finding would suggest that there is sufficient cardiac reserve to pump an increased preload. Plotting this on the Frank Starling curve (see Figure 4-2), the patient is still in the ascending portion, so an increase in volume will lead to an increase in SV and CO. The patient would likely be fluid responsive, so fluid replacement would be an acceptable intervention. If the SVI change is less than 10% of the baseline, the patient has passed the tipping point

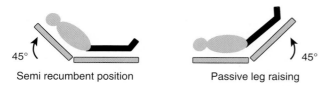

Figure 4-3. Passive leg-raising is performed by raising the patient's legs to a 45° angle while simultaneously lowering the patient's head and upper torso from a semirecumbent (head of bed elevated 45°) to a supine (flat) position. This maneuver tests for fluid responsiveness. (*Adapted with permission from Marik PE, Monnet X, Teboul JL: Hemodynamic parameters to guide fluid therapy, Ann Intensive Care. 2011 Mar 21;1(1):1.*)

on the Frank Starling curve and would not respond well to fluid administration. This indicates the need for vasopressors to maintain hemodynamic stabilization. Vasoactive medications may alter the response to the PLR. When performing the PLR, maintain a constant vasoactive infusion rate.

Determinants of Preload

Preload is determined primarily by the amount of venous return to the heart. Venous constriction, venous dilation, and alterations in the total blood volume all affect preload. Preload decreases with volume changes. This can occur in hemorrhage (traumatic, surgical, gastrointestinal [GI], postpartum), diuresis (excessive use of diuretics, diabetic ketoacidosis, diabetes insipidus), vomiting and diarrhea, third spacing (ascites, severe burns, sepsis, heart failure [HF]), redistribution of blood flow (use of vasodilators, neurogenic shock, severe sepsis), and profound diaphoresis. Venous dilation also results in diminished preload. Etiologies that increase venous pooling and result in decreased venous return to the heart include hyperthermia, septic shock, anaphylactic shock, and medication administration (nitroglycerin, nitroprusside) (Table 4-2).

Factors leading to increased preload include excessive administration of crystalloids or blood products and the presence of renal failure (oliguric phase and/or anuria). Venous constriction results in the shunting of peripheral blood to the central organs (heart and brain). The increased venous return results in an increased preload. This may occur in hypothermia, some forms of shock (classic shock states: hypovolemic, cardiogenic, and obstructive) and with administration of medications that stimulate the alpha receptors (epinephrine, dopamine at doses greater than 10 mcg/kg/min, norepinephrine) (see Table 4-2).

Clinical Indicators of Preload

The right ventricle pumps blood into the pulmonary circulation and the left ventricle ejects blood into the systemic circulation. Both circulatory systems are affected by preload, afterload, and contractility. These are discussed here and, when appropriate, the clinical indicators are differentiated by right or left heart.

RIGHT VENTRICULAR PRELOAD OR RIGHT ATRIAL PRESSURE (CVP OR RAP)

Normal right ventricular (RV) preload is 2 to 8 mm Hg or 2 to 10 cm H_2O (CVP = central venous pressure; RAP = right atrial pressure). Right atrial pressures are measured to assess right ventricular function, intravascular volume status, and the response to fluid and medication administration. CVP/RAP pressures increase because of intravascular volume overload, cardiac tamponade (effusion, blood, and the like), restrictive cardiomyopathies, and RV failure. There are three etiologies of RV failure: (1) intrinsic disease such as RV infarct or cardiomyopathies; (2) secondary factors that increase pulmonary vascular resistance (PVR) such as pulmonary arterial hypertension, pulmonary embolism, hypoxemia, chronic obstructive pulmonary disease (COPD), acute

TABLE 4-2.   HEMODYNAMIC EFFECTS OF CARDIOVASCULAR AGENTS

Drug	CO	PAOP	SVR	MAP	HR	CVP	PVR
Norepinephrine (Levophed)	↑ (slight)	↑	↑	↑	↔,↑	↑	↑
Phenylephrine (Neosynephrine)	↔,↓	↑	↑	↑	↔,↓	↑	↑
Epinephrine (Asthmahaler)	↑	↑	↑	↑	↑	↑	↑
Dobutamine	↑	↓	↓	↑	↔,↑	↓	↓
(Dobutrex)				(with ↑ CO)	(slight)		↑
Dopamine (Intropin)	↑	↑	↑	↑			↔
< 5 mcg/kg/min	↑	↑↑	(slight)	(slight)	↑	↑↑	↑
> 5 mcg/kg/min			↑↑	↑↑			
Digoxin (Lanoxin)	↑	↔	↔	↔	↓	↔	↔
Isoproterenol (Isuprel)	↑	↓	↓	↓	↑	↓	↓
Levosimendan (Simdax)	↔,↓ (related to ↑ SVR)	↑	↑	↑	↔,↓	↑	↑
Vasopressin	↔, ↓ (related to ↑ SVR)	↑	↑	↑	↔,↓	↑	↑
Milrinone (Primacor)	↑	↓	↓	↔ (↓ in preload-sensitive patient)	↔ (↑ in preload-sensitive patient)	↓	↓
Nitroglycerin (Tridil)	↔	↓	↔	↔	↔	↓	↔
20-40 mcg/min	↑	↓	↓	↓	↑	↓	↓
50-250 mcg/min							
(max dose)							
Nitroprusside (Nipride)	↑	↓	↓	↓	↑	↓	↓

respiratory distress syndrome (ARDS), sepsis; and (3) severe LV dysfunction as seen in mitral stenosis/insufficiency or LV failure. In contrast, the only clinically significant reason for a decreased CVP/RAP is hypovolemia. CVP/RAP is a late indicator of alterations in RV function therefore limiting its value in clinical decision making.

ESSENTIAL CONTENT CASE

Hypovolemia

A 67-year-old woman is admitted to the progressive care unit with the diagnosis of hypotension secondary to presumed gastrointestinal bleeding. A history of melena for 3 days was provided by her daughter on admission. She is presently unresponsive but is breathing spontaneously. Breath sounds are clear, urine output is 15 mL in 8 hours, and her skin is cool. Laboratory work is pending and 3 U of packed red blood cells have been ordered stat. Findings from the Focused Assessment with Sonography in Trauma (FAST) examination are inconclusive so a CV catheter is inserted to aid in the provision of fluids, blood, and medications, and to help interpret the situation. The following data are available:

BP	86/54 mm Hg
HR	118/min
RR	30 breaths/min
T	37.3°C
CVP	3 mm Hg

Case Question 1. What findings reinforce that the patient is hypovolemic?

Case Question 2. Which hemodynamic findings are abnormal?

Case Question 3. What treatments are warranted in this patient?

Answers

1. The history of melena for the past 3 days, urinary output 15 mL in 8 hours, altered mental status and BP 86/54 mm Hg. Reviewing the patient's BP history would be important—does she usually have a systolic BP less than 90? Lab tests that can be used to trend the volume status include BUN and Hct. CBC would be especially important in this patient.

2. BP 86/54 mm Hg, PR 118/min, RR 30 breaths/min, CVP 3 mm Hg.

3. The data, including the CVP indicate that the patient needs fluid resuscitation, and possibly blood transfusion. Fluid challenges are considered the cornerstone of resuscitation in acutely ill patients. However, clinical studies have demonstrated that only about 50% of hemodynamically unstable patients are volume responsive. Increasing evidence suggests that excess fluid resuscitation is associated with increased mortality. Static pressure (CVP, PAOP) and echocardiographic (IVC diameter) parameters are not reliable predictors of volume responsiveness. Dynamic parameters (SPV, PPV, SVV) are reliable predictors of fluid response and are measured based on evaluating arterial pressure data as it changes over the course of the respiratory cycle in a patient on positive pressure mechanical ventilation. In spontaneously breathing patients, the passive leg raise test is highly predictive of volume responsiveness.

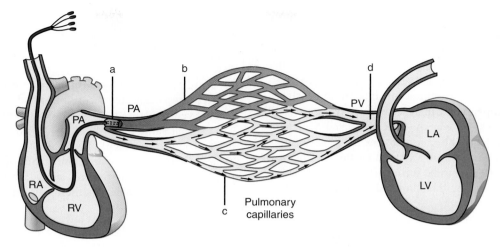

Figure 4-4. Schematic representation of the PA in the wedge position. From its position in small, occluded segment of the pulmonary circulation, the PA catheter in the wedged position allows the electronic monitoring equipment to "look through" a nonactive segment of the pulmonary circulation to the hemodynamically active pulmonary veins and left atrium. (*Reproduced with permission from Darovic GO:* Hemodynamic Monitoring: Invasive and Noninvasive Clinical Application. *Philadelphia, PA: WB Saunders; 2002.*)

LEFT VENTRICULAR PRELOAD (PAOP, PCWP, PAWP, OR LAP)

Normal LV preload is 8 to 12 mm Hg (see Table 4-1) and is measured with a PA catheter. There are many names that are synonymous with left atrial pressure (LAP) and they include: PCWP = pulmonary capillary wedge pressure; PAOP = pulmonary artery occlusion pressure; and PAWP = pulmonary artery wedge pressure. The most commonly used term is PAOP. The normal PAOP is 8 to 12 mm Hg. The pressure is measured by inserting a small amount of air into the balloon port of the PA catheter: the balloon becomes lodged in a portion of the PA that is smaller than the balloon. This occludes blood flow distal to the catheter tip. The pressure in the left atrium is sensed at the catheter tip. When the mitral valve is open during ventricular diastole, the pressure that is sensed is that of the left ventricle, the LV end-diastolic pressure (LVEDP) or LV preload (Figure 4-4).

Pulmonary artery occlusion pressure (PAOP) increases because of conditions such as intravascular volume overload, cardiac tamponade (blood, effusion, etc), impaired ventricular relaxation (diastolic dysfunction, restrictive cardiomyopathy, and constrictive pericarditis), and LV dysfunction. Common etiologies of LV dysfunction include mitral stenosis/insufficiency, aortic stenosis/insufficiency, and diminished LV compliance (ischemia, fibrosis, hypertrophy). The most clinically significant reason for a decreased PAOP is hypovolemia.

Afterload

Afterload is the resistance to ventricular emptying during systole. It is the pressure or resistance that the ventricles must overcome to open the aortic and pulmonary valves and to pump blood into the systemic and pulmonary vasculature. Vascular resistance is determined by the length of a vessel, its diameter or radius, and the viscosity of the blood. The length of the vessel is a constant. The viscosity of the blood is relatively constant except when gross volume changes occur (eg, hemorrhage) or in polycythemia. Therefore, conditions that alter the diameter of the vessels, or the outflow tract, have a primary effect on the afterload of the ventricles.

As afterload increases, due to vasoconstriction or obstruction of the outflow tract, the heart must work harder to eject the volume. Afterload affects the isovolumetric contraction phase of the cardiac cycle. During this phase, the ventricular pressure rises so the ventricles are able to overcome the existing vascular resistance, open the semilunar valves, and eject blood. Once the pressure within the ventricle is higher than the pressure in the aorta/pulmonary system, the valves open and the blood is ejected from the heart. With increased afterload, the heart works harder to eject the contents, leading to increased consumption of oxygen by the heart (increase in MVO_2). This is a crucial period of myocardial susceptibility to ischemic injury and is a major reason to consider afterload reduction therapies.

Common causes of increased afterload include aortic/pulmonic stenosis, hypothermia, hypertension, compensatory response to hypotension and decreased CO, classic shock states (hypovolemic, cardiogenic, and obstructive), and response to drugs that stimulate the alpha receptors (epinephrine, norepinephrine, dopamine, phenylephrine) (see Table 4-2). Decreased afterload is seen in hyperthermia, the distributive shocks (septic, anaphylactic, and neurogenic), and after administration of vasodilating medications (nitroprusside, nitroglycerin at higher doses, calcium channel blockers, beta-blockers, and the like) (see Table 4-2).

Clinical Indicators of Afterload

Afterload cannot be directly measured. It is evaluated with a PA catheter and is a derived value (ie, is calculated based on other measured variables). Formulas for some common derived variables are listed in Table 4-1.

Systemic Vascular Resistance

Systemic vascular resistance is normally between 800 and 1200 dynes-s/cm^{-5}. If the SVR is elevated, the left ventricle faces an increased resistance to the ejection of blood; in other words, an increased afterload. SVR is elevated in hypertension. A low CO, such as would occur in some shock states, may lead to a compensatory increase in SVR. It is important for the clinician to know why the SVR is elevated; for example, if the SVR is elevated because of systemic hypertension, afterload-reducing agents are a critical part of the therapy. However, if the SVR is elevated secondary to a compensation for low CO, therapy should be directed toward the primary goal of improving CO.

A low SVR is a pathologic response that reduces the resistance to the ejection of blood from the left ventricle. Sepsis causes a low SVR due to widespread vasodilation that is part of the dysregulated immune response. SVR is also reduced in hepatic disease due to increased collateral circulation or in neurogenic shock due to vasodilation mediated by the central nervous system. Generally, if the SVR is low, administration of fluids and/or vasopressor medications is considered while the cause is determined and corrected. If the underlying condition is not treated, the use of vasopressors provides only short-term success.

Pulmonary Vascular Resistance

Pulmonary Vascular Resistance (PVR) is lower than SVR. Normal PVR is about 100 to 250 dynes-s/cm^{-5} (see Table 4-1). An elevated PVR produces a strain on the right ventricle, in other words, an increased afterload for the right ventricle. If this strain is unrelieved, the right ventricle eventually fails. Failure of the right ventricle results in less blood entering the lungs and the left ventricle. Systemic hypotension follows due to RV dysfunction. The most common causes of an increase in PVR include pulmonary hypertension, hypoxia, end-stage COPD (cor pulmonale), and pulmonary emboli.

Contractility

Contractility is the strength of the myocardial contraction, or the degree of myocardial fiber shortening with contraction independent of preload and afterload. Contractility contributes significantly to CO. If the other determinants of CO were constant, then a heart with a greater contractile force would produce a greater CO. However, contractility depends on many variables including preload (Frank-Starling law of the heart) and afterload. The preload and afterload may be within normal limits and the patient can still have impaired contractility.

Electrolyte levels also have a major impact on the contractility of the heart. Monitoring and treating abnormal calcium, sodium, magnesium, potassium, and phosphorus levels are essential to ensure optimal contractility. Other factors that contribute to contractility include myocardial oxygenation (ischemia), amount of functional myocardium

(infarction, cardiomyopathy), and administration of positive and negative inotropic medications.

Clinical Indicators of Contractility

Myocardial contractility is reflected indirectly in the SVI, which is the SV adjusted according to body size, and the right and left ventricular stroke work index (RVSWI and LVSWI). The normal value for SVI is 33 to 47 mL/beat/m^2; RVSWI is 5 to 10 gm/m/m^2, and LVSWI is 50 to 62 gm/m/m^2 (see Table 4-1). These are not direct indicators of contractility, but can be used to identify patients at risk for poor contractility and to monitor the effects of therapeutic management.

ESSENTIAL CONTENT CASE

Decreased Afterload

A 65-year-old man is developing hypotension on the acute care floor. He had femoral-popliteal bypass surgery 4 days earlier and was doing well until yesterday. He began to complain of generalized malaise with the following vital signs:

BP:	102/58 mm Hg
RR:	27 breaths/min
PR:	110/min
T:	38.1°C

His wound site is reddened but has no drainage. He does not complain of any discomfort or shortness of breath. His lung sounds are clear and he has a pulse oximeter value of 99%.

Case Question 1. What data suggest that the patient has an inflammatory response?

Case Question 2. What are the treatment priorities at this time?

Case Question 3. If the BP drops to 80/50 mm Hg, what is the significance? What would be the priorities of treatment?

Answers
1. Tachycardia (HR = 110 beats/min) and fever (temperature 38.1°C) both suggest an inflammatory response.
2. Culture any area suspected of infection. In this patient, culture blood, sputum, urine, and wound site. Start empiric antimicrobials. A fluid bolus followed by further assessment in the form of a CVP or a passive leg raise test would help determine if the patient requires additional fluid.
3. If the BP drops to 80/50 mm Hg, the patient is now in shock (MAP 62 mm Hg). This is a critical drop in BP and requires immediate fluid resuscitation with normal saline (NS). If the patient remains hypotensive after fluid resuscitation, further fluids or the addition of a vasopressor(s) are appropriate. The recommended agents are norepinephrine and vasopressin. These medications require continuous monitoring so transfer to the critical care unit is warranted.

BASIC COMPONENTS OF HEMODYNAMIC MONITORING SYSTEMS

The basic components of hemodynamic monitoring systems include an indwelling catheter connected to a pressure transducer and flush system and a bedside monitor. All components that come in contact with the vascular system must be sterile, with meticulous attention paid to maintaining a closed sterile system during use.

Pulmonary Artery Catheter

The PA catheter is a multilumen catheter inserted into the pulmonary artery (Figures 4-4 and 4-5). Each lumen or "port" has specific functions. The PA catheter typically is inserted through an introducer sheath (large-diameter, short catheter with a diaphragm) placed in a major vein. Veins used for PA catheter insertion include the internal jugular, subclavian, femoral, and less commonly, the brachial vein. More information on the PA catheter is found in *AACN Essentials of Critical Care Nursing*.

Arterial Catheter

The arterial catheter, or "A-line," has only one lumen, which is used for measuring arterial pressures, hemodynamic parameters, and for drawing arterial blood samples (Figure 4-6). Arterial catheters are inserted in any major artery, with the most common sites being the radial and femoral arteries.

Pressure Tubing

The pressure tubing is a key component of any hemodynamic monitoring system (see Figure 4-6). It is a stiff (noncompliant) tubing to ensure accurate transfer of intravascular pressures to the transducer. The pressure tubing connects the intravascular catheter to the transducer. Many pressure tubings have stopcocks in line to facilitate blood sampling and zeroing the transducer. Normally, the pressure tubing is kept as short as possible (no more than 3-4 ft), with a minimal number of stopcocks, to increase the accuracy of pressure measurements. Inclusion of a blood-conserving device in the existing monitoring circuit may affect its dynamic response characteristics. The systolic pressure generally shows more variability than the mean arterial pressure.

Pressure Transducer

The pressure transducer is a small electronic sensor that converts a mechanical pressure (vascular pressure) into an electrical signal (see Figure 4-6). This electrical signal can then be displayed on the pressure amplifier.

Pressure Amplifier

The pressure amplifier, or "bedside monitor," augments the signal from the transducer and displays the converted vascular pressure as an electrical signal (see Figure 4-6). This

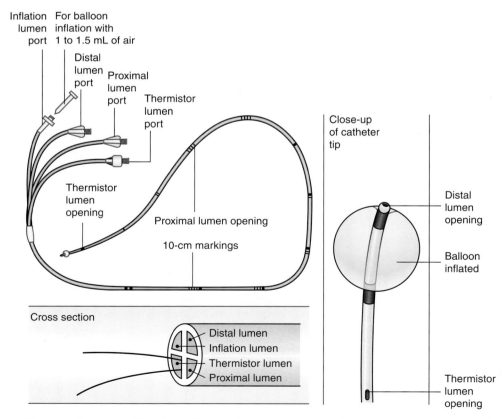

Figure 4-5. Flow-directed PA catheter (Swan-Ganz). (*Reproduced with permission from Visalli F, Evans P. The Swan-Ganz catheter: a program for teaching safe, effective use*, Nursing *1981 Jan;11(1):42-47.*)

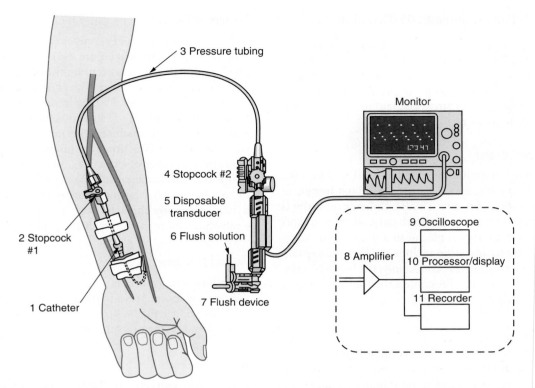

Figure 4-6. Components of a hemodynamic monitoring system. (*Reproduced with permission from Shoemaker WC, Ayers S, Grenvik A, et al: Textbook of Critical Care, 3rd ed. Philadelphia, PA: WB Saunders; 1995.*)

signal is used to display a continuous waveform on the oscilloscope of the monitor and to provide a numerical display of the pressure measurement. Most bedside monitors also have a graphic recorder to print out the pressure waveform.

Pressure Bag and Flush Device

In addition to being attached to the pressure amplifier, the transducer is connected to an intravenous (IV) solution, which is placed in a pressure bag (Figure 4-7). The IV

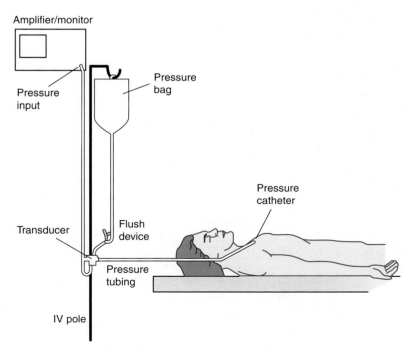

Figure 4-7. Pressure bag and flush device connected to a pressure transducer and monitoring system. (*Reproduced with permission from Ahrens TS, Taylor L: Hemodynamic Waveform Analysis. Philadelphia, PA: WB Saunders; 1992.*)

solution is normally 500 to 1000 mL of NS, although 5% dextrose in water (D_5W) can be used. The IV solution is placed under 300 mm Hg of pressure to provide a slow, continuous infusion of fluid through the vascular catheter.

The IV solution is placed under pressure for another reason. Included in most pressure systems is a flush device (see Figure 4-7). The flush device regulates fluid flow through the pressure tubing at a slow, continuous rate to prevent occlusion of the vascular catheter. Normally, the flush device restricts fluid flow to approximately 2 to 4 mL/h. If the flush device is activated, normally by squeezing or pulling the flush device, a rapid flow of fluid enters the pressure tubing. Flush devices are activated for two reasons: to rapidly clear the tubing of air or blood and to check the accuracy of the tubing/catheter system (square wave test). Measuring the fluid in the IV solution should be done on every shift to determine the amount of fluid infused from the pressure bag. Depending on hospital procedures, unfractionated heparin may be added to the IV solution to aid in keeping the system patent.

Alarms

Bedside monitors have alarms for each of the hemodynamic pressures being monitored. Normally, every parameter that is being monitored has high and low alarms, which can be set to detect variations from the current value. Alarm limits are generally set to detect significant decreases or increases in pressures or rates, typically ±10% of the current values. When alarm limits are too narrow, the frequency of monitor alarms will increase. Studies show that when alarms are frequent and do not accurately indicate a change in a patient's condition, response times increase, placing patients at risk. Setting alarm limits at liberal levels also creates a risk to patient safety, as the monitor may not alarm when in fact, there is a change in condition that warrants intervention. Progressive care nurses, in collaboration with providers, clinical engineers, and other members of the healthcare team can contribute to establishing appropriate procedures for setting alarm limits.

OBTAINING ACCURATE CVP AND ARTERIAL VALUES

The information obtained from hemodynamic monitoring technology must be verified for accuracy by the bedside clinician.

Zeroing the Transducer

A fundamental step in obtaining accurate hemodynamic values is to zero the transducer amplifier system. Zeroing is the act of electronically compensating for any offset (distortion) in the transducer. This is normally done by exposing the transducer to air and pushing an automatic zero button on the bedside monitor. This step is performed at least once before obtaining the first hemodynamic reading after catheter insertion. Because it is an electronic function, it normally has to be performed only once when the transducer and amplifier are first attached to the in situ catheter.

Leveling the Transducer to the Catheter Tip

Leveling is the process of aligning the transducer with the anatomical reference that represents the position of the atria (central BP). Leveling minimizes the effect of hydrostatic pressure on the transducer, improving the accuracy of the readings. If the transducer is positioned too low, the fluid within the tubing above the transducer exerts a greater pressure on the transducer and results in an abnormally high pressure value. If the transducer is positioned too high, the fluid within the tubing above the transducer exerts a lower pressure and results in an abnormally low pressure value. The reference point is the phlebostatic axis and is found at the intersection between the fourth intercostal space (ICS) and half the AP diameter of the chest (Figure 4-8).

There are two basic methods for leveling. When the transducer and stopcocks are mounted on a pole close to the bed, the pole height is adjusted to have the stopcock opening horizontal to the external reference point (Figure 4-9). To ensure horizontal positioning, a carpenter's level (or a similar device) is usually necessary. Each time the bed height or patient position is altered, this leveling procedure must be repeated (Figure 4-10).

The other method for leveling places the transducer and stopcock at the correct location on the chest wall or arm (Figure 4-11). Taping or strapping the transducer to the appropriate location on the body eliminates the need for repeating the leveling procedure when bed heights are changed. As long as the transducer/stopcock position remains horizontal to the external reference location, no releveling is required.

Leveling must be performed prior to obtaining the first set of values and any time the transducer is no longer horizontal to the external reference location. When obtaining the first set of readings, zeroing and leveling are frequently

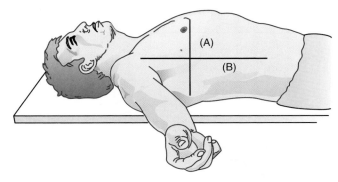

Figure 4-8. Referencing and zeroing the hemodynamic monitoring system in a supine patient. The phlebostatic axis is determined by drawing an imaginary vertical line from the fourth ICS on the sternal border to the right side of the chest. **(A)** A second imaginary line is drawn horizontally at the level of the midpoint between the anterior and posterior surface of the chest. **(B)** The phlebostatic axis is located at the intersection of points A and B. (*Reproduced with permission from Keckeisen M, Chulay M, Gawlinski A: Pulmonary artery pressure monitoring. In: Hemodynamic Monitoring Series. Aliso Viejo, CA: AACN; 1998.*)

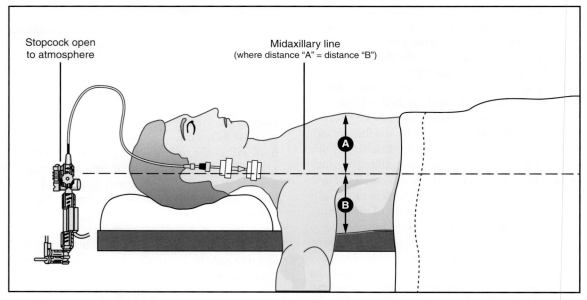

Figure 4-9. Typical leveling of CVP catheter with stopcock attached to the transducer for mounting on a pole. The stopcock close to the transducer is opened to atmospheric pressure (air) horizontal to the fourth ICS at the midaxillary line.

performed simultaneously. After this initial combined effort, zeroing does not need to be performed when leveling is done.

Ensuring Accurate Waveform Transmission

For hemodynamic monitoring to provide accurate information, the vascular pressure must be transmitted back to the transducer unaltered and then converted accurately into an electrical signal. For this waveform to be transmitted unaltered, no obstructions or distortions to the signal should be present along the transmission route. Distortion of the waveform leads to inaccurate pressure interpretations. A variety of factors can cause distortions to the waveform, including catheter obstructions (eg, clots, catheter bending, blood or air in tubing), excessive tubing or connectors, and transducer damage. Verification of an accurate transmission of the waveform to the transducer is checked by the bedside nurse by performing a square wave test. This occurs at the beginning of each shift and any time the waveform configuration changes.

Square Wave Test

The square wave test is performed on all hemodynamic pressure systems before assuming that the waveforms and pressures obtained are accurate. The square wave test is performed by recording the pressure waveform while fast flushing the catheter (Table 4-3A). The fast-flush valve is pulled or

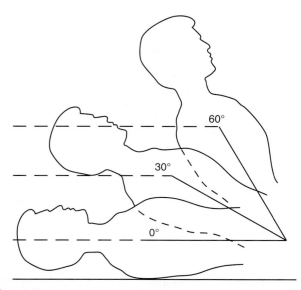

Figure 4-10. The level of the phlebostatic axis as the patient moves flat to a higher level of backrest. The level of the axis for referencing and zeroing the air-fluid interface rotates on the axis and remains horizontal as the patient moves from flat to increasingly higher backrest positions. For accurate hemodynamic pressure readings at different backrest elevations, the air-fluid interface must be at the level of the phlebostatic axis. (*Reproduced with permission from Bridges EJ, Woods SL. Pulmonary artery pressure measurement: state of the art,* Heart Lung *1993 Mar-Apr;22(2):99-111.*)

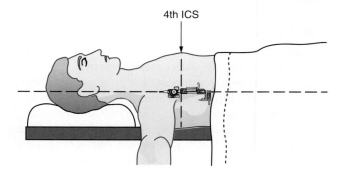

Figure 4-11. Leveling a transducer for mounting on the chest wall at the fourth ICS at the midaxillary line.

TABLE 4-3A, B, C. ASSESSING DAMPING CONCEPTS FROM SQUARE WAVE TEST

Square Wave Test	Clinical Effect	Corrective Action
A. Optimally damped system. When the fast flush of the continuous flush system is activated and quickly released, a sharp upstroke terminates in a flat line at the maximal indicator on the monitor and hard copy. This is followed by an immediate and rapid downstroke extending below the baseline with just 1 or 2 oscillations within 0.12 second (minimal ringing) and a quick return to baseline. The patient's pressure waveform is also clearly defined with all components of the waveform, such as the dicrotic notch on an arterial waveform, clearly visible. Intervention: There is no adjustment in the monitoring system required. (*Reproduced with permission from Darovic GO:* Hemodynamic Monitoring: Invasive and Noninvasive Clinical Application, *2nd ed. Philadelphia, PA: WB Saunders Co; 1995.*) Optimally damped Observed waveform	Produces accurate waveform and pressure.	None required.
B. Overdamped system. The upstroke of the square wave appears somewhat slurred, the waveform does not extend below the baseline after the fast flush, and there is no ringing after the flush. The patient's waveform displays a falsely decreased systolic pressure and a falsely high diastolic pressure as well as poorly defined components of the pressure tracing such as a diminished or absent dicrotic notch on arterial waveforms. Interventions: To correct the problem—(1) check for the presence of blood clots, blood left in the catheter following blood sampling, or air bubbles at any point from the catheter tip to the transducer and eliminate them as necessary; (2) use low compliance (rigid), short (< 3-4 ft) monitoring tubing; (3) ensure there are no loose connections; and (4) check for kinks in the line. (*Reproduced with permission from Darovic GO:* Hemodynamic Monitoring: Invasive and Noninvasive Clinical Application, *2nd ed. Philadelphia, PA: WB Saunders Co; 1995.*) Overdamped Observed waveform	Produces a falsely low systolic and high diastolic value.	Check the system for air, blood, loose connections, or kinks in the tubing or catheter. Verify extension tubing has not been added.
C. Underdamped system. The waveform is characterized by numerous amplified oscillations above and below the baseline following the fast flush. The monitored pressure wave displays falsely high systolic pressure (overshoot), possibly falsely low diastolic pressures, and "ringing" artifacts on the waveform. Intervention: To correct the problem, remove all air bubbles in the fluid system. Use large bore, shorter tubing, or a damping device. (*Reproduced with permission from Darovic GO:* Hemodynamic Monitoring: Invasive and Noninvasive Clinical Application, *2nd ed. Philadelphia, PA: WB Saunders Co; 1995.*) Underdamped Observed waveform	Produces a falsely high systolic and low diastolic value.	Remove unnecessary tubing and stopcocks. Add a damping device.

squeezed, depending on the model and then rapidly released. The tracing should show a rapid rise in the waveform to the top of the graph paper, with a square pattern. Release of the flush device should show a rapid decrease in pressure below the baseline of the pressure waveform (undershoot), followed immediately by a small increase above the baseline (overshoot) prior to resumption of the normal pressure waveform. Square wave tests with these characteristics are called *optimally damped tests* and represent an accurate waveform transmission.

The square wave test is the best method available to the clinician to check the accuracy of hemodynamic monitoring equipment. For example, if an arterial line is to be examined for accuracy, a square wave test is done. Do not compare the arterial line pressure with an indirect BP reading with a sphygmomanometer. If the square wave test indicates optimal damping, then the arterial line pressure is accurate.

Two problems may exist with waveform transmissions, and are referred to as *overdamping* and *underdamping* (see Table 4-3B, C).

Overdamping

If something absorbs the pressure wave (like air or blood in the tubing, stopcocks, or connections), it is said to be *overdamped*. Overdamping decreases systolic pressures and increases diastolic pressures. An overdamped square wave test reflects the obstruction in waveform transmission. Characteristics of overdamping include a loss of the undershoot

TABLE 4-4. SUMMARY OF METHODS FOR ASSESSING AND ENSURING ACCURACY OF HEMODYNAMIC MONITORING SYSTEMS[a]

Method	When Performed
Zero transducer	Should only be performed once. If the transducer zeros properly, a waveform should be visible on the monitor.
Level the transducer	Leveling should be done prior to each pressure reading and with any substantive change in pressures.
Square wave test	Should be performed prior to every reading and after blood has been withdrawn from the catheter.

[a]If a transducer has been zeroed, leveled, and has an optimally damped square wave test, the monitor display is accurate.

and overshoot waves after release of the flush valve and a slurring of the downstroke (Table 4-3 [Figure B]).

Underdamping

If something accentuates the pressure wave (like excessive tubing), it is said to be *underdamped*. Underdamping increases systolic pressures and decreases diastolic pressures (Table 4-3 [Figure C]). An underdamped square wave test reflects the amplification of pressure waves and includes large undershoot and overshoot waves after the release of the flush valve. Table 4-4 summarizes the methods of assessing and ensuring the accuracy of hemodynamic monitoring systems.

Care of the Tubing/Catheter System

Nosocomial infections related to the tubing/catheter system are usually caused by the entry of organisms through stopcocks. Stopcocks are opened for blood sampling and zeroing the transducer only when necessary. Closed, needleless systems are used whenever feasible to decrease the risks to the patient and clinician.

Tubing changes, including flush device, transducer, and flush solution, occur every 72 hours or in accordance with institutional policy. The frequency of catheter device changes is controversial, but must occur whenever the catheter is suspected as a source of infection or by institutional policy.

Length/duration of indwelling catheter use varies depending upon the need for use, site accessed, patient clinical status, catheter type, and antibiotic coating (if any). There are widespread variations in site care techniques and materials used across hospitals. Current Centers for Disease Control and Prevention (CDC) recommendations state central lines should be removed as soon as their exclusive use is no longer required. An intraprofessional approach to tracking "line days" with removal as soon as possible is supported by many professional organizations. Nurses adhere to unit policy and work with the care team to remove invasive lines as soon as feasible.

INSERTION AND REMOVAL OF CATHETERS

Central Venous Catheters

Central venous catheters are used in acutely ill patients to infuse fluids, vasoactive or other intravenous medications,

and total parenteral nutrition. When attached to a transducer, central venous catheters can also be used to monitor CVP and provide additional data about the patient's hemodynamic status.

Insertion

Central venous catheters can be inserted into most large-diameter veins, with the internal jugular and subclavian veins being the most common insertion sites. Typically, the CVP catheter is advanced into the superior vena cava to a level above the right atrium. Following placement, location is verified with a chest radiograph to rule out the presence of a pneumothorax, kinking of the catheter, or other complications.

The waveform configuration associated with the CVP is readily identifiable (described later) and in combination with the value allows the clinician to monitor the patient's status and response to interventions.

Removal

Removing the CVP catheter, and/or discontinuing monitoring the CVP value is a clinical decision based on the assessment that the data from the catheter are no longer necessary for care management. This decision may be made anywhere from a few hours to several days after insertion. The removal of the CVP catheter is normally performed by a provider; although in some institutions nurses perform this task. Nurses must be aware of their specific hospital and unit policies regarding removal of the CVP catheter.

Following the discontinuance of IV fluids, all stopcocks to the patient are turned off to avoid air entry into the vascular bed during catheter removal. The patient is placed in a supine position with the head of the bed flat. While the catheter is being gently withdrawn, the patient is instructed to exhale or hold his or her breath to further decrease the chance of air embolus. Resistance during catheter withdrawal may indicate catheter knotting (very rare). A chest x-ray is necessary to confirm the problem and special removal procedures are performed to avoid structural damage to the vessels.

Complications

Complications associated with CVP catheters include those associated with insertion, maintenance, and removal of the device. These include bleeding, pneumothorax or air emboli, and introduction of microorganisms and subsequent infection.

Arterial Catheters

BP measurement with the indirect method (sphygmomanometer or oscillometric method) may not be as accurate as direct BP measurement, particularly during conditions of abnormal blood flow (high or low CO states) and extremes of SVR. The presence of these conditions in acutely ill patients may necessitate insertion of an arterial catheter to directly measure BP.

Insertion

Arterial catheters are short (< 4 in) catheters that can be inserted into radial, brachial, axillary, femoral, or pedal arteries. The most common site is the radial artery. Arterial catheters can be placed by cut down or with percutaneous insertion techniques, the latter being the most common insertion method.

General insertion steps for percutaneous insertion are similar to IV catheter insertion. Prior to insertion of a radial artery catheter; however, an Allen test is performed to verify the adequacy of circulation to the hand in the event of radial artery thrombosis. The Allen test is performed by completely obstructing blood flow to the hand by compressing the radial and ulnar arteries for a minute or two. If adequate collateral blood flow exists, there will be rapid return of color to the hand upon release of the ulnar artery (Figure 4-12).

During insertion, care is exercised not to damage the arterial vessel by excessive probing or movement of the needle. Bleeding into the tissues occurs quite easily if the vessel is damaged, causing obstruction to distal blood flow and nerve pressure. Following artery cannulation, the catheter is connected to the pressure transducer and a high-pressure infusion system to prevent blood from backing up into the tubing and fluid container (see Figure 4-6).

Removal

The removal of the arterial catheter is warranted when an accurate BP can be obtained via noninvasive methods, the BP is no longer labile, or when frequent arterial blood samples are no longer indicated. Removal of arterial catheters is commonly performed by the nurse using procedures similar to IV catheter removal, but because the catheter is in an artery, greater attention to achieving hemostasis is required. Following catheter removal, firm direct pressure is maintained over the site for at least 5 minutes or until hemostasis occurs. This prevents bleeding and hematoma formation. For patients with coagulation abnormalities, manual pressure may need to be applied for 10 minutes or longer. Pressure dressings, rather than manual pressure, at the site are not recommended as a means to achieve hemostasis. Once hemostasis is achieved, a pressure dressing may be used but is generally not needed.

Frequent assessment of the site after catheter removal is recommended to identify rebleeding and thrombosis of the artery. Checking the extremity for the presence of pulses, circulation, and bleeding is recommended for a few hours after catheter removal.

Complications

A variety of complications are associated with arterial catheters (Table 4-5). The most serious are related to bleeding from the arterial catheter and loss of arterial flow to the extremity from thrombus formation. Loose connections in the arterial system can lead to rapid and massive blood loss. The morbidity and mortality associated with these complications require stringent safeguards (Luer-Lock connections, minimum number of stopcocks, pressure alarm system activated at all times) to prevent bleeding and to rapidly identify disruptions in the arterial system. The catheters are removed as early as possible to prevent the potential for thrombus formation.

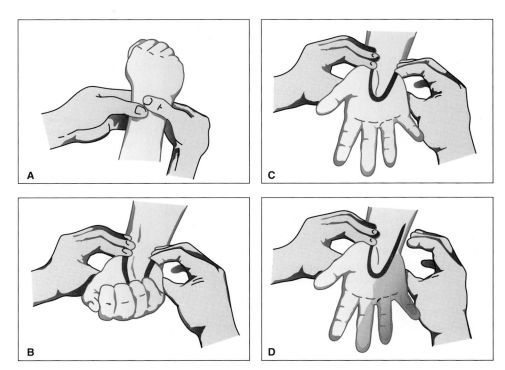

Figure 4-12. The Allen test. (*Reproduced with permission from DeGroot KD, Damato MB. Monitoring intra-arterial pressure. Crit Care Nurs. 1986;Jan-Feb;6[1]:74-78.*)

TABLE 4-5. PROBLEMS ENCOUNTERED WITH ARTERIAL CATHETERS

Problem	Cause	Prevention	Treatment[a]
Hematoma after withdrawal of needle	Bleeding or oozing at puncture site.	Maintain firm pressure on site during withdrawal of catheter and for 5-15 minutes (as necessary) after withdrawal. Apply elastic tape (Elastoplast) firmly over puncture site. For femoral arterial puncture sites, leave a sandbag on site for 1-2 hours to prevent oozing. If patient is receiving unfractionated heparin, discontinue 2 hours before catheter removal.	Continue to hold pressure to puncture site until oozing stops. Apply sandbag to femoral puncture site for 1-2 hours after removal of catheter.
Decreased or absent pulse distal to puncture site	Spasm of artery.	Introduce arterial needle cleanly, nontraumatically.	Inject lidocaine locally at insertion site and 10 mg into arterial catheter.
	Thrombosis of artery.	Use 1 U unfractionated heparin to 1 mL IV fluid.	Arteriotomy and Fogarty catheterization both distally and proximally from the puncture site result in return of pulse in > 90% of cases if brachial or femoral artery is used.
Bleedback into tubing, dome, or transducer	Insufficient pressure on IV bag.	Maintain 300 mm Hg pressure on IV bag.	Replace transducer. "Fast-flush" through system.
	Loose connections.	Use Luer-Lock stopcocks; tighten periodically.	Tighten all connections.
Hemorrhage	Loose connections.	Keep all connecting sites visible. Observe connecting sites frequently. Use built-in alarm system. Use Luer-Lock stopcocks.	Tighten all connections.
Emboli	Clot from catheter tip into bloodstream.	Always aspirate and discard before flushing. Use continuous flush device. Use 1 U unfractionated heparin to 1 mL IV fluid. Gently flush < 2-4 mL.	Remove catheter.
Local infection	Forward movement of contaminated catheter.	Carefully secure catheter at insertion site.	Remove catheter.
	Break in sterile technique.	Always use aseptic technique.	Prescribe antibiotic.
	Prolonged catheter use.	Remove catheter as early as possible. Inspect and care for insertion site daily.	
Sepsis	Break in sterile technique.	Use percutaneous insertion.	Remove catheter.
	Prolonged catheter use.	Always use aseptic technique. Remove catheters as early as possible.	Prescribe antibiotic.
	Bacterial growth in IV fluid.	Change transducer, stopcocks, and tubing every 72 hours. Do not use IV fluid containing glucose. Use a closed-system flush system rather than an open system. Carefully flush remaining blood from stopcocks after blood sampling.	

[a]Please note, many of the treatments necessitate orders or direct intervention by providers or physicians. Please refer to your institutions policies and procedures.
Adapted with permission from Lough ME. Hemodynamic Monitoring Emerging Technologies and Clinial Practice. St Louis, MO: Elsevier; 2016 and Wiegand, DL. Procedure Manual for High Acuity, Progressive and Critical Care. St Louis, MO: Elsevier; 2017.

OBTAINING AND INTERPRETING HEMODYNAMIC WAVEFORMS

To obtain hemodynamic values, interpretation of waveforms is necessary. A multichannel strip recorder, which provides both an electrocardiographic (ECG) and pressure tracing, is the required element (Figure 4-13). Many institutions also use respiratory pressure waveforms, graphed simultaneously with the ECG, CVP, and arterial waveforms. The larger the scale, the easier is the interpretation of the wave. All waveforms are easily obtained simply by activating the record function of the bedside monitor. When obtaining waveforms for interpretation, make sure the calibration scales on the left side of the paper are properly aligned with the paper grid.

Improperly aligned calibration marks increase the difficulty in reading the waveform and increase potential errors in interpretation.

Patient Positioning

The patient is placed in the supine position, with the backrest elevated anywhere from 0° to 60° (see Figure 4-10). Accurate readings can also be achieved when the patient is in a 20°, 30°, or 90° lateral position, with the HOB flat and in the prone position. When using prone position, it is important to allow adequate stabilization time after changing position (30-60 minutes) to ensure that arterial and CVP readings are

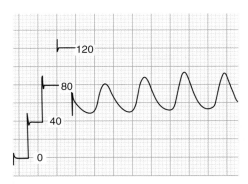

Figure 4-13. Graphic tracing of an arterial waveform preceded by calibration scale markings (0/40/80/120 mm Hg). Note how the scale markers line up with the heavy line of the tracing paper. Each 1-mm line represents 4 mm Hg in this scale.

accurate. (Figure 4-14). Improper leveling affects accurate atrial and venous pressure readings.

It is important to remember that patient comfort is a key issue when obtaining waveform readings. Do not position a spontaneously breathing patient with dyspnea flat for the sole reason of obtaining the readings. It is best to obtain values in the position in which the patient is most comfortable. If a patient demonstrates position-related changes, it is important to always measure in that position and to document the position to ensure consistency.

Interpretation

Correct interpretation of waveforms involves careful assessment of venous and arterial pressure waveforms. Normal values for each of the hemodynamic pressures are listed in Table 4-1.

Central Venous Pressure

The CVP (also known as right atrial pressure) is important because it is used to approximate the right ventricular end-diastolic pressure (RVEDP) and preload. A normal CVP is between 2 and 8 mm Hg. Low CVP values typically reflect hypovolemia or decreased venous return. High CVP values reflect volume overload, increased venous return, or right-sided cardiac failure. The CVP is not evaluated in isolation, but rather relative to other clinical data, including BP, HR, the

impact of a fluid challenge, results from bedside ultrasound, physical examination data such as capillary refill, and passive leg raise testing. Measurement of CVP is done simultaneously with the ECG. Using the ECG allows the identification of the point where the CVP best correlates with the RVEDP.

The CVP is read by one of two techniques. The first technique is to take the mean (average) of the "a" wave of the CVP waveform (Figure 4-15). Although three waves normally exist on atrial waveforms (a, c, and v waves), the mean of the "a" wave most closely approximates ventricular end-diastolic pressure. The "a" wave of the CVP waveform starts just after the P wave on the ECG is observed and represents atrial contraction. By taking the reading at the highest point of the "a" wave, adding it to the reading at the lowest point of that "a" wave, and dividing by 2, the average or mean CVP reading is obtained (generally a line is drawn though the middle of the "a" waves to derive a number).

A second method, the Z-point technique, also can be used to estimate ventricular end-diastolic pressures (Figure 4-16). The Z-point is taken just before the closure of the tricuspid valve. This point is located on a CVP tracing in the mid to late QRS complex area (0.08 seconds after the onset of the QRS complex). The Z-point technique is especially useful when an "a" wave does not exist; for example, in atrial fibrillation when atrial contraction is absent.

By isolating the "a" wave or using the Z-point technique, atrial pressures can reasonably estimate ventricular end-diastolic pressure. It is helpful to read these values off a multichannel strip recorder and not the digital display on the bedside monitor.

Central Venous Pressure: Abnormal Venous Waveforms

Two types of abnormal CVP waveforms are common. Large A waves (also called cannon A waves) occur when the atrium contracts against a closed tricuspid value (Figure 4-17). This occurs most commonly with arrhythmias like premature ventricular contractions (PVCs) or third-degree heart block. Giant V waves are common in conditions such as tricuspid insufficiency or ventricular failure. Using the Z-point for CVP readings prevents incorrect interpretations associated with the use of large A or V waves.

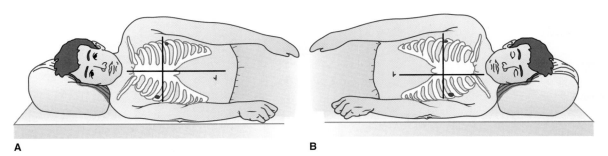

A   **B**

Figure 4-14. Referencing and zeroing the hemodynamic monitoring system in a patient in the lateral position. **(A)** For the right lateral position, the reference point is at the intersection of the fourth ICS and the midsternum. **(B)** For the left lateral position, the reference point is the intersection of the fourth ICS and the left parasternal border. *(Reproduced with permission from Keckeisen M, Chulay M, Gawlinski A: Pulmonary artery pressure monitoring.* In: Hemodynamic Monitoring Series. *Aliso Viejo, CA: AACN; 1998.)*

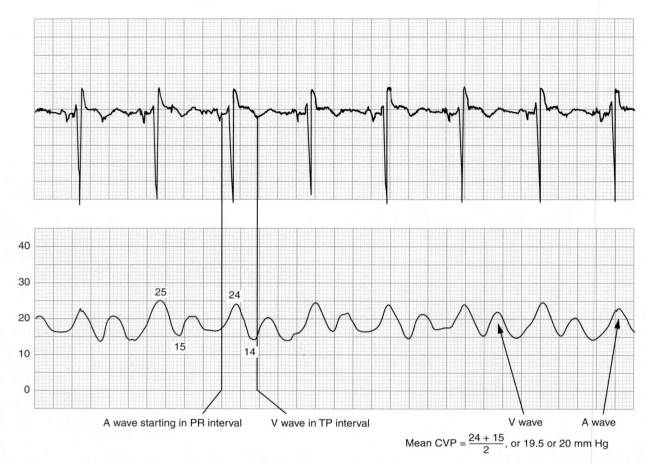

A wave starting in PR interval   V wave in TP interval   V wave   A wave

$$\text{Mean CVP} = \frac{24 + 15}{2}, \text{ or } 19.5 \text{ or } 20 \text{ mm Hg}$$

Figure 4-15. Reading a CVP waveform by averaging the A wave. (*Reproduced with permission from Ahrens TS, Taylor L.* Hemodynamic Waveform Analysis. *Philadelphia, PA: WB Saunders; 1992.*)

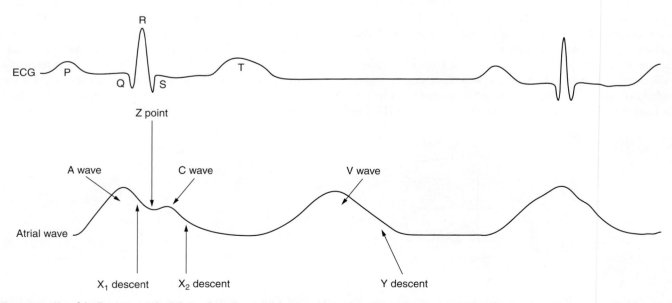

Figure 4-16. Use of the Z-point to read a CVP waveform. (*Reproduced with permission from Ahrens TS, Taylor L.* Hemodynamic Waveform Analysis. *Philadelphia, PA: WB Saunders; 1992.*)

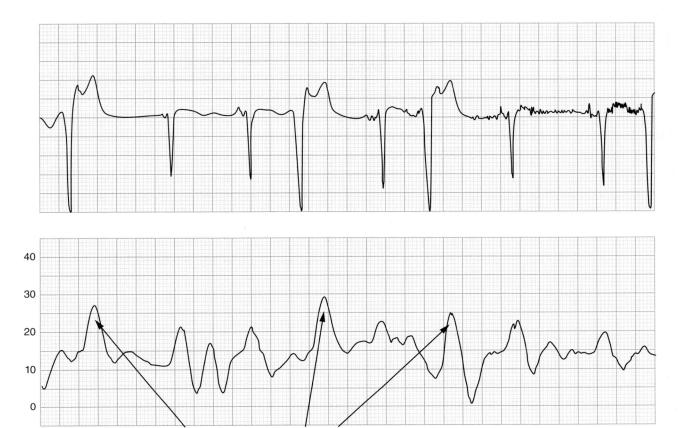

Large A waves follow each PVC

Figure 4-17. Giant A waves with loss of atrioventricular synchrony. (*Reproduced with permission from Ahrens TS, Taylor L.* Hemodynamic Waveform Analysis. *Philadelphia, PA: WB Saunders; 1992.*)

Arterial Waveforms

An arterial waveform, such as seen in systemic tracings, has three common characteristics: rapid upstroke, dicrotic notch, and progressive diastolic runoff (Figure 4-18). Diastole is read near the end of the QRS complex with systole read before the peak of the T wave. The mean arterial pressure can be calculated (see Table 4-1) or obtained from the digital display on the bedside monitor.

Systemic Arterial Pressures

Direct measurement of systemic arterial pressures is obtained when the transducer is leveled to the phlebostatic axis (see Figure 4-11), with pressure waveforms interpreted as described. Normal pressures are generally in the region of 100 to 120 mm Hg systolic, 60 to 80 mm Hg diastolic, and 70 to 105 mm Hg mean (see Table 4-1).

Systemic arterial pressures are not interpreted without other clinical information. In general, however, hypotension

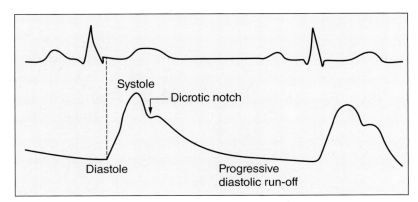

Figure 4-18. Characteristics of an arterial waveform. (*Reproduced with permission from Ahrens TS, Prentice D.* Critical Care: Certification Preparation and Review, *3rd ed. Stamford, CT: Appleton & Lange; 1993.*)

is assumed if the mean arterial pressure drops below 65 mm Hg. Hypertension is assumed if the systolic blood pressure (SBP) is greater than 140 to 160 mm Hg or the diastolic pressure exceeds 90 mm Hg.

The arterial pressure is one of the most commonly used parameters for assessing the adequacy of blood flow to the tissues. BP is determined by two factors, CO and SVR. BP does not reflect early clinical changes in hemodynamics because of the interaction with CO and SVR.

In addition, the CO consists of HR and SV. These two interact to maintain a normal CO. Subsequently, if the SV begins to fall due to loss of volume (hypovolemia) or dysfunction (LV failure), the HR increases to offset the decrease in SV. The net effect is to maintain the CO at near normal levels. If the CO does not change, then there is no change in the BP.

A key point for the nurse to consider is that because of these compensatory mechanisms, BP may not signal early clinical changes in hemodynamic status. If a patient begins to bleed postoperatively, the BP generally does not reflect this change until compensation is no longer possible. In addition, hypotension is sometimes difficult to evaluate. It is possible that true hypotension exists only when tissue hypoxia is present and end organs are affected. Although tradition dictates

that we identify hypotension using predefined levels of BP, other measures such as mixed venous saturation of hemoglobin (Svo_2) and lactate levels may be better indicators of tissue perfusion. Svo_2 monitoring is described later in the section Continuous Mixed and Central Venous Oxygen Monitoring ($Svo_2/Scvo_2$).

Although studies identify the role of hypertension in circulatory damage, the specific level of hypertension that results in the damage is unclear. Therefore, any SBP over 140 is considered potentially injurious to the vasculature.

Artifacts in Hemodynamic Waveforms: Respiratory Influence

Respiration can physiologically change hemodynamic pressures. Spontaneous breathing augments venous return and slightly increases resistance to left ventricle filling. Mechanical ventilation does the opposite, potentially reducing venous return and reducing the resistance on the heart. The effect of mechanical ventilation on an arterial pressure is seen in Figure 4-19. The effect of spontaneous breathing on a CVP is noted in Figure 4-20.

A spontaneous breath or a patient-initiated ventilator breath produces a drop in the waveform because of the decrease in pleural pressure. A ventilator breath produces an upward distortion of the baseline due to an increase in

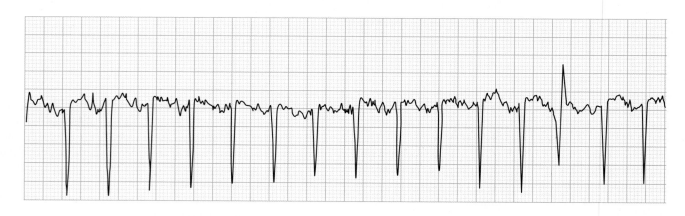

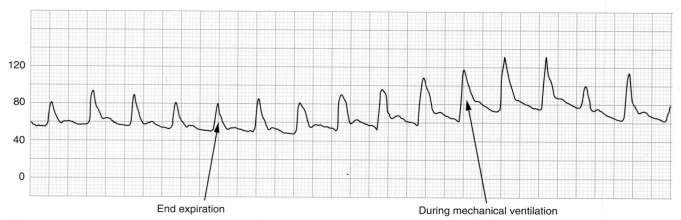

Figure 4-19. Effect of respiration on arterial pressures. (*Reproduced with permission from Ahrens TS, Taylor L. Hemodynamic Waveform Analysis. Philadelphia, PA: WB Saunders; 1992.*)

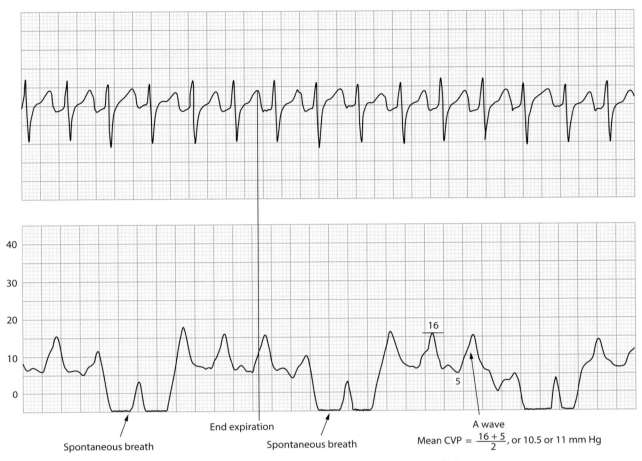

Figure 4-20. Effect of a spontaneous breath on a CVP waveform. (*Reproduced with permission from Ahrens TS, Taylor L.* Hemodynamic Waveform Analysis. *Philadelphia, PA: WB Saunders; 1992.*)

pleural and intrathoracic pressure. The key to reading the waveform correctly is to isolate the point where pleural pressure is closest to atmospheric pressure. This point is usually at end expiration, just prior to inspiration (Figure 4-20).

Functional Hemodynamics
To determine fluid responsiveness, progressive care nurses and providers may also assess dynamic parameters. The aim of these measurements is to determine the patient's position on the Frank-Starling curve (see Figure 4-2). If the patient is situated on the ascending portion of the Frank-Starling curve, an increase in preload via a fluid bolus results in an increase of SV (preload-dependent situation). If the patient is on the plateau portion of the Frank-Starling curve, a variation of preload does not alter SV (preload-independent situation). Ventilator-induced changes in systolic pressure, pulse pressure or SV can reflect the heart's ability to respond to a fluid bolus and are more accurate than static measures such as CVP and PAOP. If the functional indicator is below its threshold, administering additional fluid will not result in an increase in SV and may even result in fluid overload. See Table 4-6 for a description of functional hemodynamic measurements.

The traditional approach to fluid resuscitation consisted of measuring a pressure parameter such as the central venous pressure (CVP) or pulmonary artery occlusion pressure (POAP) together with a CO determination. A "fluid challenge" and reassessment of the parameter(s) were then made.

TABLE 4-6. FUNCTIONAL HEMODYNAMIC MEASUREMENTS

Variable	Equation	Threshold for Responders
Formulas		
SPV (Systolic pressure variation)	$SBP_{max} - SBP_{min}$	> 10 mm Hg
SPV % (Percent variation in SPV)	$[(SBP_{max} - SBP_{min})/(SBP_{max} + SBP_{min}/2)] \times 100$	> 10%
PPV % (Pulse pressure variation)	$[(PP_{max} - PP_{min})/(PP_{max} + PP_{min}/2)] \times 100$	> 12.5%
SVV % (Stroke volume variation)	$[(SV_{max} - SV_{min})/(SV_{max} + SV_{min}/2)] \times 100$	> 12%
PVI (Pleth variability index)	Derived from oximeter perfusion index	12%-16%

Bridges EJ, presenter. Live Q&A: Functional Hemodynamic Monitoring. Table: Functional Hemodynamic Measurements. AACN Webinar Series. Aliso Viejo, CA: AACN. ©2015 by the American Association of Critical-Care Nurses. Used with permission.

This approach has been largely discredited by the data suggesting a poor or no correlation between the CVP or PAOP and volume responsiveness. Dynamic parameters, listed in Table 4-6, appear to be more reliable. Patients who demonstrate a ventilator induced change in systolic pressure, pulse pressure or SV that is above the threshold are likely to respond to a fluid bolus. These measures, like the Passive Leg Raise Maneuver described earlier, are noninvasive assessments of hemodynamic status.

CONTINUOUS MIXED AND CENTRAL VENOUS OXYGEN MONITORING (Svo_2/$Scvo_2$)

Svo_2/$Scvo_2$ Monitoring Principles

Mixed venous oxygen saturation (Svo_2) monitoring is generally done in a critical care unit and uses a specialized PA catheter. While a comprehensive discussion of the technology is not within the scope of this book, the associated concepts are important and are briefly discussed below.

Svo_2 catheters are different from other PA catheters in that they have two special fiber-optic bundles within the catheter that determine the oxygen saturation of hemoglobin by measuring the wavelength (color) of reflected light. Light is transmitted from the tip of the PA catheter down one bundle and is reflected off the oxygen-saturated hemoglobin, returning up the other bundle. This information is quantified by the bedside computer and numerically displayed as the percentage of saturation of the mixed venous blood.

The measurement of central venous oxygen saturation ($Scvo_2$) requires the placement of a central venous catheter, which has fewer complications than a PA catheter. Theoretically, it measures the degree of oxygen extraction from the brain and upper body and trends well with Svo_2. The goal for $Scvo_2$ is greater than 70%. The $Scvo_2$ is usually less than the Svo_2 except in shock states. This occurs because of redistribution of blood flow in classic shock states.

Continuous Svo_2 monitoring is used as a diagnostic tool. It provides early warning of alterations in hemodynamic status and a continuous monitor of the relationship between oxygen delivery and consumption. Many therapeutic strategies are added and adjusted in response to the changes in the Svo_2. If a BP is considered low but the Svo_2 is above 60%, then the BP is not contributing to a decrease in tissue perfusion. However, if the BP and Svo_2 are low, interventions to improve perfusion are essential.

Svo_2 monitoring is used to continuously monitor how well the body's demand for oxygen is being met under different clinical conditions. To understand this concept, an understanding of how the tissues are supplied with oxygen is necessary.

Blood leaves the left heart 100% saturated with oxygen and is transported to the tissues for cellular use based on the amount of perfusion (CO). Under normal conditions, only about 25% of the oxygen available on the hemoglobin

is extracted by the tissues, with blood returning to the right heart with approximately 75% of the hemoglobin saturated with oxygen. Normal values for mixed venous oxygen saturation are 60% to 80%.

In situations where tissue demands for oxygen increase, the oxygen saturation of blood returning to the right heart will be lower than 70%. Clinical situations of increased tissue demand for oxygen include fever, pain, anxiety, infection, seizures, and some "routine" nursing activities like turning and suctioning. In contrast, hypothermia dramatically decreases oxygen consumption by the tissues. Interventions, then, are directed at decreasing or increasing the oxygen requirements as needed.

The concept of oxygen utilization is often referred to as supply and demand (or more accurately consumption) and is the essential concept inherent in Svo_2 monitoring. Because tissue oxygenation depends on hemoglobin level, saturation of hemoglobin, oxygen consumption, and CO, the saturation of blood returning to the PA tells us much about the interaction of these four variables and can be used to assess the adequacy of interventions.

MINIMALLY INVASIVE HEMODYNAMIC MONITORING

In some acute care units, new noninvasive technology may be used periodically to assess CO and other hemodynamic parameters. While further research is needed to determine the efficacy of the devices, the noninvasive nature of the technologies makes them attractive for use in the progressive care setting. Two, thoracic bioimpedance/bioreactance and pulse contour measurement, are described here.

Thoracic Bioimpedance/Bioreactance

The resistance of current flow (impedance) across the chest is inversely related to the thoracic fluid. Using a current that flows from the electrodes on the chest and neck, the SV can be determined. Changes in impedance occur with changes in blood flow and velocity through the ascending aorta. The impedance changes reflect aortic flow, which is directly related to ventricular function (contractility).

Variables that change the bioimpedance and alter the relationship between impedance and SV are changes in hematocrit, lung water, lead contact, shivering, mechanical ventilation, and rhythm changes. Thoracic bioimpedance is a useful method for trend analysis but to date is not accurate enough for diagnostic interpretation. Its major application has been outside the critical care setting (HF clinics, emergency department, pacemaker clinics).

A method that has evolved from bioimpedance is bioreactance. Bioreactance provides continuous, totally noninvasive CO measurement by analyzing phase shifts of an oscillating current as it travels through the thoracic cavity (NICOM system; Cheetah Medical Inc., Portland, OR, USA)

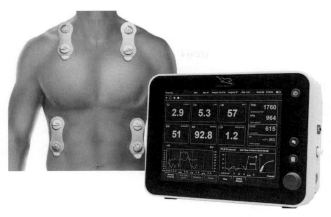

Figure 4-21. Electrode placement for bioreactance. (NICOM system). (*Used with permission from Cheetah Medical Inc, Portland, OR, USA.*)

(Figure 4-21). The hemodynamic parameters measured by this device are CO/CI, SVI, and SV variation (SVV) (see Table 4-1). It has been found to provide reliable CO measurements when compared with thermodilution in a variety of clinical settings including post-cardiac surgery and in patients with pulmonary hypertension.

Pulse Contour Measurement

Pulse contour measurement of hemodynamic parameters can be achieved invasively with an arterial line (PiCCO, LiDCO, Flotrac) and noninvasively with a finger pneumatic cuff (Nexfin). Various formulas are used to compute CO values from the BP waveform.

The device provides a continuous beat-by-beat finger BP measure through the volume-clamp method (Figure 4-22). It then transforms the finger BP curve into a brachial arterial BP waveform and calculates CO from the brachial pressure pulse contour.

Hemodynamic parameters that can be measured with the noninvasive system are CO/index, systolic/diastolic BP, mean arterial pressure, HR, SV, stroke volume variation, pulse pressure variation, and SVR. It also includes pulse oximetry and noninvasive hemoglobin. The hemodynamic parameters will allow for the calculation of oxygen delivery.

The technology has been validated for measuring arterial pressure and has been found especially useful in cardiology clinics during tilt-test to detect orthostatic hypotension. It has also been used successfully in the perioperative management of patients. However, studies are needed to test the reliability of the measurement of CI in critically ill patients. The sensor should only be continuously used on a finger for an 8-hour period then moved to another finger.

Ambulatory Pulmonary Artery Pressure Monitoring

Ambulatory PA pressure monitoring measured by the CardioMEMS™ device correlates with PAP measurements by a PA catheter and echocardiography (Figure 4-23). The device is used in patients with heart failure NYHA class III who are on optimal therapy. The trial showed a 28% reduction of HF hospitalization in 6 months and 37% reduction in 15 months.

ESSENTIAL CONTENT CASE

Ambulatory PA Pressure Monitoring

A 75-year-old male diagnosed with heart failure with reduced EF (HFrEF) has been admitted to hospital three times in the past 6 months with progressively worsening heart failure. He is admitted for the placement of a CardioMems PA pressure monitoring device. Other comorbidities include diabetes, atrial fibrillation, CAD, COPD, and gout.

Medications included valsartan, carvedilol CR, spironolactone, furosemide, allopurinol, digoxin, warfarin, insulin, and metformin. Initial hemodynamic findings are:

EF	25%
CO	3.2 L/min
PA	65/32 mm Hg

Following implantation of the device, he has no further hospitalizations for a period of 1 year and six months. Adjustment of medications is made remotely.

Case Question 1. What is a normal PA systolic, diastolic, and mean?

Case Question 2. What is the benefit of ambulatory PA pressure monitoring?

Answers

1. A normal PA systolic is 15-35 mm Hg; PA diastolic is 10-15 mm Hg; PA mean is 15-20 mm Hg.
2. Ambulatory PA pressure monitoring allows the HCP to identify periods of nonadherence remotely. It allows for same day or next day medication adjustments to prevent decompensation. It greatly reduces readmission of patients for heart failure decompensation providing a more proactive approach to medical management.

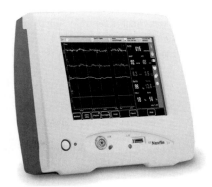

Figure 4-22. Nexfin System for noninvasive continuous hemodynamic monitoring. (*Used with permission from Edwards Lifesciences.*)

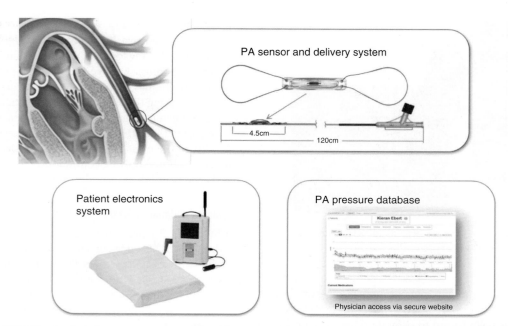

Figure 4-23. CardioMEMS HF system including pressure sensor and external measurement unit. CardioMEMS™ (*Cardio MEMS, Champion and St. Jude Medical are trademarks of St. Jude Medical, LLC or its related companies. Reproduced with permission of St. Jude Medical, ©2018. All rights reserved.*)

SELECTED BIBLIOGRAPHY

Hemodynamic Monitoring

AACN webinar: Integrating Functional Hemodynamics at the Point of Care, 2014. https://www.aacn.org/education/webinar-series/wb0014/integrating-functional-hemodynamics-at-the-point-of-care. Accessed March 20, 2018.

AACN webinar series: Live Q &A Functional Hemodyanmic Monitoring, 2015. https://www.aacn.org/education/webinar-series/wb0024/live-qa-functional-hemodynamic-monitoring. Accessed March 20, 2018.

Abraham WT, Adamson PB, Bourge RC, et al. Wireless pulmonary artery haemodynamic monitoring in chronic heart failure: a randomised controlled trial. *Lancet*. 2011;377(9766):658-666.

Ahrens TS. *Hemodynamic Waveform Recognition*. Philadelphia, PA: WB Saunders; 1993.

Ahrens TS, Taylor L. *Hemodynamic Waveform Analysis*. Philadelphia, PA: WB Saunders; 1992.

Alhashemi JA, Cecconi M, Hofer CK. Cardiac output monitoring: an integrative perspective. *Crit Care*. 2011;15(2):214.

Bernards J, Mekeirele M, Hoffmann B. Hemodynamic monitoring: to calibrate or not to calibrate? Part 2 – Non-calibrated techniques. *Anaesthesiol Intensive Ther*. 2015;47(5):501-516.

Casserly B, Read R, Levy MM. Hemodynamic monitoring in sepsis. *Crit Care Nurs Clin North Am*. 2011;23(1):149-169.

Cecconi M, Johnston E, Rhodes A. What role does the right side of the heart play in circulation? *Crit Care*. 2006;10(Suppl 3):S5.

Daily EK. Hemodynamic waveform analysis. *J Cardiovasc Nurs*. 2001;15(2):6-22.

de Waal EE, Wappler F, Buhre WF. Cardiac output monitoring. *Curr Opin Anaesthesiol*. 2009;22(1):71-77.

Glickman SW, Cairns CB, Otero RM, et al. Disease progression in hemodynamically stable patients presenting to the emergency department with sepsis. *Acad Emerg Med*. 2010;17(4):383-390.

Huygh J, Peeters Y, Bernards J. Hemodynamic monitoring in the critically ill: an overview of current cardiac output monitoring methods. *F1000Res*. 2016;5(F1000 Faculty Rev):2855.

Kanat N, Nichols M. CardioMEMS for effective management of heart failure: reducing healthcare utilization and 30 day readmissions. *Heart & Lung*. 2017;46(2017):211-214.

Kim HK, Pinsky MR. Effect of tidal volume, sampling duration, and cardiac contractility on pulse pressure and stroke volume variation during positive pressure ventilation. *Crit Care Med*. 2008;36(10):2858-2862.

Kim SH, Lilot M, Sidhu KS, et al. Accuracy and precision of continuous noninvasive arterial pressure monitoring compared with invasive arterial pressure: a systematic review and meta-analysis. *Anesthesiology*. 2014;120(5):1080-1097.

Langwieser N, Prechtl L, Meidert AS, et al. Radial artery applanation tonometry for continuous noninvasive arterial blood pressure monitoring in the cardiac intensive care unit. *Clin Res Cardiol*. 2015;104(6):518-524.

Latham HE, Rawson ST, Dwyer TT, et al. Peripherally inserted central catheters are equivalent to centrally inserted catheters in intensive care unit patients for central venous pressure monitoring. *J Clin Monit Comput*. 2012;26(2):85-90.

Lough ME. *Hemodynamic Monitoring: Evolving Technologies and Clinical Practice*. St Louis, MO: Elsevier; 2016.

Payen D, Gayat E. Which general intensive care unit patients can benefit from placement of the pulmonary artery catheter? *Crit Care*. 2006;10(Suppl 3):S7.

Peeters Y, Bernards J, Mekeirele M, et al. Hemodynamic monitoring: to calibrate or not to calibrate? Part 1 – Calibrated techniques. *Anaesthesiol Intensive Ther*. 2015;47(5):487-500.

Perel A, Habicher M, Sander M. Bench-to-bedside review: functional hemodynamics during surgery – should it be used for all high-risk cases? *Crit Care*. 2013;17(203):1-8.

Pinksy MR. Functional hemodynamic monitoring. *Curr Opin Crit Care*. 2014;20(3):288-293.

Pinksy MR. Functional hemodynamic monitoring. *Crit Care Clin.* 2015;31(1):89-111.

Pinksy MR. Understanding preload reserve using functional hemodynamic monitoring. *Intensive Care Med.* 2015;41(8):1480-1482.

Plante A, Ro E, Rowbottom JR. Hemodynamic and related challenges: monitoring and regulation in the postoperative period. *Anesthesiol Clin.* 2012;30(3):527-554.

Preister S, Case L, Deibert J. Pulmonary artery sensor (CardioMEMS) effect on hospital admissions and emergency department visits. *Heart & Lung.* 2017;46:215-219.

Quaal SJ. Improving the accuracy of pulmonary artery catheter measurement. *J Cardiovasc Nurs.* 2001;15(2):71-82.

Raina A, Benza RL. Ambulatory hemodynamic monitoring in the management of pulmonary arterial hypertension. *Adv Pulm Hypertens.* 2014;13(2):81-85.

Rajaram SS, Desai NK, Kalra A, et al. Pulmonary artery catheters for adult patients in intensive care. *Cochrane Database Syst Rev.* 2013;28(2):CD003408.

Reinhart K, Bloos F. The value of venous oximetry. *Curr Opin Crit Care.* 2005;11:259-263.

Richard C, Monnet X, Teboul JL. Pulmonary artery catheter monitoring in 2011. *Curr Opin Crit Care.* 2011;17(3):296-302.

Robin E, Costecalde M, Lebuffe G, Vallet B. Clinical relevance of data from the pulmonary artery catheter. *Crit Care.* 2006;10 (Suppl 3):S3.

Saggar R, Sitbon O. Hemodynamics in pulmonary arterial hypertension: current and future perspectives. *Am J Cardiol.* 2012;110(6 Suppl):9S-15S.

Sakka SG. Hemodynamic monitoring in the critically ill patient – current status and perspective. *Front Med (Lausanne).* 2015;2:44.

Sakka SG, Reuter DA, Perel A. The transpulmonary thermodilution technique. *J Clin Monit Comput.* 2012;26(5):347-353.

Saugel B, Malbrain ML, Perel A. Hemodynamic monitoring in the era of evidence-based. *Crit Care.* 2016;20:401.

Sauld C, Pedersen R, Sulemanjee N. Remote hemodynamic monitoring program: a single center experience in reducing heart failure admissions. *Heart & Lung.* 2017;46:215-219.

Sivarajan VB, Bohn D. Monitoring of standard hemodynamic parameters: heart rate, systemic blood pressure, atrial pressure, pulse oximetry, and end-tidal CO_2. *Pediatr Crit Care Med.* 2011;12(4 Suppl):S2-S11.

Tucker D, Hazinski MF. The nursing perspective on monitoring hemodynamics and oxygen transport. *Pediatr Crit Care Med.* 2011;12(4 Suppl):S72-S75.

Vakily A, Parsaei H, Movahhedi M, Sahmeddini M. A system for estimating and monitoring cardiac output via arterial waveform analysis. *J Biomed Phys Eng.* 2017;7(2):181-190.

Minimally Invasive Hemodynamic Monitoring

Aherns T, Sona C. Capnography application in acute and critical care. *AACN Clin Issues.* 2003;14(2):123-132.

Asamoto M, Orli R, Otsuji M, Bougaki M, Imai Y, Yamada Y. Reliability of cardiac output measurements using LiDCOrapid™ and FloTrac/Vigileo™ across broad ranges of cardiac output values. *J Clin Monit Comput.* 2017;31(4):709-716.

Avolio AP, Butlin M, Walsh A. Arterial blood pressure measurement and pulse wave analysis—their role in enhancing cardiovascular assessment. *Physiol Meas.* 2010;31(1):R1-47.

Bayram M, Yancy CW. Transthoracic impedance cardiography: a noninvasive method of hemodynamic assessment. *Heart Fail Clin.* 2009;5(2):161-168.

Bogert LW, van Lieshout JJ. Non-invasive pulsatile arterial pressure and stroke volume changes from the human finger. *Exp Physiol.* 2005;90(4):437-446.

Boyd JH, Walley KR. The role of echocardiography in hemodynamic monitoring. *Curr Opin Crit Care.* 2009;15(3):239-243.

Camporota L, Beale R. Pitfalls in hemodynamic monitoring based on the arterial pressure waveform. *Crit Care.* 2010;14(2):124.

Compton F, Schäfer JH. Noninvasive cardiac output determination: broadening the applicability of hemodynamic monitoring. *Semin Cardiothorac Vasc Anesth.* 2009;13(1):44-55.

de Jong RM, Westerhof BE, Voors AA, van Veldhuisen DJ. Noninvasive haemodynamic monitoring using finger arterial pressure waveforms. *Neth J Med.* 2009;67(11):372-375.

Fellahi JL, Caille V, Charron C, Deschamps-Berger PH, Vieillard-Baron A. Noninvasive assessment of cardiac index in healthy volunteers: a comparison between thoracic impedance cardiography and Doppler echocardiography. *Anesth Analg.* 2009;108(5):1553-1559.

Franchi F, Silvestri R, Cubattoli L, et al. Comparison between an uncalibrated pulse contour method and thermodilution technique for cardiac output estimation in septic patients. *Br J Anaesth.* 2011;107(2):202-208.

Ghanayem NS, Wernovsky G, Hoffman GM. Near infrared spectroscopy as a hemodynamic monitor in critical illness. *Pediatr Crit Care Med.* 2011;12(4 Suppl):S27-S32.

Hett DA, Jonas MM. Non-invasive cardiac output monitoring. *Intensive Crit Care Nurs.* 2004;20(2):103-108.

Horster S, Stemmler HJ, Sparrer J, et al. Mechanical ventilation with positive end-expiratory pressure in critically ill patients: comparison of CW-Doppler ultrasound cardiac output monitoring (USCOM) and thermodilution (PiCCO). *Acta Cardiol.* 2012;67(2):177-185.

Lima A, Bakker J. Noninvasive monitoring of peripheral perfusion. *Intensive Care Med.* 2005;31:1316-1326.

Lima MV, Ochiai ME, Vieira KN, et al. Continuous noninvasive hemodynamic monitoring in decompensated heart failure. *Arq Bras Cardiol.* 2012;99(3):843-847.

Magder S. Central venous pressure: a useful but not so simple measurement. *Crit Care Med.* 2006;34(8):2224-2227.

Marik P, Levitov A, Young A, et al. The use of bioreactance and carotid Doppler to determine volume responsiveness and blood flow redistribution following passive leg raising in hemodynamically unstable patients. *Chest.* 2013;143(2):364-370.

Marik PE. Noninvasive cardiac output monitors: a state-of the-art review. *J Cardiothorac Vasc Anesth.* 2013;27:121-34.

Marik PE. Regional carbon dioxide monitoring to assess the adequacy of tissue perfusion. *Curr Opin Crit Care.* 2005;11:245-251.

Marino R, Magrini L, Ferri E, Gagliano G, Di Somma, S. B-type natriuretic peptide and non-invasive haemodynamics and hydration status assessments in the management of patients with acute heart failure in the emergency department. *High Blood Press Cardiovasc Prev.* 2010;17(4):1-7.

Marquél S, Cariou A, Chiche JD, Squara P. Comparison between flotrac-vigileo and bioreactance, a totally noninvasive method for cardiac output monitoring. *Crit Care.* 2009;13(3):R73.

Mesquida J, Gruartmoner G, Espinal C. Skeletal muscle oxygen saturation (StO₂) measured by near-infrared spectroscopy in the critically ill patients. *Biomed Res Int.* 2013;2013:502194.

Middleton PM, Davies SR. Noninvasive hemodynamic monitoring in the emergency department. *Curr Opin Crit Care.* 2011;17(4):342-350.

Napoli AM. Physiologic and clinical principles behind noninvasive resuscitation techniques and cardiac output monitoring. *Cardiol Res Pract.* 2012;2012:531908.

Napoli AM, Machan JT, Corl K, Forcada A. The use of impedance cardiography in predicting mortality in emergency department patients with severe sepsis and septic shock. *Acad Emer Med.* 2010;17(4):452-455.

Nardi O, Polito A, Aboab J, et al. StO₂ guided early resuscitation in subjects with severe sepsis or septic shock: a randomised trial. *J Clin Monit Comput.* 2013;27(3):215-221.

Nelson MR, Stepanek J, Cevette M, et al. Noninvasive measurement of central vascular pressures with arterial tonometry: clinical revival of the pulse pressure waveform? *Mayo Clin Proc.* 2010;85(5):460-472.

Nguyen HB, Banta DP, Stewart G, et al. Cardiac index measurements by transcutaneous Doppler ultrasound and transthoracic echocardiography in adult and pediatric emergency patients. *J Clin Monit Comput.* 2010;24(3):237-247.

Nicklas JY, Saugel B. Non-invasive hemodynamic monitoring for hemodynamic management in perioperative medicine. *Front Med (Lausanne).* 2017;23(4):209.

Noritomi DT, Vieira ML, Mohovic T, et al. Echocardiography for hemodynamic evaluation in the intensive care unit. *Shock.* 2010;34(Suppl 1):59-62.

Nowak RM, Sen A, Garcia AJ, et al. The inability of emergency physicians to adequately clinically estimate the underlying hemodynamic profiles of acutely ill patients. *Am J Emerg Med.* 2012;30(6):954-960.

Ospina-Tascon GA, Cordioli RL, Vincent JL. What type of monitoring has been shown to improve outcomes in acutely ill patients? *Intensive Care Med.* 2008;34(5):800-820.

Sakka SG. Hemodynamic monitoring in the critically ill patient – current status and perspective. *Front. Med (Lausanne).* 2015;2:44.

Silver MA, Cianci P, Brennan S, Longeran-Thomas H, Ahmad F. Evaluation of impedance cardiography as an alternative to pulmonary artery catheterization in critically ill patients. *Congest Heart Fail.* 2004;10(Suppl 2):17-21.

Temporelli PL, Scapellato F, Eleuteri E, Imparato A, Giannuzzi P. Doppler echocardiography in advanced systolic heart failure: a noninvasive alternative to Swan-Ganz catheter. *Circ Heart Fail.* 2010;3(3):387-394

Truijen J, van Lieshout JJ, Wesselink WA, Westerhof BE. Noninvasive continuous hemodynamic monitoring. *J Clin Monit Comput.* 2012;26(4):267-278.

van der Spoel AG, Voogel AJ, Folkers A, Boer C, Bouwman RA. Comparison of noninvasive continuous arterial waveform analysis (Nexfin) with transthoracic Doppler echocardiography for monitoring of cardiac output. *J Clin Anesth.* 2012;24(4):304-309.

van Genderen ME, van Bommel J, Lima A. Monitoring peripheral perfusion in critically ill patients at the bedside. *Curr Opin Crit Care.* 2012;18(3):273-279.

Yung GL, Fedullo PF, Kinninger K, Johnson W, Channick RN. Comparison of impedance cardiography to direct Fick and thermodilution cardiac output determination in pulmonary arterial hypertension. *Congest Heart Fail.* 2004;10(2 Suppl 2):7-10.

Zhang X, Xuan W, Yin P, et al. Gastric tonometry guided therapy in critical care patients: a systematic review and meta-analysis. *Crit Care.* 2015;19:22.

Zhang Z, Xu X, Yao M, et al. Use of PiCCO system in critically ill patients with septic shock and acute respiratory distress syndrome. *Trials.* 2013;14:32.

Zimlichman E, Szyper-Kravitz M, Shinar Z, et al. Early recognition of acutely deteriorating patients in non-intensive care units: assessment of an innovative monitoring technology. *J Hosp Med.* 2012;7(8):628-633.

Therapeutics

Bentzer P, Griesdale DE, Boyd J, et al. Will this hemodynamically unstable patient respond to a bolus of intravenous fluids? *JAMA.* 2016;316(12):1298-1309.

Biais M, Ouattara A. Janvier G, Sztark F. Case scenario: respiratory variations in arterial pressure for guiding fluid management in mechanically ventilated patients. *Anesthesiology.* 2012;116(6):1354-1361.

Bridges E. Using functional hemodynamic indicators to guide fluid therapy. *Am Jour Nurs.* 2013;113(5):42-50.

Buerke M, Lemm H, Dietz S, Werdan K. Pathophysiology, diagnosis, and treatment of infarction–related cardiogenic shock. *Herz.* 2011;36(2):73-83.

Cecconi M, Arulkumaran N, Kilic J, Ebm C, Rhodes A. Update on hemodynamic monitoring and management in septic patients. *Minerva Anestesiol.* 2014;80(6):701-711.

Cecconi M, Monge Garcia MI, Gracia Romero M, et al. The use of pulse pressure variation and stroke volume variation in spontaneously breathing patients to assess dynamic arterial elastance and to predict arterial pressure response to fluid administration. *Anesth Analg.* 2015;120(1):76-84.

Cherpanath TG, Hirsch A, Geerts BF, et al. Predicting fluid responsiveness of passive leg raising: a systematic review and meta-analysis of 23 clinical trials. *Crit Care Med.* 2016;44(5):981-991.

De Backer D, Creteur J, Dubois M, et al. The effects of dobutamine on microcirculatory alterations in patients with septic shock are independent of its systemic effects. *Crit Care Med.* 2006;34(2):403-408.

Deedwania PC, Carbajal E. Evidence-based therapy for heart failure. *Med Clin North Am.* 2012;96(5):915-931.

Dellinger RP, Levy MM, Rhodes A, et al. Surviving sepsis campaign: international guidelines for management of severe sepsis and septic shock, 2012. *Intensive Care Med.* 2013;39(2):165-228.

Dellinger RP, Levy MM, Rhodes A, et al. Surviving sepsis campaign: international guidelines for management of severe sepsis and septic shock: 2012. *Crit Care Med.* 2013;41(2):580-637.

Di Giantomasso D, Morimatsu H, May CN. Increasing renal blood flow: low-dose dopamine or medium-dose norepinephrine. *Chest*. 2004;125(6):2260-2267.

Faybik P, Hetz H, Baker A. Iced versus room temperature injectate for assessment of cardiac output, intrathoracic blood volume, and extravascular lung water by single transpulmonary thermodilution. *J Crit Care*. 2004;19(2):103-107.

Felker GM, Lee KL, Bull DA, et al. Diuretic strategies in patients with acute decompensated heart failure. *N Engl J Med*. 2011;364(9):797-805.

Fellahi JL, Brossier D, Dechanet F, et al. Early goal-directed therapy based on endotracheal bioimpedance cardiography: a prospective, randomized controlled study in coronary surgery. *J Clin Monit Comput*. 2015;29(3):351-358.

Ferguson-Myrthil N. Vasopressor use in adult patients. *Cardiol Rev*. 2012;20(3):153-158.

Havel C, Arrich J, Losert H, et al. Vasopressors for hypotensive shock. *Cochrane Database Syst Rev*. 2011;11(5):CD003709.

Heart Failure Society of America, Lindenfield J, Albert NM, et al. HFSA 2010 Comprehensive Heart Failure Practice Guideline. *J Card Fail*. 2010;16:e1.

Hollenberg SM. Inotrope and vasopressor therapy of septic shock. *Crit Care Clin*. 2009;25(4):781-802.

Honore PM, Spapen HD. Passive leg raising test with minimally invasive monitoring: the way forward for guiding septic shock resuscitation? *J Intensive Care*. 2017;5(36):1-3.

Howell MD, Davis AM. Management of sepsis and septic shock. *JAMA*. 2017;317(8):847-848.

Jansen TC, van Bommel J, Mulder PG, et al. The prognostic value of blood lactate levels relative to that of vital signs in the pre-hospital setting: a pilot study. *Crit Care*. 2008;12:R160.

Kampmeier TG, Rehberg S, Westphal M, Lange M. Vasopressin in sepsis and septic shock. *Minerva Anestesiol*. 2010;76(10):844-850.

Kapoor PM, Kakani M, Chowdhury U, et al. Early goal-directed therapy in moderate to high-risk cardiac surgery patients. *Ann Card Anaesth*. 2008;11(1):27-34.

Kelm DJ, Perrin JT, Cartin-Ceba R, et al. Fluid overload in patients with severe sepsis and septic shock treated with early goal-directed therapy is associated with increased acute need for fluid-related medical interventions and hospital death. *Shock*. 2015;43(1):68-73.

Khot UN, Novaro GM, Popović ZB. Nitroprusside in critically ill patients with left ventricular dysfunction and aortic stenosis. *N Engl J Med*. 2003;348(18):1756-1763.

Klijn E, van Velzen MHN, Lima PA. Tissue perfusion and oxygenation to monitor fluid responsiveness in critically ill, septic patients after initial resuscitation: a prospective observational study. *J Clin Monit Comput*. 2015;29:707-712.

Krejci V, Hiltebrand LB, Sigurdsson GH. Effects of epinephrine, norepinephrine and phenylephrine on microcirculatory blood flow in the gastrointestinal tract in sepsis. *Crit Care Med*. 2006;34(5):1456-1463.

Landoni G, Biondi-Zoccai G, Greco M, et al. Effects of levosimendan on mortality and hospitalization. A meta-analysis of randomized controlled studies. *Crit Care Med*. 2012;40(2):634-646.

Lewis SR, Butler AR, Brammar A, et al. Perioperative fluid volume optimization following proximal femoral fracture. *Cochrane Database Syst Rev*. 2016;3:CD003004.

Li C, Lin FQ, Fu SK, et al. Stroke volume variation for prediction of fluid responsiveness in patients undergoing gastrointestinal surgery. *Int J Med Sci*. 2013;10(2):148-155.

Liu SS, Monti J, Kargbo HM, et al. Frontiers of therapy for patients with heart failure. *Am J Med*. 2013;126(1):6-12.

Malliotakis P, Xenikakis T, Linardakis M, Hassoulas J. Haemodynamic effects of levosimendan for low cardiac output after cardiac surgery: a case series. *Hellenic J Cardiol*. 2007;48(2):80-88.

Mangi MA, Rehman H, Rafique M, et al. Ambulatory heart failure monitoring: a systemic review. *Cureus*. 2017;9(4):e1174.

Marik PE, Cavallazzi R. Does the central venous pressure predict fluid responsiveness? An updated meta-analysis and a plea for some common sense. *Crit Care Med*. 2013;41:1774-1781.

Monnet X, Teboul JL. Passive leg raising: five rules, not a drop of fluid! *Crit Care*. 2015;19(18):1-3.

Myburgh J. Norepinephrine: more of a neurohormone than a vasopressor. *Crit Care*. 2010;14(5):196.

O'Connor CM, Starling RC, Hernandez AF, et al. Effect of nesiritide in patients with acute decompensated heart failure. *N Engl J Med*. 2011;365(1):32-43.

Osawa EA, Rhodes A, Landoni G, et al. Effect of perioperative goal-directed hemodynamic resuscitation therapy on outcomes following cardiac surgery: a randomized clinical trial and systematic review. *Crit Care Med*. 2016;44(4):724-733.

Parissis JT, Rafouli-Stergiou P, Stasinos V, et al. Intropes in cardiac patients: update 2011. *Curr Opin Crit Care*. 2010;16(5):432-441.

Pearse RM, Harrison DA, MacDonald N, et al. Effect of a perioperative, cardiac output-guided hemodynamic therapy algorithm on outcomes following major gastrointestinal surgery: a randomized clinical trial and systematic review. *JAMA*. 2014;311(21):2181-2190.

Pickett JD, Bridges E, Kritek PA. Passive leg-raising and prediction of fluid responsiveness: systematic review. *Crit Care Nurse*. 2017;37(2):32-48.

Pinto BB, Rehberg S, Ertmer C, Westphal M. Role of levosimendan in sepsis and septic shock. *Curr Opin Anaesthesiol*. 2008;21(2):168-177.

Puskarich MA. Emergency management of severe sepsis and septic shock. *Curr Opin Crit Care*. 2012;18(4):295-300.

Richards AM, Troughton RW. Use of natriuretic peptides to guide and monitor heart failure therapy. *Clin Chem*. 2012;58(1):62-71.

Rivers E, Nguyen B, Havestad S, et al. Early goal-directed therapy on the treatment of severe sepsis and septic shock. *NEJM*. 2001;345(19):1368-1377.

Ruggiero M. Effects of vasopressin in septic shock. *AACN Adv Crit Care*. 2008;19(3):281-287.

Russell JA. Bench-to-bedside review: vasopressin in the management of septic shock. *Crit Care*. 2011;15(4):226.

Sandifer JP, Jones AE. Dopamine versus norepinephrine for the treatment of septic shock EBEM commentators. *Ann Emerg Med*. 2012;60(3):372-373.

Shoemaker WC, Wo CC, Yu S. Invasive and noninvasive hemodynamic monitoring of acutely ill sepsis and septic shock patients in the emergency department. *Eur J Emerg Med.* 2000;7(3):169-175.

Teerlink JR, Metra M, Zacà V, et al. Agents with inotropic properties for the management of acute heart failure syndromes. Traditional agents and beyond. *Heart Fail Rev.* 2009;14(4):243-253.

Vollman KM. Understanding critically ill patients hemodynamic response to mobilization: using the evidence to make it safe and feasible. *Crit Care Nurs Q.* 2013;56(1):17-27.

Wohlfahrt P, Melenovsky V, Redfield MM, et al. Aortic waveform analysis to individualize treatment in heart failure. *Circ Heart Fail.* 2017;10:e003516.

Zafir B, Amir O. Beta blocker therapy, decompensated heart failure, and inotropic interactions: current perspectives. *Isr Med Assoc J.* 2012;14(3):184-189.

Zanotti Cavazzoni SL, Dellinger RP. Hemodynamic optimization of sepsis-induced tissue hypoperfusion. *Crit Care.* 2006;10 (Suppl 3):S2.

Evidence-Based Practice Guidelines

AACN Practice Alert: Alarm Management. 2013. https://www .aacn.org/clinical-resources/practice-alerts/alarmmanagement. Accessed February 27, 2018.

AACN Practice Alert: Pulmonary Artery/Central Venous Pressure Monitoring in Adults. 2016. https://www.aacn.org/ clinical-resources/practice-alerts/pulmonary-artery-pressure-measurement. Accessed June 30, 2017.

Cecconi M, De Backer D, Antonelli M, et al. Consensus on circulatory shock and hemodynamic monitoring. Task force of the European Society of Intensive Care Medicine. *Intensive Care Med.* 2014;40:1795-1815.

Rauen CA, Makic MB, Bridges E. Evidence-based practice habits: transforming research into bedside practice. *Crit Care Nurse.* 2009;29:46-59.

AIRWAY AND VENTILATORY MANAGEMENT

5

Robert E. St. John and Maureen A. Seckel

KNOWLEDGE COMPETENCIES

1. Interpret normal and abnormal arterial blood gas (ABG) results and determine common management strategies for treatment.

2. Identify indications, complications, and management strategies for artificial airways, oxygen delivery, and monitoring devices.

3. Identify pulmonary and nonpulmonary factors important to the promotion of positive weaning

outcomes in long-term mechanically ventilated (LTMV) patients.

4. Describe the concepts of respiratory muscle fatigue, rest, and conditioning as they relate to the mechanically ventilated weaning patient.

5. Identify essential components for the successful design and use of weaning predictors, protocols for weaning trials, and multidisciplinary institutional approaches to the care of LTMV patients.

DIAGNOSTIC TESTS, MONITORING SYSTEMS, AND RESPIRATORY ASSESSMENT TECHNIQUES

Arterial Blood Gas Monitoring

Arterial blood gas (ABG) monitoring may be used to assess acid-base balance, ventilation, and oxygenation. An arterial blood sample is analyzed for oxygen tension (Pao_2), carbon dioxide tension ($Paco_2$), and pH using a blood gas analyzer. From these measurements, several other parameters are calculated by the blood gas analyzer, including base excess (BE), bicarbonate (HCO_3), and oxygen saturation (Sao_2). Fractional arterial Sao_2 can be directly measured if a co-oximeter is available. Normal ABG values are listed in Table 5-1.

ABG samples are obtained by direct puncture of an artery, usually the radial artery, or by withdrawing blood through an indwelling arterial catheter system. A heparinized syringe is used to collect the sample to prevent clotting of the blood prior to analysis. Blood gas samples are kept on ice unless there is the ability to immediately analyze to prevent the continued transfer of CO_2 and O_2 in and out of the red blood cells. ABG analysis equipment is often kept in or near progressive care units to maximize accuracy and decrease the

time for reporting of results. Additionally, portable point-of-care devices are available at many hospitals that allow measurement at the bedside. Regardless of the method used to obtain the ABG sample, practitioners should wear gloves and follow standard precautions to prevent exposure to blood during the sampling procedure.

Techniques
Indwelling Arterial Catheters
Pressure monitoring systems used with indwelling arterial catheters have sites where samples of arterial blood can be withdrawn for ABG analysis or other laboratory testing (Figure 5-1). Using the stopcock closest to the catheter insertion site, or the indwelling syringe or reservoir of the needleless systems, a 3- to 5-mL sample of blood is withdrawn to clear the catheter system of any flush system fluid. A 1-mL sample for ABG analysis is then obtained in a heparinized syringe. Any air remaining in the syringe is then removed, an airtight cap is placed on the end of the syringe, and the sample is placed on ice to ensure accuracy of the measurement. The arterial catheter system is then flushed to clear the line of any residual blood.

TABLE 5-1. LABORATORY AND CALCULATED RESPIRATORY VALUES

Parameter	Value
Arterial Blood Gases	
• pH	7.35-7.45
• $Paco_2$	35-45 mm Hg
• HCO_3^-	22-26 mEq/L
• Base excess	− 2 to + 2 mEq/L
• Pao_2	80-100 mm Hg (normals vary with age and altitude)
• Sao_2	> 95% (normals vary with age and altitude)
Mixed Venous Blood Gases	
• pH	7.32-7.42
• $Pmvco_2$	40-50 mm Hg
• $Pmvo_2$	35-45 mm Hg
• Svo_2	60%-80%
Respiratory Parameters	
• Tidal volume (V_T)	6-8 mL/kg
• Respiratory rate	8-16/min
• Respiratory static compliance	70-100 mL/cm H_2O
• Inspiratory force (IF)	≤ − 20 cm H_2O
Respiratory Calculations	
• Alveolar gas equation (Pao_2)	$Pao_2 = Fio_2(P_{ATM} - PH_2O)$ $- \dfrac{Paco_2}{RQ \text{ (Respiratory quotient)}}$
• Static compliance	$V_T/$(Plateau pressure − PEEP)

Complications associated with this technique for obtaining ABG samples include infection and hemorrhage. Any time an invasive system is used, the potential exists for contamination of the sterile system. The use of needleless systems on indwelling catheter systems decreases patients' risk for infection, as well as the progressive care practitioners' risk for accidental needlestick injuries, and should be used whenever feasible. Hemorrhage is a rare complication, occurring when stopcocks are inadvertently left in the wrong position after blood withdrawal or when the tubing is disconnected. These complications can be avoided by carefully following the proper technique during blood sampling, limiting sample withdrawal to experienced practitioners, assuring connections are tight, and keeping the pressure alarm system of the bedside monitoring system activated at all times.

Arterial Puncture

When indwelling arterial catheters are not in place, ABG samples are obtained by directly puncturing the artery with a needle and syringe. The most common sites for arterial puncture are the radial, brachial, and femoral arteries. Similar to venipuncture, the technique for obtaining an ABG sample is relatively simple, but success in obtaining the sample requires experience.

An Allen test is performed prior to obtaining an ABG by puncture and prior to the insertion of an arterial line into the radial artery. The Allen test requires that the ulnar and radial pulses be occluded for a brief period of time with the forearm held upward to facilitate blood emptying from the hand. Once blanching of the hand is observed, the forearm is placed in a downward position, the ulnar artery is released, and the hand is observed for flushing. If the hand flushes, it is clear that the ulnar artery is capable of supplying blood to the fingers should the radial artery be damaged.

Following location of the pulsating artery and antiseptic preparation of the skin, the needle is inserted into the artery at a 45° angle with the bevel facing upward. The needle is slowly advanced until arterial blood appears in the syringe barrel or the insertion depth is below the artery location. If blood is not obtained, the needle is pulled back to just below the skin and relocation of the pulsating artery is verified prior to advancing the needle again.

As soon as the 1-mL sample of arterial blood is obtained, the syringe is withdrawn and firm pressure quickly applied to the insertion site with a sterile gauze pad. Handheld pressure is maintained for at least 5 minutes and the site inspected for bleeding or oozing. If present, pressure is reapplied until all evidence of oozing has stopped. Pressure dressings are not applied until hemostasis has been achieved.

As described, all air must be removed from the ABG syringe and an airtight cap applied to the end (remove the needle first). Given the importance of maintaining pressure at the puncture site, it is sometimes helpful to have another practitioner assisting during arterial puncture to ensure appropriate handling of the blood sample.

Complications associated with arterial puncture include arterial vessel tears, air embolism, hemorrhage, arterial obstruction, loss of extremity, and infection. Using a proper technique during sampling can dramatically decrease the incidence of these complications. Damage to the artery may be decreased by using a small diameter needle (21-23 gauge in adults) and by avoiding multiple attempts at the same site. After one or two failed attempts at entering the artery, a different site is selected or another experienced practitioner enlisted to attempt the ABG sampling. All facilities have specific policies and procedures providing guidance on sample acquisition and handling of ABGs and the reader is encouraged to follow their institutional guidelines.

Hemorrhage can occur easily into the surrounding tissues if adequate hemostasis is not achieved with direct pressure following the puncture. Bleeding into the tissue can range from small blood loss with minimal local damage to large blood loss with loss of distal circulation and even exsanguination. Large blood loss is more commonly seen with femoral punctures and is often the result of inadequate pressure on the artery following needle removal. Bleeding from the femoral artery is difficult to visualize, so significant blood loss can occur before practitioners are alerted to the problem. For this reason, the femoral site is the least preferred site for ABG sampling and is used only when other sites are not accessible.

The need for frequent ABG sampling for ventilation and oxygenation assessment and management may require the insertion of an arterial catheter and monitoring

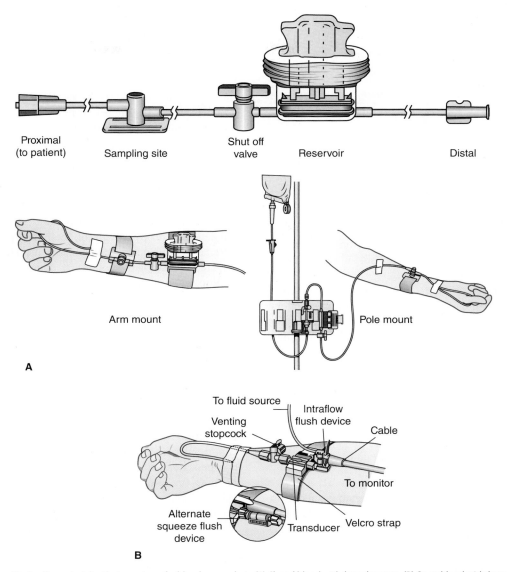

Proximal (to patient)   Sampling site   Shut off valve   Reservoir   Distal

Arm mount   Pole mount

A

To fluid source
Venting stopcock
Intraflow flush device
Cable
To monitor
Alternate squeeze flush device
Transducer   Velcro strap

B

Figure 5-1. Examples of indwelling arterial catheter systems for blood gas analysis. **(A)** Closed blood withdrawal system. **(B)** Open blood withdrawal system. (*Used with permission from Edwards Lifesciences [A].*)

system to decrease the risks associated with repetitive arterial punctures.

Analysis

The best approach to analyzing the results of ABGs is a systematic one. Analysis is accomplished by evaluating acid-base and oxygenation status. Upon receipt of ABG results, the practitioner first identifies any abnormal values (see Table 5-1). Then a systematic evaluation of acid-base and oxygenation status is done.

Acid-Base Analysis

Optimal cellular functioning occurs when the pH of the blood is between 7.35 and 7.45. Decreases in pH below 7.35 are termed *acidemia*, and increases in pH above 7.45 are termed *alkalemia*. When the amount of acids or bases in the body increases or decreases, the pH changes if the

ratio of acids to bases is altered. For example, if acid production increases, and there is no change in the amount of base production, pH decreases. If the base production were to increase as well, as a response to increased acid production, then no change in pH would occur because the ratio of acids to bases would be maintained. Because the body functions best at a pH in the 7.35 to 7.45 range, there are strong systems in place to maintain the balance between acids and bases, even if one of those components is functioning abnormally. Although a variety of regulatory systems are involved in acid-base balance, the bicarbonate ((HCO_3^-)) and carbon dioxide (CO_2) levels are the primary regulators.

- *Metabolic component*: HCO_3^- levels are controlled primarily by the kidneys and are called the metabolic component of the acid-base system. By increasing or decreasing the amount of HCO_3^- excreted in the

TABLE 5-2. ACID-BASE ABNORMALITIES

Acid-Base Abnormality	Primary ABG Abnormalities			ABG Changes With Compensation (If Present)	
	pH	$Paco_2$	(HCO_3^-)	Respiratory ($Paco_2$)	Metabolic (HCO_3^-)
Alkalemia					
Metabolic	↑		↑	↑	
Respiratory	↑	↓			↓
Acidemia					
Metabolic	↓		↓	↓	
Respiratory	↓	↑			↑

kidneys, the pH of the blood can be increased or decreased. Changes in HCO_3^- excretion may take up to 24 hours or longer to accomplish, but can be maintained for prolonged periods.

- *Respiratory component:* CO_2 levels are controlled primarily by the lungs and are called the respiratory component of the acid-base system. By increasing or decreasing the amount of CO_2 excreted by the lungs, the pH of the blood can be increased or decreased. Changes in CO_2 excretion can occur rapidly, within a minute, by increasing or decreasing the rate or depth of respiration (minute ventilation). Compensation by the respiratory system is difficult to maintain over long periods of time (24 hours).
- *Acid-base abnormalities:* A variety of conditions may result in acid-base abnormalities (Tables 5-2 and 5-3).

Metabolic alkalemia is present when the pH is above 7.45 and the HCO_3^- is above 26 mEq/L. In metabolic alkalosis, there is either a primary increase in hydrogen ion (H_1) loss or HCO_3^- gain. The respiratory system attempts to compensate for the increased pH by decreasing the amount of CO_2 eliminated from the body (alveolar hypoventilation). This compensatory attempt by the respiratory system results in a change in pH, but rarely to a normal value. Clinical situations or conditions that cause metabolic alkalemia include loss of body acids (nasogastric suction of HCl, vomiting, excessive diuretic therapy, steroids, hypokalemia) and ingestion of exogenous bicarbonate or citrate substances. Management of metabolic alkalosis is directed at treating the underlying

cause, decreasing or stopping the acid loss (eg, use of anti-emetic therapy for vomiting), and replacing electrolytes.

Metabolic acidemia is present when the pH is below 7.35 and the HCO_3^- is below 22 mEq/L. In metabolic acidosis, there is excessive loss of HCO_3^- from the body by the kidneys or the accumulation of acid. The respiratory system attempts to compensate for the decreased pH by increasing the amount of CO_2 eliminated (alveolar hyperventilation). This compensatory attempt by the respiratory system results in a change in pH toward normal. Clinical situations or conditions that cause metabolic acidosis include increased metabolic formation of acids (diabetic ketoacidosis, uremic acidosis, lactic acidosis), loss of bicarbonate (diarrhea, renal tubular acidosis), hyperkalemia, toxin ingestion (salicylates overdose, ethylene and propylene glycol, methanol, paraldehyde), and adrenal insufficiency. Management of metabolic acidosis is directed at treating the underlying cause, decreasing acid formation (eg, decreasing lactic acid production by improving cardiac output [CO] in shock), decreasing bicarbonate losses (eg, treatment of diarrhea), and removal of toxins through dialysis or cathartics. When metabolic acidosis is severe and the underlying cause is not amenable to rapid correction, administration of sodium bicarbonate ($NaHCO_3$) may be considered.

Respiratory alkalemia occurs when the pH is above 7.45 and the $Paco_2$ is below 35 mm Hg. In respiratory alkalosis, there is an excessive amount of ventilation (alveolar hyperventilation) and removal of CO_2 from the body. If these changes persist for 24 hours or more, the kidneys attempt to compensate for the elevated pH by increasing the excretion of HCO_3^- until normal or near-normal pH levels occur. Clinical situations or conditions that cause respiratory alkalosis include neurogenic hyperventilation, interstitial lung diseases, pulmonary embolism, asthma, acute anxiety/stress/fear, hyperventilation syndromes, excessive mechanical ventilation, and severe hypoxemia. Management of respiratory alkalosis is directed at treating the underlying cause and decreasing excessive ventilation, if possible.

Respiratory acidemia occurs when the pH is below 7.35 and the $Paco_2$ is above 45 mm Hg. In respiratory acidosis, there is an inadequate amount of ventilation (alveolar hypoventilation) and removal of CO_2 from the body. If these changes persist for 24 hours or more, the kidneys attempt to

TABLE 5-3. EXAMPLES OF ARTERIAL BLOOD GAS RESULTS

ABG Analysis	pH	$Paco_2$ (mm Hg)	HCO_3^- (mEq/L)	Base Excess	Pao_2 (mm Hg)	Sao_2 (%)
Normal ABG	7.37	38	24	−1	85	96
Respiratory acidosis, no compensation, with hypoxemia	7.28	51	25	−1	63	89
Metabolic acidosis, no compensation, without hypoxemia	7.23	35	14	−12	92	97
Metabolic alkalosis, partial compensation, without hypoxemia	7.49	48	37	+11	84	95
Respiratory acidosis, full compensation, with hypoxemia	7.35	59	33	+6	55	86
Respiratory alkalosis, no compensation, with hypoxemia	7.52	31	24	0	60	88
Metabolic acidosis, partial compensation, with hypoxemia	7.30	29	16	−9	54	85
Laboratory error	7.31	32	28	0	92	96

compensate for the decreased pH by increasing the amount of HCO_3^- in the body (decreased excretion of HCO_3^- in the urine) until normal or near-normal pH levels occur. Clinical situations or conditions that cause respiratory acidosis include hypoventilation associated with respiratory failure (eg, acute respiratory distress syndrome [ARDS], severe asthma, pneumonia, chronic obstructive pulmonary diseases [COPD], and sleep apnea), pulmonary embolism, pulmonary edema, pneumothorax, respiratory center depression, and neuromuscular disturbances in the presence of normal lungs, and inadequate mechanical ventilation. Management of respiratory acidosis is directed at treating the underlying cause and improving ventilation.

Mixed (combined) disturbance is the simultaneous development of a primary respiratory and metabolic acid-base disturbance. For example, metabolic acidosis may occur from diabetic ketoacidosis, with respiratory acidosis occurring from respiratory failure associated with aspiration pneumonia. Mixed acid-base disturbances create a more complex picture when examining ABGs and are beyond the scope of this text.

Oxygenation

After determining the acid-base status from the ABG, the adequacy of oxygenation is assessed. Normal values for PaO_2 depend on age and altitude. Lower levels of PaO_2 are acceptable as normal with increasing age and altitude levels. In general, PaO_2 levels between 80 and 100 mm Hg are considered normal on room air.

SaO_2 levels are also affected by age and altitude, with values above 95% considered normal. Hemoglobin saturation with oxygen is primarily influenced by the amount of available oxygen in the plasma (Figure 5-2). The S shape to the normal oxyhemoglobin dissociation curve emphasizes that as long as PaO_2 levels are above 60 mm Hg with an arterial

pH above 7.35, 90% or more of the hemoglobin is bound or saturated with O_2. Factors that can shift the oxyhemoglobin curve to the right and left include temperature, pH, $PaCO_2$, and abnormal hemoglobin conditions. In general, shifting the curve to the right (reducing the pH) decreases the affinity of oxygen for hemoglobin, resulting in an increase in the amount of oxygen released to the tissues. Shifting of the curve to the left (increasing the pH) increases the affinity of oxygen for hemoglobin, resulting in a decreased amount of oxygen released to the tissues.

A decrease in PaO_2 below normal values is *hypoxemia*. A variety of conditions cause hypoxemia:

- *Low inspired oxygen:* Usually, the fraction of inspired oxygen concentration (FiO_2) is reduced at high altitudes or when toxic gases are inhaled. Inadequate or inappropriately low FiO_2 administration may contribute to hypoxic respiratory failure in patients with other cardiopulmonary diseases.
- *Overall hypoventilation:* Decreases in tidal volume (V_T), respiratory rate, or both reduce minute ventilation and cause hypoventilation. Alveoli are underventilated, leading to a fall in alveolar oxygen tension (PaO_2) and increased $PaCO_2$ levels. Causes of hypoventilation include respiratory center depression from drug overdose, anesthesia, excessive analgesic administration, neuromuscular disturbances, and fatigue.
- *Ventilation-perfusion mismatch:* When the balance between adequately ventilated and perfused alveoli is altered, hypoxemia develops. Perfusion of blood past underventilated alveoli decreases the availability of oxygen for gas exchange, leading to poorly oxygenated blood in the pulmonary vasculature. Examples of this include bronchospasm, atelectasis, secretion retention, pneumonia, pulmonary embolism, and pulmonary edema.
- *Diffusion defect:* Thickening of the alveolar-capillary membrane decreases oxygen diffusion and leads to hypoxemia. Causes of diffusion defects are chronic disease states such as pulmonary fibrosis and sarcoidosis. Hypoxemia usually responds to supplemental oxygen in conditions of diffusion impairment (eg, interstitial lung disease).
- *Shunt:* When blood bypasses or shunts past the alveoli, gas exchange cannot occur and blood returns to the left side of the heart without being oxygenated. Shunts caused anatomically include pulmonary arteriovenous fistulas or congenital cardiac anomalies of the heart and great vessels, such as tetralogy of Fallot. Physiologic shunts are caused by a variety of conditions that result in closed, nonventilated alveoli such as seen in ARDS.
- *Low mixed venous oxygenation:* Under normal conditions, the lungs fully oxygenate the pulmonary arterial blood and mixed venous oxygen tension ($PmvO_2$)

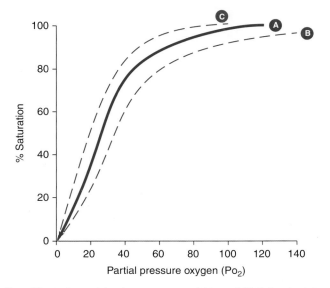

Figure 5-2. Oxyhemoglobin dissociation curve. **(A)** Normal. **(B)** Shift to the right. **(C)** Shift to the left.

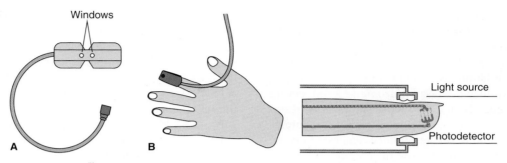

Figure 5-3. Pulse oximeter. **(A)** Sensor. **(B)** Schematic of sensor operation on finger.

does not affect PaO_2 significantly. However, a reduced $PmvO_2$ can lower the PaO_2 significantly when either ventilation-perfusion mismatch or right to left intrapulmonary shunting is present. Conditions that can contribute to low mixed venous oxygenation include low CO, anemia, hypoxemia, and increased oxygen consumption. Improving tissue oxygen delivery by increasing CO or hemoglobin usually improves mixed venous oxygen saturation.

Venous Blood Gas Monitoring

Analysis of oxygen and carbon dioxide levels in the venous blood provides additional information about the adequacy of perfusion and oxygen use by the tissues. Venous blood gas analysis, also referred to as a *mixed venous blood gas sample*, is obtained from the distal tip of a pulmonary artery (PA) catheter or from a central venous pressure (CVP) catheter. Normal values for venous blood gas results are listed in Table 5-1. Central venous oxygen saturation ($ScvO_2$) can be obtained from any central venous catheter with the tip positioned in the superior vena cava. Mixed venous oxygen saturation ($SmvO_2$ or SvO_2) can only be obtained from a PA or specialized catheter generally only be used in a critical care unit. More information on SvO_2 and $ScvO_2$ monitoring is found in Chapter 4, Hemodynamic Monitoring.

Pulse Oximetry

Pulse oximetry is a common method for the continuous, noninvasive monitoring of SaO_2. A reuseable multi-patient sensor or disposable single patient use adhesive sensor is applied to skin over areas with strong arterial pulsatile blood flow, typically a finger or toe (Figure 5-3). Alternative sites include the bridge of the nose, ear, and the forehead (Figure 5-4). The forehead sensor is a reflectance sensor and provides a central monitoring site location. Sensors are typically sized according to body weight and intended sensor placement location. It is critical to place sensors on the manufacturer-approved anatomic locations for which they were designed and Food and Drug Administration (FDA) approved. For example, a pulse oximeter sensor designed and intended to be place on a finger should not be placed on the ear or forehead. While the monitor may display an oxygen saturation value,

the accuracy of this value is questionable. The SaO_2 sensor is connected to a pulse oximeter monitor unit via a cable. Light-emitting diodes (LEDs) on one side of the sensor transmit light of two different wavelengths (infrared [IR] and red [R]) through arterial blood flowing under the sensor. Depending on the level of oxygen saturation of hemoglobin in the arterial blood, different amounts of IR and R light are absorbed and detected on the other side of the sensor (transmission) or via scattered light on the same side of the light emitters (reflectance). The sensor uses photo-detection to transmit the ratio of IR and R light information during the pulsatile and nonpulsatile intervals of the cardiac cycle to the microprocessor within the monitor, which then uses various internal software algorithms and sensor calibration curve information to calculate the oxygen saturation and pulse rate.

When blood perfusion is adequate and SaO_2 levels are greater than 70%, depending on the type of sensor being used and monitoring site, there is generally a close correlation

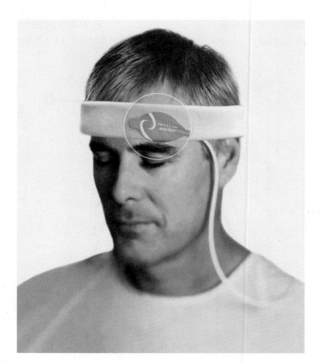

Figure 5-4. Forehead reflectance pulse oximeter sensor. (©*2018 Medtronic. All rights reserved. Used with the permission of Medtronic.*)

between the saturation reading from the pulse oximeter (SpO_2) and SaO_2 directly measured from ABGs. In situations where perfusion to the sensor is markedly diminished (eg, peripheral vasoconstriction due to disease, medications, or hypothermia), the ability of the pulse oximeter to detect a signal may be less than under normal perfusion conditions. Newer generation pulse oximeters have the ability to detect signals during most poor perfusion conditions, as well as certain other sources of signal interference, such as motion or other conditions, which create potential for artifact.

Pulse oximetry has several advantages for respiratory monitoring. The ability to have continuous information on the SaO_2 level of patients without the need for an invasive arterial punctures decreases infection risks and blood loss

from frequent ABG analysis. In addition, these monitors are easy to use, well tolerated by most patients, and portable enough to use during transport.

The major disadvantage of pulse oximeters for assessing oxygen status is that accuracy depends on having an adequate arterial pulsatile signal in order for the pulse oximeter to properly function. Clinical situations that decrease the accuracy of the device include:

- Hypotension
- Low CO states
- Vasoconstriction or vasoactive medications
- Hypothermia
- Movement of the sensor and/or poor skin adherence

ESSENTIAL CONTENT CASE

Respiratory Failure-Asthma

A 35-year-old woman with a history of asthma was admitted to the emergency department with an asthma exacerbation secondary to a viral pneumonia. Vital signs and laboratory tests on admission were:

Temperature:	38.1°C (oral)
HR:	110/min, slightly labored
BP:	148/90 mm Hg

Lung sounds: pronounced wheezing noted in all lung fields.

ABGs on room air were:

pH:	7.45
$PaCO_2$:	35 mm Hg
HCO_3:	23 mEq/L
BE:	0 mEq/L
PaO_2:	53 mm Hg

She is started on oxygen therapy via a nonrebreather mask at 100% O_2. IV fluids, steroids, and albuterol continuous nebulizers are also initiated along with empiric antibiotics. Within 30 minutes her BP, HR, and RR decrease to normal values, with improvement in her PaO_2 level (81 mm Hg). She is transferred to the progressive care unit 3 hours later. The patient is stable until approximately 6 hours following her admission to the hospital. At that time she begins experiencing increased shortness of breath, wheezing, and increased HR, BP, and RR. ABGs show a respiratory acidosis with partial compensation and hypoxemia despite 4 L of O_2 by nasal cannula:

pH:	7.31
$PaCO_2$:	55 mm Hg
HCO_3:	26.8 mEq/L
BE:	0.9 mEq/L
PaO_2:	48 mm Hg

The patient is intubated with a 7.5-mm oral ET tube without difficulty and placed on a ventilator (mode, SIMV; rate, 15/min; V_T, 600 mL; FiO_2, 0.5; PEEP, 5 cm H_2O). Immediately after intubation and initiation of mechanical ventilation,

her BP drops to 90/64 mm Hg. Following a 500-mL bolus of IV fluids, her BP returns to normal values (118/70). ABGs 15 minutes after intubation are as follows:

pH:	7.36
$PaCO_2$:	47 mm Hg
HCO_3:	27.3 mEq/L
BE:	2.1 mEq/L
PaO_2:	65 mm Hg

Case Question 1. Why do you think the patient's BP decreased after intubation?

Case Question 2. What ventilator changes if any would you anticipate?

Answers

1. Hypotension post-intubation is multifactorial. The increased intrathoracic pressure caused by positive end-expiratory pressure (PEEP) and positive-pressure ventilation can cause a decrease in venous return to the heart along with decrease in CO, which may be additionally exaggerated in a patient with hypovolemia. For this patient with severe asthma, hemodynamic stability is further compromised by lung hyperinflation and auto-PEEP. Other potential causes of post-intubation hypotension may include hemothorax, pneumothorax, or the sequela of medications used to intubate.

2. (A) Increase FiO_2: the patient is on 50% O_2 and her PaO_2 is only 65. She is likely experiencing a late asthmatic response. Once her bronchoconstriction is improved with more bronchodilators and her hyperinflation is decreased, the FiO_2 requirements will be less.

   (B) Initiate interventions to decrease auto-PEEP and dynamic hyperinflation. A likely cause of hypotension in this patient is hyperinflation and auto-PEEP associated with her history of asthma. There are several strategies to prevent further complications. Auto-PEEP and plateau pressure measurements should be performed. Low tidal volumes, low ventilator rates, short inspiratory times, and long expiratory times may help to prevent hyperinflation. Ensure adequate exhalation time to minimize hyperinflation and auto-PEEP if present.

TABLE 5-4. TIPS TO MAXIMIZE SAFETY AND ACCURACY OF PULSE OXIMETRY

- Apply sensor to dry finger of nondominant hand according to manufacturer's directions and observe for adequate pulse wave generation or signal on pulse oximeter unit.
- Avoid tension on the sensor cable.
- Rotate application sites and change sensor according to manufacturer's directions whenever adherence is poor.
- In children and elderly patients, assess application sites more often and carefully assess skin integrity when using adhesive sensors.
- Never use pulse oximeter sensors on non-approved monitoring site locations; such as finger or digit sensor use on the ear or forehead.
- If pulse wave generation is inadequate or a signal alert message is displayed check for proper adherence to skin and position. Apply a new sensor to another site, if necessary.
- Compare pulse oximeter displayed Sao_2 values with ABGs periodically, when changes in the clinical condition may decrease accuracy and/or when values do not fit the clinical situation.

Additionally, other sources of potential interference may include venous pulsation, bone and tendon, sensor movement, direct exposure to ambient light, and certain nail polish applications and treatments. Because these conditions are commonly encountered in any patient connected to a pulse oximeter, caution is exercised when using pulse oximetry in progressive care units. Proper use (Table 5-4) and periodic validation of the accuracy of the devices with ABG analysis using a co-oximeter instrument is essential to avoid erroneous patient assessment. Routinely used pulse oximeters measure light absorbance at only two wavelengths of light. As such, dyshemoglobinemias such as methemoglobinemia (Met-Hgb) and carboxyhemoglobinemia (CO-Hgb) cannot be measured. Further, the presence of such elevations may cause errors in interpretation of pulse oximetry. Although there are noninvasive devices available for detecting such dyshemoglobinemias, the most widely used and recognized "gold standard" technique for determining the presence of dyshemoglobinemias is co-oximetry via invasive ABG analysis.

Assessing Pulmonary Function

A variety of measurements in addition to ABG analysis can be used to further evaluate the acutely ill patient's respiratory system.

Measurement of selected lung volumes can be easily accomplished at the bedside. Tidal volume (V_T), exhaled minute ventilation (V_E), and negative inspiratory pressure (NIP) are measured with portable, handheld equipment (spirometer and NIP meter, respectively). Lung compliance and alveolar oxygen content can be calculated with standard formulas (see Table 5-1). Frequent trend monitoring of these parameters provides an objective evaluation of the patient's response to interventions.

ABG analysis for arterial partial pressure of carbon dioxide ($Paco_2$) is an important parameter in critically ill patients for assessment of ventilation. To limit invasive procedures or for more continuous monitoring or $Paco_2$, clinicians may sometimes rely on venous blood gases or capnography. Each of these techniques for assessing ventilation status has certain advantages and limitations. Central venous Pco_2 allows accurate estimation of $Paco_2$, so long as CO is relatively normal. Pco_2 measured from a central vein is normally approximately 4 mm Hg higher than $Paco_2$. However, peripheral venous Pco_2 is a poor predictor of $Paco_2$. Capnography offers measurement of the partial pressure of end-tidal Pco_2 ($PetCO_2$), a value that is close to $Paco_2$ when the lung is healthy. It has the advantages of being noninvasive and can be monitored continuously.

End-Tidal Carbon Dioxide Monitoring

Carbon dioxide is a by-product of cellular metabolism and is transported via the venous blood to the lungs where it is eliminated by the lungs during exhalation. End-tidal CO_2 (also referred to as partial pressure of end-tidal CO_2: $PetCO_2$) is the concentration of CO_2 present at the end of exhalation and is expressed either as a percentage ($PetCO_2\%$) or partial pressure ($PetCO_2$ mm Hg). The normal range for $PetCO_2$ is typically 35 to 45 mm Hg and 2 to 5 mm Hg less than the arterial carbon dioxide tension or $Paco_2$. For this reason, clinicians have sought to use this noninvasive monitoring method for assessing ventilation status over time. Thus, under conditions of normal ventilation and perfusion ($\dot{V}/\dot{Q}$) matching, the relationship between $PetCO_2$ and $Paco_2$ is relatively close. However, when $\dot{V}/\dot{Q}$ relationships are abnormal, this gradient may be as high as 20 mm Hg or more, limiting the use of this technology to accurately reflect $Paco_2$. However, in most clinical circumstances, an increase in $PetCO_2$ above normal can be interpreted as a sign of hypoventilation. Assessing the arterial to end-tidal CO_2 gradient as a trend also may be useful. An increasing gradient reflects a worsening condition and a narrowing gradient may reflect improved ventilation/perfusion matching.

Currently available end-tidal CO_2 monitoring devices fall into one of several categories: colorimetric, capnometric (numeric display only), or capnographic (numeric and graphical display). Colorimetric devices are pH-sensitive, colored paper strips that change color in response to different concentrations of carbon dioxide (Figure 5-5). They are typically used for either initial or intermittent monitoring purposes such as verifying endotracheal tube (ET) placement in the trachea following intubation or in some cases, to rule out inadvertent pulmonary placement of enteral feeding tubes following insertion. A capnometer provides a visual analog or digital display of the concentration of the $PetCO_2$. Capnography includes both capnometry plus the addition of a calibrated graphic recording of the exhaled CO_2 on a breath-by-breath basis and is perhaps the most common instrument used for continuous monitoring. Figure 5-6 demonstrates the various phases of a normal carbon dioxide waveform during exhalation.

Capnography devices measure exhaled carbon dioxide using one of several different techniques: infrared spectrography, Raman spectrography, mass spectrometry, or a laser-based technology called molecular correlation spectroscopy

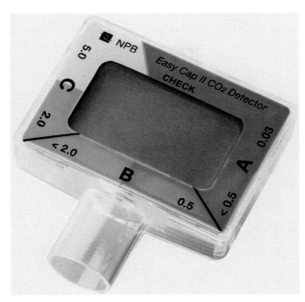

Figure 5-5. Colorimetric carbon dioxide detector. (©2018 Medtronic. All rights reserved. Used with the permission of Medtronic.)

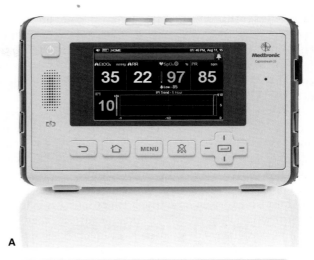

A

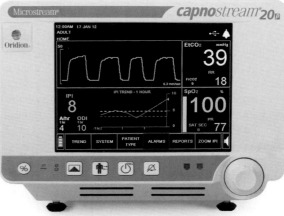

B

Figure 5-7. Handheld **(A)** and Bedside **(B)** combined capnography (sidestream) and pulse oximetry instruments. (©2018 Medtronic. All rights reserved. Used with the permission of Medtronic.)

as the infrared emission source. The laser creates an infrared emission precisely matching the absorption rate spectrum of CO_2 and eliminates the need for moving parts. A capnography device using this technology is shown in Figure 5-7. All capnographs sample and measure expired gases either directly at the patient-ventilator interface (mainstream analysis) or are collected and transported via small-bore tubing to the sensor in the monitor (sidestream analysis). Each technique has advantages and disadvantages and the user should strictly follow manufacturer recommendations for optimal performance.

Clinical application of capnography includes assessment of endotracheal or tracheostomy tube placement, gastric or small bowel tube placement, pulmonary blood flow, and alveolar ventilation, provided $\dot{V}/\dot{Q}$ relationships are normal. The 2015 American Heart Association (AHA) Guidelines for Advanced Cardiovascular Life Support (ACLS) recommend using quantitative waveform capnography during ET placement and in intubated patients during CPR. Waveform

capnography allows nurses and other caregivers to monitor CPR quality, optimize chest compressions, and detect return of spontaneous circulation (ROSC) during chest compressions. High quality chest compressions are achieved when the end-tidal CO_2 value is at least 10 to 20 mm Hg. An abrupt

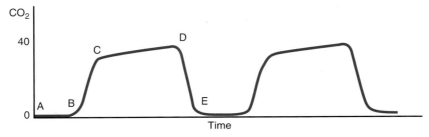

Figure 5-6. Capnogram waveform phases. Phase A to B: Early exhalation. This represents anatomic dead space and contains little carbon dioxide. Phase B to C: Combination of dead space and alveolar gas. Phase C to D: Exhalation of mostly alveolar gas (alveolar plateau). Phase D: End-tidal point, that is, exhalation of carbon dioxide at maximum point. Phase D to E: Inspiration begins and carbon dioxide concentration rapidly falls to baseline or zero. (©2018 Medtronic. All rights reserved. Used with the permission of Medtronic.)

increase in the PetCO$_2$ to 35 to 40 mm Hg is reasonable to consider as an indication of ROSC. In intubated patients, failure to achieve a PetCO$_2$ of greater than 10 mm Hg by waveform capnography after 20 minutes of CPR may be considered as one component of a multimodal approach to decide when to end resuscitative efforts.

Assessment of the capnographic waveform alone can yield useful information in detecting ventilator malfunction, response to changes in ventilator settings and weaning attempts in intubated patient. It should be noted that capnography can also be used to monitor nonintubated patients via a modified nasal/oral sampling cannula. Patients at high risk for respiratory compromise, such as those with known or suspected obstructive sleep apnea, acute exacerbation of asthma or COPD, and in particular, patients receiving opioids or other related CNS depressant medications all face a risk for impaired ventilation. While pulse oximetry is a very useful tool for assessing oxygenation status, it is a poor ventilation monitor, especially in patients receiving supplemental oxygen. Whenever clinicians use capnography in the clinical setting, it is important to follow manufacturer recommendations regarding set-up, maintenance, and troubleshooting of equipment. Institutional policies and protocols regarding clinical management for patient care should also be followed.

AIRWAY MANAGEMENT

Maintaining an open and patent airway is an important aspect of progressive care management. Patency can be ensured through conservative techniques such as coughing, head and neck positioning, and alignment. If conservative techniques fail, insertion of an oral or nasal airway or endotracheal intubation may be required.

Oropharyngeal Airway

The oropharyngeal airway, or oral bite block, is an airway adjunct used to relieve upper airway obstruction caused by tongue relaxation (eg, postanesthesia or during unconsciousness), secretions, seizures, or biting down on oral ETs (Figure 5-8A). Oral airways are made of rigid plastic or rubber material, semicircular in shape, and available in sizes ranging from infants to adults. The airway is inserted with the concave curve of the airway facing up into the roof of the mouth. The oral airway is then rotated down 180° during insertion to fit the curvature of the tongue and ensure the tongue is not obstructing the airway. The tip of the oropharyngeal airway rests near the posterior pharyngeal wall. For this reason, oral airways are not recommended for use in alert patients because they may trigger the gag reflex and cause vomiting. Oropharyngeal airways are temporary devices for achieving airway patency.

Management of oropharyngeal airways includes frequent assessment of the lips and tongue to identify pressure injuries. At least every 24 hours, the airway is removed, lips and tongue assessed, and oral care provided.

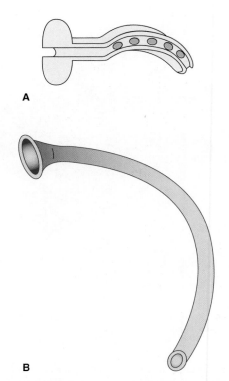

Figure 5-8. (A) Oropharyngeal and **(B)** nasopharyngeal airways.

Nasopharyngeal Airway

The nasopharyngeal airway, or nasal trumpet, is another type of airway adjunct device used to help maintain airway patency, especially in the semiconscious patient (Figure 5-8B). The nasopharyngeal airway is also used to facilitate nasotracheal suctioning. Made of soft malleable rubber or soft plastic, the nasal airway ranges in sizes from 26 to 35 Fr. Depending on hospital policy, a topical anesthetic (such as viscous lidocaine) may be applied to the nares prior to insertion of the airway. The nasopharyngeal airway, lubricated with a water-soluble gel, is then gently inserted into one of the nares. To assess the patency of the airway, listen for or feel for air movement during expiration. The airway is secured to the nose with a small piece of tape to prevent displacement. Complications of these airways include bleeding, sinusitis, and erosion of the mucous membranes.

Care of the patient with a nasal airway includes frequent assessment for pressure injuries and occlusion of the airway with dried secretions. Sinusitis has been documented as a complication. The continued need for the nasal airway is assessed daily and rotation of the airway from nostril to nostril is done on a daily basis. When performing nasotracheal suctioning through the nasal airway, the suction catheter is lubricated with a water-soluble gel to ease passage. Refer to the following discussion on suctioning for additional standards of care.

Laryngeal Mask Airway

The laryngeal mask airway (LMA) is an ET tube with a small mask on one end that can be passed orally over the larynx to provide ventilatory assistance and prevent aspiration. Placement of the LMA is easier than intubation using a standard ET tube. Commonly used as the primary airway device in the operating room for certain types of surgical procedures, it is a temporary airway for patients who require ventilatory support. LMA is often used for difficult intubations, particularly "unable to intubate" or "unable to ventilate" clinical scenarios.

Esophageal Tracheal Airway

Esophageal tracheal airways are double-lumen airways that can be rapidly established through either esophageal or tracheal placement. They are used primarily for difficult or emergency intubation and the design permits blind placement without the need for a laryngoscope. The multifunction design permits positive-pressure ventilation, but an ET tube or tracheostomy is eventually needed. The primary advantages to using these airways include less training required to use than standard intubation, no special equipment required, and the cuff provides some protection against aspiration of gastric contents. The tube is contraindicated in responsive patients with intact gag reflexes, patients with known esophageal pathology, and patients who have ingested caustic substances. The tube is sized to the patient's height.

Artificial Airways

Artificial airways (oral and nasal ET tubes, tracheostomy tubes) are used when a patent airway cannot be maintained with an adjunct airway device, when patients require mechanical ventilation, or to manage severe airway obstruction. The artificial airway also provides some protection for the lower airway from aspiration of oral or gastric secretions and allows for easier secretion removal.

Types of Artificial Airways and Insertion

Endotracheal and tracheostomy tubes are made of either polyvinyl chloride or silicone and are available in a variety of sizes and lengths (Figure 5-9). Standard features include a 15-mm adapter at the end of the tube for connection to life-support equipment such as mechanical ventilation circuits, closed-suction catheter systems, swivel adapters, or a manual resuscitation bag (MRB). Tubes may be cuffed or uncuffed. For cuffed tubes, air is manually injected into the cuff located near the distal tip of the ET tube through a small one-way pilot valve and inflation lumen. Distance markers are located along the side of the tube for identification of tube position. A radiopaque line is also located on all tubes so as to aid in determining proper position radiographically.

ETs are inserted into the patient's trachea either through the mouth or nose (Figures 5-10 and 5-11). Orally inserted ET tubes are more common than the nasal route because nasal intubation is associated with sinus infections and are considered an independent risk factor for developing ventilator-associated pneumonia (VAP). With use of the laryngoscope, the upper airway is visualized and the tube is inserted

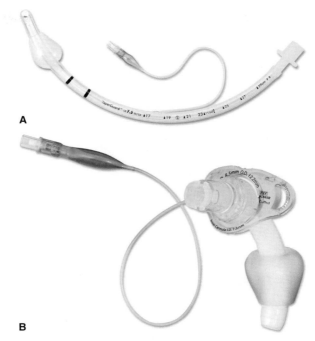

Figure 5-9. Artificial airways. **(A)** Cuffed endotracheal tube. **(B)** Cuffed tracheostomy tube. (*©2018 Medtronic. All rights reserved. Used with the permission of Medtronic.*)

through the vocal cords into the trachea, 2 to 4 cm above the carina. The presence of bilateral breath sounds, along with equal chest excursion during inspiration and the absence of breath sounds over the stomach, preliminarily confirms proper tube placement. An end-tidal CO_2 monitor with waveform verification is used as an immediate assessment for determining tracheal placement. If not available, a colorimetric CO_2 detector may be used. A portable chest x-ray verifies proper tube placement. Once proper placement is confirmed, the tube is anchored with either tape or a special ET tube fixation device (Figure 5-12) to prevent movement. The centimeter marking of the ET tube at the lip is documented and checked during each shift to monitor proper tube placement.

ET sizes are typically identified by the tubes' internal diameter in millimeters (mm ID). The size of the tube is printed on the tube and generally also on the outside packaging. Knowledge of the tube ID is critical; the smaller the mm ID, the higher the resistance to breathing through the tube, thus increasing the work of breathing (WOB). The most common ET tube sizes used in adults are 7.0 to 9.0 mm ID.

Complications of ET intubation are numerous and include laryngeal and tracheal damage, laryngospasm, aspiration, infection, discomfort, sinusitis, and subglottic injury. ETs can in some situations be safely left in place for up to 2 to 3 weeks, but tracheostomy is often considered following 10 to 14 days of intubation or less if a prolonged recovery is anticipated. The decision to place a tracheostomy ideally also takes into account the patient's goals of care and the disease prognosis.

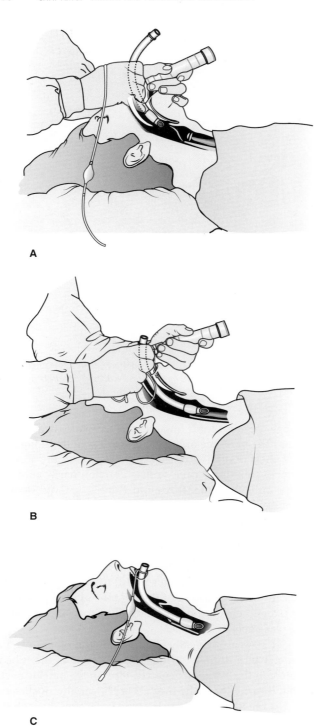

A

B

C

Figure 5-10. Oral intubation with an endotracheal (ET) tube. **(A)** Insertion of ET tube through the mouth with the aid of a laryngoscope. **(B)** ET tube advanced through the vocal cords into the trachea. **(C)** ET tube positioned with the cuff below the vocal cords. (*Reproduced with permission from Boggs Wooldridge-King M. AACN Procedure Manual for Progressive Care. 3rd ed. Philadelphia, PA: WB Saunders; 1993.*)

The majority of tracheostomy tubes used in acutely ill patients are made of medical-grade plastic or silicone and come in a variety of sizes (see Figure 5-9B). Tracheostomy

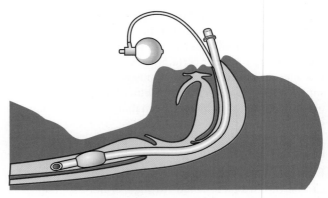

Figure 5-11. Nasal endotracheal tube. (*©2018 Medtronic. All rights reserved. Used with the permission of Medtronic.*)

tubes may be cuffed or uncuffed. As with ET tubes, a standard 15-mm adapter at the proximal end ensures universal connection to MRBs and ventilator circuits. Tracheostomy tubes may be inserted as an elective procedure using a standard open surgical technique in the operating room or at the bedside via a percutaneous insertion. This technique involves a procedure in which a small incision is made in the neck and a series of dilators are manually passed into the trachea over a guide wire, creating a stoma opening through which the tracheostomy tube is inserted. Bedside placement obviates the need for general anesthesia and for patient transport out of the unit.

Tracheostomies are secured with cotton twill tape or latex-free Velcro tube holders attached to openings on the neck flange or plate of the tube. Many tracheostomy tubes have inner cannulae that can be easily removed for periodic cleaning (reusable) or replacement (disposable). Some tracheostomy tubes incorporate an additional opening along the outer tube cannula referred to as a fenestration. A fenestrated tracheostomy tube is sometimes used as an aid for facilitating vocalization by allowing airflow upward and through the vocal cords. A fenestration is not necessary to be able to talk with a tracheostomy tube. Patients generally tolerate tracheostomy and find them more comfortable than oral or nasal ET tubes. Further, there are more nutrition and communication options available to patients with tracheostomy tubes than with ET tubes.

Complications of tracheostomies include hemorrhage from erosion of the innominate artery; tracheal stenosis, malacia, or perforation; laryngeal nerve injury; aspiration; infection; air leak; device-related pressure injuries; and mechanical problems. Most complications rarely occur with proper management.

Cuff Inflation

Following insertion of an endotracheal or tracheostomy tube, the cuff of the tube is inflated with just enough air to create an effective seal. The cuff is typically inflated with the lowest possible pressure that prevents air leak during mechanical ventilation and decreases the risk of pulmonary aspiration. Cuff

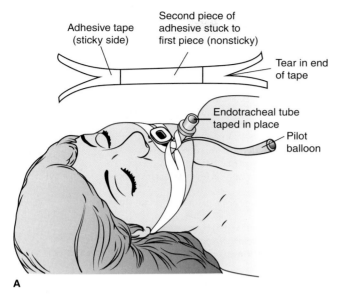

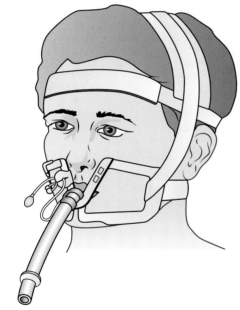

minimal occlusive volume techniques (MLT and MOV, respectively). The minimal leak technique involves listening over the larynx during positive pressure breaths with a stethoscope while slowly inflating the tube cuff in 1- to 2-mL increments. Inflation continues until only a small air leak, or rush of air, is heard over the larynx during peak inspiration. The MLT should result in no more than a 50- to 100-mL air loss per breath during mechanical ventilation. The cuff pressure and amount of air instilled into the cuff are recorded following the maneuver.

The MOV cuff inflation technique is similar to the MLT. Cuff inflation continues, however, until the air leak completely disappears. The amount of air instilled and the cuff pressure are recorded during cuff inflation and periodically to ensure an intracuff pressure of less than 25 mm Hg (30 cm H_2O). Manual palpation of the tube pilot balloon does not ensure optimal inflation assessment.

Cuff Pressure Measurement

The connection of the ET tube pilot balloon to an intracuff measuring manometer device, such as a manual handheld cuff inflator, allows for the simultaneous measurement of pressure during inflation or periodic checking (Figure 5-13). The need for excessive pressures to properly seal the trachea

Figure 5-12. Methods for anchoring an endotracheal tube to prevent movement. **(A)** Taping of an oral ET tube. (*Reproduced with permission from Boggs R, Wooldridge-King M. AACN Procedure Manual for Critical Care. 3rd ed. Philadelphia, PA: WB Saunders; 1993.*) **(B)** Use of a special fixation device. (*Reproduced with permission from Kaplow R, Bookbinder M. A comparison of four endotracheal tube holders. Heart Lung. 1994 Jan-Feb;23(1):59-66.*)

pressure is maintained at less than 25 mm Hg (30 cm H_2O). Excessive cuff pressure causes tracheal ischemia, necrosis, and erosion, as well as overinflation-related obstruction of the distal airway from cuff herniation. It is important to recognize that even a properly inflated cuffed artificial airway does not completely protect the patient from aspiration.

There are two common techniques to ensure proper cuff inflation without overinflation: the minimal leak and

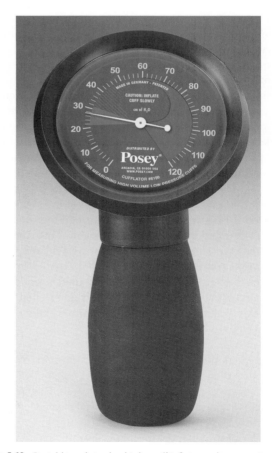

Figure 5-13. Portable endotracheal tube cuff inflator and manometer. (*Used with permission from Posey Company, Arcadia, CA.*)

may indicate that the ET tube diameter is too small for the trachea. In this case, the cuff is inflated to properly seal the trachea until the appropriately sized ET tube can be electively reinserted. At present, evidence of long-term outcomes is lacking to warrant mandatory cuff pressure monitoring. Untill a more definitive statement may be made, the clinician is encouraged to follow tube manufacturer and hospital policy. Current available evidence from clinical and laboratory testing suggests that intracuff pressure may be an important contributing factor to the development of complications related to cuffed endotracheal and tracheostomy tubes so attention to proper inflation is encouraged.

Endotracheal Suctioning

Pulmonary secretion removal is normally accomplished by coughing. An effective cough requires a closed epiglottis so that intrathoracic pressure can be increased prior to sudden opening of the epiglottis and secretion expulsion. The presence of an artificial airway such as an ET tube prevents glottic closure and effective coughing, necessitating the use of periodic endotracheal suctioning to remove secretions.

Currently, two methods are commonly used for ET tube suctioning: the closed and open methods. *Closed suctioning* means the ventilator circuit remains closed while suctioning is performed, whereas *open suctioning* means the ventilator circuit is opened, or removed, during suctioning. The open method requires disconnection of the ET tube from the mechanical ventilator or oxygen therapy source and insertion of a suction catheter each time the patient requires suctioning. The closed method refers to an in-line suction catheter device that remains attached to the ventilator circuit, allowing periodic insertion of the suction catheter through a diaphragm to suction without removing the patient from the ventilator. Following suctioning, the catheter is withdrawn into a plastic sleeve where it is stored until the next suctioning procedure.

Indications

The need for ET suctioning is determined by a variety of clinical signs and symptoms, such as coughing, increased inspiratory pressures on the ventilator, and the presence of adventitious sounds (rhonchi, gurgling) during chest auscultation. Suctioning may also be performed periodically to ensure airway patency. Suctioning is only done when there is a clinical indication and never on a routine schedule.

Procedure

Hyperoxygenation with 100% O_2 for a minimum of 30 seconds is provided prior to each suctioning episode, whether using an open or closed technique (Table 5-5). Hyperoxygenation helps to prevent decreases in arterial oxygen levels after suctioning. Hyperoxygenation can be achieved by increasing the Fio_2 setting on the mechanical ventilator or by using the "suction" button or temporary oxygen-enrichment function available on most microprocessor ventilators. Manual

TABLE 5-5. STEPS FOR SUCTIONING THROUGH AN ARTIFICIAL AIRWAY

1. Assess for signs and symptoms of airway obstruction:
   ◦ Secretions in the airway
   ◦ Suspected aspiration
   ◦ Upper airway secretions
   ◦ Decreased breath sounds, inspiratory wheezes, or expiratory crackles
   ◦ Increase in peak airway pressures
   ◦ Restlessness or decreased level of consciousness
   ◦ Ineffective or frequent cough
   ◦ Tachypnea, shallow respirations or decreased respirations
   ◦ Gradual or sudden decrease in Pao_2, Sao_2, or Spo_2
   ◦ Sudden onset of respiratory distress
2. Hyperoxygenate with 100% oxygen for minimum of 30 seconds with one of the following:
   ◦ Press the suction hyperoxygenation button to increase the Fio_2 to 1.0 (100%) on the ventilator (preferred), or
   ◦ Manually increase the Fio_2 to 1.0 (100%), or
   ◦ Disconnect from the ventilator and manually ventilate with MRB
3. Insert catheter (closed or open system) gently until resistance is met, then pull back
4. Place the non-dominant thumb over the control vent of the suction catheter to apply continuous or intermittent suction as the catheter is completely withdrawn.
   NOTE: Suction should be applied only as needed and for as short a time as possible.
5. Hyperoxygenate for 30 seconds as described in step 2.
6. Repeat steps 3, 4, and 5 as needed if secretions remain and patient is tolerating the procedure.
7. Monitor cardiopulmonary status before, during, and after suctioning for the following:
   ◦ Decreased arterial or mixed venous oxygen saturation
   ◦ Decreased oxygenation
   ◦ Cardiac dysrhythmias
   ◦ Bronchospasms
   ◦ Respiratory distress
   ◦ Cardiac arrest
   ◦ Hypertension or hypotension
   ◦ Increased ICP
   ◦ Decreased Svo_2
   ◦ Anxiety, agitation, pain, or change in level of consciousness
   ◦ Increased peak airway pressure
   ◦ Pulmonary hemorrhage or bleeding
   ◦ Increased work of breathing

Data from Wiegand DL, ed. AACN Procedure Manual for Critical Care. 7th ed. St. Louis. MO: Elsevier Saunders; 2016.

ventilation of the patient using an MRB is not recommended as the best choice and has been shown to be ineffective for providing delivered Fio_2 of 1.0. If no other alternative is available to hyperoxygenate, then an MRB can be used. At least 30 seconds of manual breaths with 100% Fio_2 are provided before and after each pass of the suction catheter. In spontaneously breathing patients, encourage several deep breaths of 100% O_2 before and after each suction pass. Usually, two or three suction passes are sufficient to clear the airway. The mechanical act of inserting the suction catheter into the trachea can stimulate the vagus nerve and result in bradycardia or asystole. Because of this risk, suction passes stop once the airway is clear, and each pass of the suction catheter is 10 seconds or less.

The instillation of 5 to 10 mL of normal saline during ET tube suctioning has risks and no documented benefits and therefore, is not recommended. This practice was previously thought to decrease secretion viscosity and increase secretion removal during ET tube suctioning. Bolus saline instillation has not been shown to be beneficial and is associated with SaO_2 decreases and bronchospasm.

Complications

A variety of complications are associated with ET tube suctioning. Decreases in PaO_2 are well documented when no hyperoxygenation therapy is provided prior to suctioning. Serious cardiac arrhythmias can occur with suctioning, including bradycardia, asystole, ventricular tachycardia, and heart block. Less severe arrhythmias frequently occur with suctioning and include premature ventricular contractions, atrial contractions, and supraventricular tachycardia. Other complications associated with suctioning include increases in arterial pressure and intracranial pressure, bronchospasm, tracheal wall damage, and nosocomial pneumonia. Many of these complications can be minimized by using sterile technique, vigilant monitoring during and after suctioning, and hyperoxygenation before and after each suction pass.

Extubation

The reversal or significant improvement of the underlying condition(s) that led to the use of artificial airways usually signals the readiness for removal of the airway. Common indicators of readiness for artificial airway removal include the patient's ability to:

- maintain spontaneous breathing and adequate ABG values with minimal to moderate amounts of O_2 administration ($FiO_2 < 0.50$),
- protect their airway, and
- clear pulmonary secretions.

Removal of an artificial airway usually occurs following weaning from mechanical ventilatory support (see the discussion on weaning later in this chapter). Preparations for extubation include an explanation to the patient and family of what to expect, the need to cough, medication for pain as needed, setting up the appropriate method for delivering O_2 therapy (eg, face mask, nasal cannula), and positioning the patient with the head of the bed elevated at 30° to 45° to improve diaphragmatic function. Suctioning of the artificial airway is performed prior to extubation, if clinically indicated. Obtaining a baseline cardiopulmonary assessment also is important for later evaluation of the response to extubation. Extubation is best performed when full ancillary staff is available to assist if reintubation is required.

Hyperoxygenation with 100% O_2 is provided for 30 to 60 seconds prior to extubation in case respiratory distress occurs immediately after extubation and reintubation is necessary. The artificial airway is then removed following complete deflation of the ET or tracheostomy cuff, if present. Immediately apply the oxygen delivery method and encourage the patient to take deep breaths.

Monitor the patient's response to the extubation. Changes in heart rate, respiratory rate, and/or blood pressure of more than 10% of baseline values may indicate respiratory compromise, necessitating more extensive assessment and possible reintubation. Pulmonary auscultation is also performed.

Complications associated with extubation include aspiration, bronchospasm, and tracheal damage. Monitor the patient's vital signs, listen for stridor in the upper airway and encourage coughing and deep breathing. Inspiratory stridor occurs from glottic and subglottic edema and may develop immediately or take several hours. If the patient's clinical status permits, 2.5% racemic epinephrine (0.5 mL in 3 mL of normal saline) is administered via an aerosol delivery device. If the upper airway obstruction persists or worsens, reintubation is generally required. A reattempt at extubation is usually delayed for 24 to 72 hours following reintubation for upper airway obstruction to allow further assessment and treatment of any swelling.

OXYGEN THERAPY

Oxygen is used for any number of clinical problems (Table 5-6). The goals for oxygen use include increasing alveolar O_2 tension (PAO_2) to treat hypoxemia, decreasing the WOB, and maximizing myocardial and tissue oxygen supply.

Complications

As with any drug, oxygen is used cautiously. The hazards of oxygen misuse include alveolar hypoventilation, absorption atelectasis, and oxygen toxicity and can be life threatening.

Alveolar Hypoventilation

Alveolar hypoventilation is underventilation of alveoli, and it is a side effect of great concern in patients with COPD with

---

TABLE 5-6. COMMON INDICATIONS FOR OXYGEN THERAPY

- Decreased cardiac performance
- Increased metabolic need for O_2 (fever, burns)
- Acute changes in level of consciousness (restlessness, confusion)
- Acute shortness of breath
- Decreased O_2 saturation
- $PaO_2 < 60$ mm Hg or $SaO_2 < 90\%$
- Normal PaO_2 or SaO_2 with signs and symptoms of significant hypoxia
- Acute myocardial infarction with $SpO_2 < 90\%$, respiratory distress, or signs of hypoxemia
- Carbon monoxide (CO) poisoning
- Methemoglobinemia (a form of hemoglobin where ferrous iron is oxidized to ferric form, causing a high affinity for O_2 with decreased O_2 release at tissue level)
- Acute anemia
- Cardiopulmonary arrest
- Reduced cardiac output
- Consider in the presence of hypotension, tachycardia, cyanosis, chest pain, dyspnea, and acute neurologic dysfunction
- During stressful procedures and situations, especially high-risk patients (eg, ET suctioning, bronchoscopy, thoracentesis, PA catheterization, travel at high altitudes)

carbon dioxide retention. It was once thought that because the patient with COPD adjusts to chronically high levels of $Paco_2$, the chemoreceptors in the medulla of the brain lost responsiveness to high $Paco_2$ levels and hypoxemia becomes the primary stimulus for ventilation. However, there are several other physiologic mechanisms in the patient with COPD that also contribute to increased $Paco_2$ levels including inability to increase minute ventilation and lack of hypoxic vasoconstriction, which leads to increased dead space ventilation.Correction of hypoxemia in the patient with COPD remains important with a target Pao_2 of 55 to 60 mm Hg ($Sao_2 \geq 90\%$), despite the presence of hypercapnia. (refer to Chapter 10, Respiratory System).

Absorption Atelectasis

Absorption atelectasis results when high concentrations of O_2 (> 90%) are given for long periods of time and nitrogen is washed out of the lungs. The nitrogen in inspired gas is approximately 79% of the total atmospheric gases. The large partial pressure of nitrogen in the alveoli helps to maintain open alveoli because it is not absorbed. When the inspired gas is 90% to 100% oxygen, alveolar closure occurs because oxygen readily diffuses into the pulmonary capillary.

Oxygen Toxicity

The toxic effects of oxygen are targeted primarily to the pulmonary and central nervous systems (CNSs). CNS toxicity usually occurs with hyperbaric oxygen treatment. Signs and symptoms include nausea, anxiety, numbness, visual disturbances, muscular twitching, and grand mal seizures. The physiologic mechanism is not understood fully but is probably related to subtle neural and biochemical changes that alter the electric activity of the CNS.

Pulmonary oxygen toxicity may lead to ARDS or bronchopulmonary dysplasia. Two phases of lung injury occur with prolonged exposure to high Fio_2 levels. The first phase occurs after 1 to 4 days of exposure to higher O_2 levels and is manifested by decreased tracheal mucosal blood flow and tracheobronchitis. Vital capacity decreases due to poor lung expansion and progressive atelectasis persists. The alveolar capillary membrane becomes progressively impaired, decreasing gas exchange. The second phase occurs after 12 days of high exposure. The alveolar septa thicken and an ARDS picture develops, with associated high mortality.

Caring for the patient who requires high levels of oxygen requires astute monitoring as well as interventions to promote oxygen delivery and reduce oxygen demand. Monitor those patients at risk for absorption atelectasis and oxygen toxicity. Signs and symptoms include nonproductive cough, substernal chest pain, general malaise, fatigue, nausea, and vomiting.

An oxygen concentration of 100% ($Fio_2 = 1.0$) is regarded as safe for short periods of time (< 24 hours). Oxygen concentrations greater than 60% for more than 24 to 48 hours may damage the lungs and worsen respiratory

problems. Fio_2 levels are decreased as soon as Pao_2 levels reach clinically acceptable levels (> 60 mm Hg or higher).

Oxygen Delivery

Noninvasive Devices

Face masks and nasal cannulas are standard oxygen delivery devices for the spontaneously breathing patient (Figure 5-14). Oxygen can be delivered with a high- or low-flow device, with the concentration of O_2 delivered ranging from 21% to approximately 100% (Table 5-7). An example of a high-flow device is the Venturi mask system that can deliver precise concentrations of oxygen (Figure 5-15). The usual Fio_2 values delivered with this type of mask are 24%, 28%, 31%, 35%, 40%, and 50%. Often, Venturi masks are useful in patients with COPD and hypercapnia because the clinician can titrate the Pao_2 to minimize carbon dioxide retention.

An example of a low-flow system is the nasal cannula or prongs. Nasal prongs flow rate ranges are limited to 6 L/min. Flow rates less than 4 L/min need not be humidified. The main advantage of nasal prongs is that the patient can drink, eat, and speak during oxygen administration. The disadvantage is that the exact Fio_2 delivered is unknown, because it is influenced by the patient's peak inspiratory flow demand and breathing pattern. As a general guide, 1 L/min of O_2 flow is an approximate equivalent to an Fio_2 of 24%, and each additional liter of oxygen flow increases the Fio_2 by approximately 4%.

Simple oxygen face masks can provide an Fio_2 of 34% to 50% depending on fit at flow rates from 5 to 10 L/min. Flow rates should be maintained at 5 L/min or more in order to avoid rebreathing exhaled CO_2 that can be retained in the mask. Limitations of using a simple face mask include difficulty in delivering accurate low concentrations of oxygen and long-term use can lead to skin irritation and potential pressure breakdown.

Nonrebreathing masks can achieve higher oxygen concentrations (approximately 60%-80%) than partial rebreathing systems. A one-way valve placed between the mask and reservoir bag with a nonrebreathing system prevents exhaled gases from entering the bag, thus maximizing the delivered Fio_2.

A variation of the nonrebreathing mask without the one-way valves is called a partial rebreathing mask. Oxygen should always be supplied to maintain the reservoir bag at least one-third to one-half full on inspiration. At a flow of 6 to 10 L/min, the system can provide 40% to 70% oxygen. High-flow delivery devices such as aerosol masks or face tents, tracheostomy collars, and t-tube adapters can be used with supplemental oxygen systems. A continuous aerosol generator or large-volume reservoir humidifier can humidify the gas flow. Some aerosol generators cannot provide adequate flows at high oxygen concentrations.

Unlike conventional low-flow nasal cannulae and oxygen masks, which are constrained by flow, humidity, and accuracy of delivered inspired oxygen, the reintroduction of

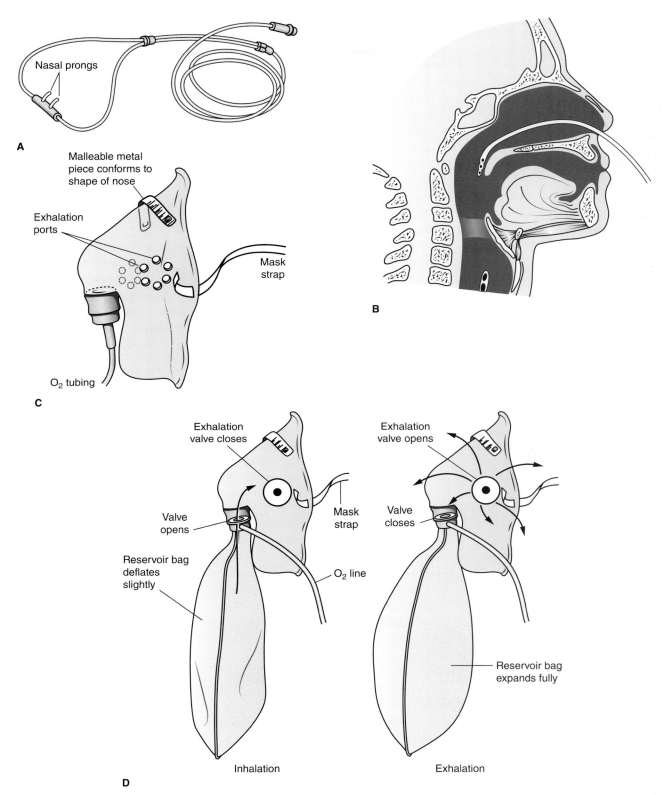

Figure 5-14. Noninvasive and invasive methods of O$_2$ delivery. **(A)** Nasal prongs. **(B)** Nasal catheter. **(C)** Face mask. **(D)** Nonrebreathing mask. (*Reproduced with permission from Kersten L. Comprehensive Respiratory Nursing. Philadelphia, PA: WB Saunders; 1989.*)

TABLE 5-7. APPROXIMATE OXYGEN DELIVERY WITH COMMON NONINVASIVE AND INVASIVE OXYGEN DEVICES[a]

Device	% O$_2$
Nasal Prongs/Cannula	
• 2 L/min	28
• 4 L/min	36
• 5 L/min	40
High-Flow Nasal Cannula	
• 1-60 L/min	21-100[b]
Face Mask	
• 5 L/min	30
• 10 L/min	50
Nonbreathing Mask 10 L/min	60-80
Partial Rebreathing Mask 6-10 L/min	40-70
Venturi Mask	
• 24%	24
• 28%	28
• 35%	35
Manual Resuscitation Bag (MRB)	
• Disposable MRB	Dependent on model

[a]Actual delivery dependent on minute ventilation rates except for Venturi mask.
[b]Actual oxygen concentration dependent on oxygen blender setting.

high-flow nasal cannula (HFNC) oxygen devices are capable of delivering well-humidified blended and actively warmed oxygen (using vapor) across a wide range of oxygen concentrations. These devices are useful in those patients who require a higher flow of oxygen than can be delivered with traditional low-flow oxygen devices. HFNC can provide oxygen at very high-flow rates between 30 and 60 L/min and

a moderate PEEP. Improved outcomes in patients placed on HFNC following a period of mechanical ventilation are due to a controlled oxygen concentration which may reduce transient hypoxemic episodes, and high flows which wash nasopharyngeal dead space, thus reducing CO_2 rebreathing, respiratory rate, and minute ventilation. Lastly, the small amount of PEEP generated with HFNC may help reduce lung collapse and enable improved gas exchange and reduce the WOB.

Invasive Devices

Manual Resuscitation Bags

Manual resuscitation bags provide 40% to 100% O_2 at adult V_T and respiratory rates when attached to an ET tube or tracheostomy tube.

Mechanical Ventilators

The most common method for delivering oxygen invasively is with a mechanical ventilator. Oxygen can be accurately delivered from 21% to 100% O_2. Mechanical ventilation is discussed below in more detail.

Transtracheal Oxygen Therapy

Transtracheal oxygen therapy is a method of administering continuous oxygen to patients with chronic hypoxemia. The therapy requires the percutaneous placement of a small plastic catheter into the trachea. The catheter is inserted directly into the trachea above the suprasternal notch under local anesthesia in an outpatient setting. This device allows for low O_2 flow rates (< 1-2 L/min) to treat chronic hypoxemia. Advantages of this method for chronic O_2 delivery include

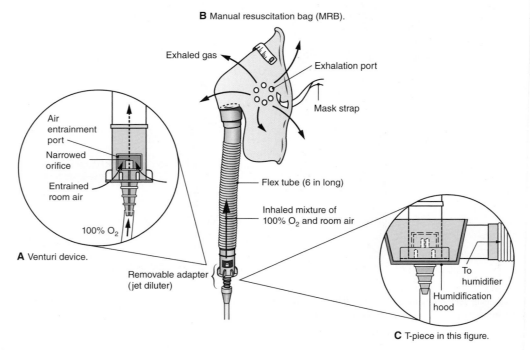

Figure 5-15. (A) Venturi device. **(B)** Manual resuscitation bag (MRB). **(C)** T-piece. (*Reproduced with permission from Kersten L. Comprehensive Respiratory Nursing. Philadelphia, PA: WB Saunders; 1989.*)

improved mobility and patient aesthetics because the tubing and catheter, unlike the nasal cannula or face mask, can often be hidden from view. Transtracheal oxygen also avoids the nasal and ear irritation common with nasal cannulas, decreases O_2 requirements, and corrects refractory hypoxemia.

Typically, these patients are managed in the outpatient setting, but occasionally they may be in progressive care units. It is important to maintain the catheter unless specifically ordered to discontinue its use. The stoma formation process takes several weeks and if the catheter is removed, the stoma is likely to close. The catheter is cleaned daily to prevent the formation of mucous plugs. Refer to the manufacturer's guidelines for further recommendations on care of the catheter while the patient is hospitalized.

T-Piece

Oxygen can also be provided directly to an ET or tracheostomy tube with a T-piece, or blow by, in spontaneously breathing patients who do not require ventilatory support. The T-piece is connected directly to the ET tube or tracheostomy tube 15-mm adapter, providing 21% to 80% O_2.

BASIC VENTILATORY MANAGEMENT

Indications

Mechanical ventilation is indicated when noninvasive management modalities fail to adequately support oxygenation and/or ventilation. The decision to initiate mechanical ventilation is based on the ability of the patient to support their oxygenation and/or ventilation needs. The inability of the patient to maintain clinically acceptable CO_2 levels and acid-base status is recognized as one type of *respiratory failure* and is a common indicator for mechanical ventilation. *Refractory hypoxemia,* which is the inability to establish and maintain acceptable arterial oxygenation levels despite the administration of oxygen-enriched breathing environments, is another type of *respiratory failure* and also a common reason for mechanical ventilation. Table 5-8 presents a variety of

physiologic indicators for initiating mechanical ventilation. By monitoring these indicators, it is possible to differentiate stable or improving values from continuing decompensation. The need for mechanical ventilation may then be anticipated to avoid emergent use of ventilatory support.

Depending on the underlying cause of the respiratory failure, different indicators may be assessed to determine the need for mechanical ventilation. Many of the causes of respiratory failure, however, are due to inadequate alveolar ventilation and/or hypoxemia, with abnormal ABG values and physical assessment as the primary indicators for ventilatory support.

General Principles

Mechanical ventilators are designed to partially or completely support ventilation. Two different categories of ventilators are available to provide ventilatory support. Negative-pressure ventilators (NPVs) decrease intrathoracic pressure by applying negative pressure to the chest wall, typically with a shell placed around the chest (Figure 5-16A). The decrease in intrathoracic pressure causes atmospheric gas to be drawn into the lungs. Positive-pressure ventilators deliver pressurized gases into the lung during inspiration (Figure 5-16B). Positive-pressure ventilators can dramatically increase intrathoracic pressures during inspiration, potentially decreasing venous return and CO.

NPVs are rarely used to manage acute respiratory problems in progressive care. These devices are typically used for long-term noninvasive ventilatory support when respiratory muscle strength is inadequate to support unassisted, spontaneous breathing. Since the emergence of other, noninvasive modes of positive pressure (eg, bilevel positive airway pressure [BiPAP] or Bilevel, described later in this chapter), negative-pressure ventilators are infrequently selected.

While rarely encountered, there is still a role for NPV in select patients with chronic respiratory failure who are unable to tolerate noninvasive positive-pressure ventilation as well as in those patients who are unable to use a facial mask because of facial deformity, claustrophobia, and excessive

TABLE 5-8. INDICATIONS FOR MECHANICAL VENTILATION

Basic Physiologic Impairment	Best Available Indicators	Approximate Normal Range	Values Indicating Need for Ventilatory Support
Apnea	Neuromuscular and/or cardiovascular collapse		
Acute ventilatory failure (hypercarbic respiratory failure)	$Paco_2$ mm Hg elevated above normal or patient baseline with decrease in pH (acidosis)	35-45 7.35-7.45	$Paco_2$ > 50 with pH ≤ 7.25
Impending ventilatory failure	Serial decrement of arterial blood gas values Symptoms of increased work of breathing		
Hypoxemia (acute oxygenation failure)	Pao_2 < 50 mm Hg on room air Pao_2/Fio_2 ratio, mm Hg	85-100 mm Hg < 300	< 50 mm Hg
Respiratory muscle fatigue	Respiratory muscles are not contracting optimally due to fatigue with resulting hypercarbia Tidal volume, mL/kg Vital capacity, mL/kg Respiratory rate, breaths/min (adult)	5-7 65-75 10-20	< 5 < 10-12 < 10 or > 35

Reproduced with permission from Wiegand DL, ed. AACN Procedure Manual for Critical Care. 7th ed. St. Louis, MO: Elsevier Saunders; 2016.

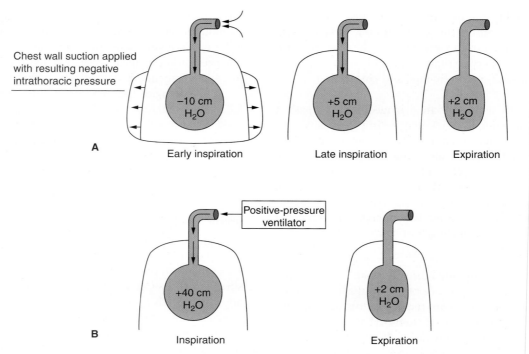

Figure 5-16. Principles of mechanical ventilation as provided by **(A)** negative-pressure and **(B)** positive-pressure ventilators.

airway secretions. There are also some polio patients who have suffered resultant paralysis and successfully used these ventilators for years. However, because of the rarity of this type of ventilator, and access to same, this chapter focuses only on the use of positive-pressure ventilators for ventilatory support.

Patient-Ventilator System

Positive-pressure ventilatory support can be accomplished invasively or noninvasively. Invasive mechanical ventilation is still widely used in most hospitals for supporting ventilation, although noninvasive technologies, which do not require the use of an artificial airway, are becoming more popular. To provide invasive positive-pressure ventilation, intubation of the trachea is required via an ET tube or tracheostomy tube. The ventilator is then connected to the artificial airway with a tubing circuit to maintain a closed delivery system (Figure 5-17). During the inspiratory cycle, gas from the ventilator is directed through a heated humidifier or a heat and moisture exchanger (HME) prior to entering the lungs through the ET tube or tracheostomy tube. Contraindications to HME use are listed in Table 5-9. At the completion of inspiration, gas is passively exhaled through the expiratory side of the tubing circuit.

Ventilator Tubing Circuit

The humidifier located on the inspiratory side of the circuit is necessary to overcome two primary problems. First, the presence of an artificial airway allows gas entering the lungs to bypass the normal upper airway humidification process. Second, the higher flows and larger volumes typically administered during mechanical ventilation require additional humidification to avoid excessive intrapulmonary membrane drying.

Pressure within the ventilator tubing circuit is continuously monitored to alert clinicians to excessively high or low airway pressures. Airway pressure is dynamically displayed on the front of the ventilator control panel.

Traditionally, ventilator circuits have incorporated special water collection cups in the tubing to prevent the condensation from humidified gas from obstructing the tubing. Other ventilator circuits contain heated wires that run through the inspiratory and expiratory limbs of the circuit. These wires maintain the temperature of the gas at or close to body temperature, significantly reducing the condensation and rainout of humidity in the gas, eliminating the need for in-line water traps. Certain medications, such as bronchodilators or steroids, can also be administered via metered dose inhaler (MDI) or nebulized into the lungs through a low volume aerosol-generating device located in the inspiratory side of the circuit.

The ventilator tubing circuit is maintained as a closed circuit as much as possible to avoid interrupting ventilation and oxygenation to the patient, as well as to decrease the potential for VAP. Avoiding frequent or routine changes of the ventilator circuit also decreases the risk of VAP (see Chapter 10, Respiratory System).

Ventilator Control Panel

The user interface or control panel of the ventilator usually incorporates three basic sections or areas: (1) control settings for the type and amount of ventilation and oxygen delivery,

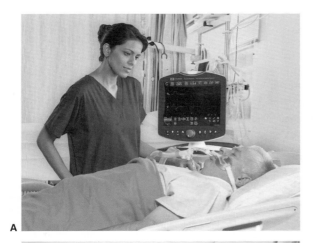

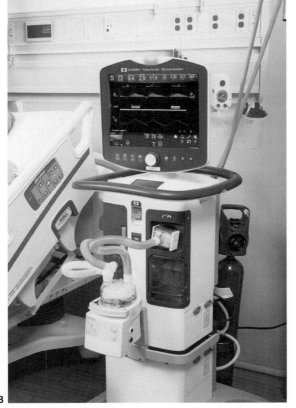

Figure 5-17. Typical setup of a ventilator with a closed system tubing circuit connected to an ET tube **(A)**, and common ventilator components **(B)** including display panel, humidifier, and inspiratory gas filter. (©2018 Medtronic. All rights reserved. Used with the permission of Medtronic.)

TABLE 5-9. CONTRAINDICATIONS TO USE OF HEATED MOISTURE EXCHANGER (HME)

1. Frank bloody or thick, copious secretions
2. Patients with large bronchopleural fistulas
3. Uncuffed or malfunctioning ET tube cuffs
4. During lung protective strategies such as patients with ARDS
5. Patients with body temperature < 32°C

Data from American Association for Respiratory Care. AARC clinical practice guideline: humidification during invasive and noninvasive mechanical ventilation, Resp Care *2012;57:782-788.*

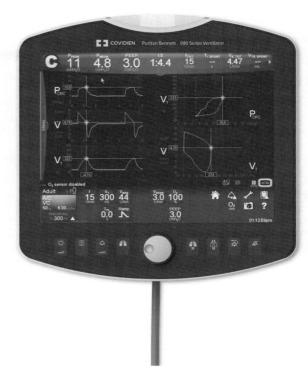

Figure 5-18. Ventilator visual display control panel for setting and adjusting ventilator parameters and alarms used in the assessment of patient-ventilator interaction and synchrony. (*©2018 Medtronic. All rights reserved. Used with the permission of Medtronic.*)

(2) alarm settings to specify desired high and low limits for key ventilatory measurements, and (3) visual displays of monitored parameters (Figure 5-18). The number and configuration of these controls and displays vary from ventilator model to model, but their function and principles remain essentially the same.

Control Settings

The control settings area of the user interface allows the clinician to set the mode of ventilation, volume, pressure, respiratory rate, Fio_2, PEEP level, inspiratory trigger sensitivity or effort, and a variety of other breath delivery options (eg, inspiratory flow rate, inspiratory waveform pattern).

Alarm Settings

Alarms, which continuously monitor ventilator function, are essential to ensure safe and effective mechanical ventilation. Both high and low alarms are typically set to identify when critical parameters vary from the desired levels. Common alarms include low exhaled V_T, high or low exhaled minute volume, low Fio_2 delivery, high or low respiratory rate, and high or low airway pressures (Table 5-10).

Visual Displays

Airway pressures, respiratory rate, exhaled volumes, and the inspiratory to expiratory (I:E) ratio are among the most common visually displayed breath-to-breath values on the

TABLE 5-10. TRADITIONAL VENTILATOR ALARMS

Disconnect Alarms (Low-Pressure or Low-Volume Alarms)
- It is essential that when disconnection occurs, the clinician be immediately notified. Generally, this alarm is a continuous one and is triggered when a preselected inspiratory pressure level or minute ventilation is not sensed. With circuit leaks, this same alarm may be activated even though the patient may still be receiving a portion of the preset breath. Physical assessment, digital displays, and manometers are helpful in troubleshooting the cause of the alarms.

Pressure Alarms
- *High-pressure alarms* are set with volume modes of ventilation to ensure notification of pressures exceeding the selected threshold. These alarms are usually set 10-15 cm H_2O above the usual peak inspiratory pressure (PIP). Some causes for alarm activation (generally an intermittent alarm) include secretions, condensate in the tubing, biting on the endotracheal tubing, increased resistance (ie, bronchospasm), decreased compliance (eg, pulmonary edema, pneumothorax), and tubing compression.
- *Low-pressure alarms* are used to sense disconnection, circuit leaks, and changing compliance and resistance. They are generally set 5-10 cm H_2O below the usual PIP or 1-2 cm H_2O below the PEEP level or both.
- *Minute ventilation alarms* may be used to sense disconnection or changes in breathing pattern (rate and volume). Generally, low-minute ventilation and high-minute ventilation alarms are set (usually 5-10 L/min above and below usual minute ventilation). When stand-alone pressure support ventilation (PSV) is in use, this alarm may be the only audible alarm available on some ventilators.
- *Fio_2 alarms* are available when the ventilator circuit has a sensor to detect when the provided Fio_2 differs from the programmed Fio_2 setting.
- *Alarm silence or pause.* Because it is essential that alarms stay activated at all times, ventilator manufacturers have built-in silence or pause options so that clinicians can temporarily silence alarms for short periods (ie, 20 seconds). The ventilators "reset" the alarms automatically. Alarms provide important protection for ventilated patients. However, inappropriate threshold settings decrease usefulness. When threshold gradients are set too narrowly, alarms occur needlessly and frequently. Conversely, alarms that are set too loosely (wide gradients) do not allow for accurate and timely assessments.

Reproduced with permission from Kinney MR, et al, eds. AACN Clinical Reference for Critical Care Nursing, 4th ed. St Louis, MO: CV Mosby; 1998.

ventilator. Airway pressures are monitored during inspiration and exhalation and are often displayed as peak pressure, mean pressure, and end-expiratory pressure. A breath delivered by the ventilator produces higher airway pressures than an unassisted, spontaneous breath by the patient (Figure 5-19). The presence of PEEP is identified by a positive value at the end of expiration rather than 0 cm H_2O. Careful observation of the airway pressures provides the clinician with a great deal of information about the patient's

respiratory effort, coordination with the ventilator, and changes in lung compliance.

The display of the patient's exhaled V_T reflects the amount of gas that is returned to the ventilator via the expiratory tubing with each respiratory cycle. Exhaled volumes are measured and displayed with each breath. The patient's total exhaled minute volume is also often displayed. Exhaled V_Ts for ventilator-assisted mandatory breaths should be similar (± 10%) to the desired V_T setting selected on the control panel. The V_T of spontaneous breaths, or partially ventilator-supported breaths, however, may be different from the V_T control setting.

Modes

The *mode* of ventilation refers to one of the several different methods by which a ventilator supports ventilation. Modes are often classified as invasive (via an ET tube or tracheostomy tube) or noninvasive (via a face or nasal interface). These modes generate different levels of airway pressures, flow rate, volumes, and patterns of respiration and, therefore, different levels of support. The greater the level of ventilator support, the less muscle work performed by the patient. This "work of breathing" varies considerably with each of the modes of ventilation and is discussed later in this chapter in the section on respiratory muscle fatigue.

The different modes of ventilation used to support ventilation depend on the underlying respiratory problem and clinical preferences. A brief description of the basic invasive and noninvasive modes of mechanical ventilation follows.

Control Ventilation

The control mode of ventilation ensures that patients receive a predetermined number and volume of breaths each minute. No deviations from the respiratory rate or V_T settings are

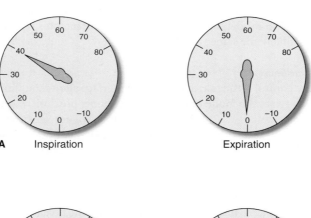

A   Inspiration   Expiration

B   Inspiration   Expiration

Figure 5-19. Typical airway pressure gauge changes during **(A)** ventilator-assisted breath and **(B)** spontaneous breath (cm H_2O).

delivered with this mode of ventilation. Generally the patient is heavily sedated and possibly paralyzed with neuromuscular blocking agents and in the ICU or the operating room when they are on this mode of ventilation. Occasionally, the "control" mode might be used in the patient who is paralyzed from a spinal cord injury or has a neuromuscular condition that precludes spontaneous breathing but is otherwise physiologically stable.

Assist-Control Ventilation

Similar to control ventilation, the assist-control or volume-controlled mode of ventilation (eg, A/C, VC, or AMV) provides a predetermined number and volume of breaths each minute should the patient not initiate respirations at that rate or above. In this mode, however, if the patient attempts to initiate breaths at a rate greater than the set minimum value, the ventilator delivers the spontaneously initiated breaths at the prescribed V_T; the patient may determine the total rate. WOB with this mode is variable mainly due to the ventilator delivering a fixed inspiratory flow rate that may not meet the patient's demand. In these circumstances, other modalities are now available which target a prescribed V_T but have the capability to generate a variable flow rate to better meet patient demand, thus reducing patient WOB.

Assist-control ventilation is often used when the patient is initially intubated (because minute ventilation requirements can be determined by the patient), for short-term ventilatory support such as postanesthesia, and as a support mode when high levels of ventilatory support are required. Excessive ventilation can occur with this mode in situations where the patient's spontaneous respiratory rate increases for nonrespiratory reasons (eg, pain, CNS dysfunction). The increased minute volume may result in potentially dangerous respiratory alkalosis. Changing to a different mode of ventilation or addressing the underlying cause of tachypnea may be necessary in these situations.

Synchronized Intermittent Mandatory Ventilation

The synchronized intermittent mandatory ventilation (SIMV) mode of ventilation ensures (or mandates) that a predetermined number of breaths at a selected V_T are delivered each minute. Any additional breaths initiated by the patient are allowed but, in contrast to the assist-control mode, the ventilator does not deliver these breaths. The patient is allowed to spontaneously breathe at the depth and rate desired until it is time for the next ventilator-assisted, or mandatory, breath. Mandatory breaths are synchronized with the patient's inspiratory effort, if present, to optimize patient-ventilator synchrony. The spontaneous breaths taken during SIMV are at the same FiO_2 as the mandatory breaths.

Originally designated as a ventilator mode for the gradual weaning of patients from mechanical ventilation, the use of a high-rate setting of SIMV can provide total ventilatory support. Reduction of the number of mandatory breaths allows the patient to slowly resume greater responsibility for

spontaneous breathing. SIMV can be used for similar indications as the assist-control mode, as well as for weaning the patient from mechanical ventilatory support. It is common to add pressure support (PS) to SIMV as a means of decreasing the WOB associated with spontaneous breathing.

The WOB with this mode of ventilation depends on the V_T and rate of the spontaneous breaths. When the mandatory, intermittent breaths provide the majority of minute volume, the WOB by the patient may be less than when spontaneous breathing constitutes a larger proportion of the patient's total minute volume.

Although strong clinician and institutional biases exist regarding whether to use SIMV or other modes for ventilatory support, little data exist to clarify which mode of ventilation is best. Close observation of the physiologic and psychological response to the ventilatory mode is required, and consideration is given to trials on alternative modes if warranted.

Spontaneous Breathing

Many ventilators have a mode that allows the patient to breathe spontaneously without ventilator. This is similar to placing the patient on a T-piece or blow-by oxygen setup, except it does have the benefit of providing continuous monitoring of exhaled volumes, airway pressures, and other parameters along with a closed circuit. The patient performs all the WOB. Use of the ventilator rather than the T-piece during spontaneous breathing actually may slightly increase the WOB. This occurs because of the additional inspiratory muscle work that is required to trigger flow delivery for each spontaneous breath. The amount of additional work required varies with different ventilator models.

This mode of ventilation is often identified as continuous positive airway pressure (CPAP), flow-by, or spontaneous (SPONT) on the ventilator. CPAP is a spontaneous breathing setting with the addition of PEEP during the breathing cycle.

Some ventilators have an additional adjunct that compensates for the resistance secondary to airway tube diameter. It is called automatic tube compensation (ATC). ATC can be used with ventilatory support or alone with spontaneous breathing.

Pressure Support

Pressure support is a spontaneous breathing mode, available in SIMV and SPONT modes, which maintain a set positive pressure during the spontaneous inspiration. The volume of a gas delivered by the ventilator during each inspiration varies depending on the level of PS and the demand of the patient. The higher the PS level, the higher the amount of gas delivered with each breath. Higher levels of PS can augment the spontaneous V_T and decrease the WOB associated with spontaneous breathing. At low levels of support, it is primarily used to overcome the airway resistance caused by breathing through the artificial airway and the breathing circuit. The airway pressure achieved during a PS breath is the result of the PS setting plus the set PEEP level.

Positive End-Expiratory Pressure/Continuous Positive Airway Pressure

Positive end-expiratory pressure is used in conjunction with any of the ventilator modes to help stabilize alveolar lung volume and improve oxygenation. The application of positive pressure to the airways during expiration may keep alveoli open and prevent early closure during exhalation. Lung compliance and ventilation-perfusion matching are often improved by prevention of early alveolar closure. If alveolar recruitment is not needed and excessive PEEP/CPAP is applied, it may result in adverse hemodynamic (ie, hypotension) or respiratory compromise (ie, auto-PEEP) and lung trauma (ie, barotrauma).

PEEP/CPAP is indicated for hypoxemia, which is secondary to diffuse lung injury (eg, ARDS, interstitial pneumonitis). PEEP/CPAP levels of 5 cm Hg or less are often used to provide "physiologic PEEP." The presence of the artificial airway allows intrathoracic pressure to fall to zero, which is below the usual level of intrathoracic pressure at end expiration (2 or 3 cm H_2O).

Use of PEEP may increase the risk of barotrauma due to higher mean and peak airway pressures during ventilation, especially when peak pressures are greater than 40 cm H_2O. High intrathoracic pressures also decrease venous return and CO. If CO decreases with PEEP/CPAP initiation and oxygenation is improved, a fluid bolus to correct hypovolemia may improve CO. Other potential complications of PEEP/CPAP include increases in intracranial pressure, decreased renal perfusion, increased hepatic congestion, and worsening of intracardiac shunts.

Bilevel Positive Airway Pressure

Bilevel positive airway pressure (ie, BiPAP) is a noninvasive mode of ventilation that combines two levels of positive pressure (PSV and PEEP) by means of a full face mask, nasal mask (most common), or nasal pillows. The ventilator is designed to compensate for leaks in the set-up, and a snug fit is needed, usually requiring head or chin straps. This form of therapy can be very labor intensive, requiring frequent assessment of patient tolerance. Full face mask ventilation is cautiously used because the potential for aspiration is high. If full face mask ventilation is chosen, the patient should be able to remove the mask quickly if nausea occurs or vomiting is imminent. The patient must be able to protect their airway during the use of BiPAP. For this reason, BiPAP is not used with patients who are obtunded patients and those with excessive secretions.

A number of options are available with BiPAP and include a spontaneous mode where the patient initiates all the pressure-supported breaths; a spontaneous-timed option, similar to PSV with a backup rate (some vendors call this A/C); and a control mode. The control mode requires the selection of a control rate and inspiratory time. A newer BiPAP mode adjusts pressure-supported breaths to maintain a targeted tidal volume and is known as average volume-assured pressure support (AVAPS).

Bilevel positive airway pressure is used successfully in a wide variety of progressive care patients such as those with sleep apnea, some patients with chronic hypoventilation syndromes, and also to prevent intubation and reintubation following extubation. Use of BiPAP in patients with COPD and heart failure is associated with decreased mortality and need for intubation. These patients are often difficult to wean from conventional ventilation given their underlying disease processes. Study results also demonstrate that outcomes in immunocompromised patients may also be better with non-invasive ventilation.

Complications of Mechanical Ventilation

Significant complications can arise from the use of mechanical ventilation and can be categorized as those associated with the patient's response to mechanical ventilation or those arising from ventilator malfunctions. Although the approach to minimizing or treating the complications of mechanical ventilation relate to the underlying cause, it is critical that frequent assessment of the patient, ventilator equipment, and the patient's response to ventilatory management be accomplished. Many clinicians participate in activities to assess the patient and ventilator, but the ultimate responsibility for ensuring continuous ventilatory support of the patient falls to the progressive care team including the bedside nurse and the respiratory therapist. Critically evaluating clinical indicators such as pH, $PaCO_2$, PaO_2, SpO_2, heart rate, BP, and so on, in conjunction with patient status and ventilatory parameters, is essential to decrease complications associated with this highly complex technology.

Patient Response

Hemodynamic Compromise

Normal intrathoracic pressure changes during spontaneous breathing are negative throughout the ventilatory cycle. Intrapleural pressure varies from about +5 cm H_2O during exhalation to –8 cm H_2O during inhalation. This decrease in intrapleural pressure during inhalation facilitates lung inflation and venous return. Thoracic pressure fluctuation during positive-pressure ventilation is opposite to those that occur during spontaneous breathing. The mean intrathoracic pressure is usually positive and increases during inhalation and decreases during exhalation. The use of positive-pressure ventilation increases peak airway pressures during inspiration, which in turn, increases mean airway pressures. This increase in mean airway pressure can impede venous return to the right atrium, thus decreasing CO. In some patients, this decrease in CO can be clinically significant, leading to increased heart rate and decreased blood pressure and impaired perfusion to vital organs.

Whenever mechanical ventilation is instituted or when ventilator changes are made, it is important to assess the patient's cardiovascular response. Approaches to managing hemodynamic compromise include increasing the preload of the heart (eg, fluid administration), decreasing the airway pressures exerted during mechanical ventilation by ensuring appropriate airway management techniques (suctioning, positioning, etc), and by judiciously setting ventilator parameters.

Barotrauma and Volutrauma

Barotrauma describes damage to the pulmonary system due to alveolar rupture from excessive airway pressures or overdistention of alveoli. Alveolar gas enters the interstitial pulmonary structures causing pneumothorax, pneumomediastinum, pneumoperitoneum, or subcutaneous emphysema. Because pneumothorax can lead to cardiovascular collapse, prompt recognition and management is essential. Pneumothorax should be considered whenever airway pressure rises acutely, breath sounds are diminished unilaterally, or blood pressure falls abruptly.

Patients with obstructive airway diseases (eg, asthma, bronchospasm), unevenly distributed lung disease (eg, lobar pneumonia), or hyperinflated lungs (eg, emphysema) are at high risk for barotrauma. Techniques to decrease the incidence of barotrauma include the use of small V_Ts, cautious use of PEEP, and the avoidance of high airway pressures and development of auto-PEEP in high-risk patients.

Volutrauma describes alveolar damage that results from high pressures resulting from large-volume ventilation in patients with ARDS. A common technique to reduce this risk is the use of smaller V_Ts (4-6 mL/kg of ideal body weight) and sometimes this is described as the "low stretch" protocol or low tidal volume ventilation. Different from barotrauma, this damage results in alveolar fractures and flooding of alveoli. It is linked to the use of V_Ts greater than 6 mL/kg in patients with ARDS.

Auto-PEEP occurs when a delivered breath is incompletely exhaled before the onset of the next inspiration. This gas trapping increases overall lung volumes, inadvertently raising the end-expiratory pressure in the alveoli. The presence of auto-PEEP increases the risk for complications from PEEP. Ventilator patients with COPD (eg, asthma, emphysema) or high respiratory rates are at increased risk for the development of auto-PEEP.

Auto-PEEP, also termed *intrinsic* PEEP, is difficult to diagnose because it cannot be observed on the airway pressure display at end expiration. The technique for assessment for auto-PEEP varies with different ventilator models and modes, but typically involves measuring the airway pressure close to the artificial airway during occlusion of the expiratory ventilator circuit during end expiration. This method requires that the patient be completely passive and not trigger a breath; it is not possible to measure auto-PEEP by this method in actively breathing patients. Another technique of monitoring auto-PEEP in actively breathing patients is the use of the flow-time curve displayed by the ventilator. If flow does not return to baseline at the end of exhalation before the next breath starts, the patient has auto-PEEP. Auto-PEEP can be minimized by:

- Maximizing the length of time for expiration (eg, increasing inspiratory flow rates by shortening inspiratory times)
- Decreasing obstructions to expiratory flow (eg, using larger diameter ET tubes, eliminating bronchospasm and secretions)
- Avoiding overventilation

Ventilator-Associated Pneumonia

Ventilator-associated pneumonia is a hospital-acquired complication that is associated with increased patient morbidity and mortality. Prevention includes evidence-based practices to limit the use of invasive ventilation, promote patient safety while undergoing invasive ventilation, and effective protocols for ventilator liberation. Interventions during ventilation are aimed at avoiding colonization and subsequent aspiration of bacteria into the lower airway. Elevation of the head of the bed to 30° to 45° helps minimize aspiration of oral and gastric secretions. A specially designed ET tube (Figure 5-20) incorporates a dedicated suction lumen above the ET cuff, which permits continuous low suction pressure (–20 mm Hg) or intermittent suctioning of subglottic secretions pooled above the cuff. Removal of the accumulated secretions may be particularly helpful before cuff deflation or manipulation. Studies have demonstrated that the application of continuous aspiration of subglottic secretions with ET tubes only may prevent or delay the onset of VAP. Although subglottic suctioning is now available in some tracheostomy tubes, there are currently no recommendations for the use of subglottic suctioning in these tubes. In addition, oral care protocols including chlorhexidine gluconate 0.12% mouth rinse and tooth brushing to remove plaque are important adjuncts in VAP prevention. See Chapter 10, Respiratory System: Preventing Hospital-Acquired Pneumonia for complete discussion.

Positive Fluid Balance and Hyponatremia

Hyponatremia is a common occurrence following the institution of mechanical ventilation and develops from several factors, including applied PEEP, humidification of inspired gases, hypotonic fluid administration and diuretics, and increased levels of circulating antidiuretic hormone.

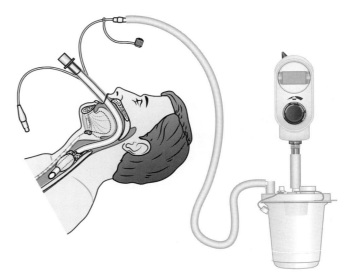

Figure 5-20. Cuffed endotracheal tube with dedicated lumen for continuous aspiration of subglottic secretions accumulated immediately above cuff. The dedicated lumen connector is attached to wall suction. (©2018 Medtronic. All rights reserved. Used with the permission of Medtronic.)

Upper Gastrointestinal Hemorrhage

Upper gastrointestinal (GI) bleeding may develop secondary to ulceration or gastritis. In some patients the use of proton-pump inhibitors, H$_2$ receptor antagonists, antacids, or cytoprotective agents is appropriate to prevent bleeding (see Chapter 7, Pharmacology and Chapter 14, Gastrointestinal System, for discussions of GI prophylaxis).

Ventilator Malfunction

Problems related to the proper functioning of mechanical ventilators, although rare, may have devastating consequences for patients. Many of the alarm systems on ventilators are designed to alert clinicians to improperly functioning ventilatory systems. These alarm systems must be activated at all times if ventilator malfunction problems are to be quickly identified and corrected, and untoward patient events avoided (see Table 5-10).

Many of the "problems" identified with ventilatory equipment are actually related to inappropriate setup or use of the devices. Examples of operator-related issues include ventilator circuits that are not properly connected, alarm systems that are set improperly, or inadequate ventilator settings for a particular clinical condition.

There are occasions, however, when ventilator systems do not operate properly. Examples of ventilator malfunctions include valve mechanisms sticking and obstructing gas flow, inadequate or excessive gas delivery, electronic circuit failures in microprocessing-based ventilators, failures with complete shutdown, and power failures or surges in the institution.

The most important approach to ventilator malfunction is to maintain a high level of vigilance to determine if ventilators are performing properly. Ensuring that alarm systems are set appropriately at all times, providing frequent routine assessment of ventilator functioning, and the use of experienced support personnel to maintain the ventilator systems are some of the most crucial activities necessary to avoid problems. In addition, whenever ventilator malfunction is suspected, the patient should be immediately removed from the device and temporary ventilation and oxygenation provided with an MRB or another ventilator until the question of proper functioning is resolved. Any sudden change in the patient's respiratory or cardiovascular status alerts the clinician to consider potential ventilator malfunction as a cause.

Weaning From Short-Term Mechanical Ventilation

The process of transitioning the ventilator-dependent patient to unassisted spontaneous breathing is *weaning from mechanical ventilation*. This is a period of time where the requirement for oxygenation and ventilation is decreased, either gradually or abruptly, while monitoring the patient's response to the resumption of spontaneous breathing. A standardized approach along with weaning readiness criteria has been shown to reduce ventilator days and improve outcomes. Weaning or "liberation" is considered to be complete, or successful, when the patient has been extubated successfully and does not require reintubation within 48 hours. The majority of patients intubated and ventilated for short periods of time (< 72 hours) are successfully weaned with the first spontaneous breathing trial (SBT) in the ICU. Additionally, there is a subset of patients with long-term tracheostomy tubes who may require short-term ventilation who are able to wean quickly once the clinical issue requiring mechanical ventilation is resolved. Approximately 30% of patients, however, require extended time periods for successfully weaning, and some remain unable to breathe without partial or complete support from mechanical ventilation.

Weaning proceeds when the underlying cause of respiratory failure is addressed and the patient is breathing spontaneously, maintaining adequate gas exchange, and protecting their own airway. Unnecessary delays in weaning from mechanical ventilation increase the likelihood of complications such as ventilator-induced lung injury, pneumonia, discomfort, and increases in hospitalization costs. Thus, aggressive and timely weaning trials such as SBT are encouraged.

Steps in the Weaning Process
Assessment of Readiness

Readiness to wean from short-term mechanical ventilation (STMV) may be assessed with a wide variety of criteria. However, in most institutions, for short-term ventilator patients, assessment of readiness to wean includes just three or four criteria. Examples of these criteria include:

- ABGs within normal limits on minimal to moderate amounts of ventilatory support (Fio$_2$ ≤ 0.50, minute ventilation ≤ 10 L/min, PEEP ≤ 5 cm H$_2$O)
- NIP that is more negative than −20 cm H$_2$O
- Spontaneous V$_T$ ≥ 5 mL/kg
- Vital capacity ≥10 mL/kg
- Respiratory rate < 30 breaths/min
- Spontaneous rapid-shallow breathing index < 105 breaths/min/liter

An effective measure of weaning readiness can be incorporated into a bundled approach that includes both a daily safety screen and a collaborative weaning protocol. The "ABCDEF" bundle incorporates sedation awakening trials, SBTs, and other evidence-based practices for ICU management (Table 5-11). Bundles are a structured method of improving patient care processes and when collectively performed, have resulted in improved patient outcomes. Interventions such as minimizing sedation, assessing for delirium, promoting early mobility, and involving the family contribute to prompt ventilator liberation. Protocols that incorporate these elements of care can decrease practice variation and improve patient outcomes.

Following selection of the method for weaning (see the discussion below), the actual weaning trial can begin. It is important to prepare both the patient and the progressive

TABLE 5-11. ABCDEF BUNDLE AND COMPONENTS

Requires a coordinated effort between the healthcare team

A—Assess, Prevent and Manage Pain
- See Chapter 6 for more on the management of pain

B—Both Spontaneous Awakening Trials (SAT) and Spontaneous Breathing Trials (SBT)
1. Spontaneous Awakening Trial
   - Daily assessment of SAT safety screen to turn off sedation
   - Daily awakening, sedation vacation, or daily interruption of sedation trial
2. Spontaneous Breathing Trial
   - Daily assessment of SBT safety screen
   - Daily spontaneous breathing trial

C—Choice of Analgesia and Sedation
- Assessment of Pain and Sedation using validated tool
- See chapter 6 for more on management of sedation

D—Delirium: Assess, Prevent and Manage
1. Routine Assessment of Delirium using validated tool
   - Confusion assessment method for the ICU (CAM-ICU)
   - Intensive care delirium screening checklist (ICDSC)
2. Stop
   - Evaluate risk factors for delirium
3. THINK pneumonic to evaluate causes of delirium
   - T–Toxic situations
     - CHF, shock, dehydration
     - Medications
     - New organ failure
   - H–Hypoxemia
   - I–Infection/sepsis
   - N–Nonpharmacologic interventions
     - Hearing aids, glasses, reorientation, sleep protocols, music, noise control, ambulation, family
   - K+ –electrolyte problems
4. Medicate if needed

E—Early Mobility and Exercise
- Early Mobility Protocol
- Daily assessment of mobility readiness
- **Mobility program**

F—Family Engagement and Empowerment
- Patient and family centered care

Data from Society of Critical Care Medicine. ICU Liberation: ABCDEF Bundles. http://www.iculiberation.org/SiteCollectionDocuments/Bundles-ICU-Liberation-ABCDEF.pdf. Accessed June 6, 2017.

care environment properly to maximize the chances for weaning success.

During an SBT, interventions include appropriate explanations of the process to the patient, positioning and medication to improve ventilatory efforts, and the avoidance of unnecessary activities during the weaning trial. Throughout the weaning time, continuous monitoring for signs and symptoms of respiratory distress or fatigue is essential. They include dyspnea, tachypnea, chest abdominal dyssynchrony, anxiety, tachycardia, changes in blood pressure, and changes in oxygenation or ventilation. Many of these indicators are subtle, but careful monitoring of baseline levels before weaning progresses and throughout the trial provides objective indicators of the need to return the patient to previous levels of ventilator support.

The need to temporarily stop the weaning trial is not viewed as, or termed, a failure. Instead it simply suggests that more time needs to be provided to ensure success. A full evaluation of the multiple reasons for inability to wean is necessary, however.

Weaning Trials

SBTs for patients undergoing short-term mechanical ventilation are usually done on T-piece or on the ventilator using CPAP or a low level of PS. Recent guidelines recommend that the initial SBT be implemented on the ventilator with CPAP or low level of PS. Readiness for weaning is assessed daily using a "safety screen" which includes such factors as hemodynamic stability, oxygenation status, and improvement in the condition that necessitated the use of mechanical ventilation. Weaning protocols also include a daily trial of minimal sedation, sometimes called a spontaneous awakening trial (SAT) which is done prior to or concurrently with the SBT (Figure 5-21). Once the patient is assessed as "ready," the SBT is initiated for a duration of at least 30 minutes but no more than 120 minutes. The trial is stopped if the patient shows signs of distress and/or deterioration. A decision to extubate is made with the conclusion of a successful trial. The need for reintubation is associated with increased mortality. Thus, premature attempts at extubation are to be avoided. Recent guidelines suggest that the use of noninvasive positive-pressure ventilation via face or nasal mask immediately after extubation may be useful for patients who have been receiving mechanical ventilation for more than 24 hours and are at high risk for re-intubation after passing a successful SBT.

Methods

A variety of methods are available for weaning patients from mechanical ventilation. To date, research on these techniques has not clearly identified any one method as optimal for weaning from short-term mechanical ventilation. Most institutions, however, use one or two approaches routinely. A body of research has demonstrated that the outcomes of patients managed with protocols driven by nonphysician clinicians were better than those managed with standard physician-directed care. Most experts on weaning believe that, with short-term ventilator-dependent patients, the actual method used to wean the patient is less important to weaning success than using a consistently applied protocol strategy. In addition, there are some ventilators that have automated weaning systems that adapt to the patient's clinical needs. Additional research is needed to determine automated ventilator weaning efficacy over clinician-driven protocols.

- *T-piece, blow by, or trach collar:* The T-piece method of weaning involves removing the patient from the mechanical ventilator and attaching an oxygen source to the artificial airway with a "T" piece for an SBT. A trach collar also provides oxygen but attaches by an elastic strap around the neck instead of directly to the artificial airway. No ventilatory support occurs with this device, the patient breaths spontaneously

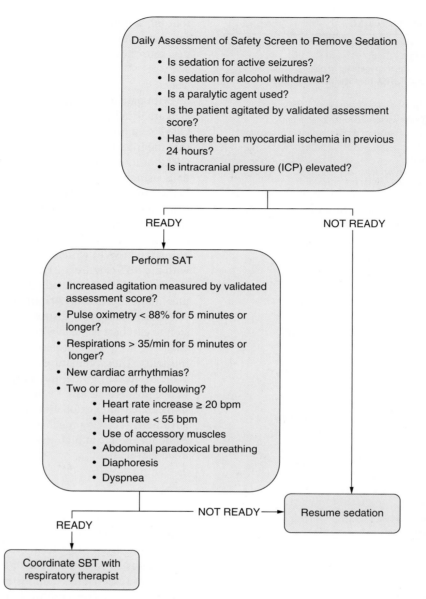

Figure 5-21. Spontaneous awakening trial–SAT. (*Data from Balas MC, Vasilevskis EE, Burke WJ, et al. Critical care nurses' role in implementing the "ABCDE Bundle" into practice.* Crit Care Nurse. *2012;32(5):35-38.*)

the entire time this device is connected. The advantage of this method of weaning is that the resistance to breathing is low, because no special valves need to be opened to initiate gas flow. Rapid assessment of the patient's ability to spontaneously breathe is another purported advantage. Limitations of this SBT are that it may cause ventilatory muscle overload and fatigue. When this occurs, it usually appears early in the SBT, so the patient must be closely monitored during the initial few minutes. A PEEP valve can be added to the T piece; however, similar to trach collar weaning, there are no alarms or backup systems to support the patient if ventilation is inadequate. It is critical to recognize that this technique relies on the clinician to monitor for signs and symptoms of respiratory difficulty and fatigue. Frequently, the Fio_2 is increased by at least 10% over the Fio_2 setting on the ventilator to prevent hypoxemia resulting from the lower V_T of spontaneous breaths. Patients who are unable to tolerate an SBT should receive a stable, nonfatiguing, comfortable form of ventilatory support following the trial.

- *CPAP:* The use of the ventilator to allow spontaneous breathing periods without mandated breaths, similar to the T-piece, can be done with the CPAP mode. With this approach, ventilator alarm systems can be used to monitor spontaneous breathing rates and volumes, and a small amount of continuous pressure (5 cm H_2O) can be applied if needed. The disadvantage of this approach is that the WOB resulting from the need to open the demand valve to receive gas flow for the breath is higher than with the T-piece. For most patients, this slight additional WOB is not likely to be a critical factor to their weaning success or failure unless the trial is unduly long. If needed, a low level of PS (eg, 5-7 cm H_2O) may also be added to offset this workload (CPAP + PS). In some ventilators, an additional feature, ATC, can offset the additional workload imposed by the ventilator circuit and the ET.

- *Pressure support:* Another method for weaning from mechanical ventilation is the use of low level PS ventilation. With this method, patients can spontaneously breathe on the ventilator with a small amount of ventilator *support* to augment their spontaneous breaths. This technique overcomes some of the resistance to breathing associated with ET tubes and demand valves. The main disadvantage with this approach is that clinicians may underestimate the degree of support that is provided and prematurely stop the weaning process.
- *SIMV:* One of the most popular methods of weaning patients in the past, this modality has recently been shown to prolong the duration of mechanical ventilation in comparison to weaning with SBT or PS. By progressively decreasing the number of mandated breaths delivered by the ventilator, the patient performs more and more of the WOB by increasing spontaneous breathing. Advantages to the SIMV mode are the presence of built-in alarms to alert clinicians when ventilation problems occur and, in some modes, the guarantee of a minimum minute ventilation. The disadvantage of SIMV is that each spontaneous breath requires some additional WOB to open a valve, which allows gas flow to the patient for the spontaneous breath. SIMV is used either alone or in conjunction with pressure support (SIMV + PS).

Weaning From Long-Term Mechanical Ventilation

In contrast to patients who require short-term (< 3 days) ventilation, those who require long-term mechanical ventilation (LTMV) (defined as > 3 days) may take days, weeks, or even months to liberate from the ventilator. In these LTMV patients, the weaning process varies and consists of four stages. The first stage is marked by instability and high ventilatory support requirements. During the second stage, called the prewean stage, many physiologic factors continue to require attention, and the patient's overall status may fluctuate. Ventilatory requirements are less and adjustments are made to maintain oxygenation and acid-base status as well as provide ventilatory muscle conditioning. The third, or weaning stage, is evident when the patient is stable, and rapid progress with weaning trials is possible. Finally, the last stage is called the outcome stage, which consists of successful extubation, or provision of partial or full ventilatory support.

Long-term mechanical ventilation is associated with high morbidity and mortality rates, and institutions lose money on patients ventilated long-term because reimbursement rarely covers the associated costs. As a result, clinicians, scientists, and institutions are interested in testing methods of care delivery that improve the clinical and financial outcomes. Research in the area of weaning offers some guidance to clinicians working with these patients. The following discussions of weaning patients from LTMV address weaning readiness assessment, wean planning, and weaning modes and methods, including comprehensive institutional approaches.

Wean Assessment

Traditionally, the decision about when to begin the weaning process is determined once the condition that necessitates mechanical ventilation is improved or resolved. In the past, "traditional" weaning predictors were used in an attempt to determine the optimal timing for extubation. More recently, investigators combined pulmonary assessments to improve predictive ability in LTMV patients. An example is the index of rapid shallow breathing, also known as the frequency (f_X)/tidal volume (V_T) index, which integrates rate and tidal volume. Unfortunately, these measures have not accurately predicted success in weaning. This is in part because they focus exclusively on pulmonary components to the exclusion of important nonpulmonary factors that influence a patient's ability to breath independently (Table 5-12). Although the standard weaning criteria are not predictive, the components are helpful for assessing the patient's overall condition and readiness for weaning.

As noted, assessment of weaning potential starts with an evaluation of the underlying reason for mechanical ventilation (sepsis, pneumonia, trauma, and the like). Resolution of the underlying cause is necessary before gains in the weaning process can be expected. However, it is important to remember that resolution alone is frequently not sufficient to ensure successful weaning. Patients who require prolonged mechanical ventilation, sometimes referred to as the "chronically, critically ill," often suffer from a myriad of conditions that impede weaning. Even with resolution of the acute disease or condition that necessitated mechanical ventilation, the patient's overall functional status is often below baseline (weak, malnourished, etc). Therefore, a

TABLE 5-12. PULMONARY SPECIFIC WEAN CRITERIA THRESHOLDS

Traditional Weaning Criteria
- Negative inspiratory pressure (NIP) ≤ −20 cm H_2O
- Positive expiratory pressure (PEP) ≥ + 30 cm H_2O
- Spontaneous tidal volume (SV_T) ≥ 5 mL/kg
- Vital capacity (VC) ≥ 15 mL/kg
- Fraction of inspired oxygen (FiO_2) ≤ 50%
- Minute ventilation (MV) ≤ 10 L/min

Integrated Weaning Criteria
- Index of rapid shallow breathing or frequency tidal volume ratio (f_X/V_T) ≤ 105

TABLE 5-13. BURNS' WEAN ASSESSMENT PROGRAM (BWAP)^A

I. General Assessment

Yes	No	Not Assessed	
____	____	_____	1. Hemodynamically stable (pulse rate, cardiac output)?
____	____	_____	2. Free from factors that increase or decrease metabolic rate (seizures, temperature, sepsis, bacteremia, hypo/hyperthyroid)?
____	____	_____	3. Hematocrit > 25% (or baseline)?
____	____	_____	4. Systemically hydrated (weight at or near baseline, balanced intake and output)?
____	____	_____	5. Nourished (albumin > 2.5, parenteral/enteral feedings maximized)? *If albumin is low and anasarca or third spacing is present, score for hydration should be "no."
____	____	_____	6. Electrolytes within normal limits (including Ca^{++}, Mg^+, PO_4)? *Correct Ca^{++} for albumin level.
____	____	_____	7. Pain controlled (subjective determination)?
____	____	_____	8. Adequate sleep/rest (subjective determination)?
____	____	_____	9. Appropriate level of anxiety and nervousness (subjective determination)?
____	____	_____	10. Absence of bowel problems (diarrhea, constipation, ileus)?
____	____	_____	11. Improved general body strength/endurance (ie, out of bed in chair, progressive activity program)?
____	____	_____	12. Chest x-ray improving?

II. Respiratory Assessment

Yes   No   Not Assessed

Gas Flow and Work of Breathing

Yes	No	Not Assessed	
____	____	_____	13. Eupneic respiratory rate and pattern (spontaneous RR < 25, without dyspnea, absence of accessory muscle use)? *This is assessed off the ventilator while measuring #20-23.
____	____	_____	14. Absence of adventitious breath sounds (rhonchi, rales, wheezing)?
____	____	_____	15. Secretions thin and minimal?
____	____	_____	16. Absence of neuromuscular disease/deformity?
____	____	_____	17. Absence of abdominal distention/obesity/ascites?
____	____	_____	18. Oral ETT > #7.5 or trach > #6.5?

Airway Clearance

| ____ | ____ | _____ | 19. Cough and swallow reflexes adequate? |

Strength

| ____ | ____ | _____ | 20. NIP < 20 (negative inspiratory pressure)? |
| ____ | ____ | _____ | 21. PEP > 30 (positive expiratory pressure)? |

Endurance

| ____ | ____ | _____ | 22. STV > 5 mL/kg (spontaneous tidal volume)? |
| ____ | ____ | _____ | 23. VC > 10-15 mL/kg (vital capacity)? |

ABGs

____	____	_____	24. pH 7.30-7.45?
____	____	_____	25. $Paco_2$, 40 mm Hg (or baseline) with mV < 10 L/min? *This is evaluated while on ventilator.
____	____	_____	26. Pao_2 60 on Fio_2 < 40%?

^{a}The BWAP score is obtained by dividing the total number of BWAP factors scored as "yes" by 26. © Burns 1990.

systematic, comprehensive approach to weaning assessment is important. One example of a tool that encourages such an approach is the Burns Wean Assessment Program (BWAP) (Table 5-13). The BWAP score is used to track the progress of the patient and keep care planning on target. Factors important to weaning are listed in the BWAP bedside checklist.

Wean Planning

Once impediments to weaning are identified, plans that focus on addressing the impediments are made in collaboration with an intraprofessional team. A collaborative approach to assessment and planning greatly enhances positive outcomes in the LTMV patient. However, for care planning to

be successful, it must also be systematic. The wean process is dynamic and regular reassessment and adjustment of plans are necessary. Tools like the BWAP can be used to routinely assess and track weaning progress. Clinical pathways, protocols for weaning, and institution-wide approaches to managing and monitoring the patients are also effective strategies that ensure consistency in care and promote better outcomes.

Weaning Trials, Modes, and Methods

A wide variety of weaning modes and methods are available for weaning the patient ventilated short term as described earlier. To date, no data support the superiority of any one mode for weaning those requiring LTMV; however, methods using

ESSENTIAL CONTENT CASE

Long-Term Weaning

A 75-year-old man with COPD and oxygen dependence was admitted to the ED in respiratory distress. He was intubated and placed on the ventilator secondary to profound hypercarbia and respiratory acidosis and then transferred to the MICU for management of respiratory failure and right upper lobe pneumonia. In the ICU, the intensive care team anticipates that this patient will need long-term weaning and so a tracheostomy tube is placed on day 4 to increase his comfort and mobility.

After 7 days of treatment with mechanical ventilation, the patient is transferred to the respiratory step-down unit for further management and weaning. Major impediments to weaning as assessed by the unit team include:

- Poor nutritional status (albumin < 1.8 g/dL)
- Anxiety and agitation
- Debilitation and inability to ambulate
- Persistent upper lobe infiltrate
- Copious secretions
- NIP < 15 cm H_2O
- Minute ventilation > 15 L/min with a $Paco_2$ of 50 mm Hg

The team recognizes that these factors contributed to his high WOB (secretions, respiratory rate, minute ventilation) and his overall weak and debilitated state (nutrition, immobility, NIP). They acknowledge that these factors must be addressed before successful weaning.. Based on these factors, prolonged mechanical ventilation is likely. After 2 days of "complete rest," a ventilatory mode is selected that allows for gradual respiratory muscle conditioning while overall improvement in physical status is addressed. PSV is selected at PSV max (which in this case was 20 cm H_2O). This setting resulted in a respiratory rate of 16 breaths/min, a tidal volume of 8 mL/kg, and a eupneic respiratory pattern. PSV max is used for rest during the day and at night. For gradual conditioning trials, the PSV level is decreased in increments of 5 cm H_2O as defined by the PSV protocol.

Case Question 1. What other weaning modality could have been used in this patient and why?

Case Question 2. What components of the ABCDEF protocol were used for this patient?

Answers

1. As the research has not demonstrated any mode or method to be superior for a patient weaning with a tracheostomy, progressively longer SBTs may be used effectively. The modes can vary and include using trach collar or low levels of PSV with intermittent rest periods on the ventilator (with support settings such as AC or a higher level of PSV). When the patient is able to sustain spontaneous breathing for a full 12 hours during the day, the nighttime ventilator support (at the "rest" level) may then be reduced, or if clinically appropriate, curtailed. The next steps would be to work on removal of the tracheostomy tube following downsizing and or use of a talking trach to determine tolerance. This stepwise approach allows the patient to gradually transition to liberation from the ventilator.

2. The patient received daily spontaneous awakening and assessment for readiness to wean (B). His delirium was addressed by using a modified sleep protocol and by using the family (F) to reorient the patient as well as encouraging the use of personal items when possible (D). Early exercise was implemented in the ICU and continued after transfer and integrated into his daily routine (E).

   Three days later, the patient is sitting in a chair at the bedside and beginning to ambulate with the help of the nurse and physical therapist. Enteral nutrition is provided via a small-bore nasal gastric tube. Serial BWAP assessments demonstrate improvement (47%-55%) but the team recognizes that his recovery would likely take weeks. After 2 more weeks of this routine, the patient is able to tolerate a PSV of 5 (the lowest level of the plan), and the team initiates tracheostomy collar trials. Night rest continues until the patient tolerates 12 hours without signs of intolerance. He is decannulated and sent home with his family 1 week later.

protocols and other systematic, intraprofessional approaches do appear to make a difference and are to be encouraged. These methods are described following a discussion of respiratory muscle fatigue, rest, and conditioning because the concepts are integrated into the section on protocols.

Respiratory Fatigue, Rest, and Conditioning

Respiratory muscle fatigue is common in ventilated weaning patients and occurs when the respiratory workload is excessive. When the workload exceeds metabolic stores, fatigue and hypercarbic respiratory failure ensue. Examples of those at risk include patients who are hypermetabolic, weak, or malnourished. Signs of encroaching fatigue include dyspnea, tachypnea, chest-abdominal asynchrony, and elevated $Paco_2$ (a late sign). These signs and symptoms indicate a need for increased ventilatory support. Once fatigued, the

muscles require 12 to 24 hours of rest to recover, which is accomplished through the selection of appropriate modes of ventilation.

For the respiratory muscles to recover from fatigue, the inspiratory workload must be decreased. In the case of volume ventilation (eg, assist-control, intermittent mandatory ventilation), this means complete cessation of spontaneous effort, but in the case of pressure ventilation, a high level of PSV may accomplish the necessary "unloading." Generally, this means increasing the PSV level to attain a spontaneous respiratory rate of 20 breaths/min or less and the absence of accessory muscle use. However, in patients with obstructive diseases (eg, asthma and COPD), this higher level of support may result in further hyperinflation and adverse clinical outcomes. If the technique is used in these patients, it should be done cautiously.

Respiratory muscle conditioning employs concepts borrowed from exercise physiology. To condition muscles and attain an optimal training effect from exercise, the concepts of endurance and strength conditioning may be considered. With strength training, a large force is moved a short distance. The muscles are worked to fatigue (short duration intervals) and rested for long periods of time. SBTs on T-piece or CPAP both mimic this type of training because they employ high pressure and low-volume work.

Endurance conditioning, which requires that the workload be increased gradually, is easily accomplished with PSV because the level of support can be decreased over time. This kind of endurance training employs low pressure and high-volume work. Central to the application of both conditioning methods is the provision of adequate respiratory muscle rest between trials. Prolonging trials once the patient is fatigued serves no useful purpose and may be extremely detrimental physiologically and psychologically.

Wean Trial Protocols

Study results suggest that no mode of ventilation is superior for weaning; however, research does show that the process of weaning, specifically the use of protocols, decreases variations in care and improves outcomes. Protocols clearly delineate the actions caregivers take to promote successful weaning. The protocol components consist of weaning readiness criteria (wean screens), weaning trial method and duration (ie, CPAP, T-piece, or PSV), and parameters for assessing intolerance and providing respiratory muscle rest.

Spontaneous breathing trials (described earlier), using CPAP or T-piece, are commonly used for weaning trials. The duration of such trials is generally between 30 minutes and 2 hours, although in those patients with tracheotomy tubes, the duration may be much longer. While CPAP or T-piece are most often used for weaning trials, other protocols may include the use of PSV (an endurance mode) and CPAP (a strengthening mode) and providers may individualize to meet specific patient requirements. One example is that of patients with heart failure. In these patients, the sudden transition from ventilator support to the use of T-piece or CPAP for an SBT may result in an increased venous return during the wean trial that overwhelms the heart's ability to compensate. Until appropriate preload and after-load reduction is addressed in these patients, PSV may be a gentler method of weaning. Another example is that of patients with profound myopathies or extremely debilitated states that may benefit from more gradual increases in work such as provided by PSV. Some new pressure modes such as proportional assist ventilation and adaptive support ventilation may potentially decrease the patient's workload during weaning. More on advanced modes of ventilation, including these, may be found in the *AACN Essentials of Critical Care Nursing*, Chapter 20: Advanced Respiratory Concepts.

A popular and common sense approach to wean trial progression is to attempt weaning trials during the daytime,

TABLE 5-14. GENERAL WEANING GUIDELINES FOR LONG-TERM MECHANICALLY VENTILATED PATIENTS

Active Weaning Should Occur
- When patient is stable and reason for mechanical ventilation is resolved or improving
- When the "wean screen protocol criteria" are attained. A temporary hold and even an increase in support may be necessary when setbacks occur
- During the daytime, not at night (to allow respiratory muscle rest)

Considerations for Temporary Hold
- With acute changes in condition
- During procedures that require that the patient be flat or in the Trendelenburg position (ie, during line insertion)
- During "road trips" (consider increased ventilatory support to protect the patient while off the unit)
- If suctioning is excessive (every half hour)
- When febrile, bacteremic, septic, or with *Clostridium difficile* disease

Rest and Sleep
- Rest is important for psychological and physiologic reasons. Complete rest in the mechanically ventilated patient is defined as that level of ventilatory support that offsets the work of breathing and decreases fatigue (refer to detailed description in text). Decisions about when rest is important include the following:
- When an acute event has occurred (ie, hypercarbic respiratory failure, pulmonary embolus, pulmonary edema)
- A reasonable approach for the chronic or nonacute patient is to work on active weaning trials during the day with rest at night until most of the daytime wean is accomplished (≥ 10 hours). Then, nighttime wean trials can be accomplished fairly rapidly. At night, the patient is allowed to sleep—if work of breathing is high, sleep is not possible. Ventilator rate should be high enough to allow for relaxation and optimal resting. If night sleeping aids are used, administer them early in the night to enhance sleep and ventilatory synchronization so that the drugs can be metabolized before the daytime trials begin.

allowing the patient to rest with increased ventilator support at night until the protocol threshold for extubation is reached. In the case of the patient with a tracheostomy, progressively longer episodes of spontaneous breathing, usually on tracheostomy collar or T-piece, are accomplished until tolerated for a specified amount of time. Then, decisions about discontinuation of ventilation and tracheostomy downsizing or decannulation may be made. Clearly communicating the wean plans to all members of the healthcare team, and especially the patient and family ensures team acceptance and consistency. The aim is that the plan be sufficiently aggressive but safe and effective in meeting the patient's goals. Table 5-14 describes some general mechanical ventilator weaning philosophy concepts.

Other Protocols for Use

Patients who require LTMV often face a variety of clinical conditions that not only prolong ventilator duration, but also affect other outcomes such as length of stay and mortality. Research has demonstrated that outcomes of critically ill patients are improved with protocol-directed management. The "ABCDEF" bundle, for instance, is effective in short term mechanical ventilation and the principles of the bundle may also be useful in the LTMV patient. More research is needed on protocol-directed management in the subset of patients who require prolonged mechanical ventilation (greater than 21 days).

Critical Pathways

Critical pathways are used to ensure that evidence-based care is provided and that variation in care delivery is reduced. Some pathways can be very directive, such as those for patients undergoing hip replacements, where clinical progression can be anticipated by hours or days. However, such specificity is not possible in the ventilated patient. Instead, pathways for the LTMV patient combine elements of care by specific time intervals (ie, begin deep vein thrombosis prophylaxis by day one) with those that are designated by the stage of illness (ie, patient up to the chair during the prewean stage). In addition to providing an evidence-based blueprint for a wide variety of care elements, the pathways encourage intraprofessional input and collaboration. Ideally, they are incorporated into systematic institutional approaches to care of the LTMV patient population.

Systematic Institutional Initiatives for the Management of the LTMV Patient Population

Given the importance of systematic assessment and care planning, it is not surprising that many institutions have taken a very comprehensive approach to the care of patients who require LTMV. Solutions to reduce variation and promote standardization of care are implemented to ensure adherence to best practices.

In one study, an algorithmic approach to weaning was instituted in three adult ICUs and nurses managed the process. In another study, advanced practice nurses called "outcomes managers" managed and monitored long-term ventilated patients using an intraprofessional clinical pathway and protocols for the management of sedation and weaning trials. The two studies demonstrated that statistically significant positive differences in most variables of interest such as ventilator duration, ICU and hospital lengths of stay (LOS), mortality rate, and cost savings were attainable with the approaches.

The healthcare environment is often chaotic. Short LOS and decreased staffing levels affect the continuity of care and contribute to gaps in practice and care planning. Given the complexity of the care of the ventilated patient, it is clear that approaches to care that decrease variation and promote coordination may improve patient outcomes and are to be encouraged.

Troubleshooting Ventilators

The complexity of ventilators and the dynamic state of the patient's clinical condition, as well as the patient's response to ventilation, create a variety of common problems that may occur during mechanical ventilation. It is crucial that progressive care clinicians be expert in the prevention,

identification, and management of ventilator-associated problems in ventilated patients.

During mechanical ventilation, sudden changes in the clinical condition of the patient, particularly respiratory distress, as well as the occurrence of ventilator alarms or abnormal functioning of the ventilator, require immediate assessment and intervention. A systematic approach to each of these situations minimizes untoward ventilator events (Figure 5-22).

The first step is to determine the presence of respiratory distress or hemodynamic instability. If either is present, the patient is removed from the mechanical ventilator and manually ventilated with an MRB and 100% O_2 for a few minutes. During manual ventilation, a quick assessment of the respiratory and cardiovascular system is made, noting

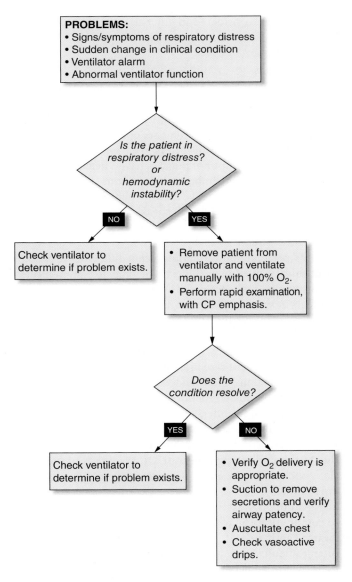

Figure 5-22. Algorithm for management of ventilator alarms and/or development of acute respiratory distress.

changes from previous status. Clinical improvement rapidly following removal from the ventilator suggests a ventilator problem. Manual ventilation is continued while another clinician corrects the ventilator problem (eg, tubing leaks or disconnections, inaccurate gas delivery) or replaces the ventilator. Continuation of respiratory distress after removal from the ventilator and during manual ventilation suggests a patient-related cause.

Oral Feedings

Being able to eat "regular food" enhances the ventilated patient's sense of well-being and optimism and can help address nutritional needs. However, evaluation of the patient's ability to swallow is essential prior to oral feeding following extubation (especially in those ventilated long term) and in those who have a tracheostomy tube in place. "Swallow studies" are commonly done in these patients and should also be considered in any patient with a history of aspiration.

Communication

Mechanically ventilated patients are unable to speak and communicate verbally due to the presence of a cuffed ET tube or tracheostomy tube. The inability to speak is frustrating for the patient, nurse, and members of the healthcare team. Impaired communication results in patients experiencing anxiety and fear, symptoms that can have a deleterious effect on their physical and emotional conditions. Patients interviewed after extubation reveal how isolated and alone they felt because of their inability to speak.

Common Communication Problems

Patients' perceptions of communication difficulties related to mechanical ventilation include: (1) inability to communicate, (2) insufficient explanations, (3) inadequate understanding, (4) fears related to potential dangers associated with the inability to speak, and (5) difficulty with communication methods. Except for the problem of inability to vocalize, all of the problems cited by ventilated patients may be resolved easily by progressive care practitioners. For instance, "insufficient explanations" and "inadequate understanding" can be remedied by frequent repetition of all plans and procedures in language that is understandable to a nonmedical person and that takes into account that attention span and cognitive abilities, especially memory, are frequently diminished due to the underlying illness or injury, effects of medications and anesthesia, and the impact of the progressive care environment.

Although most messages the ventilated patient needs to communicate lie within a narrow range ("pain," "hunger," "water," and "sleep"), communicating these basic needs is often difficult. Most adults are accustomed to attending to their own basic needs, but in the progressive care unit, not only are they unable to physically perform certain activities, they also may not be able to communicate their needs

effectively. Basic needs include such activities as elimination, bathing, brushing teeth, combing hair, eating, drinking, and sleeping. Other examples include simple requests or statements such as "too hot," "too cold," "turn me," "up," "down," "straighten my legs," "my arm hurts," "I can't breathe," and "moisten my lips."

Patients have described difficulties with communication methods while being mechanically ventilated. This also can be avoided by assessing the patient's communication abilities. Is the patient alert and oriented? Can the patient answer simple yes and no questions? Does the patient speak English? Can the patient use at least one hand to gesture? Does the patient have sufficient strength and dexterity to hold a pen and write? Are the patient's hearing and vision adequate? Knowledge of the patient's communication abilities assists the clinician to identify appropriate communication methods.

Once the most successful communication methods have been identified for a particular patient, they should be written into the plan of care. Continuity among healthcare professionals in their approach to communication with nonvocal patients improves the quality of care and increases patient satisfaction.

Methods to Enhance Communication

A variety of methods for augmenting communication are available and can be classified into two categories: nonvocal treatments (gestures, lip reading, mouthing words, paper and pen, alphabet/numeric boards, flashcards, computers, tablets, etc) and vocal treatments (talking tracheostomy tubes and speaking valves). The best way to communicate with the patient who has an artificial airway or who is being mechanically ventilated is still unknown.

Nonvocal Treatments

Individual patient needs vary and it is recommended that the nurse use a variety of nonvocal treatments (eg, gestures, alphabet board, and paper and pen). Success with communication interventions varies with the diagnosis, age, type of injury or disease, type of respiratory assist devices, and psychosocial factors. For instance, lip reading can be successful in patients who have tracheostomies because the lips and mouth are visible, but in a patient with an ET tube, where tape and tube holders limit lip movement and visibility, lip reading may be less successful.

WRITING

Typically, the easiest, most common method of communication readily available is the paper and pen. However, the supine position is not especially conducive to writing legibly. In addition, the absence of proper eyeglasses, an injured or immobilized dominant writing hand, or lack of strength also can make writing difficult for mechanically ventilated patients. Writing paper should be placed on a firm writing surface (eg, clipboard) with an attached felt-tipped pen that writes in any position. Strength, finger flexibility, and dexterity are required to grasp a pen. Some patients prefer to use a pressure sensitive, inexpensive toy writing screen that is easy to use and easy to erase, allowing for privacy. Their low cost is an advantage, if isolation precludes reuse. Although costly, computer keyboards or touchscreen tablets may also facilitate written communication, particularly in patients who used these devices prior to their illness.

GESTURING

Another nonvocal method of communication that can be very effective is the deliberate use of gestures. Gestures are best suited for the short-term ventilated patient who is alert and can move at least one hand, even if only minimally. Generally, well-understood gestures are emblematic, have a low level of symbolism, and are easily interpreted by most people.

For example, ventilated patients often indicate that they need suctioning by curving an index finger (to resemble a suction catheter), raising a hand toward the ET tube, and moving their hand back and forth. This is known as an idiosyncratic gesture, a gesture that is used by a particular community, namely, the nurse and the ventilated patient. Other idiosyncratic gestures include "ice chips," "moisten my mouth," "spray throat," "fan," and "doctor."

One important aspect of communicating by gesture is to "mirror" the gesture(s) back to the patient, at the same time verbalizing the message or idea conveyed by the patient's gesture. This mirroring ensures accuracy in interpretation and assists the clinician and patient to form a repertoire to be used in future gestural conversations. When observing a patient's gestures, stand back from the bed, and watch his or her arms and hands. Most gestures are easily understood, especially those most frequently used by patients (eg, the head nod, indicating "yes" or "no"). Practitioners should ask simple yes-and-no questions but avoid playing "twenty questions" with ventilated patients because this can be very frustrating. Before trying to guess the needs of ventilated patients, give them the opportunity to use gestures to communicate their needs.

ALPHABET BOARD/PICTURE BOARD

For patients who face a language barrier, a picture board is sometimes useful along with well-understood gestures. Picture boards have images of common patient needs (eg, bedpan, glass of water, medications, family, doctor, nurse) that the patient can point to. Picture boards, although commercially available, can be made easily and laminated to more uniquely meet the needs of a specific progressive care population.

Another approach is the use of flash cards that can be purchased or made. Language flash cards contain common words or phrases in the patient's preferred language.

Vocalization Techniques

If patients with tracheostomy tubes in place have intact organs of speech, they may benefit from vocal treatment strategies like pneumatic and electrical devices, fenestrated tracheostomy tubes, talking tracheostomy tubes, and tracheostomy speaking valves. Several conditions preclude use of vocalization devices, such as neurologic conditions that impair vocalization (eg, Guillain-Barré syndrome), severe upper airway obstruction (eg, head/neck trauma), or vocal cord adduction (eg, presence of an ET tube).

A number of vocal treatments for patients with tracheostomies exist. Generally, they require that the cuff be completely deflated to allow for air to be breathed in and out through the mouth and nose as well as around the sides of the tracheostomy. On exhalation, the gases pass through the vocal cords allowing for speech. Some use one-way speaking valves (eg, Passy-Muir valve, shown in Figure 5-23) to allow for air to be inhaled through the valve but close during exhalation to direct air up past the vocal cords. A fenestrated tracheostomy tube (Figure 5-24) also allows passage of air

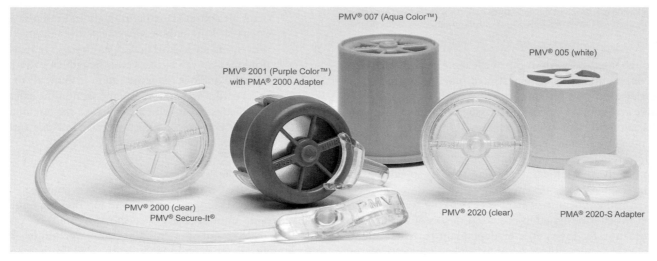

Figure 5-23. Passy-Muir speaking valves. (*Used with permission from Passy-Muir, Inc., Irvine, CA.*)

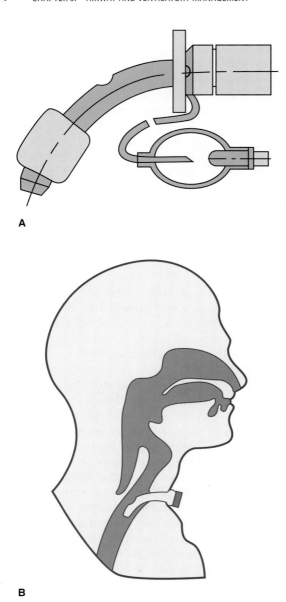

Figure 5-24. **(A)** Fenestrated tracheostomy tube. **(B)** Opening above the cuff site allowing gas, flow past the vocal cords during inspiration and expiration. (*©2018 Medtronic. All rights reserved. Used with the permission of Medtronic.*)

through the vocal cords. A cap or speaking valve may be used in conjunction with the fenestrated tube to ensure that all exhaled air moves through the vocal cords for vocalization. There are reports of granuloma tissue developing at the site adjacent to the fenestration, which resolves after removal of the tube. In addition, fenestrated ports often become clogged with secretions, again preventing the production of sound. It is imperative that if the tracheostomy tube is capped, the cuff of the tracheostomy be completely deflated.

Another vocal treatment is the talking tracheostomy tube, which is designed to provide a means of verbal communication for the ventilator-dependent patient. Patients who seem to be unable to wean may take a renewed interest in the weaning process, and successfully wean upon hearing

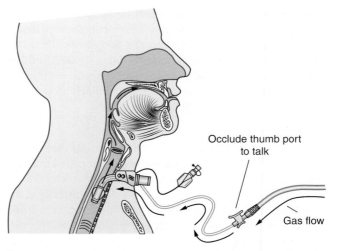

Figure 5-25. Tracheostomy tube with side port to facilitate speech. (*Used with permission from Smith Medical, Keen, NH.*)

their own voice. Currently, there are two talking tracheostomy tubes available that maintain a closed system with cuff inflation but differ in how they function.

1. *The Portex tracheostomy* operates by gas flowing (4-6 L/min) through an airflow line, which has a fenestration just above the tracheostomy tube cuff (Figure 5-25). The air flows through the glottis, thus supporting vocalization if the patient is able to form words with their mouth. However, an outside air source must be provided, which is usually not humidified and the trachea can become dry and irritated. The line for this air source requires diligent cleaning and flushing of the air port to prevent it from becoming clogged. The patients or staff must be able to manually divert air through the tube via a thumb port control.
2. *The Blom tracheostomy tube system* (Figure 5-26) uses a two-valve system in a specialized speech inner cannula that redirects air and does not require use of an air source. During inhalation, the flap valve opens and the bubble valve seals the fenestration preventing air leak to the upper airway. On exhalation, the flap valve closes and the bubble valve collapses to unblock the fenestration to allow air to the vocal cords. An additional component is the exhaled volume reservoir, which attaches to the circuit and returns volume to minimize false low expiratory minute volume alarms.

Teaching Communication Methods

The progressive care environment presents many teaching and learning challenges. Patients and families are under a considerable amount of stress, so the nurse must be a very creative teacher and offer communication techniques that are simple, effective, and easy to learn. The desire to communicate with loved ones, however, often makes the family

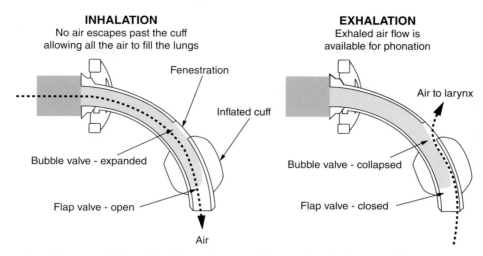

INHALATION
No air escapes past the cuff
allowing all the air to fill the lungs

Fenestration

Inflated cuff

Bubble valve - expanded

Flap valve - open

Air

EXHALATION
Exhaled air flow is
available for phonation

Air to larynx

Bubble valve - collapsed

Flap valve - closed

Figure 5-26. Tracheostomy tube with inner cannula for speaking (Blom tracheostomy tube system). (*Used with permission from Pulmodyne, Indianapolis, IN [http://www.dolema.com/uploads/6869E_Blom_Brochure.pdf]*)

very willing to learn. Frequently, it is the family who makes up large-lettered communication boards, purchases a Magic Slate, or brings in a laptop computer or tablet for the patient to use. Suggesting that families do this is usually very well received, because loved ones want so desperately to help in some way.

All patients should be informed prior to intubation that they will be unable to speak during the intubation period. A flipchart illustrating what an endotracheal tube or tracheostomy tube is like, with labeling in simple words, may be shown to patients who will be electively intubated (eg, for planned surgery). Practicing with a few nonverbal communication techniques before intubation (eg, gestures, alphabet boards, flash cards) is also beneficial. Another important point to emphasize with patients is that being unable to speak is usually temporary, just while the breathing tube is in place. If preintubation explanations are not feasible or possible, provide these explanations to the intubated patient.

PRINCIPLES OF MANAGEMENT

The majority of interventions related to mechanical ventilation focus on maximizing oxygenation and ventilation, and preventing complications associated with artificial airways and the sequelae of assisting the patient's ventilation and oxygenation with an invasive mechanical device.

Maximizing Oxygenation, Ventilation, and Patient-Ventilator Synchrony

- Provide frequent explanations of the purpose of the ventilator.
- Monitor the patient's response to ventilator therapy and for signs that the patient is dyssynchronous with the ventilator respiratory pattern. The use of graphic displays, common on many ventilator systems, is often a helpful aid to patient assessment.

- Consider ventilator setting changes to maximize synchrony (eg, changes in flow rates, respiratory rates, sensitivities, and/or modes).
- Administer the minimal dose of sedative agents required to enhance patient/ventilator synchrony.

Maintain a Patent Airway

- Suction the airway only when clinically indicated according to patient assessment.
- Maintain adequate hydration and humidification of all inhaled gases to reduce secretion viscosity.
- Monitor for signs and symptoms of bronchospasm and administer bronchodilator therapy as appropriate.
- Prevent obstruction of oral ET tubes by using an oral bite block, if necessary.

Monitor Oxygenation and Ventilation Status Frequently

- Collect arterial blood for ABG analysis as appropriate (eg, after some ventilator changes, with respiratory distress or cardiovascular instability, or with significant changes in clinical condition).
- Use a noninvasive SpO_2 monitor continuously. Validate noninvasive measures with periodic ABG analysis (see Table 5-4).
- Observe for signs and symptoms of decreased PaO_2, increased $PaCO_2$, and respiratory distress. Indications of respiratory distress require immediate intervention (see Figure 5-22).
- Reposition the patient frequently and develop a mobilization plan to improve ventilation-perfusion relationships and prevent atelectasis.
- Aggressively manage pain, particularly chest and upper abdominal pain, to increase mobility, deep breathing, and coughing (see Chapter 6, Pain and Sedation Management).

Physiotherapy and Monitoring

- Administer chest physiotherapy for selected clinical conditions (eg, large mucus production, lobar atelectasis).
- Monitor oxygenation status closely during chest physiotherapy for signs and symptoms of hypoxemia.

Maintain Oxygenation and Ventilatory Support at All Times

- Assess ventilator settings, alarm activation, and devise functioning every 1 to 2 hours to ensure proper operation of the mechanical ventilator.
- During even brief periods of removal from mechanical ventilation, maintain ventilation and oxygenation with an MRB. During intrahospital transport, verify adequacy of ventilatory support equipment, particularly the maintenance of PEEP (when > 10 cm H_2O is required) as well as ensuring adequate portable oxygen supply tank pressure. When possible, a portable mechanical ventilator should be used versus MRB.
- Keep emergency sources of portable oxygen readily available in the event of loss of wall oxygen capabilities.

Weaning From Mechanical Ventilation

- Systematically assess wean potential and address factors impeding weaning.
- Use a weaning protocol with a "wean screen." Ensure that the patient, family, and key caregivers are aware of weaning trials.
- Stop weaning trial, if signs of intolerance emerge.
- Promote the consistent use of an evidence-based intraprofessional approach to weaning.

Preventing Complications

- Maintain ET or tracheostomy cuff pressures less than 25 mm Hg (30 cm H_2O).
- Maintain artificial airway position by securing with a properly fitting holder device or selected tapes. Frequently, verify proper ET position by noting ET marking at lip or nares placed after intubation.
- Ensure tape or devices used to secure the artificial airway are properly applied and are not causing pressure injury. Periodic repositioning of ET tubes may be required to prevent skin integrity problems.
- Use a bite block with oral ET tubes if necessary to prevent accidental biting of the tube.
- Provide frequent mouth care and assess for development of pressure areas from ET tubes. Move the ET from one side of the mouth to the other daily or more frequently if necessary.
- Assess for signs and symptoms of sinusitis with nasal ET tube use (eg, pain in sinus area with pressure, purulent drainage from nares, fever, increased white blood cell count).

Maximizing Communication

- Assess communication abilities and establish an approach for nonverbal communication. Assist family members in using that approach with the patient.
- Anticipate patient needs and concerns in the planning of care.
- Ensure that call lights, bells, or other methods for notifying unit personnel of patient needs are in place at all times.
- Frequently, repeat information about communication limitations and how to use different nonverbal communication methods.

Reducing Anxiety and Providing Psychosocial Support

- Maintain a calm, supportive environment to avoid unnecessary escalation of anxiety. Provide brief explanations of activities and procedures. The vigilance and presence of healthcare providers during periods of anxiety is crucial to avoid panic by patients and visiting family members.
- Teach the patient relaxation techniques to control anxiety.
- Administer low doses of anxiolytics, if needed, that do not depress respiration (see Chapter 6, Pain and Sedation Management and Chapter 9, Cardiovascular System).
- Encourage the family to stay with the patient as much as desired and to participate in caregiver activities as appropriate. Presence of a family member provides comfort to the patient and assists the family member to better cope with the illness.
- Promote sleep at night by decreasing light, noise, and unnecessary patient interruptions.

SELECTED BIBLIOGRAPHY

General Critical Care

Ahrens T, Sona C. Capnography application in acute and progressive care. *AACN Clin Issues.* 2003;14:123-132.

Balas MC, Devlin JW, Verceles AC, Morris P, Ely EW. Adapting the ABCDEF bundle to meet the needs of patients requiring prolonged mechanical ventilation in the long-term acute care hospital setting: historical perspectives and practical implications. *Semin Respir Crit Care Med.* 2016;37:119-135.

Balas MC, Olsen Km, Cohen MZ, et al. Effectiveness and safety of the awakening and breathing coordination, delirium monitoring/management, and early exercise/mobility bundle. *Crit Care Nurse.* 2014;42:1024-1036.

Balas MC, Vasilevskis EE, Burke WJ, et al. Critical care nurses' role in implementing the "ABCDE Bundle" into practice. *Crit Care Nurse.* 2012;32:35-47.

Berry E, Zecca H. Daily interruptions of sedation: a clinical approach to improve outcomes in clinically ill patients. *Crit Care Nurse.* 2012;32:43-51.

Blissitt PA. Sleep and mechanical ventilation in critical care. *Crit Care Nurs Clin North Am.* 2016;28:195-203.

Bounds M, Kram S, Speroni KG, et al. Effect of ABCDE bundle implementation on prevalence of delirium in intensive care unit patients. *Am J Crit Care*. 2016;25:535-544.

Branson RD, Mannheimer PD. Forehead oximetry in critically ill patients: the case of a new monitoring site. *Respir Care Clin N Am*. 2004;10(3):359-367.

Dolovich MB, Ahrens RC, Hess DR, et al. Device selection and outcomes of aerosol therapy: evidence-based guidelines. *Chest*. 2006;127:335-371.

El-Rabbany M, Zaghol N, Bhandari M, Azarpazhooh A. Prophylactic oral health procedures to prevent hospital-acquired and ventilator-associated pneumonia: a systemic review. *Int J Nurs Stud*. 2015;52:452-464.

Faust AC, Echevarria KL, Attridge RL, Shepherd L, Restrepo MI. Prophylactic acid-suppression therapy in hospitalized adults: indications, benefits, and infectious complications. *Crit Care Nurse*. 2017;37:18-29.

Fernandez R, Subira C, Frutos-Vivar F, et al. High-flow nasal cannula to prevent postextubation respiratory failure in high-risk non-hypercapnic patients: a randomized multicenter trial. *Ann Intensive Care*. 2017;7:47-52.

Gonzalez S. Permissive hypoxmia versus normoxemia for critically ill patients receiving mechanical ventilation. *Crit Care Nurse*. 2015;35:80-81.

Grant M. Resolving communication challenges in the intensive care unit. *AACN Adv Crit Care*. 2015;26:123-130.

Hernandez G, Vaquero C, Colinas L. Effect of postextubation high-flow nasal cannula vs noninvasive ventilation on reintubation and postextubation respiratory failure in high-risk patients: a randomized clinical trial. *JAMA*. 2016;316:1565-1574.

Jongerden IP, Rovers MM, Grypdonck MH, Bonten MJ. Open and closed endotracheal suction systems in mechanically ventilated intensive care patients: a meta-analysis. *Crit Care Med*. 2007;35:260-270.

Kazmarek RM, Stoller JK, Heur AJ. *Egan's Fundamentals of Respiratory Care*. 11th ed. St. Louis, MO: Elsevier Mosby; 2016.

Kjonegaard R, Fields W, King ML. Current practice in airway management: a descriptive evaluation. *Am J Crit Care*. 2009;doi: 10.4037/ajcc2009803.

Klompas M, Anderson D, Trick W, et al. The preventability of ventilator-associated events. The CDC prevention epicenters wake-up and breathe collaborative. *Am J Resp Crit Care Med*. 2015;191:292-301.

Klompas M, Branson R, Eichenwald EC, et al. Strategies to prevent ventilator-associated pneumonia in acute care hospitals: 2014 update. *Inf Cont Hosp Epidemiol*. 2014;35:915-936.

Klompas M, Speck K, Howell MD, Greene LR, Berenholtz SM. Reappraisal of routine oral care with chlorhexidine gluconate for patients receiving mechanical ventilator: systemic review and meta-analysis. *JAMA Intern Med*. 2014;174:751-761.

Link MS, Berkow LC, Kudenchuk PJ, et al. 2015 American Heart Association guidelines update for cardiopulmonary resuscitation and emergency cardiovascular care. Part 7: adult advanced cardiovascular life support. *Circulation*. 2015;132:S444-S464.

MacLeod DB, Cortinez LI, Keifer JC, et al. The desaturation response time of finger pulse oximeters during mild hypothermia. *Anaesthesia*. 2005;60(1):65-71.

Malinoski DJ, Todd SR, Slone S, Mullins RJ, Schreiber MA. Correlation of central venous and arterial blood gas measurements in mechanically ventilated trauma patients. *Arch Surg*. 2005;140:1122-1125.

Morris LL, Whitmer A, McIntosh E. Tracheostomy care and complications in the intensive care unit. *Crit Care Nurse*. 2013;33:18-30.

Munro CL, Grap MJ, Jones DJ, et al. Chlorhexidine, toothbrushing, and preventing ventilator-associated pneumonia in critically ill adults. *Am J Crit Care*. 2009;18:428-437.

Munro N, Ruggiero M. Ventilator-associated pneumonia bundle. *AACN Adv Crit Care*. 2014;25:163-175.

Nassar BS, Schmidt GA. Estimating arterial partial pressure of carbon dioxide in ventilated patients: how valid are surrogate measures? *Ann Am Thorac Soc*. 2017;14:1005-1014.

Raoof S, Baumann MH. Ventilator-associated events: the new definition. *Am J Crit Care*. 2014;23:7-9.

Rose L, Burry L, Mallick R, et al. Prevalence, risk factors, and outcomes associated with physical restraint use in mechanically ventilated adults. *J Crit Care*. 2016;31:31-35.

Schallom L, Sona C, McSweeney M, et al. Comparison of forehead and digit oximetry in surgical/trauma patients at risk for decreased peripheral perfusion. *Heart Lung*. 2007;36:188-194.

Seckel MA. Ask the experts: does the use of a closed suction system help to prevent ventilator-associated pneumonia? *Crit Care Nurse*. 2008;28(1):65-66.

Seckel MA. Ask the experts: normal saline and mucous plugging. *Crit Care Nurse*. 2012;32:66-68.

Seckel MA, Schulenburg K. Ask the experts: eating while receiving mechanical ventilation. *Crit Care Nurse*. 2011;31:95-97.

Siobal MS. Monitoring exhaled carbon dioxide. *Respir Care*. 2016;61:1397-1416.

Smith SG. Ask the experts: best method for securing an endotracheal tube. *Crit Care Nurse*. 2016;36:78-80.

St John RE, Malen JF. Airway management. *Crit Care Nurs Clin North Am*. 2004;16:413-430.

Stonecypher K. Ventilator-associated pneumonia: the importance of oral care in intubated adults. *Crit Care Nurs Q*. 2010;33(4):339-347.

Toftegaard M, Rees SE, Andreassen S. Correlation between acid–base parameters measured in arterial blood and venous blood sampled peripherally, from vena cavae superior, and from the pulmonary artery. *Eur J Emerg Med*. 2008;15:86-91.

Valdez-Lowe C, Ghareeb SA, Artinian NT. Pulse oximetry in adults. *AJN*. 2009;109(6):52-59.

Wang C, Tsai J, Chen S, et al. Normal saline instillation before suctioning: a meta-analysis of randomized controlled trials. *J Australian Crit Care*. 2016. http://dx.doi.org/10.1016/j.aucc.2016.11.001

Ventilator Management

Burns SM. Pressure modes of mechanical ventilation: the good, the bad, and the ugly. *AACN Adv Crit Care*. 2008;19:399-411.

Hess D, Kacmarek KM. *Essentials of Mechanical Ventilation*. 3rd ed. New York, NY: McGraw-Hill; 2014.

Kane C, York NL. Understanding the alphabet soup of mechanical ventilation. *Dimens Crit Care Nurs*. 2012;31:217-222.

Restrepo RD, Walsh BK. Humidification during invasive and noninvasive mechanical ventilation: 2012. *Resp Care*. 2012;57:782-788.

Seckel MA. Mechanical ventilation and weaning. In: Good VS, Kirkwood PL, eds. *Advanced Critical Care Nursing*. 2nd ed. St Louis, MO: Elsevier; 2018.

Tobin MJ. *Principles and Practice of Mechanical Ventilation*. 3rd ed. New York, NY: McGraw-Hill; 2013.

Unroe M, Kahn JM, Carson SS, et al. One-year trajectories of care and resource utilization for recipients of prolonged mechanical ventilation: a cohort study. *Ann Intern Med*. 2010;153:167-175.

Walkey AJ, Wiener RS. Use of noninvasive ventilation in patient with acute respiratory failure, 2000-2009. *Annals ATS*. 2013;10:10-17.

White AC. Long-term mechanical ventilation: management strategies. *Resp Care*. 2012;57:889-897.

Weaning From Mechanical Ventilation

Bell L. Safe weaning from mechanical ventilation. *Am J Crit Care*. 2015;24:130.

Blackwood B, Burns KE, Cardwell CR, O'Halloran P. Protocolized versus non-protocolized weaning for reducing duration of mechanical ventilation in critically ill adult patients. *Cochrane Database Syst Rev*. 2014;11:CD006904. doi: 10.1002/14651858. CD006904.pubs.MJ. 2011;342c7237.doi:1-.1136/bmj.b7237.

BouAki I, Bou-Khalil P, Kanazi G. Weaning from mechanical ventilation. *Curr Opin Anesthesiol*. 2012;25:42-47.

Burns SM. Weaning from mechanical ventilation: where were we then, and where are we now? *Crit Care Nurs Clin N Am*. 2012;24:457-458.

Burns SM, Fisher C, Tribble SS, et al. The relationship of 26 clinical factors to weaning outcome. *Am J Crit Care*. 2012;21:52-58.

Girard TD, Kress JP, Fuchs BD, et al. Efficacy and safety of a paired sedation and ventilator weaning protocol for mechanically ventilated patients in intensive care (Awakening and Breathing Controlled trial): a randomised controlled trial. *Lancet*. 2008;371:126-134.

Gupta P, Geihler K, Walters RW, Meyerink K, Modrykamien AM. The effect of mechanical ventilation discontinuation protocol in patients with simple and difficult weaning: impact on clinical outcomes. *Resp Care*. 2014;59:170-177.

Haas CF, Loik PS. Ventilator discontinuation protocols. *Resp Care*. 2012;57:1649-1662.

MacIntyre NR. Evidence-based assessments in the ventilator discontinuation process. *Resp Care*. 2012;57:1611-1618.

McConville JF, Kress JP. Current concepts: weaning patients from the ventilator. *N Engl J Med*. 2012;367:2233-2239.

Mendes-Tellez PA, Needham DM. Early physical rehabilitation in the ICU and ventilator liberation. *Resp Care*. 2012;57:1663-1669.

Olff C, Clark-Wadkins C. Tele-ICU partners enhanced evidence-based practice: ventilator weaning initiative. *AACN Adv Crit Care*. 2012;23:312-322.

Rose L, Schultz MJ, Cardwell CR, et al. Automated versus non-automated weaning for reducing the duration of mechanical ventilation for critically ill adults and children: a Cochrane systematic review and meta-analysis. *Crit Care*. 2015;48:doi: 10.1186/s13054-015-0755-6.

Communication

Colandrea M, Eckardt P. Improving tracheostomy care delivery: instituting clinical care pathways and nursing education to improve patient outcomes. *ORL Head Neck Nurs*. 2016;34:7-16.

Grossbach I, Stranberg S, Chlan L. Promoting effective communication for patients receiving mechanical ventilation. *Crit Care Nurse*. 2011;31:46-61.

Happ MB, Garrett K, DiVirgilio D, et al. Nurse-patient communication interactions in the intensive care unit. *Am J Crit Care*. 2011;20:e28-e40.

Morris LL, Bedon AM, McIntosh E, Whitmer A. Restoring speech to tracheostomy patients. *Crit Care Nurse*. 2015;35:13-27.

Rodriquez CS, Rowe M, Thomas L, et al. Enhancing the communication of suddenly speechless critical care patients. *Am J Crit Care*. 2016;25:e40-e47.

Evidence-Based Resources

American Association of Critical Care Nurses (AACN). *Practice Alert: Alarm Management*. Alisio Veijo, CA: AACN; 2013. www.aacn.org. Accessed June 10, 2017.

American Association of Critical Care Nurses (AACN). *Practice Alert: Assessment and Management of Delirium Across the Lifespan*. Alisio Viejo, CA: AACN; 2016. www.aacn.org. Accessed June 10, 2017.

American Association of Critical Care Nurses (AACN). *Practice Alert: Prevention of Aspiration in Adults*. Alisio Viejo, CA: AACN: 2016. www.aacn.org. Assessed June 11, 2017.

American Association of Critical Care Nurses (AACN). *Practice Alert: Prevention of Ventilator Associated Pneumonia*. Alisio Veijo, CA: AACN; 2017. www.aacn.org. Accessed June 10, 2017.

American Association of Critical Care Nurses (AACN). *Practice Alert: Oral Care for Acute and Critically Ill Patients*. Alisio Veijo, CA: AACN; 2017. www.aacn.org. Accessed June 10, 2017.

American Association of Respiratory Care. AARC clinical practice guideline: capnography/capnometry during mechanical ventilation: 2011. *Resp Care*. 2011;56:503-509.

American Association for Respiratory Care. AARC clinical practice guideline: care of the ventilator circuit and its relation to ventilator-associated pneumonia. *Resp Care*. 2003;48:869-879.

American Association of Respiratory Care. AARC clinical practice guideline: effectiveness of nonpharmacolgoic airway clearance therapies in hospitalized patients. *Resp Care*. 2013;58:2187-2193.

American Association of Respiratory Care. AARC clinical practice guideline: effectiveness of pharmacologic airway clearance therapies in hospitalized patients. *Resp Care*. 2015;60(7):1071-1077.

American Association of Respiratory Care. AARC clinical practice guideline: endotracheal suctioning of mechanically ventilated patients with artificial airway. *Resp Care*. 2010;55:758-764.

American Association for Respiratory Care. AARC clinical practice guideline: removal of the endotracheal tube-2007 revision and update. *Resp Care*. 2007:52;81-93.

American Thoracic Society and the Infectious Diseases Society of America. Guidelines for the management of adults with hospital-acquired, ventilator-associated, and healthcare-associated pneumonia. *Am J Respir Crit Care Med*. 2005;171:388-416.

Barden C, Davis T, Seckel M, et al. C. AACN Tele-ICU Nursing Practice Guidelines. 2013. http://www.aacn.org/wd/practice/docs/tele-icu-guidelines.pdf.

Barr J, Fraser Gl, Puntillo K, et al. Clinical practice guidelines for the management of pain, agitation, and delirium in adult patients in the intensive care unit. *Crit Care Med*. 2013;41:263-306.

Centers for Disease Control and Prevention National Healthcare Safety Network. Ventilator-Associated Events. 2017. https://www.cdc.gov/nhsn/pdfs/pscmanual/10-vae_final.pdf. Accessed June 10, 2017.

Centers for Disease Control and Prevention. Guidelines for preventing health-care-associated pneumonia, 2003: recommendations of CDC and the Health Care Infection Control Practices Advisory Committee. *MMWR.* 2004;53(No. RR-3):1-35.

Girard TD, Alhazzani W, Kress JP, et al. An official American Thoracic Society/American College of Chest Physicians clinical practice guideline: liberation from mechanical ventilation in critically ill adults: rehabilitation protocols, ventilator liberation protocols, and cuff leak tests. *Am J Resp Crit Care Med.* 2017;195:120-133.

Good VS, Kirkwood PL, eds. *Advanced Critical Care Nursing.* 2nd ed. St. Louis, MO: Elsevier; 2018.

Klompas M, Branson R, Eichenwald EC, et al. Strategies to prevent ventilator-associated pneumonia in acute care hospitals: 2014 update. *Infect Control Hosp Epidemiol.* 2014;35(8);915-936.

Mitchell RB, Hussey HM, Setzen G, et al. Clinical consensus statement: tracheostomy care. *Otolaryngol Head Neck Surg.* 2013;148:6-20.

Ouellette DR, Patel S, Girard TD, et al. Liberation from mechanical ventilation in critically ill adults: an official American College of Chest Physicians/American Thoracic Society clinical practice guideline. Inspiratory pressure augmentation during spontaneous breathing trials, protocols minimizing sedation, and noninvasive ventilation immediately after extubation. *Chest.* 2017;151:166-180.

Raimondi N, Vial MR, Calleja J, et al. Evidence-based guidelines for the use of tracheostomy in critically ill patients. *J Crit Care.* 2017;38:304-318.

Schmidt GA, Girard TD, Kress JP, et al. Official executive summary of the American Thoracic Society/American College of Chest Physicians clinical practice guideline: liberation from mechanical ventilation in critically ill adults. *Am J Respir Crit Care Med.* 2017;195:115-119.

Society of Critical Care Medicine. ABCDEF Bundle. http://www.iculiberation.org/Bundles/Pages/default.aspx. Accessed June 10, 2017.

Vanderbilt University Medical Center. Delirium Prevention and Safety: Starting with the ABCDEF's. http://www.icudelirium.org/medicalprofessionals.html. Accessed June 11, 2017.

Wiegand DL, ed. *AACN Procedure Manual for Critical Care.* 7th ed. St. Louis, MO: Elsevier Saunders; 2016.

PAIN AND SEDATION MANAGEMENT

Yvonne D'Arcy and Sara Knippa

KNOWLEDGE COMPETENCIES

1. Describe the elements of pain assessment in progressive care patients.

2. Describe how behavioral pain scales may be used to assess pain in patients who cannot self-report.

3. Compare and contrast pain-relieving modalities for the acutely ill:
   - Nonsteroidal anti-inflammatory drugs
   - Opioids, including patient-controlled analgesia (PCA)
   - Epidural analgesia with opioids and/or local anesthetics (LAs)
   - Elastomeric pumps with LA

   - Nonpharmacologic modalities: distraction, cutaneous stimulation, imagery, and relaxation techniques

4. Identify the important elements of pain control for a patient who is an addict, dependent on opioids for pain relief, has a past history of addiction or receiving medication for control of addiction.

5. Describe special considerations for pain-management in vulnerable populations such as the older adults.

6. Identify the need for sedation, commonly used sedatives, and how to monitor and manage the patient requiring sedation.

Pain management is central to the care of the acutely ill or injured patient. In some cases, acutely ill patients are not able to self-report their pain management needs to their health-care team. Patients identify physical care that promotes pain relief and comfort as an important element of their hospitalization and recovery, especially while in the hospital environment. Providing optimum pain relief for acutely ill patients not only enhances their emotional well-being, but can also help avert additional physiologic injury. This chapter explores a multimodal approach to pain management in acutely ill patients based on the physiologic mechanisms of pain transmission and human responses to pain. Specific pharmacologic and nonpharmacologic pain management techniques are described, including the integral relationships among relaxation, sedation, and pain relief. Strategies also are presented that promote comfort and are easy to incorporate into a plan of care for progressive care patients. Finally, special considerations are delineated for vulnerable populations within the acute care setting.

PHYSIOLOGIC MECHANISMS OF PAIN

Peripheral Mechanisms

The pain response is elicited with tissue injuries, whether actual or potential. Undifferentiated free nerve endings, or nociceptors, are the major receptors signaling tissue injury (Figure 6-1). Nociceptors are polymodal and can be stimulated by thermal, mechanical, and chemical stimuli. Nociception refers to the transmission of impulses by sensory nerves, which signal tissue injury.

At the site of injury, the release of a variety of neurochemical substances potentiates the activation of peripheral nociceptors. Many of these substances are also mediators of the inflammatory response and they can facilitate or inhibit

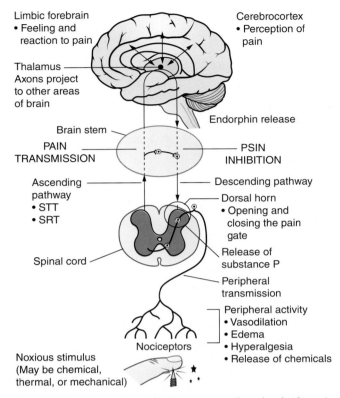

Figure 6-1. Physiologic pathway of pain transmission. (*Reproduced with permission from Copstead L, ed.* Perspectives on Pathophysiology. *Philadelphia, PA: WB Saunders;1995.*)

the pain impulse. These substances include histamine, kinins, prostaglandins, serotonin, and leukotrienes (Figure 6-2).

The nociceptive impulse travels to the spinal cord via specialized, afferent sensory fibers. Small, myelinated A-delta (Aδ) fibers conduct nociceptive signals rapidly to the spinal cord. The A-delta fibers transmit sensations that are generally localized and sharp in quality. In addition to A-delta fibers, smaller, unmyelinated C fibers also transmit nociceptive signals to the spinal cord. Because C fibers are unmyelinated, their conduction speed is much slower than their A-delta counterparts. The sensory quality of signals carried by C fibers tends to be dull and unlocalized (Figure 6-3).

Spinal Cord Integration

Sensory afferent fibers enter the spinal cord via the dorsal nerve, synapsing with cell bodies of spinal cord interneurons in the dorsal horn (see Figure 6-1). Most of the A-delta and C fibers synapse in laminae I through V in an area referred to as the substantia gelatinosa. Numerous neurotransmitters (eg, substance P, glutamate, and calcitonin gene-related peptide [CGRP]) and other receptor systems (eg, opiate, alpha-adrenergic, and serotonergic receptors) modulate the processing of nociceptive inputs in the spinal cord.

Central Processing

Following spinal cord integration, nociceptive impulses travel to the brain via specialized, ascending somatosensory

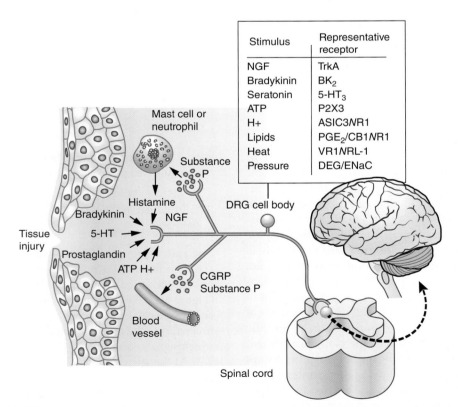

Figure 6-2. Peripheral nociceptors and the inflammatory response at the site of injury. (*Reproduced with permission from Julius D, Basbaum AI. Molecular mechanisms of nociception.* Nature. *2001; Sep 13;413(6852):203-210.*)

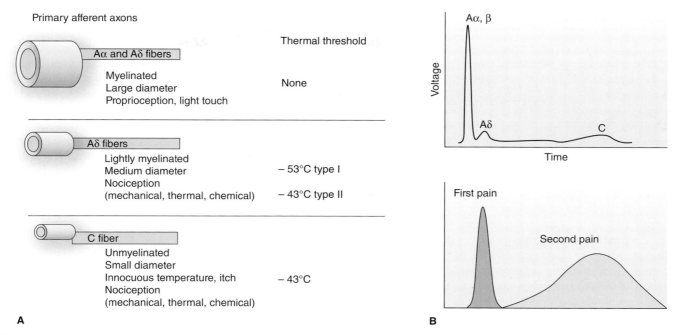

Primary afferent axons

Aα and Aδ fibers
Myelinated
Large diameter
Proprioception, light touch

Thermal threshold

None

Aδ fibers
Lightly myelinated
Medium diameter
Nociception
(mechanical, thermal, chemical)

− 53°C type I
− 43°C type II

C fiber
Unmyelinated
Small diameter
Innocuous temperature, itch
Nociception
(mechanical, thermal, chemical)

− 43°C

A

Aα, β
Voltage
Aδ
C
Time

First pain
Second pain

B

Figure 6-3. Different nociceptors detect different types of pain. **(A)** Peripheral nerves include small-diameter (Aδ) and medium- to large-diameter (Aα- β) myelinated afferent fibers, as well as small-diameter unmyelinated afferent fibers (C). **(B)** The fact that conduction velocity is directly related to fiber diameter is highlighted in the compound action potential recording from a peripheral nerve. Most nociceptors are either Aδ or C fibers, and their different conduction velocities (6-25 and ~1.0 m/s, respectively) account for the first (fast) and second (slow) pain responses to injury.

pathways (see Figure 6-1). The spinothalamic tract conducts nociceptive signals directly from the spinal cord to the thalamus. The spinoreticulothalamic tract projects signals to the reticular formation and the mesencephalon in the midbrain, as well as to the thalamus. From the thalamus, axons project to somatosensory areas of the cerebrocortex and limbic forebrain. The unique physiologic, cognitive, and emotional responses to pain are determined and modulated by the specific areas to which the somatosensory pathways project. The stimulus to the cerebrocortex can also activate the patient's previous memories of the experience of pain; for example, the thalamus regulates the neurochemical response to pain, and the cortical and limbic projections are responsible for the perception of pain and aversive response to pain, respectively. Similarly, the reticular activating system regulates the heightened state of awareness that accompanies pain. The modulation of pain by activities in these specific areas of the brain is the basis of many of the analgesic therapies available to treat pain.

RESPONSES TO PAIN

Human responses to pain can be both physical and emotional. The physiologic responses to pain are the result of hypothalamic activation of the sympathetic nervous system associated with the stress response. Sympathetic activation leads to:

- A shift in circulation away from superficial vessels and toward striated muscle, the heart, the lungs, and the nervous system
- Dilation of the bronchioles to increase oxygenation

- Increased cardiac contractility
- Inhibition of gastric secretions and contraction
- Increase in circulating blood glucose for energy

Signs and symptoms of sympathetic activation that frequently accompany nociception and pain include:

- Increased heart rate
- Increased blood pressure
- Increased respiratory rate
- Pupil dilation
- Pallor and perspiration
- Nausea and vomiting

Although patients experiencing acute pain often exhibit signs and symptoms as noted earlier, it is critical to note that the absence or presence of any or all of these signs and symptoms does not negate or confirm the presence of pain. In fact some patients, especially those who are seriously ill and have little or no compensatory reserves, may exhibit a shock-like clinical picture in the presence of pain. Patients who are accustomed to underlying chronic pain may have a decreased physiologic response to pain while the actual intensity of the pain remains high (Table 6-1).

Acutely ill patients express pain both verbally and nonverbally. The expressions can take many forms, some of which are subtle cues that could easily be overlooked (Table 6-2). Any signs that may indicate pain warrant further exploration and assessment. Although physiologic and behavioral expressions of acute pain have been described, each person's response to pain is unique.

TABLE 6-1. TYPES OF PAIN

Pain is defined as an unpleasant sensory and emotional experience associated with actual or potential tissue damage (APS, 2008). There are three main types of pain that can occur alone or in combination: • Acute pain from which the patient expects to recover   • Chronic pain that lasts beyond the normal healing period   • Neuropathic pain is a special type of chronic pain that is the result of nerve damage

PAIN ASSESSMENT

Pain assessment is a core element of ongoing surveillance of the acutely ill patient. Self-report of pain intensity and distress should be used whenever possible, especially for patients who can talk or communicate effectively. Regular documentation of pain assessment not only helps monitor the efficacy of analgesic modalities, but also helps ensure communication among caregivers regarding patient's pain. A variety of tools to assess pain intensity are available. There are three commonly used scales. The numeric rating scale (NRS) uses numbers between 0 and 10 to describe pain intensity; the anchors are "no pain to worst pain imaginable." Some patients find it easier to use adjectives to describe their pain. The verbal descriptive scale offers patients a standardized list of adjectives to describe their pain intensity. The descriptors are "none," "mild," "moderate," and "severe." With the visual analogue scale (VAS), a tool developed primarily for research, patients indicate their pain intensity by drawing a vertical line, bisecting a horizontal baseline. The baseline is anchored at either end by the terms "no pain" or "worst pain imaginable." The patient's response is converted to a numeric figure by measuring length from the left anchor to the patient's mark, in millimeters.

Any of these scales can be used with patients who are intubated or unable to speak for other medical reasons; for example, patients can be asked to use their fingers to indicate a number between 0 and 10; similarly, patients can be asked to indicate by nodding their head or pointing to the appropriate adjective or number as they either hear or read the list of choices. With the VAS, the line can be printed on a sheet of paper or dry erase board and the patient asked to mark the line to indicate their level of pain. While the VAS has been used in some acutely or critically ill patients, it may be difficult to use as it requires dexterity that may be inhibited by invasive lines, bandages, etc.

TABLE 6-2. EXAMPLES OF PAIN EXPRESSION IN CRITICALLY ILL PATIENTS

Verbal Cues	Facial Cues	Body Movements
Moaning	Grimacing	Splinting
Crying	Wincing	Rubbing
Screaming	Eye signals	Rocking
Silence		Rhythmic movement of extremity Shaking or tapping bed rails Grabbing the nurse's arm

Data from Herr K, Coyne P, Kry T, et al. Pain assessment in the nonverbal patient: position statement with clinical practice recommendations. Pain Manag Nurs. 2006 Jun;7(2):44-52.

Unfortunately, some acutely ill patients are unable to indicate their pain intensity either verbally or nonverbally. In these situations, nurses use other criteria to assess their patient's pain. Using a behavioral pain scale provides a guide for identifying and assessing pain in nonverbal patients. Two examples include the Detroit Medical Center Behavioral Pain Scale and the Behavioral Pain Assessment Tool (BPAT) (Table 6-3 and 6-4).

The Detroit behavioral pain scale measures facial signs, restlessness, muscle tone, vocalization, and consolability. The observer scores one of the three possible descriptions (0 being the absence of pain behavior and 3 being the most severe). The BPAT has recently been published. The tool measures four facial expressions, two verbal responses and two body muscle responses. The clinician records a numeric rating for each of the categories. Additional studies in varied critically and acutely ill patient populations are needed to best determine appropriate implementation of the tool.

Pain intensity may be effectively assessed by using well-developed interviewing and observational skills in conjunction with pain scales such as those described earlier.

A MULTIMODAL APPROACH TO PAIN MANAGEMENT

Today there are numerous approaches and modalities available to treat acute pain. Pharmacologic techniques traditionally have been the mainstay of analgesia, other complementary or nonpharmacologic methods are growing in their acceptance and use in clinical practice. Most modalities used in the treatment of acute pain can be used effectively in patients in progressive care units. Evidence-based practice guidelines to maximize analgesia in acutely ill patients are summarized in Table 6-5.

One of the central goals of pain management is to combine therapies or modalities that target as many of the processes involved in nociception and pain transmission as possible. Analgesic modalities, both pharmacologic and nonpharmacologic, exert their effects by altering nociception at specific structures within the peripheral or central nervous system (CNS), that is, the peripheral nociceptors, the spinal cord, or the brain or by altering the transmission of nociceptive impulses between these structures (Figure 6-4). By understanding the different sites where analgesic modalities work, nurses can select a combination of strategies to best treat the source or type of pain the patient is experiencing. A multimodal approach to pain control can achieve optimal analgesia with minimal side effects.

To assist nurses in the selection and use of analgesic modalities, the following descriptions of each modality include where and how it works, clinical situations where it can be used most effectively, and strategies for titrating it. Finally, because few modalities exert a singular effect, a summary of commonly associated secondary or side effects and strategies to minimize their occurrence are also addressed.

In response to the national opioid misuse and abuse epidemic, the Centers for Disease and Prevention drafted guidelines for managing chronic pain. These recommendations do not apply to cancer patients, or to patients who are receiving

TABLE 6-3.   DETROIT MEDICAL CENTER PAIN ASSESSMENT BEHAVIOR SCALE (NONVERBAL) FOR PATIENTS UNABLE TO PROVIDE A SELF-REPORT OF PAIN

	0	1	2	
FACE	Face muscles relaxed.	Facial muscle tension, frown, grimace.	Frequent to constant frown, clenched jaw.	**Face Score**
RESTLESSNESS	Quite, relaxed appearance, normal movement.	Occasional restless movement shifting position.	Frequent restless movement may include extremities or head.	**Restlessness Score**
MUSCLE TONE[a]	Normal muscle tone, relaxed.	Increased tone, flexion of fingers and toes.	Rigid tone.	**Muscle Tone Score**
VOCALIZATION[b]	No abnormal sounds.	Occasional moans, cries, whimpers, or grunts.	Frequent or continuous moans, cries, whimpers, or grunts.	**Vocalization Score**
CONSOLABILITY	Content, relaxed.	Reassured by touch or talk. Distractible.	Difficult to comfort by touch or talk.	**Consolability Score**
Behavioral Pain Assessment Scale Total (010)				

[a]*Assess muscle tone in patients with spinal cord lesion or injury at a level above the lesion or injury. Assess patients with hemiplegia on the unaffected side.*
[b]*This item cannot be measured in patients with artificial airways.*
How to use the pain assessment behavioral scale:
1. Observe behaviors and mark appropriate number for each category.
2. Total the numbers in the pain assessment behavioral score column.
*3. **Zero = No evidence of pain. Mild pain = 1-3. Moderate pain = 4-6. Severe uncontrolled pain is ≥ 6.***
Considerations:
4. Use the standard pain scale whenever possible to obtain the patient's self-report of pain. Self-report is the best indicator of the presence and intensity of pain.
5. Use this scale for patients who are unable to provide a self-report of pain.
6. In addition, a "proxy pain evaluation" from family, friends, or clinicians close to the patient may be helpful to evaluate pain based on previous knowledge of patient response.
7. When in doubt, provide an analgesic. "If there is reason to suspect pain, an analgesic trial can be diagnostic as well as therapeutic."
Used with permission from the Detroit Medical Center via Margaret L. Campbell, PhD, RN.

TABLE 6-4.   THE BEHAVIOR PAIN ASSESSMENT TOOL. NOTE: ACTION UNITS (AU) WERE ADDED FOR DESCRIPTION PURPOSES ONLY, BUT WERE NOT AVAILABLE TO CLINICIAN RATERS

Present	Absent	Behavior	Definition	Photos of Behaviors
		Neutral expression	Muscles relaxed	
		Grimace	A sharp contortion of the face AU4: Brow Lowering AU7: Lid Tightening AU6: Cheek Raising AU20: Mouth Stretching AU43: Eye Closing	
		Wince	To shrink away from, or start AU7: Lid Tightening AU6: Cheek Raising	
		Eyes closed	Lids are shut	
		Moaning	Low, soft indistinguishable sounds	
		Verbal complaints of pain	Words used to describe pain, e.g., *it hurts, ouch*	
		Rigid	Stiff, tensed muscles of extremities and torso	
		Clenched fists	Act of forming a fist	

Data from Gelinas C, Puntillo KA, Levin P, et al: The behavior pain assessment tool for critically ill adults: a validation study in 28 countries, Pain 2017 May;158(5):811-821.

TABLE 6-5. EVIDENCE-BASED GUIDELINES: PAIN MANAGEMENT

- Pain should be routinely monitored
- Use the behavioral pain scale BPS or critical-care pain observation tool (CPOT) for patients who cannot self-report pain
- Do not use vital signs alone for pain assessment in ICU patients
- Use preemptive analgesia prior to procedures
- Consider IV opioids as the first line to treat non-neuropathic pain
- Non-opioids and coanalgesics such as gabapentin or carbamazepine be considered for use with opioids
- Epidural analgesia is recommended for rib fractures and postoperative analgesia for abdominal aortic aneurysm

Data from Barr J, Fraser G, Puntillo K, et al. Clinical practice guidelines for the management of pain, agitation, and delirium in adult patients in the intensive care unit. Crit Care Med. 2013;41(1):263-306.

palliative care or end-of-life care. In addition these guidelines do not specifically address the management of acute pain. However, understanding these guidelines is pertinent in progressive care, as patients often have ongoing comorbidities such as fibromyalgia, arthritis, or other painful neuropathic conditions that complicate acute pain control. In addition patients may develop chronic pain as a result of trauma or surgical procedures such as amputations. Thus the CDC guidelines may be useful to consider when caring for acutely ill patients.

CDC 2016 Chronic pain guidelines summary

- Use nonpharmacologic and non-opioid medications as a first option
- If opioids are indicated use short acting opioids as the first opioid option
- Limit postoperative opioids prescriptions to 3 to 7 days
- Keep opioid equivalents to 50 morphine milligram equivalents (MME) with a maximum of 90 MME a day

Although these indications may not immediately apply to the acutely ill patient, awareness of the guidelines is helpful in considering appropriate medication use and pain management options during the recovery period.

NONSTEROIDAL ANTI-INFLAMMATORY DRUGS

Nonsteroidal anti-inflammatory drugs (NSAIDs) target the peripheral nociceptors. The NSAIDs exert their effect at the site

of injury by inhibiting the formation of the enzyme cyclooxygenase, which is responsible for the breakdown of arachidonic acid and formation of the neurotransmitter prostaglandin. By modifying and reducing the production of prostaglandin, the NSAIDs have been shown to have opioid-sparing effects and are very effective in managing pain associated with inflammation, trauma to peripheral tissues (eg, soft tissue injuries), bone pain (eg, fractures, metastatic disease), and pain associated with indwelling tubes and drains (eg, chest tubes).

One of the NSAIDs commonly used in the acute care setting is ketorolac tromethamine (Toradol). Ketorolac is currently the only parenteral NSAID preparation available in the United States and can be administered safely via the intravenous (IV) route. Intramuscular administration is not recommended due to the potential for irregular and unpredictable absorption. Recommended dosing for ketorolac is a 30-mg loading dose followed by 15 mg every 6 hours. Like all NSAIDs, ketorolac has a ceiling effect where administration of higher doses offers no additional therapeutic benefit yet significantly increases the risk of toxicity. Another non-opioid alternative to ketorolac is acetaminophen IV for patients who can tolerate the medication and do not have liver disease or other potential contraindications. The Society of Critical Care Medicine (SCCM) recommends the use of adjuvant analgesics such as NSAIDs to reduce opioid analgesic use and reduce opioid-related side effects.

Side Effects

The side effects associated with the use of NSAIDs relate to the function of prostaglandins in physiologic processes other than nociception; for example, gastrointestinal (GI) irritation and bleeding may result from NSAID use because prostaglandins are necessary for maintaining the mucous lining of the stomach. Similarly, the enzyme cyclooxygenase is needed for the eventual production of thromboxane, a key substance involved in platelet function. As a result, when NSAIDs are used chronically or in high doses, platelet aggregation may be altered, leading to bleeding problems. Prostaglandin inhibition by NSAIDs can also cause vasoconstriction of the renal afferent arterioles, reducing glomerular blood flow and contributing

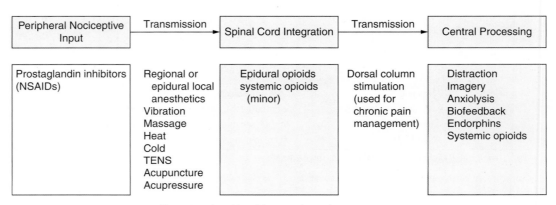

Figure 6-4. A multimodal approach to pain management.

to renal toxicity, particularly when NSAIDs are combined with other medications that affect kidney circulation. Cross-sensitivities with other NSAIDs have been documented (eg, ibuprofen, naproxen, indomethacin, piroxicam, aspirin). For these reasons, ketorolac and other NSAIDs are avoided in patients who have a history of gastric ulceration, renal insufficiency, and coagulopathies or a documented sensitivity to aspirin or other NSAIDs. In addition, NSAID use is not recommended in patients with heart disease, recent heart bypass surgery, or patients with a history of ischemic attacks or strokes.

An alternative to ketorolac for patients who are not candidates for NSAIDs is intravenous acetaminophen, as noted earlier. The severity of all NSAID-related side effects increases with high doses or prolonged use. For this reason, ketorolac and other such medications are designed for short-term modality only and should not be used for more than 5 days.

OPIOIDS

The principal modality of pain management in the acute care setting continues to be opioids. The SCCM recommends that opioids be considered as first-line treatment for non-neuropathic pain. Traditionally referred to as narcotics, opioids produce their analgesic effects primarily by binding with specialized opiate receptors throughout the CNS and thereby altering the perception of pain. Opiate receptors are located in the brain, spinal cord, and GI tract. Although opioids work primarily within the CNS, they also have been shown to have some local or peripheral effects as well. There are at least 45 variations of opiate receptors, which account for the varied response in individual patients.

Opioids are well tolerated by most acutely ill patients and can be administered by many routes including IV, IM, oral, buccal, nasal, rectal, transdermal, and intraspinal. Morphine sulfate is still the most widely used opioid and serves as the gold standard against which others are compared. Other opioids commonly used in the care of the acutely ill include hydromorphone (Dilaudid) and fentanyl. Opioid polymorphisms may cause opioids to affect patients differently, thus careful use and frequent assessment are necessary to determine optimal dosing.

Side Effects

Patient's responses to opioids, both analgesic responses and side effects, are highly individualized. Just as all the opioid agents have similar pain-relieving potential, all opioids currently available share similar side effect profiles. When side effects do occur, it is important to remember that they are primarily the result of opioid pharmacology, as opposed to the route of administration.

Nausea and Vomiting

Nausea and vomiting are distressing side effects often related to opioids that, unfortunately, many patients experience. Generally, nausea and vomiting result from stimulation of the chemoreceptor trigger zone (CTZ) in the brain and/or

from slowed GI peristalsis. Nausea and vomiting often can be managed effectively with antiemetic medications. Metoclopramide (Reglan), a procainamide derivative, works both centrally at the CTZ and on the GI tract to increase gastric motility. However, there are significant risks with metoclopramide use such as the potential for seizures and tardive dyskinesia. These conditions occur more commonly in older adults and with prolonged use.

The vestibular system also sends input to the CTZ. For this reason, movement frequently exacerbates opioid-related nausea. If patients complain of movement-related nausea, the application of a transdermal scopolamine patch can help prevent and treat opioid-induced nausea. The use of transdermal scopolamine is best avoided in patients older than 60 years because it can increase the incidence and severity of confusion in older patients.

The phenothiazines (ie, prochlorperazine [Compazine], promethazine [Phenergan]) and the butyrophenones (droperidol [Inapsine]) treat nausea through their effects at the CTZ. The serotonin antagonist ondansetron (Zofran) is also effective for treatment of opioid-related nausea. The doses required for postoperative or opioid-related nausea are significantly smaller doses (4 mg IV) than those used with emetogenic chemotherapy.

Pruritus

Pruritus is another opioid-related side effect commonly reported by patients. The actual mechanisms producing opioid-related pruritus are unknown. Although antihistamines can provide symptomatic relief for some patients, the role of histamine in opioid-related pruritus is unclear. One of the drawbacks of using antihistamine agents, such as diphenhydramine (Benadryl), is the sedation associated with their use. In addition, the use of diphenhydramine has been shown to have a 70% increase in cognitive deterioration in older adult patients. Similar to other opioid side effects, the incidence and severity of pruritus is dose-related and tends to diminish with ongoing use. Another option to treat pruritis is nalbuphine (Nubain), dosed at small doses of 2.5 to 5.0 mg IV every 6 hours as needed.

Constipation

Constipation, another common side effect, results from opioid binding at opiate receptors in the GI tract and decreased peristalsis. The incidence of constipation may be low in acutely ill patients or underreported, but it is important to remember that it is likely to be a problem for many patients following the acute initial phase of their illness or injury. The best treatment for constipation is prevention by ensuring adequate hydration, as well as by administering stimulant laxatives and stool softeners, as needed. Bulk forming laxatives are not recommended for older adults as they often do not drink enough fluid to move the medication through the GI tract. For palliative care patients with opioid-induced constipation, methylnaltrexone (Relistor) can be given as a subcutaneous injection.

Urinary Retention

Urinary retention can result from increased smooth muscle tone caused by opioids, especially in the detrusor muscle of the bladder. Opioids have no effect on urine production and neither cause nor worsen oliguria.

Respiratory Depression

Respiratory depression, the most adverse side effect of opioids, occurs due to their impact on the respiratory centers in the brain stem. Both respiratory rate and the depth of breathing can decrease as a result of opioids, usually in a dose-dependent fashion. Patients at increased risk for respiratory depression include older adults, those with preexisting cardiopulmonary diseases or sleep apnea, patients receiving other respiratory depressive medications such as benzodiazepines, and those who receive high doses. Signs and symptoms of respiratory depression include altered level of consciousness, shallow breathing, decreased respiratory rate, pupil constriction, hypoxemia, and hypercarbia. Currently, the CDC discourages concomitant use of opioids and benzodiazepines related to the increased risk of oversedation. In addition to monitoring for signs and symptoms of respiratory depression, many acute care settings are using capnography when IV opioids or PCA opioids are being used to closely monitor respiratory depression.

Clinically significant respiratory depression resulting from opiate use is usually treated with IV naloxone (Narcan). Naloxone is an opioid antagonist; it binds with opiate receptors, temporarily displacing the opioid and suspending its pharmacologic effects. As with other medications, naloxone is administered in very small doses and titrated to the desired level of alertness (Table 6-6). The half-life of naloxone is short—approximately 30 to 45 minutes. Thus ongoing assessment of the patient is essential as additional doses of naloxone may be needed.

Naloxone is used with caution in patients with underlying cardiovascular disease. The acute onset of hypertension, pulmonary hypertension, and pulmonary edema with naloxone administration has been reported. Naloxone is avoided in patients who have developed a tolerance to opioids since opioid antagonists can precipitate withdrawal or acute abstinence syndrome.

Intravenous Opioids

Many acutely ill patients are unable to use the oral route, thus the IV route is frequently used. One of the advantages of IV opioids is their rapid onset of action, allowing for easy

TABLE 6-6. ADMINISTRATION OF NALOXONE

1. Support ventilation.
2. Dilute 0.4 mg (400 mcg) ampule of naloxone with normal saline to constitute a 10-mL solution.
3. Administer in 1-mL increments, every 2-5 minutes, titrating to desired effect. Onset of action: approximately 2 minutes.
4. Continue to monitor patient; readminister naloxone as needed. Duration of action: approximately 45 minutes.
5. For patients requiring ongoing doses, consider naloxone infusion: Administer at 50-250 mcg/h, titrating to desired response.

titration. Loading doses of IV opioids are administered to achieve an adequate blood level. Additional doses are administered intermittently to maintain analgesic levels.

Progressive care patients may benefit from the addition of a continuous IV opioid infusion. Pain control in patients who may not be able to communicate their pain levels effectively, especially those that are mechanically ventilated, are candidates for continuous opioid infusions. The continuous infusion not only helps to achieve the appropriate blood levels, but also can be titrated as needed. Whenever appropriate, the maintenance dose for the infusion is based on patients' previous opioid requirements.

Patient-Controlled Analgesia

Patient-controlled analgesia (PCA) pumps can also be used effectively in the progressive care setting with alert patients able to activate the PCA button. With PCA, patients self-administer small doses of an opioid infusion using a programmable pump. PCA prescriptions typically include a bolus dose of the selected medication, a lockout or delay interval, and either a 1- to 4-hour limit; many of the PCA devices also can be programmed to deliver a basal or background infusion for patients who are opioid tolerant. The bolus dose refers to the amount of the medication the patient receives following pump activation. The initial dose usually ranges between 0.5 and 2.0 mg of morphine or its equivalent. The lockout or delay interval typically ranges between 5 and 10 minutes, which is enough time for the prescribed medication to circulate and take effect, yet allows the patient to easily titrate the medication over time. The 1- to 4-hour limit serves as an additional safety feature by regulating the amount of medication the patient can receive over this period of time.

Assessing whether an acutely ill patient is capable of using a PCA is essential in order to assure the success of this analgesic modality. PCA is not appropriate for patients unable to reliably self-administer pain medication (eg, a patient with a decreased level of consciousness). However, a cognitively intact patient, who is unable to activate the PCA button due to lack of manual dexterity or strength, may use a PCA device that has been ergonomically adapted (eg, a pressure switch pad). Patients, family members, and visitors are educated to understand that the patient is the only person to activate the PCA device. Family members and friends may think they are helping by activating the PCA device for the patient and not realize that this can produce life-threatening sedation and respiratory depression.

Titrating PCA

Patients using PCAs usually find a dose and frequency that balances pain relief with other medication-related side effects such as sedation. It is best to start a PCA only after the patient has received loading doses to achieve adequate blood levels of the prescribed opioid. For patients who continue to experience pain while using the PCA pump, the first step in titration is to give an additional loading dose and increase the bolus dose, usually by 25% to 50% depending on the pain intensity. If patients continue to have pain in spite of the increased dose, the lockout interval or delay is then reduced, if possible.

Continuous PCA infusions are no longer recommended for the majority of patients as they increase sedation and do not provide additional pain relief. However, in patients who have preexisting opioid tolerance, a continuous infusion may maintain their baseline opioid requirements while the patient-controlled bolus doses are available to help manage any new pain they experience. The hourly dose of the continuous infusion should be equianalgesic to, and calculated from, patients' preexisting opioid requirements.

Regional Analgesia

The combination of standard options such as opioids and regional analgesia is an additional method of reducing pain. This is commonly done with a block performed during surgery. A regional block may last 6 to 8 hours using local anesthetic (LA). An alternative is a continuous infusion using a small self-contained elastomeric pump. These pumps include a reservoir for the LA that resembles a filled softball, and a preset flow control that allows the LA to infuse at a selected rate. The pump is attached to a catheter that can be placed along the surgical incision in a soaker hose configuration. It can also be placed along a nerve, such as the femoral nerve, for patients undergoing such procedures as a total knee replacement where a continuous flow can be provided for a period of several days. The concentrations of regional analgesics do not cause motor blockade and are especially helpful to reduce pain associated with respiratory effort such as in thoracotomy patients.

Switching From IV to Oral Opioid Analgesia

Most often switching from IV to oral opioids is accomplished when acute pain subsides and the patient is able to tolerate oral or enteral nutrition. Patients who receive analgesics by

ESSENTIAL CONTENT CASE

Pain Management Using an Epidural Catheter

A 59-year-old man was admitted to the surgical step-down unit following a thoracotomy with wedge resection of the left lung for small-cell lung cancer. On his second postoperative day, his two left pleural chest tubes had a moderate amount of drainage and continuing air leaks. He was alert, responsive, and able to communicate his pain to the nurse. He had a thoracic epidural catheter in place (T7-T8) with a bupivacaine (0.625 mg/mL) and fentanyl (4 mcg/mL) combination infusing at 6 mL/h. He also had an elastomeric infusion device that was providing a localized block at the incision site using an LA only. When asked about his pain level, he said it was 5 on a scale of 0 (no pain) to 10 (worst pain imaginable).

His nurse noticed he was reluctant to cough and seemed to have some difficulty taking a deep breath. She also noticed his oxygen saturation was slowly drifting downward from 97% to 95%. His respiratory rate was increasing, as was his heart rate. When she listened to his breath sounds, they were bilateral and equal, but diminished throughout with scattered rhonchi. When she asked him about his pain, he said his pain was still a 5 as long as he did not move or cough. He also indicated that he tried to avoid taking a deep breath because it would make him cough and that made the pain go to an 8 or 10.

The nurse knew the patient needed to breathe deeply and cough to clear his lungs, but his pain and discomfort were limiting his ability to perform those maneuvers. He also refused to move from the bed to a chair. The nurse discussed strategies to help minimize the pain associated with activity. First, she found an extra pillow for him to use as a splint to support his incision and chest wall, but also to stabilize his chest tubes.

Then she called the anesthesiologist to confer about increasing the rate of the bupivacaine/fentanyl infusion to increase the pain relief. She also inquired about adding ketorolac or IV acetaminophen to his analgesic regimen to help with pain associated with the chest tubes. Because the patient also had an elastomeric infusion pump with LA along the surgical incision the nurse checked to make sure the clamp was open and the medication was infusing.

The anesthesiologist prescribed a bolus of 3 mL of the epidural solution via the pump and increased the continuous rate to 8 mL/h and added ketorolac, 15 mg, IV every 6 hours and a dose of IV acetaminophen. Over the course of the next 2 hours, the patient was able to cough more effectively, with less pain. His oxygen saturation returned to 97% and he was also able to sit in his chair for lunch.

Case Question 1: What are the advantages of using epidural analgesia?
(A) Local anesthetic blocks the entire surgical area.
(B) Combining an opioid with LA improves pain relief, decreases opioid needs, and can increase respiratory efforts.
(C) An epidural provides the patient with a method of continuous pain relief.
(D) Patients like epidurals because they provide superior pain relief.

Case Question 2: What is the value of adding ketorolac or acetaminophen to the pain regimen?
(A) IV medications work very quickly.
(B) The two medications do not make the patient sedated.
(C) Adding non-opioid medications can reduce opioid needs and decrease opioid-related side effects.
(D) Patients have fewer allergies to non-opioid medications.

Answers
1. B. Local anesthetics can have a short-term effect on pain relief and allow the patient to be more active and effectively cough and deep breathe. Combining the opioid and LA can have a synergistic effect increasing the overall pain relief more than using just a single medication.
2. C. Combining a non-opioid and opioid can also have a synergistic effect and decrease pain. The two different medications work on different areas of the pain mechanism. The combination can be used to help the patient become more active and if dosed at bedtime may help the patient to rest better.

ESSENTIAL CONTENT CASE

The Addicted Patient

A 22-year-old woman was admitted to the cardiovascular ICU (CVICU) following a tricuspid valve replacement related to recurrent subacute bacterial endocarditis. She has a self-reported history of heroin use (approximately 2 g/day).

She was extubated within the first 24 hours after surgery and transferred to the cardiovascular step-down unit for further management. During the unit transfer report the CVICU nurse commented "She is a constant whiner. She refuses to do anything. All she wants is to go out for a smoke and more drugs. She had 10 mg of IV morphine on my shift."

When the step-down unit nurse came into this patient's room to make her initial assessment, the patient said, "I can't take much more of this pain." The nurse probed further and asked her to use some numbers to describe her pain. She replied, "It's at 10!"

The nurse noticed that the patient was reluctant to move and refused to cough. Her vital signs were:

Heart rate	130 beats/min
BP	150/85 mm Hg
Temperature	38.5°C (orally)
Respiration rate	26 breaths/min, shallow

The nurse was concerned that due to the patient's preoperative use of heroin, she might not be receiving adequate doses of morphine to control her pain. She consulted the clinical nurse specialist for assistance in calculating an equivalent dose of morphine based on the usual heroin use. Using an estimated equivalence of heroin of 1 g = 10 to 15 mg morphine, the nurse calculated that the patient would need approximately 20 to 30 mg of morphine per day to account for her preexisting opioid tolerance. Consequently, analgesic dosing related to her surgery would also need to be relative to this baseline requirement. The patient's nurse approached the surgical team to discuss the potential benefits of using a PCA pump in addition to a continuous infusion of morphine. "By doing this," the nurse explained, "she will receive her baseline opioid requirements related to her drug tolerance. The continuous infusion will address her baseline opioid requirements while the patient-controlled boluses will allow her to treat the new surgical pain. The PCA may also offer her some control during a time in her recovery when there are few options to do so. In addition to starting the PCA with a continuous infusion, the surgical team and the primary nurse also discussed using other non-opioid agents such as NSAIDs to augment her analgesia. The team also discussed adding morphine sulfate controlled-release

(MS-Contin) to the patient's regimen once she was more comfortable on the PCA and titrating the oral medication doses up while decreasing the PCA. Once the MS-Contin was titrated to an effective dose, the PCA could be discontinued and short-acting oral breakthrough medication used for additional pain relief. The nurse noted she would also need to monitor the patient for any signs or symptoms of withdrawal.

In addition to the changes in the medications, the primary nurse worked with the patient to use relaxation techniques. The nurse explained that relaxation techniques could be thought of as "boosters" to her pain medications and were something that she could do to help control the pain. They also agreed to try massage in the evening to promote sleep and relaxation.

Case Question 1: In order to maintain adequate pain control after surgery in a patient who is addicted to heroin or takes regular opioids the nurse will need to:
(A) Provide a continuous rate on the PCA.
(B) Provide a continuous rate on the PCA to account for her presurgical heroin usage and add additional pain medications for the surgical pain.
(C) Try to limit the patient's opioid use because she is an addict.
(D) Substitute a non-opioid medication such as acetaminophen or ketorolac because the patient is an addict.

Case Question 2: The best way to control postoperative pain is to:
(A) Use opioids exclusively.
(B) Use only medications.
(C) Encourage the patient to cough and deep breathe.
(D) Use a multimodal approach with medications and complementary techniques such as relaxation.

Answers
1. B. Local anesthetics can have a short-term effect on pain relief and allow the patient to be more active and effectively cough and deep breathe. Combining the opioid and LA can have a synergistic effect increasing the overall pain relief more than using just a single medication.
2. C. Combining a non-opioid and opioid can also have a synergistic effect and decrease pain. The two different medications work on different areas of the pain mechanism. The combination can be used to help the patient become more active and if dosed at bedtime, may help the patient to rest better.

mouth or via the enteral route may experience comparable pain relief to parenteral analgesia with less risk of infection and at a lowered cost. Calculating the equianalgesic dose increases the likelihood that the transition to the oral route will be made without a change in pain control. A creative way to wean PCA is to substitute oral or enteral opioid (such as morphine or oxycodone) for one-half of the total dosage of PCA demand doses. Over the next 24 hours, reducing PCA consumption by increasing the lockout period or reducing the bolus size may help transition the patient and narrow

the "analgesic gap" between different routes. To prevent opioid overdose, controlled-release preparations of morphine and oxycodone, designed to be taken less frequently than their immediate-release counterparts, are not to be crushed, halved, or administered into enteral feeding tubes.

EPIDURAL ANALGESIA

Over the past decade the use of epidural analgesia has grown rapidly. The advantages of epidural analgesia include improved pain control with less sedation, lower overall opioid doses, and generally longer duration of pain management. Epidural analgesia has been associated with a lower morbidity and mortality in acutely ill patients. Both opioids and LAs, either alone or in combination, are commonly administered via the epidural route. Epidural analgesia may be administered by several methods, including intermittent bolus dosing, continuous infusion, or PCA technology. The mechanisms of action and the resultant clinical effects produced by epidurally administered opioids and LAs are distinct. For this reason, these agents are discussed separately, and are important to distinguish in clinical practice.

Epidural Opioids

When opioids are administered epidurally, they diffuse into the cerebrospinal fluid and into the spinal cord (Figure 6-5). There, the opioids bind with opiate receptors in the substantia gelatinosa, preventing the release of the neurotransmitter substance P, and altering the transmission of nociceptive impulses from the spinal cord to the brain. Because the opioid is concentrated in the areas of high opiate receptor density and where nociceptive impulses are entering the spinal cord, lower doses offer enhanced analgesia, with few, if any, supraspinal effects such as drowsiness.

A variety of opioids are commonly used for epidural analgesia including morphine, fentanyl, and hydromorphone. Preservative-free (PF) preparations are usually preferred because some preservative agents can have neurotoxic effects. The opioids can be administered either by intermittent bolus or continuous infusion depending on the pharmacokinetic activity of the selected agent; for example, fentanyl is generally administered via continuous infusion due to its high lipid solubility, resulting in a short duration of action. In contrast, the low lipid solubility of PF morphine results in a delayed onset of action (30-60 minutes) and a prolonged duration of action (6-12 hours). Because of the delayed onset of action, PF morphine is recommended for use as a continuous infusion but not as a patient-controlled bolus dose.

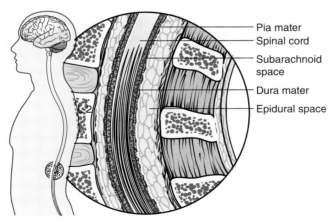

Figure 6-5. Epidural space for catheter placement.

- Pia mater
- Spinal cord
- Subarachnoid space
- Dura mater
- Epidural space

Side Effects

The side effects associated with epidural opioids are the same as those described for oral opioids. Side effects are determined primarily by the medication administered and not by the route of administration. For example, the incidence of nausea and vomiting with epidural morphine is similar to that associated with IV morphine. Although epidural opioids were once feared to be associated with a higher risk of respiratory depression, clinical studies and experience have not confirmed this risk. The incidence of respiratory depression has been reported as being no higher than 0.2%. Risk factors for respiratory depression are similar to those seen with IV opioids: increased age, high doses, underlying cardiopulmonary dysfunction, obstructive sleep apnea, obesity, and the use of perioperative or supplemental parenteral opioids or the combination of epidural opioids with other agents that cause sedation such as benzodiazepines.

Epidural Local Anesthetics

Epidural opioids can also be combined with dilute concentrations of LAs. When administered in combination, these agents work synergistically, reducing the amount of each agent that is needed to produce analgesia. Whereas epidurally administered opioids work in the dorsal horn of the spinal cord, epidural LAs exert work primarily at the dorsal nerve root by blocking the conduction of afferent sensory fibers. The extent of the blockade is dose related. Higher LA concentrations block more afferent fibers within a given region, resulting in an increased density of the blockade. Higher infusion rates of LA-containing solutions increase the extent or spread of the blockade because more afferent fibers are blocked over a broader region.

Bupivacaine is the LA most commonly used for epidural analgesia and is usually administered in combination with either fentanyl or PF morphine as a continuous infusion. The concentration of bupivacaine used for epidural analgesia usually ranges between 1/16% (0.065 mg/mL) and 1/8% (1.25 mg/mL). These concentrations are significantly lower than those used for surgical anesthesia, which usually range between 1/4% and 1/2% bupivacaine. The type and concentration of opioid used in combination with bupivacaine vary by practitioner and organizational preferences, but usually range between 2 and 5 mcg/mL fentanyl or between 0.02 and 0.04 mg/mL PF morphine. Ropivacaine, an LA alternative to bupivacaine, has less potential for creating motor block. For older patients with rib fractures or flail chest, an epidural catheter with LA only may provide positive results with less respiratory compromise and reduced pain.

Side Effects

The side effects accompanying LAs are a direct result of the conduction blockade produced by the agents. Unfortunately, the LA agents are relatively nonspecific in their capacity to block nerve conduction. That is, LAs not only block sensory afferent fibers, but also can block the conduction of motor efferent and autonomic nerve fibers within the same dermatomal regions. Side effects associated with epidural LAs include hypotension—especially postural hypotension from sympathetic blockade—and functional motor deficits from varying degrees of efferent motor fiber blockade. Sensory deficits, including changes in proprioception in the joints of the lower extremities, can accompany epidural LA administration due to the blockade of non-nociceptive sensory afferents.

The extent and type of side effects that can be anticipated with epidural LAs depend on three primary factors: (1) the location of the epidural catheter, (2) the concentration of the LA administered, and (3) the volume or rate of infusion; for example, if a patient has an epidural catheter placed within the midthoracic region, one may anticipate signs of sympathetic nervous blockade, such as postural hypotension, because the sympathetic nerve fibers are concentrated in the thoracic region. In contrast, a patient with a lumbar catheter may experience a mild degree of motor weakness in the lower extremities because the motor efferent and nerves exit the spine in the lumbar region. This usually presents clinically as either heaviness in a lower extremity or an inability to "lock" the knee in place when standing.

Both the concentration and infusion rate of the LA influence the severity and extent of side effects. The density of the blockade and intensity of observed side effects may be increased with high LA concentrations. With higher infusion volumes, greater spread of the LA can be anticipated which in turn may lead to a greater number or extent of side effects. If side effects occur, the dose of the LA often is reduced either by decreasing the concentration of the solution or by decreasing the rate. Additionally, low dose vasopressors may be used to counteract hypotension caused by LA.

Titrating Epidural Analgesia

To maximize epidural analgesia, doses may need to be adjusted. With opioids alone, the dose needed to produce effective analgesia is best predicted by the patient's age as opposed to body size. Older patients typically require lower doses to achieve pain relief than those who are younger. Small bolus doses of fentanyl (50 mcg) may help safely titrate the epidural dose or infusion to treat pain. Similarly, a small bolus dose of fentanyl may also help treat breakthrough pain that may occur with increased patient activity or procedures. For patients receiving combinations of LAs and opioids, a small bolus dose of the prescribed infusate in conjunction with an increased rate can produce pain relief. Recall, that increasing the rate of the LA infusion increases the spread of medication to additional dermatomes, whereas increasing the LA concentration increases the depth or intensity of the blockade and subsequent analgesia.

CUTANEOUS STIMULATION

One of the primary nonpharmacologic techniques for pain management used in the acute care setting is cutaneous stimulation. Cutaneous stimulation produces an analgesic effect by altering conduction of sensory impulses as they move from the periphery to the spinal cord through the stimulation of the largest sensory afferent fibers, known as the A-alpha (α) and A-beta (β) fibers. The sensory information transmitted by these large fibers is conducted more rapidly than that carried by their smaller counterparts (A-delta [δ] and C fibers) (see Figure 6-3). As a result, nociceptive input from the A-delta and C fibers can be preempted by the sensory input from the non-noxious cutaneous stimuli. Examples of cutaneous stimulation include the application of heat, cold, vibration, or massage. Transcutaneous electrical nerve stimulation units produce similar effects by electrically stimulating large sensory fibers.

Cutaneous stimulation can produce analgesic effects whether used as a complementary modality with other pharmacologic treatments or as an independent treatment modality. Nurses can integrate these modalities easily and safely into analgesic treatment plans for the acutely ill, especially for patients who are unable to tolerate higher opioid doses. To apply or administer cutaneous stimulation, one simply needs to stimulate sensory fibers anywhere between the site of injury and the spinal cord, but within the sensory dermatome (Figure 6-6). Massage, especially back massage, has additional analgesic benefits; it has been shown to promote relaxation and sleep, both of which can influence patient's responses to pain.

DISTRACTION

Distraction techniques such as music, conversation, television viewing, laughter, and deep breathing for relaxation can be valuable adjuncts to pharmacologic modalities. These techniques produce their analgesic effects by sending intense stimuli through the thalamus, midbrain, and brain stem, which can increase the production of modulating substances such as endorphins. Also, because the brain can process only a limited amount of incoming signals at any given time, the input provided by distraction techniques *competes* with nociceptive inputs. This is particularly true for the reticular activating system.

When planning for and using distraction techniques, keep in mind that they are most effective when activities are interesting to the patient (eg, their favorite type of music, television program, or video) and when they involve multiple senses such as hearing, vision, touch, and movement. Flexible selection of activities that are consistent with patient's energy levels and changing requirements is essential for good outcomes.

IMAGERY

Imagery is another technique that can be used effectively with acutely ill patients, particularly during planned procedures. Imagery alters the perception of pain stimuli, promotes relaxation, and increases the production of endorphins in the brain. Patients can use imagery independently or use guided imagery where a care provider, family member, or friend helps *guide* the patient in painting an imaginary picture. There are also audio

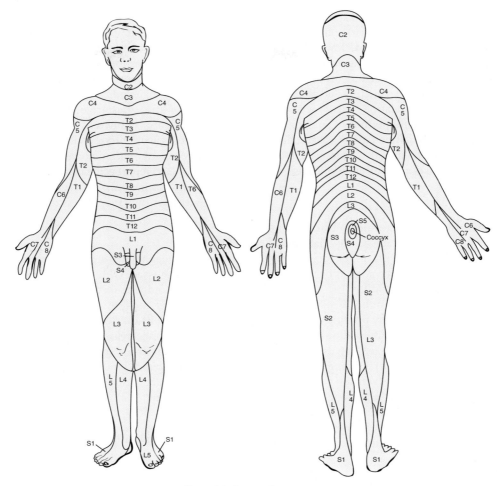

Figure 6-6. Sensory dermatomes.

recordings of guided imagery techniques that can be downloaded or played through a personal device. The more details pictured with the image, the more effective it can be. As with distraction techniques, tapping into multiple sensations is beneficial. Some patients prefer to involve the pain in their picture and imagine it melting or fading away. Other patients may prefer to paint a picture in their mind of a favorite place or activity. Strategies to help guide patients include the use of details to describe the imaginary scene (eg, "smell the fresh scent of the ocean air" or "see the intense red hue of the sun setting beyond the snow-capped mountains") and the use of relaxing sensory terms such as floating, smooth, dissolving, lighter, or melting. If patients are able to talk, it may be helpful to have them describe the image they see using appropriate detail, although some patients will prefer not to talk and instead focus on their evolving image. Again, it is important to be flexible in the approach to imagery in order to maximize its benefits.

RELAXATION TECHNIQUES

Because acutely ill patients experience numerous stressors, most patients benefit from the inclusion of relaxation or

anxiolytics. The use of relaxation techniques can help interrupt the vicious cycle involving pain, anxiety, and muscle tension that often develops when pain goes unrelieved. The physiologic response associated with relaxation includes decreased oxygen consumption, respiratory rate, heart rate, and muscle tension; blood pressure may either normalize or decrease.

A wide variety of pharmacologic and nonpharmacologic techniques can be used safely and effectively with progressive care patients to achieve relaxation and/or sedation. Relaxation techniques are simple to use and may be particularly useful in situations involving brief procedures such as turning or minor dressing changes, and following coughing or endotracheal suctioning or other stressful events.

Deep Breathing and Progressive Relaxation

Guided deep breathing and progressive relaxation can be incorporated easily into a plan of care for the progressive care patient. Nurses can coach patients with deep breathing exercises by helping them to focus on and guide their breathing patterns. As patients begin to control their breathing, nurses can work with them to begin progressive relaxation of their muscles. To do this, the nurse can say to the patient as he or she just begins to exhale, "Now begin to relax, from the top of your head to the tips of your toes". Change the pitch of the voice to be higher for "top of your head," lower for "tips of your toes." Time it such that the final phrase ends as the patient completes exhalation. This procedure capitalizes on the positive aspects of normal body functions, as the body tends to relax naturally during exhalation. This process can and is practiced during nonstressful periods to augment its efficacy. In fact, teaching and coaching patients to use deep breathing exercises helps equip them with a lifelong skill that may be used any time stressful or painful situations arise.

Presence

Probably the single most important aspect of promoting comfort in the ill or injured is the underlying relationship between the patient, the family, and his or her care providers. Family presence at the patient's bedside has been shown to decrease anxiety and promote healing. Including the people identified by the patient as his or her family support (with a broad definition of family) may provide enormous comfort for the patient, resulting in relaxation. Presence not only refers to physically "being there," but also refers to psychologically "being with" a patient. Although presence has not been well defined as an intervention to promote comfort, patients have described the importance of nurses simply "being there" and "being with" them. Nonpharmacologic methods of pain control have little known side effects and in some instances have demonstrated effectiveness and increased patient satisfaction.

SPECIAL CONSIDERATIONS FOR PAIN MANAGEMENT IN OLDER ADULTS

Misperceptions about older adults' experience of pain abound. Some believe that older patients have less pain because their extensive life experiences have equipped them to cope with discomfort more effectively. This may be true for some individuals but to accept this as fact for all older adults is short sighted and incorrect. In fact, the incidence of and morbidity associated with pain is higher in older adults than in the general population. Many older adults continue to experience chronic pain in addition to any acute pain associated with their illness or injury. Major sources of underlying pain in older adults include low back pain, arthritis, headache, chest pain, and neuropathies.

Assessment

Older patients often report pain very differently from younger patients due to physiologic, psychological, and cultural changes accompanying age. Some patients may fear loss of control, loss of independence, or being labeled as a "bad patient" if they report pain-related concerns. Also, for some patients the presence of pain may be symbolic of impending death, especially in the acute care setting. In such cases, a patient may be reticent to report pain to a care provider or family member as if to deny pain is to deny death. For reasons such as these, it is important for nurses to explain the importance of reporting any discomfort. Nurses may also use a variety of pain assessment strategies to incorporate behavioral or physiologic indicators of pain.

Similar strategies are often needed to assess pain in persons who are cognitively impaired. Preliminary reports from ongoing work among nursing home patients suggest that many patients with moderate to severe cognitive impairment are able to report acute pain reliably at the time they are asked. For these patients, pain recall and integration of pain experience over time may be less reliable.

Interventions

Acutely ill older adults can benefit from any of the analgesic therapies discussed. Older patients may tolerate opioids if the doses are individualized and the patient is monitored for effect. However, medication requirements may be reduced in some older adults due to age-related renal insufficiency and the potential for decreased renal clearance. In addition, older adults have a reduced muscle to body fat ratio that affects the way that opioids bind and activate in the body. Analgesic requirements are highly individualized and doses should be carefully titrated to achieve pain relief.

Principles of Pain Management

- Pain is a common occurrence in acutely ill patients either from trauma, surgery, procedures, and/or a painful comorbidity.
- In order to enhance healing, adequate pain relief using a multimodal approach with medications, interventional techniques, and nonpharmacologic methods is encouraged.
- Pain assessment is the key to adequate pain relief and there are a variety of tools that may be used to effectively assess and manage pain in the acutely ill patient.
- Treating pain in older patients may be more difficult as they may misunderstand the goals of pain assessment and the need for pain medications.

SEDATION

The progressive care environment can be uncomfortable and anxiety provoking for patients. Once pain is addressed, anxiolysis may be appropriate to enhance comfort, decrease anxiety or agitation, and induce sleep. In some cases, the use of sedatives may be necessary to ensure tolerance of medical interventions, clinical stability, and to protect patients from inadvertent self-harm. While the treatment of anxiety is an important aspect of acute care, frequent dosing methods (infusions or IV boluses) intended to induce a depressed sensorium (ie, amnesia) in these patients are discouraged. The use of sedation infusions in mechanically ventilated patients has been associated with negative outcomes such as prolonged mechanical ventilation, increased lengths of stay, and even death. To that end, in critical care and progressive care units where mechanically ventilated patients are cared for, nursing care aims to minimize infusion use.

Daily interruptions of sedation infusions have been associated with improved outcomes and do not appear to incur additional psychological stress. This finding is in direct opposition to the previously held philosophy that amnesia protects patients from the psychological stress induced by critical or acute care environments. Further, there is a strong association between sedation infusion use and delirium. Compounding the issue is the fact that those who develop delirium are then at risk for the development of long-term cognitive dysfunction. Because of this finding and other studies demonstrating the positive effect of less sedation in ventilated patients, SCCM evidence-based guidelines recommend treating pain first, light sedation if necessary, and the use of nonpharmacologic means of promoting sleep. To ensure that appropriate and adequate anxiolysis is achieved in the acutely ill patient, the nurse must be able to identify the reason for sedation, the medications most commonly used, the level of sedation required, and how to monitor and manage the sedated patient. Clear identification of the reason for sedation is the first step in the process.

Reasons for Sedation

Amnesia

One of the most common reasons for sedative use is to ensure amnesia. Many of the procedures and interventions performed in acute care units may potentially cause pain and anxiety. In anticipation of this, sedatives are proactively administered, often concomitantly with analgesics. Moderate sedation (also called conscious sedation) is commonly employed in these situations; it is discussed later in this chapter.

Ventilator Tolerance

Ineffective, dyssynchronous, and excessive respiratory efforts result in increased work of breathing and oxygen consumption. The reason for the dyssynchronous breathing should be quickly assessed and managed. Efforts should be made to improve tolerance by first treating potential pain and adjusting the ventilator to optimize patient-ventilator interaction. Sedative use in severe cases of patient/ventilator dyssynchrony may also be necessary, and in some cases, lifesaving. These patients are generally transferred to a critical care unit. For more in-depth information on advanced modes of ventilation see Chapter 20 in the *AACN Essentials of Critical Care Nursing, 4th edition.*

Anxiety and Fear

Anxiety and fear are symptoms that can be experienced by acutely ill patients. However, these symptoms may be difficult to assess, especially if patients are unable to adequately communicate their feelings secondary to the underlying condition, the presence of an artificial airway, or a reduced sensorium.

When the patient can identify anxiety or fear, the treatment goals are clear. However, in the patient who cannot, the presence of behaviors and signs that are associated with anxiety and/or fear are used as evidence and are the reason sedatives are provided. Manifestations of severe anxiety and/or fear include nonspecific signs of distress such as agitation, thrashing, diaphoresis, facial grimacing, blood pressure elevation, and increased heart rate. These nonspecific signs may also be indicative of pain or may be due to delirium. Pain management requirements must be addressed prior to the administration of sedation in such cases as well as assessing the patient for potential delirium.

Patient Safety and Agitation

Agitation includes any activity that appears unhelpful or potentially harmful to the patient. The patient may be aware of the activity and be able to communicate the reason for the activity; more commonly they are not aware, making it difficult to identify the reason for the agitation. The patient appears distressed and the associated activity includes episodic or continuous nonpurposeful movements, severe thrashing, attempts to remove tubes, efforts to get out of bed, or other behaviors which may threaten patient or staff safety. Reasons for agitation include pain and anxiety, delirium, preexisting conditions that require pharmacologic interventions (ie, preexisting psychiatric history), withdrawal from certain medications such as benzodiazepines (especially if they have been on them for a long time), and delirium tremens secondary to alcohol withdrawal (see Chapter 11, Multisystem Problems, section on withdrawal). Patients who experience inadequately controlled agitation face a high risk of morbidity and mortality. Thus, potential reasons for the agitation are explored so that appropriate therapy may be initiated.

Sleep Deprivation

Sleep deprivation is common among hospitalized patients. Although patients may appear restful, physiologically they may never experience the stages of sleep that provide a restorative state (ie, rapid eye movement sleep, and stages 3 and 4). These restorative stages of sleep are adversely affected by many factors, including a wide variety of medications. Sleep deprivation is also common among those with pain, discomfort, and anxiety. Additionally, sleep deprivation may be a result of the increased auditory, tactile, and visual stimuli ubiquitous to the hospital environment. The SCCM guidelines recommend the use of nonpharmacologic interventions to promote sleep when possible.

Delirium

Delirium is more prevalent in acutely ill patients than previously assumed. Patients are especially at risk if they have been on sedatives, especially by infusion for longer than 24 hours, are older, have preexisting dementia, a history of hypertension, and high severity of illness at admission. Coma is an independent risk factor for the development of delirium. As noted earlier, the risk of long-term cognitive dysfunction is increased in patients who experience delirium. There are three types of presentations of acute delirium: (1) hypoactive, (2) hyperactive, or (3) mixed. In the past, delirium was commonly associated with hyperactivity or agitation. In fact, the agitated presentation of delirium accounts for less than 5% of those who experience the condition. Most patients with delirium have the hypoactive (calm, quiet) or mixed presentation of the condition. The hypoactive category is underdiagnosed and the associated outcomes are worse than for those with the agitated/active form of delirium. The hallmarks of the condition are disorientation and disorganized thinking. Awareness of the potential for delirium and early recognition are essential for effective management and prevention of undesirable outcomes. Routine assessment of delirium with a valid and reliable delirium-monitoring tool such as the confusion assessment method for the ICU (CAM-ICU) is a common strategy for recognizing the condition. The medications of choice for delirium in the acute care setting are described later in this chapter under "Medications for Delirium" and further discussed in Chapter 7, Pharmacology.

Sedatives

After ensuring that the presence of pain is either ruled out or addressed with the appropriate administration of analgesics, sedatives may be selected based on patient-specific factors such as the level and duration of sedation required. Sedative category summaries follow and comprehensive descriptions of the medications are discussed in Chapter 7, Pharmacology.

Short-Term Sedatives

These sedatives have a rapid onset of action and a short duration of effect.

- *Dexmedetomidine* is a centrally acting alpha-2 receptor agonist that has sedative and anesthetic properties. It is short acting and is often used in an IV infusion. Dexmedetomidine has become one of the preferred short-acting sedatives in the critically ill over benzodiazepines. The medication may be used for sedation in mechanically ventilated patients and does not produce respiratory depression when used as designed (ie, boluses are not recommended). Side effects include hypotension, bradycardia, sinus arrest, or transient hypertension. In some institutions, dexmedetomidine can be infused in the progressive care unit while in other institutions, it is used primarily in critical care.
- *Midazolam* is a popular benzodiazepine that fits in this category. It can be administered intermittently in a bolus IV form or as a continuous infusion. Generally continuous infusions of midazolam are reserved for the critical care unit.

- *Ketamine* is an IV *general* anesthetic that produces analgesia, anesthesia, and amnesia without loss of consciousness. It may be given in an IV bolus form, intranasally, or orally. Although contraindicated in those with elevated intracranial pressure, its bronchodilatory properties make it a good choice in those with asthma. A well-known side effect of ketamine is hallucinations; however, these may be prevented with concurrent use of benzodiazepines. Ketamine is rarely a first-line sedative of choice, but is commonly used in patients requiring painful, frequent skin debridement procedures (eg, burn patients). The nurse needs to be aware of the hospital policy for use of this medication as some hospitals allow it only in specific circumstances.

Intermediate-Term Sedatives

These medications have an intermediate onset of action and duration of effect. However, when given as infusions they may last much longer as they are lipophilic. Generally, continuous infusions of these medications are reserved for the critical care unit.

- *Lorazepam* is the most common benzodiazepine in acute care and can be administered orally and IV as an intermittent bolus or continuous infusion. When given orally or in a bolus intermittent form, the effect is intermediate; however, when used as a continuous infusion (24 hours), its effect is more long term and awakening may take hours to days to accomplish. Lorazepam, if given frequently or by infusion, may accumulate in those with decreased metabolic function such as older adults or those with hepatic dysfunction.

Long-Acting Sedatives

- *Diazepam,* a long-acting benzodiazepine, and *chlordiazepoxide* are infrequently used in acute care; however, they may be selected for treatment of severe alcohol withdrawal. They may be given orally or as an IV bolus.

Medications for Delirium

In the past, the medication of choice for treatment of delirium was haloperidol. However, no evidence to date supports the use of haloperidol to reduce the duration of delirium. Haloperidol was popular in the past because it sedates without significant respiratory depression and is not associated with the development of tolerance or dependence. It, however, has potential adverse side effects that must be closely monitored. Extrapyramidal reactions such as dystonia and neuroleptic malignant syndrome are possible. Another adverse effect of haloperidol is prolonged QTc intervals; QTc interval monitoring is essential and required when using this medication. Atypical antipsychotics such as risperidone and olanzapine have also been used for delirium, but little data exist to support widespread use for the treatment of delirium.

Current guidelines do not suggest the routine use of antipsychotics or dexmedetomidine for prevention of delirium. However, in patients requiring mechanical ventilation, the use of dexmedetomidine may be less likely to increase the risk for delirium than the use of benzodiazepines (see Chapter 7, Pharmacology, for more on these classes of medications). Nonpharmacologic strategies to reduce the incidence of delirium such as early mobility, family involvement in care, correction of sensory deficits with glasses and hearing aids, and ensuring adequate sleep are also appropriate. Further research on medication management to reduce the incidence and severity of delirium is needed.

Goals of Sedation, Monitoring, and Management

After identification the rationale for sedative use (anxiety, sleep, ventilator tolerance, amnesia, etc) target level of sedation is determined and a medication plan established which includes dose adjustments according to patient response.

Moderate or Conscious Sedation

A technique referred to as "moderate sedation" (also known as conscious or procedural sedation) is common in progressive, acute care, and special procedure units (interventional radiology, endoscopy, etc). It refers to the use of a combination of analgesics and sedatives to minimize discomfort during a procedure while assuring that the patient can communicate and maintain ventilation throughout the procedure. Amnesia is anticipated and often desired. The patient's ability to maintain a patent airway is central to the decision to use moderate sedation. Patients considered "lowest risk" are generally those who are recommended for the technique, although higher risk individuals may also undergo moderate sedation based on consultation with the healthcare team. The American Society of Anesthesiology Patient Classification Status is used to guide the level of sedation (Table 6-7). Institutional guidelines for the use of moderate sedation vary somewhat; however, they generally include the use of continuous real-time monitoring such as respiratory rate and pattern, pulse oximetry, capnography, and heart rhythm in addition to very frequent (ie, every 5 minutes during the procedure) assessment of vital signs and evaluation of level of consciousness.

Sedation Scales: Goals and Monitoring

In contrast to moderate sedation goals, there are times when sedation is used to produce deeper sedation as in the case of an agitated ventilated patient with oxygenation problems. These patients may require transfer to a critical care unit for vigilant monitoring. Sedation scales have been developed in an effort to assist with the management of sedation in these cases, especially if the sedation requirements are anticipated to last for longer than a few hours.

Sedation scales allow the healthcare team to select a target level of sedation for the patient. Descriptors of each level of sedation are provided so that the sedative may be adjusted appropriately. When patients in progressive care areas require aggressive sedation management (eg, for ventilator intolerance), the scales noted later may be helpful. Sedation monitoring in these cases is done at least hourly and the level of sedation achieved is recorded. The SCCM evidence-based guidelines recommend the use of two tested and reliable sedation scales that may be used for these patients (Table 6-8).

TABLE 6-7. ASA CONTINUUM OF DEPTH OF SEDATION: DEFINITION OF GENERAL ANESTHESIA AND LEVELS OF SEDATION/ANALGESIA

	Minimal Sedation (Anxiolysis)	Moderate Sedation/Analgesia (Conscious Sedation)	Deep Sedation/Analgesia	General Anesthesia
Responsiveness	Normal response to verbal stimulation	Purposeful[a] response to verbal or tactile stimulation	Purposeful[a] response after repeated or painful stimulation	Unarousable, even with painful stimulus
Airway	Unaffected	No intervention required	Intervention may be required	Intervention often required
Spontaneous ventilation	Unaffected	Adequate	May be inadequate	Frequently inadequate
Cardiovascular function	Unaffected	Usually maintained	Usually maintained	May be impaired

Minimal Sedation (Anxiolysis) = a drug-induced state during which patients respond normally to verbal commands. Although cognitive function and coordination may be impaired, ventilatory and cardiovascular functions are unaffected.

Moderate Sedation/Analgesia (Conscious Sedation) = a drug-induced depression of consciousness during which patients respond purposefully[a] to verbal commands, either alone or accompanied by light tactile stimulation. No interventions are required to maintain a patent airway, and spontaneous ventilation is adequate. Cardiovascular function is usually maintained.

Deep Sedation/Analgesia = a drug-induced depression of consciousness during which patients cannot be easily aroused but respond purposefully[a] following repeated or painful stimulation. The ability to independently maintain ventilatory function may be impaired. Patients may require assistance in maintaining a patent airway, and spontaneous ventilation may be inadequate. Cardiovascular function is usually maintained.

General Anesthesia = a drug-induced loss of consciousness during which patients are not arousable, even by painful stimulation. The ability to independently maintain ventilatory function is often impaired. Patients often require assistance in maintaining a patent airway, and positive pressure ventilation may be required because of depressed spontaneous ventilation or drug-induced depression of neuromuscular function. Cardiovascular function may be impaired.

Since sedation is a continuum, it is not always possible to predict how an individual patient will respond. Hence, practitioners intending to produce a given level of sedation should be able to rescue patients whose level of sedation becomes deeper than initially intended. Individuals administering Moderate Sedation/Analgesia (Conscious Sedation) should be able to rescue patients who enter a state of Deep Sedation/Analgesia, while those administering Deep Sedation/Analgesia should be able to rescue patients who enter a state of general anesthesia.

[a]*Reflex withdrawal from a painful stimulus is not considered a purposeful response.*

Reproduced with permission from American Society of Anesthesiologists Task Force on Sedation and Analgesia by Non-Anesthesiologists: Practice guidelines for sedation and analgesia by non-anesthesiologists, Anesthesiology 2002 Apr;96(4):1004-1017.

TABLE 6-8.   SEDATION ASSESSMENT SCALES WITH VALIDITY AND RELIABILITY IN ADULT PATIENTS

Sedation-Agitation Scale[a]	Richmond Agitation-Sedation Scale[b]
1. Unarousable (minimal or no response to noxious stimuli, does not communicate or follow commands)	– 5 Unresponsive (no response to voice or physical stimulation)
2. Very sedated (arouses to physical stimuli but does not communicate or follow commands; may move spontaneously)	– 4 Deep sedation (no response to voice, but any movement to physical stimulation)
3. Sedated (difficult to arouse, awakens to verbal stimuli or gentle shaking but drifts off again, follows simple commands)	– 3 Moderate sedation (any movement, but no eye contact to voice)
4. Calm and cooperative (calm, awakens easily, follows commands)	– 2 Light sedation (briefly, < 10 seconds, awakening with eye contact to voice)
5. Agitated (anxious or mildly agitated, attempting to sit up, calms down to verbal instructions)	– 1 Drowsy (not fully alert, but has sustained, > 10 seconds, awakening with eye contact to voice)
6. Very agitated (does not calm, despite frequent verbal reminding of limits; requires physical restraints, biting ET tube)	0 Alert and calm
7. Dangerous agitation (pulling at ET tube, trying to remove catheter, climbing over bed rail, striking at staff, thrashing side to side)	1. Restless (anxious or apprehensive but movements not aggressive or vigorous)
	2. Agitated (frequent nonpurposeful movement or patient-ventilator dyssynchrony)
	3. Very agitated (pulls on or removes tubes or catheters or has aggressive behavior toward staff)
	4. Combative (overly combative or violent; immediate danger to staff)

Data compiled from:
[a]Riker R, Picard J, Fraser G, et al (1994).
[b]Sessler C, Gosnet M, Grap MJ, et al (2002).

Sedation Management

Management of sedation is an essential step in attaining positive outcomes for acutely ill patients. Patients may require sedatives for the treatment of mild to moderate anxiety while in the progressive care unit. Treatment of such anxiety is appropriate and rarely results in adverse effects. Generally, the sedatives are provided orally and occasionally as an IV bolus. The doses are adjusted to prevent excessive drowsiness or respiratory depression. Appropriately dosed, use of the sedatives does not interfere with clinical progress such as weaning or rehabilitation. In contrast, it is especially important to consider the effects associated with sedation infusions on outcomes. Often, if a sedation infusion is used in a progressive care unit, its use is short lived and the patient is converted to PO or IV bolus doses as soon as possible.

In patients who require high levels of sedation to prevent self-harm, sedation infusions and/or frequent IV bolus sedation may be essential. These patients may need to be transferred to a critical care unit if the condition persists.

Principles of Management for the Use of Sedatives

- Treat pain prior to providing sedation.
- Target the lightest level of sedation that will allow individualized treatment goals to be achieved.
- Assess sedation level with a valid and reliable scale, including during moderate sedation procedures.
- Routinely monitor for and treat delirium.

ESSENTIAL CONTENT CASE

Moderate (Procedural) Sedation

A 78-year-old man with a history of mitral valve insufficiency presents to the cardiology clinic with 1 week of fatigue, dizziness, and palpitations. Electrocardiogram (ECG) reveals new atrial fibrillation with rapid ventricular response, and he is admitted to the Progressive Care Unit. The patient is hemodynamically stable with the following admission assessment data: BP 110/70 mm Hg, HR 125 beats/min and irregular, RR 14 breaths/min, SpO_2 94% on room air. An intravenous infusion of unfractionated heparin is started for anticoagulation, and the next morning the patient's activated partial thromboplastin time (aPTT) is within a therapeutic range. The team schedules a bedside trans-esophageal echocardiogram (TEE) to evaluate for atrial thrombus before deciding whether to proceed with cardioversion.

Moderate sedation is planned for the TEE with a goal level on the Richmond Agitation-Sedation Scale (RASS) of –2. After obtaining informed consent, the provider orders bolus doses of fentanyl and midazolam to be prepared. The nurse obtains these medications and also (per hospital policy) has the reversal agent's naloxone and flumazenil on hand.

Case Question 1: Which equipment should the nurse ensure is available at the bedside for the procedure?
(A) Pacemaker and suction
(B) Bag-valve mask and capnography
(C) Ventilator and defibrillator
(D) Peripheral nerve stimulator and oral airway

Answers
B. The nurse should be prepared with equipment to monitor and support the patient's ventilatory status during sedation. Capnography is an evidence-based method to detect underventilation and hypercarbia (signs of oversedation) and supplies immediately available for airway support should include suction, an oral airway, and a bag-valve mask. A defibrillator

would be used if the provider elects to perform a cardioversion while the patient is still under sedation. It is not likely that a pacemaker or ventilator would be necessary, although having them easily accessible is prudent.

The nurse obtains a baseline assessment of the patient that includes vital signs, pain level, and sedation level.

BP 115/65 mm Hg	Spo$_2$ 97% on 2 liters O$_2$	Pain level 0
Heart rate 120 beats/min, atrial fibrillation	Capnography (ETCO$_2$) 40 mm Hg	RASS score 0
Respiration rate 12 breaths/min		

The team performs a time-out and starts the procedure. The nurse gives incremental doses of 50 mcg fentanyl and 1 mg midazolam as directed by the provider, and continuously monitors the telemetry, respiratory rate and depth, and capnography waveform. Every 3 to 5 minutes, the nurse assesses the patient's blood pressure, pain level, and response to verbal stimuli.

Ten minutes into the procedure, the nurse notes the following assessment data:

BP 100/52 mm Hg	Spo$_2$ 95% on 4 liters O$_2$	Pain level 0
Heart rate 130 beats/min, atrial fibrillation	Capnography (ETCO$_2$) 50 mm Hg	RASS score −4
Respiration rate 6 breaths/min, snoring		

Case Question 2: Which would be the most appropriate response by the nurse to the assessment data?
(A) Continue to monitor the patient
(B) Replace the nasal cannula with a simple mask
(C) Verbally stimulate the patient
(D) Perform a head tilt-chin lift maneuver

Answers
D. An increase in end-tidal carbon dioxide of 10 or more mm Hg and a decrease in respiratory rate indicates that the patient is hypoventilating. The nurse should notify the provider performing the procedure and intervene early to optimize ventilation. Giving more oxygen via simple mask would not help the issue of the patient taking few, shallow breaths. Verbally stimulating the patient is not likely to be effective since patients with a RASS score of −4 respond only to painful stimulation.

After a pause for airway support and using a bag-valve mask to temporarily ventilate the patient, the procedure is completed, and the patient recovers uneventfully. There is an atrial thrombus, so the team plans for anticoagulation and medical management of the atrial fibrillation.

SELECTED BIBLIOGRAPHY

Pain Management

American Association of Critical Care Nurses. Assessing Pain in the Criticall Ill Adult, 2014. https://www.aacn.org/clinical-resources/practice-alerts/assessing-pain-in-the-critically-ill-adult. Accessed July 16, 2018.

American Pain Society. *Principles of Analgesic Use in the Treatment of Acute Pain and Cancer Pain.* 6th ed. Glenview, IL: American Pain Society; 2008.

American Society of Pain Management Nursing. *Core Curriculum for Pain Management Nursing.* Dubuque, IA: Hunt Publishing; 2009.

Barr J, Fraser G, Puntillo K, et al. Clinical practice guidelines for the management of pain, agitation, and delirium in adult patients in the intensive care unit. *Crit Care Med.* 2013;41(1):263-306.

Barthélémy O, Limbourg T, Collet J, et al. Impact of non-steroidal anti-inflammatory drugs (NSAIDs) on cardiovascular outcomes in patients with stable atherothrombosis or multiple risk factors. *Int J Cardiol.* 2013;163(3):266-271.

Bavry A, Khaliq A, Gong Y, et al. Harmful effects of NSAIDs among patients with hypertension and coronary artery disease. *Am J Med.* 2011;124:614-620.

Bennett JS, Daugherty A, Herrington D, et al. The use of non-steroidal anti-inflammatory drugs (NSAIDs): a science advisory from the American Heart Association. *Circulation.* 2005;111 (13):1713-1716.

Berry P, Covington E, Dahl J, Katz J, Miaskowski C. *Pain: Current Understanding of Assessment, Management, and Treatments.* Reston, VA: National Pharmaceutical Council, Inc., and the Joint Commission on Accreditation of Healthcare Organizations; 2006.

D'Arcy Y. *A Compact Clinical Guide to Acute Pain Management.* New York, NY: Springer Publishing; 2011.

Faucett J. Care of the critically ill patient in pain: the importance of nursing. In: Puntillo KA, ed. *Pain in the Critically Ill.* Gaithersburg, MD: Aspen; 1991.

Fine P, Portenoy R. *A Clinical Guide to Opioid Analgesia.* New York, NY: Vendome Group LLC; 2007.

Gardner DL. Presence. In: Bulechek GM, McCloskey JC, eds. *Nursing Interventions: Essential Nursing Treatments.* Philadelphia, PA: WB Saunders; 1992:316-324.

Gélinas C. Puntillo KA, Levin P, Azoulay E. The behavior pain assessment tool for critically ill adults: a validation study in 28 countries. *Pain.* 2017;158(5):811-821.

Gordon DB, Dahl J, Phillips P, et al. The use of "as-needed" range orders for opioid analgesics in the management of acute pain: a consensus statement of the American Society for Pain Management Nursing and the American Pain Society. *Pain Manag Nurs.* 2004;5:53-58.

Julius D, Basbaum AI. Molecular mechanisms of nociception. *Nature.* 2001;413:203-210.

Khatta M. A complementary approach to pain management. *Adv Pract Nurs.* 2007. https://www.cdc.gov/drugoverdose/prescribing/guideline.html. Accessed June 30, 2018.

Marmo L, D'Arcy Y. *A Compact Clinical Guide to Critical Care, ER, and Trauma Pain Management.* New York, NY: Springer – Publishing; 2013.

Melton S, Liu S. Regional anesthesia techniques. In: Fishman S, Ballantyne J, Rathmell J, eds. *Bonica's Management of Pain.* 5th ed. Philadelphia PA: Lippincott Williams and Wilkins; 2010:92-106.

Pain Management and the Opioid Epidemic: Balancing Societal and Individual Benefits and Risks of Prescription Opioid Use. National Academies Press; 2017.

Pasternak GW. Molecular biology of opioid analgesia. *J Pain Symp Manage.* 2005;29(5S):S2-S9.

Pettigrew J. Intensive nursing care: the ministry of presence. *Crit Care Nurs Clin North Am.* 1990;2(3):503-508.

Puntillo K. Advances in management of acute pain: great strides or tiny footsteps? Capsules comments. *Crit Care Nurse.* 1995;3:97-100.

Puntillo K. Pain experience in intensive care patients. *Heart Lung.* 1990;19:526-533.

Puntillo K, Weiss SJ. Pain: its mediators and associated morbidity in critically ill cardiovascular surgical patients. *Nurs Res.* 1994;43:31-36.

Puntillo KA, Morris AB, Thompson CL, et al. Pain behaviors observed during six common procedures: results from Thunder Project II. *Crit Care Med.* 2004;32(2):421-427.

Puntillo KA, White C, Morris AB, et al. Patients' perceptions and responses to procedural pain: results from Thunder Project II. *Am J Crit Care.* 2001;10(4):238-251.

Puntillo KA, Wild LR, Morris AB, et al. Practices and predictors of analgesic interventions for adults undergoing painful procedures. *Am J Crit Care.* 2002;11(5):415-429.

Puntillo KA, Wilke DJ. Assessment of pain in the critically ill. In: Puntillo KA, ed. *Pain in the Critically Ill.* Gaithersburg, MD: Aspen; 1991:45-64.

Richman JM, Liu SS, Courpas G, et al. Does peripheral nerve block provide superior pain control to opioids? A metanalysis. *Anesth Analg.* 2006;102(1):248-257.

Rose L, Smith O, Gélinas C, et al. Critical care nurses' pain assessment and management practices: a survey in Canada. *Am J Crit Care.* 2012;21(4):151-259.

Schulz-Stübner S, Boezaart A, Hata JS. Regional analgesia in the critically ill. *Crit Care Med.* 2005;33:1400-1407.

Stanik-Hutt JA, Soeken KL, Belcher AE, Fontaine DK, Gift AG. Pain experiences of traumatically injured patients in a critical care setting. *Am J Crit Care.* 2001;10:252-259.

Summer G, Puntillo K. Management of surgical and procedural pain in the critical care setting. *Crit Care Clin North Am.* 2001;13:233-242.

Wong DL, Baker CM. Pain in children: comparison of assessment scales. *Pediatr Nurs.* 1988;14(1):9-17.

Wu CL, Cohen SR, Richman JM, et al. Efficacy of postoperative patient-controlled and continuous infusion epidural analgesia versus intravenous patient-controlled analgesia with opioids: a meta-analysis. *Anesthesiology.* 2005;103(5):1079-1088.

Sedation

American Association of Critical Care Nurses. AACN Practice Alert: assessment and management of delirium across the life span. *Crit Care Nurse.* 2016;36(5):e14-e19.

Balas MC, Vasilevskis EE, Olsen KM, et al. Effectiveness and safety of the awakening and breathing coordination, delirium monitoring/management, and early exercise/mobility bundle. *Crit Care Med.* 2014;42(5):1024-1036.

Ely EW, Truman B, Shintani A, et al. Monitoring sedation status over time in ICU patients: reliability and validity of the Richmond Agitation-Sedation Scale (RASS). *JAMA.* 2003;289(22):2983-2991.

Khan BA, Guzman O, Campbell NL, et al. Comparison and agreement between the Richmond Agitation-Sedation Scale and the Riker Sedation-Agitation Scale in evaluating patients' eligibility for delirium assessment in the ICU. *Chest.* 2012;142(1):48-54.

Zaal IJ, Devlin JW, Peelen LM, Slooter AJ. A systematic review of risk factors for delirium in the ICU. *Crit Care Med.* 2015;43(1):40-47.

Evidence-Based Practice Guidelines

American Geriatric Society (AGS). Pharmacological management of persistent pain in older persons. *J Am Geriatr Soc.* 2009;57(8):1331-1346.

American Society of Anesthesiologists. Practice Guidelines for Moderate Procedural Sedation and Analgesia 2018: A Report by the American Society of Anesthesiologists Task Force on Moderate Procedural Sedation and Analgesia, the American Association of Oral and Maxillofacial Surgeons, American College of Radiology, American Dental Association, American Society of Dentist Anesthesiologists, and Society of Interventional Radiology. *Anesthesiology.* 2018;128(3):437-479.

American Society of Anesthesiologists Task Force on Acute Pain Management. Practice guidelines for acute pain management in the perioperative setting: an update report by the American Society of Anesthesiologists Task Force on Acute Pain Management. *Anesthesiology.* 2012;116:248-273.

Barr J, Fraser G, Puntillo K, et al. Clinical practice guidelines for the management of pain, agitation, and delirium in adult patients in the intensive care unit. *Crit Care Med.* 2013;41(1):263-306.

Centers for Disease Control Opioid Prescribing Guidelines for Chronic Pain, 2016. www.cdc.gov/guidelines. Accessed July 13, 2018.

Chou, Gordon DB, de Leon-Casasola OA, et al. Management of Postoperative Pain: A Clinical Practice Guideline from the American Pain Society, the American Society of Regional Anesthesia and Pain Medicine, American Society of Anesthesiologists' Committee of Regional Anesthesia, Executive Committee and Administrative Council. *J Pain.* 2016;17(2):131-157.

Herr K, Coyne P, Kry T, et al. Pain assessment in the nonverbal patient: position statement with clinical practice recommendations. *Pain Manag Nurs.* 2006;7(2):44-52.

PHARMACOLOGY

7

Earnest Alexander

KNOWLEDGE COMPETENCIES

1. Discuss advantages and disadvantages of various routes for medication delivery in acutely ill patients.

2. Identify indications for use, mechanism of action, administration guidelines, side effects, and contraindications for drugs commonly administered in acute illness.

Patients in high acuity setting often require complex medication regimens. These patients may be at risk for adverse effects from their medications because of altered metabolism and elimination that is commonly seen in the acutely ill patient. Organ dysfunction or drug interactions may produce increased serum drug or active metabolite concentrations, resulting in enhanced or adverse pharmacologic effects. Therefore, it is important to be familiar with each patient's medications, including the drug's metabolic profile, drug interactions, and adverse effect profile. This chapter reviews medications commonly used in progressive care units and discusses mechanisms of action, indications for use, common adverse effects, contraindications, and usual doses. A summary of intravenous (IV) medication information is provided in Chapter 22, Pharmacology Tables.

MEDICATION SAFETY

In the care of the acutely ill, the medication-use process (which includes prescribing, preparation, dispensing, administration, and monitoring) is particularly complex. Each step in the process is fraught with the potential for breakdowns in medication safety (ie, adverse drug events [ADEs], medication errors). Improvement in medication safety requires interdisciplinary focus and attention. The Institute for Safe Medication Practices (ISMP) has highlighted the following

key elements that must be optimized in order to maintain patient safety in the medication-use process:

- *Patient information:* Having essential patient information at the time of medication prescribing, dispensing, and administration will result in a significant decrease in preventable ADEs.
- *Drug information:* Providing accurate and usable drug information to all healthcare practitioners involved in the medication-use process reduces the amount of preventable ADEs.
- *Communication of drug information:* Miscommunication between physicians, pharmacists, and nurses is a common cause of medication errors. To minimize medication errors caused by miscommunication, it is important to always verify drug information and eliminate communication barriers.
- *Drug labeling, packaging, and nomenclature:* Drug names that look alike or sound alike, as well as products that have confusing drug labeling and non-distinct drug packaging, significantly contribute to medication errors. The incidence of medication errors is reduced with the use of proper labeling and the use of unit dose systems within hospitals.
- *Drug storage, stock, standardization, and distribution:* Standardizing drug administration times, drug concentrations, and limiting the concentration of drugs

available in patient care areas will reduce the risk of medication errors or minimize their consequences in the event an error occurs.

- *Drug device acquisition, use, and monitoring:* Appropriate safety assessment of drug delivery devices is made both prior to their purchase and during their use. Also, a system of independent double checks within the institution helps prevent device-related errors such as selecting the wrong drug or drug concentration, setting the rate improperly, or mixing the infusion line up with another.

- *Environmental factors:* A well-designed system offers the best chance of preventing errors; however, sometimes the acute care environment may contribute to medication errors. Environmental factors that can often contribute to medications errors include poor lighting, noise, interruptions, and a significant workload.

- *Staff competency and education:* Staff education focuses on priority topics, such as new medications being used in the hospital, high-alert medications, medication errors that have occurred both internally and externally, protocols, policies, and procedures related to medication use. Staff education can be an important error-prevention strategy when combined with the other key elements for medication safety.

- *Patient education:* Patients must receive ongoing education from physicians, pharmacists, and the nursing staff about the brand and generic names of medications they are receiving, their indications, usual and actual doses, expected and possible adverse effects, drug or food interactions, and how to protect themselves from errors. Patients can play a vital role in preventing medication errors when they are encouraged to ask questions and seek answers about their medications before drugs are dispensed at a pharmacy or administered in a hospital.

- *Quality processes and risk management:* The way to prevent errors is to redesign the systems and processes that lead to errors rather than focus on correcting the individuals who make errors. Effective strategies for reducing errors include making it difficult for staff to make an error and promoting the detection and correction of errors before they reach a patient and cause harm.

MEDICATION ADMINISTRATION METHODS

Intravenous

Intravenous administration is the preferred route for medications in acutely ill patients because it permits complete and reliable delivery. Depending on the indication and the therapy, medications may be administered by IV push, intermittent infusion, or continuous infusion. Typically, *IV push* refers to administration of a drug over 3 to 5 minutes;

intermittent infusion refers to 15-minute to 2-hour drug administration at set intervals throughout day, and *continuous infusion* administration occurs over a prolonged period of time.

Intramuscular or Subcutaneous

Intramuscular (IM) or subcutaneous (SC) administration of medications are rarely used in acutely ill patients. This is due to a number of factors including delayed onset of action, unreliable absorption because of decreased peripheral perfusion (particularly in patients who are hypotensive or hypovolemic), or inadequate muscle or decreased SC fat tissue. Furthermore, SC/IM administration may result in incomplete, unpredictable, or erratic drug absorption. If medication is not absorbed from the injection site, a depot of medication can develop. If this occurs, once perfusion is restored, absorption can potentially lead to supratherapeutic or toxic effects. Additionally, patients with thrombocytopenia or who are receiving thrombolytic agents or anticoagulants may develop hematomas and bleeding complications due to SC or IM administration. Finally, administering frequent IM injections may also be inconvenient and painful for patients.

Oral

Oral (PO) administration of medication in the acutely ill patient can also result in incomplete, unpredictable, or erratic absorption. This may be caused by a number of factors including the presence of an ileus impairing drug absorption, or to diarrhea decreasing gastrointestinal (GI) tract transit time and time for drug absorption. Diarrhea may have a pronounced effect on the absorption of sustained-release preparations such as calcium channel–blocking agents, resulting in a suboptimal serum drug concentration or clinical response. Several medications such as fluconazole and the fluoroquinolones have been shown to exhibit excellent bioavailability when orally administered to acutely ill patients. The availability of an oral suspension for some of these agents makes oral administration a reliable and cost-effective alternative for patients with limited IV access.

In patients unable to swallow, tablets are often crushed and capsules opened for administration through nasogastric or orogastric tubes. This practice is time consuming and can result in blockage of the tube, necessitating removal of the clogged tube and insertion of a new tube. If enteral nutrition is being administered through the tube, it often has to be stopped for medication administration, resulting in inadequate nutrition for patients. Also, several medications (eg, phenytoin, carbamazepine, and warfarin) have been shown to compete, or interact, with enteral nutrition solutions. This interaction results in decreased absorption of these agents, or complex formation with the nutrition solution leading to precipitation and clogging of the feeding tube. To avoid reduced medication absorption, enteral nutrition may be held before and after administration of these medications. In these instances, caloric intake will be reduced unless feeding rates are adjusted accordingly.

Liquid medications may circumvent the need to crush tablets or open capsules, but have their own limitations. An example is ciprofloxacin (Cipro) oral suspension, which is an oil-based preparation that is not given via feeding tube because of the high probability of clogging. Many liquid dosage forms contain sorbitol as a flavoring agent or as the primary delivery vehicle. Sorbitol's hyperosmolarity is a frequent cause of diarrhea in acutely ill patients, especially in patients receiving enteral nutrition. Potassium chloride elixir is extremely hyperosmolar and requires dilution with 120 to 160 mL of water before administration. Administering undiluted potassium chloride elixir can result in osmotic diarrhea.

Lastly, sustained-release or enteric-coated preparations are difficult to administer to acutely ill patients. When sustained-release products are crushed, the patient absorbs the entire dose immediately as opposed to gradually over a period of 6, 8, 12, or 24 hours. This results in supratherapeutic or potentially toxic effects soon after the administration of the medication, with subtherapeutic effects at the end of the dosing interval. Sustained-release preparations must be converted to equivalent daily doses of immediate-release dosing forms and administered at more frequent dosing intervals. Enteric-coated dosage forms that are crushed may be inactivated by gastric juices or may cause stomach irritation. Enteric-coated tablets are specifically formulated to pass through the stomach intact so that they can enter the small intestine before they begin to dissolve.

Sublingual

Because of the high degree of vascularity of the sublingual mucosa, sublingual administration of medication often produces serum concentrations of medication that parallel IV administration, and an onset of action that is often faster than orally administered medications.

Traditionally, nitroglycerin has been one of the few medications administered sublingually (SL) to acutely ill patients. Several oral and IV medications, however, have been shown to produce therapeutic effects after sublingual administration. Captopril reliably and predictably lowers blood pressure in patients with hypertensive urgency. Oral lorazepam tablets can be administered SL to treat patients in status epilepticus; preparations of oral triazolam and IV midazolam have been shown to produce sedation after sublingual administration.

Intranasal

Intranasal administration is a way to effectively administer sedative and analgesic agents. The high degree of vascularity of the nasal mucosa results in rapid and complete absorption of medication. Agents that have been administered successfully intranasally include meperidine, fentanyl, sufentanil, butorphanol, ketamine, midazolam, and naloxone.

Transdermal

Transdermal administration of medication is of limited value in acutely ill patients. Although nitroglycerin paste is extremely effective as a temporizing measure before IV access is established in the acute management of patients with angina, heart failure (HF), pulmonary edema, or hypertension, nitroglycerin transdermal patches are of limited benefit in this population because of their slow onset of activity and their inability for dose titration. Also, patients with decreased peripheral perfusion may not sufficiently absorb transdermally administered medications to produce the desired therapeutic effect. Transdermal preparations of clonidine, nitroglycerin, or fentanyl may be beneficial in patients who have been stabilized on IV or oral doses, but require chronic administration of these agents. Chronic use of nitroglycerin transdermal patches is further complicated by the development of tolerance. However, the development of tolerance can be avoided by removing the patch at bedtime, allowing for an 8- to 10-hour "nitrate-free" period.

A eutectic mixture of local anesthetic (EMLA) is a combination of lidocaine and prilocaine. This local anesthetic mixture can be used to anesthetize the skin before insertion of IV catheters or the injection of local anesthetics that may be required to produce deeper levels of topical anesthesia.

Although transdermal administration of medications is an infrequent method of drug administration in acutely ill patients, its use should not be overlooked as a potential cause of adverse effects in this patient population. Extensive application to burned, abraded, or denuded skin can result in significant systemic absorption of topically applied medications. Excessive use of viscous lidocaine products or mouthwashes containing lidocaine to provide local anesthesia for mucositis or esophagitis also can result in significant systemic absorption of lidocaine. Lidocaine administered topically to the oral mucosa has resulted in serum concentrations capable of producing seizures. The diffuse application of topical glucocorticosteroid preparations also can lead to absorption capable of producing adrenal suppression. This is especially true with the high-potency fluorinated steroid preparations such as betamethasone dipropionate, clobetasol propionate, desoximetasone, or fluocinonide.

CENTRAL NERVOUS SYSTEM PHARMACOLOGY

Sedatives

Sedatives can be divided into four main categories: benzodiazepines, barbiturates, neuroleptics, and miscellaneous agents. Benzodiazepines are commonly used sedatives in acutely ill patients. Neuroleptics have a limited use in patients who manifest a psychological or behavioral component to their sedative needs, as indiscriminant use is largely discouraged. Barbiturates are reserved for patients with refractory status epilepticus, head injuries, and increased intracranial pressure. Propofol is a short-acting IV general anesthetic that is approved for use as a sedative for mechanically ventilated patients. Dexmedetomidine is another short-acting IV general anesthetic used for light sedation. Dosing of sedatives is guided by frequent assessment of the level of sedation with a valid and reliable sedation assessment scale (see Chapter 6, Pain Management/Sedation).

Benzodiazepines

Benzodiazepines are frequently used agents for sedation in acutely ill patients. These agents provide sedation, decrease anxiety, have anticonvulsant properties, possess indirect muscle-relaxant properties, and induce anterograde amnesia. Benzodiazepines bind to gamma-aminobutyric acid (GABA) receptors located in the central nervous system, modulating this inhibitory neurotransmitter. These agents have a wide margin of safety as well as flexibility in their routes of administration.

Benzodiazepines are often used to provide short-term sedation and amnesia during imaging procedures, other diagnostic procedures, and invasive procedures such as central venous catheter placement or bronchoscopy. A common long-term indication for using benzodiazepines is sedation and amnesia during mechanical ventilation.

Excessive sedation and confusion can occur with initial doses, but these effects diminish as tolerance develops during therapy. Older adult and pediatric patients may exhibit a paradoxical effect manifested as irritability, agitation, hostility, hallucinations, and anxiety. Respiratory depression may be seen more commonly in patients receiving concurrent narcotics, as well as in elderly patients and patients with chronic obstructive pulmonary disease (COPD) or obstructive sleep apnea (OSA). Benzodiazepines have also been associated with the development of delirium, which has been linked with worse clinical outcomes, and a resultant decrease in usage overall. Additionally, there is a trend toward more bolus dosing and less continuous infusions. This trend is likely aimed at reducing the level of sedation and the duration of mechanical ventilation but comparative trials are needed to demonstrate the best dosing strategy.

Patients with histories of prior benzodiazepine or chronic alcohol use may require higher benzodiazepine doses.

Monitoring Parameters

- Mental status, level of consciousness, respiratory rate, and level of comfort are monitored in any patient receiving a benzodiazepine.
- Signs and symptoms of withdrawal reactions are monitored for patients receiving short-acting agents (ie, midazolam).
- Monitor level of sedation and use the lowest dose that produces the desired effect.

Midazolam

Midazolam is a short-acting, highly lipophilic (at physiologic pH) benzodiazepine that may be administered IV, IM, SL, PO, intranasally, or rectally. Clearance of midazolam has been shown to be extremely variable in acutely ill patients.

The elimination half-life can be increased by as much as 6 to 12 hours in patients with liver disease, shock, or concurrently receiving enzyme-inhibiting drugs such as erythromycin or fluconazole, and hypoalbuminemia. Midazolam's two primary metabolites, 1-hydroxymidazolam and 1-hydroxymidazolam glucuronide, have been shown to accumulate in acutely ill patients, especially those with renal dysfunction, contributing additional pharmacologic effects. Older adult patients demonstrate prolonged half-lives secondary to age-related reduction in liver function.

Dose

- *IV bolus:* 0.025 to 0.05 mg/kg
- *Continuous infusion:* 0.5 to 5 mcg/kg/min

Lorazepam

Lorazepam is an intermediate-acting benzodiazepine that offers the advantage of not having its metabolism affected by impaired hepatic function, age, or interacting drugs. Glucuronidation in the liver is the route of elimination of lorazepam. Because lorazepam is relatively water insoluble, it must be diluted in propylene glycol, and it is propylene glycol that is responsible for the hypotension that may be seen after bolus IV administration. Large volumes of fluid are required to maintain the drug in solution, so that only 20 to 40 mg can be safely dissolved in 250 mL of dextrose-5%-water (D_5W). In-line filters are recommended when administering lorazepam by continuous infusion because of the potential for the drug to precipitate. Finally, lorazepam's long elimination half-life of 10 to 20 hours limits its dosing flexibility by continuous infusion. Patients requiring high-dose infusions may be at risk for developing propylene glycol toxicity, which is manifested as a hyperosmolar state with a metabolic acidosis.

Dose

- *IV bolus:* 0.5 to 2 mg q1-4h
- *Continuous infusion:* 0.06 to 0.1 mg/kg/h
- *Oral:* 1 to 10 mg daily divided 2 to 3 times/day

Diazepam

Diazepam is a long-acting benzodiazepine with a faster onset of action than lorazepam or midazolam. Although its duration of action is 1 to 2 hours after a single dose, it displays cumulative effects because its active metabolites contribute to its pharmacologic effect. Desmethyldiazepam has a half-life of approximately 150 to 200 hours, so it accumulates slowly and then is slowly eliminated from the body after diazepam is discontinued. Diazepam metabolism is reduced in patients with hepatic failure and in patients receiving drugs that inhibit hepatic microsomal enzymes. Diazepam may be used for one or two doses as a periprocedure anxiolytic and amnestic, but not used for routine sedation of mechanically ventilated patients.

Dose

- *IV bolus:* 2.5 to 10 mg q2-4h
- *Continuous infusion:* Not recommended
- *Oral:* 2 to 10 mg bid-qid

Benzodiazepine Antagonist

Flumazenil

Flumazenil is a specific benzodiazepine antagonist indicated for the reversal of benzodiazepine-induced moderate sedation, recurrent sedation, and benzodiazepine overdose. It is used with caution in patients who have received benzodiazepines for an extended period of time to prevent the precipitation of withdrawal reactions.

Dose

- *Reversal of conscious sedation:* 0.2 mg IV over 2 minutes, followed in 45 seconds by 0.2 mg repeated every minute as needed to a maximum dose of 1 mg. Reversal of recurrent sedation is the same as for conscious sedation, except doses may be repeated every 20 minutes as needed.
- *Benzodiazepine overdose:* 0.2 mg over 30 seconds followed by 0.3 mg over 30 seconds; repeated doses of 0.5 mg can be administered over 30 seconds at 1-minute intervals up to a cumulative dose of 3 mg. With a partial response after 3 mg, additional doses up to a total dose of 5 mg may be administered. In all of the above-mentioned scenarios, no more than 1 mg is administered at any one time, and no more than 3 mg in any 1 hour.
- *Continuous infusion:* 0.1 to 0.5 mg/h (for the reversal of long-acting benzodiazepines or massive overdoses).

Monitoring Parameters

- Level of consciousness and signs and symptoms of withdrawal reactions

Neuroleptics

Haloperidol

Haloperidol is a major tranquilizer that has commonly been used for the management of agitated or delirious patients who fail to respond to nonpharmacologic interventions or other sedatives. It is important to note that despite the common usage of this agent to treat delirium, there is no published evidence that haloperidol reduces the duration of delirium. The lack of supporting evidence is leading to the reconsideration of the role of haloperidol in this setting compared with other potentially more well-tolerated agents with fewer side effects (ie, atypical antipsychotics). Prolonged corrected QT interval (QTc) is a significant adverse reaction and the risk for dysrhythmia must be carefully weighed against the potential benefit of haloperidol. Advantages of haloperidol are that it causes limited respiratory depression and has little potential for the development of tolerance or dependence. Although its exact mechanism of action is unknown, it probably involves dopaminergic receptor blockade in the central nervous system, resulting in central nervous system depression at the subcortical level of the brain.

IV haloperidol is the most frequently used neuroleptic for controlling agitation in acutely ill patients. Initial doses of 2 to 5 mg may be doubled every 15 to 20 minutes until the patient is adequately sedated. Single IV doses as large as 150 mg as well as total daily doses of approximately 1000 mg have been safely administered to patients. As soon as the patient's symptoms are controlled, the total dose required to calm the patient is divided into four equal doses and administered every 6 hours on a regularly scheduled basis. When the patient's symptoms are stable, the daily dose is rapidly tapered to the smallest dose that controls the patient's symptoms. Continuous IV infusions have also been advocated to allow flexible dosing titration to control patient's symptoms. Higher doses and IV administration of haloperidol may prolong the QTc interval in patients, especially those patients receiving haloperidol by IV injection or continuous infusions or concomitant administration with other medications that prolong QTc. Monitoring the QTc interval is mandatory for all patients receiving haloperidol by IV injection or continuous infusion.

Another major side effect of haloperidol is its extrapyramidal reactions, such as akathisia and dystonia. These reactions usually occur early in therapy and may resolve with dose reduction or discontinuation of the drug. However, in more severe cases, diphenhydramine, 25 to 50 mg IV, or benztropine, 1 to 2 mg IV, may be required to relieve the symptoms. Extrapyramidal reactions appear to be more common after oral haloperidol than after IV haloperidol administration. Neuroleptic malignant syndrome may also be seen with this agent, manifested by hyperthermia, severe extrapyramidal reactions, severe muscle rigidity, altered mental status, and autonomic instability. Treatment involves supportive care and the administration of dantrolene. Cardiovascular side effects include hypotension.

Dose

- *IV or IM bolus:* 1 to 10 mg (titrated up as clinically indicated)
- *Continuous infusion:* 10 mg/h (not generally recommended)

Monitoring Parameters

- Mental status, blood pressure, electrocardiogram (ECG), bedside delirium monitoring, and electrolytes (especially with continuous infusions), signs of extrapyramidal reaction

Atypical Antipsychotics

Atypical antipsychotic agents such as quetiapine, olanzapine, risperidone, and ziprasidone have been suggested as possible alternatives to haloperidol, due to their similar mechanism of action and more favorable side effect profile, including reduced incidence of extrapyramidal reactions and QT prolongation. The use of atypical antipsychotics to manage ICU delirium has increased during recent years with reported usage as high as 40% in some studies. Despite these increases, additional well-controlled studies are warranted as their efficacy remains uncertain.

Monitoring Parameters

- Mental status, level of consciousness, ECG, bedside delirium monitoring

Quetiapine

Quetiapine is the most well studied of these agents to this point, with a randomized, placebo-controlled trial demonstrating a reduction in duration of delirium. Quetiapine can be administered as a scheduled dosing, with additional doses of haloperidol as needed. Dose escalation of the scheduled quetiapine may be required in 50-mg increments in patients still requiring breakthrough management with haloperidol. Sedation is the most commonly associated adverse effect. A limitation of quetiapine is that it is only available as an oral preparation.

Dose
- *PO or per tube*: 50 to 200 mg q12h

Monitoring Parameters
- Mental status, level of consciousness, ECG, bedside delirium monitoring

Miscellaneous Agents
Propofol

Propofol is an IV general anesthetic that has become popular for sedation of mechanically ventilated patients. The use of propofol is limited to 3 days or less because of the rapid development of tolerance and an increased risk of adverse events with prolonged use. The agent is often used as the primary sedative in daily awakening protocols. The advantages of propofol are its rapid onset and short duration of action compared to the benzodiazepines. Propofol is associated with pain on injection, respiratory depression, and hypotension in acutely ill patients, especially those who are hypotensive or hypovolemic. Hypotension can be avoided by limiting bolus doses to 0.25 to 0.5 mg/kg and the initial infusion rate to 5 mcg/kg/min. The fat-emulsion vehicle of propofol has been shown to support the growth of microorganisms. The manufacturer recommends changing the IV tubing of extemporaneously prepared infusions every 6 hours, or every 12 hours if the infusion bottles are used. Propofol is formulated in a fat-emulsion vehicle that provides 1.1 kcal/mL and its infusion rate must be accounted for when determining a patient's nutrition support regimen because the fat-emulsion base can be considered as a calorie source. High infusion rates can be a cause of hypertriglyceridemia. This agent can also cause a rare but serious adverse effect known as propofol related-infusion syndrome (PRIS). PRIS is associated with the use of propofol for more than 48 hours and at doses greater than 75 mcg/kg/min. Hyperkalemia, tachyarrythmia, bradycardia, rhabdomyolysis, and lactic acidosis combined with hypertriglyceridemia as previously described are common signs of PRIS. The bedside nurse monitors closely for these signs as discontinuance of therapy may avoid the serious outcomes of PRIS: myocardial failure, metabolic acidosis, rhabdomyolysis, dysrhythmias, and renal failure. Propofol is available in 50- and 100-mL infusion vials. To decrease waste, 50-mL vials may be used when changing vials in patients who are scheduled for IV line changes, extubation from mechanical ventilation, and low infusion rates.

Dose
- *IV bolus:* 0.25 to 0.5 mg/kg
- *Continuous infusion:* 5 to 50 mcg/kg/min

Monitoring Parameters
- Level of consciousness, blood pressure, lactic acid, creatinine kinase, and serum triglyceride level, especially at high infusion rates

Ketamine

Ketamine is an analog of phencyclidine that is commonly used as an IV general anesthetic. It is an agent that produces analgesia, anesthesia, and amnesia without the loss of consciousness. The sedation noted with this agent is dissociative and dose-dependent. Doses of 0.1 to 0.5 mg/kg provide analgesia only with no sedation, while doses greater than 0.5 mg/kg provide some degree of sedation. The onset of anesthesia after a single 0.5- to 1.0-mg/kg bolus dose is within 1 to 2 minutes and lasts approximately 5 to 10 minutes. Ketamine causes sympathetic stimulation that normally increases blood pressure and heart rate while maintaining cardiac output. This may be important in patients with hypovolemia. Ketamine is useful in patients who require repeated painful procedures such as wound debridement. The bronchodilatory effects of ketamine may be beneficial in patients experiencing status asthmaticus. However, ketamine may increase intracranial pressure and is avoided or used with caution in patients with head injuries, space-occupying lesions, or any other conditions that may cause an increase in intracranial pressure. Emergence reactions or hallucinations, commonly seen after ketamine anesthesia, may be prevented with the concurrent use of benzodiazepines.

Dose
- *IV bolus:* 0.1 to 1 mg/kg
- *Continuous infusion:* 0.05 to 3 mg/kg/h
- *Oral:* 10 mg/kg diluted in 1 to 2 oz of juice
- *Intranasal:* 5 mg/kg

Monitoring Parameters
- Levels of sedation and analgesia, heart rate, blood pressure, and mental status

Dexmedetomidine

Dexmedetomidine is a relatively selective alpha-2-adrenergic agonist with sedative properties indicated for light sedation of intubated and mechanically ventilated patients. Dexmedetomidine is not associated with respiratory depression but has been associated with reductions in heart rate and blood pressure. Some patients may complain of increased awareness while receiving this drug. Dexmedetomidine has minimal amnestic properties and most patients require breakthrough doses of sedatives and analgesics while receiving the drug. The agent has been evaluated for longer term sedation, up to 28 days in a limited number of patients. In this setting, a reduction of the loading infusion or elimination altogether is advised to minimize cardiovascular depression. However, a higher maintenance infusion (up to 1.5 mcg/kg/h) may be required compared to short-term sedation. Patients receiving prolonged infusions of dexmedetomidine may be at risk for withdrawal symptoms, reflex tachycardia, and neurologic manifestations (eg, agitation, irritability, speech abnormalities), following abrupt discontinuation. Patients are monitored for 12 to 24 hours following discontinuation. To prevent withdrawal, dexmedetomidine can be tapered in patients who have received therapy greater than 24 hours (eg, infusion reduced by 0.1 mcg/kg/h every 12-24 hours).

Dexmedetomidine is the preferred sedative compared with benzodiazepines for reducing the duration of delirium in adult ICU patients with delirium unrelated to alcohol or benzodiazepine withdrawal.

Dose
- *IV bolus:* 1 mcg/kg over 10 minutes
- *Continuous infusion:* 0.2 to 1.5 mcg/kg/h

Monitoring Parameters
- Levels of sedation and analgesia, heart rate, and blood pressure

Analgesics
Opioids
Opioids, also known as narcotics, produce their effects by reversibly binding to the mu, delta, kappa, and sigma opiate receptors located in the central nervous system. Mu-1 receptors are associated with analgesia, and mu-2 receptors are associated with respiratory depression, bradycardia, euphoria, and dependence. Delta receptors have no selective agonist and modulate mu-receptor activity. Kappa receptors function at the spinal and supraspinal levels and are associated with sedation. Sigma receptors are associated with dysphoria and psychotomimetic effects.

Monitoring Parameters
- Level of pain or comfort, blood pressure, renal function, hepatic function, and respiratory rate

Morphine
Morphine is a commonly used narcotic analgesic. Morphine is hepatically metabolized to several metabolites, including morphine-6-glucuronide (M6G), which is approximately 5 to 10 times more potent than morphine. M6G is renally eliminated and after repeated doses can accumulate in patients with renal dysfunction, producing enhanced pharmacologic effects. Morphine's clearance is reduced in acutely ill patients due to increased protein binding, decreased hepatic blood flow, reduced renal function, or reduced hepatocellular function. Morphine possesses vasodilatory properties and can produce hypotension because of either direct effects on the vasculature or histamine release.

Dose
- *IV bolus:* 2 to 5 mg
- *Continuous infusion:* 2 to 30 mg/h
- *Oral:* 10 to 30 mg q3-4h prn

Patient-Controlled Analgesia (PCA)
- *IV bolus:* 0.5 to 3 mg
- *Lockout interval:* 5 to 20 minutes

Meperidine
Meperidine is a short-acting opioid that has one-seventh the potency of morphine. It is hepatically metabolized to normeperidine, which is eliminated through the kidneys, and is also a neurotoxin. Normeperidine can accumulate in patients with renal dysfunction, resulting in seizures. Meperidine is avoided in patients taking monoamine oxidase inhibitors because of the potential for development of a hypertensive crisis when these agents are administered concurrently. The role of this agent as an analgesic has been reduced dramatically due to seizure potential. In many institutions, the agent has been limited to serve as an adjunctive therapy to minimize shivering in hypothermic patients.

Dose
- *IV bolus:* 25 to 100 mg
- *Oral:* 50 to 150 mg q2-4h prn

Fentanyl
Fentanyl is an analog of meperidine that is 100 times more potent than morphine. After single doses, its duration of action is limited by its rapid distribution into fat tissue. However, after repeated dosing or continuous infusion administration, fat stores become saturated, thereby prolonging its terminal elimination half-life to more than 24 hours. Fentanyl does not have active metabolites, although accumulation can occur in hepatic dysfunction. Unlike morphine, fentanyl does not cause histamine release.

Dose
- *IV bolus:* 25 to 100 mcg q1-2h
- *Continuous infusion:* 50 to 300 mcg/h
- *Transdermal:* Patients not previously on opioids: 25 mcg/h
- *Opioid-tolerant patients:* 25 to 100 mcg/h

Patient-Controlled Analgesia
- *IV bolus:* 25 to 100 mcg
- *Lockout interval:* 5 to 10 minutes

Opioid Antagonist
Naloxone
Naloxone is a pure opiate antagonist that displaces opioid agonists from the mu-, delta-, and kappa-receptor–binding sites. Naloxone reverses narcotic-induced respiratory depression, producing an increase in respiratory rate and minute ventilation, a decrease in arterial P_{CO_2}, and normalization of blood pressure if reduced. Narcotic-induced sedation or sleep is also reversed by naloxone. Naloxone reverses analgesia, increases sympathetic nervous system activity, and may result in tachycardia, hypertension, pulmonary edema, and cardiac arrhythmias. Naloxone administration produces withdrawal symptoms in patients who have been taking narcotic analgesics chronically. In non-life-threatening

situations (eg, postsurgical patient with respiratory depression, but not in cardiac or respiratory arrest), diluting and slowly administering naloxone in incremental doses can prevent the precipitation of acute withdrawal reactions as well as prevent the increase in sympathetic stimulation that may accompany the reversal of analgesia. One 0.4-mg ampule is diluted with 0.9% NaCl (saline) to 10 mL to produce a concentration of 0.04 mg/mL. Sequential doses of 0.04 to 0.08 mg are administered slowly until the desired response is obtained. A more aggressive dosing approach may be warranted in life-threatening situations. Because its duration of action is generally shorter than that of opiates, the effect of opiates may return after the effects of naloxone dissipate, approximately 30 to 120 minutes. To combat this, continuous infusions may be required in situations of overdose with extended release opioid formulations.

Dose

- *Opiate depression:* Initial dose: 0.1 to 0.2 mg given at 2- to 3-minute intervals until the desired response is obtained. Additional doses may be necessary depending on the response of the patient and the dose and duration of the opiate administered.
- *Known or suspected opiate overdose:* Initial dose: 0.4 to 2.0 mg administered at 2- to 3-minute intervals, if necessary. If no response is observed after a total of 10 mg has been administered, other causes of the depressive state are explored.
- *Continuous infusion:* Initial infusion rates can be customized based on calculating two-thirds of the initial effective intermittent dosing, given hourly. Typical rates range 2.5 to 5 mcg/kg/h, titrated to the patient's response.

Monitoring Parameters

- Signs and symptoms of withdrawal reactions, respiratory rate, blood pressure, mental status, level of consciousness, and pupil size

Nonsteroidal Anti-Inflammatory Drugs

Ketorolac

Ketorolac is a nonsteroidal anti-inflammatory drug (NSAID) that is indicated for the short-term treatment of moderate to severe acute pain that requires analgesia at the opioid level. The drug exhibits anti-inflammatory, analgesic, and antipyretic properties. Its mechanism of action is thought to be due to inhibition of prostaglandin synthesis by inhibiting cyclooxygenase, an enzyme that catalyzes the formation of endoperoxidases from arachidonic acid. NSAIDs are more efficacious in the treatment of prostaglandin-mediated pain. Ketorolac is the only currently available NSAID approved for IM, IV, and oral administration, and it is often used in combination with other analgesics because pain often involves multiple mechanisms. Combination therapy may be more efficacious than single-drug regimens, and combinations with narcotics can decrease narcotic requirements, minimizing narcotic side effects.

Ketorolac is associated with the same adverse effects as orally administered NSAIDs, such as reversible platelet inhibition, GI bleeding, and reduced renal function. Ketorolac is contraindicated in patients with advanced renal failure and in patients at risk for renal failure due to volume depletion. Therefore, volume depletion is corrected before administering ketorolac. Because of the potential for significant adverse effects, the maximum combined duration of parenteral and oral use is limited to 5 days.

Dose

- *Loading dose:* Less than 65 years: 60 mg; more than 65 years or less than 50 kg: 30 mg
- *Maintenance dose:* Less than 65 years: 30 mg q6h; more than 65 years or less than 50 kg: Less than 15 mg q6h

Monitoring Parameters

- Renal function and volume status

Acetaminophen

Acetaminophen is an analgesic and antipyretic available in a number of dosage forms, including an IV formulation. IV acetaminophen is indicated for the management of mild to moderate pain, and management of moderate to severe pain with adjunctive opioid analgesics. The preferred route of administration for acetaminophen continues to be oral, but the IV route has proven beneficial in the perioperative setting when oral therapy is not feasible. The IV form of this agent is not cost-effective as an antipyretic because equally effective and less expensive options exist (eg, acetaminophen rectal suppositories). Use of IV acetaminophen is restricted to postsurgical patients who are unable to take oral or rectal acetaminophen.

Dose

- *IV bolus:* 1 g IV every 6 hours for 24 to 48 hours postoperative (maximum of 4 g in 24 hours)

Monitoring Parameters

- Liver function test, pain control, blood pressure

Anticonvulsants

Hydantoins

Phenytoin

Phenytoin is an anticonvulsant used for the acute control of generalized tonic clonic seizures, following the administration of benzodiazepines, and for maintenance therapy once the seizure has been controlled. Phenytoin stabilizes neuronal cell membranes and decreases the spread of seizure activity. Phenytoin may inhibit neuronal depolarizations by blocking sodium channels in excitatory pathways and prevent increases in intracellular potassium concentrations and decreases in intracellular calcium concentrations.

The bioavailability of oral phenytoin is approximately 90% to 100%. Dissolution is the rate-limiting step in phenytoin absorption with peak serum concentrations occurring 1.5 hours (eg, oral liquid and immediate release) to

12 hours (eg, Dilantin Kapseal capsules) after a dose. The rate of absorption is dose dependent, with increasing times to peak concentration with increasing doses. In addition, the dissolution and absorption rates depend on the phenytoin formulation administered. The Dilantin Kapseal brand of phenytoin capsules has the dissolution characteristics of an extended-release preparation, whereas generic phenytoin products possess rapid-release characteristics and are absorbed more quickly. Extended-release and rapid-release products are not interchangeable and only extended-release products may be administered in a single daily dose.

Phenytoin is 90% to 95% bound to albumin. In acutely ill patients, the pharmacologically free fraction is highly variable and ranges between 10% and 27% of the total serum concentration. The free fraction has been shown to increase by more than 100% from baseline during the first week of illness and is generally associated with a significant reduction in serum albumin concentration. Alterations in albumin binding also may be seen in hypoalbuminemia (< 2.5 g/dL), major trauma, sepsis, burns, malnutrition, and surgery, as well as liver or renal disease, and may result in an increase in a free concentration with potentially toxic effects. Significant alterations in phenytoin metabolism usually do not occur until the serum albumin falls below 2.5 g/dL. Equations used to normalize the phenytoin concentration in patients with hypoalbuminemia are usually unreliable, and direct measurement of the free phenytoin concentration is used to adjust therapy.

Phenytoin is metabolized by the cytochrome P-450 enzyme system to its inactive primary metabolite 5-(p-hydroxyphenyl)-5-phenylhydantoin, which is glucuronidated and renally eliminated. Phenytoin undergoes dose-dependent metabolism such that proportional increases in the dose may result in greater than proportional increases in the serum concentration. It is difficult to predict the concentration at which a patient's metabolism will become saturated, so that any changes in dose above 400 to 500 mg/day need to be carefully monitored. Because phenytoin displays nonlinear metabolism, *half-life* is an inappropriate term to describe phenytoin elimination. Phenytoin metabolism is usually referred to as the time it takes to eliminate 50% (t_{50}) of a given daily dose. In normal patients taking 300 mg/day, the t_{50} is about 22 hours. As the dose is increased, the t_{50} increases, with the time to reach steady state becoming progressively longer. The time to steady state may vary from several days to several weeks depending on the dose and the patient's ability to metabolize the drug.

Other medications can affect phenytoin metabolism by inducing or inhibiting its metabolic pathway. The effects of enzyme induction can occur within 2 days to 2 weeks after starting an agent. Inhibition usually occurs within 1 to 2 days after a drug is started and its effects usually last until the inhibiting drug is eliminated from the body. Phenytoin clearance is increased in acutely ill patients, resulting in subtherapeutic serum concentrations less than 10 mg/L. The

mechanism for the increase in clearance is unclear, but may be caused by changes in protein binding, induction in phenytoin metabolism, or a stress-related transient increase in hepatic metabolic function.

Phenytoin precipitates in dextrose-containing solutions and is only be mixed in 0.9% sodium chloride solutions. Because of its short-stability, it should be administered within 4 hours of compounding. To prevent phlebitis, the maximum concentration for peripheral administration is 10 mg/mL; a final concentration of 20 mg/mL may be used if the dose is being administered through a central venous catheter. Phenytoin solution must be administered through an in-line 1.2- or 5.0-μ filter to prevent the administration of phenytoin crystals into the systemic circulation. Phenytoin doses are not administered at a rate faster than 50 mg/min because hypotension and arrhythmias may occur, with hypotension likely related to propylene glycol diluent. The infusion rate is decreased by 50%, if hypotension or arrhythmias develop.

Oral administration is not usually recommended in acutely ill patients because of the risk of erratic or incomplete absorption. Phenytoin oral suspension may adhere to the inside walls of oro- or nasogastric tubes, reducing the dose delivered to the patient. If phenytoin is administered through a feeding tube, the tube is flushed with 30 to 60 mL of 0.9% sodium chloride before and after administering the dose. After the dose is administered, the feeding tube should be clamped for an hour before restarting the feeding solution. Oral absorption may be impaired by concomitant administration with enteral nutrition solutions, reducing its bioavailability and resulting in erratic serum concentrations with seizures occurring as a result of subtherapeutic serum concentrations. Phenytoin oral solution must be shaken prior to use to ensure uniformity in the distribution of the phenytoin particles throughout the suspension. If the suspension is not shaken before obtaining a dose, the phenytoin powder settles to the bottom of the bottle producing subtherapeutic doses when the bottle is first opened and toxic doses as the bottle is used.

Hemodialysis and hemofiltration have no effect on phenytoin clearance. Early adverse effects that may be associated with increasing serum concentrations are nystagmus (> 20 mg/L), ataxia (> 30 mg/L), and lethargy, confusion, and impaired cognitive function (> 40 mg/L).

The normal therapeutic range for the total phenytoin serum concentration is 10 to 20 mg/L with the free fraction therapeutic range of 1 to 2 mg/L. Serum concentration of 20 to 30 mg/L may be required in patients who are having seizures. Phenytoin serum concentrations can be obtained 30 to 60 minutes after the IV loading dose is infused to assess the adequacy of the dose. Trough concentrations are monitored 2 to 3 times a week, particularly after the first week of therapy. Measurement of free phenytoin concentrations may be indicated in acutely ill patients, patients with serum albumin concentrations less than 2.5 g/dL, renal failure, or receiving drugs known to displace phenytoin from albumin-binding sites. Other monitoring parameters include the patient's seizure activity and medication profile for agents known to alter phenytoin's metabolism.

Dose

- *Loading dose:* 15 to 20 mg/kg IV (18-20 mg/kg for status epilepticus or 15-18 mg/kg for seizure prophylaxis). An additional IV loading dose of up to 10 mg/kg can be given to status epilepticus patients refractory to the initial loading dose.
- *Maintenance dose:* 5 to 7.5 mg/kg/day IV or PO (5-6 mg/kg/day in typical adults or 6-7.5 mg/kg/day may be required in acutely ill or neurotrauma). IV doses administered every 6 to 8 hours.

Monitoring Parameters

- Seizure activity, electroencephalogram (EEG), serum phenytoin concentration (free phenytoin concentration if applicable), albumin, liver function, infusion rate, blood pressure, ECG with IV administration, and IV injection site

Fosphenytoin

Fosphenytoin is a phenytoin prodrug with good aqueous solubility that was developed to be a water-soluble alternative to phenytoin. In patients unable to tolerate oral phenytoin, equimolar doses of fosphenytoin have been shown to produce equal or greater plasma phenytoin concentrations. Although phenytoin sodium 50 mg is equal to fosphenytoin sodium 75 mg, fosphenytoin doses are converted to an equivalent phenytoin dose known as phenytoin equivalents (PEs) on a milligram-per-milligram basis. Thus, a phenytoin 300 mg dose is equal to fosphenytoin 300 mg PE.

Fosphenytoin, administered IM or IV, is rapidly and completely converted to phenytoin in vivo, resulting in essentially 100% bioavailability. The conversion half-life to phenytoin is about 33 minutes following IM administration and about 15 minutes after IV infusion. After IM administration, peak plasma fosphenytoin concentrations occur approximately 30 minutes postdose, with peak phenytoin concentrations occurring in about 3 hours. Fosphenytoin's peak concentration following IV administration occurs at the end of the infusion, with peak phenytoin concentrations occurring in approximately 40 to 75 minutes. In patients with renal or hepatic dysfunction or hypoalbuminemia, there is enhanced conversion to phenytoin without an increase in clearance. Fosphenytoin is 90% to 95% bound to plasma proteins and is saturable with the percent of bound fosphenytoin decreasing as the fosphenytoin dose increases.

The maximum total phenytoin concentration increases with increasing fosphenytoin doses, but the total phenytoin concentration is less affected by increasing fosphenytoin infusion rates. Maximum free phenytoin concentrations are nearly constant at infusion rates up to 50 mg phenytoin equivalents (PEs)/min, whereas they increase with faster infusion rates secondary to phenytoin displacement from albumin-binding sites in the presence of high fosphenytoin concentrations.

For the treatment of status epilepticus, the recommended loading dose of IV fosphenytoin is 15 to 20 PE/kg, and it is not to be administered faster than 150 mg PE/min because of the risk of hypotension. Fosphenytoin 15 to 20 mg PE/kg infused at 100 to 150 mg PE/min yields plasma-free phenytoin concentrations over time that approximate those achieved when an equimolar dose of IV phenytoin is administered at 50 mg/min. In the treatment of status epilepticus, total phenytoin concentrations greater than 10 mg/L and free phenytoin concentrations greater than 1 mg/mL are achieved within 10 to 20 minutes after starting the infusion.

In nonemergent situations, loading doses of 10 to 20 PE/kg administered IV or IM are recommended. In nonemergent situations, IV administration of infusion rates of 50 to 100 mg PE/min may be acceptable, but results in slightly lower and delayed maximum free phenytoin concentrations as compared with administration at higher infusion rates. The initial daily maintenance dose is 4 to 6 mg PE/kg/day. Dosing adjustments are not required when IM fosphenytoin is substituted temporarily for oral phenytoin. However, patients switched from once-daily extended-release phenytoin capsules may require twice-daily or more frequent administration of fosphenytoin to maintain similar peak and trough phenytoin concentrations.

The incidence of adverse effects tends to increase as both dose and infusion rate are increased. At doses above 15 mg PE/kg and infusion rates higher than 150 mg PE/min, transient pruritus, tinnitus, nystagmus, somnolence, and ataxia occur more frequently than at lower doses or infusion rates. Severe burning, itching, and paresthesias of the groin are commonly associated with infusion rates greater than 150 mg PE/min. Slowing or temporarily stopping the infusion can minimize the frequency and severity of these reactions. Continuous cardiac rate and rhythm, blood pressure, and respiratory function are monitored throughout the fosphenytoin infusion and for 10 to 20 minutes after the end of the infusion.

Following fosphenytoin administration, phenytoin concentrations are not monitored until the conversion to phenytoin is complete. This occurs within 2 hours after the end of an IV infusion and 5 hours after an IM injection. Prior to complete conversion, commonly used immunoanalytic techniques such as fluorescence polarization and enzyme-mediated assays may significantly overestimate plasma phenytoin concentrations because of cross-reactivity with fosphenytoin. Blood samples collected before complete conversion to phenytoin are collected in tubes containing ethylenediamine tetraacetic acid (EDTA) as an anticoagulant to minimize the ex vivo conversion of fosphenytoin to phenytoin. Monitoring is similar to phenytoin. In acutely ill patients with renal failure receiving fosphenytoin, one or more metabolites of adducts of fosphenytoin accumulate and display significant cross-reactivity with several phenytoin immunoassay methods.

Pyrrolidine Derivatives

Levetiracetam

Levetiracetam is a second-generation antiepileptic drug with increasing usage in acute care settings. The agent leads to selective prevention of burst firing and seizure activity. Levetiracetam is commonly prescribed for adjunctive treatment of partial onset seizures with or without secondary generalization. Other approved indications include monotherapy treatment of partial onset seizures with or without secondary generalization, and adjunctive treatment of myoclonic seizures associated with juvenile myoclonic epilepsy, and primary generalized tonic-clonic (GTC) seizures associated with idiopathic generalized epilepsy. Seizure prophylaxis in posttraumatic brain injury patients is also an established role for levetiracetam.

Levetiracetam lacks cytochrome P450 isoenzyme-inducing potential and is not associated with clinically significant interactions with other drugs, including other antiepileptic drugs. Sedation is the most common adverse effect noted.

Dose
- *Maintenance dose*: 250 mg to 1000 mg q12 IV or PO

Monitoring Parameters
- Seizure activity, EEG, sedation

Benzodiazepines

Benzodiazepines are the primary agents in the management of status epilepticus. These agents suppress the spread of seizure activity but do not abolish the abnormal discharge from a seizure focus. Although IV diazepam has the fastest onset of action, lorazepam or midazolam are equally efficacious in controlling seizure activity. They are the agents of choice to temporarily control seizures and to gain time for the loading of phenytoin or phenobarbital.

Monitoring Parameters
- Seizure activity, EEG, and respiratory rate and quality

CARDIOVASCULAR SYSTEM PHARMACOLOGY

Miscellaneous Agents

Nesiritide

Nesiritide is a recombinant human b-type natriuretic peptide, which is a cardiac hormone that regulates cardiovascular homeostasis and fluid volume during states of volume and pressure overload. The agent has a limited role in practice and is effective in reducing pulmonary capillary wedge pressure and improving dyspnea symptoms in patients with acutely decompensated HF who have dyspnea at rest or with minimal activity. The most common adverse effects include hypotension, tachycardia, and/or bradycardia.

Dose
- *IV bolus:* 2 mcg/kg
- *Continuous infusion:* 0.01 mcg/kg/min

Monitoring Parameters
- Blood pressure, heart rate, urine output, and hemodynamic parameters

Parenteral Vasodilators

Nitrates

Sodium Nitroprusside

Sodium nitroprusside is a balanced vasodilator affecting the arterial and venous systems. Blood pressure reduction occurs within seconds after an infusion is started, with a duration of action of less than 10 minutes once the infusion is discontinued. Sodium nitroprusside was previously considered the agent of choice in acute hypertensive conditions such as hypertensive encephalopathy, intracerebral infarction, subarachnoid hemorrhage, carotid endarterectomy, malignant hypertension, microangiopathic anemia, and aortic dissection, and after general surgical procedures, major vascular procedures, or renal transplantation. However, usage of this agent has been severely restricted due to significant cost increases compared with effective, safer, and less costly alternatives.

If sodium nitroprusside is used for longer than 48 hours, there is the risk of thiocyanate toxicity. However, this may only be a concern in patients with renal dysfunction. In this setting, thiocyanate serum concentrations are monitored to ensure that they remain below 10 mg/dL. Other potential side effects include methemoglobinemia and cyanide toxicity. Nitroprusside is used with caution in the setting of increased intracranial pressure, such as head trauma or postcraniotomy, where it may cause an increase in cerebral blood flow. Nitroprusside's effects on intracranial pressure may be attenuated by a lowered $PaCO_2$ and raised PaO_2. In pregnant women, nitroprusside is reserved only for refractory hypertension associated with eclampsia, because of the potential risk to the fetus.

Dose
- *Continuous infusion:* 0.5 to 10 mcg/kg/min

Monitoring Parameters
- Blood pressure, renal function, thiocyanate concentration (prolonged infusions), acid-base status, and hemodynamic parameters

Nitroglycerin

Nitroglycerin is a preferential venous dilator affecting the venous system at low doses, but relaxes arterial smooth muscle at higher doses. The onset of blood pressure reduction after starting a nitroglycerin infusion is similar to sodium nitroprusside, approximately 1 to 3 minutes, with duration of action of less than 10 minutes. Headaches are a common adverse effect that may occur with nitroglycerin therapy and can be treated with acetaminophen. Tachyphylaxis can be seen with the IV infusion, similar to what is seen after the chronic use of topical nitroglycerin preparations. In patients receiving unfractionated heparin in addition to nitroglycerin, increased doses of unfractionated heparin may be required to maintain a therapeutic partial thromboplastin time (PTT). The mechanism by which nitroglycerin causes unfractionated heparin resistance is unknown. However, the PTT is closely monitored in patients receiving nitroglycerin and unfractionated heparin concurrently.

Nitroglycerin is the preferred agent in the setting of hypertension associated with myocardial ischemia or infarction because its net effect is a reduction in oxygen consumption.

Dose
- *Continuous infusion:* 10 to 300 mcg/min
- *Oral:* 2.5 to 9 mg bid-qid

Monitoring Parameters
- Blood pressure, heart rate, signs and symptoms of ischemia, hemodynamic parameters (if applicable), and PTT (in patients receiving unfractionated heparin concurrently)

Arterial Vasodilating Agents
Hydralazine

Hydralazine reduces peripheral vascular resistance by directly relaxing arterial smooth muscle. Blood pressure reduction occurs within 5 to 20 minutes after an IV dose and lasts approximately 2 to 6 hours. Common adverse effects include headache, nausea, vomiting, palpitations, and tachycardia. Reflex tachycardia may precipitate anginal attacks. Co-administration of a beta-receptor antagonist can decrease the incidence of tachycardia.

Dose
- 10 to 25 mg IV q2-4h
- *Oral:* 10 to 125 mg bid-qid

Monitoring Parameters
- Blood pressure and heart rate

Diazoxide

Diazoxide is used intravenously in hypertensive crisis to reduce peripheral vascular resistance by directly relaxing arterial smooth muscle. Side effects such as hypotension, nausea and vomiting, dizziness, weakness, hyperglycemia, and reflex tachycardia have been associated with the use of the higher than 300-mg dosing regimen. Using lower dose regimens produces similar but less severe side effects. Caution is used when diazoxide is administered with other antihypertensive agents because excessive hypotension may result.

Blood pressure reduction occurs within 1 to 2 minutes and lasts 3 to 12 hours after a dose. Blood pressure is monitored frequently until stable, and then monitored hourly.

Dose
- *IV bolus:* 50 to 150 mg q5min
- *Continuous infusion:* 7.5 to 30 mg/min
- *Oral:* 3 to 8 mg/kg/day divided 2 to 3 times/day

Monitoring Parameters
- Blood pressure, heart rate, and serum glucose

Alpha- and Beta-Adrenergic Blocking Agents
Labetalol

Labetalol is a combined alpha- and beta-adrenergic blocking agent with a specificity of beta receptors to alpha receptors of approximately 7:1. Labetalol may be administered parenterally by escalating bolus doses or by continuous infusion. The onset of action after the administration of labetalol is within 5 minutes with a duration of effect from 2 to 12 hours. Because labetalol possesses beta-blocking properties, it may produce bronchospasm in individuals with asthma or reactive airway disease. It also may produce conduction system disturbances or bradycardia in susceptible individuals, and its negative inotropic properties may exacerbate symptoms of HF.

Labetalol may be considered as an alternative to sodium nitroprusside in the setting of hypertension associated with head trauma or postcraniotomy, spinal cord syndromes, transverse lesions of the spinal cord, Guillain-Barré syndrome, or autonomic hyperreflexia, as well as hypertension associated with sympathomimetics (eg, cocaine, amphetamines, phencyclidine, nasal decongestants, or certain diet pills) or withdrawal of centrally acting antihypertensive agents (eg, beta-blockers, clonidine, or methyldopa). It also may be used as an alternative to phentolamine in the setting of pheochromocytoma because of its alpha- and beta-blocking properties.

Dose
- *IV bolus:* 10 to 20 mg over 2 minutes, then 40 to 80 mg IV q10min to a total of 300 mg
- *Continuous infusion:* 1 to 4 mg/min and titrate to effect
- *Oral:* 100 to 400 mg bid

Monitoring Parameters
- Blood pressure, heart rate, ECG, and signs and symptoms of HF or bronchospasm (if applicable)

Alpha-Adrenergic Blocking Agents
Phentolamine

Phentolamine is an alpha-adrenergic blocking agent that may be administered parenterally by bolus injection or continuous infusion. Onset of action is within 1 to 2 minutes, with a duration of action of 3 to 10 minutes. Potential adverse effects that may occur with phentolamine include tachycardia, GI stimulation, and hypoglycemia.

Phentolamine is considered the drug of choice for the treatment of hypertension associated with pheochromocytoma because of its ability to block alpha-adrenergic receptors. Also, it is the primary agent used to treat acute hypertensive episodes in patients receiving monoamine oxidase inhibitors.

Dose
- *IV bolus:* 5 to 10 mg q5-15min
- *Continuous infusion:* 1 to 10 mg/min

Monitoring Parameters
- Blood pressure and heart rate

Beta-Adrenergic Blocking Agents

Beta-adrenergic blocking agents available for IV delivery include propranolol, atenolol, esmolol, and metoprolol.

Propranolol and metoprolol may be administered by bolus injection or continuous infusion. Atenolol typically is administered by bolus injection, and esmolol is administered by continuous infusion. A continuous infusion of esmolol may or may not be preceded by an initial bolus injection.

Esmolol has the fastest onset and shortest duration of action, approximately 1 to 3 minutes and 20 to 30 minutes, respectively. Propranolol and metoprolol have similar onset times, but durations of action vary between 1 and 6 hours. The duration of action after a bolus dose of atenolol is approximately 12 hours.

All agents may produce bronchospasm in individuals with asthma or reactive airway disease and may produce conduction system disturbances or bradycardia in susceptible individuals. Also, because of their negative inotropic properties, they may exacerbate symptoms of HF.

Beta-blocking agents typically are used as adjuncts with other agents in the treatment of acute hypertension. They may be used with sodium nitroprusside in the treatment of acute aortic dissections. They are administered to patients with hypertension associated with pheochromocytoma only after phentolamine has been given. Also, they are the agents of choice in patients who have been maintained on beta-blocking agents for the chronic management of hypertension but who have abruptly stopped therapy.

Beta-blocking agents are avoided in patients with hypertensive encephalopathy, intracranial infarctions, or subarachnoid hemorrhages because of their central nervous system depressant effects. They also are avoided in patients with acute pulmonary edema because of their negative inotropic properties. Finally, beta-blocking agents are avoided in hypertension associated with eclampsia and renal vasculature disorders.

Dose
- *Esmolol:* IV bolus 500 mcg/kg; continuous infusion: 50 to 400 mcg/kg/min
- *Metoprolol:* IV bolus: 5 mg IV q2min; or maintenance 1.25 to 5 mg IV q6-12h. Oral: 25 to 450 mg daily divided 2 to 3 times/day
- *Propranolol:* IV bolus: 0.5 to 1 mg q5-15min; continuous infusion: 1 to 4 mg/h. Oral: 30 to 320 mg daily divided 2 to 4 times/day

Monitoring Parameters
- Blood pressure, heart rate, ECG, and signs and symptoms of HF or bronchospasm (if applicable)

Angiotensin-Converting Enzyme Inhibitors
Angiotensin-converting enzyme (ACE) inhibitors competitively inhibit ACE, which is responsible for the conversion of angiotensin I to angiotensin II (a potent vasoconstrictor). In addition, ACE inhibitors increase the availability of bradykinin and other vasodilatory prostaglandins, and reduce plasma aldosterone concentrations. The net effect is

a reduction in blood pressure in hypertensive patients and a reduction in afterload in patients with HF.

ACE inhibitors are indicated in the management of hypertension and HF. ACE inhibitors currently available in oral formulations include quinapril, ramipril, benazepril, captopril, enalapril, fosinopril, and lisinopril. Adverse effects associated with ACE inhibitors include rash, taste disturbances, and cough. Additionally, ACE inhibitors can cause drug-induced angioedema, which most often usually affects the lips, tongue, face, and upper airway, and more rarely is associated with abdominal symptoms (eg, pain with diarrhea). Initial-dose hypotension may occur in patients who are hypovolemic, hyponatremic, or who have been aggressively diuresed. Hypotension may be avoided or minimized by starting with low doses or withholding diuretics for 24 to 48 hours. Worsening of renal function may occur in patients with bilateral renal artery stenosis. Additionally, hyperkalemia is also a possible complication of ACE inhibitor therapy.

Enalapril
Enalapril is unique among ACE inhibitors, as it is a prodrug that is converted in the liver to its active moiety, enalaprilat, a long-acting ACE inhibitor. Enalapril is available in an oral dosage form, and enalaprilat is available in the IV form. Following an IV dose of enalaprilat, blood pressure lowering occurs within 15 minutes and lasts 4 to 6 hours.

Dose
- *Enalaprilat:* IV bolus: 0.625 to 1.25 mg over 5 minutes q6h; continuous infusion: not recommended
- *Enalapril:* Oral: 2.5 to 40 mg qd

Monitoring Parameters
- Blood pressure, heart rate, renal function, and electrolytes

Angiotensin Receptor Blockers
Angiotensin receptor blockers (ARBs) selectively block the binding of angiotensin II (a powerful vasoconstrictor in vascular smooth muscle) to the receptors in tissues such as vascular smooth muscle and the adrenal gland. This receptor blockade results in vasodilation and decreased secretion of aldosterone, which leads to increased sodium excretion and potassium-sparing effects. ARBs are indicated for both hypertension and HF. ARBs currently available in oral formulations include valsartan, candesartan, irbesartan, azilsartan, eprosartan, losartan, telmisartan, and olmesartan. The most common adverse effects of ARBs are hypotension, dizziness, and headache. Although rare, cough can also be associated with ARBs. This cough can be reversed by discontinuance of therapy. Overall, these agents are relatively well-tolerated and thus used quite commonly for the chronic management of stages 1 and 2 hypertension. The role in acute blood pressure lowering is limited due to the lack of a parenteral formulation.

Monitoring Parameters
- Blood pressure and heart rate, and electrolytes

Calcium Channel–Blocking Agents

Calcium channel–blocking agents may be used as alternative therapy in the treatment of hypertension resulting from hypertensive encephalopathy, myocardial ischemia, malignant hypertension, or eclampsia, or after renal transplantation.

Nicardipine

Nicardipine is an IV calcium channel–blocking agent that is primarily indicated for the treatment of hypertension. Onset is within 5 minutes with duration of approximately 30 minutes. Nicardipine also is available in an oral dosage form so that patients started on IV therapy can convert to oral therapy when indicated.

> #### Dose
> - *Continuous infusion:* 5 mg/h, increase every 15 minutes to a maximum of 15 mg/h
> - *Oral:* 20 to 40 mg q8h
>
> #### Monitoring Parameters
> - Blood pressure and heart rate

Clevidipine

Clevidipine is an IV calcium channel–blocking agent that is also indicated for the treatment of hypertension. An onset of 2 minutes is faster than nicardipine with a shorter duration of 10 minutes. Clevidipine is delivered as an injectable lipid emulsion (20%), similar to intralipids, and is not available in an oral dosage form. Similar to propofol, vials of clevidipine and IV tubing must be changed every 12 hours during therapy because the phospholipids support microbial growth.

> #### Dose
> - *Continuous infusion:* 1 to 2 mg/h, increase by doubling dose every 90-second interval initially to achieve blood pressure reduction. As the blood pressure approaches goal, increase dose less aggressively every 5 to 10 minutes. Maximum recommended dose of 32 mg/h, with an average rate of 21 mg/h
>
> #### Monitoring Parameters
> - Blood pressure and heart rate

Central Sympatholytic Agents

Clonidine

Clonidine is an oral agent that stimulates alpha-2-adrenergic receptors in the medulla oblongata, causing inhibition of sympathetic vasomotor centers. Although clonidine typically is used as maintenance antihypertensive therapy, it can be used in the setting of hypertensive urgencies or emergencies. Its antihypertensive effects may be seen within 30 minutes and last 8 to 12 hours. Once blood pressure is controlled, oral maintenance clonidine therapy may be started.

Centrally acting sympatholytics rarely are indicated as first-line agents except when hypertension may be due to the abrupt withdrawal of one of these agents.

> #### Dose
> - *Hypertensive urgency:* 0.2 mg PO initially, then 0.1 mg/h PO (to a maximum of 0.8 mg)
> - *Transdermal:* Transdermal therapeutic system (TTS)-1 (0.1 mg/day) to TTS-3 (0.3 mg/day) topically q1wk
>
> #### Monitoring Parameters
> - Blood pressure, heart rate, and mental status. Monitor for syncope with first dose

Antiarrhythmics

Antiarrhythmic agents are divided into five classes. Dosage information for individual antiarrhythmic agents is listed in Chapter 22, Pharmacology Tables (see Table 22-4).

Class I Agents

Class I agents are further divided into three subclasses: Ia (procainamide, quinidine, disopyramide), Ib (lidocaine, mexiletine), and Ic (flecainide, propafenone). All class I agents block sodium channels in the myocardium and inhibit potassium-repolarizing currents to prolong repolarization.

Class Ia Agents

Class Ia agents inhibit the fast sodium channel (phase 0 of the action potential), slow conduction at elevated serum drug concentrations, and prolong action potential duration and repolarization. Class Ia agents can cause proarrhythmic complications by prolonging the QT interval or by depressing conduction and promoting reentry.

> #### Monitoring Parameters
> - ECG (QRS complex, QT interval, arrhythmia frequency)

Class Ib Agents

Class Ib agents have little effect on phase 0 depolarization and conduction velocity, but shorten the action potential duration and repolarization. QT prolongation typically does not occur with class Ib agents. Class Ib agents act selectively on diseased or ischemic tissue where they block conduction and interrupt reentry circuits.

> #### Monitoring Parameters
> - ECG (QT interval, arrhythmia frequency), hepatic function

Class Ic Agents

Class Ic agents inhibit the fast sodium channel and cause a marked depression of phase 0 of the action potential and slow conduction profoundly, but have minimal effects on repolarization. The dramatic effects of these agents on conduction may account for their significant proarrhythmic effects, which limit their use in patients with supraventricular arrhythmias and structural heart disease.

> #### Monitoring Parameters
> - ECG (PR interval and QRS complex, arrhythmia frequency)

Class II Agents

Beta-blocking agents inactivate sodium channels and depress phase 4 depolarization and increase the refractory period of the atrioventricular node. These agents have no effect on repolarization. Beta-blockers competitively antagonize catecholamine binding at beta-adrenergic receptors.

Beta-blocking agents can be classified as selective or nonselective agents. *Nonselective agents* bind to beta-1 receptors located on myocardial cells and beta-2 receptors located on bronchial and skeletal smooth muscle. Stimulation of beta-1 receptors causes an increase in heart rate and contractility, whereas stimulation of beta-2 receptors results in bronchodilation and vasodilation. Selective beta-blocking agents block beta-1 receptors in the heart at low or moderate doses, but they become less selective with increasing doses.

Class II agents are used for the prophylaxis and treatment of both supraventricular arrhythmias and arrhythmias associated with catecholamine excess or stimulation, slowing the ventricular response in atrial fibrillation, lowering blood pressure, decreasing heart rate, and decreasing ischemia. Esmolol is useful especially for the rapid, short-term control of ventricular response in atrial fibrillation or flutter.

Nonselective beta-blocking agents are avoided or used with caution in patients with HF, atrioventricular nodal blockade, asthma, COPD, peripheral vascular disease, Raynaud phenomenon, and diabetes. Beta-1 selective beta-blocking agents are used with caution in these populations.

Monitoring Parameters
- ECG (heart rate, PR interval, arrhythmia frequency)

Class III Agents

Class III agents (amiodarone, dofetilide, and sotalol) lengthen the action potential duration and effective refractory period and prolong repolarization. Additionally, amiodarone possesses alpha- and beta-blocking effects and calcium channel–blocking properties and inhibits the fast sodium channel. Sotalol possesses nonselective beta-blocking properties. Although torsades de pointes is relatively rare with amiodarone, precautions are taken to prevent hypokalemia- or digitalis-toxicity–induced arrhythmias. Sotalol may be associated with proarrhythmic effects in the setting of hypokalemia, bradycardia, high sotalol dose, and QT-interval prolongation, and in patients with preexisting HF. Sotalol is also contraindicated in patients with severe renal impairment.

Amiodarone

The antiarrhythmic effect of amiodarone is due to the prolongation of the action potential duration and refractory period, and secondarily through alpha-adrenergic and beta-adrenergic blockade. In patients with recent-onset (< 48 hours) atrial fibrillation or atrial flutter, IV amiodarone has been shown to restore normal sinus rhythm within 8 hours in approximately 60% to 70% of treated patients. Although IV amiodarone has been associated with negative inotropic effects, minimal side effects are associated with its short-term administration.

Amiodarone is recommended as an option for the treatment of wide-complex tachycardia; stable, narrow-complex supraventricular tachycardia; stable, monomorphic or polymorphic ventricular tachycardia; atrial fibrillation and flutter; ventricular fibrillation; and pulseless ventricular tachycardia.

Monitoring Parameters
- ECG (PR and QT intervals, QRS complex, arrhythmia frequency)
- Longer-term toxicities monitored by liver function tests, thyroid function tests, pulmonary function tests, that are taken at baseline and monitored through the course of therapy

Dofetilide

Dofetilide is a class III antiarrhythmic (potassium channel blocker) agent used for rhythm conversion in patients with atrial fibrillation. Prior to 2016, the agent was Food and Drug Administration (FDA) approved with substantial restrictions, as prescribers were required to undergo drug-specific training before being permitted to prescribe it. Initiation of drug therapy was also limited to hospitalized patients with continuous ECG monitoring and dosing based on a prespecified dosing algorithm. These restrictions were based on substantial adverse events associated with dofetilide administration including proarrhythmic events and sudden cardiac death. Since 2016, these restrictions have been lifted. The dose is now adjusted according to QT prolongation and creatinine clearance. If the QTc is greater than 440 milliseconds (or > 500 milliseconds in the setting of ventricular conduction abnormality), dofetilide is contraindicated. Dofetilide is also contraindicated in patients with severe renal impairment.

Dose
- Modified based on creatinine clearance and QT or QTc interval. The usual recommended oral dose is 250 mcg bid.

Monitoring parameters
- Renal function and QTc interval

Ibutilide

Ibutilide is a class III antiarrhythmic agent indicated for the conversion of recent-onset atrial fibrillation and atrial flutter to normal sinus rhythm. Ibutilide prolongs the refractory period and action potential duration, with little or no effect on conduction velocity or automaticity. Its electrophysiologic effects are predominantly derived from activation of a slow sodium inward current. Ibutilide can cause slowing of the sinus rate and atrioventricular node conduction, but has no effect on heart rate, PR interval, or QRS interval. The drug is associated with minimal hemodynamic effects with no significant effect on cardiac output, mean pulmonary arterial pressure, or pulmonary capillary wedge pressure. Ibutilide has not been shown to lower blood pressure or worsen HF.

Ibutilide has been shown to be more effective than procainamide and sotalol in terminating atrial fibrillation and atrial flutter. In addition, ibutilide has been shown to decrease the amount of joules required to treat resistant atrial fibrillation and atrial flutter during cardioversion. Depending on the duration of atrial fibrillation or flutter, ibutilide has an efficacy rate of 22% to 43% and 37% to 76%, respectively, for terminating these arrhythmias. Ibutilide is only available as an IV dosage form and cannot be used for the long-term maintenance of normal sinus rhythm.

Sustained and nonsustained polymorphic ventricular tachycardia is the most significant adverse effect associated with ibutilide. The overall incidence of polymorphic ventricular tachycardia diagnosed as torsades de pointes was 4.3%, including 1.7% of patients in whom the arrhythmia was sustained and required cardioversion. Ibutilide administration is avoided in patients receiving other agents that prolong the QTc interval, including class Ia or III antiarrhythmic agents, phenothiazine antipsychotic, antidepressants, haloperidol, and some antihistamines. Before ibutilide administration, patients are screened carefully to exclude high-risk individuals, such as those with a QTc interval greater than 440 millisecond or bradycardia. Serum potassium and magnesium levels are measured and corrected before the drug is administered. The ibutilide infusion is stopped in the event of nonsustained or sustained ventricular tachycardia or marked prolongation in the QTc interval. Patients are monitored for at least 4 hours after the infusion or until the QTc returns to baseline, with longer monitoring if nonsustained ventricular tachycardia develops.

Dose
- *Greater than or equal to 60 kg:* 1 mg over 10 min; wait 10 min; then prn
- *Less than 60 kg:* 0.01 mg/kg over 10 min; wait 10 min; then prn

Monitoring Parameters
- ECG (heart rate, PR interval, ST segment, T wave, arrhythmia frequency)

Class IV Agents
Calcium channel–blocking agents inhibit calcium channels within the atrioventricular node and sinoatrial node, prolong conduction through the atrioventricular and sinoatrial nodes, and prolong the functional refractory period of the nodes, as well as depress phase 4 depolarization. Class IV agents are used for the prophylaxis and treatment of supraventricular arrhythmias and to slow the ventricular response in atrial fibrillation, flutter, and multifocal atrial tachycardia. These agents include: diltiazem and verapamil.

Monitoring Parameters
- ECG (PR interval, arrhythmia frequency)

Class V Agents
Adenosine, digoxin, and atropine possess different pharmacologic properties but ultimately affect the sinoatrial node or atrioventricular node.

Monitoring Parameters
- ECG (heart rate, PR interval, ST segment, T wave, arrhythmia frequency)

Adenosine
Adenosine depresses sinus node automaticity and atrioventricular nodal conduction. Adenosine is indicated for the acute termination of atrioventricular nodal and reentrant tachycardia, and for supraventricular tachycardias, including Wolff-Parkinson-White syndrome. Some side effects of adenosine include flushing, chest tightness, and a brief asystole or bradycardia that can occur shortly after rapid administration.

Atropine
Atropine increases the sinus rate and decreases atrioventricular nodal conduction time and effective refractory period by decreasing vagal tone. The major indications for the use of atropine include symptomatic sinus bradycardia and type I second-degree atrioventricular block.

Digoxin
Digoxin slows the sinoatrial node rate of depolarization and conduction through the atrioventricular node primarily through vagal stimulating effects. Digoxin is indicated for the treatment of supraventricular tachycardia and for controlling ventricular response associated with supraventricular tachycardia.

Vasodilators and Remodeling Agents
Idiopathic pulmonary arterial hypertension (IPAH), formerly called primary pulmonary hypertension, is characterized by elevations in pulmonary arterial pressure in the absence of a demonstrable cause. Vasoconstriction in the pulmonary vasculature is thought to play an important role in the pathogenesis of IPAH. This vasoconstriction occurs secondary to either impaired production of endogenous vasodilators (prostacyclin and nitric oxide), or from increased production of endothelin, an endogenous vasoconstrictor. Thus, treatment strategies target these three pathways (nitric oxide, prostacyclin, and endothelin) and fit into corresponding categories.

Nitric Oxide
Nitric oxide is an odorless, and tasteless gas with vasodilator properties that is administered by respiratory therapists via continuous inhalation using a closed system for targeted pulmonary hypertensive patients (acute pulmonary hypertension in postoperative setting or prior to initiation of chronic therapies). The goal of inhaled nitric oxide is to improve oxygenation and reduce the need for extracorporeal membrane oxygenation. This is a restricted therapy considering the high cost and potential risk of occupational gas exposure to clinicians. Given these risks, clear institutional policies, procedures, and guidelines are essential to identify appropriate patients who meet the criteria for this therapy, and ensure a closely monitored system to eliminate unintended exposure to this gas.

Prostacyclin Analogues

Epoprostenol (Flolan, Veletri), treprostinil (Remodulin, Tyvaso), and iloprost (Ventavis) are potent vasodilators, which also inhibit platelet aggregation and smooth muscle proliferation and are the mainstay of IPAH therapy. Epoprostenol is delivered intravenously via continuous infusion, and also via inhalation. For acute treatment, continuous inhalation therapy is being used more frequently. In these instances, protocols and procedures to optimize the administration of this agent are essential. For long-term therapy, a permanently implanted central venous catheter and portable infusion pump are used. Side effects include jaw pain, diarrhea, and arthralgias. The doses are typically titrated based on impact on systemic blood pressure; therefore, monitoring is recommended whenever therapy is initiated. Treprostinil has several routes of administration. This agent can be administered via continuous IV infusion. Also, treprostinil has an advantage of continuous SC delivery, a longer half-life (possibly less immediately life threatening if interrupted), and the lack of a need for refrigeration. A major disadvantage of treprostinil is the high rate of significant infusion site discomfort, if the SC route is used. Additionally, treprostinil is available as a solution for inhalation administered using the Tyvaso Inhalation System. Iloprost is an aerosolized preparation which is delivered via a specialized nebulizer device.

Endothelin Receptor Antagonist

Bosentan (Tracleer), ambrisentan (Letairis), and macitentan (Opsumit) work by blocking the vasoconstrictive properties of endothelin and are available orally. The main adverse event associated with these therapies is elevations in liver enzymes; therefore, close monitoring of liver function tests is required. These agents are often combined with prostacyclin analogues to treat refractory cases of IPAH.

Phosphodiesterase 5 Inhibitors

Numerous studies of patients with IPAH have demonstrated improvements in pulmonary hemodynamics after treatment with sildenafil (Viagra, Revatio). Tadalafil (Cialis) and vardenafil (Levitra) have similar mechanisms of action; however, there appear to be some differences in the degree of phosphodiesterase inhibition, leading to questions of whether these agents are interchangeable. Sildenafil is the most widely studied and therefore the most commonly prescribed phosphodiesterase inhibitor. Similar to bosentan, sildenafil's most prominent role appears to be in combination with prostacyclin analogues.

Calcium Channel Blockers

Nifedipine (Procardia, Adalat), amlodipine (Norvasc), and diltiazem (Cardizem) all have proven beneficial in IPAH therapy due to vasodilatory properties. Relatively high doses are required to see responses, with systemic hypotension and edema being the most significant adverse effects in these patients. The historical role for these agents has been first-line management; however, many clinicians currently opt for prostacyclin therapy or phosphodiesterase therapy initially.

Soluble Guanylate Cyclase Stimulators

Riociguat (Adempas) is an oral soluble guanylate cyclase (sGC) stimulator and is indicated for the treatment of adults with IPAH, and patients with persistent/recurrent chronic thromboembolic pulmonary hypertension (CTEPH) after surgical treatment or inoperable CTEPH. Riociguat is the first FDA-approved agent showing efficacy for patients with CTEPH. The sGC stimulators relax arteries to increase blood flow thereby decreasing blood pressure. Riociguat is an FDA pregnancy category X drug and is therefore, only available to female patients through a special restricted distribution program called the Adempas Risk Evaluation Mitigation Strategies (REMS) program.

Vasopressor Agents

The 2016 Surviving Sepsis Campaign international guidelines for management of sepsis and septic shock continue to recommend norepinephrine as the first-choice vasopressor in this setting. It is recommended that vasopressor therapy initially target a mean arterial pressure (MAP) of 65 mm Hg. Norepinephrine is a direct-acting vasoactive agent. It possesses alpha- and beta-adrenergic agonist properties producing mixed vasopressor and inotropic effects. Dopamine is recommended as an alternative vasopressor agent to norepinephrine only in highly selected patients (eg, patients with low risk of tachyarrhythmias and absolute or relative bradycardia). Dopamine is both an indirect-acting and a direct-acting agent. Dopamine works indirectly by causing the release of norepinephrine from nerve terminal storage vesicles as well as directly by stimulating alpha and beta receptors. Dopamine is unique in that it produces different pharmacologic responses based on the dose infused. Doses between 5 and 10 mcg/kg/min are typically associated with an increase in inotropy resulting from stimulation of beta receptors in the heart, and doses above 10 mcg/kg/min stimulate peripheral alpha-adrenergic receptors, producing vasoconstriction and an increase in blood pressure.

Dopamine and norepinephrine are both effective for increasing blood pressure. Dopamine raises cardiac output more than norepinephrine, but its use is limited by tachyarrhythmias. Norepinephrine may be a more effective vasopressor in some patients, thus the first-line designation. The 2012 and 2016 Surviving Sepsis Campaign international guidelines highlighted epinephrine as an option in patients whose hypotension is refractory to norepinephrine. Epinephrine possesses alpha- and beta-adrenergic effects, increasing heart rate, contractility, and vasoconstriction with higher doses. Epinephrine's use is reserved for when other vasoconstrictors are inadequate. Adverse effects include tachyarrhythmias; myocardial, mesenteric, renal, and extremity ischemia, and hyperglycemia.

Phenylephrine is not recommended in the treatment of septic shock except in the following circumstances: (a) norepinephrine is associated with serious arrhythmias, (b) cardiac output is known to be high and blood pressure persistently low, or (c) as salvage therapy when combined inotrope/vasopressor drugs and low-dose vasopressin have failed to achieve the MAP target. Phenylephrine is a pure alpha-adrenergic agonist. It produces vasoconstriction without a direct effect on the heart, although it may cause a reflex bradycardia. Phenylephrine may be useful when dopamine, dobutamine, norepinephrine, or epinephrine cause tachyarrhythmias and when a vasoconstrictor is required.

Vasopressin is an emerging therapeutic agent for the hemodynamic support of septic and vasodilatory shock. Vasopressin is a hormone that mediates vasoconstriction via V1-receptor activation on vascular smooth muscle. During septic shock, vasopressin levels are particularly low. Exogenous vasopressin administration is based on the theory of hormone replacement. Vasopressin (up to 0.03 unit/min) can be added to norepinephrine with the intent of raising MAP to target or decreasing norepinephrine dosage. Low-dose vasopressin is not recommended as the single initial vasopressor for treatment of sepsis-induced hypotension, and vasopressin doses higher than 0.03 to 0.04 units/min are reserved for salvage therapy (failure to achieve an adequate MAP with other vasopressor agents). It is important to note that harmful vasoconstriction of the GI vasculature will occur with dose escalation greater than 0.04 units/min.

Dose

- See Table 22-3.

Monitoring Parameters

- Blood pressure, heart rate, ECG, urine output, and hemodynamic parameters

Inotropic Agents (see Table 22-3)

Catecholamines
Dobutamine

Dobutamine produces pronounced beta-adrenergic effects such as increases in inotropy and chronotropy along with vasodilation. Dobutamine is useful especially for the acute management of low cardiac output states, as in cardiogenic shock. Adverse effects associated with the use of dobutamine include tachyarrhythmias and ischemia.

A trial of dobutamine infusion up to 20 mcg/kg/min may be administered or added to vasopressors (if in use) in the presence of: (a) myocardial dysfunction as suggested by elevated cardiac filling pressures and low cardiac output, or (b) ongoing signs of hypoperfusion, despite achieving adequate intravascular volume and adequate MAP. Norepinephrine and dobutamine can be titrated separately to maintain both blood pressure and cardiac output.

The 2016 Surviving Sepsis Campaign international guidelines provide a weak recommendation suggesting the use of dobutamine in septic patients who show evidence of persistent hypoperfusion despite adequate fluid resuscitation and use of vasopressor agents. It is important to note that more evidence is needed in this area.

Dopamine

Dopamine in the range of 5 to 10 mcg/kg/min typically produces an increase in inotropy and chronotropy. Doses above 10 mcg/kg/min typically produce alpha-adrenergic effects.

Isoproterenol

Isoproterenol is a potent pure beta-receptor agonist. It has potent inotropic, chronotropic, and vasodilatory properties. Its use typically is reserved for temporizing life-threatening bradycardia. The restrictions on this agent are further enhanced by dramatic price increases, which negate clinical benefit compared with other agents and devices (eg, pacemakers). Adverse effects associated with isoproterenol include tachyarrhythmias, myocardial ischemia, and hypotension.

Epinephrine

Epinephrine produces pronounced effects on heart rate and contractility and is used when other inotropic agents have not resulted in the desired response. Epinephrine is associated with tachyarrhythmias; myocardial, mesenteric, renal, and extremity ischemia; and hyperglycemia.

Dose

- See Table 22-3.

Monitoring Parameters

- Blood pressure, heart rate, ECG, urine output, and hemodynamic parameters

ANTIBIOTIC PHARMACOLOGY

There are a wide variety of antibiotic agents used in hospitalized patients. Commonly used antibiotic classes include beta lactams or penicillins (eg, penicillin G potassium, ampicillin ± sulbactam, oxacillin, nafcillin, ticarcillin ± clavulanic acid, and piperacillin ± tazobactam), carbapenems (eg, meropenem, doripenem, and imipenem/cilastatin), monobactams (eg, aztreonam), cephalosporins (eg, cefazolin, cefotetan, cefoxitin, cefotaxime, ceftazidime, ceftriaxone, and cefepime), fluoroquinolones (eg, levofloxacin, moxifloxacin, and ciprofloxacin), macrolides (eg, azithromycin, erythromycin), lincosamides (eg, clindamycin), nitroimidazoles (eg, metronidazole), lipopeptides (eg, daptomycin), oxazolidinones (eg, linezolid), glycopeptides (eg, vancomycin, telavancin), and aminoglycosides (eg, amikacin, tobramycin, and gentamicin). Since the development of the first antibiotic (penicillin) in 1944, microorganisms have continually evolved by developing resistance to these agents. This has led to the need for newer and more innovative classes of antibiotics with different targets and ways to avoid resistance. Selection of the correct agent(s) is a key consideration, along with correct identification of the site of infection, and knowledge of resistance patterns within your institution. In some instances, combinations of different antibiotic classes (eg, aminoglycoside + beta lactam, or fluoroquinolone + beta lactam) may be used as a strategy to address resistance patterns. This is used particularly with gram-negative organisms. Additionally, the antibiotic dose, frequency, and/or length of infusion can also be modified as well.

As noted, there are a number of factors related to optimal antibiotic therapy. A complete review of all antibiotic classes is beyond the scope of this text, and the focus of this section is on aminoglycosides and vancomycin due to the commonality of their usage and the link to therapeutic drug monitoring (TDM).

Aminoglycosides

Gentamicin, tobramycin, and amikacin are the most commonly used aminoglycoside antibiotics in acutely ill patients. These agents are typically used with antipseudomonal penicillins or third- or fourth-generation cephalosporins for additional gram-negative bacteria coverage. Occasionally, they are added to vancomycin or a penicillin for synergy against staphylococcal, streptococcal, or enterococcal organisms. Aminoglycosides are not metabolized but are cleared from the body through the kidney by glomerular filtration with some proximal tubular reabsorption occurring. The clearance of aminoglycosides parallels glomerular filtration, and a reduction in glomerular filtration results in a reduction in clearance with elevation in serum concentrations. Additional factors accounting for the reduced aminoglycoside clearance in acutely ill patients include the level of positive end-expiratory pressure and the use of vasoactive agents to maintain blood pressure and perfusion. Aminoglycosides are removed from the body by hemodialysis, peritoneal dialysis, continuous renal replacement therapy (CRRT), extracorporeal membrane oxygenation, exchange transfusion, and cardiopulmonary bypass.

The major limiting factors in the use of aminoglycosides are drug-induced ototoxicity and nephrotoxicity. Ototoxicity results from the loss of sensory hair cells in the cochlea and vestibular labyrinth. Gentamicin is primarily vestibulotoxic, amikacin primarily causes cochlear damage, and tobramycin affects vestibular and cochlear function equally. Symptoms of ototoxicity typically appear within the first 1 to 2 weeks of therapy but may be delayed as long as 10 to 14 days after stopping therapy. Early damage may be reversible, but it may become permanent if the agent is continued. Vestibular toxicity may be manifested by vertigo, ataxia, nystagmus, nausea, and vomiting, but these symptoms may not be apparent in a sedated or paralyzed, acutely ill patient. Cochlear damage occurs as subclinical high-frequency hearing loss that is usually irreversible and may progress to deafness even if the drug is discontinued. It is difficult to diagnose hearing loss in the absence of pretherapy audiograms. Risk factors for ototoxicity include advanced age, duration of therapy for more than 10 days, total dose, previous aminoglycoside therapy, and renal impairment.

Nephrotoxicity has been estimated to occur in up to 30% of acutely ill patients and typically develops 2 to 5 days after starting therapy. An increase in serum creatinine of 0.5 mg/dL above baseline has been arbitrarily defined as significant and as possible evidence of nephrotoxicity. Nephrotoxicity is associated with a reduction in glomerular filtration rate, impaired concentrating ability, increased serum creatinine, and increased urea nitrogen. In most cases, the renal insufficiency is nonoliguric and reversible. The mechanism of nephrotoxicity is possibly related to the inhibition of intracellular phospholipases in lysosomes of tubular cells in the proximal tubule, resulting in rupture or dysfunction of the lysosome, leading to proximal tubular necrosis. Risk factors for the development of aminoglycoside nephrotoxicity include advanced age, prolonged therapy, preexisting renal disease, preexisting liver disease, volume depletion, shock, and concurrent use of other nephrotoxins such as amphotericin B, cyclosporine, or cisplatin.

Aminoglycosides are effectively removed during hemodialysis. However, there is a rebound in the serum concentration within the first 2 hours after the completion of hemodialysis as the serum and tissues reach a new equilibrium. Therefore, a serum concentration is drawn at least 2 hours after a dialysis treatment. Typically a dose of 1 to 2 mg/kg of gentamicin or tobramycin (amikacin 4-8 mg/kg) is sufficient to increase the serum level into the therapeutic range after dialysis. Continuous hemofiltration is also effective at removing aminoglycosides. Up to 35% of a dose can be removed during a 24-hour period of CRRT. Initially, several blood samples may be required to determine the drug's pharmacokinetic profile for dosing regimen adjustments. If the hemofiltration rate remains constant, aminoglycoside clearance generally remains stable, permitting the administration of a stable dosing regimen. In this setting, drug concentration monitoring may only be required 2 to 3 times a week.

Vancomycin

Vancomycin is a glycopeptide antibiotic active against gram-positive and certain anaerobic organisms. It exerts its antimicrobial effects by binding with peptidoglycan and inhibiting bacterial cell wall synthesis. In addition, the antibacterial effects of vancomycin also include alteration of bacterial cell wall permeability and selective inhibition of RNA synthesis.

Vancomycin is minimally absorbed after oral administration so oral use is indicated only for intestinal infections such as *Clostridium difficile*. After single or multiple IV doses, therapeutic vancomycin concentrations can be found in ascitic, pericardial, peritoneal, pleural, and synovial fluids. Vancomycin penetrates poorly into cerebrospinal fluid (CSF), with CSF penetration being directly proportional to vancomycin dose and degree of meningeal inflammation. Vancomycin is eliminated through the kidneys primarily via glomerular filtration with a limited degree of tubular secretion. Nonrenal elimination occurs through the liver and accounts for about 30% of total clearance. The elimination half-life of vancomycin is 3 to 13 hours in patients with normal renal function and increases in proportion to decreasing creatinine clearance. In acute renal failure, nonrenal clearance is maintained but eventually declines approaching the nonrenal clearance in chronic renal failure. In ill patients with reduced renal function, the increase in half-life may be due to a reduction in clearance as well as an increase in the volume of distribution.

Vancomycin is removed minimally during hemodialysis with cuprophane filter membranes, so that dosage supplementation after hemodialysis is not necessary. Vancomycin's half-life averages 150 hours in patients with chronic renal failure. With the newer high-flux polysulfone hemodialysis filters, vancomycin is removed to a greater degree, resulting in significant reductions in vancomycin serum concentrations. However, there is a significant redistribution period that takes place over the 12-hour period after the high-flux hemodialysis procedure with postdialysis concentrations similar to predialysis concentrations. Therefore, dose supplementation is based on concentrations obtained at least 12 hours after dialysis.

Vancomycin is removed very effectively by CRRT resulting in a reduction in half-life to 24 to 48 hours. Up to 33% of a dose can be eliminated during a 24-hour hemofiltration period. Supplemental doses of vancomycin may need to be administered every 2 to 5 days in patients undergoing CRRT.

The most common adverse effect of vancomycin is the "red-man syndrome," which is a histamine-like reaction associated with rapid vancomycin infusion and characterized by flushing, tingling, pruritus, erythema, and a macular papular rash. It typically begins 15 to 45 minutes after starting the infusion and abates 10 to 60 minutes after stopping the infusion. It may be avoided or minimized by infusing the dose over 2 hours or by pretreating the patient with diphenhydramine, 25 to 50 mg, 15 to 30 minutes before the vancomycin infusion. Other rare, but reported, adverse effects include rash, thrombophlebitis, chills, fever, and neutropenia.

PULMONARY PHARMACOLOGY

Albuterol

Albuterol is a selective beta-2 agonist, used to treat or prevent reversible bronchospasm. Adverse effects tend to be associated with inadvertent beta-1 stimulation leading to cardiovascular events including tachycardia, premature ventricular contractions, and palpitations.

Monitoring Parameters
- Heart rate and pulmonary function tests

Levalbuterol

Levalbuterol is the active enantiomer of racemic albuterol. Dose ranging studies in stable ambulatory asthmatics and patients with COPD have documented that levalbuterol 0.63 mg and albuterol 2.5 mg produced equivalent increases in the magnitude of forced expiratory volume 1 (FEV_1) for a similar duration. There are no studies evaluating the efficacy of levalbuterol in hospitalized or acutely ill patients.

One study assessing the tachycardic effects of these agents in acutely ill patients showed a clinically insignificant increase in heart rate following the administration of either agent. This has led to restrictions of levalbuterol within many institutions to patients intolerant to albuterol, or with histories of tachyarrhythmias.

Monitoring Parameters
- Heart rate and pulmonary function tests

Ipratropium

Ipratropium is an inhaled anticholinergic, used most commonly as a bronchodilator for cholinergic-mediated bronchospasm associated with asthma or COPD. Ipratropium is often combined with inhaled short-acting beta-2 agonists (eg, albuterol) for the management of asthma or COPD exacerbations.

Monitoring Parameters
- Pulmonary function tests

GASTROINTESTINAL PHARMACOLOGY

Stress Ulcer Prophylaxis

Stress ulcers are superficial lesions commonly involving the mucosal layer of the stomach that appear after stressful events such as trauma, surgery, burns, sepsis, or organ failure. Risk factors for the development of stress ulcers include coagulopathy, patients requiring mechanical ventilation for more than 48 hours, patients with a history of GI ulceration or bleeding within the past year, sepsis, an ICU stay longer than 1 week, occult bleeding lasting more than 6 days, and the use of high-dose steroids (> 250 mg of hydrocortisone or the equivalent). Numerous studies support the use of antacids, H2-receptor antagonists, and sucralfate to treat stress ulcers. There are limited prospective comparative studies supporting the use of proton pump inhibitors (PPIs) for preventing stress ulcer formation in acutely ill patients. More studies are warranted to highlight the role of PPIs in this setting. The use of any therapy to prevent stress ulcer formation requires a careful assessment of individual patient risk and benefit, particularly in light of the increased risk for ventilator-associated pneumonia and C. difficile that is associated with increasing gastric pH.

H2 Antagonists

Ranitidine and famotidine essentially have replaced antacids as therapy for the prevention of stress gastritis. These agents have the benefit of requiring administration only every 6 to 12 hours or may be delivered by continuous infusion. When they are administered by continuous infusion, they may be added to parenteral nutrition solutions, decreasing the need for multiple daily doses. Each agent has been associated with thrombocytopenia and mental status changes. Mental status changes typically occur in older adults or in patients with reduced renal function when the dose is not appropriately adjusted. Also, similar to antacids, alkalinization of the GI tract with H2 antagonists may predispose patients to pneumonias with gram-negative organisms that originate in the GI tract.

Dose
- *Ranitidine:* Intermittent IV: 50 mg q8h; continuous infusion: 6.25 mg/h. Oral: 300 to 600 mg daily divided 1 to 2 times/day
- *Cimetidine:* Oral: 300 mg qid or 800 mg qhs, or 400 mg bid
- *Famotidine:* Intermittent IV: 20 mg q12h; continuous infusion: not recommended. Oral: 20 to 40 mg daily divided 1 to 2 times/day

Monitoring Parameters
- Nasogastric aspirate pH, platelet count, hemoglobin, hematocrit, and nasogastric aspirate and stool guaiac

Other Agents
Sucralfate
Sucralfate is an aluminum disaccharide compound that has been shown to be safe and effective for the prophylaxis of stress gastritis. Sucralfate may work by increasing bicarbonate secretion, mucus secretion, or prostaglandin synthesis to prevent the formation of stress ulcers. Sucralfate has no effect on gastric pH. It can be administered either as a suspension or as a tablet that can be partially dissolved in 10 to 30 mL of water and administered orally or through a nasogastric tube. Although sucralfate is free from systemic side effects, it has been reported to cause hypophosphatemia, constipation, and the formation of bezoars. Because sucralfate does not increase gastric pH, it lacks the ability to alkalinize the gastric environment and may decrease the development of gram-negative nosocomial pneumonias. Sucralfate has a limited role as an alternative to H2 antagonists in patients with thrombocytopenia or mental status changes.

Dose
- 1 g PO, NG q6h

Monitoring Parameters
- Hemoglobin, hematocrit, nasogastric aspirate, and stool guaiac

Acute Peptic Ulcer Bleeding

Proton Pump Inhibitors
Proton pump inhibitors have demonstrated efficacy in preventing rebleeding and reducing transfusion requirements in several randomized-controlled trials. The rationale for adjunctive acid-suppressant therapy is based on in vitro data demonstrating clot stability and enhanced platelet aggregation at gastric pHs more than 6. High-dose IV PPI therapy in conjunction with therapeutic endoscopy is the most cost-effective approach for the management of hospitalized patients with acute peptic ulcer bleeding.

Pantoprazole and esomeprazole are available in oral and injectable forms, while lansoprazole and omeprazole are available in oral forms only. It is advisable to transition to oral/enteral PPI therapy, if possible, after 72 hours of IV therapy. The 72-hour time period for continuous infusions is the longest duration that has been studied.

Dose
- *Pantoprazole and esomeprazole:* IV bolus dosing: 40 to 80 mg IV q12h for 72 hours; continuous infusion: 80 mg IV bolus; then 8 mg/h for 72 hours

Monitoring Parameters
- Hemoglobin, hematocrit, and stool guaiac

Variceal Hemorrhage
Upper GI bleeding is a common problem encountered in the intensive care unit. Its mortality remains around 10%. Vasoactive drugs to control bleeding play an important role in the immediate treatment of acute upper GI bleeding associated with variceal hemorrhage.

Vasopressin
Vasopressin remains a commonly used agent for acute variceal bleeding. Vasopressin is a nonspecific vasoconstrictor that reduces portal pressure by constricting the splanchnic bed and reducing blood flow into the portal system. Vasopressin is successful in stopping bleeding in about 50% of patients. Many of the adverse effects of vasopressin are caused by its relative nonselective vasoconstrictor effect. Myocardial, mesenteric, and cutaneous ischemia have been reported in association with its use. Drug-related adverse effects have been reported in up to 25% of patients receiving vasopressin. The use of transdermal or IV nitrates with vasopressin reduces the incidence of these adverse effects.

Dose
- 0.3 to 0.9 units/min

Monitoring Parameters
- Hemoglobin, hematocrit, nasogastric aspirate, stool guaiac, ECG, signs and symptoms of ischemia, blood pressure, and heart rate

Octreotide
Octreotide, the longer acting synthetic analog of somatostatin, reduces splanchnic blood flow and has a modest effect on hepatic blood flow and wedged hepatic venous pressure with little systemic circulation effects. Although octreotide produces the same results as vasopressin in the control of bleeding and transfusion requirements, it produces significantly fewer adverse effects. Continuous infusion of octreotide has been shown to be as effective as injection sclerotherapy in control of variceal hemorrhage.

Dose
- *Initial bolus dose:* 100 mcg, followed by 50 mcg/h continuous infusion

Monitoring Parameters
- Hemoglobin, hematocrit, nasogastric aspirate, and stool guaiac

Propranolol

Propranolol has been shown to reduce portal pressure both acutely and chronically in patients with portal hypertension by reducing splanchnic blood flow. The primary use of propranolol has been in the prevention of variceal bleeding. Propranolol or other beta-blockers are avoided in patients experiencing acute GI bleeding, because beta-blocking agents may prevent the compensatory tachycardia needed to maintain cardiac output and blood pressure in the setting of hemorrhage.

Monitoring Parameters
- Hemoglobin, hematocrit, heart rate, and blood pressure

RENAL PHARMACOLOGY

Diuretics

Diuretics may be categorized in a number of ways, including site of action, chemical structure, and potency. Although many diuretics are available for oral and IV administration, intravenously administered agents typically are given to acutely ill patients because of their guaranteed absorption and more predictable responses. Therefore, the primary agents used in intensive care units are the intravenously administered loop diuretics, thiazide diuretics, and osmotic agents. However, the oral thiazide-like agent, metolazone, is used commonly in combination with loop diuretics to maintain urine output for patients with diuretic resistance.

Monitoring Parameters
- Urine output, blood pressure, renal function, electrolytes, weight, fluid balance, and hemodynamic parameters (if applicable)

Loop Diuretics

Loop diuretics (furosemide, bumetanide, torsemide) act by inhibiting active transport of chloride and possibly sodium in the thick ascending loop of Henle. Administration of loop diuretics results in enhanced excretion of sodium, chloride, potassium, hydrogen, magnesium, ammonium, and bicarbonate. Maximum electrolyte loss is greater with loop diuretics than with thiazide diuretics. Furosemide, bumetanide, and torsemide have some renal vasodilator properties that reduce renal vascular resistance and increase renal blood flow. Additionally, these three agents decrease peripheral vascular resistance and increase venous capacitance. These effects may account for the decrease in left ventricular filling pressure that occurs before the onset of diuresis in patients with HF.

Loop diuretics typically are used for the treatment of edema associated with HF or oliguric renal failure, the management of hypertension complicated by HF or renal failure, in combination with hypotensive agents in the treatment of hypertensive crisis, especially when associated with acute pulmonary edema or renal failure, and in combination with 0.9% sodium chloride to increase calcium excretion in patients with hypercalcemia.

Common adverse effects associated with loop diuretic administration include hypotension from excessive reduction in plasma volume, hypokalemia and hypochloremia resulting in metabolic alkalosis, and hypomagnesemia. Reduction in these electrolytes may predispose patients to the development of supraventricular and ventricular ectopy. Tinnitus, with reversible or permanent hearing impairment, may occur with the rapid administration of large IV doses. Typically, IV bolus doses of furosemide are not administered faster than 40 mg/min.

Dose
- *Furosemide:* IV bolus: 10 to 100 mg q1-6h; continuous infusion: 1 to 15 mg/h. Oral: 20 to 600 mg daily divided 1 to 4 times/day
- *Bumetanide:* IV bolus: 0.5 to 1 mg q1-2h; continuous infusion: 0.5 to 2 mg/h. Oral: 0.5 to 5 mg qd-bid (maximum of 10 mg)
- *Torsemide:* IV bolus: 5 to 20 mg qd. Oral: 2.5 to 20 mg qd

Thiazide Diuretics

Thiazide (IV chlorothiazide) and thiazide-like (PO metolazone) diuretics enhance excretion of sodium, chloride, and water by inhibiting the transport of sodium across the renal tubular epithelium in the cortical diluting segment of the nephron. Thiazides also increase the excretion of potassium and bicarbonate.

Thiazide diuretics are used in the management of edema and hypertension as monotherapy or in combination with other agents. They have less potent diuretic and antihypertensive effects than loop diuretics. Intravenously administered chlorothiazide and oral metolazone are often used in combination with loop diuretics in patients with diuretic resistance. By acting at a different site in the nephron, this combination of agents may restore diuretic responsiveness. Thiazide diuretics decrease glomerular filtration rate, and this effect may contribute to their decreased efficacy in patients with reduced renal function (glomerular filtration rate < 20 mL/min). Metolazone, unlike thiazide diuretics, does not substantially decrease glomerular filtration rate or renal plasma flow and often produces a diuretic effect even in patients with glomerular filtration rates less than 20 mL/min.

Adverse effects that may occur with the administration of thiazide diuretics include hyponatremia, hypovolemia, hypotension, hypochloremia, and hypokalemia resulting in a metabolic alkalosis, hypercalcemia, hyperuricemia, and the precipitation of acute gouty attacks.

Dose
- *Chlorothiazide:* 500 to 1000 mg IV q12h
- *Metolazone:* 2.5 to 20 mg PO qd

Osmotic Diuretics

Mannitol

Mannitol is an osmotic diuretic commonly used in patients with increased intracranial pressure. Mannitol produces a diuretic effect by increasing the osmotic pressure of the glomerular filtrate and preventing the tubular reabsorption of water and solutes. Mannitol increases the excretion of sodium, water, potassium, and chloride, as well as other electrolytes.

Mannitol is used to treat acute oliguric renal failure, and reduce intracranial and intraocular pressures. The renal protective effects of mannitol may be due to its ability to prevent nephrotoxins from becoming concentrated in the tubular fluid. However, its ability to prevent or reverse acute renal failure may be owing to restoring renal blood flow, glomerular filtration rate, urine flow, and sodium excretion. To be effective in preventing or reversing renal failure, mannitol must be administered before reductions in glomerular filtration rate or renal blood flow have resulted in acute tubular damage. Mannitol is useful in the treatment of cerebral edema, especially when there is evidence of herniation or the development of cord compression.

The most severe adverse effect of mannitol is overexpansion of extracellular fluid and circulatory overload, producing acute HF and pulmonary edema. This effect typically occurs in patients with severely impaired renal function. Therefore, mannitol is not administered to individuals in whom adequate renal function and urine flow have not been established.

Dose
- 0.25 to 0.5 g/kg, then 0.25 to 0.5 g/kg q4h

Monitoring Parameters
- Urine output, blood pressure, renal function, electrolytes, weight, fluid balance, hemodynamic parameters (if applicable), serum osmolarity, and intracranial pressure (if applicable)

HEMATOLOGIC PHARMACOLOGY

Anticoagulants

Unfractionated Heparin

Unfractionated heparin consists of a group of mucopolysaccharides derived from the mast cells of porcine intestinal tissues. It binds with antithrombin III, accelerating the rate at which antithrombin III neutralizes coagulation factors II, VII, IX, X, XI, and XII. Unfractionated heparin is used for prophylaxis and treatment of venous thrombosis and pulmonary embolism, atrial fibrillation with embolization, and treatment of acute disseminated intravascular coagulation.

Subcutaneously administered unfractionated heparin is absorbed slowly and completely over the dosing interval. The total amount of unfractionated heparin required to achieve the same degree of anticoagulation over the same time period does not appear to differ whether the unfractionated heparin is administered subcutaneously or intravenously. The apparent volume of distribution of unfractionated heparin is directly proportional to body weight, but this process is likely saturable to some extent in obese patients. Literature describing dosing recommendations in the obese population is variable, with some suggesting ideal body weight for dosing and others proposing total body weight.

The metabolism and elimination of unfractionated heparin involves the process of depolymerization and desulfation. Enzymes reported to be involved in unfractionated heparin metabolism include heparinase and desulfatase, which cleave unfractionated heparin into oligosaccharides. The half-life of unfractionated heparin ranges from 0.4 to 2.5 hours. Patients with underlying thromboembolic disease have been shown to have shorter elimination half-lives, faster clearance, and require larger doses to maintain adequate thrombotic activity.

A weight-based nomogram is utilized with a loading dose followed by a continuous infusion. The infusion is traditionally titrated based on activated PTT monitoring. Recently some centers have used antifactor Xa monitoring. The main adverse effects may be attributed to excessive anticoagulation. Bleeding occurs in 3% to 20% of patients receiving short-term, high-dose therapy. Bleeding is increased threefold when the PTT is 2 to 2.9 times above control and eightfold when the PTT is more than 3 times the control value. Unfractionated heparin–induced thrombocytopenia may occur in 1% to 5% of patients receiving the drug.

The PTT is the most commonly used test to monitor and adjust unfractionated heparin doses. Although unfractionated heparin is typically administered as a continuous infusion, it is important that samples are collected as close to steady state as possible. After starting unfractionated heparin therapy or adjusting the dose, PTT values are drawn at least 6 to 8 hours after the change. Samples drawn too early are misleading and may result in inappropriate dose adjustments. Once the unfractionated heparin dose has been determined, daily monitoring of the PTT for minor adjustments in the unfractionated heparin dose is indicated. Large variations in subsequent coagulation tests are investigated to ensure that the patient's condition has not changed or the patient is not developing thrombocytopenia. A similar approach is used, if antifactor Xa levels are monitored in lieu of PTT.

Platelet counts are monitored every 2 to 3 days while a patient is receiving unfractionated heparin to assess for unfractionated heparin–induced thrombocytopenia, thrombosis, or hemorrhage. Hemoglobin and hematocrit are monitored every 2 to 3 days to assess for the presence of bleeding. Additionally, sputum, urine, and stool are examined for the presence of blood. Patients are examined for signs of bleeding at IV access sites and for the development of hematomas and ecchymosis. In addition, IM injections are avoided in patients receiving unfractionated heparin and elective invasive procedures are avoided or rescheduled.

Dose

- *Individualized dosing:* Bolus: 80 units/kg followed by a continuous infusion of 18 units/kg/h for the treatment of deep venous thrombosis (DVT) or pulmonary embolism, for the treatment of arterial thromboembolism including cerebral thromboembolism, or for the treatment of mural thrombosis. Lower bolus doses and initial infusion rates recommended for ST-Elevation Myocardial Infarction (STEMI), Non-ST-Elevation Myocardial Infarction (NSTEMI), and other indications. Infusion rates are adjusted to maintain a PTT between 1.5 and 2.0 times the control value, or antifactor Xa within institution-specific therapeutic range (eg, 0.3-0.7 IU/mL).

Monitoring Parameters

- PTT or antifactor Xa, hemoglobin, hematocrit, platelet count, and signs of active bleeding

Low-Molecular-Weight Heparins

Low-molecular-weight heparins have a role in the treatment of DVT, pulmonary embolism, and acute MI. Low-molecular-weight heparins are less time consuming for nurses and laboratories and more comfortable for patients by allowing them to be discharged earlier from the hospital. The use of a fixed-dose regimen avoids the need for serial monitoring of the PTT and follow-up dose adjustments. Enoxaparin is the most studied low-molecular-weight heparin. Its dose for the treatment of DVT, pulmonary embolism, and acute MI is 1 mg/kg q12h. Dalteparin is another agent that has been shown to be as effective as unfractionated heparin in the treatment of thromboembolic disease and acute MI. Dalteparin 200 units/kg once daily is the typical dose used for the treatment of thromboembolic disease; 120 units/kg followed by 120 units/kg 12 hours later has been used in patients with acute MI receiving streptokinase. Warfarin can be started with the first dose of enoxaparin or dalteparin. When used as a bridge to warfarin therapy, enoxaparin or dalteparin are continued until two consecutive therapeutic international normalized ratio (INR) values are achieved, typically in about 5 to 7 days.

Both dalteparin and enoxaparin are primarily renally eliminated with the potential for drug accumulation in patients with renal impairment. The approach for managing these patients differs between the two drugs. Because these agents work by inhibiting factor Xa activity, it is possible to monitor their anticoagulation by measuring antifactor Xa levels. This is a useful monitoring tool, particularly when compared with serum drug levels. Doses of either agent may be adjusted based on antifactor Xa levels in patients with significant renal impairment (ie, creatinine clearance < 30 mL/min). The dosing adjustment for enoxaparin in patients with creatinine clearances less than 30 mL/min is to extend the dosing interval from 12 hours to 24 hours in both prophylaxis and treatment of thrombosis. No such dosage adjustment guideline has been approved for dalteparin, thus antifactor Xa levels may be required.

Several studies have documented that acutely ill patients have significantly lower anti-Xa levels in response to single daily doses when compared to patients on general medical wards. Factor Xa activity may need to be monitored in acutely ill patients to adjust doses to ensure adequate anticoagulation to prevent deep venous clots from developing.

Dose

- *Enoxaparin:* 1 mg/kg SC q12h, for treatment of DVT, pulmonary embolism, and acute MI

Monitoring Parameters

- Hemoglobin, hematocrit, signs of active bleeding, platelet count, and antifactor Xa levels

Warfarin

Warfarin prevents the conversion of vitamin K back to its active form from the vitamin K epoxide, impairing the formation of vitamin K–dependent clotting factors II, VII, IX, X, protein C, and protein S. Warfarin is indicated in the treatment of venous thrombosis or pulmonary embolism following full-dose parenteral anticoagulant (eg, unfractionated or low-molecular-weight heparin) therapy. Warfarin is also used for chronic therapy to reduce the risk of thromboembolic episodes in patients with chronic atrial fibrillation.

Warfarin is rapidly and extensively absorbed from the GI tract. Peak plasma concentrations occur between 60 and 90 minutes after an oral dose with bioavailability ranging between 75% and 100%. Albumin is the principal binding protein with 97.5% to 99.9% of warfarin being bound.

Warfarin's metabolism is stereospecific. The R-isomer is oxidized to 6-hydroxywarfarin and further reduced to 9S, 11R-warfarin alcohols. The S-isomer is oxidized to 7-hydroxywarfarin and further reduced to 9S, 11R-warfarin alcohols. The stereospecific isomer alcohol metabolites have anticoagulant activity in humans. The warfarin alcohols are renally eliminated. The elimination half-lives of the two warfarin isomers differ substantially. The S-isomer half-life is approximately 33 hours and the R-isomer half-life is 45 hours.

Warfarin therapy may be started on the first day of unfractionated or low-molecular-weight heparin therapy. Traditionally, warfarin 5 mg daily is given for the first 2 to 3 days then adjusted to maintain the desired prothrombin time (PT) or INR. The timing of INR measurements relative to changes in daily dose is important. After the administration of a warfarin dose, the peak depression of coagulation occurs in about 36 hours. It is important to select an appropriate time during a given dosing interval and perform coagulation tests consistently at that time. After the first four to five doses, the fluctuation in the INR over a 24-hour dosing interval is minimal. The timeframe for stabilization of warfarin plasma concentrations and coagulation response during continued administration of maintenance doses is less clear. A minimum of 10 days appears to be necessary before the dose-response curve shows interval-to-interval stability. During the first week of therapy, two INR measurements are determined to assess the impact of warfarin accumulation on INR. Several factors are assessed when evaluating an unexpected response to warfarin. Laboratory results are verified to exclude inaccurate or spurious results. The medication profile is reviewed to exclude drug-drug interactions including changes in warfarin product, and the patient is evaluated for disease-drug interactions, nutritional-drug interactions, and nonadherence.

Bleeding is the major complication associated with the use of warfarin, occurring in 6% to 29% of patients receiving the drug. Bleeding complications include ecchymoses, hemoptysis, and epistaxis, as well as fatal or life-threatening hemorrhage. The effects of warfarin can be reversed with oral doses of vitamin K and with transfusion of fresh frozen plasma (FFP) to replace vitamin K-dependent clotting factors in patients without major bleed. In patients with major bleeding, 4-factor prothrombin complex concentrate (KCentra) plus vitamin K may be preferred compared with FFP, according to the 2012 American College of Chest Physicians Practice Guidelines for Oral Anticoagulant Therapy: Antithrombotic Therapy and Prevention of Thrombosis.

Dose
- 5 mg PO qd × 3 days, then adjusted to maintain the INR between 2 and 3
- To prevent thromboembolism associated with prosthetic heart valves, the dose is adjusted to maintain an INR between 2.5 and 3.5.

Monitoring Parameters
- INR, hemoglobin, hematocrit, and signs of active bleeding

Factor Xa Inhibitors

Rivaroxaban and Apixaban
Rivaroxaban and apixaban are oral factor Xa inhibitors, indicated for venous thromboembolism (VTE) prophylaxis, or prophylaxis of embolism or cerebrovascular accident (CVA) in patients with nonvalvular atrial fibrillation. The agents are also indicated for PE and DVT treatment. Presently, there are no FDA-approved reversal agents for this class of anticoagulants. Outcomes data with 4-factor prothrombin complex concentrate (KCentra) reversal in bleeding and non-bleeding factor Xa inhibitor patients are limited to case reports and case series. Although these small studies indicate there may be some benefit, more robust research is needed to evaluate if there is a clear role in this setting.

Dose
Rivaroxaban:
- *VTE prophylaxis postsurgery:* 10 mg PO qd
- *Atrial fibrillation, nonvalvular-CVA prophylaxis:* 20 mg PO qd
- *DVT or PE treatment, and secondary prophylaxis:* 15 mg PO bid × 21 days followed by 20 mg PO qd

Apixaban:
- *Atrial fibrillation, nonvalvular-CVA prophylaxis:* For most patients, 5 mg PO bid. In patients with any two of the following characteristics: age more than or equal to 80 years; body weight less than or equal to 60 kg; or serum creatinine more than or equal to 1.5 mg/dL, reduce the dose to 2.5 mg PO bid.
- *DVT or PE treatment, and secondary prophylaxis:* 10 mg PO bid × 7 days followed by 5 mg PO bid
- *VTE prophylaxis:* 2.5 mg PO bid

Monitoring Parameters
- Hemoglobin, hematocrit, renal function, and signs of active bleeding

Direct Thrombin Inhibitors

Dabigatran
Dabigatran is an oral direct thrombin inhibitor, indicated for use for stroke prevention in patients with nonvalvular atrial fibrillation. In clinical trials, dabigatran was superior to warfarin in reducing the risk for stroke and systemic embolism with lower minor bleed risk comparatively. Dabigatran also has a developing role as VTE prophylaxis after total knee or hip arthroplasty, as well as the treatment of DVT and PE. It is important to note that dabigatran capsules cannot be opened for feeding tube or oral administration. This agent can be reversed with idarucizumab (Praxbind), which works by binding to dabigatran, causing inactivation.

Dose
- 150 mg PO bid

Monitoring Parameters
- Hemoglobin, hematocrit, aPTT, ecarin clotting time (ECT), and signs of active bleeding

Bivalirudin
Bivalirudin is an anticoagulant with direct thrombin inhibitor properties. Bivalirudin, when given with aspirin, is indicated for use as an anticoagulant in patients with unstable angina undergoing coronary angioplasty. It has been used as a substitute for unfractionated heparin; potential advantages over unfractionated heparin include activity against clot-bound thrombin, more predictable anticoagulation, and no inhibition by components of the platelet release reaction. Numerous studies have compared bivalirudin to unfractionated heparin with or without a glycoprotein IIb/IIIa inhibitor, with mixed results. The most recent major clinical trial published in 2015, MATRIX, demonstrated that bivalirudin, compared to UFH with or without glycoprotein IIb/IIIa inhibitor, reduced bleeding complications, but resulted in higher rates of ischemic events, including acute stent thrombosis. Thus, bivalirudin may be considered a reasonable alternative to UFH primarily in patients at high risk of bleeding, or with a heparin allergy or heparin-induced thrombocytopenia, undergoing percutaneous coronary intervention (PCI). There is no FDA-approved reversal agent

for bivalirudin. In the event of bleeding, discontinuation of infusion is recommended and coagulation returns to baseline in approximately 1 hour following discontinuation with normal renal function. Please note that renal dysfunction will further delay clearance in this setting.

Dose
- *Bolus:* 1 mg/kg
- *Continuous infusion:* 2.5 mg/kg/h × 4 hours, if necessary 0.2 mg/kg/h for up to 20 hours

Monitoring Parameters
- Activated PTT, activated clotting time (ACT), hemoglobin, hematocrit, and signs of active bleeding

Argatroban

Argatroban is a selective thrombin inhibitor indicated for the prevention or treatment of thrombosis in unfractionated heparin–induced thrombocytopenia and for use in PCIs. It has also shown effectiveness in ischemic stroke and as an adjunct to thrombolysis in patients with acute MI. Further studies are needed to establish effectiveness for other indications. Argatroban is dosed as a continuous infusion that is titrated based on activated PTT, similar to unfractionated heparin. During PCI, the ACT may be used. A notable drug-laboratory value interaction is the increase in PT and INR values that occurs with argatroban therapy, which may complicate the monitoring of warfarin therapy once oral anticoagulation is initiated. There is no FDA-approved reversal agent for argatroban. If bleeding occurs, discontinuation of infusion is recommended and coagulation returns to baseline in approximately 4 to 6 hours following discontinuation. This may be prolonged in hepatic impairment or critically ill.

Dose
- *Percutaneous coronary intervention*: Bolus: 350 mcg/kg; continuous infusion: 25 mcg/kg/min
- *Heparin-induced thrombocytopenia with thrombosis*: continuous infusion: 2 mcg/kg/min in non-critically ill. Lowering initial doses to 0.5 to 1 mcg/kg/min in critically ill patients is recommended.

Monitoring Parameters
- Activated PTT, ACT, PT, INR, hemoglobin, hematocrit, and signs of active bleeding

Glycoprotein IIb/IIIa Inhibitor

Glycoprotein IIb/IIIa inhibitors are recommended, in addition to aspirin and unfractionated heparin, in patients with acute coronary syndrome awaiting PCI. If the glycoprotein IIb/IIIa inhibitor is started in the catheterization laboratory just before PCI, abciximab is the agent of choice.

Dose
- *Abciximab:* Bolus: 0.25 mg/kg over 1 to 5 minutes; continuous infusion: 0.125 mcg/kg/min for 12 hours (maximum infusion of 10 mcg/kg/min)

- *Tirofiban:* Bolus infusion: 25 mcg/kg within 5 minutes continuous infusion: 0.1 mcg/kg/min for 12 to 24 hours after angioplasty or atherectomy
- *Eptifibatide:* Bolus: 180 mcg/kg; continuous infusion: 2 mcg/kg/min until discharge or coronary artery bypass grafting (maximum of 72 hours)

Monitoring Parameters
- Platelet count, hemoglobin, hematocrit, and signs of active bleeding

Thrombolytic Agents

Thrombolytic agents may be beneficial as reperfusion therapy in STEMI. The 2013 American College of Cardiology Foundation/American Heart Association guidelines for the management of STEMI include the following recommendations in order from most supported by published literature (Class I) to least supported (Class III).

Class I Recommendations

- In the absence of contraindications, fibrinolytic therapy is given to patients with STEMI and onset of ischemic symptoms within the previous 12 hours when it is anticipated that primary PCI cannot be performed within 120 minutes of first medical contact.

Class IIa Recommendations

- In the absence of contraindications and when PCI is not available, fibrinolytic therapy is reasonable for patients with STEMI if there is clinical and/or electrocardiographic evidence of ongoing ischemia within 12 to 24 hours of symptom onset and a large area of myocardium at risk or hemodynamic instability.

Class III Recommendations

- Fibrinolytic therapy is not administered to patients with ST depression except when a true posterior (inferobasal) MI is suspected or when associated with ST elevation in lead aVR.

Absolute contraindications to the use of thrombolytic agents include any active or recent bleeding, suspected aortic dissection, intracranial or intraspinal neoplasm, arteriovenous malformation or aneurysms, neurosurgery or significant closed head injury within the previous 3 months, ischemic stroke within the previous 3 months (except acute ischemic stroke within 3 hours), or facial trauma in the preceding 3 months. Relative contraindications include acute or chronic severe uncontrolled hypertension, ischemic stroke more than 3 months prior, traumatic or prolonged cardiopulmonary resuscitation greater than 10 minutes in duration, major surgery within the previous 3 weeks, internal bleeding within 2 to 4 weeks, noncompressible vascular punctures, prior allergic reaction to thrombolytics, pregnancy, active peptic ulcer, and current anticoagulation (risk increasing with increasing INR).

Adverse effects include bleeding from the GI or genitourinary tracts, as well as gingival bleeding and epistaxis. Superficial bleeding may occur from trauma sites such as those for IV access or invasive procedures. IM injections, and noncompressible arterial punctures, are avoided during thrombolytic therapy.

Monitoring Parameters
- *For short-term thrombolytic therapy of MI:* ECG, signs and symptoms of ischemia, and signs and symptoms of bleeding at IV injection sites (laboratory monitoring is of little value)
- *Continuous infusion therapy:* Thrombin time, activated PTT, and fibrinogen, in addition to above-mentioned monitoring parameters

Alteplase
Alteplase (recombinant tissue-type plasminogen activator or TPA) has a high affinity for fibrin-bound plasminogen, allowing activation on the fibrin surface. Most plasmin formed remains bound to the fibrin clot, minimizing systemic effects. The risk of an intracerebral bleed is approximately 0.5%.

Dose
- *Acute MI-accelerated infusion:* Patients over 67 kg, total dose 100 mg IV (15 mg IV bolus, then 50 mg over 30 minutes, then 35 mg over 60 minutes)
- *Acute MI-accelerated infusion:* Patients 67 kg or less, (15 mg IV bolus, then 0.75 mg/kg over 30 minutes, then 0.5 mg/kg over 60 minutes); total dose not to exceed 100 mg
- *Acute MI-3-hour infusion:* Weight 65 kg or more, 60 mg IV in the first hour (6 to 10 mg of which to be given as bolus), then 20 mg over the second hour, and 20 mg over the third hour
- *Acute MI-3-hour infusion:* Weight less than 65 kg, 1.25 mg/kg IV administered over 3 hours, give 60% in the first hour (10% of which to be given as bolus), give remaining 40% over the next 2 hours
- *Pulmonary embolism:* 100 mg IV over 2 hours
- *Ischemic stroke:* 0.9 mg/kg (not to exceed 90 mg); 10% of total dose as IV bolus over 1 minute; then remaining 90% as IV infusion over 60 minutes

Tenecteplase

Tenecteplase (recombinant TNK-tissue-type plasminogen activator) has a longer elimination half-life (20-24 minutes) and is more resistant to inactivation by plasminogen activator inhibitor-1 than alteplase. Tenecteplase appears more fibrin specific than alteplase, which may account for a lower rate of noncerebral bleeding comparatively. However, there have been reports of antibody development to tenecteplase. Tenecteplase and alteplase have similar clinical efficacy for thrombolysis after MI.

Dose
- *Acute MI:* 30 to 50 mg (based on weight) IV over 5 seconds

Reteplase
Reteplase is a recombinant plasminogen activator for use in acute MI and pulmonary embolism as a thrombolytic agent. Reteplase has a longer half-life (13-16 minutes) than that of alteplase, allowing for bolus administration. The dosing regimen requires double bolus doses.

Dose
- *Acute MI and pulmonary embolism:* Two 10-unit IV bolus doses, infused over 2 minutes via a dedicated line. The second dose is administered 30 minutes after the initiation of the first injection.

IMMUNOSUPPRESSIVE AGENTS

Cyclosporine

Cyclosporine is used to prevent allograft rejection after solid organ transplantation and graft-versus-host disease in bone marrow transplant patients. Unlike other immunosuppressive agents, cyclosporine does not suppress bone marrow function. Cyclosporine inhibits cytokine synthesis and receptor expression needed for T-lymphocyte activation by interrupting signal transduction. A lack of cytokine disrupts the activation and proliferation of the helper and cytotoxic T-cells that are essential for rejection.

Cyclosporine is poorly absorbed from the GI tract with bioavailability averaging 30%. Its absorption is influenced by the type of organ transplant, time from transplantation, presence of biliary drainage, liver function, intestinal dysfunction, and the use of drugs that alter intestinal function. Cyclosporine is metabolized by cytochrome P-450 isoenzyme 3a to numerous metabolites with more than 90% of the dose excreted into the bile and eliminated in the feces. The kidneys eliminate less than 1% of the dose. There is no evidence that the metabolites have significant immunosuppressive activity compared with cyclosporine and none of the metabolites are known to cause nephrotoxicity.

Because of poor oral absorption, the oral dose is 3 times the IV dose. When converting from IV to oral administration, it is important to increase the oral dose by a factor of three to maintain stable cyclosporine concentrations. The oral solution can be administered diluted with chocolate milk or juice and administered through a nasogastric tube. The tube is flushed before and after cyclosporine is administered to ensure complete drug delivery and optimal absorption.

The microemulsion formulation of cyclosporine capsules and solution has increased bioavailability compared to the original formulation of cyclosporine capsules and solution. These formulations are not bioequivalent and cannot be used interchangeably. Converting from cyclosporine capsules and solution for microemulsion to cyclosporine capsules and oral solution using as 1:1 mg/kg/day ratio may result in lower cyclosporine blood concentrations. Conversions between formulations are made utilizing increased monitoring to avoid toxicity due to high concentrations or possible organ rejection owing to low concentrations.

Nephrotoxicity is cyclosporine's major adverse effect. Three types of nephrotoxicity have been shown to occur. The first is an acute reversible reduction in glomerular filtration; second, tubular toxicity with possible enzymuria and aminoaciduria; and third, irreversible interstitial fibrosis and arteriopathy. The exact mechanism of cyclosporine nephrotoxicity is unclear, but may involve alterations in the various vasoactive substances in the kidney. Other side effects include a dose-dependent increase in bilirubin that occurs within the first 3 months after transplantation. Hyperkalemia can develop secondary to cyclosporine nephrotoxicity. Cyclosporine-induced hypomagnesemia can cause seizures. Neurotoxic effects such as tremors and paresthesias may occur in up to 15% of treated patients. Hypertension occurs frequently and may be because of the nephrotoxic effects or renal vasoconstrictive effects of the drug. Cyclosporine is a narrow therapeutic index drug and thus levels are monitored and doses adjusted accordingly. The target levels are individualized based on type of transplant, time since transplant, and concurrent immunosuppressants.

Tacrolimus (FK506)

Tacrolimus is a macrolide antibiotic produced by the fermentation broth of *Streptomyces tsukubaensis*. Although it bears no structural similarity to cyclosporine, its mode of action parallels cyclosporine. Tacrolimus exhibits similar in vitro effects to cyclosporine, but at concentrations 100 times lower than those of cyclosporine.

Tacrolimus is primarily metabolized in the liver by the cytochrome P-450 isoenzyme 3A4 to at least 15 metabolites. There is also some evidence to suggest that tacrolimus may be metabolized in the gut. The 13-*O*-demethyl-tacrolimus appears to be the major metabolite in patient blood. Less than 1% of a dose is excreted unchanged in the urine of liver transplant patients. Renal clearance accounts for less than 1% of total body clearance. The mean terminal elimination half-life is 12 hours but ranges from 8 to 40 hours. Patients with liver impairment have a longer tacrolimus half-life, reduced clearance, and elevated tacrolimus concentrations. The elevated tacrolimus concentrations are associated with increased nephrotoxicity in these patients. Because tacrolimus is primarily metabolized by the cytochrome P-450 enzyme system, it is anticipated that drugs known to interact with this enzyme system may affect tacrolimus disposition.

In most cases, IV therapy can be switched to oral therapy within 2 to 4 days after starting therapy. The oral dose starts 8 to 12 hours after the IV infusion has been stopped. The usual initial oral dose is 150 to 300 mcg/kg/day, administered in two divided doses every 12 hours.

Nephrotoxicity is the most common adverse effect associated with the use of tacrolimus. Nephrotoxicity occurs in up to 40% of transplant patients receiving tacrolimus. Other side effects observed during tacrolimus therapy include headache, tremor, insomnia, diarrhea, hypertension, hyperglycemia, and hyperkalemia. Tacrolimus is a narrow therapeutic index drug and thus levels are monitored and doses adjusted accordingly. The target levels are individualized based on type of transplant, time since transplant, and concurrent immunosuppressants.

Sirolimus (Rapamycin)

Sirolimus is an immunosuppressive agent used for prophylaxis of organ rejection in patients receiving renal transplants. It typically is used in regimens containing cyclosporine and corticosteroids. Sirolimus inhibits T-lymphocyte activation and proliferation that occurs in response to antigenic and cytokine stimulation. Sirolimus also inhibits antibody production.

Sirolimus is administered orally once daily. The initial dose of sirolimus is administered as soon as possible after transplantation. It is recommended that sirolimus be taken 4 hours after cyclosporine modified oral solution or capsules.

Routine therapeutic drug level monitoring is not required in most patients. Sirolimus levels are monitored in patients with hepatic impairment, during concurrent administration of cytochrome P-450 cyp3a4 inducers and inhibitors, or when cyclosporine dosing is reduced or discontinued. Mean sirolimus whole blood trough concentrations, as measured by immunoassay, are approximately 9 ng/mL for the 2-mg/day dose and 17 ng/mL for the 5-mg/day dose. Results from other assays may differ from those with an immunoassay. On average, chromatographic methods such as HPLC or mass spectroscopy yield results that are 20% lower than immunoassay whole blood determinations.

SPECIAL DOSING CONSIDERATIONS

Drug Disposition in Older adults

Older adults are the fastest growing segment of the population in the United States. Older patients consume nearly 3 times as many prescription drugs as younger patients and therefore are at risk for experiencing significantly more drug-drug interactions and ADEs. The most common risk factors that contribute to adverse events include polypharmacy, low body mass, preexisting chronic disease, excessive length of therapy, organ dysfunction, and prior history of drug reaction. Often the clinical trials in which safe dosing ranges are established do not include subjects who are older adults so a usual dose in an older adult may have unintended effects. Special attention must be paid on the part of healthcare professionals when dosing medications in older adults with low body mass and potentially impaired metabolism and clearance of drug secondary to age-related organ dysfunction (eg, renal or hepatic impairment). Agents that are of particular concern include sedatives, antihypertensives, narrow therapeutic index drugs, and anti-infectives. These agents often require a decrease in dose or longer intervals between doses to facilitate drug clearance and minimize the likelihood of toxicity.

Therapeutic Drug Monitoring

Therapeutic drug monitoring (TDM) is the process of using drug concentrations, pharmacokinetic principles, and pharmacodynamics to optimize drug therapy (see Table 22-5). The goal of TDM is to maximize the therapeutic effect while avoiding toxicity. Drugs that are toxic at serum concentrations close to those required for therapeutic effect are the drugs most commonly monitored. The indications for TDM include narrow therapeutic range, limited objective monitoring parameters, potential for poor patient response, the need for therapeutic confirmation, unpredictable dose-response relationship, suspected toxicity, serious consequences of toxicity or lack of efficacy, correlation between serum concentration and efficacy or toxicity, identification of drug interactions, determination of individual pharmacokinetic parameters, and changes in patient pathophysiology or disease state.

The specific indication for TDM is important, because it affects the timing of the sample. Timing of sample collection depends on the question being asked. The timing of serum drug concentrations is critical for the interpretation of the results. The timing of peak serum drug concentrations depends on the route of administration and the drug product. Peak serum drug concentrations occur soon after an IV bolus dose, whereas they are delayed after IM, SC, or oral doses. Oral medications can be administered as either liquid or rapid- or slow-release dosage forms (eg, theophylline). The absorption and distribution phases must be considered when obtaining a peak serum drug concentration. The peak serum concentration may be much higher and occur earlier after a liquid or rapid-release dosage form compared to a sustained-release dosage form. Trough concentrations usually are obtained just prior to the next dose. Drugs with long half-lives (eg, phenobarbital) or sustained-release dosage forms (eg, theophylline) have minimal variation between their peak and trough concentrations. The timing of the determination of serum concentrations may be less critical in patients taking these dosage forms. Serum drug concentrations may be drawn at any time after achieving a steady state in a patient who is receiving a drug by continuous IV infusion. However, in patients receiving a drug by continuous infusion, the serum specimen is drawn from a site away from where the drug is infusing. If toxicity is suspected, serum drug concentrations can be obtained at any time during the dosing interval.

Appropriate interpretation of serum concentrations is the step that requires an understanding of relevant patient factors, pharmacokinetics of the drug, and dosing regimen. Misinterpretation of serum drug concentrations can result

---

ESSENTIAL CONTENT CASE

Tips for Calculating IV Medication Infusion Rates

Information Required to Calculate IV Infusion Rates to Deliver Specific Medication Doses

- Dose to be infused (eg, mg/kg/min, mg/min, mg/h)
- Concentration of IV solution (eg, dopamine 400 mg in D₅W 250 mL = 1.6 mg/mL; nitroglycerin 50 mg in D₅W 250 mL = 200 mcg/mL)
- Patient's weight

Case Question 1: Calculate the IV infusion rate in milliliters per hour for a 70-kg patient requiring dobutamine 5 mcg/kg/min using a dobutamine admixture of 500 mg in D₅W 250 mL.

- Dose to be infused: 5 mcg/kg/min
- Dobutamine concentration: 500 mg/250 mL = 2 mg/mL or 2000 mcg/mL
- Patient weight: 70 kg

Calculation:

5 mcg/kg/min × 70 kg = 350 mcg/min
350 mcg/min × 60 min/h = 21,000 mcg/h
21,000 mcg/h ÷ 2000 mcg/mL = 10.5 mL/h

Answer: Setting the infusion pump at 10.5 mL/h will deliver dobutamine at a dose of 5 mcg/kg/min.

Case Question 2: Calculate the IV infusion rate in milliliters per hour for a 70-kg patient requiring nitroglycerin 50 mcg/min in using a nitroglycerin admixture of 50 mg in D₅W 250 mL.

- Dose to be infused: 50 mcg/min
- Nitroglycerin concentration: 50 mg/250 mL = 0.2 mg/mL or 200 mcg/mL
- Patient weight: 70 kg

Calculation:

50 mcg/min × 60 min/h = 3000 mcg/h
3000 mcg/h ÷ 200 mcg/mL = 15 mL/h

Answer: Setting the infusion pump at 15 mL/h will deliver nitroglycerin at a dose of 50 mcg/min.

Case Question 3: Calculate the IV infusion rate in milliliters per hour for a 70-kg patient requiring heparin 18 units/kg/h using a heparin admixture of 25,000 units in D₅W 500 mL.

- Maintenance infusion: 18 units/kg/h
- Heparin concentration: 25,000 units/500 mL = 50 units/mL
- Patient weight: 70 kg

Calculation:

Infusion rate: Heparin 18 units/kg/h × 70 kg = 1260 units/h ÷ 50 units/mL = 25.2 mL/h

Answer: Setting the infusion pump at 25 mL/h will infuse the heparin at a dose of 18 units/kg/h.

in ineffective and, at worst, harmful dosage adjustments. Interpreting serum concentrations includes an assessment of whether the patient's dose is appropriate, if the patient is at a steady state, the timing of the blood samples, an assessment of whether the time of blood sampling is appropriate for the indication, and an evaluation of the method of delivery to assess the completeness of drug delivery. Serum drug concentrations are interpreted within the context of the individual patient's condition. Therapeutic ranges serve as guidelines for each patient. Doses are not adjusted on the basis of laboratory results alone. Individual dosage ranges are developed for each patient as various patients may experience therapeutic efficacy, failure, or toxicity within a given therapeutic range.

SELECTED BIBLIOGRAPHY

General

Clinical Pharmacology [database online]. Tampa, FL: Gold Standard, Inc. http://www.clinicalpharmacology.com. Accessed June 10, 2017.

Drug Information Handbook. 26th ed. Hudson, OH: Wolters Kluwer Clinical Drug Information, Inc; 2017.

Faust AC, Echevarria KL, Attridge RL, et al. Prophylactic acid-suppressive therapy in hospitalized adults: indications, benefits, and infectious complications. *Crit Care Nurse.* 2017;37:18-29.

Institute of Safe Medication Practices. www.ismp.org. Accessed June 2, 2017.

Martin SJ, Olsen KM, Susla GM. *The Injectable Drug Reference.* 2nd ed. Des Plaines, IL: Society of Critical Care Medicine; 2006.

Papadopoulos J. *Pocket Guide to Critical Care Pharmacotherapy.* 2nd ed. Philadelphia, PA: Springer; 2015.

Sulsa GM, Suffredini AF, McAreavey D, et al. *The Handbook of Critical Care Drug Therapy.* 3rd ed. Philadelphia, PA: Lippincott William and Wilkins; 2006.

Vincent J, Abraham E, Kochanek P, et al. *Textbook of Critical Care.* 7th ed. Philadelphia, PA: Elsevier; 2016.

Evidence-Based Practice Guidelines

Ageno WA, Gallus AS, Wittkowsky A, et al. Clinical practice guidelines for oral anticoagulant therapy: antithrombotic therapy and prevention of thrombosis. *Chest.* 2012;141:e44S-e88S.

Barr J, Fraser GL, Puntillo K, et al. Clinical practice guidelines for the management of pain, agitation, and delirium in adult patients in the intensive care unit. *Crit Care Med.* 2013;41:263-306.

Murray MJ, DeBlock H, Erstad B, et al. Clinical practice guidelines for sustained neuromuscular blockade in the adult critically ill patient. *Crit Care Med.* 2016;44:2079-2103.

O'Gara PT, Kushner FG, Ascheim DD, et al. American College of Cardiology Foundation/American Heart Association guidelines for management of ST-elevation myocardial infarction. Executive summary. *Circulation.* 2013;127:529-555.

Rhodes A, Evans LE, Alhazzani W, et al. Surviving sepsis campaign: international guidelines for management of severe sepsis and septic shock: 2016. *Crit Care Med.* 2017;45:486-552.

ETHICAL AND LEGAL CONSIDERATIONS 8

Sarah A. Delgado

KNOWLEDGE COMPETENCIES

1. Characterize the nurse's role in recognizing and addressing ethical concerns.

2. Recognize problems that warrant ethical analysis.

3. Identify the steps involved in analyzing an ethical problem.

4. Describe the influence of environment in resolving ethical problems and the nurse's contribution to the work environment.

Ethical problems are pervasive in progressive care settings. Serious illness and its treatment constrain patient autonomy and patients, families, and healthcare teams struggle to determine the ethical course of action when there is uncertainty about prognosis and patient outcomes. Healthcare team members experience moral distress when their own actions do not align with their professional values, and face ethical dilemmas when obligations to patients, employers, colleagues, and self suggest conflicting courses of action.

The first step to managing ethical problems is the recognition that they exist, referred to as ethical sensitivity. Because of the complexity of the healthcare environment, differentiating issues that require moral reasoning from other common problems such as poor communication, differences of opinion, or compassion fatigue can be challenging. Successful resolution of ethical issues depends on the ability to apply ethical decision-making skills and arrive at a conclusion about the right course of action. Whether or not that action is taken depends not only on the motivation of the individual nurse but also on the environment in which care is provided. This chapter introduces the elements that serve as a foundation for addressing ethical problems including professional codes and standards, institutional policies, and ethical principles. An approach to ethical decision making is described, and problems that commonly occur in

progressive care setting are discussed. The final section of this chapter looks at the work environment and its impact on the healthcare team's ability to navigate ethical issues.

TYPES OF ETHICAL PROBLEMS

The most often cited ethical problems in health care are ethical dilemmas, moral uncertainty, and moral distress. The problems are discussed here from the nurse's perspective but in reality, all members of the healthcare team face ethical problems. An ethical dilemma occurs when the nurse identifies two (or more) ethically acceptable but mutually exclusive courses of action. The dilemma is further complicated as either choice can be supported by a line of ethical reasoning, yet each also has undesirable consequences. In cases of moral uncertainty, a nurse recognizes that an ethical problem exists but is unable to identify the correct course of action. An analysis that includes considering all the possible actions, beyond those that conflict, can be helpful in resolving ethical dilemmas and moral uncertainty.

When the nurse experiences moral distress, on the other hand, there is little uncertainty about what course of action is correct but there is a profound inability to take that action. Internal factors such as fear of retribution and self-doubt can serve as the barrier to action. External factors that

TABLE 8-1. ETHICAL PROBLEMS

Type of Problem	Definition	Example
Ethical dilemma	The moral agent identifies two opposing but equally justifiably courses of action.	The manager asks the nurse to stay for an extra shift because someone on the next shift called out. The nurse planned to see a friend after work. On one hand, the nurse feels obligated to work the extra shift to ensure her patients are safe; at the same time, she recognizes a duty to herself and her friend to honor the prior commitment. She cannot both work the extra hours and see her friend—they are mutually exclusive but equally justifiable options.
Moral uncertainty	The moral agent is unable to determine what the right action is.	The nurse witnesses one family member verbally abusing another during their visit to a patient's room. The altercation does not affect the patient's care but does generate concern for the nurse. Is there an obligation to protect the vulnerable family member from this treatment? What action if any should be taken to prevent this from happening again?
Moral distress	A moral agent knows the right action to take but is unable to take that action.	An older adult with dementia and recurrent aspiration is scheduled for placement of a percutaneous endoscopic gastrostomy (PEG) tube for enteral nutrition. The nurse knows this treatment is inconsistent with current evidence, which shows that feeding tubes do not improve outcomes in patients with advanced dementia. However, the family has signed a consent form, the surgery is scheduled, and the nurse feels obligated to prepare the patient for the procedure.
Allocation of resources	A decision is required as to how to distribute a finite supply of goods or services across a group of people.	The principle of justice is the basis for allocation of resource problems, and organ transplantation, discussed in the section on justice, is one example of this kind of problem. Another example is when a hospital unit that provides a specific level of monitoring has one available bed and two patients, one in the operating room and one in the emergency room, who both require that level of care. Determining which patient will be admitted to the unit is an allocation of resources decision.
Locus of authority	Two or more individuals have a claim to the role of decision maker but do not agree on the course of action.	The patient's durable power of attorney for healthcare form indicates that both her adult daughters should make her healthcare decisions. They support opposing courses of treatment and it is unclear which course of action to take.

can constrain the nurse from taking action include hierarchies within the healthcare system that create power imbalances, lack of administrative support, and the presence or absence of hospital policies. While an ethical dilemma can lead the nurse to feel trapped between opposing courses of action, moral distress threatens their personal and professional integrity. Repeated episodes of moral distress can lead to the phenomenon of moral residue, in which the negative feelings engendered by an ethical problem are compounded by the unresolved feelings from past similar experiences. More research on moral residue and its effect on nurses in acute care settings are needed. Table 8-1 provides the definition and examples of other types of ethical problems encountered in healthcare settings.

ESSENTIAL CONTENT CASE

Diagnosing Moral Distress

In selecting a topic for a graduate school assignment, Karen chose idiopathic pulmonary fibrosis, inspired by a patient, Adeline, she cared for in the intermediate medical intensive care unit (IMICU), in room 576. Adeline was 66 years old and on high flow nasal cannula oxygen when Karen first met her and learned that she was a retired nurse. They chatted briefly about Adeline's career and her family while the patient awaited transfer to the operating room (OR) for a lung biopsy. Following the procedure, Adeline was intubated and sedated and Karen, rounding with the pulmonary team a few days later, learned that the biopsy showed a rare and very aggressive form of the disease. Over the subsequent week, Adeline's hypoxia worsened, and she was unable to undergo spontaneous breathing trials or sedation interruption without her oxygen saturation dropping to the low 80s. In a family conference, Adeline's sons presented the team with an advanced directive, which stated that in the event of a poor prognosis, Adeline did not desire life-sustaining measures such as mechanical ventilation.

After much discussion, the family elected to remove Adeline from the ventilator. Because she had a chance to know Adeline, even very briefly, and to relate to her, Karen feels distressed observing her adult children as they grieve their loss. "This doesn't seem right" she thinks, "it's just so sad." After tearfully describing the situation to a colleague who is kind and gives her a hug, Karen decides she wants to learn more about this disease process.

A month later, Karen is working nights and is again assigned to room 576. The patient, Gabriel, is a 55 year old who was admitted that day with a diagnosis of sepsis. The nurse from dayshift reports that she placed a urinary catheter, but no urine is draining from it. "But" she tells Karen "I know it's in, right? He's a man, after all!" After the dayshift nurse leaves, Karen finds that one of the antibiotics prescribed STAT and documented as administered is still hanging on the IV pole and has not infused. Furthermore, the patient complains of severe abdominal pain and a strong urgency to urinate.

Karen removes the catheter and a stream of blood and urine are released. Based on the patient's history, she theorizes that an enlarged prostate impeded passage of the catheter into the bladder, and the balloon was actually inflated in the urethra, causing trauma. Karen feels angry at the treatment her patient received and consults the charge nurse for guidance. The charge nurse points out that the nurse on the prior shift had a really tough day and asks that Karen not mention what happened. She advises "You know what's it like to have a bad day, don't you? You don't want her to get in trouble for that and leave and then we're short staffed!" Karen feels distressed and does not know where to go for support. She is certain that the patient was harmed by the dayshift nurse's negligence and she feels obligated to protect him and other patients from further harm, but she is compelled to remain silent based on the guidance she was given by the charge nurse.

Case question 1: How is the distress Karen experienced in these two situations different?

Case Question 2: How does identifying the form of distress help Karen?

Answers
1. In both of these cases, Karen felt a sense of distress but the source of her distress is profoundly different. In the first situation, Karen felt emotional distress witnessing the grief engendered by the untimely death of a patient whom she briefly related to through a shared profession. In acute care settings, emotionally distressing situations happen often. In the second scenario, Karen's distress was due to her inability to act in the way she felt was right (formally reporting the errors). Furthermore, because her silence about her colleague's care was inconsistent with her professional values, her integrity suffered, and shame ensued, creating an additional barrier to discussing the problem and getting support.
2. Distinguishing between emotional distress and moral distress is essential for the same reason that making an accurate diagnosis of the cause of shock is essential. The strategies to address these problems and their outcomes are very different. In the first scenario, Karen's emotional distress was alleviated by support from a friend and her own determination to learn more about the disease. Adeline's death seemed "not right" but nothing in that situation compelled Karen to act in a manner that she felt was wrong. With Gabriel, Karen felt complicit in the harm he suffered because she did not speak up about her colleague's negligence. Her professional integrity is threatened when she cannot take the action she believes to be right. Ethical analysis would not help Karen manage the emotional distress of caring for Adeline, but perhaps it could help her to navigate the moral distress she experienced with Gabriel.

THE FOUNDATION FOR ETHICAL DECISION MAKING

Professional Codes and Standards

The purpose of professional codes is to identify the moral requirements of a profession and the relationships in which they engage. The *Code of Ethics for Nurses* developed by the American Nurses Association (ANA) articulates the essential values, principles, and obligations that guide nursing actions. The nine provisions of the ANA *Code of Ethics for Nurses* identify the ethical obligations of nurses and are applicable across all nursing roles (American Nurses Association, Code of Ethics for Nurses with Interpretive Statements, 2015. http://nursingworld.org/DocumentVault/Ethics-1/Code-of-Ethics-for-Nurses.html). While these provisions do not address specific ethical problems, they do provide a framework for examining issues and understanding the nurse's role in resolving them. The nurse's primary obligation to the patient, their role in patient advocacy, their contribution to the work environment, and the duty to self are among the provisions in the *Code of Ethics for Nurses*.

In addition to the ANA *Code of Ethics for Nurses*, nurses function in accordance with particular standards of practice. Professional organizations and statutory bodies delineate the standards that govern the practice of nursing in various jurisdictions. Derived from nursing's contract with society, professional nursing standards define the criteria for the assessment and evaluation of nursing practice. External bodies, such as state boards of nursing, impose certain regulations for licensure, regulate the practice of nursing, and evaluate and monitor the actions of professional nurses. Many organizations also delineate standards of practice for registered nurses practicing in a defined area of specialty; for example, the American Association of Critical-Care Nurses (AACN) establishes expectations of performance for nurses practicing in acute and critical care and documents these in *the Scope and Standards for Acute and Critical Care Nursing Practice*.

Standards of practice outlined by statutory bodies and specialty organizations are not confined to clinical skills and knowledge. Nurses are expected to function within the profession's code of ethics and are held morally and legally accountable for unethical practice. When allegations of unsafe, illegal, or unethical practice arise, the regulatory body serves to protect the public by investigating and disciplining the culpable professional. Although specialty organizations do not have authority to retract professional licensure, issues of professional misconduct are reviewed and may result in revocation of certification and notification of external parties.

Institutional Policies

Because nurses practice within organizations, institutional policies and procedures also guide their practice. Institutional guidelines such as those for assessing decision-making capacity, caring for unrepresented patients who lack capacity, or policies for the determination of brain death are intended to guide employees of a healthcare facility when they are faced with ethical uncertainty. These policies usually reflect expectations congruent with the professional codes of ethics. However, in some circumstances, organizations may assume a particular position or value and therefore expect the employees to uphold this position; for example, some hospitals endorse particular religious values and may prohibit professional practices that violate these positions. Ideally, the nurse and institution have complementary values and beliefs about professional responsibilities and obligations.

Institutions often provide internal resources to help clinicians resolve difficult ethical issues. Ethics committees provide consultation on challenging situations and institutional policies can provide guidance and support to nurses who are uncertain about the correct action to take. Other resources for progressive care nurses include colleagues with additional training in ethics, physicians, nurse managers, and advanced practice nurses. While the ANA code states that nurses act as advocates for patients, finding support is an essential step in that process.

Legal Standards

Public policies and state and federal laws also influence the practice of healthcare professionals. Agencies such as the Centers for Disease Control and Prevention (CDC) or the Department of Health and Human Services (DHHS) generate changes in practice and in the actions of health professionals. For example, the CDC maintains and updates the list of notifiable conditions, mostly infectious diseases, so that their incidence can be tracked, and offers guidelines on the use of transmission-based precautions such as contact or droplet isolation. In addition, the Centers for Medicare and Medicaid Services (CMS), a major payer for health care, set standards for hospitals and providers that must be abided to ensure reimbursement for services. State legislation can also influence acute care nursing practice. For instance, in the event that a patient does not designate, through an advance directive, a surrogate decision maker, state law guides the selection of a family member to serve in this role. States differ in their recognition of unmarried domestic partners and the right of a partner to serve as the medical decision maker when a patient is rendered incapable by illness or injury.

The Affordable Care Act (ACA) passed in 2010 requires hospitals to report quality indicators, such as the rate of hospital-acquired infections (CMS, 2010). This legislation ties these indicators to Medicare reimbursement. The ACA thus creates financial incentives for hospital systems to implement strategies to prevent infection as a complication of hospital admission. In this way, the ACA offers a legal manifestation of the ethical principle of non-maleficence, discussed below. The Health Information Portability and Accountability Act (HIPAA) Privacy Rules similarly create a legal mandate to honor the ethical obligation of confidentiality.

When faced with an ethical problem, the professional codes, institutional policies, or legal standards can assist, and sometimes resolve, the issue. Thus, it is imperative that nurses

be familiar with these resources and how to access them. However, nurses also need to recognize that guidelines and policies and even the law do not always answer the question of what the ethical course of action is. In such situations, the nurse must be prepared to identify the ethical principles involved and follow a step-wise approach to addressing the problem.

Principles of Ethics

One of the most influential perspectives in biomedical ethics is that of principle-based ethics. This framework arose in the 1970s through the work of Beauchamp and Childress and continues to be a dominant method of bioethical thinking today. Inherent in this viewpoint is the belief that some basic moral principles define the essence of ethical obligations in human society. Four basic principles, and derivative imperatives or rules, are considered *prima facie* binding. In other words, to breach a principle is wrong unless there are prevailing and compelling reasons that outweigh the necessary infringement. The principles and rules are binding, but not absolute.

Because many approaches to ethics integrate the rules and principles outlined by the principle-oriented approach, it is helpful for nurses to understand these fundamental concepts. The primary principles used are nonmaleficence, beneficence, justice, and respect for persons (or autonomy). The derivative principles or rules include privacy, confidentiality, veracity, and fidelity.

The principles are not ordered in a particular hierarchy, but their application and interpretation are based on the specific features of the ethical problem and the values of the team members involved. Articulating the principles involved and recognizing the personal values of the providers and family members are essential steps to resolving an ethical problem.

Nonmaleficence

The principle of nonmaleficence imposes the duty to do no harm. This injunction suggests that the nurse should not knowingly inflict harm and is responsible if negligent actions result in detrimental consequences. In general, a nurse upholds the principle of nonmaleficence by maintaining competence and practicing within accepted standards of care.

When the patient's safety or well-being is threatened by the actions of others, the nurse is obligated to act. Knowledge of unsafe, illegal, or unethical practice by any healthcare provider obligates the nurse both morally and legally to intervene. The nurse must remove the immediate danger and communicate the infringement to the appropriate sources to prevent further harm. The nurse can turn to institutional policies and their state's nurse practice act for guidance on the appropriate process of reporting.

Beneficence

The ethical principle of beneficence affirms an obligation to promote good by actively helping others to advance and realize their interests. In health care, understanding the values and preferences of the patient and family is intrinsic to this principle. The duty to do good requires that the healthcare team understand the patient's interpretation of what is "good" and nurses, because of their relationship with patients and the time spent in close proximity with them and their families, are often in the best position to assess their perspective. When nurses are able to incorporate their understanding of the patient's wishes into the care they deliver, the principle of beneficence is honored.

Respect for Persons (Autonomy)

The principle of respect for persons or autonomy affirms the freedom and right of an individual to make decisions and choose actions based on that individual's personal values and beliefs. In other words, an autonomous choice is an informed decision made without coercion that reflects the individual's underlying interests and values. To respect a person's autonomy is to recognize that patients may make choices and take particular actions that are incongruent with the values of the healthcare providers. In some cases, this concept is difficult to accept and endorse, particularly when the patient's choice conflicts with the caregivers' view of what is best in this situation.

Patients in acute care settings frequently have varying degrees of autonomy. The capacity of ill patients to participate in decisions is often compromised by the severity of their disease and by its treatment. External factors, such as the hospital environment, also influence the patient's ability to make autonomous choices. The nurse advocates for the patient by limiting, as much as possible, the factors that constrain the patient's freedom to make autonomous choices. In this way, the nurse supports the principle of respect for personal autonomy.

Justice

The principle of justice is defined as fairness and is often applied to the manner in which goods, burdens, and services are distributed among a population. When resources are limited, justice demands that they be fairly allocated. There are three interpretations of the justice principle that will be described here by the following example. Imagine a population of people who have a set of goods that must be shared fairly among them. (1) *Egalitarian justice* would demand that the goods be divided into equal portions and every member of the population given the same share. (2) *Humanitarian justice* would demand that the goods be divided according to the needs of each member, with the neediest members getting larger portions. (3) *Libertarian justice* would demand the goods be distributed according to the contributions made by each member of the population; those making the greatest contributions get the greater share.

Organ transplantation offers one example of the justice principle in health care. Organs are a scarce resource and some of those listed for transplant will not survive the wait. Priority for transplant can be based strictly on time spent waiting (an egalitarian approach), or on illness severity (a humanitarian approach), or based on assessment of an individual's contributions and potential contributions to society (libertarian approach).

On a day-to-day basis, nurses make decisions involving the allocation of nursing care—which patient to assess first or how to assign patients on the unit to the staff on the next shift. The complex and competing demands for nursing resources can lead to chaotic and random decisions. The principle of justice argues for a comprehensive, thoughtful approach to address competing claims to resources.

Privacy and Confidentiality

Privacy and confidentiality are associated, but distinct, concepts that are derived from the principles of respect for autonomy, beneficence, and nonmaleficence. Privacy refers to the right of an individual to be free from unjustified or unnecessary access by others. In acute care settings, the patient's privacy is sometimes disregarded. The design of many units includes easy visualization of patient rooms, and in their focus on addressing life-limiting illness, the healthcare team may assume that open access to the patient is for the best. The principle of privacy is honored when nurses request permission from the patient or family for any bodily intrusion or physical exposure. The casual infringement of an individual's privacy erodes trusting and caring nurse-patient relationships and contributes to the view of the patient as something other than an autonomous being.

Confidentiality refers to the protection of information. When the patient shares information with the nurse or any member of the healthcare team, the information should be treated as confidential and discussed only with those directly involved in the patient's care. Exceptions to confidentiality include quality improvement activities, mandatory disclosures to public health agencies, reporting abuse, or required disclosures in a judicial setting. Intentional disclosures of information obtained in a confidential manner take place only when strong and compelling reasons to do so exist such as when there is risk of harm to others. When possible, the patient is made aware of the impending disclosure, and ideally provides permission.

Violations of patient confidentiality may occur inadvertently. Casual conversations in hallways or elevators in which patient information is shared within earshot of strangers and unauthorized release of patient information to friends or family constitute a breach in confidentiality. The electronic health record (EHR) also introduces opportunities for violations of confidentiality, such as when a user does not log out of the system and patient information displayed on the computer screen can be viewed by anyone passing by.

Fidelity

Fidelity is the obligation to be faithful to commitments and promises and uphold the implicit and explicit commitments to patients, colleagues, and employers. The concept of fidelity is particularly important in progressive care. The vulnerability of seriously ill patients increases their dependency on the relationship with the nurse, thus making the nurse's faithfulness to that relationship essential. Nurses demonstrate faithfulness by fulfilling the commitments of the relationship, which include the provision of competent care and advocacy on the patient's behalf. In addition, the nurse is obligated to demonstrate fidelity in relationships with colleagues and employers. In this way, the principle of fidelity can be difficult to uphold as institutions may have policies, such as those related to resource utilization, that the nurse finds are in conflict with the patient's best interests. When confronted with such situations, the nurse is wise to carefully weigh the ethical principles involved, to seek guidance if necessary, and to consider a role as an advocate for change if appropriate.

Veracity

The rule of veracity simply means that one should tell the truth and not lie or deceive others. Derived from the principle of respect for persons and the concept of fidelity, veracity is fundamental to relationships and society. The nurse-patient relationship is based on truthful communication and the expectation that each party will adhere to the rules of veracity. Deception, misrepresentation, or incomplete disclosure of information undermines and erodes the patient's trust in healthcare providers.

Patients expect that information about their condition will be relayed in an open, honest, and sensitive manner. Without truthful communication, patients are unable to make fully informed decisions. However, the complex nature of acute illness does not always manifest as a single truth with clear boundaries. Uncertainty about the course of the illness, the appropriate treatment, or the plan of care is common in progressive care and a single "truth" may not exist. As emphasized in patient-centered care, patients or surrogate decision makers must be kept informed of the plan of care and areas of uncertainty should be openly acknowledged. Disclosure of uncertainty enables the patient or surrogate to realistically examine the proposed plan of care and reduces the likelihood that the healthcare team will proceed in a paternalistic manner.

Paternalism

In ethics, paternalism refers to instances in which the principle of beneficence overrides that of autonomy. In such cases, healthcare providers select and implement interventions that they believe will lead to the best outcomes without (or even against) consent from the patient. There are limited instances in which these actions are appropriate. An example of paternalism in progressive care is the use of mitts to prevent removal of an intravenous line. The action of placing the mitts imposes a limitation on the patient's autonomy but is justified by the benefit of ensuring patient safety. However, interventions that restrict patient autonomy are only applied with careful consideration. In some cases, an acceptable alternative is to explain the rationale for the intervention and then seek input from the patient or family to determine if the proposed care fits with their priorities and goals.

Nurses may find the balance between the patient's autonomy and the duty to promote good difficult and confusing. In the acute care setting, it is often unclear what actions or course of treatment will most benefit the patient physiologically and which plan best reflects the patient's values. This lack of certainty may result in fragmented discussions with the patient or surrogate and a treatment plan that reflects the values of the healthcare team rather than the patient. The nurse's moral obligation is to continue to promote the patient's interests by pursuing an accurate representation of the patient's beliefs and values, and to raise concerns of conflicting interpretations to appropriate members of the healthcare team.

Frameworks for Ethical Analysis

While principle-based approaches to ethics have strong roots, there are other frameworks for examining ethical problems. A full description of these approaches is beyond the scope of this chapter; however, an awareness of the variety of approaches to ethical problems is essential to collaborative decision making. The Essential Content Case "Applying Different Approaches to Ethical Problems" and Table 8-2

TABLE 8-2. FRAMEWORKS FOR ETHICAL ANALYSIS

Name	Emphasis	Application	Example From Case
Principle-based approach	Identifying and prioritizing ethical principles	The right action is determined through detached analysis of relevant ethical principles	Both the pulmonologist and the hospitalist identify specific principles as guiding the action they believe should be taken
Duty based	Acting in a manner consistent with primary duties and obligations	The right action is the one that best upholds the primary duty of the moral agent	Pulmonologist: "My duty is to the parents and to honor their autonomy. We should allow them time to determine when to change the goals of care"
Utilitarian	Achieving the best possible outcome of the situation	The right action will result in the greatest good for the greatest number	Hospitalist: "We should initiate comfort measures so that the healthcare team is not distressed by the care they are providing"
Care based	Protecting the relationships at risk in the situation	The moral agent's best option is the action that recognizes and preserves key relationships	Nurse "We should transfer the patient to the unit that knows him and his parents best"
Feminist	Addressing power inequity in the situation	The right action will correct power imbalances and promote the interest of vulnerable parties	Social worker "We should try to transfer the patient home because the patient's mother has the least power"

provide a general overview of some common frameworks and an example of how they are applied. The nurse, as a member of the healthcare team, recognizes that other team members and patients and families may adopt different approaches when faced with the same ethical problem. Active listening and open-ended questions enable the nurse to recognize the approach adopted by another provider or family member and this recognition improves communication and ultimately promotes resolution of the ethical problem.

Ethic of Care

One framework for ethics that is viewed as an alternative to the principle-based approach and particularly resonates with nurses is the ethic of care. Rather than distinguishing the ethical dilemma as a conflict of principles, the ethic of care emphasizes the important relationships in a case and identifies the correct ethical action as the one that preserves those relationships.

Carol Gilligan (1987) first described the phenomenon of using relationships to identify moral actions by observing how children make ethical decisions. While some children adhere to rules (eg, "do not steal," "do not lie"), others consider how an action will affect others involved (eg, hurt feelings, loss of trust or respect). These ways of thinking carry through to adulthood. Most adults can view a situation through both the rules lens and the relationship lens.

The ethic of care begins from an attached, involved, and interdependent position. From this standpoint, morality is viewed as caring about others, developing relationships, and maintaining connections. Moral problems result from disturbances in interpersonal relationships and disruptions in perceived responsibilities. The resolution of moral issues emerges as the involved parties examine the contextual features and embrace the relevance of the relationship and the related responsibilities.

In contrast, a principle-oriented approach typically originates from a position of detachment and individuality. This approach recognizes the concepts of fairness, rights, and equality as the core of morality. Therefore, dilemmas arise when these elements are compromised. From this perspective, the approach to moral resolution is a reliance on formal logic, deductive reasoning, and a hierarchy of principles.

For nursing, the ethic of care provides a useful approach to moral analysis. The professional values of nursing emphasize attachment, caring, attention to context, and the development of relationships. To maintain this position, nurses develop proficiency in forming and sustaining relationships with patients and within families. The importance of relationships is also suggested in the first provision of the *Code of Ethics for Nurses*. The ethic of care legitimizes and values the emotional, intuitive, and informal interpretation of moral issues. This perspective expands the sphere of inquiry and promotes the understanding and resolution of moral issues.

ESSENTIAL CONTENT CASE

Applying Different Approaches to Ethical Problems

Pablo is a 24 year old with cystic fibrosis, who has had repeated admissions with pneumonia. He is admitted to the progressive care unit (PCU) from the general medical unit with respiratory compromise. He has been hospitalized eight times in the past year for respiratory infections, malnutrition, and other complications of his chronic disease, and on one admission was intubated for 6 days due to pneumonia. On this admission, he is found to have flu. Pablo and his parents, who are divorced and schedule their visits to avoid one another, have a longstanding relationship with a pulmonologist and during a recent outpatient visit made a collaborative decision that Pablo would not undergo intubation again, unless for the purpose of lung transplant surgery. He recollects the experience and it terrifies him. They are aware that Pablo's prognosis is increasingly poor, and though he is listed for a lung transplant, he may not survive the wait for the surgery, particularly given his nutritional state and recurrent admissions.

In the PCU, Pablo is started on noninvasive mechanical ventilation and initially improves but cannot tolerate the switch to high flow nasal cannula. After 3 days in the PCU, the hospitalist requests a meeting with Pablo's parents, and the nurse and the social worker also attend. After the hospitalist describes the measures being taken to support Pablo, the parents explain the decision they have made regarding intubation. At that point, the pulmonologist, who knows the family

well, arrives and the hospitalist states her recommendation that Pablo begin on comfort measures, including a morphine drip to address his breathlessness. Pablo's dad, who is physical therapist so has additional understanding of healthcare interventions, initially looks resigned, then slowly nods. Pablo's mother becomes upset and states "If he is really going to die, I need to take him home." To this, Pablo's father states "You always want to take him away from me, but you can't do that this time. Don't you get it? He is too sick to go anywhere!" The mother, still crying, replies angrily "You always want to make this about us, but this is about him!" and leaves the conference room. The father then turns to the team and states "I get it, he is really dying this time. But I don't think his mother will ever accept that." In a separate conversation with the patient's mother, she tells the team "we can start him on the medication if that's what's best, but I want to take him home first."

The members of the healthcare team all witness the same situation, but they interpret it through different ethical frameworks and arrive at different conclusions as to how to proceed.

Case Question 1: How would a principle-based approach apply to this situation?

Case Question 2: What is the correct action to take if this case is examined from a care-based perspective?

Answers

1. The hospitalist views the situation from a principle-based approach and considers her primary obligation to the team currently caring for Pablo. She, therefore, proposes establishing a day and time for switching to comfort measures, preferably when both parents are visiting. She believes this action is supported by several ethical principles: *beneficence*—her desire to do what is best for her patient and *nonmaleficence*—to prevent any complications of hospitalization. In addition, she notes that continuing to watch the patient, delirious, struggling to breath and becoming increasingly weak will cause distress among the healthcare team whereas initiating a morphine drip will make everyone, the patient, the parents, and the healthcare team more comfortable with his impending death. In this way, the hospitalist's perspective emphasizes principles and considers the greatest good for the greatest number, a utilitarian approach.

   The pulmonologist, who has known the family longer than anyone else, advises waiting for a few days to see if the parents can get on better terms with each other. He has seen them come together periodically throughout their son's illness and thinks this might happen again. Like the hospitalist, he feels that the principles of beneficence and nonmaleficence support initiating comfort measures. However, he believes his primary duty is to honor the parents' autonomy and that this is best accomplished by allowing them time to arrive at the appropriate decision. He is not concerned with the PCU team's distress. Because he focuses primarily on his duty to protect the parents' autonomy, he arrives at a different conclusion about the right course of action.

2. The social worker adopts a care-based perspective. He observes that the father's occupation puts him in a position to speak to the healthcare team as an equal while the

mother's relationship with the healthcare team is more tenuous. During rounds, he hears one member of the healthcare team describe the idea of transferring the patient home as "hopelessly unrealistic." His approach is to address the power imbalance in these relationships, an approach referred to as feminist ethics. He begins exploring resources to see if transferring the patient home is indeed feasible, to correct the imbalance of power in the parents' relationships with the healthcare team.

   The nurse also takes a care-based approach and she focuses on the relationships between the parents and the patient. By asking open-ended questions and actively listening, she learns that the father is unwelcome in the home his ex-wife and his son share. Pablo's mother, at the same time, feels a strong desire to honor the request her son has repeatedly made throughout his many hospital admissions: "I want to go home." After learning more about each parent's perspective, she proposes a different course of action: transfer the patient to the general medicine floor where he has been cared for during his many admissions. Both parents speak in positive terms about their relationships with the staff there, and the staff's prior knowledge enables them to accommodate the parents' mutual desire to be with their son despite the bitterness between them. While the patient will not be home, as the mother desires, this unit is closer to being a home to him than the PCU and the move to this setting does not affect the father's ability to visit.

   This case illustrates how professionals adopting different ethical frameworks can arrive at different conclusions about the right course of action. It also offers an example of ethical creativity, which is required in difficult situations, particularly in ethical dilemmas where opposing courses of action are justified. What is needed in such situations is often more options.

Patient Advocacy

Patient advocacy is an essential role of the nurse, as emphasized in provision 3 of the *Code of Ethics for Nurses*. Although there are many models for defining and interpreting the relationship between the nurse and the patient and no model can thoroughly describe its complexity and uniqueness, the patient advocacy role offers an essential description of the moral nature of this relationship.

The term advocacy refers to the use of one's own skills and knowledge to promote the interests of another. Nurses, through their education and experience, are able to interpret healthcare information and understand the impact of disease and medical interventions in a unique way. A nurse acts as a patient advocate by applying this unique understanding to ensure that the patient's beliefs and values guide the plan of care. The nurse does not impose personal values or preferences when acting as an advocate, but instead guides the patient or surrogate decision maker through values clarification, identification of the patient's best interests, and the process of communicating decisions. Thus, the patient or surrogate is empowered by the nurse to participate in the healthcare plan.

Assuming the role of patient advocate is not without risk. Nurses may find that obligations to oneself, the patient, the patient's family, other members of the healthcare team, or the institution are in conflict and have competing claims on nursing resources. These situations are intensely troubling to nurses and the support of colleagues is essential to resolving these dilemmas. In circumstances of conflict, nurses can clarify the nature and significance of the moral problem, engage in a systematic process of moral decision making, communicate concerns openly, and seek mutually acceptable resolutions. A framework within which to identify and compare options provides the necessary structure to begin the process of ethical resolution.

THE PROCESS OF ETHICAL ANALYSIS

When faced with ethical problems, nurses are more likely to achieve resolution if a consistent process is applied. A structured approach to ethical dilemmas reduces the risk of overlooking relevant contextual features and invites thoughtful reflection. While the individual nurse can hone and practice the skill of ethical analysis, a more robust process involves including others in addressing the issue. Through a casual conversation with a colleague or formal consult with an institution's ethics committee, nurses can engage others in discussing ethical problems and working toward a resolution. While there are a variety of ethical decision-making processes, the one described here mirrors the nursing process. The following steps are involved in case analysis.

Assessment

- Identify the problem. Is it an ethical dilemma? Is it moral distress? Is there moral uncertainty or a locus of authority concern? Clarify the competing ethical claims, the conflicting obligations, and the personal and professional values in contention. Acknowledge the emotional components and any communication issues. In some cases, the situation may have elements of more than one type of ethical problem. Consider using a resource, such as a colleague with experience in ethics consults or a member of the institution's ethics committee.
- Gather data. Distinguish the morally relevant facts, including any medical, nursing, legal, social, or psychological information. Clarify the patient's and family's beliefs and values.
- Identify the individuals involved in the problem. Clarify who is involved in the problem's development and who should be involved in the decision-making process. Consider any barriers the person or persons making the decision will face.

Plan

- Consider all possible courses of action and avoid restricting choices to the most obvious.
- Identify the risks and benefits likely to arise from each action.
- Analyze each course of action. In a principle-based approach, identify which principles support the alternative courses of action. In a care-based approach, consider the impact of each course of action on the existing relationships in the situation.
- Consult the *Code of Ethics for Nurses*, professional practice standards, or institutional policies for additional guidance. What action do these suggest is the right one?
- Seek input from the resources available to help with ethical problems. In many cases, this is an ethics consult service or an ethics committee. Any hospital that is accredited by the joint commission must have in place a mechanism for dealing with ethical issues.

Implementation

- Choose a plan and act. Communicate with identified sources of support and anticipate and prepare for objections from others

Evaluation

- Outline the results of the plan. Identify what harm or good occurred as a result of the action.
- Identify the necessary changes in institutional policy or other strategies to avoid similar conflicts in the future.

ESSENTIAL CONTENT CASE

Applying the Process

The patient, an 82 year old with hypertension, atrial fibrillation, multi-infarct dementia, and chronic kidney disease is admitted to the PCU following an ischemic stroke. Despite endovascular treatment, she continues to have right-sided weakness and impaired speech. The neurologist caring for her is concerned that she will not return to her baseline functional status. The patient's son with whom she lives is distraught and wants to stay at her bedside at all times. The unit has an open visitation policy but asks that all visitors wait in the waiting room during shift report, to allow nurses to exchange patient information without fearing that it will be inappropriately overheard. When asked to leave, the son becomes angry, and verbally abuses the nurse, Maria who is caring for his mother. When Maria attempts to reassure him that he can return after report, he throws the hairbrush he had been using with the patient towards her and storms out, punching the wall as he goes.

Sharon, the nurse on the next shift witnesses this behavior and becomes fearful of the patient's son. She recognizes her obligation to provide the best care possible to her patient and that best practice usually includes supporting family involvement. At the same, she notes that she has an obligation to herself, her team, and the other patients on the unit to maintain a safe and calm environment. She begins a deliberate analysis of the situation applying the nursing process.

Case Question 1: What information does Sharon need to gather?

Case Question 2: What kind of ethical problem is this?
A. Moral distress
B. Ethical dilemma
C. Ethical uncertainty
D. Locus of authority

Case Question 3: What options for action should Sharon consider?

Case Question 4: How can Sharon examine this problem using ethics?

Case Question 5: What steps are involved in implementing a chosen action?

Case Question 6: After taking action, what criteria will Sharon use to evaluate the outcome?

Answers

1. Important sources of guidance for Sharon include her unit's policy on visitation, and the institution's policy on managing potentially violent family members. Many organizations have de-escalation protocols or teams that can support nurses caring for potentially violent patients or families. Sharon can also seek input from her manager, particularly if there is no written policy that applies to this situation. Sharon can seek input from Maria about the son's behavior prior to this outburst and any assessment she has conducted regarding the son's understanding of the patient's prognosis. While the report she receives from Maria will also include clinical details, these may be less pertinent to the ethical analysis. Essentially, the patient has a poor prognosis, which is a key relevant fact. Ideally, Sharon can also gather information by asking the son questions, if he is calm and able to converse without presenting a threat.

2. Answer is option B. This problem, as Sharon frames it, is an ethical dilemma. She sees two opposing but equally justifiable options. The principle of beneficence and her obligation to provide the best possible care support allowing the son to visit the patient. However, she also has a duty to herself and to the other patients on the unit to prevent potential harm and this means asking the son not to visit. Sharon cannot both allow and not allow the son at the bedside.

3. Sharon recognizes that she must consider actions beyond the two that are in conflict. The following are some of the options she considers:
   - Tell the son he cannot visit the patient under any circumstances
   - Allow the son to visit, ignore his outbursts
   - Tell the charge nurse that she is uncomfortable with this assignment and cannot care for this patient
   - Talk to the manager about having hospital security on the unit in case the son becomes violent. Restrict the son to visiting only during hours when security is available
   - Allow the son to visit whenever he can but assess him at every point of contact for the risk of violent behavior
   - Contact the social worker for help creating a contract with the son that indicates strict parameters for his behavior. Any further violent outbursts will affect his visiting hours
   - Call a member of the pastoral care team to talk to the son about his feelings and appropriate outlets

   - Schedule a conference with members of the healthcare team and the son. Allow the son to verbalize his feelings. Offer emotional support but also explain how his behavior with Maria is inappropriate and cannot be repeated
   - Call a member of hospital administration to come to the unit and speak with the patient's son.

4. The next stage of the planning process is to examine the options through a selected framework. If Sharon adopts a principle-based approach and considers her primary duty to the patient, she may eliminate the options of telling the son he cannot visit under any circumstances or refusing to take the assignment. These options fail to meet the best interests of the patient. At the same time, simply ignoring the son's outbursts places her own safety at risk which violates her right to protection from harm. A principle-based approach may support the option of seeking a security presence on the unit or contracting with the son as these options uphold Sharon's duty to the patient and her duty to protect herself.

   A care-based perspective would examine these options based on their impact on the relationships in the situation. The relationship between the patient and the son is of course important; and is supported if this son is able to visit. The relationship between the son and the healthcare team is new and at risk due to the fear engendered by the son's outburst. Sharon determines that bringing the team together with the son is probably the best action to take to establish a better relationship. In discussing the situation with members of the healthcare team, she suggests that a family conference include assurance that the healthcare wants what is best for his mother, and a clear description of expectations with regard to his behavior.

5. In the course of applying a process for ethical analysis, taking the chosen action is an essential step. A key aspect of many of the options Sharon identified is that they involve other members of the healthcare team. Resolution of ethical problems is rarely through independent action and often involves collaboration with colleagues, patients, families, or members of the hospital administration. If Sharon is unable to take the chosen course of action due to resistance from her colleagues or other barriers, she is at risk for moral distress. Later in this chapter, there is further discussion of the work environment and its impact on achieving resolution of ethical problems.

6. Once action is taken, Sharon will evaluate the effect on all involved parties. Her goal in conducting the analysis and taking action was to provide the son appropriate access to the patient while also ensuring her own safety and the safety of her colleagues. If her evaluation shows that there are still gaps, for instance, if she or other members of the healthcare team continue to feel afraid of the son's violent behavior, additional action is needed.

CONTEMPORARY ETHICAL ISSUES

This section includes descriptions of informed consent, end-of-life care, and evolving technology which are some of the contemporary issues that generate ethical problems for the healthcare team. This is by no means an all-inclusive list but rather is intended to provide examples of how ethical analysis applies to situations that nurses working in progressive

care settings commonly encounter. Nursing interventions to respond to each issue are included.

Informed Consent

The term "informed consent" is often interpreted as the task of ensuring that the appropriate form is completed and signed. From the standpoint of bioethics, informed consent is not a task but a process by which the healthcare team honors the autonomy of patients and their families. There are four elements that encompass informed consent: disclosure, comprehension, voluntariness, and competence.

Disclosure and Comprehension

The healthcare team is obligated to disclose information about specific treatments or treatment plans in a manner in which the patient and family can understand. This can be challenging because healthcare treatments are complex and their risks and benefits are not easily understood. Furthermore, patients and families who are facing serious illness may experience anxiety that impairs comprehension. Strategies such as rewording the same information, offering written information, and asking the patient or family member to restate information in their own words can improve comprehension. Deliberating omitting information about a treatment, minimizing its risks or benefits, or failing to address questions from a patient or family threatens the integrity of the informed consent process and represents unethical professional behavior.

Voluntariness

Decisions by the patient and family must be reached voluntarily; any threat of coercion, manipulation, or duress is unethical. The language used to describe treatment options is carefully chosen to avoid subtle forms of coercion that reflect personal views and do not constitute objective descriptions of the treatment involved. Consider a family member making a decision about a do not resuscitate (DNR) order. If the provider describes cardiopulmonary resuscitation (CPR) as a potentially life-saving intervention without further details, the family member may feel compelled to refuse the DNR order. If instead, CPR is described as a violent procedure in which the patient will most assuredly suffer, the family member's inclination will be very different. To the extent possible, balanced and objective descriptions of interventions are provided to ensure the element of voluntariness in the consent provided by the patient and family.

Competence and Capacity

The final element of informed consent is competence. Competence is a legal term and reflects judicial involvement in the determination of a patient's decision-making capacity. Capacity reflects the ability of an individual to participate in the medical decision-making process. Capacity is not based on the ability to concur with healthcare providers or family members, or on cultural or religious beliefs. A functional standard that focuses on the patient's abilities as a decision maker and the consistency of their stated preferences is a better tool for measuring capacity. Many institutions have policies on determining capacity, and on managing patients who lack competence in decision making. Questioning the capacity of a patient or family member to make decisions is carefully considered, to avoid denying an autonomous individual input into decisions about their medical care.

When a patient lacks capacity due to illness or its treatment, a surrogate decision maker is assigned to provide informed consent. If the patient has assigned a friend or family member to the role of durable power of attorney for health care, that person is recognized as the surrogate decision maker. In the absence of documentation from the patient, state laws guide the designation of a family member to the role surrogate decision maker. In the event that no family is available, a guardian may be assigned to this role. The surrogate decision maker is not asked to make decisions based on their own values but rather to consider the values, goals, and preferences previously expressed by the patient and how they would respond, if they could, to the information given by the healthcare team.

In some cases, patients who have never had capacity require care: infants, children, and adults with disabilities that prevented them from expressing their preferences at any time in their lives. In those instances, the surrogate decision maker applies the best interests standard to the informed consent process, analyzing the burdens and benefits of treatment options to arrive at what is in the patient's best interests. This burden/benefit analysis includes considering the relief of suffering, restoration of function, likelihood of regaining capacity, and quality of an extended life in weighing options for treatment.

Principles of Management

Ideally, informed consent is comprised not only of documented conversations about specific treatments but also includes a series of interactions between the patient, family, and healthcare team to ensure a mutual understanding of the goals of care and strategies for achieving them. In this way, the healthcare team can disclose information at an appropriate pace, assessing the patient and family's comprehension and addressing questions as they arise.

Nursing interventions that uphold informed consent include:

- Providing and reinforcing information about disease, treatment options, risks, and benefits with patients and families.
- Honestly answering questions from patients and their families and consulting other members of the healthcare team for answers when needed.
- Using a teach back method in which decision makers are asked to restate in their own words the information given in order to assess their comprehension.
- Attending to environmental factors that impact disclosure and comprehension such as excess noise or inadequate seating. Seek private, quiet spaces for conversations about treatment options. When nurses and providers sit to talk to patients and families, they convey a willingness to listen and speak on an equal level.
- Taking time to consider and recognize personal views and opinions. If the family requests input in the form of "what would you do?" an honest answer can be

provided, but might be amended with the statement "I would make that choice because of who I am. But this is about you (or about your loved one)" to redirect the discussion around the values of the patient and their family.

- Choosing language carefully to increase comprehension and enhance voluntariness.
- Assuming that patients and families are competent to make decisions and provide support for their decision-making skills.
- Increasing interaction between the healthcare team and the patient by using alternative methods of communication with intubated patients and asking for medical translators when needed.

End-of-Life Issues

Providing end-of-life care is a common source of moral distress for nurses working in progressive care settings. When nurses participate in the use of life-sustaining measures for patients who derive little benefit from it, they may feel that they are complicit in causing harm and unable to pursue what they believe is the right course action. Conversely, patients and family members may decline treatment and generate similar distress among nurses who feel that such treatment would be of benefit to them. Ethical problems also arise when patients and families do not agree on the goals of care at end of life or when resources are not available to meet the needs of complex chronically ill patients as they approach end of life.

A wide range of circumstances contribute to the development of ethical problems during end-of-life care. This discussion reviews honoring patient preferences, decisions to forgo life-sustaining treatment, requests for potentially inappropriate care, symptom management, and decisions about resuscitation. Nursing management to promote ethical resolution is also described.

Honoring Patient Preferences

While nurses and the intraprofessional team uphold the doctrine of informed consent in all situations, discussions about end-of-life care have a unique complexity. Impending death is a source of duress for the patient, family, and healthcare team as they consider treatment options. Sometimes, seriously ill patients who are admitted to progressive care settings cannot actively participate in healthcare decisions because an altered mental status bars communication. Patients who do verbalize preferences about end-of-life care may identify specific circumstances such as who they want to be with and where they want to be, but they are less likely to speak of death itself as the desired outcome. Many times, preferences for end-of-life care are stated with the assumption that death will occur sometime in the distant future.

In addition, while some disease processes can be accurately predicted, many common chronic disorders such as heart failure, chronic obstructive pulmonary disease (COPD), and dementia impair quality of life but have an unpredictable impact on the duration of life. Healthcare teams may in fact provide end-of-life care, unwittingly, as they were not aware, until the patient's death, how near to dying the patient was. In such cases, even if the patient has established specific preferences regarding end-of-life care, the healthcare team may not recognize the appropriate point in time for altering the treatment plan to meet those goals.

Advance Directives

In addition to conversations with the healthcare team, patients also convey their preferences regarding end-of-life care through written documents such as advanced directives. Advance directives are statements made by an individual with decision-making capacity that describe the care or treatment he or she wishes to receive when no longer competent. Most states recognize two forms of advance directives, the treatment directive, or "living will," and the proxy directive. The treatment directive enables the individual to specify in advance his or her treatment choices and which interventions are desired. Usually treatment directives focus on CPR, mechanical ventilation, nutrition and hydration, and other life-sustaining technologies.

Proxy directives, also called the durable power of attorney for health care, expand the sphere of decision making by identifying an individual to make treatment decisions when the patient is unable to do so. The appointed individual, a relative or close friend, assumes responsibility for healthcare decisions as soon as the patient loses the capacity to participate in the decision-making process. Treatment decisions by the healthcare proxy are based on a knowledge and understanding of the patient's values and wishes regarding medical care. Most states have statutory provisions that recognize the legal authority of the healthcare proxy, and this individual is given complete authority to accept or refuse any procedure or treatment on behalf of a patient who lacks capacity.

The proxy directive has some important advantages over a treatment directive. Many treatment directives are valid only under certain conditions. Terminal illness or an imminent death are common requirements before the treatment directive is enacted and prognostic uncertainty may render this condition difficult to meet. Such restrictions are not relevant in proxy directives, where the sole requirement before the proxy assumes decision-making responsibility on the individual's behalf is that the patient lacks decisional capacity. Furthermore, the proxy directive enables the authorized decision maker to consider the unique features of the specific situation before arriving at a decision. A treatment directive may indicate refusal of mechanical ventilation, but a durable power of attorney speaking for the patient with a reversible acute respiratory process may consent to a trial of noninvasive ventilation. In this way, the benefits and burdens of proposed interventions are considered in partnership with the knowledge and understanding of the patient's preferences and values.

CONTEMPORARY ETHICAL ISSUES

Decisions to Forego Life-Sustaining Treatments

Grounded in the principle of patient autonomy, patients with capacity have the moral and legal right to forego life-sustaining treatments including mechanical ventilation, medications, surgery, dialysis, nutrition, and hydration. The right of a capable patient to refuse treatment, even beneficial treatment, must be upheld if the elements of informed consent are met and innocent or third parties are not injured by the refusal. Ongoing dialogue among the healthcare team, family, and patient is appropriate so that mutually satisfactory realistic goals are adopted. Patients must understand that refusal of treatment will not lead to inadequate care or abandonment by members of the healthcare team.

Conflicts regarding the discontinuation of life-sustaining treatments often reflect differences in values and beliefs. When patients or their surrogate decision makers choose to forego treatments that extend life, relinquishing the original goal of restoring health is sometimes difficult. Shifting to a paradigm that advocates for a calm and peaceful death requires the nurse to relinquish control and to change the treatment goals to promote comfort and support the grieving process. The intensity required to support the patient and family during the process of removing life-sustaining treatment must also be valued and appreciated by healthcare professionals in all settings.

Requests for Potentially Inappropriate Treatment

In some cases, surrogate decision makers request continued life-sustaining treatment which the healthcare team believes is burdensome and not beneficial for the patient. Frequently, the request for such treatment reflects the surrogate or patient's desire to be assured that "everything" is being done to manage the disease and restore health. Emotional, financial, and social concerns can motivate individuals to request nonbeneficial, and even harmful, treatments. In such situations, nurses advocate for the treatment plan that is most appropriate, based on their knowledge of the patient's prognosis, preferences, and the burdens and benefits that treatment options offer. Participating in providing care that constitutes an inappropriate treatment plan is a source of moral distress.

A complicated array of factors including advances in healthcare technology, the aging of the population, and increased attention to burn-out syndrome in clinicians have intensified efforts to address the distress that members of the healthcare team experience when they participate in providing potentially inappropriate treatment. An official policy statement from five critical care professional organizations, including AACN, offers recommendations such as proactive, routine communication with the families of critically ill patients, early consultation with palliative care or ethics services, and institutional procedures for conflict resolution when disagreements in the plan of care persist. While this statement was created to address the issue of requests for inappropriate treatment in critical care settings, the

TABLE 8-3. RECOMMENDED PRACTICES FOR IMPROVING COMMUNICATION AND SUPPORT FOR SURROGATES IN THE INTENSIVE CARE UNIT

Systems Level Interventions

Conduct regular, structured interprofessional family meetings

Integrate palliative care and/or ethics teams into care for difficult cases

Provide printed educational materials to family

Maintain dedicated meeting space for ICU family meetings (and ensure adequate seating)

Clinician-Level Skills

Coordinate an effective family meeting

Establish consensus among treating clinicians before the meeting

Use a private, quiet space for family meetings

Introduce all participants

Use patient/family-centered communication strategies (see below)

Affirm nonabandonment and support family decisions

Provide family-centered communication

Elicit surrogates' perceptions first

Use active listening skills and deliver information in small chunks

Respond to questions and check for understanding of key facts

Acknowledge and address emotion

Support religious/spiritual needs and concerns

Foster shared decision making

Assess clinical prognosis and degree of certainty

Evaluate surrogate preferences for decision-making responsibility

Elicit the patient's treatment preferences and health-related values

Data from Bosslet GT, Pope TM, Rubenfeld GD, et al: An Official ATS/AACN/ACCP/ESICM/SCCM Policy Statement: Responding to Requests for Potentially Inappropriate Treatments in Intensive Care Units, Am J Respir Crit Care Med. 2015 Jun 1;191(11):1318-1330.

recommendations are applicable to most acute care settings, including progressive care. Table 8-3 lists the system level and clinician-level recommendations from that statement.

Symptom Management

When faced with a potentially life-limiting disease process, issues regarding symptom management also arise. Although palliation, the relief of troubling symptoms, is a priority in the care of all patients, once the decision to forego life-sustaining measures is made, palliation becomes the main focus of care. In some circumstances, patients experience distressing symptoms despite the availability of pharmacologic agents to manage the uncomfortable effects of chronic and terminal illness. Whether due to a lack of knowledge, time, or a deliberate unwillingness to prescribe or administer the necessary medication, inadequate symptom management is unethical. Nurses are obligated to ensure that patients receive care and treatments that are consistent with their choices. At the same time, nurses rely on provider colleagues to prescribe medications and order consults, such as for a palliative care service. A disagreement in which the nurse believes a particular order is justified and the provider does not agree can become an ethical problem, if effective communication between the two parties is absent.

Conflict can arise when patients require large doses of medications, such as narcotics, to effectively alleviate their

ESSENTIAL CONTENT CASE

The Patient's Wishes

An 82 year-old man, Mr. Johnson, is transferred to the PCU after a protracted stay in the surgical intensive care unit (ICU). The patient underwent emergent aortic aneurysm repair 3 weeks ago and due to underlying health problems including Parkinson disease, he had a slow recovery. At the time of transfer, he has a tracheostomy and requires frequent suctioning due to a weak cough. He also has a percutaneous endoscopic gastrostomy (PEG) tube for enteral feedings and oral medications and a peripherally inserted central catheter (PICC) line for intravenous medications. In report, the ICU nurse states that Mr. Johnson follows simple commands and has tolerated sitting upright for up to 30 minutes at a time. He has one adult daughter who served as his surrogate decision maker during his ICU stay.

After getting the patient settled into his PCU bed, the nurse briefly leaves the room to enter his information into the monitoring system. When she returns, she hears his daughter saying "No Daddy, we can't take that tube away. You need that! Just be patient, you'll be all better and back home again soon." When the nurse asks the daughter if everything is okay, she replies "Oh yes. He gets confused sometimes. He was just mouthing to me that he wants me to take the tubes away. He doesn't understand that he can't live without them." The nurse asks Mr. Johnson questions which confirm that he is oriented to person, place, time, and his plan of care. She then asks if he has any pain. Mr. Johnson shakes his head to indicate no, and then points to the tracheostomy, and waves his hand away from his chest, as if to request that the tube be removed.

Case Question 1: What factors need to be considered to evaluate Mr. Johnson's capacity in requesting removal of his tracheostomy tube?

Case Question 2: What guidance can Mr. Johnson's nurse offer to his daughter to help her in her role as surrogate decision maker?

Answers

1. Knowing that Mr. Johnson is oriented and able to follow simple commands confirms his mental status but not his capacity. One way to determine capacity is to assess the consistency of behavior, values, and beliefs over time. Asking his daughter if Mr. Johnson ever expressed a view on mechanical ventilation or other forms of life support might help determine if this perceived wish for removal of the tracheostomy tube is consistent with his past views. If Mr. Johnson has written an advanced directive, that document may also be helpful in demonstrating his past views which can then be compared to his communication now. If, in fact Mr. Johnson makes similar requests repeatedly and these statements are consistent with past beliefs and values, then even if he is not oriented to place or time, he may in fact have the capacity to contribute to decisions about his care.

2. Because the nurse is meeting the daughter for the first time, providing emotional support is an important first step. Noting that the last 3 weeks must have been hard and allowing the daughter time to talk about her experiences in the ICU helps to develop a relationship between the daughter and the progressive care team. Once this is established, the nurse can offer guidance on the surrogate decision maker role. Surrogate decision makers take in the information provided by the healthcare team and view it through the lens of the patients' goals and values. While her love for her father may lead her to hope for a complete recovery, her obligation to him now includes being his voice. This means thinking about this illness from his perspective and listening to any communication he provides about his response to it. The nurse can encourage the daughter to recall conversations in which he may have indicated his preferences regarding resuscitation, life support, and the use of medical hydration and nutrition.

symptoms. Legally and ethically, nurses must refrain from actions that hasten death and the side effect of respiratory depression may have an impact on the time of death. The essential element in this situation is the nurse's intent in providing the medication. When the intent is to relieve pain and suffering, and not to deliberately hasten death, the action is morally justified. The concept that supports this reasoning is called the principle of double effect. This principle states that if an action has both a good and bad effect, a person is justified in taking that action if the intent was the good effect, the bad effect was a possible but not certain outcome of the action, and there was no additional course of action which could produce the good effect and avoid the bad one. The US Supreme Court cited the principle of double effect in a decision that distinguished palliative care from assisted suicide. A provider who assists in a patient's death intends to cause that person's death, which is ethically and legally distinct from a provider who seeks to control symptoms and gives medications that may, inadvertently, hasten death.

Resuscitation Decisions

Acute and critically ill patients are susceptible to sudden and unpredictable changes in cardiopulmonary status. The presumption exists that, unless stated otherwise, resuscitation efforts will be instituted immediately upon cardiopulmonary arrest. In-hospital resuscitation is moderately successful, and delay in efforts significantly reduces the chance of the patient's survival. The emergent nature, the questionable effectiveness, and the presumed consent for CPR contribute to the ethical dilemmas that surround this intervention.

"Do not resuscitate" or "no code" are orders to withhold CPR. Other medical or nursing interventions are not influenced by a DNR order. In other words, the decision to forego CPR is not a decision to forego any other interventions. Appropriate discussions with the patient or surrogate must occur before a resuscitation decision is made. Open communication and a shared understanding of the treatment plan are essential to understanding and responding to the patient's interests and preferences. When the issue of resuscitation status is not addressed with the patient or surrogate or the decision is not documented or communicated, then a code is initiated, risking the provision of unwanted care.

Most institutions have policies that address the process of writing and implementing a DNR order. In addition, many states have an approved process and forms to indicate a desire to forgo life support so that this wish can be conveyed across all healthcare settings. Examples of such forms include the Durable DNR form in Virginia and the Physician Order for Life-Sustaining Treatment or POLST form in California. These forms play an essential role in preventing the provision of undesired care as patients are never capable of verbally refusing in the moment when the need for resuscitation arises.

Principles of Management

The application of primary palliative care is one strategy that can help mitigate the moral distress and ethical conflicts that arise in end-of-life care. While hospice is a set of services that patients with a poor prognosis can enroll in if they meet specific criteria for insurance reimbursement, palliative care is an approach that applies to all seriously ill patients. Specialists in palliative care provide extra support to patients, families, and the healthcare team; however, in some cases a palliative approach can be adopted by the team that is responsible for the patient's care without a specialist. Palliative care emphasizes symptom management, psychosocial support, and alignment of the patients' goals of care with the treatment plan. Skills in palliative care can be applied to patients even when the prognosis is uncertain, thus circumventing the issue of identifying an appropriate time for changing the goals of care. Below is a list of nursing interventions that can be used to implement a palliative care approach and may be helpful in preventing or resolving ethical problems in end-of-life care:

- Take advantage of the close proximity that nurses have with the patient and family and seek to know the patient as a person
- Use open-ended questions and statements such as "tell me more" to clarify patient values and beliefs
- Share information about patients and families and goals of care with other members of the healthcare team
- Participate in family conferences to offer additional support to patients or their surrogate decision makers and to reinforce information about prognosis that is conveyed during the meeting
- Clarify personal preferences with regard to the use of life-sustaining treatment and listen as other healthcare team members, patients, and families explain alternative preferences
- Collaborate with other members of the healthcare team to plan for the discontinuation of life-sustaining treatment when goals of care change

- Use medications and nonpharmacologic strategies for a multimodal approach to symptom management (see Chapter 6 [Pain Management/Sedation] for more on this)
- Be aware of patients' wishes regarding resuscitation efforts whether expressed verbally, through a surrogate decision maker, or in an advanced directive, or other state-specific documentation such as a MOLST form (Medical Order for Life-Sustaining Treatment)
- Seek professional development opportunities that offer training in palliative care

Evolving Technology

Technology not only affects the care that patients receive, it also has implications for how that care is documented, and how healthcare team members communicate with each other and with patients. Because of the rapid pace of innovation, professional codes, state and federal laws, and institutional policies may not yet address all the issues that advance in technology introduce. While application of technology is an opportunity to improve the delivery of health care, the application of ethical analysis to address concerns about its use is warranted.

Advances in Healthcare Technology

All approaches to ethics seek to answer the questions "What should we then do?" and this is a particularly pertinent question when applied to healthcare technology that extends life without ensuring quality of life. Examples of past advances include hemodialysis and left ventricular assist devices (LVADs), both of which were conceived as interventions to maintain life until definitive treatment in the form of a kidney or heart transplant took place. The use of these technologies in patients as an ongoing treatment rather than a bridge to transplant means that patients experience an additional burden of treatment in order to derive the benefit of a longer lifespan. For many patients, this is tolerable, but in the event that the patient's existence with these kinds of interventions does not meet their individual definition of quality of life, they have a right to refuse such therapy or to discontinue it after it has begun. Honoring the doctrine of informed consent, the healthcare team must ensure that the patient and family understand both the risks and benefits of technology-driven care, their impact on the disease and on the patient.

In progressive care settings, patients with a complex mix of health problems often require an extensive array of healthcare technology. For instance, an older patient with coronary artery disease and chronic lung disease who develops sepsis may require invasive monitoring, mechanical ventilation, consults with specialists, and a long period of rehabilitation when the acute phase resolves. Restoration to the prior functional status may not be feasible if the patient's age and underlying health conditions have compromised his resiliency. Moral uncertainty may surface in the healthcare team around the justice of using resources in this way, particularly given the unequal distribution of healthcare resources in our society.

There is additional uncertainty around some forms of technology, such as continuous renal replacement therapy (CRRT) and extracorporeal membrane oxygenation (ECMO) because the evidence to support their use remains mixed. The application of these interventions is appropriate if they meet the mutual goals of the patient, the family, and the healthcare team, but careful consideration and extensive discussion is warranted, particularly when the patient's prognosis is poor.

Electronic Health Record

In 2011, the Medicare and Medicaid Electronic Health Record Incentive Program, established by the Centers for Medicare & Medicaid Services, began offering incentives for hospitals and providers who demonstrated meaningful use of EHRs. These incentives lead to the rapid replacement of traditional pen and paper charting with electronic documentation in most healthcare settings. The use of EHRs can improve quality of care for patients by providing some protection against errors and facilitating communication across healthcare settings. However, because incentives drove this implementation, many EHR systems were designed to meet federal requirements for meaningful use and not necessarily designed around healthcare work flow. For some members of the healthcare team, EHR implementation became a source of moral distress; they were compelled to spend their time learning and using a new system of documentation, and unable to fulfill their primary obligation to patients.

While EHR appropriately facilitates sharing patient information among the healthcare team, storing patient information electronically also creates risks. Individuals with access to the EHR who view information about patients they are not caring for are violating patient privacy, a circumstance that arises when public figures become patients. Whole groups of patients are affected when systems that house EHRs are hacked. An additional concern is the "copy forward" strategy for documentation that offers a short cut for entering patient information and introduces the risk that the note does not reflect the patient's current status but is information carried over from previous patient interactions. To address this problem, some institutions have eliminated the copy forward function completely. The EHR is thus an example of healthcare technology with the potential to improve the delivery of care and at the same time, introduce new ethical problems that require thoughtful and deliberate action.

Social Media

Another example of technology advancing before guidelines for its use are established is social media, which includes internet-based social networks, blogs, wikis, and podcasts. These forms of communication can be beneficial in allowing healthcare professionals to share ideas or patients and families to garner support from those who are geographically distant. However, the use of social media also introduces ethical problems for nurses and other members of the healthcare team. The ease of transmitting information to a large audience with a single post means that inappropriate communication about a patient or colleague has a much broader impact. Violations range from intentional bullying of colleagues to unintended disclosure of patient information when seeking emotional support after a challenging shift. The ability to create photos or videos with a smart phone also introduces a risk for violating patient privacy.

Patient and family use of social media can generate problems for the healthcare team. Reliance on blogs or wikis for health information becomes a barrier to effective patient education and impacts trust between nurse and patient. Patients and families may also seek to contact members of the healthcare team through social networks such as Facebook or Twitter. Online relationships of this kind can erode the boundaries between the nurse's personal and professional lives. Patients and families may use social media to learn private information about a nurse or they may expect the nurse to provide support that exceeds the parameters of the nurse's professional role.

Principles of Management

This discussion provides an overview of some of the ways in which technology impacts ethical problems in health care. Further innovations are likely to advance healthcare delivery but will also require careful consideration to determine the full range of impact on patients and the healthcare team. Some strategies for nurses that facilitate resolution of the ethical problems generated by evolving technology include:

- Use peer-reviewed journals and clinical practice guidelines to develop and maintain an accurate understanding of the indications for the technology you use
- Be honest with patients and families when they ask about the effectiveness of healthcare technology
- When uncertain about the use of a particular intervention or procedure, ask providers to clarify the rationale and expected outcome of the treatment
- Refer to hospital policies on the use of EHRs and avoid inappropriately accessing patient information
- Be deliberate in turning away from the computer to make eye contact with patients and families, observe their nonverbal communication, and demonstrate your interest in their needs
- Review the American Nurses' Association Social Networking Principles Toolkit which includes a poster of six key tips for guidance on the appropriate use of social media
- Avoid sharing information about specific patient situations in any electronic format other than the EHR

BUILDING AN ETHICAL ENVIRONMENT

While the information in this chapter provides the basis for recognizing and analyzing ethical problems, evidence shows that that the environment has a profound effect on nurses' ability to resolve ethical problems. A nurse may approach an ethical dilemma, such as the one described in the case "Applying the Process" above, with the intention of exploring all possible alternatives, using ethical creativity and motivated to take the action that ethical analysis supports. However, if factors within the environment such as incivility, lack of leadership, inadequate staffing, or hierarchical structures are barriers to action, the nurse's ability to preserve professional integrity is threatened. Multiple studies show that nurses who rate their work environments as unethical are more likely to experience moral distress. When nurses feel unable to take action because of features in their environment, they are at risk for moral distress whenever an ethical concern arises. Furthermore, nurses who experience moral distress repeatedly are unlikely to meet their obligation to contribute to building an ethical work environment.

Healthy Work Environments

The AACN Standards for Establishing and Sustaining Healthy Work Environments provide a framework for identifying the elements of the environment that promote effective resolution of ethical problems. As shown in the Figure 8-1, the six standards, skilled communication, true collaboration, authentic leadership, effective decisions making, meaningful recognition, and appropriate staffing are not isolated characteristics but interdependent features that collectively contribute to an environment in which members of the healthcare

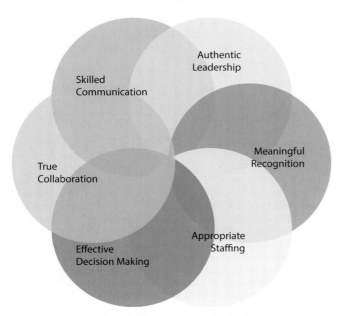

Figure 8-1. AACN's model for creating a Healthy Work Environment.

TABLE 8-4. PERCENTAGE OF RESPONDENTS WHO REPORTED EXPERIENCING MORAL DISTRESS[a]

	2006	2008	2013
Very frequently	6.8	5.6	9.4
Frequently	19.4	17.6	23.3
Occasionally	45.6	45.3	42.8
Very rarely	28.2	31.5	24.5

[a]*Because of rounding, percentages may not total 100. All changes from 2008 to 2013 are significant at P less than .05.*
Data from Ulrich B, Lavandero R, Woods D, et al: Critical Care Nurse Work Environments 2013: A Status Report, Crit Care Nurse *2014 Aug;34(4):64-79.*

team are able to make their maximum contribution to patient care. Environments in which these standards are practiced are not free of ethical problems but when those problems arise, there are mechanisms for responding. A national survey of nurses confirmed the link between moral distress and perceptions of the work environment. A troubling finding in this survey was an increase in the frequency of reported moral distress compared to similar surveys conducted in the past (Table 8-4). The essential content case "The Impact of the Environment" describes how one situation is handled differently when it occurs in different environments.

Principles of Management

The attributes of a work environment are not static; they can change over time. Furthermore, the environment is not an entity in and of itself, it is a compilation of the attitudes and behaviors of the people who work there. Provision 6 of the *Code of Ethics for Nurses* describes the nurses' obligation to contribute to an ethical work environment. Novice nurses do this by learning from their preceptors, recognizing ethical problems and seeking assistance appropriately. Experienced nurses are role models for skilled communication and true collaboration, expecting that members of the intraprofessional team will respond in kind and include them in decisions that affect their work. Below are some actions that nurses can take to help address the health of their work environment:

- Engage in values clarification to better understand what guides personal and professional commitments. Help families and patients to clarify their values as well.
- Use open-ended questions to understand the perspectives of your colleagues, patients and families. Recognize their use of different ethical frameworks and the principles they prioritize.
- Identify strategies such as journaling or talking to a friend or mentor for examining situations that lead to moral distress. There is no way to change past experiences but there may be opportunities to reframe them.
- Recognize the unique perspective that nursing brings to the healthcare team through their relationship with

The Impact of the Environment

Henrietta is a 72-year-old woman who has been transferred four times between the PCU and the cardiac ICU. In the month since her admission with a large anterolateral myocardial infarction (MI), she has suffered from heart failure, pulmonary edema, hypotension, and renal failure. While at times her cardiovascular status has improved, and she has made progress weaning from mechanical ventilation, she has also had periods of hemodynamic instability which led to transfer back to the ICU. Currently, she requires noninvasive mechanical ventilation, intermittent hemodialysis, continuous infusion of a low dose inotrope through a PICC line, and anxiolytics on an as-needed basis. She becomes hypotensive when efforts are made to address her immobility, and while she makes eye contact to her name, she does not consistently follow simple commands and will not use the communication board to convey her needs. Her husband and her son visit often and seem to be supportive but are also overwhelmed by this sudden change in her health.

The nurses caring for Henrietta in the PCU are concerned that their care is prolonging Henrietta's inevitable death. Rhonda, the patient's primary nurse on dayshift, asks the physician, Dr. Smith, if a family conference should be planned. Dr. Smith responds that he has spoken to the family several times and "They just don't seem to get it. I think it's a waste of time to schedule another meeting. We'll just keep going until she codes, I guess." Rhonda is uncomfortable with this plan. Here are two possible outcomes of this situation that differ based on the work environment:

Healthy work environment

Rhonda uses skilled communication to engage the physician in further conversation. Using a professional tone, she states "I understand that you feel that a family meeting is a bad use of time but I am concerned that we are not caring for our patient appropriately. Is this a good time for me to share my thoughts with you?" By restating what the physician has said, she demonstrates an understanding of his perspective. By referring to "we" and "our" she conveys her desire to collaborate in the management of this patient. Because Rhonda's communication is professional and clear, Dr. Smith agrees to talk further. "What are your thoughts?" he asks.

Rhonda recalls a presentation on palliative care communication skills that she attended, as part of the hospital's meaningful recognition program. She suggests "maybe instead of trying to explain to them how sick she is, we should ask them what they think she feels about all this. I think we need to better understand what the patient would want." After a 5-minute conversation, Dr. Smith and Rhonda agree to plan a family conference for the following day.

When the time for the conference arrives, Rhonda asks the charge nurse to cover for her, so they can meet in the unit conference room. The charge nurse, Susan, replies that she cannot cover Rhonda's patients, as she is already covering for a nurse who has to take a patient to radiology. Recognizing that the meeting is important to Rhonda and her patient, Susan suggests that the doctor and Rhonda speak to the family in an empty patient room. "We have an admission coming, but he won't be up for at least two more hours. That way, you can still be on the unit in case we need you." Rhonda agrees, and the charge nurse asks a nursing assistant to move extra chairs into the empty room so that Rhonda, the physician, and both family members can all sit.

Per the decision that Dr. Smith and Rhonda reached on the prior day, Rhonda starts the meeting with an open-ended question. She asks "Can you tell us a little more about Henrietta? We know about this illness but in order to make the right choices about her care we need to know more about her as a person." In prior interactions, neither man said more than a few words but with this invitation to talk about their wife and mother, they begin to speak with great affection. "You know, we've been married almost 50 years, and I've never seen her sit still for more than a few minutes. She is always on the go. You all must be giving her a lot of medicine to make her lie there all the time." The physician sees an opening to provide information about Henrietta's disease and states "The medicines can help her stay calm but she is also very sick." "Will she get better soon?" the son asks. And Rhonda, recalling another palliative care communication skill from the lecture she attended, replies "We hope she will get better, but we are worried that she will never be as healthy as she was before the heart attack." The husband, tears in his eyes, asks "So you're saying she might not be back to herself even after all this is over?" Rhonda instinctively takes his hand and nods "That is exactly what we are saying. And we need your help to understand what Henrietta would say about that."

Unhealthy work environment

Rhonda, having experienced moral distress when patients who clearly had a poor prognosis underwent CPR feels a surge of anxiety when the doctor suggests this will happen to Henrietta. Because other interactions between nurses and doctors in this unit have been characterized by incivility and mutual disrespect, she avoids further conversation with Dr. Smith. She continues to feel troubled by the care she is providing, however, and so decides that she will broach the issue with the family herself the following day. She wishes that she had been able to attend a conference on talking to patients about end-of-life care, but her request was denied. The nurse manager is dealing with the unit's short staffing by limiting the number of schedule requests that staff can make.

The next day, Rhonda is in the patient's room when the spouse and son arrive and ask her for an update. She wants to answer honestly and begin a discussion that will allow her to help her patient, but she is unsure how to do so. She explains the bilevel positive airway pressure (BiPAP) settings, the fluid balance, and the rate of the inotropic drip. The family nod but it is unclear how much of this information they take in. At that moment, Dr. Smith arrives and asks the family to wait in the waiting room while he examines the patient. Still troubled, Rhonda seeks the advice of the charge nurse, Susan but finds her totally overwhelmed and in need of support herself "We have a road trip today and an admission coming in a couple of hours and it's such pain that I'm in charge!" Just then the unit manager approaches to ask Rhonda why the family members are in the waiting room. "You know, we've already been written up for not adhering to the open visitation policy. You have to let the family stay in the room when they visit!" she tells Rhonda. Rhonda returns to Henrietta's room and completes her shift, mechanically providing the necessary nursing care.

Case Question 1: Which of the Healthy Work Environment standards were evident in the first version of the case?

Case Question 2: Which of the healthy work environment standards were notably absent in the second version of the case?

Answers

1. Rhonda used skilled communication when she spoke to the doctor, the charge nurse, and the family. In addition, true collaboration took place in her work with the doctor and with the charge nurse. The charge nurse demonstrated authentic leadership in supporting Rhonda's desire for the family meeting and helping her identify a strategy to have the meeting despite the staffing constraints. Rhonda experienced meaningful recognition when the hospital provided a professional development opportunity. Effective decision making occurred when the doctor invited Rhonda's input on how to approach the family meeting and they decided, together on the flow of the meeting.

2. In the second case, there is evidence that poor communication is pervasive in the unit. Rhonda has experienced this in the past, and the charge nurse demonstrates this by venting openly about her role rather than seeking honest input into how she can manage the challenges she is facing. The manager's decision to limit staff access to professional development and her reprimand of Rhonda without hearing her side of the story are evidence that authentic leadership is lacking. Rhonda's anxiety and fear, a result of negative past experiences in the work environment, are barriers to developing a collaborative relationship with the doctor. Because she does not receive the support she seeks, effective decision making is also absent.

Additional reflections:

- Imagine that you are Rhonda and reflect on how you would feel at the end of the shift in these two different versions of the story.
- Imagine that you are the patient's family and consider how the difference in work environment impacts your experience of Henrietta's illness.

the patient and family and their understanding of the impact of serious illness. Expect other members of the healthcare team to value this as well.

- Use inclusive language—"we" instead of "I" or "you" and "our" instead of "my" or "your." Such language signals a desire for shared decision making and collaborative action.
- Review the literature, attend conferences, and use resources available from professional nursing organizations to develop communication skills.
- Provide meaningful recognition when colleagues demonstrate attention to the work environment. A simple statement such as "I appreciated working with you in the care of this patient" is a clear acknowledgement of a collaborative relationship.
- Consider forming a group with your colleagues to complete AACN's Healthy Work Environment Assessment, a tool that helps identify gaps in the work environment that can then be addressed with targeted interventions.
- Work with a manager or hospital administrators on projects for formal recognition such as Magnet status through the American Nurse Credentialing Center or the Beacon Award through the American Association of Critical-Care Nurses.

SELECTED BIBLIOGRAPHY

American Journal of Nursing. State of the Science: Transfomring Moral Distress into Moral Resilience in Nursing. 2017;117 Supplement 1. https://journals.lww.com/ajnonline/toc/2017/02001.

Anderson WG, Puntillo K, Cimino J, et al. Palliative care professional development for critical care nurses: a multicenter program. *Am J Crit Care.* 2017;26:361-371.

Beauchamp TL, Childress JF. *Principles of Biomedical Ethics.* 7th ed. Oxford, England: Oxford University Press; 2012.

Centers for Medicare & Medicaid Services (2016). Electronic Health Records Incentive Program. https://www.cms.gov/Regulations-and-Guidance/Legislation/EHRIncentivePrograms/index.html?redirect=/EHrIncentivePrograms/. Accessed February 9, 2018.

DHHS Privacy Rule. http://www.hhs.gov/ocr/privacy/. Accessed February 15, 2018.

Doherty RF, Purtilo RB. *Ethical Dimensions in the Health Professions.* 6th ed. St. Louis, MO: Elsevier Saunders; 2016.

Epstein EG, Delgado S. Understanding and addressing moral distress. *Online J Issues Nurs.* 2010;15(3), Manuscript 1. http://www.nursingworld.org/mainmenucategories/ethicsstandards/courage-and-distress/understanding-moral-distress.html.

Gilligan C. Moral orientation and moral development. In: Kittay EF, Meyers DT, eds. *Women and Moral Theory.* New York: Rowman & Littlefield Publishers, Inc; 1987:19-33.

Hamric AB, Wocial LD, Epstein EG. Transforming moral distress into moral agency. Panel presentation. Minneapolis, MN: ASBH Annual Conference; 2011.

Hiler C, Hickman R, Reimer A, Wilson K. Predictors of moral distress in a US sample of critical care nurses. *Am J Crit Care.* 2018;27(1):59-66.

Kon AA, Davidson JE, Morrison W, et al. Shared decision making in ICUs: an American College of Critical Care Medicine and American Thoracic Society Policy Statement. *Crit Care Med.* 2016;44:188-201.

Lachman V. Social media: managing the ethical issues. *Medsurg Nurs.* 2013;22(5):326-329. http://www.nursingworld.org/MainMenuCategories/EthicsStandards/Resources/Social-Media-Ethical-Issues.pdf.

McBride S, Tietze M, Robichaux C, Stokes L, Weber E. Identifying and addressing ethical issues with use of electronic health records. *Online J Issues Nurs.* 2018;23(1), Manuscript 5. doi: 10.3912/OJIN.Vol23No01Man05.

Robichaux C, ed. *Ethical Competence in Nursing Practice*. New York: Springer Publishing Company; 2016.

Rushton CH. Moral resilience: a capacity for navigating moral distress in critical care. *Adv Crit Care*. 2016;27(1):111-119.

Ulrich B, Lavandero R, Woods D, Early S. Critical care nurse work environments 2013: a status report. *Crit Care Nurse*. 2014;34(4):64-79.

Ulrich C, Grady C, eds. *Moral Distress in the Health Professions*. New York: Springer International Publishing; 2017. https://link.springer.com/book/10.1007%2F978-3-319-64626-8.

Watcher R. *The Digital Doctor: Hope, Hype and Harm at the Dawn of Medicine's Computer Age*. New York: McGraw Hill; 2015.

Wocial LD, Hancock M, Bledsoe PD, Chamness AR, Helft PR. An evaluation of unit-based ethics conversations. *JONA's Healthc Law Ethics Regul*. 2010;12(2):48-54.

Professional Codes, Standards, and Position Statements

American Association of Critical-Care Nurses. AACN Scope and Standards for Acute and Critical Care Nursing. Aliso Viejo, CA: AACN. 2015. https://www.aacn.org/nursing-excellence/standards/aacn-scope-and-standards-for-acute-and-critical-care-nursing-practice.

American Association of Critical-Care Nurses. AACN Standards for Establishing and Sustaining Healthy Work Environments. 2nd ed. 2016. https://www.aacn.org/~/media/aacn-website/nursing-excellence/standards/hwestandards.pdf.

American Nurses Association. *Code of Ethics for Nurses*. 2015. http://www.nursingworld.org/MainMenuCategories/EthicsStandards/CodeofEthicsforNurses.

American Nurses' Association Social Networking Principles. http://www.nursingworld.org/FunctionalMenuCategories/AboutANA/Social-Media/Social-Networking-Principles-Toolkit.

Evidence-Based Guidelines

Bosslet GT, Pope TM, Rubenfeld GD, et al. An Official ATS/AACN/ACCP/ESICM/SCCM Policy Statement: Responding to Requests for Potentially Inappropriate Treatments in Intensive Care Units. *Am J Respir Crit Care Med*. 2015;191(11) 1318-1330. https://www.atsjournals.org/doi/abs/10.1164/rccm.201505-0924ST.

Davidson J, Aslakson RA, Long AC, et al. Guidelines for family-centered care in the neonatal, pediatric and adult ICU. *Crit Care Med*. 2017;45(1):103-128. https://journals.lww.com/ccmjournal/Fulltext/2017/01000/Guidelines_for_Family_Centered_Care_in_the.12.aspx.

National Consensus Project for Quality Palliative Care. *Clinical Practice Guidelines for Quality Palliative Care*. 3rd ed. Pittsburgh, PA; 2013. https://www.hpna.org/multimedia/NCP_Clinical_Practice_Guidelines_3rd_Edition.pdf.

Online References of Interest: Related to Legal and Ethical Considerations

American Association of Critical Care Nurses Webinar Series: "Palliative Care in the ICU: Critical Communication Skills. https://www.aacn.org/education/webinar-series?topic=PalliativeEOL.

American Nurses Association Ethics Resources. http://www.nursingworld.org/ethics/. Accessed February 16, 2018.

The Hastings Center. http://www.thehastingscenter.org/. Accessed February 15, 2018.

U.S. National Library of Medicine, Bioethics Information Resources. https://www.nlm.nih.gov/bsd/bioethics.html. Accessed February 15, 2018.

PATHOLOGIC CONDITIONS

II

CARDIOVASCULAR SYSTEM

9

Barbara Leeper

KNOWLEDGE COMPETENCIES

1. Identify indications for, complications of, and nursing management of patients undergoing coronary angiography and percutaneous coronary interventions.

2. Describe the etiology, pathophysiology, clinical presentation, patient needs, and principles of management of patients with ischemic heart disease.

3. Discuss the indications for, complications of, and management of patients undergoing electrophysiology studies.

4. Discuss the etiology, pathophysiology, clinical presentation, patient needs, and principles of management of patients in shock, heart failure, and hypertensive crisis.

SPECIAL ASSESSMENT TECHNIQUES, DIAGNOSTIC TESTS, AND MONITORING SYSTEMS

Assessment of Chest Pain

Obtaining an accurate assessment of chest pain is an important aspect of differentiating cardiac chest pain from other sources of pain (eg, musculoskeletal, respiratory, anxiety). Ischemic chest pain, caused by lack of oxygen to the myocardium, must be quickly identified for therapeutic interventions to be effective. The most important descriptors of ischemic pain include precursors of pain onset, quality of the pain, pain radiation, severity of the pain, what relieves the pain, and timing of onset of the current episode of pain that brought the patient to the hospital. Each of these descriptors can be assessed using the "PQRST" nomogram (Table 9-1). This nomogram prompts the clinician to ask a series of questions to help identify the characteristics of the chest pain.

Coronary Angiography

Coronary angiography is a common and effective method for visualizing the anatomy and patency of the coronary arteries. This procedure, also known as cardiac catheterization, is used to diagnose atherosclerotic lesions or thrombus in the coronary vessels. Cardiac catheterization is also used for evaluation of valvular heart disease, including stenosis or insufficiency, atrial or ventricular septal defects, congenital anomalies, and cardiac wall motion abnormalities (Table 9-2).

Procedure

Prior to cardiac catheterization, the patient is kept NPO for at least 6 hours, to minimize the risk of aspiration in the event that emergency intubation is required during the procedure. NPO may indicate everything except medications, which are taken with small sips of water the day of the procedure. Typically, if the patient is on insulin or taking oral hypoglycemics the doses may need to be adjusted or held the day of the procedure. There are other medications that may need to be held. Benadryl may be administered prior to beginning the procedure as a precautionary measure against allergic reaction to the dye. Unfractionated heparin and platelet inhibitor agents (including aspirin, glycoprotein IIb/IIIa receptor inhibitors, and/or clopidogrel) may be administered to prevent catheter-induced platelet aggregation during the procedure. Typically, patients remain awake during the procedure, allowing them to facilitate the catheterization process by controlling respiratory patterns (eg, breath

213

TABLE 9-1. CHEST PAIN ASSESSMENT

	Ask the Question	Examples
P (Provoke)	What *provokes* the pain or what precipitates the pain?	Climbing the stairs, walking; or may be unpredictable—comes on at rest
Q (Quality)	What is the *quality* of the pain?	Pressure, tightness; may have associated symptoms such as nausea, vomiting, diaphoresis
R (Radiation)	Does the pain *radiate* to locations other than the chest?	Jaw, neck, scapular area, or left or right arm
S (Severity)	What is the *severity* of the pain (on a scale of 1-10)?	On a scale of 1-10, with 10 being the worst, how bad is your pain?
T (Timing)	What is the *time of onset* of this episode of pain that caused you to come to the hospital?	When did this episode of pain that brought you to the hospital start? Did this episode wax and wane or was it constant? For how many days, months, or years have you had similar pain?

holding during injection of radiopaque dye to improve the quality of the image). An anxiolytic agent, such as diazepam, is frequently administered during the procedure to decrease anxiety or restlessness.

An intracoronary catheter is inserted through a "sheath" or vascular introducer placed in a large artery, most commonly the femoral artery (Figure 9-1A). In recent years there has been an increase in the use of the radial artery as catheters have been made smaller, allowing easier access to the vessel. If inserted via the femoral artery the catheter is then advanced into the ascending abdominal aorta, across the aortic arch, and into the coronary artery orifice located at the base of the aorta (Figure 9-1B). Ionic dye, visible to the observer or operator under fluoroscopy (x-ray), is then injected into the coronary arterial tree by the catheter. If the cardiac valves, septa, or ventricular wall motion is being evaluated, the catheter is advanced directly into the left ventricle, followed by injection of dye (Figure 9-1C). During a right heart catheterization, the catheter is inserted into the

TABLE 9-2. INDICATIONS FOR CARDIAC CATHETERIZATION

Right Heart
- Measurement of right-sided heart pressures:
  - Suspected cardiac tamponade
  - Suspected pulmonary hypertension
- Evaluation of valvular disease (tricuspid or pulmonic)
- Evaluation of atrial or ventricular septal defects
- Measurement of A-VO$_2$ difference

Left Heart
- Diagnosis of obstructive coronary artery disease
- Identification of lesion location prior to CABG surgery
- Measurement of left-sided heart pressures: Suspected left heart failure or cardiomyopathy
- Evaluate for wall motion abnormalities
- Evaluation of valvular disease (mitral or aortic)
- Evaluation of atrial or ventricular septal defects

venous system via the femoral vein and advanced into the inferior vena cava, passed through the right ventricle, and advanced into the pulmonary artery.

Interpretation of Results

The coronary vascular tree consists of a left and a right system (Figure 9-2). The left system consists of two main branches, the left anterior descending (LAD) artery and the left circumflex (LCx) artery. The right system has one main branch, the right coronary artery (RCA). Both systems have a number of smaller vessels that branch off these three primary arterial vessels. An obstruction of 75% or more in a major coronary artery or one of its major branches is considered clinically significant stenosis. If there is significant disease in only one of the major arteries, the patient is said to have single-vessel disease. If two major vessels are affected, the patient has two-vessel disease. If significant disease exists in all three major coronary arteries then the patient has three-vessel disease. Frequently, the microvasculature, or smaller vessels branching off the major coronary artery, may also have blockages. It is common to refer to these multiple lesions as diffuse disease.

A cineventriculogram is obtained by radiographic imaging during the injection of dye after advancing the catheter from the aorta, through the aortic valve, and into the left ventricle (see Figure 9-1C). The cineventriculogram provides information on ventricular wall motion, ejection fraction, and the presence and severity of mitral regurgitation and aortic regurgitation. Ejection fraction, or the percentage of blood volume ejected from the left ventricle with each contraction, is the gold standard for determining left ventricular function and is helpful in selecting treatment strategies. A left ventricular ejection fraction (LVEF) normal value is 55% to 70%. The LVEF is one of the most important predictors of long-term outcome following acute myocardial infarction (AMI). Patients with ejection fractions less than 20% have nearly 50% 1-year mortality. Another important measurement is the pressure in the left ventricle at the end of diastole. This is called "left ventricular end-diastolic pressure (LVEDP)." It, too, is an important determinant of ventricular function and is considered to be a predictor of morbidity and mortality in patients with heart failure (HF) and those undergoing cardiac surgery. The normal LVEDP is 6 to 12 mm Hg.

Complications

During cardiac catheterization, a number of complications may occur, including dysrhythmia; coronary artery vasospasm; coronary artery dissection; allergic reaction to the dye; atrial or ventricular perforation resulting in pericardial tamponade; embolus to an extremity, a lung, or, rarely, the brain; acute closure of the left main coronary; myocardial infarction (MI); or death. Common management and prevention strategies for catheterization complications are summarized in Table 9-3.

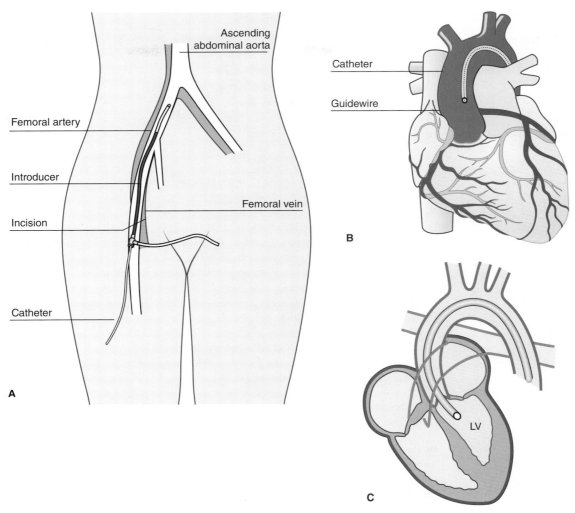

Figure 9-1. Coronary angiography. **(A)** Insertion of the coronary catheter into the femoral artery through a percutaneously inserted introducer sheath. **(B)** Coronary catheter advancement into the aorta and the left coronary artery. **(C)** Catheter advancement into the left ventricle.

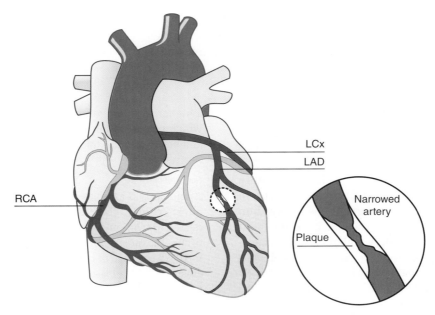

Figure 9-2. Coronary artery circulation with a coronary vessel narrowed by plaque formation.

TABLE 9-3. CARDIAC CATHETERIZATION: COMMON COMPLICATIONS AND NURSING INTERVENTIONS

Complication	Intervention
Local bleeding due to catheter site artery damage (hematoma, hemorrhage, pseudoaneurysm)	Keep patient flat; head of bed (HOB) < 30°.
	Discontinue unfractionated heparin infusion if present.
	Compress the artery just above the incision (pedal pulse should be faint).
	Monitor for hypotension, tachycardia, or arrhythmia.
	Embolectomy or vascular repair may be deemed necessary following groin ultrasound.
Coronary artery dissection	Stent will typically be placed during procedure.
	Monitor for arrhythmia or tamponade.
	Administer unfractionated heparin.
Tamponade due to perforation of the heart or bleeding due to antiplatelet medications	Typically this will be evident in the catheter laboratory at the time of perforation.
	Hypotension after procedure completed—often earliest sign.
	Monitor patient for equalization of cardiac pressures.
	Emergency surgery may be required for repair.
Peripheral thromboembolism	Extremity will exhibit pain, pallor, pulselessness, paresthesias, and paralysis; may also be cool to touch.
	Unfractionated heparin or other anticoagulant should be continued.
	Thrombolytic therapy may be administered directly to the clot using a tracking catheter.
	Surgical intervention may be necessary.
Thromboembolism: CVA due to embolus	Monitor for signs and symptoms of neurologic compromise including speech patterns, orientation, vision, equal grips and pedal pushes, and sensation.
Pulmonary embolism	Provide supplemental O_2.
	Monitor for adequate arterial oxygen saturation and respiratory rate.
	Continue administration of unfractionated heparin or other anticoagulant IV.
	Direct thrombolytic therapy may be administered using a tracking catheter; direct extraction of the clot may also be attempted.
	Ventilation-perfusion scan, computed tomography scan or pulmonary arteriograms may be done to verify thrombus location.
Arrhythmia	Direct irritation of the ventricular wall by the catheter tip poses the greatest risk; post-procedure risk is extremely low.
	Monitor the patient in lead V_1.
Infection	Use aseptic technique for all dressing changes.
	Monitor catheter insertion sites for erythema, inflammation, heat, or exudate.
	Monitor patient temperature trends.
Pulmonary edema due to recumbent position, stress of angiographic contrast, or poor left ventricular function	Elevate HOB 30°.
	Administer diuretics as necessary.
	Consider use of flexible sheath or brachial access.
Acute tubular neurosis and renal failure	Hydrate patient well prior to and following procedure with continuous infusion of normal saline (typically 8 hours before and 8 hours after at 100 mL/h).
	Monitor for elevations in serum creatinine.
Vasovagal reaction	Administer pain medications prior to sheath removal.
	Monitor BP and heart rate before and after sheath removal, then every 15 minutes for four times after removal.

Percutaneous Coronary Interventions

Percutaneous coronary interventions (PCIs) include percutaneous transluminal coronary angioplasty (PTCA), insertion of one or more stents, and coronary atherectomy. PTCA, also termed angioplasty or balloon angioplasty, is a cardiac catheterization with the addition of a balloon apparatus on the tip of the catheter for revascularizing the myocardium (Figure 9-3). The catheter tip is advanced, generally over a guidewire, into the coronary artery until the balloon is positioned across the atherosclerotic lesion in the vessel. Once properly positioned, the balloon is inflated to stretch the vessel wall, resulting in fracture and compression of the atherosclerotic plaque improving blood flow through the vessel. As a result, the degree of stenosis is reduced. This allows a higher rate and volume of blood flow through the vessel, which translates clinically into fewer symptoms of angina and better exercise tolerance.

Complications

Angioplasty is associated with the same complications found during cardiac catheterization. In addition, complications related to manipulation of the coronary artery itself may also occur. The most common serious complications include a 2% to 10% incidence of complete occlusion of the vessel (abrupt closure), AMI (1%-5% incidence), and the need for emergency coronary artery bypass surgery (1%-2% incidence). The most important predictor of complications of MI and abrupt vessel closure is reduced coronary flow through the lesion prior to the procedure. A universal scale, the TIMI Scale, is used to quantify this rate of coronary flow. The scale rates coronary blood flow as follows: no perfusion, penetration without perfusion, partial perfusion, and complete perfusion.

Other Percutaneous Coronary Interventions

In addition to balloon angioplasty, a number of other devices are commonly used for percutaneous coronary revascularization. Intracoronary stents are small metallic mesh tubes placed across the stenotic area and expanded with an angioplasty balloon (Figure 9-4). Once expanded, the tube is permanently anchored in the vessel wall. Stents are effective in decreasing the rate of abrupt vessel closure seen with traditional PTCA. Some stents are coated with a drug that is bonded to a material on the stent causing the drug to be released directly onto the arterial wall over several months to years. These drug-coated stents have been shown to significantly reduce the restenosis rate associated with metal stents. Atherectomy catheters and lasers are used infrequently; however, patient outcomes are not significantly better than those achieved with traditional balloon catheters and stent deployment and may result in higher rates of complication, including AMI. Each of these devices may offer advantages over traditional balloon angioplasty catheters in situations involving specific vascular anatomy (eg, ostial lesions) or lesion morphology (eg, high degree of calcified plaque).

PATHOLOGIC CONDITIONS

Acute Ischemic Heart Disease

Myocardial ischemia is the lack of adequate blood supply to the heart, resulting in an insufficient supply of oxygen to meet the demands of the heart muscle. This supply-demand

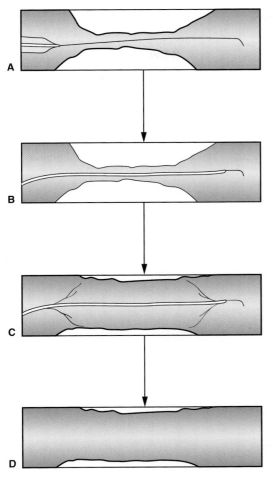

Figure 9-3. Percutaneous transluminal coronary angioplasty (PTCA). **(A)** PTCA catheter being advanced into the narrowed coronary artery over a guidewire. **(B)** Catheter position prior to balloon inflation. **(C)** Balloon inflation. **(D)** Coronary vessel following catheter removal.

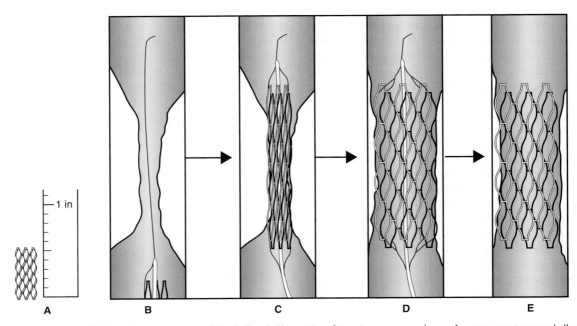

Figure 9-4. Intracoronary stent. **(A)** Size of stent device when fully deployed. **(B)** Insertion of stent into a narrowed area of a coronary artery on a balloon-inflatable catheter. **(C)** Inflation of the balloon catheter to expand the stent. **(D)** Inflation complete with stent fully expanded. **(E)** Stent following removal of balloon catheter.

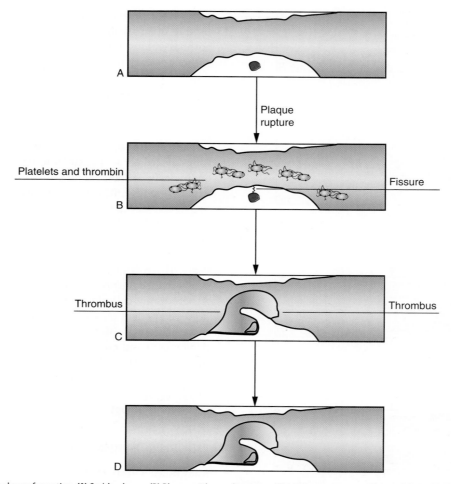

Figure 9-5. Atherosclerotic plaque formation. **(A)** Stable plaque. **(B)** Plaque with cap disruption. **(C)** Moderate amount of layered thrombus. **(D)** Occlusive thrombus.

mismatch, known as ischemia, is most often caused by thrombus formation at a site of atherosclerotic plaque rupture within a coronary artery. Decreased oxygen supply to myocardial tissue may cause a variety of symptoms such as chest discomfort (angina), shortness of breath, diaphoresis, and nausea. Unstable angina, defined as angina that is of new onset, increasing in frequency, or occurring at rest, and AMI are referred to as the acute coronary syndromes (ACSs), which form the spectrum of acute ischemic heart disease.

Etiology and Pathophysiology

Intracoronary thrombus formation, and the resulting obstruction of coronary blood flow, is the pathophysiologic mechanism of acute ischemic heart disease. Preexisting atherosclerosis and spasm of the smooth muscle wall of the coronary arteries, termed fixed obstructions, may also contribute to reduced flow. In some situations, coronary artery spasm may play a major role, unrelated to underlying atherosclerosis, causing MI. These occurrences are sometimes associated with cocaine abuse seen in MI in young patients.

Thrombus formation in the coronary arteries begins with the fissuring and rupture of atherosclerotic plaque in the vessel wall of the coronary artery (Figure 9-5). A continuous, dynamic process occurs whereby plaque may become unstable during periods of active accumulation of more lipid into the core of the plaque. The plaque then ruptures, dispelling its contents into the lumen of the coronary artery and causing activation of clotting factors at the site of plaque rupture. The rupture of plaque and resultant thrombus formation may eventually occlude the coronary artery.

Although most people have some degree of atherosclerotic plaque formation by age 30, the vast majority of these plaques are considered "stable." The smooth fibrous caps that cover these plaques allow adequate blood flow through the coronary arteries, and are not prone to development of unstable angina or MI. In young, growing plaques, the fibrous cap may become thin and rupture, resulting in unstable angina, ischemia, or MI.

A variety of factors predispose a plaque to fissure and rupture. Characteristics of plaque at increased risk for rupture include:

- *Location of the lesion in the vascular tree:* Areas of greater turbulence of flow and dynamic activity during the cardiac cycle are at higher risk.

- *Size of the lipid pool within the plaque:* A large amount of lipid inside the plaque core is more likely to be associated with plaque disruption.
- *Infiltration of the plaque with macrophages:* Macrophages are thought to weaken the integrity of the fibrous cap of the plaque, making it more susceptible to rupture.

Clinical assessment, stress testing, and even cardiac catheterization do not provide information about the contents of the plaque and therefore identification of the risk of

ESSENTIAL CONTENT CASE

Unstable Angina

A 62-year-old man presents to the emergency department (ED) with complaints of pain in his chest and jaw. The pain, originally occurring only with exertion and resolving with rest, became increasingly persistent over the past 2 to 3 days. On the evening of his arrival, the patient experienced a 15-minute episode of severe pain while watching television. This episode he characterized as a "tight, burning feeling in my chest, and an aching in my jaw" that did not vary with respiratory effort and was accompanied by diaphoresis, nausea, and shortness of breath.

On arrival to the ED, his pain and nausea had resolved, pulse oximetry showed oxygen saturation of 98% on room air, and his vital signs were:

BP	148/86 mm Hg
HR	90 beats/min
RR	18 breaths/min
T	37.6°C orally

On physical examination, heart sounds were normal, without S_3, S_4, or murmurs. Initial diagnostic tests revealed:

- Electrocardiogram (ECG): Normal sinus rhythm with non-specific ST-T wave changes
- Chest x-ray: Normal cardiac silhouette, clear lungs

A more detailed assessment of his history revealed increasing dyspnea on exertion and fatigue for the previous 6 months. Despite these symptoms, he had continued his daily 2.5-mile walking routine, sometimes experiencing shortness of breath several times during the walk. The patient reported smoking cigarettes in the past, one pack per day for 20 years, but quit 25 years ago. No ankle swelling, nocturnal dyspnea, or orthopnea were reported, nor was he aware of any family history of cardiac problems, coronary artery disease (CAD), diabetes, or hypertension.

He was started on aspirin based on his history and the likelihood of underlying CAD. He was then admitted for observation and evaluation of cardiac enzymes (see section on cardiac enzymes discussed here).

	CK-MB	Troponin I
ED	6% (3%-5%)	0.4 ng/mL (< .06 ng/mL)
4 hours later	6% (3%-5%)	0.4 ng/mL (< .06 ng/mL)

Six hours after presenting to the ED, the patient had recurrent tightness in his chest. An ECG showed T-wave inversion in the anterior leads. Sublingual nitroglycerin 0.4 mg was administered every 5 minutes with complete relief of the pressure following the second tablet. An unfractionated heparin drip was started. Subsequent cardiac enzymes showed:

	I CK-MB	Troponin I
8 hours	5% (< 5%)	0.4 ng/mL (< .06 ng/mL)
12 hours	5% (< 5%)	0.4 ng/mL (< .06 ng/mL)

Other laboratory results were normal with the exception of elevated cholesterol and triglycerides on the lipid panel. Following receipt of these results, he was scheduled for an exercise tolerance test.

The ECG recorded a heart rate of 118 beats/min after 6 minutes of exercise. Onset of chest tightness during the last minute of exercise was described as similar to that which brought him to the hospital and correlated with 1.5-mm ST depression in leads V_4 to V_6. A cardiac catheterization was scheduled.

Coronary angiography showed a 75% obstruction of the LAD artery and 90% obstruction of the diagonal branch of the same artery. LVEF was 55%. A coronary angioplasty (PTCA) was performed on both lesions.

Case Question 1: What monitoring is the highest priority during the patient's ED stay?
- (A) Obtain repeat ECGs every 4 hours
- (B) Monitor the patient's ECG continuously with continuous ST-segment monitoring
- (C) Monitor platelet levels every 6 hours
- (D) Assess breath sounds every 2 hours

Case Question 2: What diagnosis is suggested by the finding of ST-segment depression and T-wave inversion?
- (A) Non–ST-segment elevation MI
- (B) ST-segment elevation MI
- (C) Coronary spasm
- (D) Pericarditis

Case Question 3: Following the PTCA, what critical complication is the patient at risk for?
- (A) Increased heart rate of 115 beats/min
- (B) Hypotension
- (C) 4 mm ST-segment elevation in leads V_3-V_4
- (D) All of the above

Answers
1. B is the correct answer. Continuous ST-segment monitoring will reveal ischemic changes sooner when compared to intermittent ECGs.
2. A is the correct answer. Non–ST-segment MI is characterized by ST-segment depression and/or T wave inversion in the setting of chest pain and increased cardiac biomarkers. Both coronary spasm and pericarditis can cause ST-segment changes on the ECG.
3. C is the correct answer. The new onset of 4 mm ST-segment elevation in leads V_3-V_4 is an indication of acute coronary closure following the interventional procedure. Hypotension and sinus tachycardia may also be present but are non-specific signs.

TABLE 9-4. HORMONAL AND ENVIRONMENTAL TRIGGERS OF PLAQUE RUPTURE

Acute	Chronic
Hemodynamic Reactivity	**Basal Hemodynamic Forces**
• Morning increase in BP	• Increased resting BP
• Morning increase in heart rate	• Increased resting heart rate
• Physical exertion	**Basal Hemostatic Variables**
• Emotional stress	• Location of the plaque
• Exposure to cold	• Size of the lipid pool within the core plaque
Hemostatic Reactivity	• Degree of macrophage infiltration of the plaque
• Increased coronary blood flow velocity	**Chronic Risk Factors**
• Increased viscosity of blood	• Gender (male > female)
• Decreased tPA activity	• Increasing age
• Increased platelet aggregation	• Diabetes mellitus
Vasoreactivity	• Hypercholesterolemia
• Increased plasma epinephrine	• Cigarette smoking
• Increased plasma cortisol	

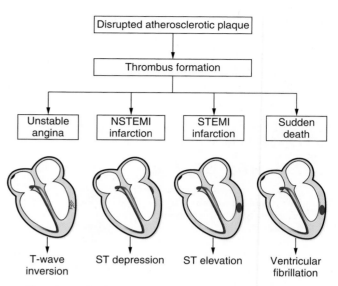

Figure 9-6. Pathophysiologic steps leading to acute coronary events.

rupture is challenging. Plaque rupture may be caused by a number of environmental or hormonal factors, known as triggers (Table 9-4). These triggers may disrupt the plaque and precipitate an acute coronary event. Some of the triggers for atherosclerotic plaque rupture can be manipulated or controlled, such as blood pressure (BP), blood glucose level, and stress. In the clinical setting, management of these variables may decrease the risk for AMI, reinfarction, and reocclusion. They are closely monitored.

When these triggers combine to cause plaque rupture, the lipid pool is exposed and a rough surface on the intima of the vessel wall occurs, stimulating the local effects of hormonal and immune factors and initiating thrombus formation. At the same time, the fibrinolytic system is stimulated, creating a dynamic process of simultaneous attempts to form and dissolve the clot. Because of the dynamic nature of the clotting process, the thrombus may be completely or only partially obstructive, or may fluctuate intermittently between the two stages. Regardless of the maturity of the clot, the process of thrombus formation may lead to obstruction of blood flow, diminishing oxygen delivery to distal myocardium and creating a mismatch between the supply of and demand for oxygen.

Because the underlying pathology of the ischemia-related diagnoses is the same (plaque rupture and thrombus formation), ischemic heart disease encompasses the entire spectrum of ischemic coronary events that are referred to as ACS. ACS represents a continuum of clinical events that may result from the supply-demand mismatch including unstable angina, non–ST-segment elevation myocardial infarction (NSTEMI), or ST-segment elevation myocardial infarction (STEMI) (Figure 9-6).

Following a decrease in oxygen supply to the myocardium, the cell membranes lose their integrity and fluid moves into the cell. The cell is no longer able to regulate its internal and external environment. The cell dies, releasing cytotoxic substances into the bloodstream. When they die, cardiac myocytes release significant amounts of myoglobin,

troponin I and T, as well as cardiac-specific creatine kinase (CK-MB). Laboratory testing that shows elevate levels of these cardiac markers confirms the MI diagnosis.

Clinical Presentation
Clinical presentation across the spectrum of ACS is similar, with slight differences depending on the involved vessels (Table 9-5).

1. Pain or discomfort, usually in the chest (see Table 9-1)
   • Pressure or tightness in the chest
   • Jaw or neck pain
   • Left arm ache or pain
   • Epigastric discomfort
   • Scapular back pain
2. Nausea/vomiting
3. Hemodynamic instability
   • Hypotension (systolic BP < 90 mm Hg or 20 mm Hg below baseline)
   • Skin cool, clammy, diaphoretic
4. Dyspnea
5. Dysrhythmia/conduction defects
   • Left bundle branch block (LBBB)
   • Tachycardia/bradycardia
   • Frequent premature ventricular contractions
   • Ventricular fibrillation
6. Anxiety, sense of impending catastrophe
7. Denial

Some patient populations are predictably different in their description of chest discomfort, such as women and diabetics. Women frequently present with symptoms that are more vague such as feeling tired, short of breath, and lack of energy. Women may deny their symptoms for longer periods of time than men, delaying their arrival to the ED and often

TABLE 9-5. CLINICAL PRESENTATION OF MYOCARDIAL ISCHEMIA AND INFARCTION

Type MI	Arterial Involvement	Muscle Area Supplied	Assessment
Anteroseptal wall	LAD	Anterior LV wall, Anterior LV septum Apex LV Bundle of His Bundle branches	↓ LV function → ↓ CO, ↓ BP ↑ PAD, ↑ PAOP S₃ and S₄, with HF Rales with pulmonary edema
Posterior septal lateral	RCA circumflex branches (right and left)	Posterior surface of LV SA node 45% AV node 10% Left atrium Lateral wall of LV	Murmurs indicating VSD (septal) PA catheter to assess R to L shunt in VSD Signs/symptoms of LV aneurysm with lateral displaced PMI leading to signs and symptoms of mitral regurgitation
Inferior or "diaphragmatic"	RCA	RV, RA SA node 50% AV node 90% RA, RV Inferior LV Posterior VI septum Posterior LBBB Posterior LV	Symptomatic bradycardia: ↓ BP, LOC changes, diaphoresis ↓ CO, ↑ PAD, ↑ PAOP Murmurs: associated with papillary muscle dysfunction mid/holosystolic rates, pulmonary edema, nausea
Right ventricular infarction	RCA	RA, RV, inferior LV SA node AV node Posterior IV septum	Kussmaul sign JVD Hypotension ↑ SVR, ↓ PAOP, ↑ CVP S₃ with noncompliant RV Clear breath sounds initially Hepatomegaly; peripheral edema; cool, clammy, pale skin

TABLE 9-5. CLINICAL PRESENTATION OF MYOCARDIAL ISCHEMIA AND INFARCTION (CONTINUED)

ECG Changes	Likely Arrhythmias	Possible Complications
Indicative ST elevation with or without abnormal Q waves in V$_{1-4}$ Loss of R waves in precordial leads **Reciprocal** ST depression in II, III, aVF	RBBB, LBBB AV blocks Atrial fibrillation or flutter Ventricular tachycardia (VT) Tachycardia (septal)	Cardiogenic shock VSD Myocardial rupture Heart blocks may be permanent (LBBB) High mortality associated with this location of MI
Lateral Indicative ST elevation I, aVL, V$_{5-6}$ Loss of R wave and ↑ ST in I, aVL, V$_{5-6}$ **Posterior Indicative** Tall, broad R waves (> 0.04 second) in V$_{1-3}$ ↑ ST V$_4$R (right-sided 12 lead, V$_4$ position) **Posterior Reciprocal** ST depression in V$_{1,2,}$ upright T wave in V$_{1,2}$ (Note: Posterior MI diagnosed by reciprocal changes)	Bradycardia Mobitz I (posterior)	RV involvement Aneurysm development Papillary muscle dysfunction Heart blocks frequently resolve
Indicative ↑ ST segments in II, III, aVF Q waves in II, III, aVF **Reciprocal** ST depression in I, aVL, V$_{1-4}$	AV blocks; often progress to CHB which may be transient or permanent; Wenckebach; bradyarrhythmias	Hiccups Nausea/vomiting Papillary muscle dysfunction MR Septal rupture (0.5%-1.0%) RV involvement associated with atrial infarcts especially with atrial arrhythmias
Indicative 1- to 2-mm ST-segment elevation in V$_4$R ST- and T-wave elevation in II, III, aVF Q waves in II, III, aVF ST-elevation decreases in amplitude over V$_{1-6}$	First-degree AV block Second-degree AV block, type I Incomplete RBBB Transient CHB Atrial fibrillation VT/VF	Hypotension requiring large volumes initially to maintain systemic pressure. Once RV contractility improves fluids will mobilize, possibly requiring diuresis

rendering them ineligible for thrombolytic therapy. In addition, women are typically postmenopausal when signs and symptoms of atherosclerotic disease become apparent. This predominantly older patient population may face additional challenges such as fear of the inability to care for oneself following MI, and additional chronic health problems.

Diabetics are another patient population with atypical symptoms when experiencing an MI. Patients with diabetes often develop atherosclerotic disease early and their experience of pain may be altered due to neuropathy. CAD in this patient population is diffuse, and poor distal vascular anatomy is common. Lesion morphology in diabetic patients is also more difficult to revascularize, either using percutaneous or surgical methods.

Diagnostic Tests
Unstable Angina

1. *12-lead ECG:* Transient changes may occur and resolve; most commonly T-wave inversion or ST-segment depression.
2. *Cardiac enzymes (Troponin [I or T], myoglobin, and CK-MB):* Normal
3. *Cardiac catheterization:* Not recommended in the acute setting, except in the case of continued pain/discomfort without relief from nitroglycerin.

Catheterization results may be normal, or with visible atherosclerotic disease, but without a complete occlusion or thrombus.

Myocardial Infarction

1. *12-lead ECG:* Thirty-five percent of patients with AMI have ST-segment elevation on their initial ECG (see Chapter 18, Advanced ECG Concepts). The label "STEMI" is used in this situation. Approximately 65% of those with AMI have no ECG or other diagnostic changes.
2. *Creatine kinase (CK and CK-MB):* (Figure 9-7).
   - Total CK > 150 to 180 mcg/L
   - MB band > 10 ng/mL or >5% of total.
   - Peaks at 12 hours after symptom onset.
   - CK-MB isoforms have better sensitivity and specificity for detecting MI within the first 6 hours.
3. *Troponin T:* Compare to laboratory reference range
   - Begins to increase 3 to 5 hours after symptom onset
   - Remains elevated for 14 to 21 days
4. *Troponin I:* Compare to laboratory reference range
   - Begins to increase 3 hours after onset of myocardial ischemia
   - Peaks at 14 to 18 hours
   - Remains elevated for 5 to 7 days

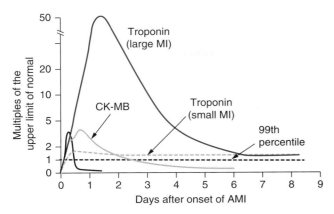

Figure 9-7. Timing and levels of biomarkers associated with heart injury. (*Data from Antman EM. Decision making with cardiac troponin tests. N Engl J Med. 2002;346:2079; and Jaffe AS, Babiun L, Apple FS. Biomarkers in acute cardiac disease: the present and the future. J Am Coll Cardiol. 2006;48:1.*)

5. *Myoglobin:* Present in serum, 17.4 to 105.7 ng/mL.
   - Released from myocardium within 2 hours of coronary occlusion
   - Peaks in 6 to 7 hours
   - Better marker for early detection of MI; better negative indicator if negative
6. *Cardiac catheterization:* Ventricular wall motion abnormalities (also may be seen by echocardiography); total occlusion of one or more coronary arteries.

Principles of Management of Acute Ischemic Heart Disease

Because most complications of acute ischemic heart disease directly result from reduced coronary flow, a primary objective in patient management is to optimize blood flow to the myocardium. Additional goals are to prevent complications of ischemia and infarction, alleviate chest discomfort/pain, and reduce anxiety.

Optimize Blood Flow to the Myocardium

Regardless of whether a patient presents with unstable angina or AMI, restoration and maintenance of coronary blood flow is important to improve patient outcomes. Interventions to optimize blood flow to the myocardium include pharmacologic measures, such as antiplatelet or antithrombin agents, and mechanical measures, such as percutaneous coronary revascularization (eg, angioplasty, stent, or other) or coronary artery bypass grafting (CABG). Refer to Table 9-6 for evidence-based guidelines for AMI. The intervention selected and the optimal timing of the intervention depends on whether the occlusion of the artery is total or partial. This determination must be made as accurately and as quickly as possible, as a totally occluded artery will soon result in tissue necrosis or MI (Figure 9-8 for algorithm on acute chest pain management). All unstable arteries benefit from the following interventions to stabilize the artery and optimize coronary perfusion.

TABLE 9-6. EVIDENCED-BASED PRACTICE: ACUTE CORONARY SYNDROME— ST-ELEVATION MI AND NON–ST-ELEVATION MI

Diagnosis
- Diagnosis of AMI is based on two of three findings:
  1. History of ischemic-like symptoms
  2. Changes on serial ECGs
  3. Elevation and fall in level of serum cardiac biomarkers
- Of AMI patients, 50% do not present with ST-segment elevation. Other indicators:
  1. ST-segment depression may indicate NSTEMI
  2. New LBBB
  3. ST-segment depression that resolves with relief of chest pain
  4. T-wave inversion in all chest leads may indicate NSTEMI with a critical stenosis in the proximal LAD

Acute Management
- Optimal time for initiation of therapy is within 1 hour of symptom onset. Rarely feasible due to delay in treatment-seeking behavior[a]
- Initial ECG should be obtained within 10 minutes of emergency department arrival
- Oxygen if $Sao_2 < 90\%$, nitroglycerin, and aspirin should be administered if not contraindicated
- Reperfusion strategy: STEMI only:
  1. If non-PCI capable hospital, fibrinolytic agent should be initiated within 30 minutes of arrival if no contraindication
  2. If PCI capable hospital, primary PCI to be done, culprit vessel should be opened within 90 minutes of arrival
- Reperfusion strategy for NSTEMI:[b]
  1. Fibrinolytics not recommended
  2. PCI to be done within 24 hours of arrival
- Weight-based heparin or low-molecular-weight heparin[a]
- Antiplatelet therapy
- IV beta-blocker should be given within 12 hours of arrival[a]
- Lipid-lowering agent should be initiated[a]

Adapted from [a]O'Gara, Kushner, Ascheim, et al. (2013); [b]Amsterdam et al. (2014).

MEDICAL MANAGEMENT

1. Decrease activity of coagulation system with pharmacologic therapy (Figure 9-9).
   - Antiplatelet agents: Aspirin, glycoprotein IIb/IIIa receptor blocking agents (eg, abciximab [ReoPro®], eptifibatide [Integrilin®], and tirofiban [Aggrastat®]), thienopyridine agents (eg, clopidogrel [Plavix®] or ticagrelor [Brilinta])
   - Antithrombin agents: Indirect (eg, unfractionated heparin, low-molecular-weight heparin), direct (eg, bivalirudin [Angiomax®])
2. Increase ventricular filling time (decrease heart rate):
   - Beta-blockers
   - Bed rest for 24 hours
3. Decrease preload:
   - Nitrates
   - Diuretics
   - Morphine sulfate
4. Decrease afterload:
   - Angiotensin-converting enzyme (ACE) inhibitors or angiotensin receptor blockers (ARBs) if EF ≤ 40%
   - Hydralazine
5. Decrease myocardial oxygen consumption (MVO_2):
   - Beta-blockers
   - Bed rest for 24 hours

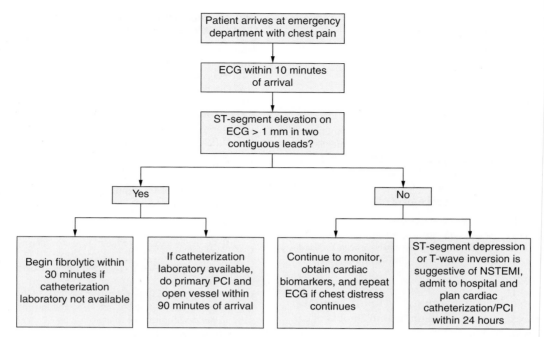

Figure 9-8. Algorithm for management of acute chest pain.

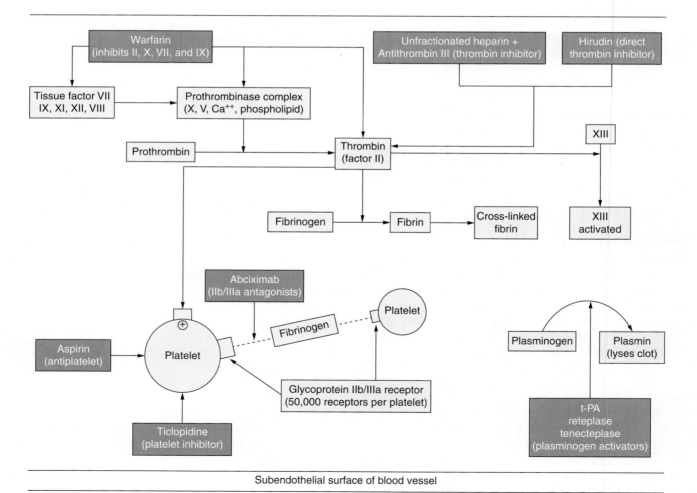

Figure 9-9. Coagulation sequence and site of antithrombotic/antiplatelet activity.

TABLE 9-7. INDICATIONS AND CONTRAINDICATIONS FOR FIBRINOLYTIC THERAPY

Indications
- Chest pain > 20 minutes, but typically < 12 hours
- ST elevation ≥ 1 mm in two contiguous leads
- LBBB
- High-risk patients with chest pain > 12 hours in duration may still be candidates if pain persists

Absolute Contraindications
- Active internal bleeding
- History of intracranial bleeding, cerebral neoplasm, or other intracranial pathology
- Stroke or head trauma within 3 months
- Intracranial or spinal surgery in the last 2 months
- Severe uncontrolled hypertension, unresponsive to treatment
- Suspected aortic dissection
- Known allergy to the drug chosen

Relative Contraindications
- Dementia
- Ischemic stroke > 3 months ago
- Active peptic ulcer
- Prolonged traumatic CPR > 10 minutes
- Major surgery < 3 weeks ago
- Traumatic puncture of noncompressible vessel
- Pregnancy or 1 month postpartum
- History of uncontrolled hypertension
- Significant hypertension systolic > 180 or diastolic > 110

TABLE 9-8. COMPLICATIONS OF FIBRINOLYTIC THERAPY

Complication	Percentage Occurrence
Groin bleeding, local (compressible external)	25-45
Intracerebral bleeding	1.45
Retroperitoneal bleeding (noncompressible internal)	1
Gastrointestinal bleeding	4-10
Genitourinary bleeding	1-5
Other bleeding	1-5

6. Reduce risk for sudden cardiac death due to ventricular tachycardia/ventricular fibrillation.
   - Beta-blockers

In addition to the interventions listed above, totally occluded arteries require immediate reperfusion therapy, such as fibrinolysis, angioplasty or CABG to effectively restore blood flow to the coronary artery. In the event of left main coronary artery stenosis or three-vessel disease, urgent or emergent CABG is usually considered. In the acute setting, for STEMI fibrinolytic therapy is often the fastest, most universally available method for reperfusion if a catheterization laboratory is not available or operational 24 hours a day. The indications, contraindications, and common complications of fibrinolytic therapy are listed in Tables 9-7 and 9-8. In those settings where the catheterization laboratory is operational 24 h/day, primary PCI is indicated. Studies have indicated that primary PCI may be associated with better outcomes and fewer complications than with the use of fibrinolytic agents.

SURGICAL MANAGEMENT

CABG is one method of revascularization generally used in patients with atherosclerosis of three or more coronary vessels or in the case of significant left main CAD. CABG is performed both electively, as well as emergently, and may be performed either prior to or following an MI. The CABG procedure in which a graft is placed in the coronary arterial tree to perfuse the area beyond the occlusion requires induction with general anesthesia, and possible initiation of cardiopulmonary bypass (blood is diverted outside of the body to a pump that mechanically oxygenates the blood before returning it to the arterial circulation) (Figure 9-10).

The use of stabilizer devices permits CABG to be performed on some patients without cardiopulmonary bypass.

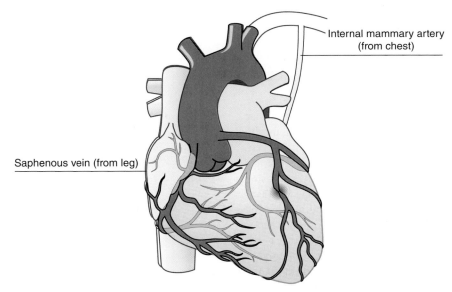

Internal mammary artery (from chest)

Saphenous vein (from leg)

Figure 9-10. Coronary artery bypass grafting (CABG).

The heart continues to beat while the surgeon places a device over the coronary artery site where the bypass graft is to be anastomosed, which stabilizes the small area allowing for suturing to occur. This is often referred to as "beating heart surgery" or "off pump" coronary artery bypass (OPCAB). The graft, generally a leg vein, left internal mammary artery, or radial artery, is inserted past the distal end of the blockage in the coronary artery and, in the case of a leg vein graft and radial artery graft, anastomosed to the aorta. Multiple grafts may be inserted based on the number of blockages present and the availability of viable insertion sites in the patient's native coronary tree.

INDICATIONS

The indications for CABG and long-term patient outcome following this procedure have been intensively reviewed over the past decade. In general, patients with three-vessel disease, poor LVEF (< 35%), or significant disease in the left main coronary artery have lower long-term morbidity and mortality with surgical revascularization (CABG) compared to medical therapy or percutaneous interventions such as angioplasty or stent. Diabetics with multivessel disease also fare better following CABG than following percutaneous interventions including drug-eluting stents. CABG may also be indicated as an emergent "rescue" procedure in patients whose coronary artery severely dissects or fractures during an attempted percutaneous procedure.

CONTRAINDICATIONS

Several populations of patients may be considered poor candidates for coronary bypass, including the very elderly, debilitated patients, patients with severely diseased distal coronary vasculature (eg, some diabetics), and patients with extremely low LVEF (eg, < 5%-15%). Patients with low ejection fractions often have difficulty being weaned from cardiopulmonary bypass following the procedure. Other contraindications are those related to general anesthesia risk, including severe chronic obstructive pulmonary disease, pulmonary edema, or pulmonary hypertension.

POSTOPERATIVE MANAGEMENT

The following is a general overview of the early postoperative management of CABG patients:

1. *Maintain hemodynamic stability:* A variety of cardiac medications are administered to maintain hemodynamic stability in the first 24 hours postoperatively. Hemodynamic monitoring may be invasive using a pulmonary artery catheter, minimally invasive using a central line or arterial line, or completely noninvasive. Interpretation of postoperative hemodynamic status is best done with the patient's preoperative hemodynamic status in mind, as some of the values may be significantly elevated or abnormal at the patient's baseline. The following hemodynamic values may serve as guides for inotropic and vasopressor administration along with intravascular fluid

therapy. In general, values greater or lower than the following require intervention:
   - Mean arterial pressure: 70 to 80 mm Hg
   - CI: 2.0 to 3.5 L/min/m^2
   - Central venous pressure (CVP): 5 to 10 mm Hg (may be used to evaluate need for volume replacement; however, research has demonstrated that there is not a relationship between pressures and the intravascular volume status)
   - HR: Intrinsic or paced rhythm in the range of 80 to 100 beats/min to keep CI $\geq$ 2.0
   - If radial artery graft used, monitor for arterial spasm. Use a prophylactic nitroglycerin drip and nitro paste if indicated

2. *Maintain ventilation and oxygenation:* Ventilation and oxygenation are maximized in the early postoperative period with mechanical ventilation. Within 2 to 12 hours, most patients have recovered from the anesthesia effects and are sufficiently stable to allow weaning from mechanical ventilation and extubation. Individuals with preexisting pulmonary problems may require longer periods of intubation until weaning can be successfully accomplished. Following weaning and extubation, supplemental O_2 therapy usually is required for 1 to 2 days to maintain PaO_2 or SaO_2 in normal ranges. Postoperative atelectasis and pleural effusions are a common occurrence after cardiopulmonary bypass, requiring frequent pulmonary interventions (eg, coughing and deep breathing, incentive spirometry, ambulation) to maintain ventilation and oxygenation.

3. Prevention of postoperative complications:
   - *Bleeding from vascular graft anastomosis sites:* Frequent monitoring of mediastinal tube drainage, hematocrit, and coagulation status; avoidance of even brief periods of hypertension.
   - *Cardiac tamponade:* Frequent assessment for signs and symptoms of tamponade which include tachycardia, SOB, anxiety/decreased level of consciousness (LOC), pulsus paradoxus, sinus tachycardia, decreased mediastinal tube drainage, increased CVP, pulmonary artery diastolic (PAD), and pulmonary artery occlusion pressure (PAOP) (note: these are often within 2-3 mm Hg of each other, which is called equalization of pressures or diastolic plateau), muffled heart sounds, decreased BP, and cardiac output.
   - *Infection:* Antibiotics may be used prophylactically for 48 hours; temperature spike within 24 hours postoperatively is not abnormal.
   - *Cardiac dysrhythmias:* ECG and continuous ST-segment monitoring, treat unstable rhythms, maintain K^+ and Mg^+ within normal limits with IV replacement.
   - *Relief of postoperative pain and anxiety:* Analgesic administration is typically required to ensure pain

relief, especially to facilitate ambulation, coughing, and deep breathing.

- If median sternotomy performed ensure sternal precautions are implemented, for example, avoid hyperextension of chest (arms and shoulders pulled posteriorly).

Preventing Complications Associated With Coronary Obstruction

Complications associated with acute ischemic syndromes include recurrent ischemia, infarction or reinfarction, onset of HF, and dysrhythmias.

1. Prevent recurrent ischemia, infarction, or reinfarction: Continue pharmacologic interventions such as antiplatelet and antithrombin agents to inhibit prothrombotic events, including ischemia and infarction. Assess for recurrent angina with frequent chest pain assessment and serial 12-lead ECG and continuous ST-segment ischemia monitoring (see AACN Practice Alert: Ensuring accurate ST-segment Monitoring).
2. Continuously monitor for dysrhythmias: Monitor for 24 to 72 hours following an ischemic episode.
3. Minimize potential for HF: Minimize myocardial oxygen consumption with the administration of beta-blockers, limit physical activity, and avoid increases in metabolic rate (eg, fever). Reduce left ventricular afterload with the administration of ACE inhibitors or ARBs and hydralazine.

Alleviating Pain

Pain relief improves coronary flow by decreasing the level of circulating catecholamines, thereby decreasing BP (afterload) and heart rate (myocardial oxygen consumption). Nitrates typically relieve anginal pain by dilating coronary arteries and increasing blood flow, thereby improving myocardial oxygenation and directly treating the source of the pain. Another pharmacologic intervention commonly used to relieve pain in ischemia is morphine sulfate. Although morphine is a potent narcotic that has been criticized for masking cardiac pain, it is also a potent vasodilator and effectively vasodilates coronary as well as peripheral arteries, resulting in mild afterload reduction. Severe pain, unrelieved with nitrates or a combination of nitrates and morphine, is typically an indication for immediate PCI if available or transfer to a referring institution for emergency PCI.

Reducing Anxiety

The reduction of anxiety in ischemic heart disease is important for a number of reasons. The most important physiologically is the reduction of catecholamine secretion and decrease in sympathetic tone following relaxation in the anxious patient. This effect has been shown to decrease the incidence of dysrhythmia and promote vasodilation and afterload reduction. Decreasing anxiety may also increase the patient's ability to process new information regarding his or her diagnosis, and to better understand instructions for tests or procedures that will be done.

Relief of pain typically is most effective in reducing patient anxiety. In the event that pain is not relieved with nitroglycerin, or fibrinolytics in the initial treatment of ischemia, pain relievers such as morphine sulfate or anxiolytics such as midazolam or lorazepam (short- or intermediate-acting benzodiazepines respectively) are usually effective.

A number of interventions may be done at the bedside to promote relaxation, including specific relaxation and imagery techniques, meditation, music therapy, and the use of relaxation applications or audio files. Providing the patient and family with adequate information regarding unfamiliar surroundings, when the provider may be available to speak with them, possible "unknowns" such as tests or procedures, and important expectations such as visitation guidelines helps provide a sense of security and facilitates relaxation by increasing the patient's level of comfort with the situation. Offering the patient opportunities for control in the acute setting also alleviates anxiety. Examples include the timing of simple activities such as visitor presence, bathing, and eating.

Electrophysiology Studies

In the past 25 years, the cardiology subspecialty of electrophysiology (EP) has grown significantly and continues to expand. An EP study involves the insertion of several catheters with multiple electrodes on each into the right atrium and ventricle, the coronary sinus and, in some cases across the intra-atrial septum (trans-septal) into the left atrium. The multiple electrode locations (Figure 9-11) are used to record the impulse initiative and/or the conduction of the electrical waveform (depolarization process) through the myocardial tissue. Reasons for EP studies include: (1) to identify the site of origin for a dysrhythmia like atrial fibrillation or ventricular tachycardia (VT); (2) to map the conduction pathway

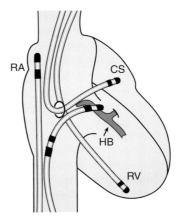

Figure 9-11. Electrophysiology study: Multiple catheters with electrodes are threaded into the right side of the heart. This allows for local monitoring and recording of the electrical activity as the heart depolarizes and repolarizes. The recordings help to locate the origin of the dysrhythmia or conduction abnormality across the anomalous pathway. *Abbreviations: CS, coronary sinus; HB, his bundle; RA, right atrium; RV, right ventricle. (Reproduced with permission of Medtronic, Inc.)*

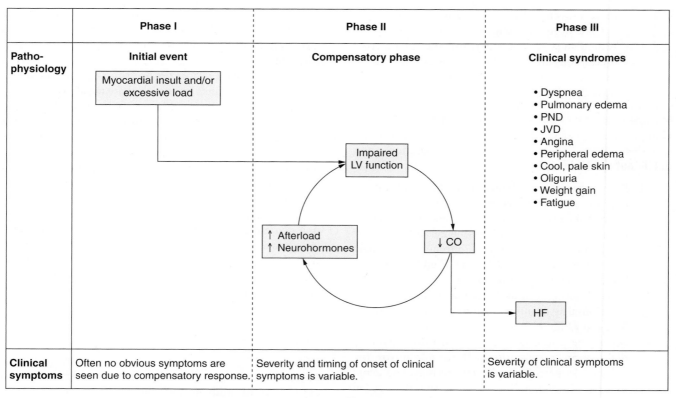

	Phase I	Phase II	Phase III
Patho-physiology	**Initial event** Myocardial insult and/or excessive load	**Compensatory phase** Impaired LV function ↑ Afterload ↑ Neurohormones ↓ CO HF	**Clinical syndromes** • Dyspnea • Pulmonary edema • PND • JVD • Angina • Peripheral edema • Cool, pale skin • Oliguria • Weight gain • Fatigue
Clinical symptoms	Often no obvious symptoms are seen due to compensatory response.	Severity and timing of onset of clinical symptoms is variable.	Severity of clinical symptoms is variable.

Figure 9-12. Pathophysiology of heart failure during phases I, II, and III.

to identify the location of a conduction disturbance; (3) to identify the presence of an anomalous pathway which may be seen with Wolf-Parkinson-White Syndrome; (4) to determine the need for an implantable device for instance a pacemaker, or cardioverter defibrillator (ICD or PCD). If the study identifies the site of origin for a dysrhythmia or abnormal pathway, the EP physician is able to use radiofrequency (electricity) ablation or cryoablation (extreme cold) to destroy the site or the abnormal pathway. Following the procedure, the patient needs to be monitored for similar groin complications as seen with cardiac catheterization. Additional monitoring includes observing for the onset of AV blocks as the AV node and/or bundle of His tissue might have been injured during ablation of the anomalous pathway. If there is evidence of the AV block during the EP study, a pacemaker will be implanted at that time.

Heart Failure

Heart failure is a broad term referring to the inability of the heart to eject an adequate cardiac output to meet the oxygen and metabolic requirements of the body. A number of underlying disease processes may contribute to this "weak pump" syndrome, with coronary atherosclerosis, valvular heart disease, hypertension, and cardiomyopathy as the most common causes. Although the underlying causes are diverse, the progressive process which occurs in response to one of these initiating events is the same.

Etiology, Risk Factors, and Pathophysiology

Although HF refers to any cardiac insufficiency, left ventricular systolic dysfunction is the most common disorder. The pathophysiology of HF is a three-stage process, beginning with an initial insult to the myocardium (phase I), followed by a response phase (phase II), and resulting in the clinical syndrome known as HF, characterized by exhaustion of compensatory mechanisms (phase III) (Figure 9-12). Regardless of the precipitating event, the physiologic progression of the syndrome, once initiated, is the same.

Phase I

Phase I of HF is characterized by an initiating event (eg, MI, viral infection, chemotherapeutic agents, valvular heart disease, hypertension, idiopathic cardiomyopathy), which causes loss of myocytes. This cell loss or permanent damage to the myocytes can be either localized or diffuse, resulting in compromised ventricular function. To date, over 700 initiating factors, such as acute ischemic damage, viruses, and toxins, have been isolated as contributors to myocardial insult and HF.

- *Result of phase I:* Decreased stroke volume/cardiac output secondary to an initial insult to the myocardium.

Phase II

A number of adaptive mechanisms occur in response to the initial insult in an effort to maintain adequate cardiac output

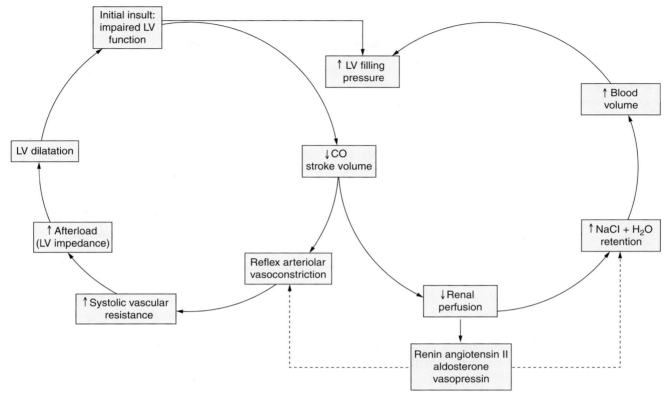

Figure 9-13. Compensatory mechanisms of heart failure.

to meet the body's needs. This phase is sometimes referred to as the compensatory phase (Figures 9-12 and 9-13). These compensatory mechanisms or responses include the Frank-Starling response, myocardial remodeling, and the neurohormonal response.

Frank-Starling Response

As cardiac output decreases and the sympathetic nervous system is activated, alpha-1 receptors are stimulated, resulting in arteriolar and venous vasoconstriction. This adaptive response initially results in increased venous return to the ventricle, increased ventricular end-diastolic volume, stretching of the ventricular myocytes, and improved stroke volume. Later, as overstretching of the ventricle occurs, this compensatory mechanism is lost, resulting in left ventricular decompensation and myocardial hypertrophy (Figure 9-14). Additionally, there is increased expression of granules in the left ventricle causing an increased release of brain natriuretic peptide (BNP). Increased BNP levels in the serum are used as markers of severity of ventricular failure.

Myocardial Hypertrophy (Remodeling)

In response to increased vascular volume and decreased myocardial function (loss of the Frank-Starling response), the left ventricle dilates and hypertrophies. This distortion of the normal left ventricular anatomy causes mitral

regurgitation and further left ventricular dilatation. Activation of angiotensin II, a by-product of the renin-angiotensin-aldosterone system, directly induces myocyte hypertrophy as well. The result of these factors is decreased left ventricular reserve (stretch), increased preload (high residual volume in the ventricle following systole), and further mitral regurgitation.

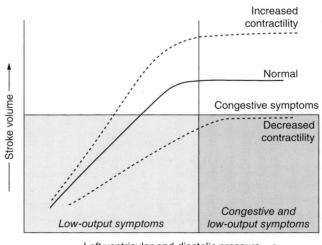

Figure 9-14. Frank-Starling curve.

ESSENTIAL CONTENT CASE

Heart Failure

A 75-year-old man presents to the ED with diaphoresis and severe dyspnea. Initial assessment revealed the following:

RR	32 breaths/min
BP	110/90 mm Hg
HR	110 beats/min, irregular
JVD	Bilateral 7-mm elevation
Lungs	Bibasilar crackles throughout the lower lobes
Cardiovascular	S_1, S_2 with an S_3

A pulse oximeter revealed 83% oxygen saturation.

Laboratory work, including an arterial blood gas sample, was done with the following results:

Pao_2	60 mm Hg
$Paco_2$	28 mm Hg
pH	7.51
Sao_2	93%

Oxygen was initiated at 4 L/min via nasal cannula. An ECG was done and showed left ventricular hypertrophy, and left bundle branch block. His chest x-ray showed an enlarged cardiac silhouette and bilateral infiltrates.

A dobutamine infusion was started at 2.5 mcg/kg/min, and furosemide 40 mg IV was given. Cardiac catheterization was performed the next morning with the following findings:

LAD	95% occlusion
RCA	50% occlusion
LCx	75% occlusion
EF	28%

Impaired myocardial contractility

Case Question 1: What effect will the dobutamine infusion and the dose of furosemide have?
(A) Increase myocardial contractility and reduce ventricular preload

(B) Increase myocardial contractility and reduce ventricular afterload
(C) Reduce myocardial contractility and increase ventricular preload
(D) Increase myocardial contractility and increase ventricular afterload

Case Question 2: What changes in the patient's clinical status will indicate that the treatment is effective?
(A) HR 120 beats/min; RR 36 breaths/min; Spo_2 83%
(B) HR 110 beats/min; RR 24 breaths/min; Spo_2 95%
(C) HR 95 beats/min; JVD Bilateral 7-mm elevation; RR 32 breaths/min
(D) BP 105/80 mm Hg; HR 130 beats/min; Spo_2 75%

Case Question 3: Based on the ECG and cardiac catheterization results, what additional intervention would benefit this patient?
(A) Implantation of a HeartMate II LVAD as destination therapy
(B) Ventricular aneurysmectomy/reconstruction surgery
(C) Mitral valve repair
(D) Insertion of a dual-chamber biventricular pacemaker

Answers
1. A is the correct answer. Dobutamine is a positive inotrope and will increase myocardial contractility and cardiac output. It has some vasodilator effects and may cause the diastolic pressure to drop. Furosemide will reduce preload by promoting diuresis. All of this will reduce the amount of work the heart has to do.
2. B is the correct answer. He has diuresed, cleared some of the fluid in his lungs and his respiratory rate is slowing and pulse oximetry is improving.
3. D is the correct answer. Left bundle branch block causes ventricular dyssynchrony, indicating the ventricles do not contract simultaneously causing the cardiac output to decrease. Implanting a biventricular pacemaker will cause the ventricles to contract simultaneously and improve cardiac output. He is not a candidate for a left ventricular device at this time and a surgical procedure is not indicated.

NEUROHORMONAL RESPONSE

In response to decreased stroke volume and decreased renal perfusion, several neurohormonal systems are activated to compensate for the decrease in stroke volume. These include:

1. *Adrenergic nervous system:* Adrenergic nervous system activity is heightened in the setting of impaired ventricular function as a direct result of baroreceptor stimulation. These baroreceptors mediate the sympathetic nervous system, which in turn stimulates the beta-1 receptors. This results in an increase in heart rate and contractility.
2. *Renin-angiotensin-aldosterone system:* Decreased renal perfusion stimulates the release of renin, increasing the production of angiotensin I and II, and the release of aldosterone. This causes arteriolar vasoconstriction, decreased cardiac output, increased arterial BP and peripheral resistance, increased ventricular filling pressures, sodium and potassium retention (imbalance), increased volume overload, increased left ventricular wall stress, increased ventricular dilation and hypertrophy, and increased sympathetic nervous system arousal.
3. *Arginine vasopressin (AVP) system:* AVP is a potent vasoconstrictor that is normally inhibited by stretch receptors in the atria during atrial distension. In HF, these receptors are less sensitive, causing a decrease in AVP inhibition. AVP activation leads to systemic vasoconstriction, and increased afterload which is the

pressure the ventricle must work against to eject blood out to the system. Increased AVP activity also inhibits free water excretion causing hypo-osmolarity, and impairs autoregulation of further AVP production.

4. *Atrial natriuretic peptide (ANP):* ANP is a counter-regulatory hormone that opposes all three of the above systems, resulting in vasodilation and sodium excretion. ANP is produced in response to atrial distension and results in decreased formation of renin, decreased effects of angiotensin II, decreased release of aldosterone and vasopressin, and enhanced renal excretion of sodium and water. In chronic HF, the levels of ANP remain elevated, but are less so than in the acute decompensation phase (phase III).

The effects of the compensatory mechanisms in phase II lead to an increase in circulating volume and perfusion to vital organs. These mechanisms are self-limiting and a vicious cycle of increased afterload and volume overload results. The neurohormonal response is no longer beneficial in the chronic state but, as seen in phase III, becomes detrimental leading to changes in the myocyte DNA, resulting in programmed cell death (apoptosis) and further loss of myocytes.

- *Result of phase II:* Ventricular hypertrophy, weakened myocytes, increased arteriolar resistance, increased vascular volume, and increased ventricular wall stress occur in an effort to maintain adequate cardiac output.

Phase III

When the adaptive mechanisms of phase II fail, the clinical syndrome of HF follows. This third phase of HF is extremely variable in onset and presentation. The clinical expression and course of the disease is determined by the extent of the initial insult and myocyte damage, the severity of hemodynamic burden (volume overload), and the patient's individual neurohormonal response to these changes. Phase III is characterized by a progressive deterioration of cardiovascular functioning due to the relationship between compromised left ventricular function and excessive cardiac afterload (Figure 9-15). As ventricular dilation occurs, BNP levels in the serum increase.

- *Result of phase III:* Clinical signs and symptoms of HF are evident, resulting in decreased functional status and activity intolerance for the patient.

Clinical Presentation

Regardless of the underlying cause of the weak pump, patients with HF present with clinical signs and symptoms of intravascular and interstitial volume overload, as well as manifestations of inadequate tissue perfusion. Common findings in HF include:

- Dyspnea (especially with exertion, commonly severe in the acute setting)
- Paroxysmal nocturnal dyspnea

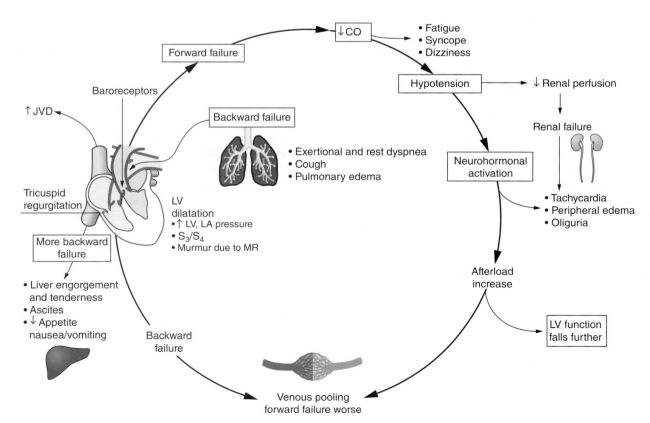

Figure 9-15. Clinical features of heart failure.

TABLE 9-9. CLINICAL SIGNS AND SYMPTOMS SPECIFIC TO RIGHT- AND LEFT-SIDED HEART FAILURE

Right Heart Failure	Left Heart Failure
Signs and Symptoms of Hepatic Congestion	**Signs and Symptoms of Pulmonary Congestion**
JVD	Pulmonary edema
Liver enlargement and tenderness	Rales
Positive hepatojugular reflex (pressure on liver increases JVD)	Atrial fibrillation or other atrial arrhythmias secondary to atrial distension
Dependent edema	Pulsus alternans (every other beat diminished)
Ascites	Dyspnea
Decreased appetite, nausea, vomiting	Cough
Cardiac Pressures	Hyperventilation
Increased RV pressure	Dizziness, syncope, fatigue
Increased RA pressure	**Cardiac Pressures**
Heart Sounds	Increased LV and LA pressure
S_3 (early sign)	Increased pulmonary artery pressures
S_4 (may also present)	**Heart Sounds**
Wide split S_2	S_3 and (occasionally) S_4
Pansystolic murmur at lower left sternal border secondary to stretching of tricuspid ring	Pansystolic murmur at apex secondary to mitral regurgitation

- Pulmonary edema (pronounced crackles)
- Jugular venous distention (JVD)
- Chest discomfort or tightness
- Peripheral edema
- Cool, pale, cyanotic skin
- Oliguria
- Reported weight gain
- Fatigue

More specific physical signs and symptoms of heart failure may vary in individuals depending on which ventricle is primarily involved. A summary of clinical findings specific to left and right ventricular failure is presented in Table 9-9.

Because subjective assessment of symptoms and their severity may vary from clinician to clinician, classification systems are used to standardize symptom severity as well as the evolution and progression of HF. The American College of Cardiology and the American Heart Association developed a staging system that addresses the evolution and progression of HF. A second system, known as the New York Heart Association (NYHA) Functional Classification System, is used to provide systematic assessment of patient status and to benchmark improvement or deterioration from initial evaluation (Table 9-10).

A number of conditions, both cardiac and non-cardiac, are similar to HF in their clinical presentation and are ruled out as possible diagnoses in the initial assessment. These conditions include MI, pulmonary disease, dysrhythmias, anemia, renal failure, nephrotic syndrome, and thyroid disease.

Diagnostic Tests

- *12-lead ECG:* Acute ST-T wave changes, low voltage, left ventricular hypertrophy, atrial fibrillation or other tachyarrhythmias, bradyarrhythmias, Q waves from previous MI, LBBB

TABLE 9-10. CLASSIFICATION OF CARDIOVASCULAR DISEASE

AHA/ACC Stages of Heart Failure	
Stage A:	Patients at high risk for HF due to the presence of conditions strongly associated with the development of HF. Asymptomatic.
Stage B:	Patients with structural disease, such as previous MI, but have never shown signs or symptoms of HF.
Stage C:	Patients with structural heart disease who have current or prior symptoms of HF.
Stage D:	Patients with advanced structural heart disease and marked symptoms at rest in spite of optimal medical therapy and who require specialized interventions.
New York Heart Association Functional Classification	
Class	
I	Patients with cardiac disease but without resulting limitations of physical activity. Ordinary physical activity does not cause undue fatigue, palpitation, dyspnea, or anginal pain.
II	Patients with cardiac disease resulting in slight limitation of physical activity. They are comfortable at rest. Ordinary physical activity results in fatigue, palpitation, dyspnea, or anginal pain.
III	Patients with cardiac disease resulting in marked limitation of physical activity. They are comfortable at rest. Less than ordinary physical activity causes fatigue, palpitations, dyspnea, or anginal pain.
IV	Patient with cardiac disease resulting in inability to carry on any physical activity without discomfort. Symptoms of cardiac insufficiency or of the anginal syndrome may be present even at rest. If any physical activity is undertaken, discomfort is increased.

- *Chest x-ray:* Cardiomegaly, cardiothoracic ratio more than 0.5
- *Complete blood count:* Low red cell count (anemia)
- *Urinalysis:* Proteinuria, red blood cells, or casts
- *Creatinine:* Elevated
- *Albumin:* Decreased
- *Serum sodium and potassium:* Decreased
- *CI:* less than 2.0 L/min/m^2
- *BNP:* Elevated
- *Echocardiography:* Dilated left ventricle, right ventricle, or right atria; hypertrophied left ventricle; AV valve incompetence; diffuse or segmental hypocontractility; atrial thrombus; pericardial effusion; LVEF less than 40%
- *Radionuclide ventriculography:* More precise measure of right ventricular dysfunction and LVEF

Principles of Management for Heart Failure

Acute management of HF has changed dramatically over the past decade, from an emphasis on the micromanagement of hemodynamic parameters, primarily using positive inotropes, to an emphasis on functional capacity and long-term survival with the use of neurohormonal blocking agents. This shift is due to a better understanding of the neurohormonal response and the dependence of the body on these mechanisms for compensation in low-output states. Goals of patient management in HF revolve around four general principles: (1) treatment of the underlying cause (eg, ischemia, valvular dysfunction), (2) management of fluid volume overload, (3) improvement of ventricular function, and (4) patient and family education.

Limiting the Initial Insult and Treating the Underlying Cause
The most effective, but often the most difficult, management strategy for HF is to limit the damage done by the initial insult. This limitation of myocardial damage and cell loss maximizes the amount of viable ventricular muscle, myocardial contractility, and overall ventricular function.

- Patients with AMI receive immediate treatment either with fibrinolytic therapy if eligible or transfer to the cardiac catheterization laboratory for primary PCI (see the previous section on acute ischemic heart disease).
- Patients with persistent ischemia may benefit from revascularization as a preventive measure against eventual tissue necrosis.
- Valve replacement or repair or other surgical corrections (ventricular reconstruction surgery) are undertaken as soon as possible to prevent prolonged overstretching of the ventricular myocardium.

Management of Fluid Volume Overload
Decrease preload by administering diuretic therapy, limiting dietary sodium, and restricting free water.

- Diuretics are initiated according to the severity of the patient's signs and symptoms. More severe symptoms require intravenous therapy and loop diuretics, and less severe symptoms may be managed adequately on loop diuretics. Thiazide diuretics may be added later if the patient does not respond to the loop diuretics. Caution must be taken not to diurese the patient too fast as rapid loss of fluid can lead to activation of the renin-angiotensin system.
- Sodium and fluid intake are monitored carefully, with sodium not exceeding 2 g/day and free water not exceeding 1500 mL in a 24-hour period. Obtain nutrition consult to reinforce sodium and water restrictions. Educate the patient and family about restricting sodium and free water after discharge.
- Serum sodium and potassium are monitored on a regular basis to prevent inadvertent electrolyte imbalances (each day or two in the acute setting, depending on the aggressiveness of therapy).
- Use daily weights to evaluate for changes in fluid status

Improvement of Left Ventricular Function
Improvement in left ventricular function is accomplished by decreasing the workload on the heart with preload and afterload reduction and by augmenting ventricular contractility. Ventricular function may be measured directly in the acute setting by monitoring CI using a noninvasive cardiac output monitor. As has been demonstrated by a number of large clinical trials, traditional micromanagement of hemodynamic variables, such as CI with inotropic agents, may be detrimental to long-term patient outcome. Current recommendations do not advocate this as an initial management strategy.

- Decrease preload (discussed earlier in section on fluid overload).
- Decrease afterload by administration of pharmacologic therapy, including ACE inhibitors and vasodilators. ACE inhibitors are recommended in all HF patients with an LVEF less than 40% unless otherwise contraindicated or not tolerated. Contraindications to ACE inhibitor therapy include previous intolerance, potassium greater than 5.5 mEq/L, hypotension with systolic blood pressure less than 90 mm Hg, and serum creatinine greater than 3.0 mg/dL. Cautious initiation of low-dose therapy in patients with contraindications may still be considered. If the patient is ACE inhibitor intolerant (eg, experiences a cough), an ARB may be administered. Vasodilators may also be used in conjunction with diuretics and ACE inhibitors if further afterload reduction is necessary. Nitrates are often used concomitantly with ACE inhibitors and diuretics to augment afterload reduction, especially in the case of underlying atherosclerotic disease, still the largest single contributor to HF. ARBs may be used if the patient does not tolerate the side effects of an ACE inhibitor (eg, cough).
- ACE inhibitors and beta-blockers are considered cornerstone therapy for HF in an effort to reverse the remodeling of the left ventricle. Aldosterone antagonists may be used as add on therapy. Isosorbide dinitrate and hydralazine may be effective, particularly in black patients. Digoxin has been shown to improve symptoms but is no longer considered to be first-line therapy unless paroxysmal atrial fibrillation or atrial flutter is present. Digoxin may be used to control the ventricular rate in this situation.
- A newer class of medications called angiotensin receptor neprilysin inhibitors (ARNI) are used for the management of heart failure with reduced ejection fraction. Sacubitril/valsartan (Entresto) is an example of this class of medications. It contains an ARB and a neprilysin inhibitor. The neprilysin inhibitor improves renal blood flow and promotes the loss of sodium. The ARB lowers blood pressure and reduces myocardial workload. Studies have demonstrated this medication reduces morbidity and mortality in heart failure as well as reduces hospital readmissions related to heart failure.
- Beta-blockers are also used to reduce the incidence of ventricular tachycardia and ventricular fibrillation, the most common cause of death in HF patients. Recommended beta-blockers for the management of HF

include carvedilol, metoprolol, and bisoprolol. Caution is indicated when initiating a beta-blocker in a patient with reactive airway disease.

- BNP (nesiritide [Natrecor®]) may be used to manage decompensated HF. Nesiritide's effects include promoting diuresis and vasodilation, thereby decreasing ventricular preload and afterload. The agent may also inhibit angiotensin II as well as some of the other neuroendocrine compensatory mechanisms associated with HF. Nesiritide® is recommended for acutely decompensated ventricular failure.

- *Dual-chamber biventricular pacemaker/implantable cardioverter defibrillator (ICD):* Approximately 60% of patients with dilated cardiomyopathy develop LBBB. In the presence of LBBB, the right and left ventricles no longer contract simultaneously but in a series causing the intraventricular septum to shift inappropriately, interfering with the aortic and mitral valve functioning. There have been several studies demonstrating significantly improved outcomes (quality of life, survival rates, etc) with the use of a dual-chamber biventricular pacemaker. This technology stimulates both ventricles simultaneously, causing both to contract at the same time resulting in a narrowing of the QRS complex and improved myocardial contractility and cardiac output. Often the pacing technology is combined with an ICD because sudden cardiac death related to ventricular tachycardia/fibrillation is the most common cause of death in these patients.

- Cardiac assist devices (left ventricular, right ventricular, or both) can provide temporary maintenance or preservation of ventricular function, especially as a bridge to recovery, bridge to cardiac transplantation, or as destination therapy (discharge to home). These devices may be inserted percutaneously via the femoral artery or femoral vein or surgically using the medial sternotomy or thoracotomy approach (see Chapter 19, Advanced Cardiovascular Concepts). Left ventricular apical cannulation allows ambulation and physical rehabilitation. Technological developments have contributed to the development of small axial flow pumps allowing many to be implanted with the drive line (power source) exiting the skin. Risks related to insertion of these devices include infection, peripheral embolization including stroke, and, for some, long-term weaning difficulties in the event that an organ donor is not available. Presently, the Heart Mate II® is approved for destination therapy (a replacement for heart transplant).

- *Intra-aortic balloon pump (IABP):* Femoral artery cannulation with the IABP allows for ventricular support, but restricts the patient to bed rest and compromises arterial flow to the cannulated limb. These patients will be in the intensive care unit (ICU).

- *Minimally invasive catheter-based micro-axial flow ventricular assist devices:* These are frequently used to reduce either left or right ventricular afterload and myocardial work. They may be inserted through the femoral artery across the aortic valve into the left ventricle or introduced via the femoral vein into the right atrium and through an atrial septostomy, and positioned in the left atrium. The device used to reduce right ventricular afterload is introduced into the right ventricle via the femoral vein and passed across the pulmonic valve. As with the IABP, the patient is restricted to bed rest.

- *Ventricular reconstruction:* Many patients with end-stage HF have a previous history of CAD and MI resulting in the development of a ventricular aneurysm on the anterior wall of the left ventricle. A surgical procedure can be performed removing the aneurysm, reducing the size of the ventricle resulting in increased contractility and cardiac output. Studies have shown that some patients experience improvement in physical functioning and NYHA Functional Class following this procedure.

- *Extracorporeal membrane oxygenation (ECMO):* In recent years, the use of ECMO has become more common for severely decompensated HF patients who are in cardiogenic shock. This is used as a bridge to recovery, a link to a ventricular assist device (VAD), or a bridge to transplant. The use of this technology is limited to the ICU.

Patient Education

Patients who present with HF to the progressive care unit have high acuity levels, require more pharmacological interventions, and have an increased need for emotional support surrounding the serious nature of the hospital admission. Previous admissions for HF make patients more aware of the serious nature of acute episodes. Patient education, which is appropriately addressed in the acute-care setting, includes the following:

- Both patient and family may require crisis interventions. The nurse may help by encouraging the verbalization of fears related to role adaptations or changes in family responsibility, lifestyle alterations and limitations, and death and dying. The completion of advanced directives and discussion of goals of care is initiated if not previously addressed.

- Family involvement in the acute-care phase is strongly encouraged, including assistance with activities of daily living such as bathing, and "patterning" of daily activities to allow for frequent periods of rest and spacing of exertional activity. In addition, family involvement in reading or other leisure activity with the patient is often restful and relaxing, and may be useful as a diversional activity. If possible, the family is also present for reinforcement of patient teaching regarding the medical regimen, the importance of fluid and sodium restriction, and the need for daily weights.

Shock

Shock is the inability of the circulatory system to deliver enough blood to meet the oxygen and metabolic requirements of body tissues. This clinical syndrome may result from ineffective pumping of the heart (cardiogenic shock), insufficient volume of circulating blood (hypovolemic shock), or massive vasodilation of the vascular bed causing maldistribution of blood (distributive shock). Although strategies for patient management vary according to the underlying pathophysiology, the basic definition of shock as ineffective or insufficient oxygen delivery to meet the needs of body tissues remains consistent.

Etiology, Risk Factors, and Pathophysiology

The ineffective delivery of oxygen to the tissues leads to cellular dysfunction, rapidly progressing to organ failure and finally to total body system failure. The cause of the initial onset of the shock syndrome may be from any number of underlying problems, including heart problems, fluid loss,

and trauma. Because the body responds in the same way, differences between cardiogenic, hypovolemic, and distributive shock are obvious to the clinician only after the initial assessment has provided key information about the patient's acute illness. Given the history and physical examination data, the clinician can classify shock into one of three major pathologic groups and proceed to further determine the patient's needs with the help of diagnostic testing. Interventions to treat shock are directed at the cause, so identifying the underlying pathophysiology is an essential step.

Cardiogenic Shock

In cardiogenic shock, the heart is unable to pump enough blood to meet the oxygen and metabolic needs of the body. Pump failure is caused by a variety of factors, the most common being CAD. A number of other factors may cause pump failure, however, and are typically categorized as coronary or noncoronary causes (Table 9-11).

In all cardiogenic shock cases, the heart ceases to function effectively as a pump, resulting in decreases in stroke

---

ESSENTIAL CONTENT CASE

Shock Following AMI

A 49-year-old man was found slumped in his living room chair, cool and clammy but still breathing. His wife called 911. The EMS arrived and transported him to the local emergency room. On arrival, his vital signs were as follows:

BP	68/44 mm Hg
HR	122 beats/min
RR	33 breaths/min
T	36.1°C, orally
Sao$_2$	91%

Oxygen at 60% by face mask had been initiated in the ambulance, as well as intravenous normal saline running wide open, 450 mL having already infused. Norepinephrine was started at a rate of 0.05 mcg/kg/min. A stat ECG showed "tombstone" ST elevation in anterior leads (V$_2$, V$_3$, V$_4$), with reciprocal changes in leads II, III, and aVF. The patient was taken for immediate PCI: angioplasty with a stent. In the laboratory, cardiac catheterization findings were as follows:

LAD	99% proximal lesion
RCA	70% mid lesion
LCx	Normal
LVEF	13%
Wall motion	Left ventricular akinesis

On return to the progressive care unit, the nurse obtained hemodynamic parameters as follows:

CO	4.0 L/min
CI	1.5 L/min/m^2

Case Question 1: What is the most likely cause of the patient's shock?
(A) Hypovolemic
(B) Distributive
(C) Cardiogenic
(D) Neurogenic

Case Question 2: Following the interventional procedure the primary goal for this patient is to:
(A) Reduce myocardial workload
(B) Dilate the pulmonary vascular bed
(C) Administer a diuretic
(D) Intubate the patient to improve oxygen delivery

Case Question 3: You anticipate the next intervention for this patient will be:
(A) Initiate a vasodilator to reduce afterload
(B) Give volume to improve preload
(C) Titrate the dopamine infusion up to 7.5 mcg/kg/min
(D) Prepare patient for transport to the cath lab for IABP insertion

Answers
1. C is the correct answer. Based on his clinical presentation and the "tombstone" ECG changes, he has had an anterior wall infarction and is in cardiogenic shock.
2. A is the correct answer. The primary goal is to reduce myocardial workload allowing the heart to recover.
3. D is the correct answer. Based on the low cardiac output, insertion of an IABP will help reduce his cardiac workload and improve coronary perfusion. Giving volume at this point is not necessary and dopamine may cause his heart to work harder.

TABLE 9-11. CAUSES OF CARDIOGENIC SHOCK

Coronary Causes
- MI with resultant cell death in a significant portion of the ventricle
- Rupture of ventricle or papillary muscle secondary to MI
- Dysfunctional ischemic—"shock ventricle"—which occurs as a result of myocardial ischemia, not involving cell death, and is therefore transient

Noncoronary Causes
- Myocardial contusion
- Pericardial tamponade
- Ventricular rupture
- Arrhythmia (PEA—pulseless electrical activity)
- Valvular dysfunction resulting in ventricular congestion
- Cardiomyopathies
- End-stage HF

volume and cardiac output. This leads to a decrease in blood pressure and tissue perfusion. The inadequate emptying of the ventricle increases left atrial pressure, which then increases pulmonary venous pressure. As a result, pulmonary capillary pressure increases, resulting in pulmonary edema.

Hypovolemic Shock

Hypovolemic shock occurs when there is inadequate volume in the vascular space. This volume depletion may be caused by blood loss, either internal or external, or by the vascular fluid volume shifting out of the vascular space into other body fluid spaces (Table 9-12). The loss of vascular volume results in insufficient circulating blood to maintain tissue perfusion.

The pathophysiology of hypovolemic shock is related directly to a decreased circulating blood volume. When an insufficient amount of blood is circulating, the venous blood returning to the heart is insufficient. As a result, right and left ventricular filling pressures are insufficient, decreasing stroke volume and cardiac output. As in cardiogenic shock, when cardiac output is decreased, BP is low and tissue perfusion is poor.

Distributive Shock

Distributive shock is characterized by an abnormal placement or distribution of vascular volume. There are three primary causes of distributive shock: (1) sepsis, (2) neurologic damage, and (3) anaphylaxis. In each of these situations, the pumping function of the heart and the total blood volume

TABLE 9-12. CAUSES OF HYPOVOLEMIC SHOCK

Sources of External Loss of Body Fluid
- Hemorrhage (loss of whole blood)
- Gastrointestinal tract (vomiting, diarrhea, ostomies, fistulas, nasogastric suctioning)
- Renal (diuretic administration, diabetes, insipidus, Addison disease, hyperglycemic osmotic diuresis)

Sources of Internal Loss of Body Fluid
- Internal hemorrhage
- Movement of body fluid into interstitial spaces ("third spacing," often the result of bacterial toxin, thermal injury, or allergic reaction)

are normal, but the blood is not appropriately distributed throughout the vascular bed. Massive vasodilation occurs in each of these situations for various reasons, causing the vascular bed to be much larger than normal. In this enlarged vascular bed, the usual volume of circulating blood (approximately 5 L) is no longer sufficient to fill the vascular space, causing a decrease in blood pressure and inadequate tissue perfusion. For this reason distributive shock is also referred to as relative hypovolemic shock.

Of the distributive shock syndromes, septic shock is most commonly seen in the acute care setting. In the field or emergency department setting, anaphylaxis and neurogenic shock are also common and typically result from allergic reactions and trauma-related spinal cord injury.

Stages of Shock

Regardless of underlying etiology, all three types of shock (cardiogenic, hypovolemic, distributive) activate the sympathetic nervous system, which in turn initiates neural, hormonal, and chemical compensatory mechanisms in an attempt to improve tissue perfusion (Figure 9-16). Cellular changes that occur as a result of these compensatory mechanisms are similar in all types of shock. Progression of these cellular changes follows a predictable, four-stage course.

Initial Stage

The initial stage of shock represents the first cellular changes resulting from the decrease in oxygen delivery to the tissue. These changes include decreased aerobic and increased anaerobic metabolism, leading to increase in serum lactic acid. No obvious clinical signs and symptoms are apparent during this stage of shock.

Compensatory Stage

The compensatory stage is composed of a number of physiologic events that represent an attempt to compensate for decrease in cardiac output and restore adequate oxygen and nutrient delivery to the tissues (Figure 9-17). These events can be organized into neural, hormonal, and chemical responses. Neural responses involve the baroreceptors in the aortic arch and carotid arteries, detecting changes in the arterial BP, and responding by activating the vasomotor center of the medulla. Hypovolemia and resultant hypotension lead to activation of the sympathetic nervous system. The sympathetic nervous system initiates compensatory mechanisms causing peripheral vasoconstriction and elevation of the BP. The sympathetic nervous system activation produces vasoconstriction of the peripheral circulation, shunting blood to vital organs (autoregulation). Vasoconstriction of the peripheral circulation shunts blood to the vital organs, reducing renal blood flow, which activates the hormonal response.

Hormonal responses include increased production of catecholamines and adrenocorticotropic hormone (ACTH) and activation of the renin-angiotensin-aldosterone system.

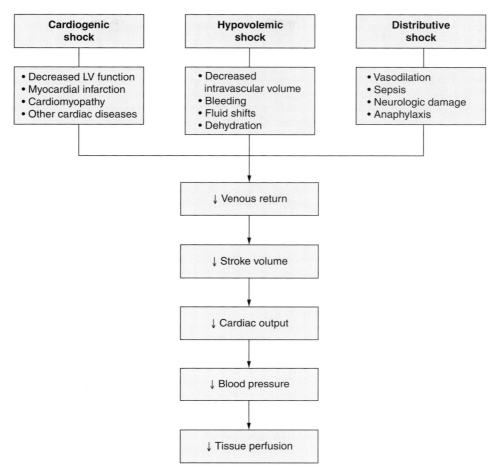

Figure 9-16. Pathophysiology of shock.

As a direct result of decreased renal blood flow, renin is released from the juxtaglomerular cells in the kidney, combining with angiotensinogen from the liver resulting in the production of angiotensin I. Angiotensin I, circulating in the blood, is converted to angiotensin II in the lungs. As was discussed in more detail in the HF section, this hormonal response results in direct peripheral vasoconstriction, as well as release of aldosterone from the adrenal cortex and antidiuretic hormone (ADH) from the pituitary gland. Sodium and potassium retention, in conjunction with increased ADH, ACTH, and circulating catecholamines, effectively increases intravascular volume, heart rate, and blood pressure, and decreases urine output.

Chemical responses during the compensatory stage are related to the respiratory ventilation-perfusion imbalance, which occurs as a result of sympathetic stimulation, redistribution of blood flow, and decreased pulmonary perfusion. A respiratory alkalosis ensues, adversely affecting the patient's level of consciousness, and causing restlessness, and agitation.

These compensatory mechanisms are effective for finite periods of time, which may vary depending on the individual and presence of comorbidities. Younger and healthier patients are more likely to survive a prolonged episode of shock. In the absence of vascular volume replacement, these intrinsic vasopressors eventually fail as a compensatory mechanism, and the patient enters the progressive, and finally refractory, stages of shock, usually resulting in death.

Progressive Stage

The progressive stage is characterized by end-organ failure due to cellular damage from prolonged compensatory changes. The compensatory changes, which supported blood pressure and therefore tissue perfusion, are no longer effective and severe hypoperfusion ensues. Impaired oxygen delivery to the tissues results in multiple organ system failure—typically beginning with gastrointestinal and renal failure—followed by respiratory and/or cardiac failure and loss of liver and cerebral function (see Chapter 11, Multisystem Problems, for more on sepsis).

Refractory Stage

The refractory stage, as its name implies, is the irreversible stage of shock. At this stage, cell death has progressed to such a point as to be irreparable, and death is imminent.

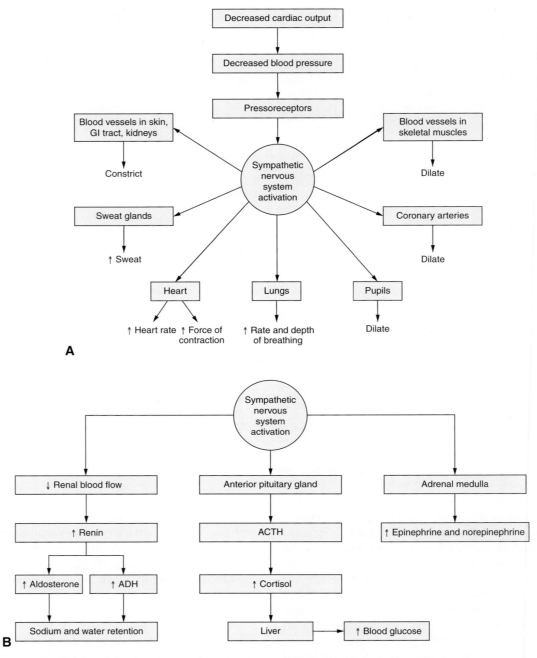

Figure 9-17. Compensatory response to shock. **(A)** Neural compensation. **(B)** Hormonal compensation.

Clinical Presentation

Clinical signs and symptoms vary depending on the underlying cause of shock and the stage of shock in which the patient presents.

- *Initial stage:* No visible signs and symptoms evident from ongoing cellular changes
- *Compensatory stage:*
  - Consciousness: Restless, agitated, confused
  - Blood pressure: Normal or slightly low
  - Heart rate: Increased (though neurogenic distributive shock causes bradycardia)

- Respiratory rate: Increased (> 20 breaths/min)
- Skin: Cool, clammy, may be cyanotic—though massive vasodilation in distributive shock may mean that these symptoms are absent
- Peripheral pulses: Weak and thready
- Urine output: Concentrated and scant (< 30 mL/h)
- Bowel sounds: Hypoactive, possible abdominal distension
- Laboratory results:
  - Glucose: Increased
  - Sodium: Increased

- Pao$_2$: Decreased
- Paco$_2$: Decreased
- pH: Increased
- *Progressive stage:*
  - Consciousness: Unresponsive to verbal stimuli
  - Blood pressure: Inadequate (< 90 mm Hg systolic)
  - Heart rate: Increased greater than 90/min
  - Respiratory rate: Increased, shallow
  - Skin: Cold, cyanotic, mottled
  - Peripheral pulses: Weak and thready, may be absent
  - Urine output: Scant (< 20 mL/h) and concentrated
  - Bowel sounds: Absent
  - Laboratory results:
    - Amylase: Increased
    - Lipase: Increased
    - SGPT/SGOT: Increased
    - Lactate: Increased
    - CPK: Increased
    - Creatinine: Increased
    - Blood urea nitrogen: Increased
    - Pao$_2$: Decreased
    - Paco$_2$: Increased
    - pH: Decreased
    - HCO$_3$: Decreased

Diagnostic Tests
- *Cardiogenic*
  - ECG: Tachycardia
  - Pulmonary arterial pressure: PAD/PAOP high (> 12 mm Hg), RAP high (> 8 mm Hg)
  - Echocardiogram: Ventricular wall motion abnormalities, cardiac tamponade, ventricular rupture
- *Hypovolemic*
  - Pulmonary arterial pressure: PAD/PAOP low (< 8 mm Hg), RAP low (< 5 mm Hg), right ventricular end-diastolic volume index low
  - Ultrasound: Groin or retroperitoneal hemorrhage
- *Distributive*
  - Septic: WBC ≥ 12,000 or ≤ 4,000 neutrophils > 10%, serum lactate > 4 mmol/L, positive blood cultures (in 50% of patients)
  - Anaphylactic: History of allergen exposure, and arterial blood gas shows inadequate oxygenation
  - Neurogenic: Computed tomography (CT) scan and magnetic resonance imaging (MRI) show spinal cord damage

Principles of Management for Shock
Differences in the underlying cause of shock lead to some variation in the principles of management. The basic goals of therapy for all forms of shock, however, include the need to correct the underlying cause of shock, improvement of oxygenation, and restoration of adequate tissue perfusion. Often, a patient in shock will be transferred to the critical care unit for management of their shock state.

Correction of the Underlying Cause of Shock
- *Cardiogenic:* Remove coronary obstruction or correct tamponade, if present, and support ventricular contractility to increase cardiac output.
- *Hypovolemic:* Identify source and stop bleeding if possible; correct fluid shunting or third spacing with electrolyte management.
- *Distributive*
  - Anaphylactic: Intubate for oxygenation and treat the underlying allergic reaction using antidote or steroid therapy.
  - Septic: Administer fluid resuscitation, draw blood cultures and serum lactate; give broad spectrum antibiotics and 30 mL/kg of fluid for hypotension; identify likely sources including consideration of any invasive lines or devices (see Chapter 11, Multisystem Problems, for more on sepsis).
  - Neurogenic: Severing of the cord may be irreversible; however, intubation provides respiratory support while the underlying cause is identified.

Improve Oxygenation
- Assess for patent airway and intubate if necessary.
- Administer oxygen to maintain Pao$_2$ > 60-70 mmHg.

Restore Adequate Tissue Perfusion
- Administer fluid volume expanders (normal saline, lactated Ringer solution, or plasmanate) in large rapid boluses. Type and cross-match for blood type and administer blood as necessary for hypovolemic shock.
- Initiate vasoactive therapy.

Hypertension
Hypertension is typically a chronic disease of BP elevation that is often masked, especially in the early years of onset, by lack of warning signs or symptoms. Hypertensive crisis is an acute episode or exacerbation, occurring infrequently in a small percentage of hypertensive patients and characterized by the pivotal effect the particular episode and its treatment may have on the patient's long-term outcome. In most cases, the numerical or absolute value of the arterial BP is less important than its impact on the individual's underlying risk of target organ damage, specifically cerebrovascular, coronary, and renal diseases.

Etiology, Risk Factors, and Pathophysiology
Although a number of clinical syndromes commonly are associated with hypertension and many underlying etiologies may contribute to the progression of hypertensive disease, the pathophysiology of hypertension is similar regardless of the underlying cause.

An acute hypertensive crisis begins with elevation of the systolic or diastolic BP causing a threat, direct or indirect, to an organ or body system. Acute, severe increases in pressure

TABLE 9-13.   CLASSIFICATION OF BLOOD PRESSURE FOR ADULTS

Blood Pressure Classification	SBP (mm Hg)	DBP (mm Hg)
Normal	< 120	And < 80
Elevated	120-129	< 80
Stage 1 hypertension	130-139	80-89
Stage 2 hypertension	≥ 140	≥ 90

Abbreviations: DBP, diastolic blood pressure; mm Hg, millimeters of mercury; SBP, systolic blood pressure.

may cause serious, life-threatening cerebrovascular and cardiovascular compromise. Prolonged hypoperfusion of an organ system leads to ischemia, necrosis, and organ system failure.

Classification

Because of the increased risk of such events in all hypertensive patients, morbidity and mortality directly related to hypertension is high, and long-term, consistent therapy in all stages of hypertension is necessary. Hypertension can be described in stages, or classified according to the value of the blood pressure. Table 9-13 refers to the classification of blood pressure for adults.

- *Elevated blood pressure:* Current guidelines define an elevated blood pressure as a SBP 120-29 and DBP < 80 mm Hg.
- *Stage 1 hypertension:* Hypertension is characterized by an elevated systolic blood pressure 130-139 mm Hg or 80-89 mm Hg diastolic in adults.
- *Stage 2 hypertension:* Hypertension is defined as a systolic BP ≥ 140 mm Hg or a diastolic BP ≥ 90 mm Hg.
- *Hypertensive crisis:* Hypertensive crisis has been subdivided into "Urgencies" and "Emergencies." Hypertensive urgency is characterized by a systolic BP > 180 mm Hg and/or a diastolic BP > 120 mm Hg. Many of these patients are found to be nonadherent with their antihypertensive therapy. Generally they do not have clinical evidence of new or worsening target organ damage. Hypertensive emergency is defined by a systolic BP > 180 mm Hg associated with target end-organ damage and/or a diastolic BP > 120 mm Hg associated with target end-organ damage. Both of these groups require immediate lowering of their blood pressure.
- *Special populations:* In pregnant women and in children a less severe elevation in blood pressure may result in significant end-organ damage and is therefore considered to be a "hypertensive crisis" at values much lower than would be expected to be problematic in the average adult. The absolute value of the blood pressure varies significantly depending on the situation and the individual involved; for example, preeclampsia, considered to be a hypertensive crisis in pregnancy, may occur at pressures as low as 130/100 to 160/100 mm Hg.

Clinical Presentation

Patients experiencing a hypertensive crisis may have the following signs and symptoms:

- Headache
- Blurred vision
- Nosebleed
- Dizziness or vertigo
- Transient ischemic attack
- Diminished peripheral pulses or bruits
- Carotid or abdominal bruit
- Heart sounds with S_3 and/or S_4
- Systolic and/or diastolic murmurs
- Gastrointestinal bleeding
- Pulmonary edema
- Shortness of breath
- Fatigue
- Malaise
- Weakness
- Nausea and vomiting
- Hematuria
- Dysuria
- *Funduscopic findings:* Arteriovenous thickening, arteriolar narrowing, hemorrhage, papilledema, or exudates

Diagnostic Tests

- *Chest x-ray:* Myocardial hypertrophy, pulmonary infiltrates
- *Computed tomography:* Arteriolar narrowing and arteriovenous thickening
- Specific tests to target organ damage
- Renal angiography
- Coronary angiography
- Carotid/cerebral angiography
- *Magnetic resonance imaging:* Cerebral vascular malperfusion

Principles of Management for Hypertension

Management of the patient with acute exacerbation of hypertension, or hypertensive crisis, revolves around three primary objectives: (1) reduction of arterial pressure, (2) evaluation and treatment of target organ damage, and (3) preparation and planning for continuous and consistent outpatient follow-up.

Reduction of Arterial Pressure

Ascertain correct arterial blood pressure. Verify arterial blood pressure, being sure to assess bilateral measurements with the correct cuff size if using sphygmomanometry, as well as orthostatic pressures if possible (lying and sitting up, if standing is not possible). Each measurement is 2 minutes apart and both right and left measurements are documented. If differences between the right and left measurements are greater than 10 mm Hg, the higher reading is used to gauge therapy. In most acute situations, priority is given to

TABLE 9-14. COMMON DRUGS USED TO MANAGE ACUTE HYPERTENSIVE EPISODES

Nitroprusside	• Dilates arterioles and veins. • Administer IV at 0.5-10.0 mcg/kg/min (mix in normal saline only; 100 mg in 500 mL). Cover bottle with foil to avoid light exposure. • Titrate up to desired BP, recognizing that the effect will be evident within 1 minute of change in dose.
Nicardipine	• Calcium channel blocker. • Administer 5 mg/h initially, titrate 2.5 mg/h at 5- to 15-minute intervals to a maximum dose of 15 mg/h.
Nitroglycerin	• Dilates veins more than arterioles. • Administer IV at a rate of 5-100 mcg/min. Mix 100 mg in 100 mL NS or D_5 IV.
Esmolol	• Beta-1 selective blocker and at higher doses inhibits B2 receptors in the blood vessels. • Useful for treating hypertension • Administer 0.5 mg/kg over 1 minute loading dose followed by 50 mcg/kg/min infusion. • Titrate to achieve desired lower BP • Onset of action within minutes • Peak effect in less than 5 minutes
Enalapril	• An ACE inhibitor. • Administer IV at a rate of 5 mg/min.
Labetalol	• Beta-receptor agonist (beta-blocker). • Particularly indicated in patients with suspected MI or angina. • Administer 5 mg bolus over 5 minutes and repeat three times. IV drip may then be started.

establishing a stable arterial access site for direct, invasive monitoring of BP.

Initiate pharmacologic intervention. For acute high arterial pressure, intravenous pharmacologic intervention is the fastest, most effective means of reducing arterial blood pressure. A number of agents are used in the acute setting for management of hypertensive crisis (Table 9-14). Aggressiveness of pharmacologic intervention is based on the severity of blood pressure elevation (immediate risk of stroke), the immediate risk of irreversible target organ damage (renal and hepatic function related to medication metabolism and clearance is also considered), and any confounding conditions or risk factors that are present (eg, the fetus in preeclampsia). In general, acute, severe hypertensive crises are treated as quickly and aggressively as can be tolerated by the patient in order to prevent the immediate risk of hypertensive encephalopathy, dissecting aortic aneurysm, MI, or intracranial hemorrhage. Maintenance of cerebral perfusion pressure is imperative during treatment, and overly aggressive pharmacologic management poses the threat of cerebrovascular compromise due to a sudden drop in arterial pressure and inability of the autoregulatory mechanism to adjust. Other organ systems dependent on higher pressure for perfusion include the renal and coronary systems. A sudden, severe drop in systemic arterial pressure may result in ischemic episodes or acute renal failure.

For non-acute hypertension, dietary alteration and relaxation, or biofeedback techniques may be used in addition to pharmacologic measures to reduce the morbidity and mortality of hypertension. Although these measures are most effective when employed long term as part of a cohesive outpatient follow-up program, initiating these strategies in the acute setting may help emphasize their importance.

Evaluation and Treatment of Target Organ Disease

Concomitant to initiation of pharmacologic intervention, the assessment and prevention of target organ disease is important to avoid irreversible damage. Target organs typically at risk include the brain, heart, kidneys, and eyes. Strategies to prevent damage to these organ systems during hypertensive crisis include the following:

- *Brain:* Reduce diastolic pressure by one-third (not to go < 95 mm Hg) using aggressive pharmacologic measures (see Table 9-14).
- *Heart:* Reduce diastolic and systolic pressure by one-third; administer combination therapy if possible (vasodilator and beta-blocker) or ACE inhibitor for afterload reduction; monitor for ischemic changes on ECG.
- *Kidneys:* Reduce systolic and diastolic BP using pharmacologic measures; monitor serum creatinine and urine specific gravity as well as proteinuria and hematuria; for patients with severe existing renal impairment, use of ACE inhibitors may exacerbate their renal compromise and is therefore contraindicated in patients with bilateral renal artery stenosis; administer diuretics to maintain serum sodium and adequate diuresis.
- *Eyes:* Reduce systolic and diastolic BP; observe retina for evidence of hemorrhage, exudate, or papilledema; instruct the patient with blurring of vision regarding his or her environment, especially location of the call bell.

Patient Education on Lifestyle Modification and Follow-Up

Following control of hypertension in the acute phase, patient education is initiated regarding the serious and chronic nature of the disease. Often, the clinician may have an opportunity in the acute stage to make an impact regarding the seriousness of uncontrolled hypertension and its potentially debilitating effects. Prior to beginning the educational process, assessment includes:

1. Family history of hypertension, cardiovascular disease, CAD, stroke, diabetes mellitus, and hyperlipidemia
2. Lifestyle history including weight gain, exercise, and smoking habits
3. Dietary patterns including high sodium, alcohol, and dietary fat intake or low potassium intake
4. Knowledge of hypertension and impact of previous medical therapy for hypertension (compliance, side effects, results, or efficacy)

ESSENTIAL CONTENT CASE

Thinking Critically

A 52-year-old man, 4 days post-anterior MI, is transferred to the progressive care unit from a medicine floor with severe shortness of breath. The initial assessment reveals the following:

HR	128 beats/min
BP	110/82 mm Hg
RR	36 breaths/min
T	37.6°C, orally
Pulse oximetry	88%
Lung sounds	Coarse, bilateral crackles in lower lobes, poor respiratory effort
Heart sounds	S_1, S_2, S_3
Skin	Flushed, diaphoretic, 2+ pedal edema
ECG	Sinus tachycardia, with tall R-waves in V_5-V_6 indicating left ventricular hypertrophy

Case Question 1: What is the first priority in the care of this patient?
(A) Obtain an arterial blood gas measurement
(B) Initiate a nesiritide infusion
(C) Prepare to intubate the patient
(D) Call a Code Blue

Case Question 2: What is the most likely underlying cause for this patient's respiratory compromise?
(A) Acute decompensated HF with pulmonary edema
(B) Abrupt onset of septic shock with ARDS

(C) Acute anxiety attack
(D) Hypovolemic shock

Case Question 3: Management of this condition would most likely include what interventions?
1. Administration of a diuretic to reduce preload
2. Initiation of a dobutamine infusion at 5 mcg/kg/min
3. Repeat arterial blood gas
4. Administration of 30 mL/kg crystalloid

(A) 1 and 3
(B) 1 and 2
(C) 3 and 4
(D) 4

Answers
1. C is the correct answer. Intubation is necessary based on his high respiratory rate (36/min) and pulse oximetry of 88%. Calling a Code Blue at this time is not necessary. Obtaining an arterial blood gas following intubation is recommended.
2. A is the correct answer. Given his recent anterior MI, decompensated heart failure and acute pulmonary edema is the most likely cause of his respiratory distress.
3. B is the correct answer. The diuretic will help reduce preload and pulmonary congestion. Dobutamine will improve myocardial contractility and improve cardiac output.

SELECTED BIBLIOGRAPHY

General Cardiovascular

Mann DL, Zipes DP, Libby P, eds. *Braunwald's Heart Disease: A Textbook of Cardiovascular Medicine*. 10th ed. Philadelphia, PA: Saunders Elsevier; 2015.
Morton PG, Fontaine DK. *Critical Care Nursing: A Holistic Approach*. 11th ed. Philadelphia, PA: Wolters Kluwer; 2017.
Pickett JD, Bridges E, Kritek PA, Whitney JD. Passive leg-raising and prediction of fluid responsiveness: systematic review. *Crit Care Nurse*. 2017;37(2):32-47.

Coronary Revascularization

Hardin S, Kaplow R. *Cardiac Surgery Essentials for Critical Care Nursing*. 2nd ed. Dudbury, MA: Jones & Bartlett Publishing; 2015.
South T. Coronary artery bypass surgery. *Crit Care Nurs Clin North Am*. 2011;23(4):573-586.

Acute Ischemic Heart Disease

Carey MG. Acute coronary syndrome and ST segment monitoring. *Crit Care Nurs Clin North Am*. 2016;(3):347-356.
Pelter MM, Kozik TM, Al-Zaiti SS, Carey MC. Differential diagnoses for suspected ACS. *Am J Crit Care*. 2016;25(4):377-378.

Thygesen K, Alpert JS, Jaffe AS, et al. Third universal definition of myocardial infarction. *Circulation*. 2012;126(16):2020-2035.

Heart Failure

Albert NM. Fluid management strategies in heart failure. *Crit Care Nurse*. 2012;32(2):20-33.
Doty D. Ventricular assist device and destination therapy candidates from preoperative selection through end of hospitalization. *Crit Care Nurs Clin North Am*. 2015;27(4):551-564.
Lee CS, Auld J. Heart failure: a primer. *Crit Care Nurs Clin North Am*. 2015;27(4):413-425.
O'Shea G. Ventricular assist devices: what intensive care unit nurses need to know about post-operative management. *AACN Adv Crit Care*. 2012;23(1):69-83.

Hypertension

Taylor DA. Hypertensive crisis: a review of pathophysiology and treatment. *Crit Care Nurs Clin North Am*. 2015;27(4):439-448.
Whelton PK, Appel LJ, Sacco RL, et al. Sodium, blood pressure, and cardiovascular disease: further evidence supporting the American Heart Association sodium reduction recommendations. *Circulation*. 2012;126(24):2880-2889.

Evidence-Based Practice Guidelines

American Association of Critical-Care Nurses. *AACN Practice Alert: Ensuring Accurate ST-Segment Monitoring.* Aliso Viejo, CA: American Association of Critical-Care Nurses; 2016, December.

American Association of Critical-Care Nurses. AACN Practice Alert: Obtaining Accurate Noninvasive Blood Pressure Measurements in Adults. *Crit Care Nurse.* 2016;36(3):e12-e16.

Amsterdam EA, Wenger NK, Brindis RG, et al. 2014 AHA/ACC guideline for the management of patients with non-ST-elevation acute coronary syndromes: executive summary: a report from the American College of Cardiology/American Heart Association Task Force on Practice Guidelines. *Circulation.* 2014;130(25):2354-2394.

Hillis LD, Smith PK, Anderson JL, et al. 2011 ACCF/AHA guideline for coronary artery bypass surgery: executive summary: a report of the American College of Cardiology Foundation/American Heart Association Task Force on Practice Guidelines. *Circulation.* 2011;124(23):e652-e735.

James PA, Oparil S, Carter BL, et al. 2014 evidence-based guideline for the management of high blood pressure in adults. Report from the panel members appointed to the Eighth Joint National Committee (JNC 8). *JAMA.* 2014;311(5):507-520. doi:10.1001/jama.2013.284427.

Levine GN, Bates ER, Blankenship JC, et al. 2010 ACCF/AHA/SCAI guidelines for percutaneous coronary intervention: a report of the American College of Cardiology Foundation/American Heart Association Task Force on Practice Guidelines and the Society for Cardiovascular Angiography and Interventions. *Circulation.* 2011;124:e574-e651.

O'Gara PT, Kushner FG, Ascheim DD, et al. 2013 ACCF/AHA guideline for the management of ST-elevation myocardial infarction: executive summary: a report of the American College of Cardiology Foundation/American Heart Association Task Force on Practice Guidelines. *Circulation.* 2013;127(4):529-555.

Peura JL, Colvin-Adams M, Francis GS, et al. Recommendations for the use of mechanical circulatory support: device strategies and patient selection: a scientific statement from the American Heart Association. *Circulation.* 2012;126:2648-2667.

Rhodes A, Evans LE, Alhazzani W, et al. Surviving sepsis campaign: international guidelines for management of sepsis and septic shock: 2016. *Crit Care Med.* 2017;45(3):486-552.

Welton PK, Carey RM, Aronow WS, et al. 2018 ACC/AHA/AAPA/ABC/ACPM/AGS/APhA/ASH/ASPC/NMA/PCNA guideline for prevention, detection, evaluation, and management of high blood pressure in adults. A report of the American College of Cardiology/American Heart Association Task Force on Clinical Practice Guidelines. *Hypertension.* 2018;70(6):1269-1324.

Yancy CW, Jessup M, Bozkurt B, et al. 2013 ACCF/AHA guideline for the management of heart failure: executive summary. A report of the American Colleege of Cardiology Foundation/American Heart Association Task Force on Practice Guidelines. *Circulation.* 2013;128(16):1810-52. doi: 10.1161/CIR.0b013e31829e8807.

Yancy CW, Jessup M, Bozkurt B, et al. 2017 ACC/AHA/HFSA focused update on the 2013 ACCF/AHA/guideline for the management of heart failure: a report of the American College of Cardiology/American Heart Association Task Force on Clinical Practice Guidelines and the Heart Failure Society of America. *Circulation.* 2017;8;136(6):e137-e161.

RESPIRATORY SYSTEM

Maureen A. Seckel

10

KNOWLEDGE COMPETENCIES

1. Identify various radiologic and pulmonary anatomic features relevant to interpretation of chest x-rays.

2. Describe different systems and principles of management for chest tubes.

3. Describe the etiology, pathophysiology, clinical presentation, patient needs, and principles of management of acute respiratory failure (ARF).

4. Compare and contrast the pathophysiology, clinical presentation, patient needs, and

management approaches for common diseases leading to ARF:
- Acute respiratory distress syndrome (ARDS)
- Acute respiratory failure
- Chronic obstructive pulmonary disease (COPD) exacerbation
- Acute asthma
- Pulmonary hypertension (PH)
- Pneumonia
- Interstitial lung disease (ILD)
- Pulmonary embolism (PE)
- Venous thromboembolism (VTE)

SPECIAL ASSESSMENT TECHNIQUES, DIAGNOSTIC TESTS, AND MONITORING SYSTEMS

Chest X-Rays

Chest radiography is an important tool in respiratory assessment, providing visualization of the heart and lungs. Chest x-rays are a complement to bedside assessment. Progressive care nurses need to know basic radiographic concepts and how to optimize portable chest x-ray technique, as well as how to systematically view a chest x-ray image.

Chest x-rays are obtained as part of routine screening procedures, when respiratory disease or an acute change is suspected, to evaluate the status of respiratory abnormalities (eg, pneumothorax, pleural effusion, tumors), to confirm proper invasive tube placement (ie, endotracheal, tracheostomy, or chest tubes, and central line catheters), or following traumatic chest injury.

Basic Concepts

An x-ray is a form of electromagnetic radiation used by imaging machines to create a radiographic image. Only a

few rays are absorbed by air whereas all rays are absorbed by solid substances such as metal or bone. When nothing but air lies between the film cassette and the x-ray source, the radiographic image is blackness or radiolucency. If density increases, more beams are absorbed between the film cassette or detector and the x-ray source, and the radiographic image is whiteness or radiopacity. As the x-ray beam passes through the patient, the denser tissues absorb more of the beam, and the less dense tissues absorb less of the beam. There are four distinct radiographic densities: white, light gray, darker gray, and black. Many institutions are replacing traditional x-ray film with detectors that convert the x-ray energy to a digital radiograph. These can then be stored and distributed in a digital format.

The lungs are primarily sacs of air or gas, so normal lungs look mostly black on chest films. Conversely, the skeletal thorax appears white, because bone is very dense and absorbs the most x-rays (Table 10-1). The heart and mediastinum appear gray because those structures are made up of mostly water and muscle or tissue. Breast tissue is made

TABLE 10-1. BASIC X-RAY DENSITIES

Radiolucent (black)
Gas, air (dark or black)
• Lungs, trachea, bronchi, alveoli
Water (dark or gray)
• Heart, muscle, blood, blood vessels, diaphragm, spleen, liver
Fat (lighter or whitish-gray)
• Breasts, marrow, hilar streaking
Radiopaque (white)
Metal, bone (lightest or white)
• Ribs, scapulae, vertebrae
• Bullets, coins, teeth, ECG electrodes

up of mostly fat and it appears whitish-gray. Structures of the thorax are made radiographically visible if they are surrounded by air. Conversely, they are obscured if adjacent to consolidation or fluid.

Basic Views of the Chest

The most common method of obtaining a chest x-ray is the posterior-anterior (PA) view. PA chest x-rays are typically done in the radiology department with the machine about 6 ft away from the x-ray film cassette and the patient standing with the anterior chest wall against the x-ray plate and the posterior chest wall toward the x-ray machine. The patient is told to take a deep breath and hold it as the x-ray beam is delivered through the posterior chest wall to the x-ray film cassette. The PA view results in a very accurate, sharp picture of the chest.

Acutely ill patients are rarely able to tolerate the positioning requirements of a PA chest x-ray. Many chest x-rays in progressive care are obtained with an anterior-posterior (AP) view with the patient supine in bed, with or without back rest elevation. With portable AP chest films, the film cassette or digital sensor is placed behind the patient and the x-ray beam is delivered through the anterior chest to the film or sensor. The x-ray machine is only 3 ft away from the patient, which results in greater distortion of chest images, making the AP chest x-ray less accurate than the PA method. Of particular concern is that the heart size is enlarged on an AP film because of its anterior placement in the chest. When viewing chest x-rays, it is important to know whether a PA or an AP view was used to avoid misinterpretation of heart size as cardiomegaly.

Placing the patient in a high Fowler position, or as erect as possible, with the thorax symmetrically placed on the film or sensor can help to minimize distortions. Explain the procedure to the patient and the need to avoid movement. All mobile objects lying on the anterior chest (such as ventilator tubing, safety pins, jewelry, ECG wires, nasogastric tubes, etc) are removed or repositioned as possible. If the patient is unconscious, taping the forehead in a neutral position may be necessary, especially in the high Fowler position to avoid malpositioning of the head. If unable to leave the room, caregivers assisting with the chest x-ray need to protect themselves from radiation exposure by positioning themselves behind the x-ray machine or by using lead aprons covering

the neck, chest, and abdomen. Non-essential staff and visitors should leave the room and remain at least 6 ft from the radiation source.

Other chest x-ray views include: (1) lateral views to identify normal and abnormal structures behind the heart, along the spine, and at the base of the lung; (2) oblique views to localize lesions without interference from the bony thorax or to get a better picture of the trachea, carina, heart, and great vessels; (3) lordotic views to better visualize the apical and middle regions of the lungs and to differentiate anterior from posterior lesions; and (4) lateral decubitus (cross-table) views, done with the patient supine or side-lying, to assess for air-fluid levels or free-flowing pleural fluid.

Systematic Approach to Chest X-Ray Interpretation

A systematic approach facilitates accurate interpretation of a chest x-ray image including reviewing the results. It is important to first make sure that the report and image are properly labeled (correct name and medical record number), and to identify the right and left sides of the images. If previous images are available, place them next to the new images for comparison. View the chest x-ray from the lateral borders, moving to the medial aspects of the thorax and asking the series of questions found in Table 10-2. Begin the chest x-ray analysis by comparing the right side to the left side using the following sequence (Figures 10-1 and 10-2): (1) soft tissues—neck, shoulders, breasts, and subcutaneous fat; (2) trachea—the column of radiolucency readily visible above the clavicles; (3) bony thorax—note size, shape, and symmetry; (4) intercostal spaces (ICSs)—note width and angle; (5) diaphragm—dome-shaped with distinct margins, right dome 1 to 3 cm higher than left dome; (6) pleural surfaces—visceral and parietal pleura appear like a thin, hairlike line along the apices and lateral chest; (7) mediastinum—size varies with age, gender, and patient size; (8) hila—large pulmonary arteries and veins; (9)

TABLE 10-2. STEPS FOR INTERPRETATION OF A CHEST X-RAY FILM

Step 1
Look at the different densities (black, gray, and white), and answer the question, "What is air, fluid, tissue, and bone?"
Step 2
Look at the shape or form of each density, and answer the question, "What normal anatomic structure is this?"
Step 3
Look at both right and left sides, and answer the question, "Are the findings the same on both sides or are there differences (both physiologic and pathophysiologic)?"
Step 4
Look at all the structures (bones, mediastinum, diaphragm, pleural space, and lung tissue), and answer the question, "Are there any abnormalities present?"
Step 5
Look for all tubes, wires, and lines, and answer the question, "Are the tubes, wires, and lines in the proper place?"

Adapted with permission from Urden L, Stacy KM, Lough M. Critical Care Nursing: Diagnosis and Management. 8th ed. St Louis, MO: Elsevier Mosby; 2017.

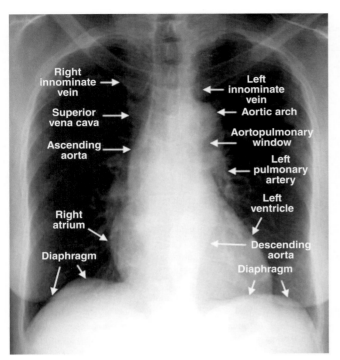

Figure 10-1. Normal chest x-ray with anatomical references. Courtesy of University of Virginia Health Sciences Center, Department of Radiology. (*Reproduced with permission from Gay SB, Olazagasti J, Higginbotham JW, et al: Introduction to Chest Radiology. University of Virginia Health Sciences Center, Department of Radiology. http://www.med-ed.virginia.edu/courses/rad/cxr/anatomy4chest.html.*)

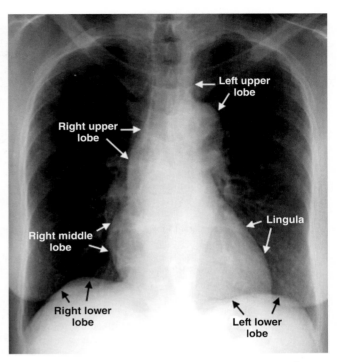

Figure 10-2. Normal chest x-ray with anatomical references. Courtesy of University of Virginia Health Sciences Center, Department of Radiology. (*Reproduced with permission from Gay SB, Olazagasti J, Higginbotham JW, et al: Introduction to Chest Radiology. University of Virginia Health Sciences Center, Department of Radiology. http://www.med-ed.virginia.edu/courses/rad/cxr/anatomy4chest.html.*)

lung fields—largest area of the chest and most radiolucent; and (10) catheters, tubes, wires, and lines.

Normal Variants and Common Abnormalities

When the soft tissues are examined, the two sides of the lateral chest should be symmetric. A mastectomy makes one lung look more radiolucent than the other due to the absence of fatty tissue. The trachea should be midline, with the carina visible at the level of the aortic knob or second ICS. The most common cause of tracheal deviation is a pneumothorax, which causes a tracheal and mediastinal shift to the area away from the pneumothorax (Table 10-3, Figures 10-3 and 10-4).

Bony thorax inspection reveals general body build. Clavicles should be symmetric and may have an irregular notch or indentation in the inferior medial aspect of the clavicle called a rhomboid fossa, a normal variant. Deformities of the thorax can be detected, such as scoliosis, pectus excavatum (also called funnel chest), or pectus carinatum (also known as pigeon chest). Decreases in the density (less white) of the spine, ribs, and other bones may indicate loss of calcium from the bones due to osteoporosis or long-term steroid dependency. Careful examination of the ICSs and rib angles may indicate pathology. Patients with chronic obstructive pulmonary disease (COPD) have widened ICS and the angle of the ribs to the spine increases to 90° instead of the normal 45° angle because of severe hyperinflation (see Figure 10-3). Conversely, narrowed ICS may be visible in patients with severe interstitial fibrosis.

Old rib fractures, if present, are commonly visible along the lateral borders of the rib cage and appear as a "callus" or thickened area of the rib where scar has developed. New rib fractures may not be as obvious unless the fracture is displaced.

Elevation of the diaphragm can be a result of abdominal distention, phrenic nerve paralysis, or lung collapse. Depression or flattening of the diaphragm is demonstrated by the presence of 11 or 12 ribs on a chest x-ray. Flattening of the diaphragm indicates hyperinflation, as in COPD or asthma. When the diaphragm is neither elevated nor flattened, 9 or 10 ribs are visible. Normal costophrenic angles can be seen where the tapered edges of the diaphragm and the chest wall meet. Because breast tissue can obscure the angles in women, these angles are more distinct in men. Obliteration or "blunting" of the costophrenic angle may occur with pleural effusion or atelectasis.

Identification of a pleural space on a chest x-ray is an abnormal finding (see Figure 10-4). The pleural space is not visible unless air (pneumothorax) or fluid (pleural effusion) enters it.

Two terms often heard regarding the appearance of the mediastinum on chest x-ray are shifting and widening. Mediastinal structures, usually the trachea, bronchi, and heart, can shift with atelectasis, with the shift directed toward the alveolar collapse. Pneumothorax shifts the mediastinum away from the area of involvement. A widening of the mediastinum can indicate several pathologic conditions, such as

TABLE 10-3. CHEST X-RAY FINDINGS

Assessed Area	Usual Adult Findings	Remarks
Trachea	Midline, translucent, tubelike structure found in the anterior mediastinal cavity	Deviation from the midline suggests tension, pneumothorax, atelectasis, pleural effusion, mass, or collapsed lung
Clavicles	Present in upper thorax and are equally distant from sternum	Malalignment or break indicates fracture
Ribs	Thoracic cavity encasement	Widening of intercostal spaces indicates emphysema; malalignment or break indicates fractured sternum or ribs
Mediastinum	Shadowy-appearing space between the lungs that widens at the hilum	Deviation to either side may indicate pleural effusion, fibrosis, or collapsed lung
Heart	Solid-appearing structure with clear edges visible in the left anterior mediastinal cavity; heart should be less than one-half the width of the chest wall on a PA film	Shift may indicate atelectasis or tension pneumothorax; if heart is greater than one-half the chest wall width, heart failure or pericardial fluid may be present
Carina	The lowest tracheal cartilage at which the bronchi bifurcate	If the end of the endotracheal tube is seen 3 cm above the carina, it is in the correct position
Main-stem bronchus	The translucent, tubelike structure visible to approximately 2.5 cm from hilum	Densities may indicate bronchogenic cyst
Hilum	Small, white, bilateral densities present where the bronchi join the lungs; left hilum should be 2-3 cm higher than the right hilum	A shift to either side indicates atelectasis; accentuated shadows may indicate emphysema or pulmonary abscess
Bronchi (other than main stem)	Not usually visible	If visible, may indicate bronchial pneumonia
Lung fields	Usually not completely visible except as fine white areas from hilum; fields should be clear as normal lung tissue is radiolucent; normal "lung markings" should be present to the periphery	If visible, may indicate atelectasis; patchy densities may be signs of resolving pneumonia, silicosis, or fibrosis; nasogastric tubes, pulmonary artery catheters, and chest tubes will appear as shadows and their positions should be noted
Diaphragm	Rounded structures visible at the bottom of the lung fields; right side is 1-2 cm higher than the left; the costophrenic angles should be clear and sharp	An elevated diaphragm may indicate pneumonia, pleurisy, acute bronchitis, or atelectasis; a unilateral flattened diaphragm suggests COPD; elevation indicates a pneumothorax or pulmonary infection; the presence of scarring or fluid causes blunting of costophrenic angles; 300-500 mL of pleural fluid must be present before blunting is seen

Reproduced with permission from Talbot I, Meyers-Marquardt M. Pocket Guide to Critical Assessment. St Louis, MO: CV Mosby; 1990.

cardiomegaly, aneurysms, or aortic disruption. Bleeding into the mediastinum, following chest trauma or cardiac surgery, also may cause widening of the mediastinum.

Heart size can be estimated easily by measuring the cardiothoracic ratio on a PA film. It is measured with a PA chest

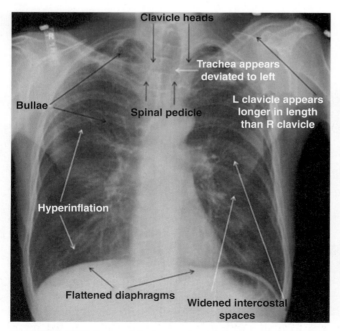

Figure 10-3. COPD, flattened diaphragms, hyperinflation, widened intercostal spaces, apical bullae, and chest rotation. (*Reproduced with permission from Siela D: Chest radiograph evaluation and interpretation, AACN Adv Crit Care 2008 Oct-Dec;19(4):444-473.*)

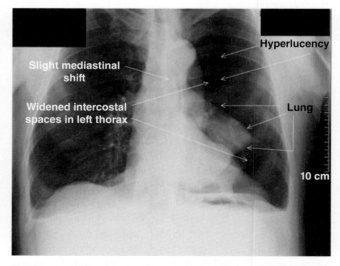

Figure 10-4. Left pneumothorax, hyperlucency, and widened intercostal spaces. (*Reproduced with permission from Siela D: Chest radiograph evaluation and interpretation, AACN Adv Crit Care 2008 Oct-Dec;19(4):444-473.*)

x-ray by comparing the ratio of the maximal horizontal cardiac diameter to the maximal horizontal thoracic diameter. A normal measurement is less than 50%. Greater percentages are indicative of cardiac enlargement. This method for determining heart size is only accurate using PA chest x-rays, and cannot be applied to AP x-rays done at the bedside.

The lung fields should be assessed for any areas of increased density (whiteness) or increased radiolucency (blackness), which can indicate an abnormality. Density increases when water, pus, or blood accumulates in the lungs, as in pneumonia (Figure 10-5). Increased radiolucency is caused by increased air in the lungs, as may occur with COPD. A fine line present on the right side of the lung at the sixth rib level (midlung) is a normal finding, representing the horizontal fissure separating the right upper and middle lobes.

Invasive Lines

Chest x-rays are frequently obtained in progressive care to confirm proper placement of invasive equipment (endotracheal tubes, central venous catheters including peripherally inserted central catheter [PICC] nasogastric or orogastric tubes, and chest tubes). All invasive tubes have radiopaque lines running the length of the tube that are visible on the x-ray (Figures 10-6 and 10-7).

All lines should be identified and followed through their paths. The nasogastric or orogastric tube should run the length of the esophagus with the tip of the tube beyond the gastroesophageal junction in the stomach. The stomach can be identified by the radiolucency just under the diaphragm on the left side, which is called the gastric air bubble. Small bore nasoenteric tubes may be positioned with the tip in the stomach or small bowel depending on whether gastric or small bowel feedings are intended. Central line catheters are properly placed when the tip can be viewed in the superior vena cava.

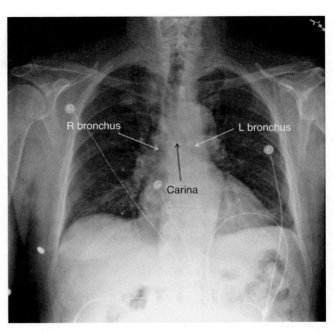

Figure 10-6. Carina and right bronchus. (*Reproduced with permission from Siela D: Chest radiograph evaluation and interpretation,* AACN Adv Crit Care *2008 Oct-Dec;19(4):444-473.*)

All items in the chest should be identified, such as temporary or permanent pacing wires, pacing generators, automatic implantable defibrillators, airway stents, tracheostomy tubes, chest tubes, and surgical wires, drains, or clips (see Figure 10-7).

Helpful Hints

Chest x-rays should be taken after every attempt to insert central venous catheters to detect the presence of an iatrogenic pneumothorax. A common error is to mistake the area above the clavicles as a pneumothorax, especially on AP views.

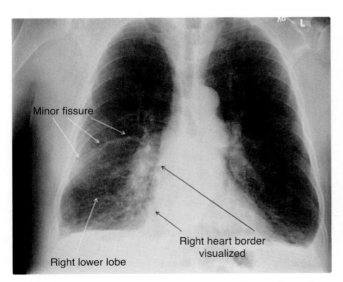

Figure 10-5. Right middle and lower lobe pneumonia with minor fissure visualized. (*Reproduced with permission from Siela D: Chest radiograph evaluation and interpretation,* AACN Adv Crit Care *2008 Oct-Dec;19(4):444-473.*)

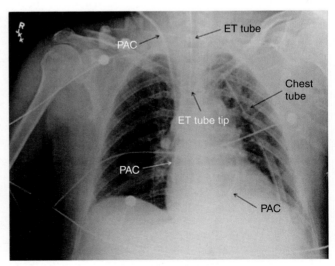

Figure 10-7. Pulmonary artery catheter, endotracheal tube, and left chest tube. (*Reproduced with permission from Siela D: Chest radiograph evaluation and interpretation,* AACN Adv Crit Care *2008 Oct-Dec;19(4):444-473.*)

Two common abnormal x-ray signs frequently discussed are the silhouette sign and the air bronchogram. For any structure to be visible, the density of its edge must contrast with the surrounding density. The loss of contrast is called the *silhouette sign*. It means that two structures of the same density have come in contact with each other and the borders are lost; for example, the heart is a muscle and water density, so if the alveoli near the left heart border fill with fluid, the two densities are the same and there is a loss of contrast and no left heart border. An air bronchogram is air showing through a greater density, such as water (Figure 10-8). The bronchi are not seen on a normal chest x-ray, except for the main-stem bronchi, because they have thin walls, contain air, and are surrounded by air in the alveoli (two structures of the same density). If water surrounds the bronchi, as in pneumonia and pulmonary edema, then the bronchi filled with air are in contrast to the water density and are visible.

Computed Tomography, Magnetic Resonance Imaging, and Bedside Ultrasonography

Computed tomography (CT) and magnetic resonance imaging (MRI) allow for the three-dimensional examination of the chest in situations where two-dimensional chest x-rays are insufficient. CT and MRI are particularly advantageous over chest x-rays to evaluate mediastinal and pleural abnormalities, particularly those with fluid collections. Pleural effusions or empyemas, malpositioned or occluded chest tubes, mediastinal hematomas, and mediastinitis are problems for which a three-dimensional view provided by CT and MRI are more sensitive than chest x-rays.

The need for transportation to the radiology department and positioning restrictions within the scanning devices pose certain risks to acutely ill patients. Of particular concern is the automatic movement of patients during the procedure into and out of the scanning device. Accidental disconnection of invasive devices can easily occur if additional tubing lengths and potential obstructions are not

considered. Decreased visualization of patients during the procedures requires vigilant monitoring of cardiovascular and respiratory parameters and devices, as well as establishing a method for conscious patients to alert nearby clinicians in case of difficulties. The strong magnetic field of MRI units may interfere with ventilator performance and a nonmagnetic ventilator is required.

MRI testing can be a frightening experience for the patient. Reactions, occurring in up to almost one-third of patients, range from mild apprehension to severe anxiety. These reactions can result in cancellation of the test or interference with its results. It is suggested that all patients receive basic information regarding the MRI procedure, including details of the small chamber they will be placed in, the noise and temperature they will experience, and the duration of the procedure. If possible, use of some form of relaxation or music tapes, ear plugs or headsets, and the presence of a family member or friend is considered. In addition, short-acting anxiolytics may be used for patients who need them.

Bedside ultrasonography is increasingly common in acute care as less expensive machines are available. Ultrasound can be performed quickly and easily and the information provided helps to confirm or rule out a suspected condition or a procedure-related complication. The transducer or probe produces sound waves along with echoes that are reflected back to produce two-dimensional images of tissue, fluid, and organs. Recent guidelines recommend ultrasound of the chest for the following situations: diagnosis of pleural effusion, identification of the location for drainage of a pleural effusion, rapid detection of pneumothorax, diagnosis of alveolar lung consolidation, and as an aide in central line insertion to prevent procedure-related complications. Advantages of ultrasound include its portability and rapid direct use at the bedside avoiding the need for patient transportation. Some disadvantages include the need for comprehensive training in obtaining and interpreting the images and the lack of availability in all acute care areas.

CTPA and V/Q Scans

Computed tomography of the pulmonary arteries (CTPAs) is the gold standard for detecting pulmonary embolism (PE). The CTPA only requires a peripheral line through which to inject the contrast material and is minimally invasive. Images are acquired following contrast material injection, with an embolus appearing as a dark filling defect in the otherwise bright white contrast dense pulmonary artery. CTPA diagnostic testing for PE has high sensitivity and specificity and has replaced the more invasive pulmonary angiography.

While less common, ventilation-perfusion (V/Q) scans may also be used to diagnose a PE. A V/Q scan is a nuclear medicine diagnostic tool that requires that medical isotopes are inhaled or injected in order to view the lungs and pulmonary arteries, respectively. Generally the perfusion (or blood circulation) part of the test is done first. If there is no defect detected, the scan is read as "low probability." If the scan detects a defect, then the inhaled (ventilation) portion of the

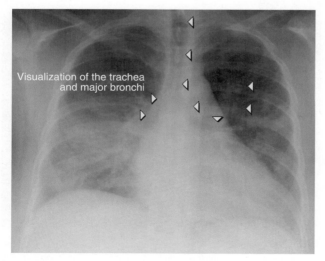

Figure 10-8. Air bronchogram. (*Used with permission from Yale School of Medicine–http://www.yale.edu/imaging/findings/air_bronchogram/index.html.*)

test is done. If no matching defect is seen in the lung, the test is interpreted as "high probability." But if a "matched defect" is noted (ie, there is a defect in the lung scan that corresponds with that of the perfusion scan), then the interpretation is "indeterminate" or "matched defect." This may be the result of an atelectasis, pneumonia, or other infiltrate where circulation to that inactive area of the lung is redistributed to other active areas thus resulting in a "matched defect." In addition to the cumbersome nature of the V/Q scan, the progressive care patient may require both tests (perfusion and ventilation) rather than just one, and the diagnostic yield is often poor.

Chest Tubes

Chest tubes are commonly used in acutely ill patients to drain air, blood, or fluid from the pleural spaces (pleural chest tubes) or from the mediastinum (mediastinal tubes). Indications for chest tube insertion are varied (Table 10-4). The only absolute contraindication is in a lung that is adherent to chest wall through the hemithorax. Relative contraindication may include patients with multiple adhesions, blebs, or coagulopathies. However, the emergent need for lung reexpansion may require careful reevaluation of risk versus benefit on an individual patient basis including reversal of any coagulopathy (if feasible). Pleural tube insertion sites vary based on the type of drainage to be removed (air: second ICS, midclavicular line; fluid: fifth or sixth ICS, midaxillary line). Mediastinal tubes are placed during surgery, exiting from the mediastinum below the xiphoid process. Types of chest tube insertions include tube thoracostomy (traditional rigid tubes) or smaller percutaneously inserted catheters (pigtails).

Following insertion, chest tubes are connected to a closed drainage collection system that uses gravity or suction to restore negative pressure in the pleural space and facilitate drainage of fluid or air (Figure 10-9). A Heimlich flutter valve is an alternative to the closed drainage system and consists of a one-way valve that allows air or drainage to collect in a vented drain bag (Figure 10-10). The PleurX® catheter also has a one-way valve and connects as needed to a drainage system (Figure 10-11). Patients may be discharged

TABLE 10-4. INDICATIONS FOR CHEST TUBE INSERTION

Pneumothorax
- Open: Both chest wall and pleural spaces are penetrated.
- Closed: Pleural space is penetrated with an intact chest wall, allowing air to enter the pleural space from the lungs.
- Tension: Air leaks into the pleural space through a tear in the lungs, with no means to escape the space, leading to lung collapse.

Hemothorax (blood)

Hemopneumothorax (blood and air)

Post-thoracostomy

Pyothorax or empyema (pus)

Chylothorax (lymph)

Cholethorax (bile)

Hydrothorax (non-inflammatory serous)

Pleural effusion (transudate or exudate)

Pleurodesis (installation of anesthetic or sclerosing agent)

Adapted with permission from Wiegand DI, ed. AACN Procedure Manual for Critical Care, 7th ed. Philadelphia, PA: Saunders; 2017.

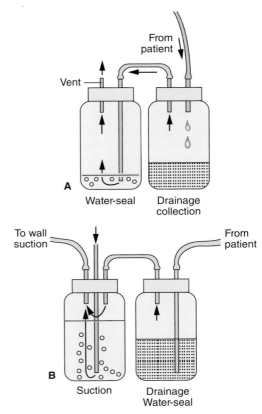

Figure 10-9. Two-bottle chest drainage system. **(A)** Drainage collection bottle and a water-seal bottle. **(B)** Water-seal/drainage collection bottle and suction control bottle. (*Reproduced with permission from Luce JM, Tyler ML, Peirson DJ. Intensive Respiratory Care. Philadelphia, PA: WB Saunders; 1984.*)

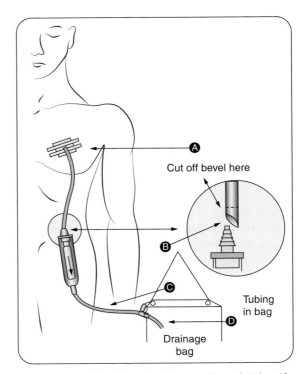

Figure 10-10. Heimlich chest drain valve with connection to drain bag. (*Courtesy and © Becton, Dickinson and Company.*)

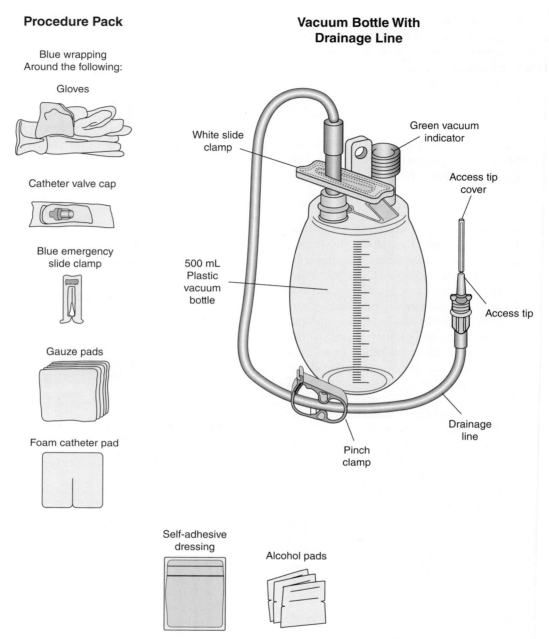

Procedure Pack

Blue wrapping
Around the following:

Gloves

Catheter valve cap

Blue emergency
slide clamp

Gauze pads

Foam catheter pad

Self-adhesive
dressing

Alcohol pads

**Vacuum Bottle With
Drainage Line**

White slide
clamp

Green vacuum
indicator

Access tip
cover

500 mL
Plastic
vacuum
bottle

Access tip

Drainage
line

Pinch
clamp

Figure 10-11. Components of a PleurX® drainage kit. (*Reproduced with permission from Elsevier Baker EM, Melander S. Management of recurrent pleural effusions with a tunneled catheter. Heart Lung. 2010; July/Aug;39(4):314-318.*)

home with either a Heimlich flutter valve or PleurX catheter for long-term use. Connections to the drainage system must be airtight and secure for proper functioning and to prevent inadvertent entry of air into the pleural space (Figure 10-12). To maintain patency of the system, inspect the tubing for kinking or clot formation. In some cases, if a clot is visualized gentle squeezing and releasing of small segments of the tubing between the thumb and the index finger can alleviate the obstruction.

Removal of the chest tube occurs when restoration of lung expansion and fluid or air removal has been accomplished and the underlying lung abnormality has resolved.

An occlusive dressing at the chest tube removal site is typically used to prevent introduction of air into the pleural space until the skin has formed a protective seal. Analgesic administration is appropriate prior to removal; discomfort associated with removal is often as much or even greater than during insertion.

THORACIC SURGERY AND PROCEDURES

Thoracic surgery and procedures are terms inclusive of a number of procedures involving the thoracic cavity and the lungs. See Table 10-5 for definitions and indications.

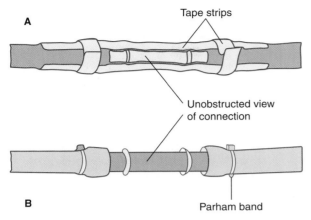

Figure 10-12. Methods for securing connections of chest tube and drainage system. **(A)** Tape. **(B)** Parham bands. (*Reproduced with permission from Kersten LD. Comprehensive Respiratory Nursing: A Decision-Making Approach. Philadelphia, PA: WB Saunders; 1989.*)

Principles of Management for Thoracic Surgery and Procedures

Management of the patient after lung surgery or post-procedure is similar to the patient with trauma to the chest. Refer to the section on thoracic trauma in Chapter 17, Trauma, with the following additions:

Pain Control

The thoracotomy incision is one of the most painful surgical incisions and pain control is an important factor in recovery and prevention of respiratory complications. The routine use of epidural catheters, intercostal blocks, intrapleural local anesthetic administration, or patient-controlled analgesia (PCA) narcotics has improved pain management significantly. Relaxation therapy, deep breathing exercises, and guided imagery may also be effective in helping to reduce pain and anxiety.

Positioning

1. It was once thought that optimal ventilation and perfusion matching occurs when the "good lung" is positioned in the dependent position. While blood flow is improved to the dependent lung, patients actually recover best when they are frequently repositioned side to side to prevent atelectasis and other complications.
2. Progressive mobility including sitting at the bedside or in a chair and assisted ambulation improves diaphragmatic excursion, enhancing ventilation and lung inflation.
3. Deep breathing and use of incentive spirometry is encouraged regularly. These activities help promote lung reexpansion of collapsed lung tissue and prevent atelectasis.

Maintenance of Chest Tube System

See section "Chest Tubes" explained earlier.

PATHOLOGIC CONDITIONS

Acute Respiratory Failure

Each of the case studies below represents a common situation in a progressive care unit—respiratory dysfunction. Rapid onset of respiratory impairment, which is severe enough to cause potential or actual morbidity or mortality if untreated, is termed acute respiratory failure (ARF). Although the origin of the respiratory failure may be a medical or surgical problem, the management approaches share similar features.

ARF is a change in respiratory gas exchange (CO_2 and O_2) such that normal cellular function is jeopardized. ARF may be primarily hypoxemia, with a Pao_2 less than 60 mm Hg or primarily hypercapnia with a $Paco_2$ greater than 50 mm Hg with a pH less than or equal to 7.30. Mixed ARF refers to situations in which both hypoxemia and hypercapnia occur. The Pao_2 and $Paco_2$ values that define ARF vary, depending on a variety of factors that influence the patient's normal (or baseline) arterial blood gas (ABG) values. Factors such as age, altitude, chronic cardiopulmonary disease, or metabolic disturbances may alter the normal blood gas values for an individual, requiring an adjustment to the classic definition of ARF; for example, if $Paco_2$ levels in a 75-year-old man with COPD are normally 56 mm Hg, ARF would not be diagnosed until pH is less than or equal to 7.30.

Etiology, Risk Factors, and Pathophysiology

Many abnormalities can lead to ARF (Table 10-6). Regardless of the specific underlying cause, the pathophysiology of ARF can be organized into four main components: impaired

TABLE 10-5. THORACIC SURGERY AND PROCEDURES

	Definitions
Thoracic Surgery	
Pneumonectomy	Removal of entire lung
Lobectomy	Resection of one or more lobes of the lung
Wedge resection	Removal of small wedge-shaped section of lung tissue
Segmental resection	Removal of bronchovascular segment of the lung lobe
Bullectomy	Resection of emphysematous bullae
Lung volume reduction surgery (LVRS)	Resection of diseased and functionless lung tissue
Open lung biopsy	Resection of portion of lung for biopsy through a thoracotomy incision
Decortication	
Video-assisted thoracic surgery (VATS)	Endoscopic procedure through small incision
Procedure	
Pulmonary stent	Device(s) placed by flexible or rigid bronchoscopes to keep airways open in the central tracheobronchial tree
Bronchoscopy (rigid or flexible)	Invasive procedure used to visualize the oropharynx, larynx, vocal cords, and tracheal bronchial tree for diagnosis and treatment

TABLE 10-6. CAUSES OF ACUTE RESPIRATORY FAILURE IN ADULT

Impaired Ventilation
- Spinal cord injury (C4 or higher)
- Phrenic nerve damage
- Neuromuscular blockade
- Guillain-Barré syndrome
- Central nervous system (CNS) depression
  Drug overdoses (narcotics, sedatives, illicit drugs)
  Increased intracranial pressure
  Anesthetic agents
- Respiratory muscle fatigue

Impaired Gas Exchange
- Pulmonary edema
- ARDS
- Aspiration pneumonia

Airway Obstruction
- Aspiration of foreign body
- Thoracic tumors
- Asthma
- Bronchitis
- Pneumonia

Ventilation-Perfusion Abnormalities
- Pulmonary embolism
- Emphysema

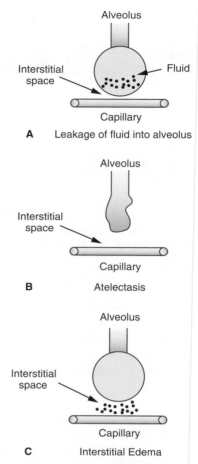

Figure 10-13. Pathophysiologic processes in ARF that impair gas exchange. **(A)** Increased alveolar membrane permeability. **(B)** Alveolar collapse from decreased surfactant production. **(C)** Increased capillary membrane permeability and interstitial edema.

ventilation, impaired gas exchange, airway obstruction, and ventilation-perfusion abnormalities.

Impaired Ventilation

Conditions that disrupt the muscles of respiration or their neurologic control can impair ventilation and lead to ARF (see Table 10-6). Decreased or absent respiratory muscle movement may be due to fatigue from excessive use, atrophy from disuse, inflammation of nerves, nerve damage (eg, surgical damage to the vagus nerve during cardiac surgery), neurologic depression, or progressive neuromuscular diseases such as Guillain-Barré or amyotrophic lateral sclerosis (ALS). Impaired respiratory muscle movement decreases movement of gas into the lungs, resulting in alveolar hypoventilation. Inadequate alveolar ventilation causes retention of CO_2 and hypoxemia.

Impaired Gas Exchange

Conditions that damage the alveolar-capillary membrane impair gas exchange. Direct damage to the cells lining the alveoli may be caused by inhalation of toxic substances (gases or gastric contents), pneumonia and/or other pulmonary conditions leading to two detrimental alveolar changes. The first is an increase in alveolar permeability, increasing the potential for interstitial fluid to leak into the alveoli and causing noncardiac pulmonary edema (Figure 10-13A). The second alveolar change is a decrease in surfactant production by alveolar type II cells, increasing alveolar surface tension, which leads to alveolar collapse (Figure 10-13B).

Another cause of impaired gas exchange occurs when fluid leaks from the intravascular space into the pulmonary interstitial space (Figure 10-13C). The excess fluid increases the distance between the alveolus and the capillary, decreasing the efficiency of the gas exchange process. Interstitial edema also compresses the bronchial airways, which are surrounded by interstitial tissue, causing bronchoconstriction. Capillary leakage may occur when pressures within the cardiovascular system are excessively high (eg, in heart failure) or when pathologic conditions elsewhere in the body release biochemical substances (eg, serotonin, endotoxin) that increase capillary permeability.

Airway Obstruction

Conditions that obstruct airways increase resistance to airflow into the lungs, causing alveolar hypoventilation and decreased gas exchange (Figure 10-14). Airway obstructions can result from conditions that: (1) block the inner airway lumen (eg, excessive secretions or fluid in the airways, inhaled foreign bodies) (Figure 10-14A), (2) increase airway wall thickness (eg, edema or fibrosis) or decrease airway circumference (eg, bronchoconstriction) as occurs in asthma (Figure 10-14B), or (3) increase peribronchial compression of the airway (eg, enlarged lymph nodes, interstitial edema, tumors) (Figure 10-14C).

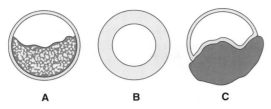

Figure 10-14. Mechanism of airway obstruction. **(A)** Fluid secretions present within airway. **(B)** Intraluminal edema narrowing airway diameter. **(C)** Peribronchial compression of airway.

Ventilation-Perfusion Abnormalities

Conditions disrupting alveolar ventilation or capillary perfusion lead to an imbalance in ventilation and perfusion. This decreases the efficiency of the respiratory gas exchange process (Figure 10-15A). In an effort to keep the ventilation and perfusion ratios balanced, two compensatory changes occur: (1) to avoid wasted alveolar ventilation when capillary perfusion is decreased (eg, with PE), alveolar collapse occurs to limit ventilation to alveoli with poor or absent capillary perfusion (Figure 10-15B); and (2) to avoid capillary perfusion of alveoli that are not adequately ventilated (eg, with atelectasis), arteriole constriction (ie, hypoxic vasoconstriction) occurs and shunts blood away from hypoventilated alveoli to normally ventilated alveoli (Figure 10-15C). As the number of alveolar-capillary units affected by these compensatory changes increases, gas exchange eventually is negatively affected.

Each of these pathophysiologic changes results in inadequate CO_2 removal, O_2 absorption, or both. The severity of ARF can be further increased when anxiety and fear of impending death develop, a common consequence of severe dyspnea and hypoxemia. These symptoms increase oxygen demand and the work of breathing, further compromising O_2 availability for crucial organ function and depleting respiratory muscle strength.

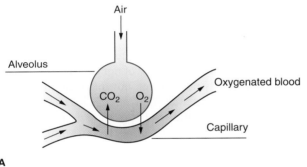

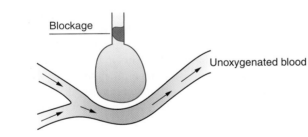

Figure 10-15. Pathophysiologic processes in ARF from ventilation-perfusion abnormalities. **(A)** Normal ventilation and perfusion relationship. **(B)** Decreased ventilation and normal perfusion. **(C)** Normal ventilation and decreased perfusion.

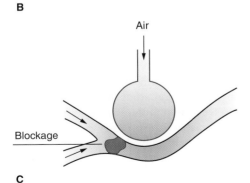

ESSENTIAL CONTENT CASE

Motor Vehicle Accident

A 22-year-old man was admitted to the progressive care unit following a motor vehicle accident in which he suffered blunt chest trauma. During his second day in the unit, his Spo_2 deteriorates and he requires increasing amounts of supplemental oxygen to maintain Pao_2 levels greater than 60 mm Hg. He is dyspneic, restless, and somewhat agitated. He verbalizes a fear of impending death.

The rapid response team is called and the patient is transferred to the ICU.

	Admission	Day 2
Respiration rate	24 breaths/min	34 breaths/min
Chest x-ray	clear	bilateral diffuse infiltrates
ABGs	40% FM	100% non-rebreather mask
Pao_2	120 mm Hg	58 mm Hg
$Paco_2$	33 mm Hg	50 mm Hg
pH	7.42	7.35
HCO_3	24 mEq/L	27 mEq/L

Case Question 1: What signs and symptoms of ARF is this patient exhibiting?

Case Question 2: What intervention do you next anticipate based on his arterial blood gases and transfer to the ICU?

Answers
1. Signs and symptoms include dyspnea, restless, agitated, fear of impending death, and hypoxemia despite increasing Fio_2 to 100% non-rebreather mask.
2. Intubation and initiation of mechanical ventilation to improve hypoxemia along with analgesia and sedation. Patient has known bilateral diffuse infiltrates by chest x-ray. See next section on Acute Respiratory Distress Syndrome.

Postanesthesia

A woman is admitted to the progressive care unit following an open lung biopsy. She is receiving oxygen by humidified face mask at 40%. A right pleural chest tube is draining minimal amounts of blood, with no evidence of air leak or obstruction.

The patient is minimally responsive to verbal and pain stimulation on admission. Her respiratory rate is 8 to 10 breaths/min with an SpO_2 of 92%. She is receiving hydromorphone by continuous PCA. She is given naloxone (Narcan) and her assessment changes as follows:

	Admission	Post-Narcan
PaO_2	70 mm Hg	140 mm Hg
$PaCO_2$	52 mm Hg	38 mm Hg
pH	7.31	7.40
HCO_3	24 mEq/L	23 mEq/L
Respiratory rate	8-10 breaths/min	22 breaths/min

Case Question 1: What was the etiology of her impaired ventilation?

Case Question 2: What is the next intervention that you anticipate?

Answers
1. Excessive use of narcotics can cause CNS depression leading to decreased ventilator muscle movement resulting in alveolar hypoventilation. Naloxone is used as a reversal agent with resulting improvement in respiratory rate and ABGs.
2. Anticipate an adjustment in the patient's narcotic dose and delivery. Due to the short half-life of naloxone as a reversal agent, careful assessment and reassessment of the patient's respiratory rate along with level of pain needs to be done. See Chapter 6, Pain Management/Sedation for additional information.

Clinical Presentation
Signs and Symptoms

- Hypoxemia (PaO_2 less than 60 mm Hg)
- SpO_2 less than 90 mm Hg
- Restlessness
- Tachypnea
- Dyspnea
- Tachycardia
- Confusion
- Diaphoresis
- Anxiety
- Hypercarbia ($PaCO_2$ more than 50 mm Hg)
- Hypertension
- Irritability
- Somnolence (late)
- Cyanosis (late)
- Loss of consciousness (late)
- Pallor or cyanosis of skin

- Use of accessory muscles of respiration
- Abnormal breath sounds (crackles, wheezes)
- Manifestations of primary disease (see description of individual diseases later on)

Diagnostic Tests

- *ABGs:* PaO_2 less than 60 mm Hg and $PaCO_2$ more than 50 mm Hg; with pH less than or equal to 7.30; or PaO_2 and $PaCO_2$ in abnormal range for that individual
- Tests specific to underlying cause (see description of individual diseases later on)

Principles of Management for Acute Respiratory Failure
The management of the patient in ARF revolves around four primary areas: improving oxygenation and ventilation, treating the underlying disease state, reducing anxiety, and preventing and managing complications.

Improving Oxygenation and Ventilation
Most causes of ARF are treatable, with a return of normal respiratory function following resolution of the pathophysiologic condition. Aggressive support of respiratory function is required until there is resolution of the underlying condition.

1. Provide supplemental O_2 to maintain PaO_2 greater than 60 mm Hg. The use of noninvasive methods for O_2 administration (high flow nasal cannula or face masks) is preferable if acceptable PaO_2 levels can be achieved. Continued hypoxemia despite noninvasive O_2 delivery methods necessitates intubation and mechanical ventilation and transfer to a critical care unit.
2. Improve ventilation with the administration of bronchodilators, suctioning, positioning, and mobilization as indicated. The routine use of chest physiotherapy has not been shown to be supported by the literature and is not recommended.
3. Intubate and initiate mechanical ventilation if noninvasive methods fail to correct hypoxemia and hypercarbia, or if cardiovascular instability develops. In patients with COPD exacerbation, a trial of noninvasive positive pressure mechanical ventilation may be appropriate prior to intubation. The mode of mechanical ventilation, rate, and tidal volume vary, depending on the underlying cause of respiratory failure and a variety of clinical factors.
4. Depending on the cause of ARF, the patient's response to treatment along with the institution's resources (specialized respiratory care units), the patient may need to be moved into intensive care for noninvasive ventilation, high flow oxygen, or intubation and mechanical ventilation.
5. If suctioning is required, closely observe for signs and symptoms of complications: drop in oxygenation (SpO_2), cardiac dysrhythmias, respiratory distress, bronchospasm, increased respiratory rate,

increased blood pressure or intracranial pressure, anxiety, pain, or change in mental status. Hyperoxygenate with 100% oxygen preferably by using the manual 100% FiO_2 button on the ventilator. An alternative is the use of a manual resuscitation bag (MRB) that delivers 100% O_2 and can be used with a positive end-expiratory pressure (PEEP) valve when ventilator PEEP levels are more than 5 cm H_2O. Suctioning is only performed when clinically indicated, and never on a routine schedule. The use of in-line suction catheters is encouraged as the catheters do not affect oxygenation as dramatically as complete disconnection, and they decrease the potential contamination of the clinician doing the suctioning.

6. Prior to intrahospital transport, verify adequacy of ventilatory support equipment to maintain cardiopulmonary stability. Verify that PEEP levels are maintained during transport equipment.

Treating the Underlying Disease State

Correction of the underlying cause of the ARF is done as soon as possible. See specific management approaches later in the chapter for selected disease states.

Reducing Anxiety

Maintain a calm, supportive environment to avoid unnecessary escalation of anxiety. Give brief explanations of activities and approaches being done to relieve ARF. Vigilance and presence of healthcare providers during anxious periods is crucial to avoid panic by patients and visiting family members.

Teach diaphragmatic breathing to slow the rate and increase the depth of respirations. Place one hand on the patient's abdomen. Instruct the patient to inhale deeply, causing the hand on the abdomen to rise. During exhalation, have the patient feel the hand on the belly sink down toward the spine. Explain that the chest should move minimally. After a minute or two, ask the patient to place his or her hands on the belly to continue the exercise.

If necessary, administer mild doses of anxiolytics (ie, lorazepam or alprazolam) that do not depress respiration. Use a validated sedation assessment tool to measure the patient's anxiety and evaluate the medication's effect.

Preventing and Managing Complications

The risk of ARF is not only the imminent danger of respiratory compromise but also the many complications that can result from the interventions required to treat ARF over a prolonged interval. Mechanical ventilation, immobility, and the use of invasive tubes and lines create risks for lung damage, pressure injury, and infection. Nursing interventions to minimize these risks include continuous monitoring, frequent repositioning, and aseptic technique. See Chapter 5, Airway and Ventilatory Management, for additional strategies to prevent the complications of mechanical ventilation; Chapter 11, Multisystem Problems, for strategies to prevent hospital-acquired conditions, and Chapter 14,

Gastrointestinal System, for preventing gastrointestinal (GI) complications.

1. *Pulmonary aspiration:* Ensure proper inflation of endotracheal tube cuff at all times. Refer to additional prevention strategies for ventilator-associated pneumonia (VAP) discussed later in this chapter.
2. *GI bleeding:* Protect gastric mucosa and increase gastric pH in ventilator patients by using stress ulcer prophylaxis and/or tube feedings after assessing the patient's risk for GI bleeding (see Chapter 14, Gastrointestinal System).
3. *Barotrauma:* Avoid unnecessary increases in airway pressures (eg, patient/ventilator dyssynchrony, excessive coughing) and assess for signs and symptoms of pneumothorax, pneumomediastinum, and other barotrauma complications.
4. *Volutrauma:* Prevent alveolar damage from excessive tidal volumes.

Acute Respiratory Distress Syndrome

The case study of the patient in a motor vehicle accident is typical of a patient who develops acute respiratory distress syndrome (ARDS). ARDS has a very high morbidity and mortality. It is characterized by noncardiac pulmonary edema caused by increased alveolar capillary membrane permeability. ARDS affects both lungs and hypoxemia refractory to oxygenation is a hallmark of the condition. ARDS is defined as "mild," "moderate," or "severe" ARDS according to the Berlin definition of ARDS. This definition considers the timing of the condition, results of chest imaging, origin of lung edema, and oxygenation status. The severity stratification of mild, moderate, and severe is based on the PaO_2/FiO_2 score and PEEP level. The PaO_2/FiO_2 ratio (also called the P/F ratio) is calculated by dividing the PaO_2 by the FiO_2 (with a decimal; 50% = 0.5).

Etiology, Risk Factors, and Pathophysiology

Risk factors for the development of ARDS can be categorized into conditions that lead to direct damage to the alveolar-capillary membrane (primary causes) and those that are thought to be mediated by cellular or humoral injury to the capillary endothelial wall (secondary causes) (Table 10-7). Whether primary or secondary causes, the pathologic processes involved in ARDS are characterized by excessive alveolar–capillary membrane permeability, interstitial edema, and diffuse alveolar injury (see Figure 10-13). Direct damage to the alveolar membrane can easily occur when toxic substances are inhaled, such as during fires or chemical spills.

Alveolar and interstitial edema, microatelectasis, and ventilation-perfusion mismatching in ARDS lead to severe hypoxemia and poor lung compliance ("stiff lungs"). In the setting of trauma and sepsis, this abnormality in microvascular permeability occurs in capillary beds throughout the body. Typically, this multisystem organ dysfunction is not clinically apparent, with clinical manifestations isolated to the respiratory system. When multiorgan dysfunction

TABLE 10-7.   PRIMARY AND SECONDARY CAUSES OF ARDS

Primary Causes (Direct Damage to the Alveolar Membrane)
- Aspiration
- Pulmonary contusion
- Near drowning
- Inhalation of smoke or toxic substances
- Pneumonia (viral and bacterial)

Secondary Causes (Mediated by Cellular or Humoral Injury to the Capillary Endothelium)
- Sepsis
- Hypovolemic shock associated with chest trauma or sepsis
- Acute pancreatitis
- Fat emboli
- Trauma
- Disseminated intravascular coagulation (DIC)
- Massive blood transfusions

syndrome does occur, it is seen in ARDS patients who develop bacterial infections and sepsis (see Chapter 11, Multisystem Problems).

The ARDS process disrupts normal macrophage function and increases the risk of infection. Mortality and long-term disability from ARDS is high.

Clinical Presentation
Signs and Symptoms

- Dyspnea
- Tachypnea (rates often more than 40 breaths/min)
- Tachycardia
- Use of accessory muscles to breathe
- Diaphoresis
- Cough
- Chest pain
- Anxiety
- Crackles and/or wheezes

Diagnostic Tests

- Chest x-ray shows new, diffuse, bilateral pulmonary infiltrates without increased cardiac size
- Pao_2/Fio_2 less than or equal to 300 mm Hg

Principles of Management for ARDS
Much of the management of ARDS relies on supportive care and the prevention of complications. To date, interventions to limit the disease progression or reverse the underlying structural defects are not known.

Improving Oxygenation and Ventilation
Interventions specific to ARDS to improve oxygenation and ventilation include the following:

1. Administer high Fio_2 levels with high-flow system or rebreathing mask if able to oxygenate noninvasively.
2. Intubate, begin mechanical ventilation, and transfer to intensive care if cardiovascular instability is present, severe hypoxemia persists, or if respiratory fatigue develops. The majority of these patients will need transfer to the ICU for additional management.

Reducing Anxiety
Same as previously described for ARF management.

Achieving Effective Communications
Refer Chapter 5, Airway and Ventilatory Management, for detailed discussion of communication techniques for intubated patients.

Maintaining Hemodynamic Stability and Adequate Perfusion

1. Minimize cardiovascular instability by careful monitoring; conservative fluid management is recommended.
2. Vasoactive drugs may be required to maintain adequate perfusion.

Preventing Complications
In addition to complications listed for ARF:

1. ARDS patients are at higher risk for development of hospital-acquired pneumonias. Follow prevention strategies described later in the chapter. Prophylactic antibiotics have not been shown to decrease hospital-acquired pneumonia rates in ARDS patients. Meticulous attention to head of bed elevation, hand washing, oral care, and removal of invasive devices as soon as possible are key prevention strategies.
2. The incidence of barotrauma is particularly high in patients with ARDS due to the stress of positive pressure ventilation on damaged alveolar membranes.
3. Delirium, deep venous thrombosis (DVT), GI bleeding, poor nutrition, pressure injury, and device-related infections are complications of ARDS as these patients often require prolonged mechanical ventilation. Assessment and preventative strategies are part of the daily plan of care.

Acute Respiratory Failure in the Patient With Chronic Obstructive Pulmonary Disease (also called COPD Exacerbation)

Individuals with COPD are at risk for exacerbations and ARF due to progressive airflow limitation with chronic inflammatory airway and lung response. Acute asthma will be discussed in the next section. Altered host defenses, increased secretion volume and viscosity, impaired secretion clearance and airway changes, and common pathophysiologic changes predispose the patient with COPD to acute exacerbations or episodes of ARF requiring hospitalizations. The etiology, clinical presentation, and management of ARF in the COPD patient vary somewhat from ARF without chronic underlying pulmonary dysfunction. This section of the chapter highlights differences in ARF management in the patient with underlying COPD.

Etiology, Risk Factors, and Pathophysiology
Any systemic or pulmonary illness can precipitate exacerbations and the development of ARF in patients with COPD. In addition to the etiologies of ARF listed in Table 10-6, diseases

TABLE 10-8. PRECIPITATING EVENTS OF ACUTE RESPIRATORY FAILURE IN COPD

Decreased Ventilatory Drive
- Oversedation
- Hypothyroidism
- Brain stem lesions

Decreased Muscle Strength
- Malnutrition
- Shock
- Myopathies
- Hypophosphatemia
- Hypomagnesemia
- Hypocalcemia

Decreased Chest Wall Elasticity
- Rib fractures
- Pleural effusions
- Ileus
- Ascites

Decreased Lung Capacity for Gas Exchange
- Atelectasis
- Pulmonary edema
- Pneumonia
- Pulmonary embolus
- Heart failure

Increased Airway Resistance
- Bronchospasm
- Increased secretions
- Upper airway obstructions
- Airway edema

Increased Metabolic Oxygen Requirements
- Systemic infection
- Hyperthyroidism
- Fever

or situations that decrease ventilatory drive, muscle strength, chest wall elasticity, or gas exchange capacity, or increase airway resistance or metabolic oxygen requirements can easily lead to ARF in patients with COPD (Table 10-8). The most common precipitating events include:

- *Respiratory infection (pneumonia, bronchitis):* This is the most frequent trigger of COPD exacerbations. Respiratory infections can be viral or bacterial. Common pathogens in patients with COPD include *Haemophilus influenzae, Streptococcus pneumoniae, Moraxella catarrhalis, and Pseudomonas aeruginosa.*
- *Pulmonary embolus:* The high incidence of right ventricular failure in COPD increases the risk of pulmonary embolus from right ventricular mural thrombi. The high incidence of PE in patients with COPD exacerbations may itself be a risk factor or an incidental finding in these patients.
- *PH:* The presence of secondary PH typically due to chronic hypoxemia, left heart failure, or sleep apnea may also be an additional risk factor.
- *Patient factors:* Other medical conditions such as heart disease or diabetes along with advanced age, previous hospitalizations, duration of COPD, productive cough, and history of antibiotic use are associated with increased risk.

The development of ARF in COPD patients places a tremendous burden on the pulmonary system. The chronic disease process leads to impaired ventilation, poor gas exchange, and airway obstruction. The additional burden of an acute disease process, even a relatively minor one, further impairs ventilation and gas exchange and increases airway obstruction. Compensatory mechanisms can easily be overwhelmed, with lethal consequences.

Clinical Presentation
Signs and symptoms are similar to ARF, but usually more pronounced.

Diagnostic Tests
- *Chest x-ray:* Evidence of COPD (flat diaphragms, hyperinflation of air fields), in addition to x-ray findings specific to the cause of the ARF (see Figure 10-3).
- *ABGs:* $Paco_2$ levels above the patient's baseline which may be greater than 50 mm Hg, during stable, chronic disease periods.

Principles of Management for ARF in Patients With COPD
The presence of chronic respiratory dysfunction and an acute respiratory problem leads to some changes in the typical management of ARF. Treatment is directed at both the acute precipitating event and the chronic airflow obstruction problems associated with COPD.

Treating the Underlying Disease State
1. Increase airway diameter with bronchodilators and reduce airway edema with corticosteroids. Short-acting beta-agonists (SABA) with or without anticholinergic agents are recommended as the initial treatment (Table 10-9). Higher than usual doses may be necessary until the precipitating event resolves. Systemic corticosteroids are used to decrease airway inflammation and thus bronchospasm, and may enhance secretion clearance as well.
2. Treat pulmonary infections with appropriate antibiotics.

TABLE 10-9. BRONCHODILATOR CATEGORIES

Category	Examples
Short-acting beta$_2$-agonists (SABA)	Albuterol (initially often given as continuous aerosol treatment)
Long-acting beta$_2$-agonists (LABA)	Salmeterol Formoterol
Short-acting anticholinergics or antimuscarinic (SAMA)	Ipratropium bromide
Long-acting anticholinergics or antimuscarinic (LAMA)	Tiotropium bromide
Combination beta$_2$-agonist (short-acting) and anticholinergic	Albuterol and ipratropium bromide
Combination beta$_2$-agonist (LABA) and corticosteroid	Salmeterol and fluticasone Vilanterol and fluticasone

3. Improve secretion removal: Strategies to improve secretion removal include adequate hydration, patient mobilization, coughing, and heated moist aerosolization. The routine use of chest physiotherapy has not been shown to be supported by the literature and is not recommended. Secretions may be thick and tenacious. Monitor response to these therapies and discontinue them if no additional benefits are observed.

Improving Oxygenation and Ventilation

1. Correct hypoxemia (oxygen saturation < 90%) with small increases in FiO_2 levels, preferably with a controlled O_2 delivery device such as a Venturi mask, biphasic intermittent positive airway pressure (BiPAP), or continuous positive airway pressure (CPAP). The goal is to maintain adequate arterial oxygenation (PaO_2 of 55-60 mm Hg or baseline values during nonacute situations) without significantly increasing $PaCO_2$ levels.

   The administration of oxygen to COPD patients was once believed to eliminate the "hypoxic drive," putting the patient at risk for hypercarbia, acidosis, and death. The hypoxic drive is responsible for only approximately 10% of the total drive to breathe. Supplemental oxygen is usually necessary to prevent the deleterious effects of hypoxia and potential organ failure. Higher than necessary FiO_2 levels are avoided. The impact of FiO_2 on $PaCO_2$ occurs by three physiologic mechanisms. (See Table 10-10.)

   Oxygen administration in COPD patients is necessary to prevent hypoxia and organ failure and are never withheld. However, titration and considerations for mechanical ventilation in the COPD patient with CO_2 retention ($PaCO_2$ > 50 mm Hg) are guided by the pH and PaO_2. These include (Figure 10-16):

   - pH less than 7.35 with PaO_2 greater than 60 mm Hg: consider noninvasive mechanical ventilation or intubation.
   - pH greater than 7.35 with PaO_2 less than 60 mm Hg: increase oxygen to increase PaO_2 to greater than 60 mm Hg. Reassess ABG.

2. Position the patient to maximize ventilatory efforts and relaxation/rest during spontaneous breathing.

A high Fowler position and leaning on an overbed table may be a position of comfort.

3. Teach relaxation techniques and diaphragmatic, pursed lip breathing to decrease anxiety and improve ventilatory patterns. Anxiolytics and other sedatives are used cautiously to avoid decreasing minute ventilation.

4. Assist with implementing noninvasive ventilation if needed. The use of noninvasive ventilation in COPD patients with ARF is preferred as the initial mode of ventilation in most patients.

5. Monitor patients managed with supplemental oxygen or noninvasive ventilation for the need for intubation. Deterioration of mental status, hemodynamic instability, and inadequate response to initial therapy are all indications that intubation and mechanical ventilation are warranted. The patient's baseline pulmonary function and functional status, and the reversibility of the condition causing ARF are also factors in the decision to intubate. Weaning from mechanical ventilation is frequently more difficult, and in some cases not possible, in the presence of COPD. Informed discussions with the patient and family regarding intubation are essential. The presence of an advanced directive and designation of a power of attorney for healthcare decisions can help in guiding clinician's actions when patients are unable to make treatment decisions themselves (see Chapter 8, Ethical and Legal Considerations).

Nutritional Support

1. Initiate enteral or oral feeding as soon as possible, once hemodynamic stability is achieved. Typically, patients with COPD have protein-calorie malnutrition, as well as low levels of phosphate, magnesium, and calcium. These chronic nutritional deficits lead to muscle weakness and may interfere with the weaning process if mechanical ventilation becomes necessary. In addition, COPD patients who are malnourished have greater air trapping, lower diffusing capacity, and are less able to mobilize (see Chapter 14, Gastrointestinal System). Early enteral feeding (oral or by feeding tube) is essential to avoid further

TABLE 10-10. PHYSIOLOGIC EFFECTS OF OXYGEN IN COPD

Haldane effect	As hemoglobin becomes desaturated with oxygen, the affinity for carbon dioxide increases. The administration of oxygen then displaces carbon dioxide on hemoglobin and increases carbon dioxide levels in the plasma. Patients with COPD are unable to increase minute ventilation or "blow off" carbon dioxide. This leads to an increase in carbon dioxide, lowering the pH and resulting in a respiratory acidosis.
Hypoxic vasoconstriction	This physiologic adaptive mechanism is a response to a decrease in alveolar oxygen and moves capillary blood flow from a closed or atelectatic alveolus to an open alveolus. In patients with COPD, this adaptive mechanism no longer occurs. As a result, dead space ventilation or decreased perfusion (see Figure 10-15C) occurs with resulting increased carbon dioxide levels.
Decreased minute ventilation	As a result of increased dead space ventilation with resulting increased carbon dioxide, some COPD patients will decrease their minute ventilation. This decrease will further limit the patient's inspiratory reserve capacity.

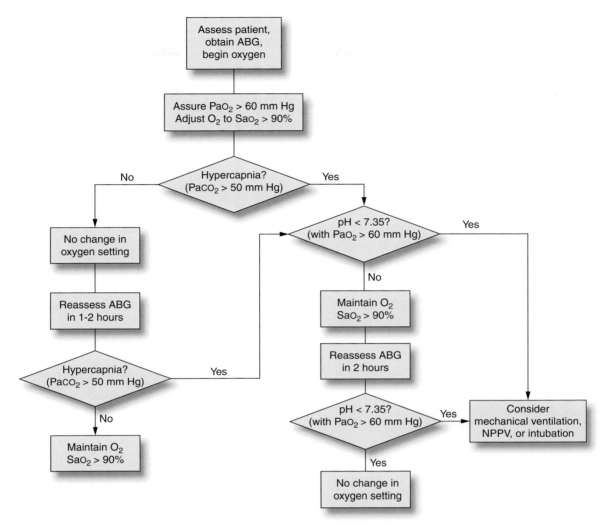

Figure 10-16. Algorithm to correct hypoxemia in an acutely ill COPD patient. ABG, arterial blood gas; NPPV, noninvasive positive pressure ventilation; O_2, oxygen; $PaCO_2$, arterial carbon dioxide tension; PaO_2, arterial oxygen tension; SaO_2, arterial oxygen saturation. (*Reproduced with permission from American Thoracic Society and European Respiratory Society. Standards for the diagnosis and management of patients with COPD, 2004 http://www.thoracic.org/sections/copd/resources.*)

deterioration in their nutritional status during the acute illness.

2. In patients who are unable to eat, use enteral feeding rather than parenteral nutrition to decrease risk of infectious complications.

3. If used, noninvasive positive pressure ventilation makes oral feeding difficult and the insertion of a small bore nasoenteric tube may be necessary.

Preventing and Managing Complications

In addition to the complications associated with ARF, the following complications are commonly observed in patients with COPD exacerbations that cause ARF:

1. *Arrhythmia:* High incidence of both atrial and ventricular arrhythmia in patients with COPD due to hypoxemia, acidosis, heart disease, medications, and electrolyte abnormalities. Cardiac monitoring and

correction of the underlying cause is the goal, with pharmacologic treatment of arrhythmia only for life-threatening situations.

2. *Pulmonary embolus:* High incidence in patients with COPD. Observe for signs and symptoms and follow the usual treatment and prevention guidelines.

3. *GI distention and ileus:* Aerophagia is common in dyspneic patients, increasing the incidence of this complication.

4. *Auto-PEEP and barotrauma* (if ventilated): High incidence, especially in the elderly and in individuals with high ventilation needs.

Patient Teaching

1. Smoking cessation continues to be the single most-effective way to stop the progression of COPD (Table 10-11).

TABLE 10-11. HELPING SMOKERS QUIT: A GUIDE FOR CLINICIANS

Ask

Ask about tobacco use at every admission.
- Implement a system in your clinical setting that ensures that tobacco-use status is obtained and recorded at every contact.

Advise

Advise tobacco users to quit.
- Tell your patient, "quitting smoking is the most important thing you can do to protect your health."

Assess

Assess readiness to quit.
- Ask every tobacco user if he or she is willing to quit at this time.
  - If willing to quit, provide resources and assistance.
  - If unwilling to quit, provide resources and help patient identify barriers to quitting.

Assist

Assist tobacco users with a plan to quit.
Advise the smoker to:
- Set a quit date, ideally within 2 weeks.
- Get support from family, friends, and coworkers.
- Review past quit attempts, what helped, what led to relapse.
- Anticipate challenges.
- Identify reasons for quitting and benefits of quitting.

Arrange

Arrange follow-up visits.
- Provide information for follow-up visits with his or her healthcare provider.

Adapted with permission from US Department of Health and Human Services, Public Health Service. Helping Smokers Quit: A Guide for Clinicians. May, 2008. https://www.ahrq.gov/sites/default/files/wysiwyg/professionals/clinicians-providers/guidelines-recommendations/tobacco/clinicians/references/clinhlpsmkqt/clinhlpsmksqt.pdf.

TABLE 10-12. INFLUENZA AND PNEUMOCOCCAL VACCINE RECOMMENDATIONS

Influenza Vaccine Recommendations
- Routine annual influenza vaccination of all persons aged ≥ 6 months without contraindications

Pneumococcal Vaccine Recommendations

Pneumococcal Conjugate Vaccine (PCV13)
- Infants and children < 2 years old (4-dose series) or 2 years through 4 years who are unvaccinated or have not completed 4-dose series
- Children 24 month through 5 years of age with certain medical conditions should get 1 or 2 doses if not completed 4-dose series
- Children 6 through 18 years of age with certain medical conditions should get 1 dose if not previously received
- Adults 19 through 65 years or older with certain medical conditions should get 1 dose if they have not previously received PCV13
- Adults 65 years or older who have not previously received PCV13

Pneumococcal Polysaccharide Vaccine (PPSV23)
- Anyone 2 through 64 years with certain chronic medical conditions
- Anyone 2 through 64 years with certain medical conditions should get 2 doses PPSV23 5 years apart
- Adults 19 through 64 years who smoke
- Adults 65 years or older should get 1 dose of PPSV23. Adults who have previously received 1-2 doses of PPSV23 before age 65 should receive 1 final dose at age 65 or older once 5 years have lapsed since most recent PPSV23 dose

Data from Grohskopf LA, Sokolow LZ, Broder KR, et al. Prevention and control of seasonal influenza with vaccines. MMWR Recomm Rep. 2016;65(No. RR-5):1-54. and Tomczyk S, Bennett NM, Stoecker C, et al. Use of 13-valent pneumococcal conjugate vaccine and 23-valent pneumococcal polysaccharide vaccine among adults aged ≥ 65 years: recommendations of the advisory committee on immunization practices (ACIP). MMWR. 2014;63:822-825.

2. Immunizations to prevent pneumococcal pneumonia (year round) and influenza (during flu season) remain important preventive measures (Table 10-12).
3. The technique used to administer inhaled medications impacts their effectiveness. Even patients who have been using inhaled medication for a long time benefit from education on the correct technique.
4. Patients discharged on home oxygen therapy need additional teaching on safe practices to prevent injury.

Acute Respiratory Failure in the Patient With Asthma (also called acute severe asthma)

Individuals with asthma are at risk for exacerbations that are characterized by a progressive increase in shortness of breath, cough, wheezing, or decrease in expiratory airflow. Acute severe asthma exacerbation, status asthmaticus, and asthma attack are also terms that have been used to describe this condition. Asthma differs from COPD in both pathophysiology and therapeutic response in that the airway restriction in asthma is usually reversible with aggressive and timely treatment whereas COPD is a progressive disorder (Figure 10-17).

Etiology, Risk Factors, and Pathophysiology

Asthma exacerbations are first and foremost due to uncontrolled airway inflammation. Severe bronchospasm and increased mucus production both contribute to airway obstruction. Triggers vary and include infection, inhaled seasonal antigens, foods, exercise, or medications to name just a few. While triggers may stimulate an exacerbation of asthma, they are not causal.

Bronchoconstriction results from mediators released from mast cells, including histamine, prostaglandins, and leukotrienes that contract the smooth muscle. Mucus plugging is thought to be because of eosinophil and shed bronchial epithelial cells as well as impaired mucus transport. Additionally, over time some patients may exhibit airway remodeling (thickening that contributes to airflow narrowing and airflow obstruction) especially if their airway inflammation is not controlled. All of these contribute to the severe and often unrelenting nature of the asthma "attack."

Some risk factors for the development of an acute severe asthma episode include frequent need for use of their "rescue" inhalers, recent illness, frequent past emergency room visits or hospitalizations, prior intubations and ICU admissions, noncompliance with medical therapy, and inadequate access to health care.

Clinical Presentation

Clinical findings are related to severe airflow obstruction and may include the inability to say a whole sentence, shortness of breath, wheezing, pulsus paradoxus, use of accessory muscles of inspiration, diaphoresis, and need to maintain upright

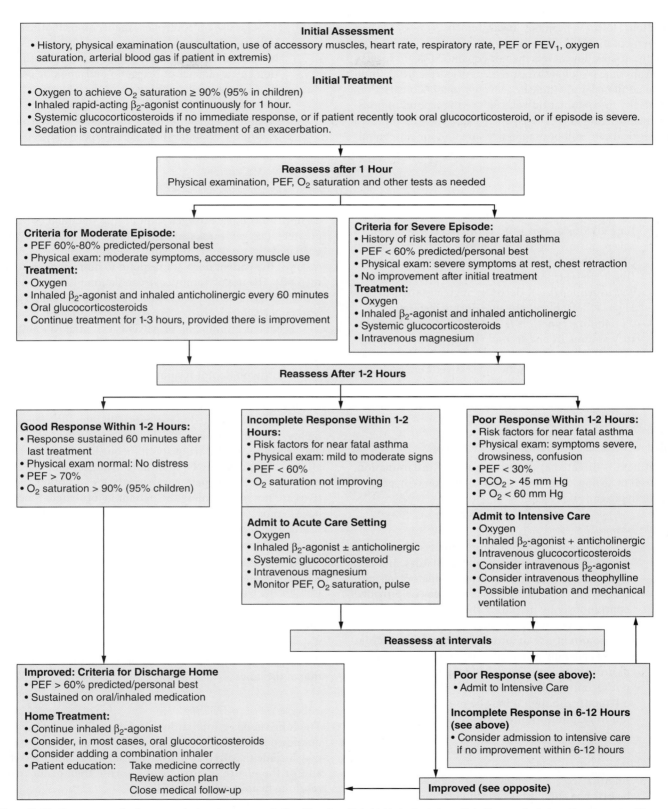

Initial Assessment
- History, physical examination (auscultation, use of accessory muscles, heart rate, respiratory rate, PEF or FEV$_1$, oxygen saturation, arterial blood gas if patient in extremis)

Initial Treatment
- Oxygen to achieve O$_2$ saturation ≥ 90% (95% in children)
- Inhaled rapid-acting β$_2$-agonist continuously for 1 hour.
- Systemic glucocorticosteroids if no immediate response, or if patient recently took oral glucocorticosteroid, or if episode is severe.
- Sedation is contraindicated in the treatment of an exacerbation.

Reassess after 1 Hour
Physical examination, PEF, O$_2$ saturation and other tests as needed

Criteria for Moderate Episode:
- PEF 60%-80% predicted/personal best
- Physical exam: moderate symptoms, accessory muscle use

Treatment:
- Oxygen
- Inhaled β$_2$-agonist and inhaled anticholinergic every 60 minutes
- Oral glucocorticosteroids
- Continue treatment for 1-3 hours, provided there is improvement

Criteria for Severe Episode:
- History of risk factors for near fatal asthma
- PEF < 60% predicted/personal best
- Physical exam: severe symptoms at rest, chest retraction
- No improvement after initial treatment

Treatment:
- Oxygen
- Inhaled β$_2$-agonist and inhaled anticholinergic
- Systemic glucocorticosteroids
- Intravenous magnesium

Reassess After 1-2 Hours

Good Response Within 1-2 Hours:
- Response sustained 60 minutes after last treatment
- Physical exam normal: No distress
- PEF > 70%
- O$_2$ saturation > 90% (95% children)

Incomplete Response Within 1-2 Hours:
- Risk factors for near fatal asthma
- Physical exam: mild to moderate signs
- PEF < 60%
- O$_2$ saturation not improving

Admit to Acute Care Setting
- Oxygen
- Inhaled β$_2$-agonist ± anticholinergic
- Systemic glucocorticosteroid
- Intravenous magnesium
- Monitor PEF, O$_2$ saturation, pulse

Poor Response Within 1-2 Hours:
- Risk factors for near fatal asthma
- Physical exam: symptoms severe, drowsiness, confusion
- PEF < 30%
- PCO$_2$ > 45 mm Hg
- P O$_2$ < 60 mm Hg

Admit to Intensive Care
- Oxygen
- Inhaled β$_2$-agonist + anticholinergic
- Intravenous glucocorticosteroids
- Consider intravenous β$_2$-agonist
- Consider intravenous theophylline
- Possible intubation and mechanical ventilation

Reassess at intervals

Improved: Criteria for Discharge Home
- PEF > 60% predicted/personal best
- Sustained on oral/inhaled medication

Home Treatment:
- Continue inhaled β$_2$-agonist
- Consider, in most cases, oral glucocorticosteroids
- Consider adding a combination inhaler
- Patient education: Take medicine correctly
                      Review action plan
                      Close medical follow-up

Poor Response (see above):
- Admit to Intensive Care

Incomplete Response in 6-12 Hours (see above)
- Consider admission to intensive care if no improvement within 6-12 hours

Improved (see opposite)

Figure 10-17.   Management of asthma exacerbations in acute care facility. (*Data from Global Initiative for Asthma. Global Strategy for Asthma Management and Prevention, updated 2018. www.ginathma.org.*)

position. However, peak flow measurement is one of the best assessment tools for determining the severity of the exacerbation. A peak flow of less than or equal to 50% of expected or an absolute peak flow measurement of less than 100 L/min in an adult generally indicates severe bronchoconstriction, especially in combination with failure to respond to bronchodilator treatments. These patients are generally admitted to a critical care unit or progressive care unit for close monitoring and urgent therapy (see Figure 10-17).

Diagnostic Tests

- *ABGs:* Initial findings may show pH greater than 7.45, $Paco_2$ less than 35 mm Hg indicating respiratory alkalosis, and mild to moderate hypoxia. In severe airflow obstruction, findings may progress to pH less than 7.35 and $Paco_2$ greater than 50 mm Hg (respiratory acidosis).
- *Pulsus paradoxus:* A decrease of greater than 10 mm Hg in systolic blood pressure during inspiration.
- *Pulmonary function tests (PFTs):* Forced expiratory volume in one second (FEV_1) of less than 20% or peak expiratory flow rate (PEFR) of less than 50% of predicted despite aggressive bronchodilator therapy.
- *Spo_2:* Observe for hypoxia. The Spo_2 should be greater than 92%.

Principles of Management for Asthma Exacerbations

Treatment is directed at decreasing airway inflammation, reversal of airflow obstruction, and correction of hypercapnia or hypoxemia if present.

Treat the Underlying Disease State

1. Reduce airway inflammation with systemic corticosteroids and inhaled bronchodilators. Inhaled short-acting beta-agonist, bronchodilators (eg, albuterol) are the drug of choice and may be provided continuously by nebulizer through a mouthpiece, mask or if ventilated, through the ventilator circuit. Concomitant use of anticholinergic bronchodilators is generally provided to enhance rapid reversal of bronchospasm. The use of magnesium sulfate is not recommended for routine use in asthma exacerbations, although it may be used in patients who fail to respond to initial treatment and persistent hypoxemia.
2. Routine use of antibiotics is not recommended unless there is strong evidence of respiratory infection.
3. Improve secretion removal: Generally secretions will be easier to mobilize as bronchodilation is enhanced. Until then, strategies are limited. Hydration with intravenous fluids is often required to correct fluid deficits and loosen secretions.
4. Provide patient education on self-management techniques to improve long-term control of the disease.

Regular use of "controller" medications to decrease inflammation, appropriate use of rescue inhalers for bronchodilation when wheezing occurs, identification and avoidance of "triggers," and smoking cessation are essential components of the education plan (see Table 10-10).

5. Administer pneumococcal and influenza (seasonal) vaccines (see Table 10-11) prior to discharge, if not already received.

Improving Oxygenation and Ventilation

Severe hypoxemia is corrected by providing high Fio_2 levels until an adequate oxygen saturation is obtained (90% or greater). Oxygen masks and high flow O_2 systems may be used to deliver oxygen. Mechanical ventilation may be necessary if the patient does not respond to more conservative methods. The use of noninvasive ventilation in an asthmatic is discouraged as it may lead to increased hyperinflation and respiratory failure.

Frequent monitoring of ABGs is essential to monitor pH and $Paco_2$. Helium-oxygen (heliox) mixtures may be used to decrease work of breathing and improve ventilation in patients who do not respond to initial therapies. Heliox can be administered via mask, or invasive ventilation. Due to the high levels of helium in the heliox mixtures, the use of heliox may be limited in patients with high Fio_2 requirements. Position the patient to maximize ventilatory efforts and relaxation/rest during spontaneous breathing. Relaxation techniques may be helpful to decrease anxiety and improve ventilatory patterns. Anxiolytics and other sedatives are not given unless the patient is intubated. Studies have demonstrated that doing so increases the potential for death. The decision to intubate and mechanically ventilate the patient may be made urgently in patients who are failing to respond to treatment and are fatiguing. If intubation is done, the patient is generally transferred to a critical care unit for management.

Interstitial Lung Disease

Interstitial lung disease is a broad category of over 130 lung disorders that are characterized by fibrosis and/or inflammation of the lungs.

Etiology, Risk Factors, and Pathophysiology

The lung tissue or interstitium is damaged by a known or unknown causes leading to inflammation. The inflammation may include the alveolar space, small airways, blood vessels, and/or the pleura. Fibrosis and scarring then occur with resulting hypoxemia and "stiff lungs."

Some known causes include:

- Occupational and environmental exposure to irritants, asbestos, and silica.
- Infections, tuberculosis.
- Medications, amiodarone, chemotherapy agents.

- Connective tissue or collagen disorders, rheumatoid arthritis, sarcoidosis, systemic sclerosis, systemic lupus erythematosis.
- Genetic/familial.

Unknown causes are classified as idiopathic pulmonary fibrosis (IPF).

Clinical Presentation
Signs and symptoms

- Dyspnea
- Dry cough
- Clubbing
- Fine crackles or "velcro lungs" on auscultation
- Signs of right-sided heart failure
- Fatigue and weakness

Diagnostic Tests

- *Chest x-ray:* May be normal or show lung volume loss
- *High resolution CT chest:* Classic description of honeycombing or "ground glass"
- *Lung biopsy:* May be indicated is some circumstances for definitive diagnosis
- *Serology:* For specific connective tissue diseases
- *PFTs:* Most of the disorders show a restrictive pattern with decreased lung volumes

Principles of Management
The management of interstitial lung disease (ILD) is similar to the management for ARF described above. Additional interventions to consider include:

1. Smoking cessation counseling and life style changes to remove inhalation exposures
2. Supplemental oxygen therapy in patients who demonstrate hypoxemia
3. Discontinue and avoid using medications that can cause lung toxicity (eg, bleomycin, cyclophosphamide, nitrofurantoin, sulfasalazine, and amiodarone)
4. Referral to pulmonary rehabilitation for monitored physical activity to prevent functional decline
5. Medications specific to disease
   - Corticosteroids
   - Cytotoxic agents
   - Recent recommendations specific to IPF include two new oral medications that target specific pulmonary vascular growth factors: nintedanib or pirfenidone
6. Referral to lung transplant center for evaluation
7. Supportive care to improve symptom control and quality of life

Pulmonary Arterial Hypertension

Pulmonary arterial hypertension (PAH) is a progressive, life-threatening disorder of the pulmonary circulation characterized by high pulmonary artery pressures (> 25 mm Hg). This persistent high pulmonary artery pressure ultimately leads to right ventricular failure. Patients with PAH or World Health Organization (WHO) Group 1 are often on a chronic regimen of therapy that is not interrupted during hospitalization. Abrupt cessation of therapy can lead to rebound PH that can be fatal.

Etiology, Risk Factors, and Pathophysiology
PAH may result from a number of etiologies (Table 10-13). The pathophysiology is multifactorial with evidence that endothelial dysfunction leads to remodeling of the pulmonary artery vessel wall causing exaggerated vasoconstriction and impaired vasodilatation. The increase in pulmonary arterial pressure causes an increase in pulmonary vascular resistance, right ventricular dilation and hypertrophy, and decreased blood flow from the right side of the heart through

TABLE 10-13. WORLD HEALTH ORGANIZATION CLASSIFICATION OF PULMONARY HYPERTENSION[a]

Group	Main Classification	Diseases Included
1.	Pulmonary arterial hypertension (PAH)	PAH: Idiopathic, heritable, drug and toxin induced, associated with connective tissue disease, associated with HIV infection, associated with portal hypertension, associated with congenital heart disease, associated with schistosomiasis, pulmonary veno-occlusive disease and/or pulmonary capillary hemangiomatosis, persistent PH of the newborn
2.	Pulmonary hypertension due to left-sided heart disease	Systolic dysfunction, diastolic dysfunction, valvular disease, congenital
3.	Pulmonary hypertension due to lung disease and/or hypoxia	Chronic obstructive pulmonary disease, interstitial lung disease, mixed restrictive and obstructive pattern, sleep disordered breathing, alveolar hypoventilation disorders, chronic exposure to high altitude, developmental abnormalities
4.	Chronic thromboembolic pulmonary hypertension	Chronic thromboembolic disease
5.	Pulmonary hypertension with unclear multifactorial mechanisms	Hematologic disorders: chronic hemolytic anemia, myeloproliferative disorders, splenectomy; systemic disorders: sarcoidosis, pulmonary histiocytosis: lymphangioleiomyomatosis, neurofibromatosis, vasculitis; metabolic disorders: glycogen storage disease, Gaucher disease, thyroid disorders; others: tumoral obstruction, fibrosing mediastinitis, chronic renal failure, segmental PH

Modified with permission from Simonneau G, Gatzoulis MA, Adatia I, et al. Updated clinical classification of pulmonary hypertension. J Am Coll Cardiol 2013 Dec 24;62(25 Suppl):D34-41.

the pulmonary vasculature. The result is a drop in the return of oxygenated blood to the left side of the heart. In PAH or WHO Class 1, the primary pathology is in the pulmonary vasculature. In PH or WHO Class 2-5, the elevation in pulmonary artery pressure is secondary to another disorder such as left-sided heart disease, lung disease, chronic thromboembolic disease, or other causes. Distinction between PAH and PH is important because the treatment differs; most of the complex medications discussed below are indicated for PAH.

Clinical Presentation

Signs and Symptoms

Signs and symptoms include pallor, dyspnea, fatigue, chest pain, and syncope. Cor pulmonale or enlargement of the right ventricle can be a result of PAH and may lead to right ventricular failure (see Table 9-10). The diagnostic strategy is related to both establishing the diagnosis of PH and if possible the underlying cause.

Diagnostic Tests

- *Echocardiogram:* Valvular heart disease, left ventricular dysfunction, and intracardiac shunts.
- *Chest x-ray:* Enlarged hilar and pulmonary arterial shadows and enlargement of the right ventricle.
- *12-lead ECG:* Right ventricular strain, right ventricular hypertrophy, and right axis deviation.
- *CTPA, ventilation-perfusion scan, or pulmonary angiogram:* These are done to rule out thromboembolism.
- *CT chest:* Assess for presence or absence of parenchymal lung disease.
- *6-minute-walk test:* Measurement of distance used to monitor exercise tolerance, response to therapy, and progression of disease.
- *Right-heart cardiac catheterization:* Gold standard for diagnosis with vasodilator (adenosine, nitric oxide, epoprostenol) testing for benefit from long-term therapy with calcium channel blockers. Positive response is a decrease in mean PAP of 10 to 40 mm Hg with an increased or unchanged CO from baseline values.
- *Serology testing:* Antinuclear antibodies.
- *Pulmonary function testing:* Used to rule out any other diseases contributing to shortness of breath.
- *Sleep study:* Done as a screen for sleep apnea, which may also contribute to the PH.

Principles of Management

Current treatment options aim to slow the progression of the disease and minimize symptoms.

1. Provide anticoagulation therapy to prevent thrombosis and patient education on the long-term use of anticoagulants.
2. Avoid beta-blockers, decongestants, or other medications that worsen PH or decrease right heart function.
3. Encourage physical activity as tolerated, alternating periods of activity with periods of rest.
4. Administer oxygen to treat hypoxemia and prevent increased pulmonary vasoconstriction due to low oxygen levels. Maintain Sao_2 greater than 90% if possible.
5. Give diuretics to control edema and ascites if right heart failure is present.
6. Use calcium channel blockers in patients who show a positive response to vasodilator during cardiac catheterization.

Medical Treatment Options

Prior to 1995, there was no medication therapy for PAH other than continuous oxygen. Epoprostenol was the first medication therapy for PAH and was approved in 1995. Patients must be preapproved through their insurance prior to starting these costly medications and be able to self-administer. In general, these medications are not stopped and require expertise in administration. There are five medication classifications. See Table 10-14 for examples.

1. Phosphodiesterase inhibitors block phosphodiesterase type 5, which is responsible for the degradation of cyclic guanosine monophosphate (cGMP). Increased cGMP concentration results in pulmonary vasculature relaxation; vasodilation in the pulmonary bed and the systemic circulation (to a lesser degree) may occur.
2. Endothelin receptor antagonists block the neurohormone endothelin from binding in the endothelium and vascular smooth muscle.
3. Prostacyclin receptor agonists stimulate the endogenous production of prostacyclin to potentiate vasodilatation.
4. Soluble guanylate cyclase stimulator acts synergistically with endogenous nitric oxide and also independently to produce vasodilatory effects, reduce

TABLE 10-14. PULMONARY ARTERIAL HYPERTENSION MEDICATIONS

Category	Examples	Route
Phosphodiesterase Inhibitor	Sildenafil	oral
	Tadalafil	oral
Endothelin Receptor Antagonist	Bosentan	oral
	Macitentan	oral
	Ambrisentan	oral
Prostacyclin Receptor Agonist	Selexipag	oral
Soluble Guanylate Cyclase Stimulator	Riociquat	oral
Prostacyclin	Epoprostenol, Epoprostenol RTS	intravenous
	Treprostinil	intravenous, subcutaneous inhaled oral
	Iloprost	inhaled

pulmonary smooth muscle proliferation, and acts against platelet inhibition.

5. Prostacyclin is a potent vasodilator of both systemic and pulmonary arterial vascular beds and is an inhibitor of platelet aggregation.

Surgical options include the following:

1. Atrial septostomy to create a right-to-left shunt to help decompress a failing right ventricle in select patients who are unresponsive to medical therapies. This also leads to significant hypoxemia in an already compromised patient.
2. Pulmonary thromboendarterectomy for those with suspected chronic thromboembolic pulmonary hypertension (CTEPH) to improve hemodynamics and functional status.
3. Lung transplantation is indicated when the PH has progressed despite optimal medical and surgical therapy.

Pneumonia

Respiratory infection is a common cause of ARF. Infections developed before hospitalization (community-acquired), during medical treatment (healthcare-acquired), and those acquired during hospitalization (hospital-acquired and ventilator-associated) can lead to significant morbidity and mortality, and require progressive care management. A variety of respiratory infections occur in acutely ill patients, including bronchitis and pneumonia. This section focuses on pneumonia, the most common respiratory infection and the most common cause of respiratory failure in acutely ill patients.

Etiology, Risk Factors, and Pathophysiology

Infants, children, older adults, those with chronic cardiopulmonary disease, and immunocompromised individuals are at increased risk for pneumonia. In addition, immobility, decreased level of consciousness, and mechanical ventilation place hospitalized patients at high risk for development of pneumonias. These latter pneumonias are most commonly referred to as ventilator-associated pneumonias or VAP.

Organisms that cause pneumonia enter the lungs by aspiration of oropharyngeal or gastric contents into the lungs, inhalation of aerosols or particles containing the organisms, or hematogenic spread of the organism into the lung from another site in the body (Figure 10-18). Most hospital-acquired pneumonias are due to aspiration of bacteria colonizing the oropharynx or upper GI tract. Pneumonia develops when the normal bronchomucociliary clearance mechanism or phagocytic cells are overwhelmed by the number or virulence of organisms aspirated or inhaled into the airways. The proliferation of organisms in the pulmonary parenchyma elicits an inflammatory response, with large influxes of phagocytic cells into the alveoli and airways and production of protein-rich exudates. This inflammatory response impairs the distribution of ventilation and decreases lung compliance, resulting in increased work of

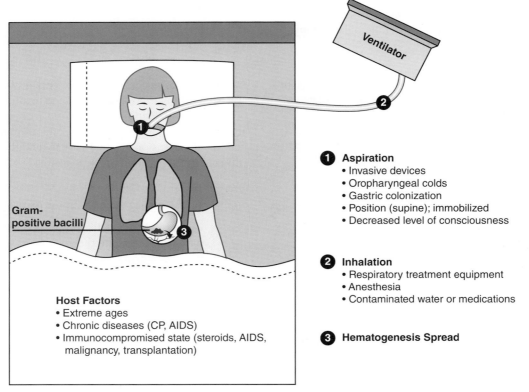

Figure 10-18. Pathogenesis of pneumonia.

breathing and leads to the sensation of dyspnea. Hypoxemia results from the shunting of blood through poorly ventilated areas of pulmonary consolidation. The inflammatory response leads to fever and leukocytosis.

Pneumonia also can develop through hematogenous spread, when organisms remote from the lungs gain access to the blood, become lodged in the pulmonary vasculature, and proliferate. Pneumonias with a hematogenous origin usually are distributed diffusely in both lung fields, rather than localized to a single lung or lobe.

Several factors present in acutely ill patients increase the risk for the development of hospital-acquired pneumonias including VAP. Aspiration of oropharyngeal and gastric secretions is increased in the presence of tracheostomy tubes, nasogastric tubes, poor GI motility, gastric distention, and immobility, all of which are common complications of acute illness. Treatments that neutralize the normally acidic gastric contents, such as antacids, H_2 blockers, or tube feeding, increase the growth of gram-negative bacteria that can be directly aspirated into the lungs or spread to the lungs via the bloodstream.

Acutely ill patients at high risk for hospital-acquired pneumonias include those who are immunocompromised from malignancy, acquired immunodeficiency syndrome (AIDS), and chronic cardiac or respiratory disease; older adults; and those with depressed alveolar macrophage function (oxygen, corticosteroids). Although a variety of similar organisms cause community-acquired and hospital-acquired pneumonias, their frequency distribution is different (Table 10-15). Of particular concern in hospital-acquired infections is the polymicrobial origin of the pneumonia and the potential for causative organisms to be resistant to antimicrobial therapy.

TABLE 10-15. INFECTIOUS ETIOLOGIC AGENTS IN SEVERE COMMUNITY-ACQUIRED PNEUMONIA REQUIRING INTENSIVE CARE SUPPORT AND HOSPITAL-ACQUIRED PNEUMONIA IN CRITICALLY ILL PATIENTS

	Etiologic Agent (Decreasing Rank)
Community-acquired pneumonias	Streptococcus pneumonia
	Staphylococcus aureus
	Legionella species
	Gram-negative bacilli
	Haemophilus influenzae
Ventilator-acquired pneumonias	Staphylococcus aureus
	Pseudomonas aeruginosa
	Klebsiella pneumoniae/oxytoca
	Enterobacter species
	Acinetobacter baumannii
	Escherichia coli
	Candida albicans
	Proteus spp
	Coagulase-negative staphylococci

Data from Mandell LA, Wunderink RG, Anzueto A, et al. Infectious Diseases Society of America/American Thoracic Society consensus guidelines on the management of community-acquired pneumonia in adults. Clin Infect Dis. 2007;44(suppl 2):S27-S72. Weiner LM, Webb AK, Limbago R, et al. Antimicrobial-resistant pathogens associated with healthcare-associated infections: summary of data reported to the National Healthcare Safety Network at the Centers for Disease Control and Prevention. 2011-2014. Infect Control Hosp Epidemiol. 2016;37:1288-1301.

Development of a hospital-acquired pneumonia is a serious complication in acutely ill patients. Increased morbidity and mortality, in addition to increases in progressive care and hospital lengths of stay and costs, make hospital-acquired pneumonias one of the most important sources of negative outcomes for acutely ill patients.

Clinical Presentation
Signs and Symptoms
- Fever
- Cough, typically productive
- Purulent sputum or hemoptysis
- Dyspnea
- Pleuritic chest pain
- Tachypnea
- Abnormal breath sounds (crackles, bronchial breath sounds)

Diagnostic Tests
- Gram stain and culture of sputum for causative organisms. May require fiberoptic bronchoscopy with brush specimen or bronchoalveolar lavage specimen retrieval in situations where pneumonia responds poorly to treatment. This may also be necessary early in admission in patients who are immunocompromised and susceptible to opportunistic infections that require very specific antibiotic coverage.
- New or progressive infiltrates on chest x-ray. Infiltrates may be either localized or diffuse in nature (see Figure 10-5).
- Elevated white blood cell (WBC).
- Abnormal ABGs (hypoxemia, hypocapnia).

Principles of Management for Pneumonia
Treating the Underlying Disease
Appropriate empirical broad-spectrum antimicrobial therapy is based on an assessment of the most likely causative organisms until definitive culture results are obtained. Fluids are administered to correct hypovolemia and hypotension, if present. Hypotension unresponsive to fluid therapy alerts the clinician to the potential for septic shock.

Improving Oxygenation and Ventilation
Similar to ARF management, with the following additions:

1. Increased PEEP in the presence of a focal pneumonia may exacerbate the associated ventilation-perfusion abnormalities by over distending unaffected alveoli leading to increased capillary resistance and redistribution of blood flow to affected alveoli. These techniques are used with caution in pneumonia.
2. Voluminous, tenacious respiratory secretions may require endotracheal intubation to assist with clearance. Chest physiotherapy may be helpful to increase secretion clearance, particularly when lobar atelectasis is present. Fiberoptic bronchoscopy may also be required to assist with secretion management.

Assessment and Surveillance

Although the signs and symptoms of VAP are known, clinical diagnosis is complicated by lack of specific and sensitive criteria. In 2013, the National Healthcare Safety Network lead by the Centers for Disease Control began collecting new surveillance criteria for ventilator-associated events (VAEs), which include ventilator-associated conditions (VACs), infection-related ventilator-associated conditions (IVACs), and VAP. These definitions were revised in 2017 and are shown in Figure 10-19. These definitions are less applicable to the clinical decisions about the care of patients with VAP and more useful for tracking rates of VAP and VAE so that the effectiveness of prevention strategies can be measured.

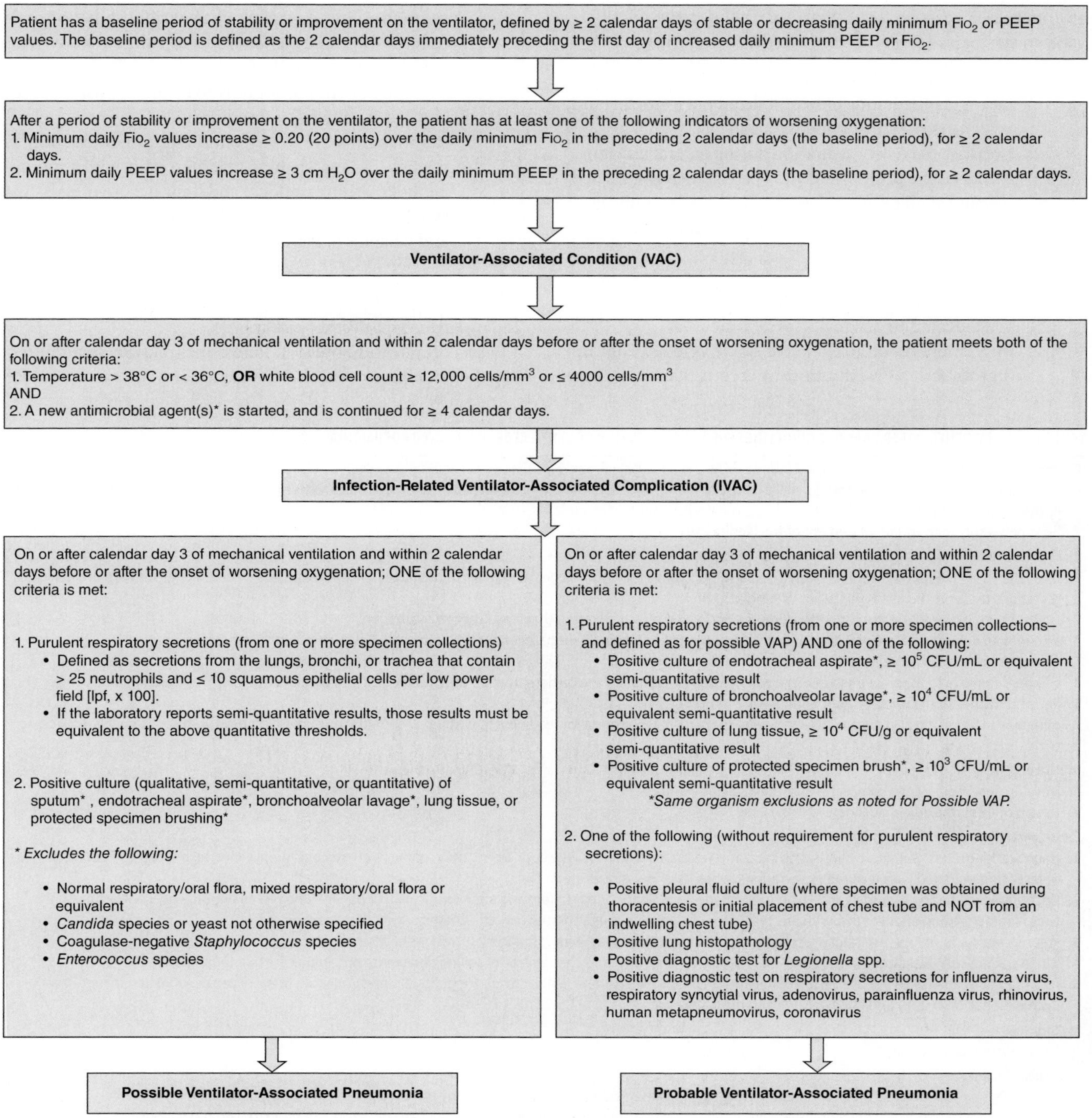

Patient has a baseline period of stability or improvement on the ventilator, defined by ≥ 2 calendar days of stable or decreasing daily minimum Fio_2 or PEEP values. The baseline period is defined as the 2 calendar days immediately preceding the first day of increased daily minimum PEEP or Fio_2.

After a period of stability or improvement on the ventilator, the patient has at least one of the following indicators of worsening oxygenation:
1. Minimum daily Fio_2 values increase ≥ 0.20 (20 points) over the daily minimum Fio_2 in the preceding 2 calendar days (the baseline period), for ≥ 2 calendar days.
2. Minimum daily PEEP values increase ≥ 3 cm H_2O over the daily minimum PEEP in the preceding 2 calendar days (the baseline period), for ≥ 2 calendar days.

Ventilator-Associated Condition (VAC)

On or after calendar day 3 of mechanical ventilation and within 2 calendar days before or after the onset of worsening oxygenation, the patient meets both of the following criteria:
1. Temperature > 38°C or < 36°C, **OR** white blood cell count ≥ 12,000 cells/mm³ or ≤ 4000 cells/mm³
AND
2. A new antimicrobial agent(s)* is started, and is continued for ≥ 4 calendar days.

Infection-Related Ventilator-Associated Complication (IVAC)

On or after calendar day 3 of mechanical ventilation and within 2 calendar days before or after the onset of worsening oxygenation; ONE of the following criteria is met:

1. Purulent respiratory secretions (from one or more specimen collections)
 • Defined as secretions from the lungs, bronchi, or trachea that contain > 25 neutrophils and ≤ 10 squamous epithelial cells per low power field [lpf, x 100].
 • If the laboratory reports semi-quantitative results, those results must be equivalent to the above quantitative thresholds.

2. Positive culture (qualitative, semi-quantitative, or quantitative) of sputum*, endotracheal aspirate*, bronchoalveolar lavage*, lung tissue, or protected specimen brushing*

* Excludes the following:
 • Normal respiratory/oral flora, mixed respiratory/oral flora or equivalent
 • *Candida* species or yeast not otherwise specified
 • Coagulase-negative *Staphylococcus* species
 • *Enterococcus* species

Possible Ventilator-Associated Pneumonia

On or after calendar day 3 of mechanical ventilation and within 2 calendar days before or after the onset of worsening oxygenation; ONE of the following criteria is met:

1. Purulent respiratory secretions (from one or more specimen collections– and defined as for possible VAP) AND one of the following:
 • Positive culture of endotracheal aspirate*, ≥ 10⁵ CFU/mL or equivalent semi-quantitative result
 • Positive culture of bronchoalveolar lavage*, ≥ 10⁴ CFU/mL or equivalent semi-quantitative result
 • Positive culture of lung tissue, ≥ 10⁴ CFU/g or equivalent semi-quantitative result
 • Positive culture of protected specimen brush*, ≥ 10³ CFU/mL or equivalent semi-quantitative result
   Same organism exclusions as noted for Possible VAP.

2. One of the following (without requirement for purulent respiratory secretions):
 • Positive pleural fluid culture (where specimen was obtained during thoracentesis or initial placement of chest tube and NOT from an indwelling chest tube)
 • Positive lung histopathology
 • Positive diagnostic test for *Legionella* spp.
 • Positive diagnostic test on respiratory secretions for influenza virus, respiratory syncytial virus, adenovirus, parainfluenza virus, rhinovirus, human metapneumovirus, coronavirus

Probable Ventilator-Associated Pneumonia

Figure 10-19. Ventilator-associated event (VAE) surveillance algorithm. (*Reproduced with permission from Centers for Disease Control and Prevention [CDC]. Device-associated module VAE. 2017. https://www.cdc.gov/nhsn/pdfs/pscmanual/10-vae_final.pdf. Accessed July 5, 2017.*)

Preventing Hospital-Acquired Pneumonias

In addition to the high morbidity and mortality associated with pneumonia in acutely ill patients, high priority must be given to strategies to prevent the development of hospital-acquired pneumonias. The development of a hospital-acquired pneumonia in an acutely ill patient increases requirements for ventilatory support (mechanical ventilation, oxygen, duration of treatment). It is estimated that a hospital-acquired pneumonia increases hospitalization 4 to 12 days, and increases costs by $20,000 to $40,000 per episode. Prevention strategies (Table 10-16) include the following:

1. Decrease the risk of cross-contamination or colonization via the hands of hospitalized personnel. Hand hygiene is the most effective strategy.
2. Decrease the risk of aspiration during enteral nutrition. Avoid supine positioning and keep the head of the bed elevated at all times, unless medically contraindicated. Assess for, and correct, gastric reflux problems.

For Patients on Mechanical Ventilation

1. Avoid supine positioning and keep the head of the bed elevated to 30° to 45° at all times.
2. Implement a comprehensive oral hygiene program that includes oral suctioning, teeth brushing, and use of oral 0.12% chlorhexidine gluconate for ventilator patients. See the AACN Practice Alert: Oral care for Acutely and Critically Ill Patients.
3. Use sterile technique for tracheal suctioning and suction only when necessary to clear secretions from large airways.
4. Maintain a closed system on ventilator/humidifier circuits and avoid pooling of condensation or secretions in the tubing. Do not routinely change the ventilator circuit, except when visibly soiled or malfunctioning. Use sterile water or saline for use with any respiratory equipment.
5. Provide nutritional support to improve host defenses and reduce the risk of pneumonia.
6. Remove invasive devices and equipment as soon as possible. Assess weaning readiness daily with a spontaneous breathing protocol and limit the use of sedatives (see Chapter 5, Airway and Ventilatory Management and Chapter 6, Pain Management/Sedation).

Pulmonary Embolism

Etiology, Risk Factors, and Pathophysiology

PE is a complication of DVT, long bone fracture, or air entering the circulatory system. There are many risk factors for PE

TABLE 10-16. EVIDENCE-BASED PRACTICE GUIDELINES FOR THE PREVENTION OF VENTILATOR-ASSOCIATED PNEUMONIA

Preventing Gastric Reflux

1. All mechanically ventilated patients, as well as those at high risk for aspiration (eg, decreased level of consciousness; enteral tube in place), should have the head of the bed elevated at an angle of 30°-45° unless medically contraindicated.[a,b,c]
2. Routinely verify appropriate placement of the feeding tube.[a]

Airway Management

1. If feasible, use an endotracheal tube with a dorsal lumen above the endotracheal cuff to allow drainage (by continuous or intermittent suctioning) of tracheal secretions that accumulate in the patient's subglottic area.[a,b]
2. Unless contraindicated by the patient's condition, perform orotracheal rather than nasotracheal intubation.[a]
3. ET cuff management: Before deflating the cuff of an endotracheal tube in preparation for tube removal, or before moving the tube, ensure that secretions are cleared from above the tube cuff.[a]
4. Use only sterile fluid to remove secretions from the suction catheter if the catheter is to be used for reentry into the patient's lower respiratory tract.[a]
5. Perform tracheostomy under aseptic conditions.[a]
6. Minimize sedation, daily spontaneous awakening trials, daily assessment for readiness to wean, pair spontaneous breathing trials with spontaneous awakening trials.[c]

Oral Care

1. Develop and implement a comprehensive oral hygiene program.[a,c]
2. Use an oral chlorhexidine gluconate (0.12%) rinse.[b,c]

Cross-Contamination

1. Hand washing: Decontaminate hands with soap and water or a waterless antiseptic agent after contact with mucous membranes, respiratory secretions, or objects contaminated with respiratory secretions, whether or not gloves are worn.[a]
2. Decontaminate hands with soap and water or a waterless antiseptic agent before and after contact with a patient who has an endotracheal or tracheostomy tube, and before and after contact with any respiratory device that is used on the patient, whether or not gloves are worn.[a]
3. Wear gloves for handling respiratory secretions or objects contaminated with respiratory secretions of any patient.[a]
4. When soiling with respiratory secretions is anticipated, wear a gown and change it after soiling and before providing care to another patient.[a]
5. Room-air humidifiers: Do not use large-volume room-air humidifiers that create aerosols (nebulizers) unless they can be sterilized or subjected to high-level disinfection at least daily and filled only with sterile water.[a]

Mobilization

1. Early exercise and mobility.[a,c]

Equipment Changes

1. Do not change routinely, on the basis of duration of use, the patient's ventilator circuit. Change the circuit when it is visibly soiled or mechanically malfunctioning. Periodically drain or discard any condensate that collects in the tubing. Do not allow condensate to drain toward the patient.[a,b,c]
2. Between use on different patients, sterilize or subject to high-level disinfection all MRBs.[a]

Data from [a]Centers for Disease Control and Prevention (2004), [b]AACN VAP Practice Alert (2016), and [c]SHEA/IDSA Practice Recommendations (2014).

TABLE 10-17. RISK FACTORS FOR THE DEVELOPMENT OF PULMONARY EMBOLISM

Thromboemboli
- Obesity
- Prior history of thromboembolism
- Advanced age
- Malignancy
- Chemotherapy
- Estrogen
- Immobility
- Acute spinal cord injury with paralysis
- Heart failure
- Trauma
- Surgery
- Trauma
- Inherited thrombophilia
- Central venous catheters
- Inflammatory bowel disease
- Nephrotic syndrome

Air Emboli
- Surgery (Neurosurgery, Cardiothoracic, Obstetrical/Gynecologic, Orthopedic, Otolaryngological)
- Pacemaker of defibrillator insertion
- Radiologic procedure
- IV contrast
- Positive pressure ventilation
- Scuba diving
- Hemodialysis
- Central venous catheter insertion or removal

Fat Emboli
- Long bone fracture and other fractures (pelvic, ribs, etc)
- Intraosseous access
- Chest compression
- Lung transplantation
- Liver disease
- Pancreatitis
- Lipid infusions
- Sickle cell crisis
- Cyclosporine administration

(Table 10-17), with acutely ill patients being especially prone due to the presence of central venous catheters, immobility, and the high rate of co-morbidities such as heart failure and cancer.

Venous Thromboembolism
Venous thrombi form at the site of vascular injuries or where venous stasis occurs, primarily in the leg or pelvic veins. Thrombi that dislodge travel through the venous circulation and can become wedged in a branch of the pulmonary circulation. Depending on the size of the thrombi, and the location of the occlusion, mild to severe obstruction of blood flow occurs beyond the thrombi.

The primary sequela, and major contributor to mortality, of the PE is circulatory impairment. The physical obstruction of the pulmonary capillary bed increases right ventricular afterload, dilates the right ventricle, and impedes coronary perfusion. This predisposes the right ventricle to ischemia and right ventricular failure (cor pulmonale).

A secondary consequence of thromboemboli is a mismatching of ventilation to perfusion in gas exchange units beyond the obstruction (see Figure 10-15C), resulting in arterial hypoxemia. This hypoxemia further compromises oxygen delivery to the ischemic right ventricle.

Air Emboli
Air or other nonabsorbable gases entering the venous system also travel to the right heart, pulmonary circulation, arterioles, and capillaries. A variety of surgical and non-surgical situations predispose patients to the development of air embolization (see Table 10-17). Damage to the pulmonary endothelium occurs from the abnormal air-blood interface, leading to increased capillary permeability and alveolar flooding. Bronchoconstriction also occurs with air embolization leading to impaired removal of carbon dioxide and hypercapnia.

Arterial embolization may occur if air passes to the left heart through a patent foramen ovale, present in approximately 30% of the population. Peripheral embolization to the brain, extremities, and coronary perfusion leads to ischemic manifestations in these organs.

Fat Emboli
Fat enters the pulmonary circulation most commonly when released from the bone marrow following long bone fractures (see Table 10-17). Nontraumatic origins of fat embolization also occur and are thought to be due to the agglutination of low-density lipoproteins or liposomes from nutritional fat emulsions. The presence of fat in the pulmonary circulation injures the endothelial lining of the capillary, increasing permeability and alveolar flooding.

Clinical Presentation
Because many of the signs and symptoms of PE are nonspecific, it is difficult to diagnosis. In acutely ill patients, diagnosis is especially difficult owing to alterations in communication and level of consciousness, and the nonspecific nature of other cardiopulmonary alterations.

Signs and Symptoms
- Dyspnea
- Pleuritic chest pain
- Cough
- Rales
- Apprehension
- Diaphoresis
- Evidence of DVT
- Hemoptysis
- Tachypnea
- Fever
- Tachycardia
- Syncope
- Hypoxia
- Hypotension

Diagnostic Tests

- *Chest x-ray:* Evaluate for basilar atelectasis, elevation of the diaphragm, and pleural effusion, although most patients with PE have nonspecific findings on chest x-ray; diffuse alveolar filling may be seen in air embolism.
- *ABG analysis:* Hypoxemia with or without hypercarbia.
- *ECG:* Signs of right ventricular strain (right axis deviation, right bundle branch block) or precordial strain; sinus tachycardia.

See earlier discussion of diagnostics for PE (CTPA and V/Q scans).

Principles of Management for Pulmonary Emboli

The key to reducing morbidity and mortality from PE is primarily prevention and secondarily early diagnosis and treatment to prevent reembolization. Goals of care include the improvement of oxygenation and ventilation, improvement of cardiovascular function, prevention of reembolization, and prevention of additional pulmonary embolus. Some facilities have recently introduced a pulmonary embolism response team (PERT) to promote rapid interprofessional decision making in the early diagnosis and treatment of PE.

Improving Oxygenation and Ventilation

Oxygen therapy is usually effective in relieving hypoxemia associated with PE. When cardiopulmonary compromise is severe, the patient may need to be moved into the ICU for intubation and mechanical ventilation to achieve optimal oxygenation.

Improving Cardiovascular Function

Controversy exists as to the benefit of vasoactive drug administration (such as norepinephrine and/or inotropic agents) to improve myocardial perfusion of the right ventricle. In severe embolic events, where cardiac failure is profound, systemic thrombolytic agents are recommended. In patients with high bleeding risk or who have failed thrombolytic therapy, catheter-directed therapies may also be warranted.

Preventing Reembolization

Several strategies are employed to prevent the likelihood of future embolization and cardiopulmonary compromise:

1. Limiting activity to prevent dislodgement of additional clots.
2. Use of initial anticoagulation therapy with unfractionated heparin to maintain a partial thromboplastin time (PTT) 1.5 to 2.5 times the control when no contraindication exists. Patients will usually transition to subcutaneous unfractionated heparin, subcutaneous low-molecular-weight heparin, oral vitamin K antagonist, or a direct oral anticoagulant (Table 10-18).

TABLE 10-18. ANTICOAGULANT AND THROMBOLYTIC MEDICATIONS

Category	Examples	Route
Unfractionated heparin	Heparin	Subcutaneous and intravenous
Low-molecular-weight heparin	Enoxaparin	Subcutaneous
	Dalteparin	Subcutaneous
Vitamin K antagonist	Warfarin	Oral
Direct oral anticoagulants	Apixaban	Oral
	Rivaroxaban	Oral
	Dabigatran	Oral
Thrombolytic	Alteplase	Intravenous

3. Insertion of vena cava filters to prevent emboli from legs, pelvis, and inferior vena cava from migrating to pulmonary circulation if anticoagulation therapy is contraindicated. Filters are placed percutaneously in the inferior vena cava if warranted.

Preventing Venous Thromboembolism

1. An important recommendation for the prevention of venous thromboembolism (VTE) is awareness and access to a hospital prevention policy including risk assessment (Table 10-19). See the AACN Practice Alert on Prevention of VTE.
2. Assess the risk for VTE on admission to the unit and daily thereafter. Discussion also includes current VTE prevention intervention, risk for bleeding, and response to treatment.

ESSENTIAL CONTENT CASE

COPD Exacerbation

A patient with COPD has the following ABGs:
- pH 7.31
- Pao_2 63 mm Hg
- $Paco_2$ 86 mm Hg

He is awake but somewhat confused and is placed on BiPAP support (inspiratory positive airway pressure [IPAP] 16 cm H_2O, expiratory positive airway pressure [EPAP] 5 cm H_2O, Fio_2 0.40).

After 2 hours he is becoming increasingly difficult to arouse. His respiration rate (RR) is 22 breaths/min and labored, and his heart rate is 122 beats/min.

Case Question: What assessment criteria lead you to suspect this patient is not tolerating noninvasive mechanical ventilation and may need to be intubated?

Answer
1. The patient's level of consciousness is decreased, and he has labored respirations, and an elevated heart rate. An ABG should be obtained, as it is likely his $Paco_2$ is high and his pH is very low. His decrease in consciousness requires that he be intubated and ventilated while further assessment is accomplished or he will likely code.

**BiPAP is contraindicated in patients with decreased mental status and inability to protect the airway (see Chapter 5, Airway and Ventilatory Management).

TABLE 10-19. RISK FACTORS, ASSESSMENT, AND THROMBOPROPHYLAXIS FOR VTE

Risk Factors	Assessment of Risk and Thromboprophylaxis
• Active malignancy	**Low Risk**
• Acute rheumatic disease	Ambulatory patients without additional risk factors or expected length of stay < 2 days
• Acute or chronic lung disease	Minor surgery without additional risk factors (same day surgery or < 30 minutes)
• Age	*Thromboprophylaxis*
• Central venous catheter	Early and aggressive ambulation
• Congestive heart failure	**Moderate Risk**
• Dehydration	Most general, open gynecologic or urologic surgery
• Impaired mobility	Patients who are neither low risk or high risk
• Inflammatory bowel disease	Medical patients who are immobile
• Known thrombophilic state	*Thromboprophylaxis*
• Moderate to major surgery	Pharmacologic prophylaxis with low-molecular-weight heparin or unfractionated heparin
• Myeloproliferative disorders	**Moderate Risk plus Bleeding Risk**
• Myocardial infarction	*Thromboprophylaxis*
• Nephrotic syndrome	Mechanical thromboprophylaxis, consider switch to pharmacologic prophylaxis when bleeding risk decreases
• Obesity	**High Risk**
• Oral contraceptives and hormone replacement therapy	Post-surgical (hip/knee, abdominal/pelvic)
• Pregnancy or postpartum with immobility	Trauma (spinal cord/multiple major trauma)
• Prior history of VTE	Hypercoagulable
• Sickle cell disease	Immobilized or limited mobility
• Smoking	Critically ill and mechanically ventilated
• Trauma	*Thromboprophylaxis*
• Varicose veins or chronic stasis	Pharmacologic prophylaxis with low-molecular-weight heparin, unfractionated heparin, oral vitamin K antagonist
	High Risk plus bleeding Risk
	Thromboprophylaxis
	Mechanical thromboprophylaxis, consider switch to pharmacologic prophylaxis (low-molecular-weight heparin or unfractionated heparin) when bleeding risk decreases

Data from Guyatt GH, Akl EA, Crowther M, et al. Antithrombotic therapy and prevention of thrombosis. 9th ed. American College of Chest Physicians practice guideline. Chest. 2012;141:7S-47S.

3. If ordered, apply graduated compression stocking or intermittent pneumatic compression (IPCs) devices (Figure 10-20; Table 10-20) and maintain their use at all times except when removed for correct fitting or skin assessment.

4. Placement of prophylactic vena cava filters in high-risk patients who have a contraindication to anticoagulation.

5. Early fixation of long bone fractures to prevent fat emboli.

6. Early mobilization. As soon as hemodynamic stability is achieved, and there are no other contraindications to mobilization, activity level increases to chair sitting several times per day and short periods of ambulation.

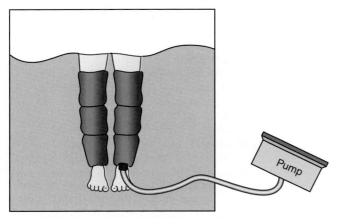

Figure 10-20. Intermittent pneumatic compression (IPC) device for prevention of DVT and PE.

TABLE 10-20. TIPS FOR SAFE AND EFFECTIVE USE OF INTERMITTENT PNEUMATIC COMPRESSION DEVICES

- Follow manufacturer recommendations for the correct fit, including patient measurement.
- Include ongoing assessment for fit as changes in weight and fluid shifts occur.
- Monitor that the devices are on the patient and in correct placement.
- Implement patient and family teaching regarding VTE and the role of mechanical prophylaxis COPD.
- Ensure that devices do not impede ambulation.

SELECTED BIBLIOGRAPHY

Critical Care Management of Respiratory Problems

Collins PF, Stratton RJ, Elia M. Nutritional support in chronic obstructive pulmonary disease: a systematic review and meta-analysis. *Am J Clin Nutr.* 2012;95:1385-1395.

Edward JA, Mandras S. An update on the management of chronic thromboembolic pulmonary hypertension. *Curr Probl Cardiol.* 2017;42:7-38.

Ferreira JL, Wipf JE. Pharmacologic therapies in anticoagulation. *Med Clin N Am.* 2016;100:695-718.

Halm MA. Relaxation: a self-care healing modality reduces harmful effects of anxiety. *Am J Crit Care.* 2009;18:169-172.

Jaber WA, Fong PP, Weisz G, et al. Acute pulmonary embolism: with an emphasis on an interventional approach. *J Am Coll Cardiol.* 2016;67:991-1002.

Kaufman JS. Acute exacerbation of COPD: diagnosis and management. *Nurs Practitioner.* 2017;42:1-7.

Klinger JR. Group III pulmonary hypertension, pulmonary hypertension associated with lung disease: epidemiology, pathophysiology, and treatments. *Cardiol Clin.* 2016;34:413-433.

Makic MB, Martin SA, Burns S, Philbrick D, Rauen C. Putting evidence into nursing practice: four traditional practices not supported by evidence. *Crit Care Nurse.* 2013;33:28-42.

Makic MBF, Rauen C, Jones K, Fisk AC. Continuing to challenge practice to be evidence based. *Crit Care Nurse.* 2015;35:39-50.

Matthay MA, Ware LB, Zimmerman GA. The acute respiratory distress syndrome. *J Clin Invest.* 2012;122:2731-2740.

McLean B. Acute respiratory failure and intensive measures. *Crit Care Nurs Clin North Am.* 2012;24:361-375.

Rauen CA, Makic MB, Bridges E. Evidence-based practice habits: transforming research into bedside practice. *Crit Care Nurse.* 2009;29:46-59.

Rigotti NA, Clair C, Munafo MR, Stead LF. Interventions for smoking cessation in hospitalized patients. *Cochrane Database Syst Rev.* 2015;5:CD001837.doi:10.1002/14651858.CDC001837.pub3.

Seckel M, Remel B. Evidence-based practice: percussion and vibration therap. *Crit Care Nurse.* 2017;37:82-83.

U.S. Department of Health and Human Services. The Health Consequences of Smoking – 50 Years of Progress: A Report of the Surgeon General. Atlanta, GA: U.S. Department of Health and Human Services, Centers for Disease Control and Prevention, National Center for Chronic Disease Prevention and Health Promotion, Office on Smoking and Health, 2014. https://www.surgeongeneral.gov/library/reports/50-years-of-progress/exec-summary.pdf. Accessed July 7, 2017.

The ARDS Definition Task Force. Acute respiratory distress syndrome; the Berlin definition. *JAMA.* 2012;307:2526-2533.

Weiner LM, Webb AK, Limbago B, et al. Antimicrobial-resistant pathogens associated with healthcare-associated infections: summary of data reported to the National Healthcare Safety Network at the Centers for Disease Control and Prevention. 2011-2014. *Infect Control Hosp Epidemiol.* 2016;37:1288-1301.

Witkin AS, Harshbarger S, Kabrhel C. Pulmonary embolism response teams. *Semin Thromb Hemost.* 2016;42:857-864.

Yokoe DS, Anderson DJ, Berenholtz SM, Calfee DP, Dubberke ER, Eilingson KD, Gerding DN et al. SHEA/IDSA PRACTICE RECOMMENDATION: EXECUTIVE SUMMARY. A Compendium of Strategies to Prevent Healthcare-Associated Infections in Acute Care Hospitals: 2014 Updates. Infect Control Hosp Epidemiol. 2014;35(8):967.

Chest X-Ray Interpretation

Connolly MA. Black, white, and shades of gray: common abnormalities in chest radiographs. *AACN Clin Issues.* 2001;12(2):259-269.

Corne J, Kumaran M. *Chest X-Ray Made Easy.* 4th ed. Edinburgh, SCT: Elsevier; 2016.

Eisenhuber E, Schaefer-Prokop CM, Prosch H, Schima W. Bedside chest radiography. *Resp Care.* 2012;57:427-443.

Godoy MC, Leitman BS, deGroot PM, Viahos J, Naidich DP. Chest radiography in the ICU: part 1; evaluation of airway, enteric, and pleural tubes. *Am J Roentgenol.* 2012;198:563-571.

Sanchez F. Fundamentals of chest x-ray interpretation. *Crit Care Nurse.* 1986;6:41-52.

Siela D. Advanced chest imaging interpretation of acute pulmonary disorders. *AACN Adv Crit Care.* 2014;25:365-374.

Evidence-Based Practice Resources

AACN Deep Vein Thrombosis Prevention Practice Alert. Aliso Viejo, CA: AACN; 2016. http://www/aacn.org. Accessed July 7, 2017.

AACN VAP Practice Alert. Aliso Viejo, CA: AACN; 2017. http://www.aacn.org. Accessed June 10, 2017.

American College of Chest Physician. Antithrombotic and thrombolytic therapy: American College of Chest Physicians evidence-based clinical practice guidelines. 2012 (9th ed). http://journal.publications.chestnet.org/issue.aspx?journalid=99&issueid=23443. Accessed July 11, 2017.

American Thoracic Society and the European Respiratory Society. International multidisciplinary consensus classification of the idiopathic interstitial pneumonias. *Am J Respir Crit Care Med.* 2002;165:277-304.

American Thoracic Society and the Infectious Diseases Society of America. Guidelines for the management of adults with hospital-acquired, ventilator-associated, and healthcare-associated pneumonia. *Am J Respir Crit Care Med.* 2005;171:388-416.

Centers for Disease Control and Prevention National Healthcare Safety Network. Ventilator-Associated Events. 2017. https://www.cdc.gov/nhsn/pdfs/pscmanual/10-vae_final.pdf. Accessed June 10, 2017.

Centers for Disease Control and Prevention. Guidelines for prevention of health-care-associated pneumonia, 2003: recommendations of CDC and the Healthcare Infection Control Practices Advisory Committee. *MMWR Recomm Rep.* 2004;53(No. RR-3):1-35.

Chung KF, Wenzel SE, Brozek JL, et al. International ERS/ATS guidelines on definition, evaluation and treatment of severe asthma. *Eur Respir J.* 2014;43:343-373.

Criner GJ, Bourbeau J, Diekemper RL, et al. Prevention of acute exacerbation of COPD: American College of Chest Physicians and Canadian Thoracic Society Guideline. *Chest.* 2015;147:883-893.

Dignani L, Toccaceli A, Lucertini C, Petrucci C, Lancia L. Sleep and quality of life in people with COPD: a descriptive-correlational study. *Clin Nurs Res.* 2016;25:432-447.

Fan E, Del Sorbo L, Goligher EW, et al. An official American Thoracic Society/European Society of Intensive Care Medicine/Society of Critical Care Medicine Clinical Practice Guideline: mechanical ventilation in adult patients with acute respiratory distress syndrome. *Am J Respir Crit Care.* 2017;195:1253-1263.

Frankel HL, Kirkpatrick AW, Elbarbary M. Guidelines for the appropriate use of bedside general and cardiac ultrasonography in the evaluation of critically ill patients-part I: general ultrasonography. *Crit Care Med.* 2015;43:2479-2502.

Global Initiative for Asthma. Global Strategy for Asthma Management and Prevention, 2017. Available from: www.ginathma.org.

Good VS, Kirkwood PL, eds. *Advanced Critical Care Nursing.* 2nd ed. St Louis, MO: Elsevier; 2018.

Kalil AC, Metersky ML, Klompas M, et al. Management of adults with hospital-acquired and ventilator-associated pneumonia: 2016 Clinical Practice Guideline by the Infectious Diseases Society of America and the American Thoracic Society. *Clin Infect Dis.* 2016;63:e61-e111.

Kearon C, Akl EA, Ornelas J, et al. Antithrombin therapy for VTE disease: CHEST Guideline and Expert Panel Report. *Chest.* 2016;149:315-352.

Mandell LA, Wunderink RG, Anzueto A, et al. Infectious Diseases Society of America/American Thoracic Society consensus guidelines on the management of community-acquired pneumonia in adults. *Clin Infect Dis.* 2007;44(suppl 2):S27-S72.

National Heart, Lung, and Blood Institute. Expert Panel Report 3: Guidelines for the Diagnosis and Management of Asthma, Full Report 2007. http://www.nhlbi.nih.gov/guidelines/asthma/asthgdln.pdf. Accessed July 10, 2017.

Parshall MB, Schwartzstein RM, Adams L, et al. An official America Thoracic Society statement: update on the mechanisms, assessment, and management of dyspnea. *Am J Respir Crit Care Med.* 2012;185:435-452.

Raghu G, Rochwerg B, Zhang Y, et al. An official ATS/ERS/JRS/ALAT clinical practice guideline: treatment of idiopathic pulmonary fibrosis. *Am J Respir Crit Care Med.* 2015;192:doi: 10.1164/rccm.201506-1063ST.

Taichman DB, Ornelas J, Chung L, et al. Pharmacologic therapy for pulmonary arterial hypertension in adults: CHEST Guideline and Expert Panel Report. *Chest.* 2014;146:449-475.

Taylor BE, McClave SA, Martindale RG, et al. Guidelines for the provision and assessment of nutrition support therapy in the adult critically ill patient. *Crit Care Med.* 2016;44:390-438.

The ARDS Definition Task Force. Acute respiratory distress syndrome: the Berlin definition. *JAMA.* 2012;307:2526-2533.

The Global Strategy for the Diagnosis, Management and Prevention of COPD. Global Initiative for Chronic Obstructive Lung Disease (GOLD) 2017. http://goldcopd.org. Accessed June 21, 2017.

US Preventive Services Taskforce (USPSTF). Screening for chronic obstructive pulmonary disease: US Preventative Services Task Force Recommendation Statement. *JAMA.* 2016;315:1372-1377.

Wedzicha JA, Miravittles M, Hurst JR, et al. Management of COPD exacerbations: a European Respiratory Society/American Thoracic Society Guideline. *Eur Respir J.* 2017;49:1600791. https://doi.org/10.1183/13993003.00791-2016.

Wiegand DL, ed. *AACN Procedure Manual for Critical Care.* 7th ed. St. Louis, MO: Elsevier Saunders; 2016.

MULTISYSTEM PROBLEMS

Julie Grishaw

11

KNOWLEDGE COMPETENCIES

1. Identify the relationship between the cellular mediators and clinical manifestations of sepsis and septic shock.

2. Describe the etiology, pathogenesis, clinical manifestations, patient needs, and principles of management of sepsis and septic shock.

3. Compare and contrast the pathogenesis, clinical manifestations, patient needs, and management

approaches for multisystem problems resulting from sepsis, septic shock, and overdoses.

4. Describe the symptoms and pharmacologic management of the patient experiencing alcohol withdrawal syndrome.

5. Describe treatment considerations for pressure injuries.

6. Identify factors related to the development of healthcare-associated infections (HAIs).

SEPSIS AND SEPTIC SHOCK

Sepsis is a serious global healthcare condition, affecting millions of patients annually. Older adults and those with underlying disease are disproportionally affected by sepsis. Despite advances in the treatment of infection, sepsis continues to be associated with high mortality rates, leading to death in 1 of every 4 patients affected and causing more than 30% of in-hospital deaths in the United States. However, early recognition and immediate treatment may reduce mortality rates significantly.

The basic elements of sepsis are infection, a dysregulated host response, and subsequent organ damage. A challenge in identifying patients with sepsis is that there is no single diagnostic test that indicates its presence. The diagnosis depends on analysis of an array of clinical data including abnormal vital signs, patient symptoms, physical examination findings, and laboratory values. Recognizing patients who are at risk for sepsis and closely monitoring their clinical status is essential to improving outcomes in the management of this disorder.

In 2016, the Third International Consensus Definitions for Sepsis and Septic Shock (Sepsis-3) defined sepsis as a dysregulated host response to an infection leading to life-threatening organ dysfunction. Septic shock, a subset of sepsis, occurs when patients with sepsis who have undergone fluid resuscitation remain hypotensive, require vasopressors, and have a serum lactate greater than 2 mmol/L. Hospital mortality from septic shock is over 40%.

Previous definitions of sepsis focused on the systemic inflammatory response syndrome (SIRS), which occurs in response to a clinical insult, such as an infection, inflammation, or injury. Research reviewed for the development of the Sepsis-3 definitions raised the concern that SIRS criteria are not specific for the dysregulated response that characterizes sepsis and septic shock. Data suggests that most patients with sepsis demonstrate SIRS criteria. However, use of SIRS to identify sepsis may result in the inclusion of patients who have an appropriate systemic inflammatory response to an infection or other insult and not a dysregulated response that extends beyond source control and leads to organ dysfunction.

Etiology, Risk Factors, and Pathogenesis

The infection that causes sepsis may be bacterial, viral, fungal, or on rare occasions, rickettsial or protozoal. Immune and inflammatory responses to infection occur as natural processes that are protective. Normally, an innate system of "checks and balances" controls these responses. In sepsis, through mechanisms that are not completely understood, the body produces a dysregulated, systemic response to an infection. This response may last even beyond achieving control over the pathogen. In some cases, microbes, such as bacteria and fungi, may exploit deficiencies in the innate host defenses. In others, the systemic response fails to destroy the organism that set it in motion. Unregulated, this response leads to life-threatening organ damage.

Figure 11-1 provides an overview of the events that comprise the dysregulated response in sepsis. While a full explanation of this response is beyond the scope of this text, it is important to understand the variety of immune mechanisms which, when unchecked, lead to organ damage. These include activation of polymorphonuclear cells (neutrophils), macrophages, platelets, and endothelial cells. These cells are either directly involved in the reaction, such as platelet aggregation which leads to microthrombi, or are stimulated to produce and release chemical mediators, such as cytokines or plasma enzymes that extend the dysregulated response.

Mediators can be divided into five groups: cytokines, plasma enzyme cascades, lipid mediators, toxic oxygen-derived metabolites, and unclassified mediators such as nitric oxide and proteases. These mediators are stimulated after cellular activation in response to an insult such as infection or trauma, and are intended to provide a protective response. Cytokines are active chemical substances secreted by cells in response to a stimulus. If secreted by lymphocytes, they are called *lymphokines,* and if secreted by monocytes or macrophages, they are called *monokines.* Examples of cytokines include tumor necrosis factor, interleukin, interferon, and colony-stimulating factors such as granulocyte colony-stimulating factor.

In addition to cytokines, there is also activation of enzymatic plasma cascades. Examples of these include the complement cascade and the coagulation cascades. Lipid mediators are also either stimulated or produced as part of a cellular destructive process. These lipid mediators include arachidonic acid metabolites, leukotrienes, prostaglandins, and platelet-activating factor. Oxygen-derived free radicals such as hydrogen peroxide and hydroxyl radical are another group of mediators in the inflammatory response. Nitric oxide and proteases are not grouped into any of the previous categories, but are also mediators of the immune and inflammatory response.

Hormonal regulation also plays a role in the inflammatory and immune response. The hormonal response is characterized by the release of stress hormones (catecholamines, glucagon, cortisol, and growth hormone), suppression of thyroid hormone, and hormonal regulation of fluid and electrolyte balance. Toll-like receptors, or transmembrane proteins that are expressed on some immune cells, such as neutrophils and macrophages, have been implicated in ischemia-reperfusion injury that can further alter perfusion and contribute to inflammation.

Research shows that the Sequential (Sepsis-related) Organ Failure Assessment Score (SOFA) and the quick SOFA (qSOFA) can be effective tools for predicting mortality in some patients with sepsis and septic shock (Tables 11-1 and 11-2). The SOFA score includes laboratory data and is a more comprehensive assessment than the qSOFA, which is

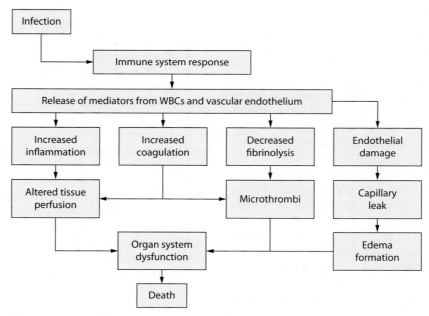

Figure 11-1. Interactive cascade of inflammation and coagulation leading to endothelium damage, diffuse thrombi, and organ system dysfunction. (*Reproduced with permission from Kleinpell R. New initiatives focus on prevention and early recognition of sepsis. Nurs Spectrum. 2004;17[12]:24-26.*)

TABLE 11-1. SEQUENTIAL (SEPSIS RELATED) ORGAN FAILURE SCORE

System	Score 0	1	2	3	4
Respiration					
Pao$_2$/Fio$_2$, mm Hg (kPa)	≥ 400 (53.3)	< 400 (53.3)	< 300 (40)	< 200 (6.7) with respiratory support	< 100 (13.3) with respiratory support
Coagulation					
Platelets, × 10^3/μL	≥ 150	< 150	< 100	< 50	< 20
Liver					
Bilirubin, mg/dL (μmol/L)	< 1.2 (20)	1.2-1.9 (20-32)	2.0-5.9 (33-101)	6.0-11.9 (102-204)	> 12.0 (204)
Cardiovascular	MAP ≥ 70 mm Hg	MAP < 70 mm Hg	Dopamine < 5 or dobutamine (any dose)[b]	Dopamine 5.1-15 or epinephrine ≤ 0.1 or norepinephrine ≤ 0.1[b]	Dopamine > 15 or epinephrine > 0.1 or norepinephrine > 0.1[a]
Central nervous system					
Glasgow Coma Scale score[b]	15	13-14	10-12	6-9	< 6
Renal					
Creatinine, mg/dL (μmol/L)	< 1.2 (110)	1.2-1.9 (110-170)	2.0-3.4 (171-299)	3.5-4.9 (300-440)	> 5.0 (440)
Urine output, mL/day				< 500	< 200

Abbreviations: Fio$_2$, fraction of inspired oxygen; MAP, mean arterial pressure; Pao$_2$, partial pressure of oxygen.

[a]Catecholamine doses are given as mcg/kg/min for at least 1 hour.

[b]Glasgow Coma scale scores range from 3 to 15; higher score indicates better neurological function.

Reproduced with permission from Vincent JL, Moreno R, Takala J, et al: The SOFA (Sepsis-related Organ Failure Assessment) score to describe organ dysfunction/failure. On behalf of the Working Group on Sepsis-Related Problems of the European Society of Intensive Care Medicine, Intensive Care Med 1996 Jul;22(7):707-710.

determined by blood pressure, respiratory rate, and mental status. Monitoring for changes in the SOFA and qSOFA scores can identify evolving organ dysfunction and mortality risk.

Risk factors for the development of sepsis include malnutrition, immunosuppression, comorbidities, and prolonged antibiotic use. The presence of invasive devices including central lines, urinary catheters, and endotracheal tubes also increase the risk for sepsis. Age is an important risk factor, as sepsis disproportionately affects the very young and the very old. A large number of infections leading to sepsis are acquired during hospitalization and may be avoided with infection prevention tactics. Hand hygiene remains the single most effective method for preventing the spread of infection. Other measures such as meticulous mouth care to prevent ventilator-associated pneumonia, prompt removal of urinary catheters, and aseptic technique when handling central lines can help prevent sepsis in hospitalized patients. Table 11-3 summarizes the nursing interventions to prevent, recognize, and ensure prompt treatment of sepsis.

Clinical Presentation

Early recognition and treatment of sepsis and septic shock are extremely important. When the nurse assessing a patient notes a change in their status that indicates infection and the

TABLE 11-2. qSOFA (QUICK SOFA) CRITERIA

Respiratory rate ≥ 22 breaths/min
Altered mentation
Systolic blood pressure ≤100 mm Hg

Data from Klein DM, Witek-Janusek L. Advances in immunotherapy of sepsis. Dimens Crit Care Nurs. 1992;11(2):75-81 and Singer M, Deutschman CS, Seymour CW, et al. The Third International Consensus Definitions for Sepsis and Septic Shock (Sepsis-3). JAMA. 2016;315(8):801-810.

onset of sepsis, further assessment and collaboration with a provider are urgent priorities. Fever and leukocytosis are classic indications of infection, but other symptoms such as altered mental state, a change in wound drainage, or a new complaint of pain may also indicate an infectious complication. The clinical manifestations of sepsis result from altered perfusion to vital organ systems, a by-product of mediator over-activation. Clinical signs of organ system dysfunction include alterations in the cardiovascular system (hypotension, tachycardia, dysrhythmias), the respiratory system (tachypnea, hypoxemia), renal function (oliguria, elevated creatinine), liver function (elevated transaminitis, jaundice, coagulopathies), the hematologic system (thrombocytopenia), the gastrointestinal system (change in bowel sounds, ileus), and cognitive function (confusion, agitation).

The prognosis of sepsis depends on the number of organ systems affected and the severity of their dysfunction. The 2016 Sepsis guidelines recommend the use of the SOFA score to predict patient outcomes from sepsis. A change of more than or equal to 2 points on the individual's baseline SOFA score is associated with organ dysfunction due to the dysregulated response of sepsis (see Table 11-1). The quick SOFA or qSOFA was designed as a quick screening tool to identify patients at risk of dying due to sepsis. It is a much shorter, modified version of the SOFA. It has three variables, respiratory rate, mentation, and systolic blood pressure (see Table 11-2). The qSOFA is considered positive if patients meet at least two of the criteria.

Diagnostic Tests

There is no single biomarker that confirms a diagnosis of sepsis. Nurses and providers caring for patients at risk for

TABLE 11-3. NURSING CARE OF PATIENTS WITH SEPSIS AND SEPTIC SHOCK

Recognize those at risk	Identify patients at risk for developing sepsis • Older adults • Immunocompromised patients • Patients undergoing surgical/invasive procedures • Patients with indwelling catheters • Mechanically ventilated patients
Monitor for sepsis	Signs of infection including • Fever or hypothermia, tachycardia, hypotension, tachypnea • Altered mental state • New compliant of pain • Adventitious breath sounds, increased oxygen requirement, new infiltrate on radiograph • Change in appearance of urine, pyuria, bacteria on urine culture • Change in wound appearance or drainage • Leukocytosis, thrombocytopenia on complete blood count (CBC) • Elevated blood glucose Signs of impaired organ perfusion • Hypotension, tachycardia, tachypnea • Elevated serum lactate • Skin mottling • Change in capillary refill • Change in renal function: drop in urine output, elevated creatinine and blood urea nitrogen (BUN) • Change in liver function: elevated transaminases • Change in clotting: bruising, bleeding, elevated international normalized ratio (INR)
Collaborate with the healthcare team to initiate immediate resuscitation	• Circulatory support with fluids and vasopressors • Empiric antibiotics • Source control • Monitor and report patient response to treatment
Provide supportive care to patients with sepsis	• Frequent monitoring of hemodynamic status to determine patient response to treatment • Use supplemental oxygen or lung protective mechanical ventilation as indicated • Apply interventions in the ABCDEF bundle to prevent delirium • Provide enteral nutrition to prevent malnutrition and lower the risk of bacterial translocation • Give ulcer prophylaxis if risk factors for GI bleeding exist • Administer pharmacologic or mechanical interventions to prevent venous thromboembolism (VTE)
Patient/family-centered care	• Promote patient comfort, assess and treat pain, use a validated scale to guide the use of sedation • Assess patient/family understanding of diagnosis and prognosis • Participate in discussions of goals of care with the healthcare team and with the patient/family

Sepsis prevention	• Hand hygiene
	• Specific measures to prevent hospital-acquired infections include:
	  • Remove urinary catheters and central lines when no longer indicated
	  • Use aseptic technique when handling lines and catheters
	  • Facilitate weaning from mechanical ventilation through the use of spontaneous breathing trials, appropriate use of sedation, and early mobility as described in Chapter 5, Airway and Ventilatory Management
	  • Adhere to transmission based precautions including the use of standard, contact, droplet, and airborne precautions as appropriate
	• Educate members of the healthcare team on prevention and recognition of sepsis

sepsis plan their care to include frequent assessment with the aim of early recognition and prompt treatment. This assessment includes attention to common sources of infection with inspection of incisions and line insertion sites, and auscultation of the chest. Screening tools that identify signs of sepsis may also be of benefit in the early recognition of this disorder.

Diagnostic and laboratory abnormalities that may occur in sepsis include:

• *Complete blood cell count:* In response to infection, the white blood cell count may rise to greater than 12,000 cells/mm^3, or fall below 4000 cells/mm^3. A rise in the percent of bands, white blood cells released from

the marrow before reaching maturity, to greater than 10%, indicates acute infection. The over-activation of platelets induced by the dysregulated response of sepsis can also lead to thrombocytopenia.

• *Serum lactate:* Tissues that are poorly perfused resort to anaerobic metabolism and produce lactate. Thus, a rise in serum lactate indicates poor perfusion. Patients with a serum lactate over 4 mmol/L and evidence of infection should undergo urgent treatment for sepsis, though patients with lower levels may also have the condition. A lactate more than 2 mmol/L after fluid resuscitation indicates septic shock.

• *Other signs of organ hypoperfusion include:* Elevated serum creatinine and transaminitis.

ESSENTIAL CONTENT CASE

Sepsis

A 67-year-old man with a 6-year history of hypertension and a 30-pack-year smoking history was admitted to the progressive care unit with a diagnosis of cirrhosis secondary to biliary obstruction. He underwent an exploratory laparotomy and cholecystectomy 3 days ago. He experienced an episode of hypotension 12 hours postoperatively, which resolved with IV crystalloid administration. He is on 6L of oxygen via nasal cannula and attempts to decrease this level have been unsuccessful.

   He currently has an arterial line, central venous catheter (CVC), T-tube drain, and an indwelling urinary catheter. He is alert and oriented, moving in bed with little assistance. Physical examination reveals that his skin is pale, but warm, pulmonary auscultation is notable for bibasilar crackles, and cardiovascular examination is positive for 1+ pedal edema bilaterally. His abdomen is soft, non-tender, nondistended, with hypoactive bowel sounds. His 5-inch midline abdominal wound requires dressing changes 3 times daily and is approximated with retention sutures. Current vital signs are:

T	38.6°C (101.0°F) core
HR	122 beats/min (Sinus tachycardia)
RR	34 breaths/min
BP	82/54 mm Hg (mean arterial pressure [MAP] 63)

Current laboratory results are:

ABG:	pH 7.30, Pao$_2$ 62, Paco$_2$ 46, HCO$_3$ 18, Sao$_2$ 94%
WBC:	22,000 (65% neutrophils, 50 segs, 12 bands)
Hemoglobin/Hematocrit:	Hct 39, Hgb 13
Platelets:	40,000 (Baseline 300,000)
BMP:	Na$^+$ 140, K$^+$ 3.5, Cl 100, CO$_2$ 20, BUN 22, Creat 1.3 (Baseline Cr 0.9)

Case Question 1: What are this patient's risk factors for sepsis?

Case Question 2: What clinical manifestations may be suggestive of sepsis?

Case Question 3: Is his qSOFA positive?

Answers

1. Postoperative status, history of tobacco abuse, invasive lines and catheters, and an abdominal wound requiring dressing changes are risk factors for sepsis in this patient.
2. Elevated temperature, leukocytosis with bandemia, sinus tachycardia, tachypnea, hypotension, thrombocytopenia, elevated creatinine, and a suspected source of infection are clinical findings consistent with sepsis.
3. Yes, he demonstrates a respiratory rate more than 22 breaths/min and a systolic blood pressure less than or equal to 100 mm Hg. (See Table 11-2 for qSOFA scoring.)

- *Chest x-ray:* May be normal or show signs of infiltrates.
- *Urinalysis:* May show pyuria and the presence of bacteria.
- *Culture and sensitivity:* Cultures of blood, urine, sputum, wound drainage, or other potential sources of infection may confirm the presence of bacteria or other pathogens.
- *CT scan, MRI, ultrasound:* May be negative or show abscess. Examples of abnormalities that may be detected include: appendicitis, diverticulitis, bowel ischemia, pancreatitis, cholecystitis.

Principles of Management of Sepsis and Septic Shock

Because sepsis is life threatening and prompt treatment impacts outcomes, the priority interventions are grouped and administered in a specific time interval. These groups of interventions are labeled "Sepsis Bundles" and can reduce the complexity and increase the rapidity of the healthcare team's response to sepsis. The Surviving Sepsis Campaign (SSC) revised the Sepsis Bundles in 2015 and further revisions are expected based on the 2016 Sepsis guidelines. The website, survivingsepsis.org, maintains a list of the most up to date information. The information below is based on evidence available at the time this text was written; however, research on sepsis management is ongoing and recommendations can change.

In general, the treatment of a patient with sepsis, or septic shock, consists of treating the underlying cause, providing fluid resuscitation, supporting dysfunctional organ systems, and applying best practices according to current evidence.

Treating the Underlying Cause

The management plan begins with source control and administration of empiric, broad-spectrum antimicrobial therapy within the first 1 hour of symptom recognition. Identifying the source of infection is paramount, as therapy will not be successful without source control. Ideally, at least two sets of blood cultures are obtained prior to administering antibiotics but a delay in culture collection should not delay treatment. Interventions beyond antibiotic therapy such as drainage of an abscess or the removal of an infected line, indwelling bladder catheter, vascular graft, or orthopedic device may be required. It is important to note that antibiotic administration must not be delayed. Even if the source of infection is not identified, antimicrobial agents should still be administered within the first hour of symptom recognition. Once the source is identified and culture results are available, antimicrobial therapy can be changed to provide more specific coverage.

Fluid Resuscitation

The 2016 SSC guidelines recommend that patients with hypotension attributed to sepsis receive a fluid bolus of

30 mL/kg of crystalloid within 3 hours of symptom recognition. Administration of fluids increases intravascular volume thereby improving organ perfusion and reducing the risk of dysfunction. The goal of initial resuscitation is to reach a mean arterial pressure (MAP) of 65 mm Hg and to achieve a normal lactate level.

While fluid resuscitation within 3 hours of onset is recommended for all patients with potential sepsis, additional consideration is warranted in patients with acute respiratory distress syndrome, heart failure, or chronic kidney disease who may develop pulmonary edema as a result of fluid administration. Patients with these comorbidities require close monitoring when given a fluid bolus. Patients who are already on high flow oxygen may require intubation and mechanical ventilation prior to fluid resuscitation. Following the initial bolus, further decisions about volume administration are based on hemodynamic assessment of the patient. The SSC guidelines emphasize that dynamic measures of a patient's hemodynamic status are preferred over static measurements. Table 11-4 provides a list of static and dynamic hemodynamic measures that are used to determine if a patient with sepsis will benefit from additional infusion of fluids. See Chapter 4 (Hemodynamic Monitoring) for a further discussion of hemodynamic monitoring.

Supporting Dysfunctional Organ Systems

While research is ongoing, there is currently no therapy available to prevent the dysregulated host response in sepsis and septic shock. Immediate administration of antibiotics and removal of the source of infection may reduce the impact and duration of this response, but once set in motion, it may continue even after source control is achieved. For this reason, interventions aimed at supporting the affected organs are essential in the management of sepsis and septic shock.

Cardiovascular Dysfunction

The impact of the dysregulated immune response on the cardiovascular system includes systemic vasodilation, increased capillary bed permeability, and microthrombi. This combination of effects can lead to peripheral edema in the setting of low intravascular volume, and poor perfusion despite a normal or elevated cardiac output. For this reason, hypotension that persists in patients who are no long responsive to fluid resuscitation is treated with intravenous vasopressors. Norepinephrine is the vasopressor of choice for sepsis and

septic shock, according to the 2016 SSC guidelines. If the goal MAP of 65 mm Hg cannot be achieved with norepinephrine, vasopressin and epinephrine can also be used.

Because vasopressors cause vasoconstriction, high doses of vasopressors in the quest to restore MAP may result in microvascular debt, impaired oxygenation and perpetuation of lactic acidosis. Patients on vasopressors require close monitoring to ensure that the minimum dose to achieve the desired effect is used. Continuous monitoring for cardiac dysrhythmias, which may occur due to sepsis or due to the use of vasopressors, and frequent assessment of perfusion including blood pressure, inspection for skin mottling, and capillary refill are also essential elements of nursing care. Passive leg raise and pulse pressure variation are noninvasive strategies for determining if further fluid resuscitation is warranted.

Pulmonary Dysfunction

The systemic inflammation of sepsis leads to pulmonary vascular leak and microthrombi, which can lodge in the small vessels of the pulmonary system. As a result, many patients with sepsis and septic shock develop acute respiratory distress syndrome (ARDS). These patients often require intubation and mechanical ventilation. The SSC guidelines support the use of low-tidal volume ventilation and positive end-expiratory pressure (PEEP) to minimize the risk of lung injury that can occur with high volumes and high Fio_2. Prone positioning may also be appropriate in septic patients with ARDS. Further discussion of the management of ARDS can be found in Chapter 10 (Respiratory System) of this book.

Because sepsis increases the demand for oxygen while ARDS reduces the supply, strategies to minimize oxygen consumption are key aspects of the nursing care. These include:

1. Controlling heart rate, respiratory rate, and temperature
2. Alleviating pain
3. Preventing shivering
4. Providing comfort measures
5. Consolidating activities
6. Placing the patient on mechanical ventilation if clinically indicated
7. Administering sedation guided by a standardized sedation assessment tool

Renal Dysfunction

Renal dysfunction is a common sequela of sepsis and septic shock. Monitoring of renal function through evaluation of creatinine and electrolytes, adjusting antibiotic doses according to renal function, and measuring urine output are all interventions to protect septic patients from kidney injury. In some situations, renal replacement therapy is required, however, the SSC guidelines suggest careful consideration in implementing this intervention based on the associated poor patient outcomes. A full discussion of renal dysfunction can be found in Chapter 15 (Renal System) of this book.

TABLE 11-4. DYNAMIC AND STATIC HEMODYNAMIC MEASUREMENTS

Dynamic Measurements	Static Measurements
Pulse pressure variation	CVP
Systolic pulse variation	PAOP
Pleth variability index	Global end diastolic volume
Stroke volume variation—via passive leg raise	Left ventricular end diastolic volume
Inferior vena cava—visualized on ultrasound	

TABLE 11-5. SUMMARY OF RECOMMENDATIONS FROM THE 2016 SURVIVING SEPSIS CAMPAIGN GUIDELINES FOR THE MANAGEMENT OF SEPSIS AND SEPTIC SHOCK

Resuscitation	Sepsis and septic shock are medical emergencies and resuscitation should begin immediately Give antibiotics within the first hour Identify and if possible, remove the source of infection as soon as logistically possible Administer a 30 mL/kg bolus of crystalloid fluid within 3 hours Administration of additional fluids is guided by frequent assessment of the patient's volume status
Goals of Resuscitation	Achieve a MAP ≥ 65 mm Hg, and normalize lactate
Use of vasopressors	Administer vasopressors, initially norepinephrine when appropriate fluid challenge fails to restore adequate blood pressure and organ perfusion If the goal MAP ≥ 65 mm Hg is not achieved with norepinephrine, administer vasopressin and then epinephrine Re-assess volume status frequently to guide further administration of fluids
Diagnosis	Obtain cultures: At least two blood cultures with one drawn percutaneously and one drawn through each vascular access device; obtain cultures of other sites such as urine, wounds, and respiratory secretions before initiating antibiotic therapy, if possible. However, antibiotic therapy should not be delayed
Antibiotic therapy	Give empirical antibiotics within 1 hour of symptom recognition, to cover the most likely pathogens Narrow antibiotic therapy when the source of infection is identified and sensitivities are available Give antibiotics for 7-10 days Assess for de-escalation of antibiotic therapy daily
Source control	Remove a potentially infected device, drain any abscess, debride infected necrotic tissue as soon as possible
Steroids	Administer steroids only to patients with septic shock who continue to be hemodynamically unstable after resuscitation and while on vasopressors
Blood product administration	Transfuse patients with a hemoglobin less than 7.0 Avoid over-transfusion
Mechanical ventilation	Provide high PEEP and low-tidal volumes to patients with sepsis-induced acute respiratory distress syndrome (ARDS) Place patients in prone position to manage persistent hypoxia due to sepsis induced ARDS (Pao_2/ Fio_2 <150) Do not use beta agonists in patients without evidence of bronchospasm and avoid use of high frequency oscillator ventilator in patients with sepsis induced ARDS
Glucose control	Apply a protocol to address hyperglycemia in patients who have two consecutive blood glucose values > 180 mg/dL Administer insulin with a goal of maintaining blood glucose < 180 mg/dL
Renal replacement	Avoid the use of renal replacement therapy for sepsis-induced acute kidney injury unless specific indications for dialysis other than oliguria and high creatinine occur (for instance, hyperkalemia, severe metabolic acidosis)
Nutrition	Avoid the use of parenteral nutrition Provide early enteral feeding and advance as tolerated
Setting goals of care	Discuss goals of care, prognosis for achieving those goals and level of certainty for the prognosis with patients and families, incorporating palliative care principles and as appropriate, end-of-life care planning as early as feasible, but no later than within 72 hours of ICU admission

Data from Dellinger RP, Schorr CA, Levy MM: A users' guide to the 2016 Surviving Sepsis Guidelines, Intensive Care Med 2017 Mar;43(3):299-303.

Best Practices Based on Current Evidence

In addition to antibiotic administration, source control, fluid resuscitation, and managing organ dysfunction, the SSC guidelines also offer additional recommendations for the care of patients with sepsis. These include managing blood glucose, judicious use of blood products, provision of enteral nutrition, and establishing goals of care with patients and families. Table 11-5 summarizes the recommendations of the 2016 SSC guidelines.

Managing Blood Glucose

Control of glucose, maintaining a blood glucose less than 180 mg/dL and more than 90 mg/dL, can improve outcomes in some acutely ill populations. The use of intravenous insulin to maintain glycemic control requires frequent monitoring of blood glucose (initially every 1-2 hours), and is a nurse-driven intervention.

Transfusions

Sufficient hemoglobin is necessary to ensure adequate oxygen-carrying capacity. The 2016 SSC guidelines suggest maintaining hemoglobin more than or equal to 7 g/dL. Higher hemoglobin goals requiring more frequent transfusion have been associated with increased morbidity and mortality in this patient population. Special exceptions may be needed for patients with significant comorbid conditions, such as an active or recent myocardial infarction.

Providing Nutritional Support

Enteral nutritional support is the gold standard and preferred route of specialized nutrition support (SNS) delivery unless contraindicated. General guidelines for nutritional support include 25 to 35 kcal/kg/day for total caloric intake and 1.5 to 2.0 g protein/kg/day. Enteral nutrition is preferred to parenteral nutrition whenever possible. It is helpful to have a nutrition specialist assist with nutritional planning. Refer to Chapter 14, Gastrointestinal System, for more on nutrition.

Providing Psychosocial Support

Chapter 1, Assessment of Progressive Care Patients and their Families, and Chapter 2, Planning Care for Progressive Care

Patients and their Families, discuss many aspects of psychosocial support. Especially important is the timely approach to goals of care discussions. The 2016 SSC guidelines recommend that a family conference to establish goals of care, and discuss prognosis be incorporated into the care of patients with sepsis and septic shock within 72 hours of admission. The use of palliative care communication skills facilitates the effectiveness of these conversations.

OVERDOSES

Drug or alcohol overdoses, as well as poisonings, can result in significant morbidity and mortality. Overdoses can be deliberate or accidental. Accidental overdose may involve one or multiple substances, and can be acute (eg, inaccurate dosing of pediatric medications) or chronic (ie, inadvertent, unnecessary dosing of asthma medications or over-the-counter medications). Data from the Centers for Disease Control and Prevention (CDC) indicates that prescription abuse is the fastest growing drug problem in the United States, with drug overdoses from opioid misuse among the highest. The level of intoxication or overdose varies with the element and amount ingested, the time until the patient is treated, the patient's age, tolerance to medications, and underlying comorbid conditions. The priority of care, as in all emergency situations, is maintenance of the patient's airway, breathing, and circulation.

Etiology, Risk Factors, and Pathophysiology
Alcohol Poisoning
Alcohol poisoning is most often seen in alcoholics, in young persons who have not yet reached legal drinking age, or in combination with other drugs as a suicide attempt. There are four types of alcohol intoxication:

1. Ethanol (ethyl or grain alcohol)
2. Methanol (wood alcohol)
3. Ethylene glycol (antifreeze)
4. Isopropyl alcohol (rubbing alcohol, solvent, and de-icer)

Alcohol dissolves readily in the lipid components of the plasma membranes of the body, and thus crosses the blood-brain barriers quickly, rapidly affecting the central nervous system. The mechanism of alcohol poisoning and withdrawal is complex. Most of the clinical effects can be explained by the interaction with neurotransmitters and neuroreceptors in the brain. In ethanol intoxication, serum levels range from 200 mg/dL (mild intoxication) to more than 500 mg/dL (coma). A serum alcohol level of 80 mg/dL is the legal upper limit for driving a car in most of the United States. In the case of methanol intoxication, serum levels range from 50 mg/dL (mild intoxication) to 100 mg/dL (severe intoxication).

While all four types of alcohol intoxication can cause metabolic acidosis with an elevated osmolal gap, only methanol and ethylene cause high anion gap acidosis. Metabolic acidosis manifests as a decreased serum bicarbonate level, and indicates that the generation of hydrogen ions exceeds the ability of the kidney to excrete them. The excess of systemic hydrogen ions leads to compensatory hyperventilation, as the body attempts to make the pH more alkaline. Refer to Chapter 5, Airway and Ventilatory Management, for further information on acid-base imbalance.

There are also differences in the way that the different types of alcohol intoxication affect patients. For instance, the metabolites generated by methanol intoxication are formaldehyde and formic acid, which cause optic nerve and central nervous system damage. Isopropyl alcohol intoxication is distinguished from other types of alcohol intoxication by the presence of ketoacids in both the urine and the serum. This usually leads to metabolic acidosis but sometimes due to rapid excretion of acetone, acidosis does not occur. Isopropyl alcohol is so rapidly absorbed that ingestion of as little as 150 mL can be fatal. The parent compound, rather than the metabolites, causes the toxicity.

Clinical Presentation
Excess ingestion of any type of alcohol may cause central nervous system symptoms such as sluggish reflexes, emotional instability, or erratic behavior. Amnesia may result for events that occurred during the period of intoxication. Unconsciousness often occurs before a person can drink enough for fatal consequences to occur; however, in some cases, the rapid consumption of alcohol leads to death from respiratory depression or aspiration during vomiting. It is estimated that there are 1.2 million hospital admissions annually for problems related to alcohol abuse with up to 5% of these patients developing severe withdrawal symptoms that require medical treatment. Over 2000 deaths each year are a result of alcohol toxicity. Signs and symptoms that are specific to each type of alcohol ingested include:

- *Acute ethanol intoxication:* Muscular incoordination, slurred speech, stupor, hypoglycemia, flushing, seizures, coma, depressed respirations, and hyporeflexia
- *Methanol intoxication:* Neurologic depression, metabolic acidosis, and visual disturbances
- *Ethylene glycol intoxication:* Neurologic depression, cardiopulmonary complications, pulmonary edema, and renal tubular degeneration
- *Isopropyl intoxication:* Neurologic depression, areflexia, respiratory depression, hypothermia, hypotension, and gastrointestinal distress

Diagnostic Tests
Excluding other potential causes of symptoms, such as hypo- or hyperglycemia, which may mimic overdose or intoxication, is an important component of the initial assessment. Because alcohol ingestion interferes with glucose production, alcohol-induced hypoglycemia in the intoxicated patient is common.

In addition to obtaining diagnostic tests, it is extremely important to obtain a history either from the patient, family member, friend, or the person who found the patient to assist with determination of the ingested substance. Diagnostic studies may aid in determining the ingested agent and determining the appropriate management. These include:

- *Ethanol and methanol serum levels:* These are elevated if these substances were ingested. Isopropyl serum levels are not performed as commonly as ethanol and methanol levels.
- *Urinalysis:* Oxalate crystals may be present in ethylene glycol intoxication and ketones may be evident in isopropyl alcohol ingestion.
- *Serum creatinine and blood urea nitrogen (BUN) levels:* These may be elevated due to renal dysfunction. These are not sensitive or specific for overdose.
- *Transaminases:* The hepatotoxic effects of certain types of alcohol may result in transaminitis. Ammonia level may also be checked if transaminases are elevated.
- *Serum glucose and electrolytes:* Patients with alcohol intoxication may develop hypoglycemia, electrolyte derangement, and metabolic acidosis as previously described. .
- *Urine drug screen:* Patients who ingest alcohol may have also ingested other substances so concurrent intoxication may contribute to the clinical presentation.
- *Serum acetaminophen and salicylate levels:* In the event that a patient with alcohol intoxication also ingests acetaminophen and salicylate, specific treatment can mitigate the toxic effects of these agents. Checking serum levels ensures prompt and appropriate management.

Treatment

The use of ethanol, or preferably fomepizole, for alcohol dehydrogenase (ADH) inhibition is a mainstay in the management of toxicity due to ingestion of methanol and ethylene glycol. Ethanol can be administered orally or intravenously to maintain a blood concentration of 100 to 150 mg/dL to prevent metabolism of alcohols to toxic metabolites. Fomepizole is much preferred as it offers a predictable decline in the ethyl glycol levels without the sedating side effects associated with ethanol. Hemodialysis is sometimes necessary to remove alcohol and toxic metabolites and is continued until metabolic acidosis resolves. Folinic acid (leucovorin) in a dose of 1 mg/kg up to 50 mg every 4 to 6 hours for 24 hours is suggested in methanol poisoning to provide the cofactor for formic acid elimination.

Isopropyl alcohol does not have a reversal agent. Toxicity caused by isopropyl alcohol is treated with supportive measures. These patients may require mechanical ventilation, intravenous fluids, and in some cases, dialysis.

TABLE 11-6. SYMPTOMS OF ALCOHOL WITHDRAWAL SYNDROME

Symptoms	Time of Appearance After Cessation Alcohol Use
Minor withdrawal symptoms: insomnia, tremulousness, mild anxiety, gastrointestinal upset, headache, diaphoresis, palpitations, anorexia	6-12 hours
Alcoholic hallucinosis: visual, auditory, or tactile hallucinations	12-24 hours[a]
Withdrawal seizures: generalized tonic-clonic seizures	24-48 hours[b]
Alcohol withdrawal delirium (delirium tremens): hallucinations (predominately visual), disorientation, tachycardia, hypertension, low-grade fever, agitation, diaphoresis	48-72 hours[c]

[a]Symptoms generally resolve within 48 hours.
[b]Symptoms reported as early as 2 hours after cessation.
[c]Symptoms peak at 5 days.
Data from Bayard M, Mcintyre J, Hill KR, et al: Alcohol withdrawal syndrome, Am Fam Physician 2004 Mar 15;69(6):1443-1450.

Alcohol Withdrawal Syndrome

Patients who experience alcohol abuse or dependence may be admitted to the hospital for management of withdrawal symptoms or they may be admitted for a different reason and develop withdrawal symptoms. Symptoms of alcohol withdrawal vary from mild anxiety to hallucinations and seizures which can be life threatening (Table 11-6). The time frame in which withdrawal symptoms emerge also varies and is influenced by the quantity and frequency of baseline alcohol consumption, comorbid conditions, older age, and concurrent liver disease. Obtain a complete history from the patient and/or family to determine the amount and frequency of alcohol ingestion. The time that alcohol was last ingested is also important to document, as this will assist in determining the most likely time frame of withdrawal symptoms. Measuring symptom severity with an alcohol withdrawal symptom assessment tool at regular intervals facilitates proactive treatment in those experiencing or at risk for withdrawal (see Figure 11-2).

Most treatment regimens include the use of fluid, electrolyte, and nutrition replacement. Administration of thiamine can prevent or treat Wernicke encephalopathy, a type of encephalopathy caused by depletion of thiamine stores which is commonly seen in patients with alcoholism or those who are severely malnourished. Multivitamins, folate, and magnesium replacement are also common elements of the treatment regimen. Benzodiazepines are given in scheduled doses or on an as needed basis to manage the symptoms of withdrawal. Intermediate-acting benzodiazepines such as lorazepam are commonly preferred in acute care settings. All benzodiazepines appear equally effective in the treatment of alcohol withdrawal syndrome. In moderate-to-severe withdrawal, long-acting agents such as diazepam are preferred over short-acting ones such as midazolam. Adjunctive medications may also be used in some cases to treat agitation (ie, haloperidol: caution, as it lowers seizure threshold and may

Clinical Institute Withdrawal Assessment of Alcohol Scale, Revised (CIWA-Ar)

Patient: _____ Date: _____ Time: _____ (24 hour clock, midnight = 00:00)

Pulse or heart rate, taken for one minute: _____ Blood pressure: _____

NAUSEA AND VOMITNG – Ask "Do you feel sick to your stomach? Have you vomited?" Observation.
0 no nausea and no vomiting
1 mild nausea with no vomiting
2
3
4 intermittent nausea with dry heaves
5
6
7 constant nausea, frequent dry heaves and vomiting

TACTILE DISTURBANCES – Ask "Have you any itching, pins and needles sensations, any burning, any numbness, or do you feel bugs crawling on or under your skin?" Observation.
0 none
1 very mild itching, pins and needles, burning or numbness
2 mild itching, pins and needles, burning or numbness
3 moderate itching, pins and needles, burning or numbness
4 moderately severe hallucinations
5 severe hallucinations
6 extremely severe hallucinations
7 continuous hallucinations

TREMOR – Arms extended and fingers spread apart. Observation.
0 no tremor
1 not visible, but can be felt fingertip to fingertip
2
3
4 moderate, with patient's arms extended
5
6
7 severe, even with arms not extended

AUDITORY DISTURBANCES – Ask "Are you more aware of sounds around you? Are they harsh? Do they frighten you? Are you hearing anything that is disturbing to you? Are you hearing things you know are not there?" Observation.
0 not present
1 very mild harshness or ability to frighten
2 mild harshness or ability to frighten
3 moderate harshness or ability to frighten
4 moderately severe hallucinations
5 severe hallucinations
6 extremely severe hallucinations
7 continuous hallucinations

PAROXYSMAL SWEATS – Observation.
0 no sweat visible
1 barely perceptible sweating, palms moist
2
3
4 beads of sweat obvious on forehead
5
6
7 drenching sweats

VISUAL DISTURBANCES – Ask "Does the light appear to be too bright? Is its color different? Does it hurt your eyes? Are you seeing anything that is disturbing to you? Are you seeing things you know are not there?" Observation.
0 not present
1 very mild sensitivity
2 mild sensitivity
3 moderate sensitivity
4 moderately severe hallucinations
5 severe hallucinations
6 extremely severe hallucinations
7 continuous hallucinations

ANXIETY – Ask "Do you feel nervous?" Observation.
0 no anxiety, at ease
1 mild anxious
2
3
4 moderately anxious, or guarded, so anxiety is inferred
5
6
7 equivalent to acute panic states as seen in severe delirium or acute schizophrenic reactions

HEADACHE, FULLNESS IN HEAD – Ask "Does your head feel different? Does it feel like there is a band around your head?" Do not rate for dizziness or lightheadedness. Otherwise, rate severity.
0 not present
1 very mild
2 mild
3 moderate
4 moderately severe
5 severe
6 very severe
7 extremely severe

AGITATION – Observation.
0 normal activity
1 somewhat more than normal activity
2
3
4 moderately fidgety and restless
5
6
7 paces back and forth during most of the interview, or constantly thrashes about

ORIENTATION AND CLOUDING OF SENSORIUM – Ask "What day is this? Where are you? Who am I?"
0 oriented and can do serial additions
1 cannot do serial additions or is uncertain about date
2 disoriented for date by no more than 2 calendar days
3 disoriented for date by more than 2 calendar days
4 disoriented for place/or person

Total **CIWA-Ar** Score _____
Rater's Initials _____
Maximum Possible Score 67

The **CIWA-Ar** *is not* copyrighted and may be reproduced freely. This assessment for monitoring withdrawal symptoms requires approximately 5 minutes to administer. The maximum score is 67 (see instrument). Patients scoring less than 10 do not usually need additional medication for withdrawal.

Figure 11-2. Revised Clinical Institute Withdrawal Assessment for Alcohol (CIWA-Ar) scale. (*Adapted with permission from Sullivan JT, Sykora K, Schneiderman J, et al: Assessment of alcohol withdrawal: the revised Clinical Institute Withdrawal Assessment for Alcohol Scale (CIWA-AR),* Br J Addict *1989 Nov;84(11):1353-1357.*)

prolong the QT interval) and to decrease autonomic symptoms (ie, dexmedetomidine and clonidine).

Many patients with chronic alcoholism have clinically significant magnesium deficiency because of malnutrition and chronic diuresis from alcohol ingestion. Electrolyte replacement is often indicated. Alcohol withdrawal management requires careful nursing assessment, including alcohol usage history, delirium management, and assessment and treatment of withdrawal symptoms.

Drug Overdose

Drug overdose may involve any type of illicit substance or medication. The majority of overdoses involve analgesics (opioids, aspirin, and acetaminophen), antidepressants, sedatives, over-the-counter medications for cough and cold, and illegal drugs, such as cocaine, heroin, or methamphetamines. Deaths from drug overdose nearly tripled between 1999 and 2014, according to a study by the CDC, and the majority of deaths were due to opioids. While illicit opioids such as heroin account for some of these deaths, the rise in opioid-related deaths correlates with a significant increase in opioid prescriptions. According to the CDC, between 1999 and 2014 sales of prescribed opioids quadrupled. Illegal diversion of prescribed opioids, accidental overdose, and suicidal intent all contribute to the epidemic of opioid overdose deaths. In response to the dramatic rise in opioid deaths, the CDC has issued opioid prescribing guidelines for primary care providers and urged increased education for patients and providers about risks of opioid use, the availability of alternative treatments for pain, and the importance of appropriately handling prescribed agents.

Acetaminophen is also a significant cause of drug overdose. Easily available as a preparation to alleviate fever or pain, acetaminophen is also present in many combination medications, both over-the-counter and prescribed. Acetaminophen can cause hepatocellular damage that may be severe enough to require liver transplantation. In 2015, concerns about acetaminophen overdose lead to changes in labeling and recommended dosing.

Illicit substances are often used to induce a relaxed state, elevate mood, or produce unusual states of consciousness. Psychoactive drugs often are chemically similar to neurotransmitters such as serotonin, dopamine, or norepinephrine, and act by either directly or indirectly altering neurotransmitter-receptor interactions. Medullary inspiratory neurons are highly sensitive to depression by drugs, especially barbiturates and morphine, and death from an overdose of these agents is often secondary to respiratory arrest.

Clinical Presentation

The specific signs and symptoms of drug overdose depend on the substance ingested. However, there are several signs and symptoms that are commonly seen, including alterations in mental status, decreased or increased level of consciousness, behavioral changes, and respiratory depression. The signs and symptoms of overdose for particular drugs are summarized in Table 11.7.

Diagnostic Tests

Diagnostic studies for patients following drug overdose may include the following:

- Toxicology screening typically consists of broad-spectrum tests and identifies the presence of substances such as amphetamines, barbiturates, benzodiazepines, and narcotics. Specific serum levels may be indicated if the substance is known. Serum acetaminophen and salicylate levels in all cases of suspected overdose as these may require specific treatments.
- Arterial blood gas and measurement of the anion gap to evaluate oxygenation, ventilation, and the acid-base status, determine the severity of metabolic derangement.
- Serum glucose and electrolytes, often abnormal as a result of overdose, are measured as they may contribute to the clinical presentation and require treatment.

Principles of Management for Overdose

The principles of management of patients following alcohol intoxication or drug overdose are similar. An initial clinical evaluation is conducted with the priority of resuscitating and

---

ESSENTIAL CONTENT CASE

Alcohol Overdose

A 19-year-old man is unresponsive after drinking at a party and his roommates bring him to the emergency department (ED). Initial assessment reveals a decreased level of consciousness (LOC), with decreased response to stimuli. His initial laboratory results reveal a serum alcohol level of 430 mg/dL. Current vital signs are:

T	36.5°C (97.8°F) rectal
HR	120 beats/min (Sinus tachycardia)
RR	16 breaths/min
BP	92/70 mm Hg

Pulse oximetry 94% on room air

Case Question 1: What are the priority interventions for this patient?

Case Question 2: What information would help in guiding treatment?

Answers
1. Maintenance of airway, hemodynamic stabilization, obtain and maintain intravenous access, administer IV fluids, and provide detoxification.
2. Amount and type of alcohol ingested and time frame since ingestion (gastric lavage is best considered within 1 hour of ingestion).

TABLE 11-7. SIGNS AND SYMPTOMS OF OVERDOSE

Opioids	• Change in level of consciousness (LOC) • Respiratory depression, aspiration • Hypotension • Miosis • Decreased gastric motility
Barbiturates	• Decreased LOC • Hypothermia • Respiratory depression
Benzodiazepines	• Altered mental status • Respiratory depression • Weakness or tremors
Cocaine	• Hyperexcitability • Headache • Hypertension • Tachycardia • Nausea/vomiting, abdominal pain • Fever • Delirium, convulsions, coma
Phencyclidine (PCP)	• Violent behavior • Hallucinations • Seizures • Rhabdomyolysis • Hypertensive crisis
Tricyclics	• Seizures • Coma • Dysrhythmias, ECG changes • Heart failure • Shock
Salicylates	• Tinnitus • Vertigo • Vomiting • Hyperthermia • Altered mental status
Acetaminophen	• GI distress • Hepatotoxicity • Hepatic necrosis

stabilizing the patient. The principles of management include maintenance of a patent airway and adequate breathing, prevention of complications, elimination of ingested substances or toxic metabolites, and maintenance of hemodynamic stability. Specific treatment depends on the agent, route, and amount of exposure, and the severity of overdose. Notification of the Poison Control Centers is essential as they often have resources which provide specific guidance regarding appropriate treatment.

Airway and Breathing

1. Maintain adequate minute ventilation. Stimulate the patient to breathe, if needed. If the patient cannot breath spontaneously and maintain adequate minute ventilation, intubation and mechanical ventilation may be required.
2. Monitor pulse oximetry and blood gas values.
3. Position the patient with the head of the bed elevated more than 30°, if tolerated.
4. Suction the patient's airway as needed.

Circulation and Maintenance of Hemodynamic Stability

1. Ensure venous access (large-bore peripheral or central access).
2. Administer isotonic fluid to maintain intravascular fluid volume. If volume expansion is not sufficient to maintain MAP more than or equal to 65, administration of vasopressors may be necessary.
3. Obtain a 12-lead ECG and maintain continuous cardiac monitoring.
4. *Treatment of dysrhythmias:* Supraventricular tachycardia with hypertension due to sympathetic nervous system response can be managed with a combination of beta-blocker and vasodilator therapy (ie, esmolol and nitroprusside), combined alpha- and beta-blocker therapy (ie, labetalol), or a calcium channel blocker (ie, verapamil or diltiazem). Amiodarone may be used for ventricular tachydysrhythmias, such as atrial fibrillation with rapid ventricular response.

Neurologic Depression

1. Measure glucose to exclude hypoglycemia and treat with 50% dextrose IV if necessary.
2. Evaluate for carbon monoxide poisoning by checking a carboxyhemoglobin level. If this is a concern, provide oxygen therapy if not already indicated.
3. Administer thiamine IV for Wernicke encephalopathy if alcohol overdose is suspected.
4. Administer naloxone IV or IM if narcotic overdose is suspected.
5. Flumazenil can be used for benzodiazepine overdose. However, this is used with caution in those who have potential for seizures. If reducing the seizure threshold is too risky, intubation for airway protection may be preferable to administration of flumazenil.

Catharsis, Clearing Drugs, and Antidotes

1. *Ipecac:* This agent is no longer recommended to induce vomiting, as there is little evidence that it improves the outcome in poisoning cases. Patients are also at increased risk for aspiration, as they may become lethargic from drug overdose before the ipecac is effective. Furthermore, there is little evidence that ipecac prevents drug absorption or systemic toxicity.
2. *Gastric lavage:* Lavage refers to utilizing a nasogastric tube to remove stomach contents and decrease absorption of an ingested substance. Significant amounts of ingested agents can be recovered if lavage is used close to the time of ingestion. This method is less effective if performed more than 1 hour after ingestion due to the timing of gastric emptying. Gastric lavage is contraindicated in the management of ingested corrosive agents due to risk of esophageal injury and gastroesophageal perforation. It is also contraindicated with hydrocarbon

ingestion because of the risk of aspiration-induced hydrocarbon pneumonitis.

3. *Activated charcoal:* Charcoal absorbs ingested toxins within the gut lumen, allowing the charcoal-toxin complex to be eliminated in the stool. Charcoal is not recommended for patients who have ingested caustic acids and alkalis, alcohols, lithium, or heavy metals. Charcoal is useful for most drug ingestions if it is used close to the time of ingestion (within 1 hour) as it only impacts the portion of drug that remains in the stomach.

4. *Hemodialysis and hemoperfusion:* Hemodialysis can be considered for severe poisoning due to methanol, ethylene glycol, salicylates, lithium, barbiturates, bromide, chloral hydrate, ethanol, isopropyl alcohol, procainamide, theophylline, salicylates, and heavy metals. Hemoperfusion, which involves the passage of blood through an absorptive-containing cartridge (usually charcoal), may be indicated for intoxications with carbamazepine, phenobarbital, phenytoin, and theophylline. Therapeutic plasma exchange has also been used to promote rapid lowering of the toxin level. Refer to Chapter 15, Renal System, for more on renal replacement therapies.

Antidotes

Antidotes help counteract the effects of poisons by neutralizing them or by antagonizing their effects. Toxins and their specific antidotes include the following:

- *Acetaminophen:* N-acetylcysteine
- *Opiates:* Naloxone
- *Benzodiazepines:* Flumazenil
- *Digoxin:* Digibind
- *Cyanide:* Kelocyanor
- *Tricyclic antidepressants:* Sodium bicarbonate
- *Beta-blockers or calcium channel blockers:* Glucagon and calcium
- *Warfarin:* Vitamin K

Preventing Complications

1. Orient the patient to their surroundings.
2. Insert a nasogastric tube for gastric decompression and for delivery of charcoal or other antidotes, if indicated.
3. Keep the head of the bed elevated more than 30°, to prevent aspiration.
4. Prevent self-injury by padding the bed's side rails and monitoring the patient's behavior closely. Use physical restraints only if other measures to prevent self-injury are ineffective or unavailable.
5. Provide support to the patient and family.

PRESSURE INJURY

Pressure injuries are troubling complications of immobility for progressive care patients. They increase length of hospitalization, recovery time, risk of infection, costs of care, and can cause discomfort for patients. Of significance to the healthcare team is that pressure injuries are thought to be preventable in most cases and are viewed as a reflection of the quality of care provided. Starting in 2008, hospitals have not received reimbursement for treatment of pressure injuries that developed during an inpatient stay. Pressure injuries cost over $9 billion per year in the United States. Medicare estimated in 2007 that each pressure injury added $43,180 in costs to a hospital stay. Because of their association with quality of care and their financial impact, documentation of the presence of pressure injuries and interventions to reduce their incidence are core elements of progressive care nursing.

A pressure injury is defined by the National Pressure Ulcer Advisory Panel (NPUAP) as an injury to the skin or tissue due to pressure and/or shear occurring in a localized area, often over a bony prominence. When a person is immobile, the soft tissue is compressed between the skin and the bone. This can lead to ischemia and tissue death. Typically, a pressure injury occurs over a bony prominence, but can occur anywhere soft tissue is compressed, such as in areas where medical devices are applied. Pressure injury prevalence rates range from 53.2% to 88% and incidence rates vary from 7% to 71.6%, depending on associated risk factors. The most common anatomical sites for pressure injuries to occur are the sacrum and heels.

There are a number of intrinsic or internal factors related to the risk of pressure injury development. In the acute care setting, sepsis, hypoxia, hypothermia, and use of vasoactive medications contribute to pressure injuries. Additionally, poor nutrition and dehydration contribute to pressure injury development because these conditions make tissue more vulnerable to damage. Older adults are at greater risk because of physiologic changes that occur to the skin and tissue with age, such as dermal thinning and the inability of tissue to distribute the mechanical load. Peripheral vasoconstriction during periods of hypotension diverts blood away from the skin to more essential organs. Additionally, malnutrition, stress, smoking, surgery, hyperthermia, and comorbid conditions such as diabetes and peripheral vascular disease may increase risk for pressure injury development.

According to the NPUAP, the six stages of pressure injuries (Table 11-8) are classified as follows:

Pressure Injury Stages

Stage 1

A stage 1 pressure injury is defined as an area of intact skin with non-blanchable erythema over a localized area, usually over a bony prominence. The area may be painful, firm, soft, warmer, or cooler when compared to adjacent tissue, but the skin remains intact. Darkly pigmented skin may not have visible blanching; its color may differ from the surrounding area, making stage 1 pressure injuries difficult to detect in

TABLE 11-8 PRESSURE INJURY CLASSIFICATION BRIEF GUIDE

Category/Stage 1 Pressure Injury	Non-blanchable erythema Intact skin
Category/Stage 2 Pressure Injury	Partial-thickness tissue loss Wound bed is pink/red
Category/Stage 3 Pressure Injury	Full-thickness tissue loss extending into the subcutaneous tissue; slough/eschar may be present in the wound bed but does not obscure depth of the wound
Category/Stage 4 Pressure Injury	Full-thickness tissue loss; the muscle, bone, or tendon may be present in the wound bed; slough/eschar may be present in the wound bed but does not obscure depth of the wound
Unstageable–Unknown Depth	Full-thickness tissue loss; unable to visualize base of the wound due to slough or eschar
Deep Tissue Injury	Purple or maroon discoloration Intact skin Non-blanchable

Data from National Pressure Ulcer Advisory Panel. NPUAP Pressure Injury Stages. https://www.npuap.org/resources/educational-and-clinical-resources/npuap-pressure-injury-stages/. Updated April, 2016.

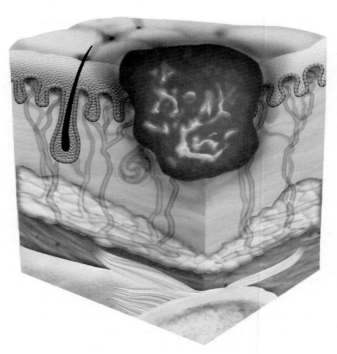

Figure 11-4. Stage 2 pressure injury.

individuals with dark skin tones. See Figure 11-3 for an illustration of stage 1 pressure injury.

Stage 2

Stage 2 pressure injuries are defined as partial-thickness loss of dermis presenting as a shallow open ulcer with a red-pink wound bed, without slough or bruising. A stage 2 pressure injury also presents as an intact or open/ruptured serum-filled blister. This stage should not be used to describe skin tears, tape burns, perineal dermatitis, maceration, or excoriation. See Figure 11-4 for an illustration of stage 2 pressure injury.

Stage 3

Stage 3 pressure injuries are defined as full-thickness tissue loss. Subcutaneous fat may be visible but bone, tendon, or muscle is not exposed. Slough may be present but does not obscure the depth of tissue loss. The wound may demonstrate undermining and tunneling. Bone/tendon is not visible or directly palpable in stage 3 pressure injury. See Figure 11-5 for an illustration of stage 3 pressure injury.

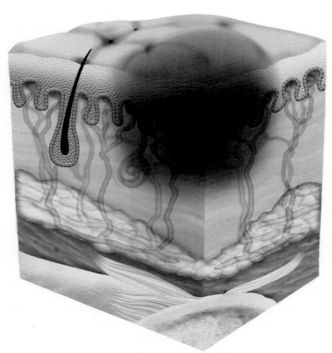

Figure 11-3. Stage 1 pressure injury.

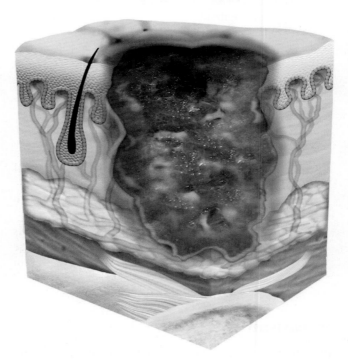

Figure 11-5. Stage 3 pressure injury.

Stage 4

Stage 4 pressure injuries are defined as full-thickness tissue loss with exposed bone, tendon, or muscle. Slough or eschar may be present on some parts of the wound. Stage 4 pressure injuries often demonstrate undermining and tunneling. The depth of stage 4 pressure injuries varies by anatomical location. Stage 4 pressure injuries can extend into muscle and/or supporting structures (ie, fascia, tendon, or joint capsules) making osteomyelitis a possible complication. Exposed bone/tendon is visible or directly palpable in stage 4 pressure injuries.

The depth of stages 3 and 4 pressure injuries varies by anatomical location. The bridge of the nose, ear, occiput, and malleolus do not have subcutaneous tissue so injury that reaches the tendon or bone occurs with shallow wounds in these areas. In areas of greater adiposity, deeper wound may not expose tendon or bone and so would be classified as a stage 3. Staging is not based on measuring the depth of the wound but rather on assessing the structures exposed by the wound. See Figure 11-6 for an illustration of stage 4 pressure injury.

Unstageable

Unstageable pressure injuries are defined as full-thickness tissue loss in which the base of the ulcer is covered by slough (yellow, tan, gray, green, or brown) and/or eschar (tan, brown, or black), making wound bed difficult to evaluate. Until enough slough and/or eschar is removed to expose the base of the wound, the true depth, and therefore stage, cannot be determined. Stable (dry, adherent, intact without erythema or fluctuance) eschar on the heels serves as a protective barrier and should not be removed.

Deep Tissue Injury

Deep tissue injury is defined as a pressure-related injury to subcutaneous tissue that occurs under intact skin. The localized area may appear as a blister or discolored, purple, maroon, or deep red. The area may appear purple, maroon, or deep red. The area does not blanche. The area may have previously demonstrated temperature changes and/or tenderness. Deep tissue injury may be difficult to detect in individuals with dark skin tones. Evolution may include a thin blister over a dark wound bed. The wound may progress to stage 3 or 4 pressure injuries. Evolution may be rapid, exposing additional layers of tissue even with optimal treatment. These injuries may occur from medical devices such as oxygen saturation probes or may occur from prolonged positioning on hard surfaces, such as on the operating room table or interventional radiology table. See Figure 11-7 for an illustration of deep tissue injury.

Principles of Management of Pressure Injury

Baseline and ongoing skin assessment, risk assessment, nutritional status assessment, and providing appropriate repositioning and support surfaces are all key pressure injury prevention strategies. The two most widely studied and validated risk assessment scales are the Braden and Norton scales. The Braden scale consists of six subcategories, sensory perception, moisture, activity, mobility, nutrition, and friction/shear. Each category is scored 1 for the (most at risk) to 4 (least at risk), with the exception of the friction and shear subcategory which is scored 1-3. The numbers are totaled, providing a score ranging from 4 to 23. A score less than 18 indicates risk for pressure injury development. The Norton score includes five parameters: physical condition,

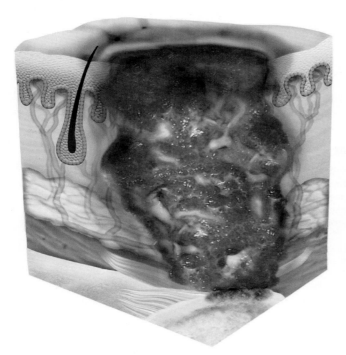

Figure 11-6. Stage 4 pressure injury.

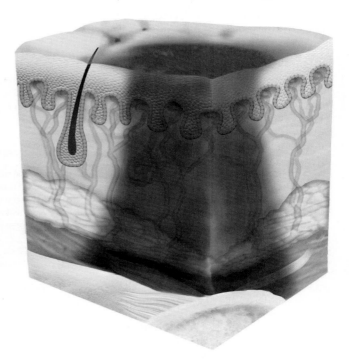

Figure 11-7. Deep tissue injury.

mental condition, activity, mobility, and continence. The rating for each category is 1-4 with a score potential of 5-20. For both the Braden and the Norton scales, a low score indicates a greater risk for pressure injury development.

Due to the significant impact on morbidity and mortality of pressure injury, coupled with the economic impact, national strategies are in place for prevention. The Agency for Healthcare Research and Quality recommends that hospitals perform routine pressure injury prevalence surveys. By carefully tracking the incidence of pressure injuries, hospitals obtain real-time information about the effectiveness of their prevention and treatment strategies.

Although the underlying relationship is uncertain, low body weight and malnutrition are risk factors for development of pressure injuries. Patients must have sufficient calories, fluid, and protein intake to reduce their risk. Evaluation and treatment for malnutrition, ideally by a registered dietician, may help prevent pressure injury development.

Repositioning should be scheduled for bed- and chair-bound patients at risk for pressure injury development. The patient's overall condition must be considered when repositioning. If the patient cannot be fully turned due to hemodynamic instability, then an advanced support surface can be used and slight adjustments in position provided. Support surfaces are used as adjunctive therapy, and do not replace turning and repositioning. A pillow or a heel elevation device can be used to suspend heels off the surface of the bed.

The treatment of pressure injuries is complex and can vary based on the types of dressings available and the patients' underlying health. Prompt recognition and treatment are essential to limit the impact of pressure injury on a patient's overall prognosis. A wound care specialist should be consulted to assist with determination of treatment and evaluating for possible debridement.

HEALTHCARE-ASSOCIATED INFECTIONS

The CDC reports that healthcare-associated infections (HAIs) occur in about 1 of every 25 inpatients on any given day. HAIs have been identified as one of the most serious patient safety issues in health care. Patients in progressive care units are at an increased risk for catheter-associated urinary tract infections (CAUTIs), central line-associated bloodstream infections (CLABSI), hospital-acquired pneumonia (HAP), ventilator-associated events (VAE), and ventilator-associated complications (VAC). The pneumonias, their etiology, identification, and management, are discussed in Chapter 10, Respiratory System.

CAUTIs result from the presence of an indwelling urinary catheter. According to the CDC, the number of hospital-acquired urinary tract infections exceeds 560,000 cases annually. The CDC also reports that catheter-associated urinary tract infection (CAUTI) is the leading cause of secondary hospital-associated bloodstream infections (BSIs). Patients that develop a bloodstream infection secondary to a CAUTI have an associated 10% mortality rate. Guidelines for the prevention of CAUTIs issued by the CDC outline several recommendations, including appropriate use of indwelling catheters, proper catheter insertion, and maintaining a closed sterile drainage system (Table 11-9).

A variety of specialized catheters have been designed to reduce the risk of CAUTI. These include antiseptic-impregnated catheters and catheters coated with silver alloy or nitrofurazone. Several systematic reviews of the use of antimicrobial urinary catheters in the prevention of CAUTI have demonstrated a reduction in catheter-associated bacteriuria, but consensus on the economic benefit compared to standard catheter use has not been reached and further research is needed.

Nursing care to reduce the risk of CAUTI includes assessment to determine if urinary catheter use is appropriate, consideration of alternative interventions such as external collection devises or in and out catheterization, strict adherence to aseptic technique in managing the catheter, monitoring patients for signs of urinary tract infection (UTI), and teaching unlicensed personnel to handle the catheter and the collection bag appropriately. Removal of catheters when their use is unnecessary is essential in preventing CAUTI.

TABLE 11-9. EVIDENCE-BASED STRATEGIES FOR URINARY TRACT INFECTION PREVENTION

- Indwelling urinary catheters should be inserted using aseptic technique and sterile equipment.
- Only hospital personnel who know the correct technique of aseptic insertion and maintenance of the catheter should handle catheters.
- Hospital personnel should be provided with periodic in-service training stressing the correct techniques and potential complications of urinary catheterization.
- Indwelling urinary catheters should be inserted only when necessary and removed when no longer necessary.
- Other methods of urinary drainage such as condom catheter drainage, suprapubic catheterization, and intermittent urethral catheterization should be considered as alternatives to indwelling urethral catheterization.
- Hand washing should be done immediately before and after any manipulation of the indwelling urinary catheter site or apparatus.
- Indwelling catheters should be properly secured after insertion to prevent movement and urethral traction.
- A sterile, continuously closed drainage system should be maintained.
- The catheter and drainage tube should not be disconnected unless the catheter is irrigated, and irrigation should be used only for suspected obstruction.
- If breaks in aseptic technique, disconnection, or leakage occur, the collecting system should be replaced using aseptic technique after disinfecting the catheter-tubing junction.
- Specimen collections should be obtained from the distal end of the catheter, preferably from the sampling port after cleansing with a disinfectant and then the urine specimen aspirated with a sterile needle and syringe.
- Consider the use of antimicrobial catheters for indwelling urinary catheters.

Data from Guideline for Prevention of Catheter Associated Urinary Tract Infections 2009 https://www.cdc.gov/infectioncontrol/guidelines/cauti/.

Nurse-driven protocols to reduce the number of days urinary catheters are in use have effectively lowered CAUTI rates and shown a financial benefit.

CVCs are frequently needed in progressive care, but have associated risks, the most common being BSI. According to the CDC, there was a 50% decrease in the incidence of CLABSI from 2009 to 2014, most likely as a result of CLABSI prevention bundles. However, CLABSI continues to be a significant cause of morbidity and mortality in hospitalized patients with thousands of patients dying from these infections on an annual basis.

A CLABSI is defined as bacteremia in a patient with an intravascular catheter with at least one positive blood culture and clinical signs of infections (ie, fever, leukocytosis, and/or hypotension), with no apparent source for the BSI except the catheter. A BSI is considered to be associated with a central line if the line was in place during the 48-hour period before development of the BSI. The most common mechanism of CLABSI is migration of the organism from the insertion site along the surface of the catheter and colonization of its distal part. CLABSIs can also occur from improper insertion techniques, lack of an occlusive dressing, or contamination of the catheter hub or of the infusate administered through the device.

Several practices have been evaluated in an attempt to reduce the incidence of CLABSI. These include using a standardized catheter insertion technique with a skin prep such as chlorhexidine and careful maintenance of the catheter. In addition, daily review of catheter necessity, the use of antimicrobial-impregnated dressings, and use of antimicrobial catheters have demonstrated reductions in incidence of CLABSI. Catheters impregnated or coated with antimicrobials or antiseptics have been shown to decrease the risk of CLABSI. Chlorhexidine-impregnated dressings have also been found to reduce the rate of CVC colonization. While evidence for the efficacy of CVCs coated with antibacterial or antiseptic agents exists, limited information exists related to their cost-effectiveness. Current CDC recommendations include use of CVCs coated with antibacterial or antiseptic agents, central line insertion bundles, daily chlorhexidine bathing of patients with CVCs, chlorhexidine-impregnated dressings, proper hand hygiene, and careful disinfecting of catheter hubs. Table 11-10 outlines evidence-based strategies for CLABSI prevention.

Nursing interventions to prevent CLABSI include maximal barrier precautions during CVC insertion; ongoing care of the insertion site including sterile dressing changes; disinfection of CVC ports during blood sampling, infusion of intravenous fluids, and medication administration; intravenous tubing changes based on protocol guidelines; and monitoring of patients with CVCs for signs of infection. Nurses also assess the need for CVC placement and advocate for removal when no longer necessary.

Selected Infectious Diseases

Multi-drug-resistant organisms, or MDROs, are bacteria resistant to traditional antibiotic therapy. MDROs can cause serious local and systemic infections that can be severely debilitating and even life threatening. The most common MDROs include methicillin-resistant *Staphylococcus aureus* (MRSA), vancomycin-resistant *enterococcus* (VRE), *Acinetobacter*, and carbapenem-resistant *enterobacteriaceae* (CRE). Hospitalization and prior use of antibiotics increases the risk for infection and colonization with MDROs. *Clostridium difficile* is often discussed with MDROs as infection with *C. diff* similarly occurs in the setting of antibiotic use, and requires special precautions to prevent transmission to other patients. According to the CDC, the prevalence of infections caused by MDROs and *C. diff* are on the rise, making early identification, treatment, and prevention of transmission an important area of focus for healthcare providers.

MRSA is a type of staphylococcal organism resistant to traditional antibiotic therapy, including methicillin, oxacillin, amoxicillin, penicillin, and cephalosporins. MRSA

TABLE 11-10. EVIDENCE-BASED STRATEGIES FOR CENTRAL LINE INFECTION PREVENTION

- Education and training should be provided for staff who insert and maintain intravenous lines.
- Maximal sterile barriers should be used during catheter insertion (cap, mask, sterile gown and gloves, and a large sterile drape).
- A 2% chlorhexidine preparation is the preferred skin antiseptic, to be applied prior to insertion.
- Antiseptic- or antibiotic-impregnated catheters should be reserved for very high-risk patients or situations in which catheter-related BSI rates are high despite careful attention to these recommendations.
- Replace peripheral intravenous sites in the adult patient population at least every 96 hours but no more frequently than every 72 hours. Peripheral venous catheters in children should be left in until the intravenous therapy is completed, unless complications such as phlebitis or infiltration occur.
- Replace intravenous tubing no more frequently than every 96 hours but at least every 7 days in patients not receiving blood, blood products, or fat emulsions.
- Replace intravenous catheters as soon as possible when adherence to aseptic technique during catheter insertion cannot be ensured (ie, prehospital, code situation).
- Central lines should not routinely be replaced at scheduled intervals.
- Consider use of a central line insertion checklist to ensure all processes related to central line insertion are executed for each line placement.
- Consider use of a central line insertion cart to avoid the difficulty of finding necessary equipment to institute maximal barrier precautions.
- Replace central line dressings whenever damp, loose, or soiled or at a frequency of every 7 days for transparent, chlorhexidine-impregnated dressings.
- Avoid use of antibiotic ointment at insertion sites because it can promote fungal infections and antibiotic resistance.
- Include daily review of line necessity.
- Assess competency of staff who insert and care for intravascular catheters.

Data from O'Grady NP, Alexander M, Burns LA, et al: Guidelines for the prevention of intravascular catheter-related infections, Clin Infect Dis *2011 May;52(9):e162-e193.*

can be transmitted via personal contact with contaminated items such as dressings or other infected materials, and can be spread due to poor hand hygiene or use of contaminated equipment, such as stethoscopes.

VRE most commonly occurs in the hospital and long-term care settings. According to the CDC, risk factors for acquiring VRE include treatment with vancomycin, immunosuppression, recent surgery, presence of invasive devices, and/or prolonged courses of antibiotics, especially while hospitalized. VRE can be transmitted from person-to-person via contact due to poor hand hygiene or by touching contaminated surfaces.

Carbapenem-resistant *enterobacteriaceae* are a growing concern in acute care settings because these bacteria do not respond to the most potent antibiotics available. While CRE can cause ventilator-associated pneumonia, BSI, and intra-abdominal abscesses, it is most commonly found as an infection of the urinary tract. The CDC estimates that up to half of patients who develop a CRE BSI will die as a result.

C. diff is also an increasing cause of HAI. A spore-forming anaerobic bacillus, *C. diff* produces endotoxins that cause diarrhea and can lead to colitis, and, in vulnerable patients, sepsis. New strains of *C. diff* cause more severe disease and are resistant to treatment. The single most important risk factor for *C. diff* is antibiotic use. Twenty percent of cases of *C. diff* resolve with antibiotic discontinuation; other cases require metronidazole or vancomycin. Particular attention to hand hygiene is essential in limiting the spread of *C. diff*. Because the spores do not die with exposure to alcohol, meticulous hand washing with soap and water and contact precautions are necessary after exposure to patients with known or suspected *C. diff*.

The CDC has identified interventions necessary to control or eradicate MDROs and *C. diff*. These include administrative support, education, MDRO surveillance, infection control precautions, environmental precautions, and decolonization. Additionally, the CDC's Campaign to Prevent Antimicrobial Resistance recommends judicious use of antibiotics and avoiding excessive duration of antibiotic therapy. General measures to prevent MDROs in healthcare settings include infection prevention measures, early detection of infections, and measures to prevent transmission.

Nurses have an important role in preventing the spread of these infections, in the acute care setting. Hand hygiene is a significant intervention that applies to all patient care activities. In addition, transmission-based precautions for patients with confirmed MDRO or *C. diff* infection include donning gowns and gloves prior to entering patients' rooms and removing them before exiting; limiting the transport of patients through the facility; using disposable equipment or disinfecting durable equipment; and frequent cleaning and disinfecting of patients' rooms. Posted signs and education of staff, patients, and visitors are also essential in reducing the spread of MDROs and *C. diff*.

SELECTED BIBLIOGRAPHY

Sepsis and Septic Shock

AACN Webinar. Updating Your Practice: The 2017 Sepsis Guidelines. https://www.aacn.org/education/webinar-series/wb0037/updating-your-practice-the-2017-sepsis-guidelines. Accessed June 21, 2017.

Balas MC, Vasilevskis EE, Burke WJ, et al. Critical care nurses role in implementing the "ABCDE bundle" into practice. *Crit Care Nurse.* 2012;32:35-47.

Barr J, Fraser GL, Puntillo K, et al. Clinical practice guidelines for the management of pain, agitation, and delirium in adult patients in the intensive care unit. *Crit Care Med.* 2013;41(1):263-306.

Davidson J, Aslakson R, Long A, et al. Guidelines for family-centered care in the neonatal, pediatric, and adult ICU. *Crit Care Med.* 2017;45(1):103-128. doi: 10.1097/CCM.0000000000002169.

Dellinger RP, Levy ML, Schorr C, Levy MM. A users' guide to the 2016 Surviving Sepsis Guidelines. *Intensive Care Med.* 2017;43:299-303. doi: 10.1007/Soo134-017-4681-8.

Gaieski DF, Edwards JM, Kallan MJ, Carr BG. Benchmarking the incidence and mortality of severe sepsis in the United States. *Crit Care Med.* 2013;41:1167-1174.

Gupta B, Agrawal P, Soni KD, et al. Enteral nutrition practices in the intensive care unit: understanding of nursing practices and perspectives. *J Anaesthesiol Clin Pharmacol.* 2012;28:41-44.

Kleinpell R, Schorr CA, Bulk R. The new sepsis definitions: implications for critical care practitioners. *Am J Crit Care.* 2016;25:457-464. http://ajcc.aacnjournals.org/content/25/5/457.full.

McClave SA, Taylor BE, Martindale RG, et al. Guidelines for the provision and assessment of nutrition support therapy in the adult critically ill patient: Society of Critical Care Medicine (SCCM) and American Society for Parental and Enteral Nutrition (A.S.P.E.N.). *JPEN J Parenter Enteral Nutr.* 2016;40(2):159-211. http://journals.sagepub.com/doi/full/10.1177/0148607115621863.

NICE-SUGAR Study Investigators. Hypoglycemia and risk of death in critically ill patients. *N Engl J Med.* 2012;367:1108-1118.

Perel P, Roberts I. Colloids versus crystalloids for fluid resuscitation in critically ill patients. *Cochrane Database Syst Rev.* 2011;(3):CD000567.

Rhodes A, Evans LE, Alhazzani W, et al. Surviving sepsis campaign: international guidelines for management of sepsis and septic shock: 2016 *Intensive Care Med.* 2017;43:304-307. doi:10.1007/s00134-017-4683-6

Rubinsky M, Clark A. Early enteral nutrition in critically ill patients. *Dimens Crit Care Nurs.* 2012;31:267-274.

Singer M, Deutschman CS, Seymour CW, et al. The Third International Consensus Definitions for Sepsis and Septic Shock (Sepsis-3). *JAMA.* 2016;315(8):801-810. doi:10.1001/jama.2016.0287.

Surviving Sepsis Campaign. http://www.survivingsepsis.org/Bundles/Pages/default.aspx. Accessed June 21, 2017.

Overdoses

Alcohol Poisoning Deaths. Centers for Disease Control and Prevention. https://www.cdc.gov/VITALSIGNS/ALCOHOL-POISONING-DEATHS/INDEX.HTML. Updated January, 2015. Accessed June 21, 2017.

Cassidy EM, O'Sullivan I, Bradshaw P, Islam T, Onovo C. Symptom-triggered benzodiazepine therapy for alcohol withdrawal syndrome in the emergency department: a comparison with the standard fixed dose benzodiazepine regimen. *Emerg Med J.* 2011;29(10):802-804.

Centers for Disease Control. 2016. https://www.cdc.gov/drugoverdose/data/prescribing.html.

Corfee FA. Alcohol withdrawal in the critical care unit. *Aust Crit Care.* 2011;24(2):110-116.

Dixon DW. Opioid abuse. *Medscape.* 2017. http://emedicine.medscape.com/article/287790-overview. Accessed July 23, 2017. Updated July 13, 2017.

Marraffa JM, Cohen V, Howland MA. Antidotes for toxicological emergencies: a practical review. *Am J Health Syst Pharm.* 2012;69(3):199-212.

Muzyk AJ, Fowler JA, Norwood DK, Chilipko A. Role of α-agonists in the treatment of acute alcohol withdrawal. *Ann Pharmacother.* 2011;45(5):649-657.

Rudd RA, Seth P, David F, Scholl L. Increases in drug and opioid-involved overdose deaths — United States, 2010-2015. *MMWR Morb Mortal Wkly Rep.* December 30, 2016;65(50-51):1445-1452.

Schutt RC, Ronco C, Rosner MH. The role of therapeutic plasma exchange in poisonings and intoxications. *Semin Dial.* 2012;25(2):201-216.

Stewart S, Swain S. Assessment and management of alcohol dependence and withdrawal in the acute hospital: concise guidance. *Clin Med.* 2012;12(3):266-271.

Taheri A, Dahri K, Chan P, et al. Evaluation of a symptom-triggered protocol approach to the management of alcohol withdrawal syndrome in older adults. *J Am Geriatr Soc.* 2014;62(8):1551-1555.

Pressure Injuries

Agency for Healthcare Research and Quality. Preventing pressure ulcers in hospitals. https://www.ahrq.gov/professionals/systems/hospital/pressureulcertoolkit/putool3a.html. Accessed July 23, 2017.

Cox J. Predictors of pressure ulcers in adult critical care patients. *Am J Crit Care.* 2011;20:364-375.

Medicare. https://www.cms.gov/Medicare/Medicare-Fee-for-Service-Payment/HospitalAcqCond/index.html?redirect=/hospitalacqcond/.

National Pressure Ulcer Advisory Panel. NPUAP Pressure Injury Stages. https://www.npuap.org/resources/educational-and-clinical-resources/npuap-pressure-injury-stages/. Updated April, 2016. Accessed June 21, 2017.

Niederhauser A, Lukas CV, Parker V, et al. Comprehensive programs for preventing pressure ulcers: a review of the literature, advances in skin and wound care. *Adv Skin Wound Care.* 2012;15:167-188.

NPUAP Clinical Practice Guidelines. 2014. http://www.npuap.org/resources/educational-and-clinical-resources/prevention-and-treatment-of-pressure-ulcers-clinical-practice-guideline/.

WOCN. Guidelines for Prevention and Management of Pressure Ulcers (Injuries). 2016. https://guideline.gov/summaries/summary/50473/guideline-for-prevention-and-management-of-pressure-ulcers-injuries. Accessed July 23, 2017.

Healthcare-Associated Infections

AACN Clinical Scene Investigator Academy. Clean Cath Club. https://www.aacn.org/clinical-resources/csi-projects/clean-cath-club. accessed July 7th, 2018.

AACN Practice Alert. Prevention of CAUTI in Adults. 2016. https://www.aacn.org/clinical-resources/practice-alerts/prevention-of-cauti-in-adults.

Centers for Disease Control and Prevention. Catheter-associated urinary tract infection. http://www.cdc.gov/HAI/ca_uti/uti.html. Accessed July 23rd, 2017.

Centers for Disease Control and Prevention. Central line-associated bloodstream infection (CLABSI). https://www.cdc.gov/hai/bsi/bsi.html. Accessed June 21, 2017.

Centers for Disease Control and Prevention. HAI data and statistics. https://www.cdc.gov/hai/surveillance/index.html. Accessed June 21, 2017.

Kleinpell RM, Munro CL, Giuliano KK. Targeting health care acquired infections: evidence based strategies. *In: Patient Safety and Quality: An Evidence Based Handbook for Nurses.* Agency for Healthcare Research and Quality. 2008. http://www.ncbi.nlm.nih.gov/books/NBK2632/. Accessed February 20, 2013.

Klompas M, Branson R, Eichenwald E, et al. Strategies to prevent ventilator-associated pneumonia in acute care hospitals: 2014 update. *Infect Control Hosp Epidemiol.* 2014;35(8):915-936. doi:10.1086/677144.

Marschall J, Mermel L, Fakih M, et al. Strategies to prevent central line–associated bloodstream infections in acute care hospitals: 2014 update. *Infect Control Hosp Epidemiol.* 2014;35(7):753-771. doi:10.1086/676533.

Richards B, Sebastian B, Sullivan H, et al. Decreasing catheter associated urinary tract infections in the neurological intensive care unit: one unit's success. *Crit Care Nurse.* 2017;37(3):42-48. doi: 10.4037/ccn2017742

Selected Infectious Diseases

Center for Disease Control and Prevention. Carbopenum resistant Enterobacteriaceae (CRE) infection: Clinician FAQs. https://www.cdc.gov/hai/organisms/cre/cre-clinicianfaq.html. Accessed November 5, 2017.

Centers for Disease Control and Prevention. *Clostridium difficile.* https://www.cdc.gov/hai/organisms/cdiff/cdiff_clinicians.html Accessed July 23, 2017.

Centers for Disease Control and Prevention. Methicillin resistant *Staphylococcus aureus.* https://www.cdc.gov/mrsa/index.html. Accessed July 23, 2017.

Centers for Disease Control and Prevention. Multidrug-resistant organism management. https://www.cdc.gov/infectioncontrol/guidelines/mdro/index.html. Accessed July 23, 2017.

Centers for Disease Control and Prevention. VRE in healthcare settings. https://www.cdc.gov/hai/organisms/vre/vre.html. Accessed July 23, 2017.

NEUROLOGICAL SYSTEM

DaiWai M. Olson and Kathrina Siaron

12

KNOWLEDGE COMPETENCIES

1. Correlate neurologic assessments to patient problems and diagnostic findings.

2. Identify indications, complications, and nursing management for commonly used neurodiagnostic tests.

3. Identify causes of increased intracranial pressure and describe strategies for management.

4. Compare and contrast the pathophysiology, clinical presentation, patient needs, and nursing management for:
   - Acute ischemic stroke
   - Hemorrhagic stroke
   - Seizure disorders
   - CNS infections
   - Selected neuromuscular diseases

SPECIAL ASSESSMENT TECHNIQUES AND DIAGNOSTIC TESTS

Although there is no single method of performing a neurologic evaluation, a systematic, orderly approach offers the best results. Knowledge of neurologic disease processes and neuroanatomy allows the progressive care nurse to tailor the assessment to individual patients. Obtaining a comprehensive past medical history that includes any preexisting neurologic conditions in addition to a thorough history of the present illness or injury is essential. The time from injury to symptom onset, and identification of the mechanism of injury have important implications for diagnostic testing and treatment. The administration of any medications that may potentially alter the neurologic examination, especially sedatives and analgesics, is also noted.

Serial assessments, coupled with accurate documentation, allow for detection of subtle changes in neurologic status. Early detection of changes permits rapid intervention and improves patient outcomes. Neurologic assessment in the progressive care unit can be broken down into the following components: level of consciousness, mental status, motor examination, sensory examination, and cranial nerve examination. A baseline examination is established and subsequent assessments are compared. Whenever a patient handover of

care occurs, the nurse should perform a neurological examination together to provide an accurate baseline for the nurse assuming care of the patient.

Level of Consciousness

There are multiple components to level of consciousness including: arousal, awareness, and responsiveness. *Arousal* refers to the state of wakefulness; *awareness* reflects the content and quality of interactions with the environment; and *responsiveness* refers to the ability to react to changes in the environment. Arousal reflects function of the reticular-activating system and brain stem, and awareness indicates functioning of the cerebral cortex. Level of consciousness is assessed on all patients. A change in level of consciousness is the most important indicator of neurologic decline. Any change in the level of consciousness requires further assessment or action from the healthcare team.

Observation of the patient's behavior, appearance, and ability to communicate is the first step in assessing level of consciousness. If the patient responds meaningfully to the examiner without the need for stimulation, then the patient is described as alert. If stimulation is required, auditory stimuli are used first. If the patient does not rouse to auditory

297

stimuli, tactile stimuli such as a gentle touch or shake are used, followed by painful stimuli if necessary to elicit a response. Accepted methods of central painful stimulus include squeezing the trapezius or other large muscle group. Care is taken to avoid causing tissue trauma. Supraorbital pressure is also an acceptable pain stimulus, but is not used if there is any suspicion of facial fracture. Use of a sternal rub may result in a motor response that is difficult to interpret and often causes bruising. Nail bed pressure is a commonly used peripheral pain stimulus. Response to central stimulus is more indicative of cerebral function than response to peripheral stimulus. Certain responses to peripheral pain, such as the triple flexion response (stereotypical flexion of the ankle, knee, and hip), can result from a spinal reflex arc and thus may remain present even following death by neurologic criteria (brain death).

Glasgow Coma Scale (GCS) and the Full Outline of Unresponsiveness (FOUR) Score

Two scales used to stratify level of neurologic function are the GCS and FOUR. Each has advantages and limitations. Table 12-1 provides a comparison of the scores.

GCS

The GCS is often used to monitor neurologic status in critically ill patients with traumatic brain injury (TBI) because it provides a standardized approach to assessing and documenting level of consciousness. Response is determined in three categories: eye opening, motor response, and verbal response. The best response in each category is scored, and the results are added to give a total GCS. Scores range from 3 to 15, with 15 indicating a patient that is alert, fully oriented, and following commands.

The eye opening score reflects the amount of stimulation that must be applied for the patient to open his eyes. Spontaneous eye opening is the best response, followed by eye opening to verbal stimulation, then eye opening to painful stimulation. Scoring of the eye opening section of the scale can be complicated by orbital trauma and swelling, and this is documented accordingly.

The verbal section of the GCS assesses a patient's ability to speak coherently and with appropriate content. Orientation to person, place, time, and situation is assessed. As mental status declines, orientation to time is lost first, followed by orientation to place. Orientation to person is seldom lost prior to loss of consciousness. Patients with an endotracheal

TABLE 12-1. COMPARISON OF GLASCOW COMA SCALE (GCS) AND FULL OUTLINE OF UNRESPONSIVENESS (FOUR) SCORES

Category	Score	GCS	FOUR Score
Eye response	4	Spontaneous eye opening	Eyelids open or opened, tracking, or blinking to command
	3	Eye opening to verbal stimuli	Eyelids open but not tracking
	2	Eye opening to painful stimuli	Eyelids closed but open to loud voice
	1	No eye opening	Eyelids closed but open to pain
	0		Eyelids remain closed with pain
Verbal	5	Oriented	
	4	Confused	
	3	Inappropriate words	
	2	Incomprehensible sounds	
	1	None	
Motor	6	Obeys commands	
	5	Localizes to pain	
	4	Withdraws to pain	Thumbs up, fist, or peace sign
	3	Flexion to pain	Localizing to pain
	2	Extension to pain	Flexion to pain
	1	No response	Extension to pain
	0		No response to pain or generalized myoclonus status
Brain stem reflexes	4		Pupil and corneal reflexes present
	3		One pupil wide and fixed
	2		Pupil or corneal reflexes absent
	1		Pupil and corneal reflexes absent
	0		Absent pupil, corneal, and cough reflexes
Respiration	4		Not intubated, regular breathing pattern
	3		Not intubated, Cheyne-Stokes breathing pattern
	2		Not intubated, irregular breathing
	1		Breaths above ventilator rate
	0		Breaths at ventilator rate or apnea

tube or tracheostomy are commonly assigned a verbal score of *T* and the total GCS is denoted as the sum of the eye opening and motor scores followed by *T*. Alternatively, the examiner assigns a verbal score based on estimation of the patient's abilities, often determined by noting the patient's response when presented with multiple choices.

The motor portion of the GCS is the most difficult to assess. Response in each extremity is tested, but only the best motor response is used in calculating a total score. The patient is first asked to follow a command such as "Hold up your thumb" or "Wiggle your toes." A patient who does not follow commands with his or her extremities is asked to look up and down. In certain neurologic disorders (such as basilar artery stroke or high cervical spinal cord injury), patients may be unable to follow commands with their extremities but still be awake and aware; assessing the ability to look up and down helps identify these individuals.

If the patient does not follow commands, the next step is to assess the response to pain stimuli in all four extremities. Upper extremity response to pain is described as localization, withdrawal, decorticate (flexor) posturing, or decerebrate (extensor) posturing. An attempt by the patient to push the stimulus away is clearly localization, but the response is not always easily apparent. Reaching across the midline of the body to a stimulus (eg, if the right arm comes up to the left shoulder when a left trapezius squeeze is applied) is scored as localization. An easy way to remember decorticate and decerebrate posturing is that decorticate is "into the core," or flexion, and decerebrate is away from the body, or extension (Figure 12-1).

Decorticate posturing signifies damage in the cerebral hemispheres or thalamus. Decerebrate posturing indicates damage to the midbrain or pons. The presence of posturing or a change from decorticate to decerebrate posturing requires immediate notification of the provider for further evaluation. Motor response to pain in the lower extremities is usually graded as withdrawal or triple flexion. In triple flexion, pain stimulus results in stereotypical flexion of the ankle, knee, and hip. This response can be differentiated from withdrawal by applying the pain stimulus to a different area of the lower extremity (eg, the medial aspect of the calf). If the response is withdrawal, the patient pulls away from the stimulus. If the response is triple flexion, the response is still stereotypical flexion at the ankle, knee, and hip.

Although the GCS is frequently used to monitor hospitalized patients, the information it provides is limited.

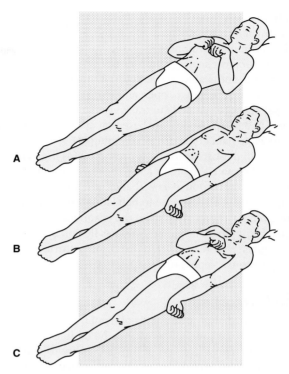

Figure 12-1. Abnormal motor responses. **(A)** Decorticate posturing. **(B)** Decerebrate posturing. **(C)** Decorticate posturing on right side and decerebrate posturing on left side of body. (*Reproduced with permission from Urden LD, Stacy KM, Lough ME:* Thelan's Critical Care Nursing: Diagnosis and Management. *St Louis, MO: Mosby; 2002.*)

Additional assessments are necessary to gain an accurate picture of neurologic functioning; these assessments are based on the type of disease process or injury and the part of the central nervous system (CNS) affected.

FOUR Score

The FOUR score is another validated tool for the assessment of neurological patients. The FOUR score assigns a value of 0 through 4 in each of four categories: eyes, motor, brain stem reflexes, and respirations. The scores in each category are added together to give a total score of 0 to 16. Table 12-2 provides an overview of the FOUR score, but complete instructions are not included; progressive care nurses who utilize this tool should seek additional information to assess verbal cognition. Because of the inclusion of brain stem reflexes and

TABLE 12-2. TESTING OF APHASIA

	Aphasia Type	Naming	Fluency	Comprehension	Repetition
Motor aphasia	Broca's	Unable	Unable	Intact	Unable
	Transcortical motor	Unable	Unable	Intact	Intact
Sensory aphasia	Wernicke's	Unable	Intact	Unable	Unable
	Transcortical sensory	Unable	Intact	Unable	Intact
Conduction aphasia		Unable	Intact	Intact	Unable
Anomic aphasia		Mixed	Intact	Intact	Intact

respiratory pattern, the FOUR score allows the clinician to identify changes in patients, such as those who are comatose with very limited responses.

The highest score given for eye response (4) indicates that the patient is able to track visual movements and also either look up and down, open and close their eyes, or both. The patient who is unable to track visual movement is given a score of 3. Lower scores are based on eye opening to command (2), to pain (1), or no eye opening (0).

The highest score for motor response (4) is given to the patient who can either make a fist, make a peace sign, or give a "thumbs up" response to verbal command. Lower scores are given based on response to pain stimulus. A score of 3 is only given if the patient touches the examiner's hand following pain stimulus. The patient who has flexion in response to pain is given a score of 2, versus extensor posturing (1), or no motor response to pain (0).

Mental Status

Although formal measurements of mental status exist, many acutely ill neurologic patients may be unable to complete these assessments because of limited ability to communicate or decreased level of consciousness. Orientation is the component of mental status most often evaluated in the progressive care unit. Other components of mental status assessment, such as attention/concentration, affect, memory and reasoning, are typically assessed informally by observing the patient throughout daily care. Short-term memory may be evaluated by giving the patient a list of three items and asking him or her to recall them later. However, deficits are often apparent in informal interactions as well.

Difficulty with speech production can be described as *dysarthria* (weakness or lack of coordination of muscles of speech). A patient with dysarthria has slurred speech and is difficult to understand, but the content of the speech is appropriate. Dysarthria represents weakness or loss of coordination of the muscles of speech versus a problem with mental status. However, dysarthria often becomes apparent during assessment of mental status and thus is included here.

Difficulty with language can be described as *aphasia*. The two major categories of aphasia are motor (Broca's aphasia and transcortical motor aphasia) and sensory (Wernicke's aphasia and transcortical sensory aphasia). Subtypes of aphasia include conduction (ie, understand but has poor speech repetition) and anomic (ie, cannot express the words they want to say). As shown in Table 12-2 testing for aphasia includes four elements: naming (can the patient name common items?); fluency (is the patient able to produce more than one or two words or sounds?); comprehension (can the patient understand the examiner?); and repetition (can the patient repeat what the examiner states?).

Delirium is an acute alteration in mental status. Delirium is usually rapid in onset, reversible, and is associated with poor clinical outcomes and increased hospitalization costs. Delirium is characterized by acute changes or fluctuations in mental status, inattention, and cognitive changes or perceptual disturbances. Delirium is described as hyperactive (restlessness, agitation) or hypoactive (flat affect, apathy, lethargy, and decreased responsiveness to the environment). Some patients present with a combination of hyperactive and hypoactive delirium.

Dementia is a progressive, irreversible loss of intellectual or cognitive abilities like reasoning, math, or abstract thinking and develops more slowly than delirium. Delirium and dementia are not mutually exclusive; a patient with mild to moderate dementia may exhibit delirium in the unfamiliar environment of the acute care hospital.

Contributing factors to the development of delirium include systemic illness (infection, fever, or metabolic dysfunction), inadequate pain control, electrolyte abnormalities, the administration of medications including benzodiazepines or opioids, sleep deprivation, and withdrawal from alcohol or other substances. Delirium is more common in older patients. The first step in treating delirium is to rule out reversible causes. Nursing strategies to prevent delirium and decrease its effects include reorientation, encouraging progressive mobility, modulating stimulation, providing appropriate cognitive activities, promoting normal sleep-wake cycles, ensuring that assistive devices such as hearing aids and glasses are available, treating pain, and facilitating family presence. Family members are educated about delirium and provided with guidance in how to interact with the patient (speak clearly and directly, provide frequent reorientation, and avoid multiple simultaneous conversations). Restraints are not used unless patient or staff safety is compromised, because they may add to the patient's confusion and apprehension. In addition to environmental controls, medications can sometimes be useful in the management of delirium.

Patients with organic brain disease, regardless of specific diagnosis, often exhibit challenging behaviors. Examples include agitation, emotional liability, and disinhibition. This can be very disconcerting to family members, especially when the patient has not exhibited these behaviors previously. Dealing with agitated, confused patients can be frustrating for staff as well. Although medication administration may be necessary to keep the patient safe, many medications alter neurologic assessment, delay recovery, or even worsen symptoms. Environmental strategies such as decreasing noise and distractions can be very effective and are always used first. If medications are required, they are combined with environmental strategies and used at the lowest dose possible for the shortest time possible.

Motor Assessment

Motor assessment includes muscle size, tone, strength, and involuntary movements such as tics or tremors. Motor function is assessed in each extremity and evaluated for symmetry. In patients who are able to follow commands, pronator drift is an excellent indicator of upper extremity motor function. To assess pronator drift, instruct the patient to close his

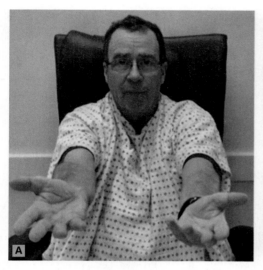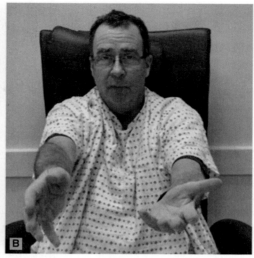

Figure 12-2. Assessment of pronator drift. Normal **(A)** and pronator drift **(B)**. The patient is asked to hold his or her arms outstretched with the palms supinated and eyes closed. If weakness is present, the weak arm gradually pronates and drifts downward.

or her eyes and raise his or her arms with the palms facing the ceiling. A normal response is for the patient to maintain this position until told to stop. An abnormal response is when the arm drifts downward, or the palms rotate inward toward the body (pronation). Depending on the severity of weakness, the affected side may drift away from its initial position quickly or slowly, or the palm may simply begin to pronate (Figure 12-2).

Further assessment of upper extremity strength involves testing the deltoids, biceps, triceps, and grips. Lower extremity testing includes the hamstrings, quadriceps, dorsiflexion, and plantar flexion. Strength is rated on a 5-point scale (Table 12-3). In patients who do not follow commands, motor assessment consists of first observing the patient for spontaneous movement. If necessary, a pain stimulus is applied and the patient's response is observed. The response is graded numerically as part of the GCS or FOUR score, but may also be described as purposeful, nonpurposeful, or no response.

In an awake, alert patient, complete motor assessment includes testing of coordination, an indicator of cerebellar function. Common testing mechanisms include assessment of rapid alternating movements, finger-to-nose testing, and the heel slide test. To test rapid alternating movements, ask

the patient to supinate and pronate his or her hands as quickly as possible. In finger-to-nose testing, the patient is instructed to alternately touch his or her nose, then the examiner's finger. To assess the lower extremities, ask the patient to run the heel of his or her foot up and down the shin of the opposite leg. Patients with cerebellar dysfunction display decreased speed and accuracy on these tests.

Sensation

Sensory assessment is performed with the patient's eyes closed. Documentation of comprehensive sensory assessment is best accomplished using a dermatome chart (Figure 12-3). Areas of abnormal sensation can be marked and tracked over time. There are three basic sensory pathways: pain/temperature, position/vibration, and light touch. Light touch is the pathway most often assessed in the progressive care unit, but may be preserved even if lesions of the spinal cord exist because of overlapping innervation. Because most patients with intracranial lesions report altered sensation in an entire extremity or one side of the body, assessment of light touch is likely to identify these patients. Ask the patient to close his or her eyes, and lightly touch each extremity working distal to proximal. Trunk and facial sensation is also assessed.

When a more comprehensive assessment is indicated, testing for pain and position sense provides useful information. A cotton tip applicator with a wooden stem can be broken and used; the end with the cotton is dull and the broken end is sharp. Touch the patient's skin lightly in a random pattern and ask the patient to identify the sensation as sharp or dull. Two seconds should elapse between stimuli. To test position sense, or proprioception, move the patient's index finger or big toe up or down by grasping the digit laterally over the joints. Provide an example of both "up" and "down"

TABLE 12-3. EVALUATION OF MUSCLE STRENGTH

Grade	Definition
0	No movement
1	Muscle contraction only (palpated or visible)
2	Active movement within a single plane (gravity eliminated)
3	Active movement against gravity
4	Active movement against some resistance
5	Active movement against full resistance (normal strength)

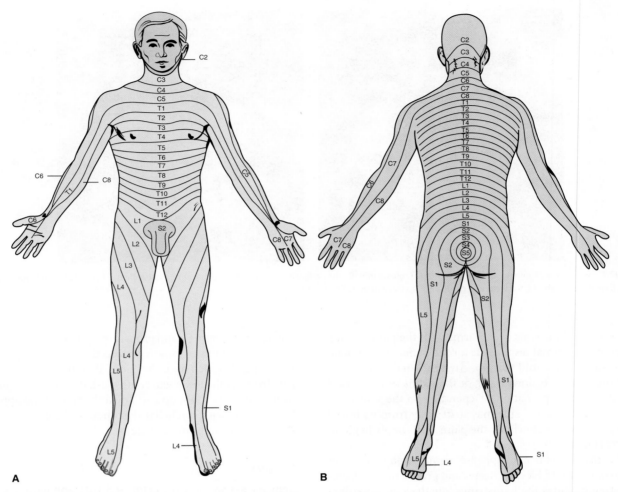

A   **B**

Figure 12-3. Dermatomes. **(A)** Anterior view. **(B)** Posterior view. (*Reproduced with permission from Urden LD, Stacy KM, Lough ME: Thelan's Critical Care Nursing: Diagnosis and Management. St Louis, MO: Mosby; 2002.*)

positions prior to testing. Repeat these movements in a random order, with the patient's eyes closed, and ask the patient to identify whether the joint is up or down. Always return to the neutral position between movements and carefully grasp the digit to avoid giving the patient clues.

Cranial Nerve Assessment and Assessment of Brain Stem Function

Assessment of the cranial nerves provides an indication of the integrity of the nerves themselves and of brain stem function. A screening examination based on pupillary response and protective reflexes (corneal, gag, cough) is conducted on all patients. Beyond that, the assessment is often customized to the individual based on pathology and the ability to participate in a more comprehensive examination. Patients with brain stem, cerebellar, or pituitary lesions merit more extensive assessment because of the proximity of the cranial nerves to these structures. The assessments noted later are the most commonly performed tests of cranial nerve function in the progressive care unit. Table 12-4 describes the primary function of the 12 cranial nerves.

TABLE 12-4. CRANIAL NERVE FUNCTION

Nerve	Function
I. Olfactory	Sense of smell
II. Optic	Visual fields, visual acuity
III. Oculomotor	Most extraocular eye movements, ability to elevate eyelid, muscular contraction of the iris in response to light
IV. Trochlear	Eye movement down and toward the nose
V. Trigeminal	Facial sensation, including cornea, nasal mucosa, and oral mucosa; muscles of chewing and mastication
VI. Abducens	Lateral eye movement
VII. Facial	Facial muscles, including eyelid closure; taste in anterior two-thirds of the tongue; secretion of saliva and tears
VIII. Vestibulocochlear	Hearing and equilibrium
IX. Glossopharyngeal	Gag reflex, muscles that control swallowing and phonation; taste in posterior third of tongue
X. Vagus	Salivary gland secretion; vagal control of heart, lungs, and gastrointestinal tract
XI. Accessory	Sternocleidomastoid and trapezius muscle strength
XII. Hypoglossal	Tongue movement

Pupil Size and Reaction to Light

Assessment of pupil size and reaction to light is performed in all patients and provides information about the function of cranial nerves II (optic) and III (oculomotor). Pupils are assessed for size (measured in millimeters), shape, and reaction to light.

The pupillary light reflex can be scored objectively using a pupillometer or subjectively by a nurse observing the pupil change in reaction to light. Assessment of pupil size and reactivity may vary depending on the person performing the test. A pupillometer can help remove the subjectivity of the test. It is a noninvasive, handheld device that is used to provide an objective measurement of pupil size before and after a light stimulus, as well as the pupillary reactivity to light. The pupillometer is capable of providing automated measurement of one pupil at a time and therefore may not be an adequate substitute for evaluating the presence of anisocoria (unequal pupils). However, after completing paired measurements of both pupils within 30 seconds, the device displays data that allow for comparison of pupillary size and reaction.

Both eyes are tested for direct and consensual response. To test direct pupillary response, shine a light directly into one eye and observe the response of the pupil in that eye. A normal response is brisk constriction followed by brisk dilation when the light is withdrawn. To test for consensual pupillary response, shine a light into one eye and observe the pupil of the other eye. It should constrict and dilate similarly. Assessing both direct and consensual response provides information about which cranial nerve (optic or oculomotor, and left or right) is affected. Certain medications can affect pupil size and reactivity; for example, atropine can dilate the pupils and narcotics can cause them to become very constricted. Pupillary changes are often seen late in the course of neurologic decline as increased intracranial pressure (ICP) leads to compression or stretching of cranial nerve III.

Corneal Reflex or Facial Movement/Sensation

The corneal reflex evaluates cranial nerves V (trigeminal) and VII (facial). This test is classically performed by assessing if the patient blinks when the examiner rapidly moves a finger toward the face (a.k.a., blink to threat). A drop of sterile saline applied to the eye can also be used as a stimulus; cotton wisps are avoided to reduce the risk of corneal abrasions. In alert patients, assessment of facial movement and sensation indicate deficits in cranial nerves V and VII. Movement is assessed by asking the patient to smile, puff out his cheeks with air, and raise his eyebrows. Assessment of facial sensation includes all three branches of cranial nerve V (the trigeminal nerve). Touching the forehead, cheek, and mandible can test the three distributions. Patients with cranial nerve VII dysfunction are unable to close the eyelid on the affected side. Strategies to prevent corneal injury in such patients include the use of lubricating drops and ointments or taping the lid closed.

Gag and Cough Reflexes

The ability to swallow and the gag reflex are controlled by cranial nerves IX (glossopharyngeal) and X (vagus). To assess the gag reflex in a conscious patient, first explain the procedure and be sure the patient does not have a full stomach. Ask the patient to open his mouth and protrude his tongue (this also provides partial assessment of cranial nerve XII, the hypoglossal nerve). Observe the palate for bilateral elevation when the patient says "ahhh." If the palate does not elevate symmetrically, lightly touch the back of the throat with a tongue blade and observe the response. Both the left and right sides should be tested. To assess the gag reflex in an unconscious patient, use a bite block to keep the patient's teeth separated, then stimulate the back of the throat with a suction catheter or tongue blade. Forward thrusting of the tongue and sometimes the head indicates an intact gag reflex. The cough reflex is also controlled by cranial nerves IX and X, and can be assessed by noting spontaneous cough or cough in response to suctioning.

Extraocular Eye Movements

Extraocular eye movements are controlled by muscles innervated by cranial nerves III, IV, and VI. To test extraocular movements, the patient is asked to follow an object (usually the examiner's finger) through six positions (Figure 12-4). A normal response consists of the eyes moving in the same direction, at the same speed, and in constant alignment (conjugate eye movement). Abnormal eye movements include nystagmus (a jerking, rhythmical movement of one or both of the eyes) or an extraocular palsy (eye movement in one or both eyes is inhibited in a certain direction). Mild nystagmus with extreme lateral gaze may be normal. Dysconjugate gaze, in which the eyes are not aligned, is an abnormal finding.

Vital Sign Alterations in Neurologic Dysfunction

Vital sign changes due to central nervous system dysfunction occur because of direct brain stem injury, decreased cerebral perfusion, or interruption of nerve pathways. Decreased perfusion causes ischemia and the body's response is to increase the blood pressure in an attempt to provide more nutrients to the brain. Hypotension is rarely seen as an early response to the primary brain injury. However, hypotension is observed in the terminal stages of brain stem dysfunction and in patients with spinal cord injury due to of loss of sympathetic tone. Abnormalities in heart rate and rhythm are common, and can be a cause of neurologic decline due to clot formation or inadequate cardiac output, or be a symptom of neurologic dysfunction (such as ST-segment abnormalities following subarachnoid hemorrhage). Respiratory patterns vary widely. Some of the more common patterns are shown in Figure 12-5. It is more important to determine if the patient is ventilating adequately than to determine the specific pattern. Temperature is carefully monitored in patients with acute neurologic dysfunction, because hyperthermia (regardless of infectious or noninfectious etiology)

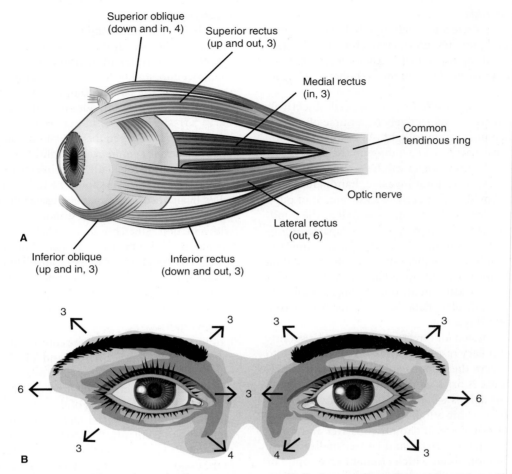

Figure 12-4. Extraocular eye movements. **(A)** Extraocular muscles. The eye movement controlled by the muscle is noted in parentheses, along with the associated cranial nerve supply. **(B)** The six cardinal directions of gaze and associated cranial nerves. (*Reproduced with permission from Urden LD, Stacy KM, Lough ME:* Thelan's Critical Care Nursing: Diagnosis and Management. *St Louis, MO: Mosby; 2002.*)

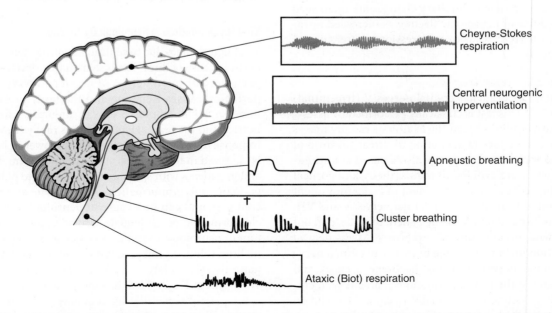

Figure 12-5. Abnormal respiratory patterns associated with increased ICP. Cheyne-Stokes respiration, arising from deep inside the cerebral hemispheres and basal ganglia; central neurogenic hyperventilation, from lower midbrain to middle pons; apneustic breathing, from middle to lower pons; cluster breathing, from upper medulla; and ataxic (Biot) respiration, from medulla. (*Reproduced with permission from Barker E:* Neuroscience Nursing: A Spectrum of Care. *St Louis, MO: Mosby; 2002.*)

causes increased cerebral metabolic demand. Hypothermia can result from injury to the brain stem or spinal cord.

Cushing response refers to a triad of vital sign changes seen late in the course of neurologic deterioration. The classic triad is marked by widened pulse pressure, bradycardia, and an irregular respiratory pattern. Cushing response is of minimal value in identifying early, significant changes in the patient's condition, but it is useful to be alert for components of Cushing response (eg, systolic hypertension or change in respiratory pattern).

DIAGNOSTIC TESTING

Diagnostic testing includes imaging, laboratory testing, ultrasound, electroencephalography, direct measurement, and the physical examination. The three most common forms of imaging include computed tomography (CT), magnetic resonance imaging (MRI), and angiography.

Computed Tomography (CT)

Head (brain) and neck CT is a common diagnostic tool when neurologic dysfunction is suspected. An x-ray beam moves in a 360° arc and a detector measures penetration of the x-ray beam into tissue. Penetration of the x-ray beams vary based on tissue density. The computer translates the collected x-ray beams into a series of finely cut pictures showing bony structures, CSF, and brain tissue. Bone appears white because it is most dense. CSF and air appear black because of their low density. Brain tissue appears in varying shades of gray. The appearance of recent intracranial bleeding is white; over time the color darkens as the blood breaks down. CT scans are quick, noninvasive, and easy to perform, and can identify most causes of acute neurologic deterioration, including bleeding, significant edema, and hydrocephalus. Acute bleeding and bony abnormalities such as fractures are better visualized with CT versus MRI.

Computed tomography scanning can be performed with a contrast medium to allow for better visualization of lesions such as tumors, abscesses, or vascular abnormalities. CT angiography (CTA) uses scanning during intravenous (IV) contrast administration to allow visualization of cerebral blood vessels. CTA is useful in the diagnosis of cerebral vascular anomalies, such as aneurysms or narrowed vessels. A three-dimensional reconstruction of the cerebrovasculature can be created from the images by using a special computer program.

During CT, the patient is placed on a narrow table that is moved up into a donut-shaped gantry. Patient movement causes blurry images; therefore, sedation may be required for patients who are unable to lie still. In patients who receive contrast, assessment of renal function (blood urea nitrogen, creatinine, glomerular filtration rate) is essential because the contrast agent can cause acute kidney injury, especially if the patient is dehydrated or has preexisting renal compromise, or is receiving other nephrotoxic agents. Because the administration of iodinated contrast medium has been associated with lactic acidosis, metformin is discontinued if contrast administration is anticipated.

The primary risks of CT scans result from the use of contrast. Patients with a history of allergic reaction to contrast or iodine require premedication. If contrast dye is administered, IV fluids are given before and after the study to decrease the risk of contrast-induced nephropathy (CIN). For more on CIN see Chapter 15, Renal System.

Magnetic Resonance Imaging

Magnetic resonance imaging offers greater anatomic detail than CT scanning without using ionized radiation. The patient is placed in a strong magnetic field and controlled bursts of radio pulse waves are delivered, causing protons within atomic nuclei to resonate. The radiofrequency signals emitted by the resonating nuclei are measured and used to construct images. Cross-sectional images can be obtained in coronal, sagittal, and oblique planes. A contrast agent is sometimes administered, and highlights areas where the blood-brain barrier is disrupted. MRI scans are useful in diagnosing disorders of the brain stem, posterior fossa, and spinal cord, areas that are difficult to fully evaluate with CT. MRI also offers an advantage over CT in the identification of demyelinating disorders such as multiple sclerosis (MS) or neurodegenerative diseases. Specific MRI sequences can be used to detect suspected lesions that cannot be seen on CT, such as early cerebral infarction and intramedullary tumors. Magnetic resonance angiography (MRA) uses a specialized computer program to highlight the cerebral vasculature. MRA is useful in the evaluation of suspected arteriovenous malformations (AVMs), aneurysms, and cavernous angiomas. The time requirement for MRI scans is typically longer than that of CT scans, which can be a disadvantage when results are needed to make urgent treatment decisions. In addition, access to the patient is significantly limited during an MRI.

All patients must be screened for the presence of implanted or embedded metal prior to MRI. Metallic objects inside the body may become dislodged or slip in the large magnetic tube and can cause patient injury. Most aneurysm clips are now made of nonferrous material and are safe for MRI; it is important to obtain additional information about the device, including when and where it was placed. Orthopedic hardware may also be safe, depending on the part of the body being imaged and the length of time since the hardware was placed. Patients who are either unable to reliably complete the MRI screening or who have a history of impaled metal fragments or shrapnel must have radiographs taken prior to MRI. The MRI magnet can also damage internally magnetized units, such as cardiac pacemakers, causing them to malfunction. An MRI-safe pacemaker is now available. Programmable shunts, frequently used for long-term management of hydrocephalus, are affected by the MRI and must be reprogrammed following the procedure. Devices such as medication pumps and nerve/spinal cord stimulators may or may not be MRI safe. At minimum, they need to be turned off before and reprogrammed after the procedure. With all devices and implants, it is important to obtain as much information as possible about the device type and when it was placed, and to report this information to the MRI technologist. Many IV pumps and other types of medical equipment contain metal and cannot be taken into the room where the MRI machine is located.

Of note, the same screening precautions apply to the staff member who accompanies the patient to MRI. Any card with a magnetic strip, such as a credit card or even an employee ID, will be damaged by the MRI magnet and is removed. Patient education is important prior to scanning. Patients must be screened closely for any contraindications. In addition, all metal objects, such as jewelry, nonpermanent dentures, prostheses, hairpins, clothing with snaps or zippers, and electrocardiogram (ECG) electrodes with metal snaps must be removed. Transdermal medication patches may also need to be removed. Patients should be advised of the loud "booming" noise of the scanner. Inform patients that the nurse or technician is in full view of them in the scanner and that they can talk to them if they feel uncomfortable on the table. Ensure the safety and comfort of the patient with safety belts and blankets for positioning. Patients who are claustrophobic may need sedation. Open-sided MRI machines are available at some institutions and decrease feelings of claustrophobia. There are no postprocedure interventions associated with MRI. Gadolinium-based contrast agents are sometimes administered in MRI and have been associated with nephrogenic systemic fibrosis (NSF) when given to patients with severe renal insufficiency, so renal function is assessed prior to administration. NSF causes fibrotic changes in the skin and other organs.

Lumbar Puncture

Lumbar puncture (LP) can be performed for diagnostic or therapeutic purposes. Diagnostic indications for LP include measurement of cerebrospinal fluid (CSF) pressure as an estimation of ICP and sampling of CSF for analysis when central nervous system (CNS) infection, inflammation, or subarachnoid hemorrhage is suspected. Therapeutic indications for LP include drainage of CSF and the placement of tubes for medication administration or ongoing CSF drainage. Examples of disease processes in which LP is used for diagnostic or therapeutic purposes include meningitis, MS, Guillain-Barré syndrome (GBS), hydrocephalus, and subarachnoid hemorrhage. Increased ICP is a theoretical contraindication to LP because of the risk for downward herniation of brain tissue due to the pressure gradient created when CSF is removed from the lumbar space. When increased ICP is suspected, a CT scan is performed prior to proceeding with the LP. Other contraindications include coagulopathy or infection in the area of skin through which the needle will be introduced. Although recommendations about duration vary based on the specific medication, anticoagulant and antiplatelet medications are often held when LP is planned.

When performing an LP, the clinician locates the L3 to L4 or L4 to L5 intervertebral space and injects a local anesthetic, then inserts a hollow needle with a stylet into the spinal subarachnoid space. The risk of spinal cord injury is minimal because the actual cord ends at L1 and only nerve roots continue below. Proper patient positioning is very important and patients may require sedation if they are unable to remain still. The LP may be performed with the patient sitting up and leaning forward, but a lateral decubitus position is used for most acutely ill patients. The patient lies on his side with his neck flexed forward and his knees pulled up toward the chest. This position widens the intervertebral space, allowing the needle to pass through more easily. The needle is inserted and the stylet is removed. Flow of CSF confirms that the needle is in the spinal subarachnoid space. A manometer is attached to the needle and used to measure an opening pressure. Pressures greater than 20 cm (200 mm) H_2O are considered abnormal. The amount of CSF drained varies based on the indication for the procedure, with smaller volumes needed for laboratory analysis than for treatment of hydrocephalus. If the purpose of the procedure is administration of medications or placement of a lumbar drain, the medications will be given or the drain will be placed once needle placement is confirmed by CSF flow.

Normal CSF is clear and colorless. Infection and blood can change the appearance of CSF. In infection, CSF may be cloudy owing to white blood cells and bacteria. Blood causes the CSF to be pink, red, or brown. Although some blood may be present if a small vessel was traumatized during needle insertion, this blood clears as more CSF is drained. Blood due to CNS hemorrhage does not clear. Common tests performed on CSF include analysis of cell counts with differential, glucose, protein, lactate, Gram stain, and culture with sensitivities. Special assays may be requested to look for specific inflammatory or demyelinating disease processes. Once the needle is removed, a small self-adhesive bandage is placed over the insertion site.

Postprocedure care varies with practitioner preference, hospital protocol, and whether or not the patient complains of headache, but always includes monitoring the insertion site for bleeding, drainage, or hematoma development. Patients may complain of headache (due to loss of CSF), local pain at the insertion site, or pain radiating to the thigh (if a nerve root was hit during the procedure). Flat positioning and increased fluid intake are sometimes recommended after LP but have not been shown to reduce the incidence of post-LP headache. If headache does occur, these strategies are used in combination with analgesic administration. If the headache persists despite positioning and fluids, an autologous blood patch may be used to stop continued CSF leakage.

Cerebral (Catheter) Angiography

Although CTA and MRA are commonly used to assess the cerebrovasculature, catheter angiography is the standard. Digital subtraction angiography (DSA) is angiography of the cerebral vasculature and is similar to cardiac catheterization. Angiography can be performed for both diagnostic purposes and therapeutic intervention. Blockages or abnormalities of the cerebral circulation can be visualized, aiding in the diagnosis of vascular malformations (such as aneurysms or AVMs) and arterial stenosis. Angioplasty (with or without stent placement) can be performed for narrowed cerebral vessels. Blood vessels can also be therapeutically embolized; this is sometimes done to decrease blood supply to a tumor prior to surgical resection or as treatment for an aneurysm.

During cerebral angiography, a catheter is placed in the femoral or brachial artery and threaded up into the carotid or vertebral arteries, and a radiopaque contrast material is injected. The flow of the contrast material is tracked using radiographic films and fluoroscopy. Patients are kept NPO for 6 hours prior to nonemergent angiography. Coagulation studies are checked on all patients because coagulopathy is a relative contraindication to cerebral angiography. Many patients require sedation during the procedure. General anesthesia may be needed for uncooperative patients because the risk of vessel injury is increased if the patient moves his or her head during the procedure.

Potential complications include neurologic deficit due to injury to an intracranial vessel, allergic reaction to contrast, hematoma formation at the site of catheter insertion, vessel injury (dissection), retroperitoneal bleeding, and vessel spasm following injection of contrast. All patients undergoing cerebral angiography receive hydration because of the large amount of contrast agent used.

Following angiogram, patients are typically kept on bed rest with the head of bed flat to help prevent hematoma formation at the puncture site. In some cases, a special arterial closure device is used to promote clot formation and allow quicker mobilization, typically after about 2 hours. The amount of time the patient must remain flat is reflected in the post-angiography orders. The arterial puncture site is monitored frequently for development of a hematoma, and the neurovascular status of the limb is also checked. Careful monitoring of vital signs and neurologic examination aids in the detection of intra- or extracranial emboli or hemorrhage.

Transcranial Doppler Ultrasound

Transcranial Doppler (TCD) ultrasound studies allow the practitioner to measure the velocity of blood flow. TCD uses ultrasonic waves projected through the thinner parts of the skull bone and directed toward the major vessels. Structures within the skull are differentiated based on how much of the wave is reflected back to the probe. A Doppler effect is created when the probe detects moving structures, like red blood cells in a blood vessel. The velocity of blood flow can be calculated. TCDs are noninvasive and can be done at the patient's bedside. TCDs are used at many institutions to aid in the detection of vasospasm after aneurysmal subarachnoid hemorrhage.

Electroencephalography

The electroencephalogram (EEG) is a measurement of the brain's electrical activity. EEG is performed by attaching a number of electrodes to standard locations on the scalp. These electrodes are attached to a recorder, which amplifies and records the activity. EEG is useful in identifying seizure disorders, determining the anatomic origin of seizures, and evaluating causes of coma (structural vs metabolic).

A routine EEG usually lasts 40 to 60 minutes with a portable machine for bedside use. The patient is instructed to lie still with his or her eyes closed. A mild sedative may be prescribed for restless or uncooperative patients, but the interpreter of the EEG must be aware of this because medications may cause changes in the recording. Documentation during the study is done by the technician and may include changes in blood pressure, changes in level of consciousness, medications the patient is currently taking or has taken within 48 hours, patient movement or posturing, and any noxious stimuli introduced. It is best to plan nursing care around the time of the test so that no interventions are done during this examination. When the EEG is complete, the electrodes are removed and any medications that were held prior to the study are resumed.

In patients with symptoms that suggest seizure activity, such as intermittent twitching or fluctuating mental status, a prolonged EEG may be ordered in an attempt to correlate the symptoms with EEG findings. This type of EEG often lasts up to 24 hours and requires the nurse to note any occurrences of the symptom or behavior thought to represent possible seizure activity.

Continuous EEG monitoring is used to guide treatment in patients with status epilepticus. Patients with status epilepticus are transferred to the intensive care unit for management because invasive airway management and continuous infusions of medications are typically required. Continuous EEG monitoring is also used in the diagnosis and management of intractable or difficult-to-control seizures, usually in conjunction with video monitoring. Continuous monitoring can also be helpful in identifying non-epileptic seizures.

Electromyography/Nerve Conduction Studies

Electromyography (EMG) evaluates the electrical activity of skeletal muscle during movement and rest. Nerve conduction studies (NCSs) evaluate peripheral nerve function by measuring the transmission of electrical impulses after stimulation. Conditions in which EMG may aid diagnosis include myopathies and neuropathies, myasthenia gravis (MG) (in which the neuromuscular junction is affected), and GBS. The patient may experience some pain related to insertion of the needle electrodes.

INTRACRANIAL PRESSURE

The skull in adults is a partially closed, nondistensible compartment that contains three components: brain parenchyma

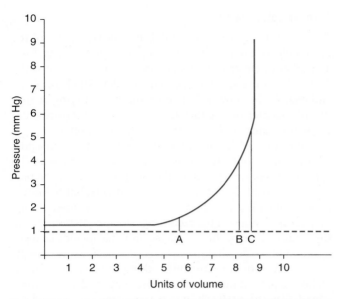

Figure 12-6. Intracranial volume-pressure curve. **(A)** Pressure is normal, and increases in intracranial volume are tolerated due to compensatory mechanisms. **(B)** Increases in volume may cause increases in pressure. **(C)** Small increases in volume may cause large increases in pressure (compensatory mechanisms have been exceeded). (*Reproduced with permission from Urden LD, Stacy KM, Lough ME: Thelan's Critical Care Nursing: Diagnosis and Management. St Louis, MO: Mosby; 2002.*)

(80%), blood (10%), and CSF (10%). The Monro-Kellie hypothesis suggests that to maintain a constant intracranial volume, an increase in any of the three components must be accompanied by a decrease in one or both of the other components. If this reciprocal decrease does not occur, ICP rises. Neuroscience researchers have questioned this hypothesis. The body is able to partially compensate for an increase in intracranial volume by displacement of intracranial venous blood, decreased production of CSF, arterial vasoconstriction, or displacement of CSF into the spinal subarachnoid space. ICP rises when these compensatory mechanisms fail (Figure 12-6).

Compliance, also called cerebral autoregulation, refers to the change in volume needed to result in a given change in pressure and reflects the effectiveness of the compensatory mechanisms. With decreased compliance, a small increase in volume results in a large increase in ICP. Compliance is based on several factors, including the amount of volume increase and the time over which the increase occurs. Smaller increases in volume result in less increase in pressure. Increases in volume that occur over a long period of time are better tolerated than rapid increases because there is time for compensation to occur. Older adults typically have increased compliance because of cerebral atrophy. Increased ICP can result in cerebral hypoperfusion, ischemia, herniation, and eventually death.

Causes of Increased Intracranial Pressure

Increased ICP occurs as a result of cerebral edema, mass lesions, increased intracranial blood volume, or increased

amounts of CSF. These factors often occur in combination. Pain, poor patient positioning (head and neck alignment), and nursing interventions such as suctioning have been associated with an increase ICP.

Cerebral Blood Flow

The brain cannot store oxygen or glucose in significant quantities. Therefore, constant blood flow is required to maintain cerebral metabolism. If cerebral blood flow (CBF) is insufficient, brain cells do not receive sufficient substrate to function and will eventually die. CBF is determined by blood pressure and cerebral vascular resistance.

Autoregulation refers to the ability of cerebral blood vessels to maintain consistent CBF by dilating or constricting in response to changes in blood pressure. Vasodilation occurs in response to decreased blood pressure; increased blood pressure results in vasoconstriction. In persons without neurologic disease, autoregulation allows consistent CBF when mean arterial pressure is 60 to 160 mm Hg. In the injured brain, the autoregulatory response becomes less predictable. When autoregulation is impaired, CBF becomes dependent on systemic arterial pressure.

Cerebral vascular resistance can also be altered through chemoregulatory processes. An increase in the pressure of arterial carbon dioxide ($Paco_2$) produces a lower extracellular pH and causes dilation of cerebral vessels. Conversely, a decrease in $Paco_2$ raises pH and results in cerebral vasoconstriction. Vasodilation also results from Pao_2 levels less than 50 or a buildup of metabolic by-products such as lactic acid. Other factors can decrease cerebral vascular resistance and thus alter CBF, including certain anesthetic agents (halothane, nitrous oxide), sodium nitroprusside, and some histamines.

Cerebral perfusion pressure (CPP) is a measurement of the pressure at which blood reaches the brain. CPP is an indirect reflection of CBF. It is calculated by subtracting ICP from MAP (CPP = MAP − ICP). Decreased CPP occurs as the result of an increase in ICP, a decrease in MAP, or both. A CPP of at least 50 to 70 mm Hg is necessary for adequate cerebral perfusion in adults. There is ongoing debate about where the arterial line transducer should be leveled when managing CPP. Some practitioners level the arterial line transducer at the foramen of Monro when calculating CPP to reflect the MAP in the cerebral vasculature versus systemic MAP, while others level the transducer at the phlebostatic axis. Follow institutional procedure to ensure consistency.

Cerebral Edema

Cerebral edema is an abnormal accumulation of water or fluid in the intracellular or extracellular space, resulting in increased brain volume. Vasogenic edema results from increased capillary permeability of the vessel walls, which allows plasma and protein to leak into the extracellular space. Cytotoxic edema occurs when fluid collects inside the cells due to failure of cellular metabolism. This causes further breakdown of the cell membrane. Cytotoxic edema can lead to capillary damage, which then results in vasogenic edema.

Mass Lesion
Mass lesions (space-occupying lesions) in the brain parenchyma include brain tumors, hematomas, and abscesses. In addition to raising ICP, mass lesions contribute to ischemia by compression of cerebral vessels.

Increased Blood Volume
Venous outflow obstruction can result from compression of the jugular veins (neck flexion, hyperextension, rotation), causing an increase in intracranial blood volume. Increased intrathoracic pressure or increased intra-abdominal pressure (Trendelenburg position, prone position, extreme hip flexion, Valsalva maneuver, coughing, tracheal suctioning) also results in venous outflow obstruction. As discussed previously, cerebral vasodilation occurs due to hypoxia, hypercapnia, increased

metabolic demands, drug effects, or increased systemic blood pressure combined with autoregulatory failure; these factors cause an overall increase in intracranial blood volume.

Increased Cerebrospinal Fluid Volume
Approximately 500 mL of CSF is produced every day. CSF normally flows through the ventricular system into the subarachnoid space where it is absorbed by the arachnoid granulations (Figure 12-7). Obstruction of CSF flow, decreased reabsorption of CSF, or increased production leads to increased intracranial CSF volume (hydrocephalus). Hydrocephalus is referred to as communicating or noncommunicating (also called obstructive). In meningitis or subarachnoid hemorrhage, the arachnoid granulations may become clogged with cellular debris; this impairs CSF absorption and leads to communicating hydrocephalus. An example of noncommunicating hydrocephalus is obstruction of CSF flow due to a tumor or cyst in the third ventricle of the brain.

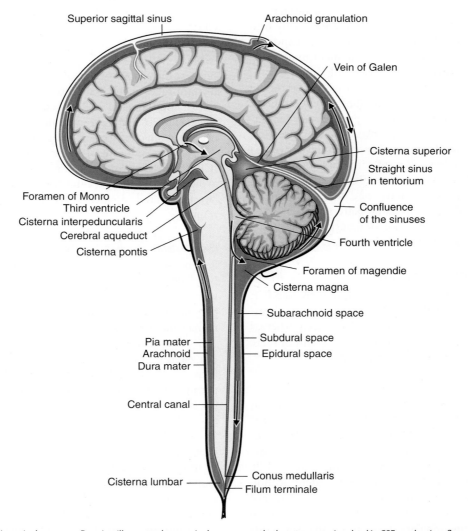

Figure 12-7. Flow of CSF/ventricular system. Drawing illustrates the ventricular system and other structures involved in CSF production, flow, and reabsorption. Arrows indicate the normal direction of flow of CSF. (*Reproduced with permission from Novack CR, Demarest RJ. Meninges, ventricles, and cerebrospinal fluid. In: The Nervous System: Introduction and Review. New York, NY: McGraw-Hill; 1986.*)

Clinical Presentation

Early signs of increased ICP include confusion, restlessness, lethargy, disorientation, headache, nausea and/or vomiting, and visual abnormalities such as diplopia. Change in level of consciousness is the most important indicator of elevated ICP. The patient may become unable to follow commands and develop motor deficits; abnormal posturing is an ominous sign. Changes in vital signs may occur. Increased systolic blood pressure is the body's attempt to maintain cerebral perfusion. As ICP worsens, alterations in heart rate or respiratory pattern may also emerge. Pupillary changes are usually late signs of increased ICP. Any of these signs and symptoms require immediate provider notification. Unless the cause of elevated ICP is known, a CT scan is ordered to evaluate for mass lesions (tumor, blood clot) or hydrocephalus. Invasive ICP monitoring devices are discussed in Chapter 20, Advanced Neurologic Concepts.

Herniation

Prolonged elevation of ICP may result in cerebral herniation. Folds in the dura mater divide the intracranial cavity into several compartments. Herniation is the distortion and displacement of the brain from one compartment to another, which damages structures and decreases CBF through compression. Classic signs associated with herniation reflect pressure on the brain stem and surrounding structures. Level of consciousness deteriorates, and the patient may demonstrate decorticate or decerebrate posturing. Compression or stretching of the oculomotor nerves (cranial nerve III) impairs pupil constriction and results in a large nonreactive pupil on one side. As compression continues, the other pupil also becomes large and nonreactive and vital sign changes (Cushing response, altered respiratory pattern) occur. When any of these classic signs are noted, emergency action is needed to prevent brain death from occurring.

Principles of Management of Increased ICP

Management focuses on early recognition of increased ICP. Interventions to reduce ICP are typically tiered. Mild or non-acute ICP elevations may be treated less aggressively, whereas aggressive treatment is required if ICP rises suddenly or there is a change in the neurological examination.

Monitoring Neurologic Status

Assess baseline neurologic signs, then reassess frequently and compare to previous findings. Include level of consciousness, coma score, pupillary size and reaction to light, eye movement, and motor and sensory function. Assess vital signs and compare with previous findings to identify trends. Close monitoring of neurologic status facilitates the identification and treatment of complications, such as the development of an epidural or subdural hematoma. In these cases, surgical evacuation of the hematoma may be required. In cases of diffuse cerebral edema, a portion of the skull may be removed to increase compliance and allow the brain to swell outside the contained area of the skull. This procedure is referred to as a craniectomy or decompressive hemicraniectomy.

Adequate Oxygenation and Ventilation

Both hypoxemia and hypercarbia can result in cerebral vasodilation and increased ICP. Hyperventilation is not routinely used to decrease ICP because the resulting decrease in $Paco_2$ may lead to vasoconstriction, reduced cerebral perfusion, and ultimately worsen cerebral ischemia. Controlled hyperventilation is sometimes still used in the setting of impending herniation to "buy time" for other measures to be implemented and take effect.

Blood Pressure and Fluid Management

Management of blood pressure is determined by the level of ICP and CPP. Blood pressure and CPP goals vary slightly based on disease process; in general, the goal is to maintain a CPP of at least 50 to 70 mm Hg. If the patient is hypotensive, infusions of non–glucose-containing fluids are preferred to ensure euvolemia. Vasopressors may be required to maintain CPP.

Positioning

Because the venous system of the brain is valveless, increased intrathoracic or intra-abdominal pressure reduces venous return and increases ICP. In general, the head of the bed is elevated to 30°. Hip flexion is minimized. A bowel regimen is used to avoid constipation and abdominal bloating.

Neck positioning affects venous drainage and can raise ICP. The head and neck are maintained in a neutral position, avoiding flexion, hyperextension, or rotation. Cervical collars are carefully applied to avoid decreasing jugular venous return.

Preventing Increased Cerebral Metabolic Demand

Seizure activity increases cerebral metabolic demand and ICP. The prophylactic use of anticonvulsants during the first week of admission is common in neurologically impaired patients at risk for seizures. Additional information on the management of seizures is included later in this chapter.

Fever increases ICP by increasing metabolic demand. For each elevation of 1°C, cerebral metabolic demand increases by approximately 6%. Methods to normalize temperature include antipyretics and air-or water-filled cooling blankets. Shivering increases metabolic demand and is avoided.

Agitation also increases cerebral metabolic demand. Work with other healthcare providers and the patient's family to maintain a calm, quiet environment. Agitation due to pain is avoided through the use of analgesics. If analgesics or sedatives are used, short-acting agents are preferred because of the importance of ongoing neurological assessment. Careful monitoring of respiration is indicated due to the effect of these medications on ventilation; hypoventilation may cause increased ICP if neurons are deprived of oxygen and glucose.

Cerebrospinal Fluid Drainage

Although CSF drainage via an intraventricular catheter is often used as an intervention to lower ICP, there are no randomized controlled trials supporting this intervention. Additional information on the use of intraventricular catheters for CSF drainage can be found in Chapter 20, Advanced Neurologic Concepts.

Medications to Decrease Cerebral Edema

Osmotic diuretics reduce cerebral edema by pulling extracellular fluid from brain tissue into the blood vessels. Mannitol is the most commonly used agent and is given as a bolus dose of 0.25 to 1 g/kg body weight. Mannitol is administered using a filter because it crystallizes easily. Euvolemia is maintained and electrolytes are closely monitored. Many practitioners also use hypertonic saline (1.8% NaCl or 3% NaCl) to increase serum osmolality and pull water into the vascular space.

Corticosteroids are useful in decreasing cerebral edema associated with intracranial tumors. Steroids are generally not useful in the management of cerebral edema related to TBI or stroke. Potential complications of steroid therapy include gastric irritation or hemorrhage and hyperglycemia.

Additional Treatments for Elevated Intracranial Pressure

Other measures to decrease ICP include continuous infusion of analgesics, sedatives, and/or anesthetic agents, the use of neuromuscular blocking (NMB) agents, and induced barbiturate coma. Patients requiring these interventions are transferred to the intensive care unit for management.

ACUTE ISCHEMIC STROKE

Etiology, Risk Factors, and Pathophysiology

Stroke is now the fifth leading cause of death in the United States and remains one of the top causes of disability worldwide. The brain cannot store oxygen or glucose and therefore requires a constant flow of blood to supply these nutrients. The blood supply to the brain can be altered through several different processes. These include embolism, thrombosis, hemorrhage, and compression or spasm of the vessels. Ischemic stroke due to embolism or thrombus formation accounts for approximately 85% of all strokes. Edema occurs in the area of ischemic or infarcted tissue and contributes to further neuronal cell death.

If ischemia is not reversed, neuronal cell death and infarction of brain tissue occurs. The penumbra is the area of tissue that surrounds the core ischemic area. The penumbra receives some blood flow from adjacent vessels but perfusion is marginal. If CBF is improved, the penumbra may recover.

Risk factors for stroke include hypertension, cardiac disease (coronary artery disease, heart failure, atrial fibrillation, endocarditis, patent foramen ovale, myocardial infarction, carotid artery disease), diabetes, increased age, race (African American), male gender, prior stroke, family

---

ESSENTIAL CONTENT CASE

Acute Ischemic Stroke

A 52-year-old teacher was recently admitted to the progressive care unit for treatment of new onset atrial fibrillation. She has a history of diabetes controlled with diet and oral medications. At 7:15 in the morning, during bedside hand-off of care, the nurses find her slumped against the right bedrail. She lifts her head to look at them when they call her name, but is unable to speak, follow commands, or move her right arm.

The patient's blood glucose is 142. Her vital signs are: HR 110 beats/min and irregular, BP 158/92 mm Hg, RR 16 breaths/min, oxygen saturation 96% on room air.

Case Question 1: What actions should the nurses take?
The night shift nurse last checked on the patient about an hour ago, at 6:15 AM. After obtaining a stat head CT, which revealed no bleeding and reviewing inclusion/exclusion criteria, the acute stroke team determines that the patient is an appropriate candidate for recombinant tissue plasminogen activator (rtPA). The initial bolus is administered at 8:00 AM, followed by the infusion.

Case Question 2: How often should VS and neurological assessment be performed for a patient who has received rtPA for acute ischemic stroke?
About 30 minutes after starting the rtPA infusion, a bed becomes available in the ICU and the patient is transferred for continued monitoring. She continues to have aphasia, but her arm weakness is resolving (strength 3/5).

Answers
1. The patient appears to be breathing well and is alert, so the first step is to follow institutional guidelines for summoning the acute stroke team. Other priorities include checking a blood glucose level, taking vital signs, and determining the last time that the patient was seen normal.
2. Every 15 minutes for 2 hours after rtPA is administered, then every 30 minutes for an additional 6 hours, then every hour until 24 hours have passed since rtPA was given.

---

history, dyslipidemia, hypercoagulability (cancer, pregnancy, high RBCs, sickle cell disease), smoking, obesity, physical inactivity, alcohol or illicit drugs, and some forms of hormone therapy.

Transient ischemic attack (TIA) is an important warning sign for stroke. With a TIA, the patient develops stroke symptoms that resolve without tissue infarction. Although most resolve within minutes, an extensive workup to identify treatable causes is warranted with any TIA.

The pathophysiology of stroke varies based on the precipitating event. Thrombosis and embolism formation, described later, result in acute ischemic stroke.

Thrombosis

Thrombosis is the most common cause of ischemic stroke and is usually due to atherosclerosis and the formation of plaque within an artery. A thrombus then forms at the site of the plaque and causes brain tissue ischemia along the course of the affected vessel, which results in infarct if not quickly reversed.

Thrombosis because of atherosclerosis of large cerebral vessels results in large areas of infarct. Considerable edema often develops, further increasing ischemia by compressing areas surrounding the infarct. Significant functional deficits are common. If thrombus forms in a smaller branching artery, a lacunar infarct develops. Lacunar infarcts result in smaller areas of neuronal cell death. Deficits are less apparent, unless the infarct is in a crucial area, such as the internal capsule. Patients with a history of atherosclerosis or arteritis are at highest risk for thrombotic strokes. Thrombotic strokes tend to develop during periods of sleep or inactivity, when blood flow is less brisk.

Embolism

Embolism refers to the occlusion of a cerebral vessel, most often by a blood clot but also by infectious particles, fat, air, or tumor fragments. Embolism is often associated with heart disease that results in bacterial vegetations or blood clots; these vegetations or clots are easily detached from the wall or valves of the heart and then travel to the brain, lodging in a cerebral vessel. Chronic atrial fibrillation, valvular disease, prosthetic valves, cardiomyopathy, and atherosclerotic lesions of the proximal aorta are common causes of embolism. Less common causes include atrial myxomas, patent foramen ovale, and bacterial endocarditis. The fragmented substance easily lodges at the bifurcation of the middle cerebral artery, sometimes breaking apart and traveling further into the cerebral vascular system. The onset of an embolic occlusion is rapid, with symptoms that develop without warning.

Clinical Presentation

Symptoms of stroke range from very mild to significant loss of functional abilities. Common signs and symptoms include weakness in an extremity or on one side of the body, sensory changes, difficulty speaking or understanding speech, facial droop, headache, and visual changes. Clinical presentation of stroke varies based on the area of ischemia or infarction. The National Institute of Health Stroke Scale (NIHSS) is often used to evaluate and monitor patients after stroke. NIHSS scores are predictive of stroke severity and outcomes. An overview of the NIHSS scoring system is presented in Table 12-5.

Stroke in a Cerebral Hemisphere

Signs and symptoms occur on the side of the body contralateral to the stroke. Weakness or paralysis occurs in one or both extremities, and sensory loss may be noted. Visual field deficits are also contralateral to the lesion. The patient often displays an ipsilateral gaze preference, in effect "looking to the lesion." The left hemisphere is dominant in nearly 95% of right-handed individuals and over 80% of left-handed individuals. As the

TABLE 12-5. NATIONAL INSTITUTES OF HEALTH STROKE SCALE (NIHSS)

Tested Item	Title	Response and Scores
1A	Level of Consciousness	0—Alert 1—Drowsy 2—Obtunded 3—Coma/unresponsive
1B	Orientation Questions (2)	0—Answers both correctly 1—Answers 1 correctly 2—Answers neither correctly
1C	Response to Commands (2)	0—Performs both tasks correctly 1—Performs 1 task correctly 2—Performs neither
2	Gaze	0—Normal horizontal movements 1—Partial gaze palsy 2—Complete gaze palsy
3	Visual Fields	0—No visual field defect 1—Partial hemianopia 2—Complete hemianopia 3—Bilateral hemianopia
4	Facial Movement	0—Normal 1—Minor facial weakness 2—Partial facial weakness 3—Complete unilateral palsy
5	Motor Function (arm) a. Left b. Right	0—No drift 1—Drift before 5 seconds 2—Falls before 10 seconds 3—No effort against gravity 4—No movement
6	Motor Function (leg) a. Left b. Right	0—No drift 1—Drift before 5 seconds 2—Falls before 5 seconds 3—No effort against gravity 4—No movement
7	Limb Ataxia	0—No ataxia 1—Ataxia in 1 limb 2—Ataxia in 2 limbs
8	Sensory	0—No sensory loss 1—Mild sensory loss 2—Severe sensory loss
9	Language	0—Normal 1—Mild aphasia 2—Severe aphasia 3—Mute or global aphasia
10	Articulation	0—Normal 1—Mild dysarthria 2—Severe dysarthria
11	Extinction or Inattention	0—Absent 1—Mild (loss 1 sensory modality lost) 2—Severe (loss 2 modalities lost)

Additional information is available at: http://www.ninds.nih.gov/disorders/stroke/strokescales .htm.
(Data from Jauch EC, Saver JL, Adams HP, et al: Guidelines for the early management of patients with acute ischemic stroke: a guideline for healthcare professionals from the American Heart Association/American Stroke Association, Stroke 2013 Mar;44(3):870-947.)

dominant hemisphere, it controls language functions and language-dependent memory. Dominant hemisphere strokes often produce receptive, expressive, or global aphasia. Nondominant hemisphere strokes often cause neglect syndromes in which the patient becomes unaware of the environment and even his or her own body on the contralateral side.

Cerebellar or Brain Stem Stroke

Motor and sensory function may be impaired on one or both sides of the body. Loss of equilibrium, decreased fine motor abilities, and nausea/vomiting are typical. Cranial nerve deficits are common and include dysarthria, nystagmus, dysphagia, and decreased cough reflex. Careful evaluation of airway protection and swallowing ability is essential to determine aspiration risk. Patients with severe deficits often require a feeding tube and potentially a tracheostomy. Because cortical injury is not present, patients maintain a normal mental status and level of alertness unless pressure in the posterior fossa leads to disruption of the reticular activating system.

In patients with cerebellar stroke, obstructive hydrocephalus may occur due to occlusion of the ventricular drainage system by edema. This is considered a medical emergency and surgical decompression of the posterior fossa may be necessary and an external ventricular drain may be placed.

Brain stem stroke owing to basilar artery occlusion may result in quadriplegia and loss of facial movements (locked-in syndrome). Cognition is intact, and vertical gaze is maintained. These patients will be able to follow commands to look up or down. Early consultation with a speech language pathologist is recommended for alternative communication strategies.

Diagnostic Tests

The goal of initial diagnostic testing in acute stroke is to rule out intracranial hemorrhage, because treatments for hemorrhagic and ischemic stroke differ significantly. This is typically accomplished by obtaining a noncontrast head CT, which can be quickly and easily obtained, although some centers use MRI for initial testing. Specialized MRI scans (diffusion-weighted imaging, perfusion-weighted imaging) can detect areas of ischemia before they are apparent on CT. MRA detects areas of vascular abnormality, as might be seen with clot due to arterial dissection. Other tests that may be done acutely include cerebral angiography and carotid ultrasound. Transthoracic or transesophageal echocardiography is used to assess cardiac causes of stroke. Hypercoagulable states are detected through laboratory work. All patients who present with stroke receive an ECG, are placed on cardiac monitoring for at least 24 hours, and undergo laboratory evaluation of cardiac biomarkers because of the correlation between cerebrovascular and cardiovascular disease. In addition, conditions that mimic stroke, such as hypoglycemia, must be ruled out.

Principles of Management of Acute Ischemic Stroke

Stroke is a medical emergency and is treated with the same urgency as acute myocardial infarction. Just as "time is muscle" when the heart is ischemic, "time is brain" when cerebral ischemia occurs. The goals of treatment are to restore circulation to the brain when possible, stop the ongoing ischemic process, and prevent secondary complications. Management principles include the following:

Evaluation of Conditions That Mimic Acute Ischemic Stroke

Other conditions may mimic acute ischemic stroke and must be ruled out. The common causes of conditions that may present with stroke signs and symptoms (a.k.a. "stroke mimic") include: seizure, systemic infection (urinary tract infection [UTI] in the elderly), brain neoplasm, hyponatremia, hypo-/hyperglycemia, migraine, and conversion disorders. Hypoglycemia may cause stroke-like symptoms and is easily detected by using a bedside monitor to check blood glucose. Radiologic tests are performed on all patients with signs and symptoms of stroke to rule out intracranial bleeding. Other conditions that may mimic acute ischemic stroke include toxic or metabolic disorders, migraines, seizures, mass lesions such as brain tumors or abscesses, and psychological disorders.

Fibrinolytic Therapy

Fibrinolytic therapy is administered in an attempt to restore perfusion to the affected area. IV administration of rtPA is considered in all patients who meet the inclusion/exclusion criteria (Table 12-6) and can be treated within 3 hours of the onset of symptoms. Patients who can be treated between 3 and 4.5 hours after symptom onset can also receive rtPA, although there are several additional exclusion criteria.

The recommended dose for rtPA is 0.9 mg/kg, with 10% of the total dose given as a bolus over 1 to 2 minutes followed by the remainder of the dose as an infusion over 1 hour. The maximum dose recommended is 90 mg. In a large-scale study, rtPA administration resulted in improved outcomes at 3 months poststroke. There is an increased risk of intracerebral hemorrhage (ICH) following rtPA administration so frequent neurologic assessments are essential. Vital signs and neurologic checks are done every 15 minutes for the first 2 hours, then every 30 minutes for 6 hours, and then hourly until 24 hours following initial treatment. If neurologic deterioration occurs, rtPA is stopped if still infusing, the provider is notified, and a head CT is performed to assess for bleeding. Following rtPA administration, antiplatelet or anticoagulant medicines are avoided for 24 hours. Placement of nasogastric tubes, bladder catheters, and invasive lines is delayed to decrease the risk of hemorrhage.

Endovascular Treatment

Endovascular treatment is an option for the management of acute ischemic stroke at some centers. However, the possibility of intra-arterial treatment should not delay the use of IV rtPA in patients who are eligible to receive it. Available endovascular therapies include intra-arterial fibrinolysis and mechanical clot extraction or disruption. These treatments, guided by cerebral angiography, must be performed by a physician specially trained in interventional neuroradiology and are not available at all centers. Although rtPA is not Food and Drug Administration (FDA) approved for intra-arterial administration, it is sometimes used for patients with middle cerebral artery occlusion who can be treated within 6 hours of the onset of symptoms and are not able to receive IV rtPA. Because medication can be infused directly into the thrombus,

TABLE 12-6. INCLUSION AND EXCLUSION CRITERIA FOR TREATMENT WITH rtPA AFTER ACUTE ISCHEMIC STROKE

Inclusion criteria
- Diagnosis of ischemic stroke causing measurable neurological deficit
- Last known well or symptom onset < 4.5 hours
- Aged ≥ 18 years

Exclusion criteria
- Significant head trauma or prior stroke (< 3 months)
- History of Ischemic Stroke (< 6 weeks)
- Frank hypodensity on CT head scan (≥ 1/3 of the cerebral hemisphere)
- Clinical presentation suggestive of subarachnoid hemorrhage
- History of previous intracranial hemorrhage within 3 months or current intracranial hemorrhage
- Elevated BP (systolic ≥ 185 mm Hg or diastolic ≥ 110 mm Hg) despite aggressive treatment with IV antihypertensive agents (IV nicardipine, IV labetalol, IV hydralazine)
- Therapeutic LMWH dose within 48 hours of stroke symptoms and/or Anti-Xa > 0.3 (DVT prophylaxis dose is not a tPA contraindication)
- Platelet count < 75, 000/mm^3
- INR > 1.7, PT > 15, PTT > 40
- Presence of intra-axial intracranial neoplasm
- Use of direct thrombin inhibitors or direct factor Xa inhibitors within 48 hours of stroke symptoms
- Recent intracranial or intraspinal surgery (< 30 days ago)
- Blood glucose concentration **< 50 mg/dL without correction**

Relative exclusion criteria/Special consideration
- Only minor, non-disabling, and/or rapidly improving stroke symptoms (clearing spontaneously)
- History of stroke between 6 weeks and 3 months with limited parenchymal injury
- Hypodensity on CT head < 1/3 of the cerebral hemisphere
- Pregnancy
- Renal and/or liver disease without abnormal coagulation factors
- Seizure at onset with postictal residual neurological impairments
- Major surgery or serious trauma within previous 14 days
- Recent gastrointestinal or urinary tract hemorrhage (within previous 21 days)
- Recent acute myocardial infarction (within previous 3 months)
- Arterial puncture at a non-compressible site in previous 7 days (example: axillary or subclavian arteries)
- Systemic malignancy with metastasis
- Acute or known bleeding diathesis
- Persistent neurological deficit after correction of hypoglycemia
- Aged < 18 years
- Presence of extra-axial intracranial neoplasm (ie, meningioma)
- Presence of one or more AVMs without evidence of recent bleeding (past 4 weeks) or evidence of mass effect causing focal symptoms
- Cerebral aneurysms > 10 mm in size
- Other known, un-ruptured, or untreated intracranial vascular malformation

Abbreviations: AVM, arteriovenous malformation; BP, blood pressure; CT, CAT scan; INR, international normalized ratio; IV, intravenous; LMWH, low-molecular-weight heparin; PT, prothrombin time; PTT, partial thromboplastin time. New guidelines for ischemic stroke were published in February 2017 but over 90 pages were subsequently retracted in April 2017. Thus, the recommendations published here do not reflect the the 2017 guidelines. The reader is encouraged to update practice recommendations when definitive guidelines for the management of ischemic stroke are published.
Data from Powers WJ, Derdeyn CP, Biller J, et al: 2015 American Heart Association/American Stroke Association Focused Update of the 2013 Guidelines for the Early Management of Patients With Acute Ischemic Stroke Regarding Endovascular Treatment: A Guideline for Healthcare Professionals From the American Heart Association/American Stroke Association, Stroke 2015 Oct;46(10):3020-3035.

smaller doses can be used, making this a treatment option for certain patients with exclusion criteria for IV rtPA (eg, major surgery in the previous 14 days). Mechanical thrombectomy using a special device may improve recanalization rates when used alone or in combination with fibrinolysis. Care of the patient following endovascular treatment for stroke includes standard post-angiogram monitoring, stroke-specific care, and other interventions as ordered by the provider.

Blood Pressure Management

Blood pressure management is essential after acute ischemic stroke because a marked or sudden decrease in blood pressure may significantly decrease cerebral perfusion. The provider may elect to hold the patient's home antihypertensive medications to maximize CBF, especially in the first 24 hours after stroke. For patients who are not eligible for fibrinolytic therapy, blood pressure is not treated emergently unless the systolic blood pressure exceeds 220 mm Hg or the diastolic blood pressure exceeds 120 mm Hg. Because of the risk of hemorrhage, blood pressure management is more stringent in patients who are eligible for or who have received fibrinolytic therapy (Table 12-7).

Management of Increased ICP

Cerebral edema occurs in the area of infarct and may lead to increased ICP. For further discussion of treatment options, refer to the section on ICP. Osmotic diuresis using mannitol and hypertonic saline (up to 23.4% NaCl) may be used to reduce cerebral edema. Hemicraniectomy may be used to allow for expansion of cerebral edema and alleviate increased ICP in patients with large infarcts, particularly those in the area of the middle cerebral artery. Normothermia and mild hypothermia are treatment options depending on resources. However, aggressive treatment of fever is warranted to avoid increases in cerebral metabolic demand.

TABLE 12-7. APPROACH TO BLOOD PRESSURE MANAGEMENT AFTER ACUTE ISCHEMIC STROKE IN PATIENTS WHO ARE CANDIDATES FOR REPERFUSION THERAPY

Patient otherwise eligible for acute reperfusion therapy except that BP is > 185/110 mm Hg
- Labetalol 10-20 mg IV over 1-2 minutes, may repeat 1 time; or
- Nicardipine 5 mg/h IV, titrate up by 2.5 mg/h every 5-15 minutes, maximum 15 mg/h; when desired BP reached, adjust to maintain proper BP limits; or
- Other agents (hydralazine, enalaprilat, etc) may be considered when appropriate
- If BP is not maintained at or below 185/110 mm Hg, do not administer rtPA.

Management of BP during and after rtPA or other acute reperfusion therapy to maintain BP at or below 180/105 mm Hg
Monitor BP every 15 minutes for 2 hours from the start of rtPA therapy, then every 30 minutes for 6 hours, and then every hour for 16 hours.
If systolic BP > 180-230 mm Hg or diastolic BP > 105-120 mm Hg:
- Labetalol 10 mg IV followed by continuous IV infusion 2-8 mg/min; or
- Nicardipine 5 mg/h IV, titrate up to desired effect by 2.5 mg/h every 5-15 minutes, maximum 15 mg/h
If BP not controlled or diastolic BP > 140 mm Hg, consider IV sodium nitroprusside

New guidelines for ischemic stroke were published in February 2017 but over 90 pages were subsequently retracted in April 2017. Thus, the recommendations published here do not reflect the 2017 guidelines. The reader is encouraged to update practice recommendations when definitive guidelines for the management of ischemic stroke are published.
(Data from Jauch EC, Saver JL, Adams HP, et al: Guidelines for the early management of patients with acute ischemic stroke: a guideline for healthcare professionals from the American Heart Association/American Stroke Association, Stroke 2013 Mar;44(3):870-947.)

Glucose Management

Hyperglycemia is associated with worse outcomes after stroke and TBI. Although ongoing research seeks to define the optimal blood glucose target, current recommendations support lowering blood glucose to 140 to 180 mg/dL. Hypoglycemia is deleterious and must be avoided.

Preventing and Treating Secondary Complications

Patients are at significant risk for aspiration following stroke due to difficulty protecting their airway. Decreased level of consciousness, facial weakness, and cranial nerve deficits contribute. Endotracheal intubation is sometimes necessary during the acute phase, and some patients may need a tracheostomy. Dysphagia is very common after stroke, so careful assessment of swallowing ability is indicated before any oral intake. Most hospitals now have dysphagia screening protocols in place that support initial dysphagia screening by nursing staff. Consultation with the speech language pathologist is indicated for patients who fail a nursing bedside dysphagia examination. Placement of a feeding tube may be necessary if the patient is unable to swallow safely.

Deep venous thrombosis (DVT) is a common complication in stroke patients and may lead to pulmonary embolism. Strategies to decrease risk include elastic compression stockings, intermittent pneumatic compression devices, subcutaneous administration of low-dose anticoagulants, and early progression in activity.

In addition to pneumonia and DVT, patients with stroke are at risk for UTI. To reduce this risk, indwelling catheters are used only when medically necessary, the need is assessed daily, and they are removed as soon as possible. In patients without indwelling catheters, urinary retention may occur; methods of evaluation include bedside bladder scanning or catheterization for post-void residual volumes.

Preventing Recurrent Stroke

The use of antiplatelet and anticoagulant medications varies depending on the size of the infarct, presumed etiology, and whether or not the patient received fibrinolytic therapy. Patients are commonly placed on aspirin within 24 to 48 hours after the initial event and the decision to use other antiplatelet or anticoagulant medications is made on an individual basis. Anticoagulation is typically not used in the acute phase of treatment because it increases the risk of hemorrhagic conversion (development of bleeding within the infarcted tissue), but may be used in certain circumstances.

Carotid endarterectomy is the most common surgical procedure to prevent further ischemic strokes, but is not typically performed in the time period immediately following a stroke due to the risk of reperfusion injury and hemorrhage. Stenosis may also be treated with angioplasty, with or without stent placement.

Other strategies to prevent recurrent stroke include statins for dyslipidemia and behavior modification to address risk factors.

HEMORRHAGIC STROKE

Etiology, Risk Factors, and Pathophysiology

Approximately 15% of all strokes are hemorrhagic; either subarachnoid hemorrhage or ICH. In subarachnoid hemorrhage, bleeding into the subarachnoid space occurs, usually as the result of a ruptured aneurysm. Although subarachnoid hemorrhage is a type of stroke, management issues differ significantly from ischemic stroke. Subarachnoid hemorrhage is discussed in Chapter 20, Advanced Neurologic Concepts. Here, hemorrhagic stroke refers to intraparenchymal bleeding (also called ICH).

Hypertension is the most common cause of ICH. Other causes include vascular malformations (AVMs or cavernous malformations), coagulopathy, amyloid angiopathy, tumor, vasculitis, venous infarction, and illicit drug abuse. Amyloid angiopathy is most common in patients older than the age of 70. It is a presumed diagnosis in older patients with repeated ICH, but can only be definitively diagnosed by deposits of beta-amyloid protein found in the vessel walls (usually on autopsy). AVM is a common cause of ICH in younger patients (ages 20-40). AVMs are congenital abnormalities in which a tangled mass of blood vessels is present. Within the AVM, the arterial circulation and venous circulation connect without going through a capillary system. Following resolution of the acute ICH, AVMs are treated with endovascular embolization, surgical resection, or stereotactic radiosurgery.

In addition to direct tissue injury, the hematoma formed by ICH displaces nearby brain tissue and causes ischemia through compression. Edema occurs around the site of hemorrhage. If the ICH occurs deep within the cerebral hemispheres, it can rupture into the ventricle (intraventricular hemorrhage). The mortality rate is higher in hemorrhagic stroke than ischemic stroke.

Clinical Presentation

Intracerebral hemorrhage most often presents with an acute onset of focal neurologic deficits often associated with a sudden severe headache (frequently described as a "thunderclap" headache or the "worst headache of my life"), nausea/vomiting, decreased consciousness, and sometimes seizures. Neurologic deficits vary based on the area of the brain affected and are similar to the focal deficits experienced by patients with acute ischemic stroke.

Diagnostic Tests

Intracerebral hemorrhage is diagnosed using CT scanning or, less commonly, MRI. Tests that may be performed to determine the etiology of the hemorrhage include CTA, MRA, and cerebral angiography.

Principles of Management of Intracerebral Hemorrhage

Initial priorities of care for the patient with ICH include blood pressure control and correction of coagulopathy.

Bleeding can continue or recur for several hours after the initial event, so prompt action is essential. IV medications are often required to treat elevated blood pressure and may be administered intermittently or continuously. Generally the goal is to keep the systolic blood pressure below 140 to 160 mm Hg. Treatment of coagulopathy is based on the underlying cause of abnormal clotting. Fresh frozen plasma, platelets, vitamin K, or prothrombin complex concentrate may be ordered; regardless of the agent used, the goal is rapid correction of coagulopathy.

Operative management may or may not be indicated based on size and location of hemorrhage. Cerebellar hemorrhage may require a suboccipital craniectomy to evacuate the clot and decrease pressure on vital structures. Intraventricular hemorrhage may cause hydrocephalus, which is treated by placement of an external ventricular drain. Antiepileptic medications are recommended for patients who experience a seizure or who show electrographic evidence of seizure on EEG. These agents may also be administered to prevent seizures if the hemorrhage is in a part of the brain associated with seizure risk such as the temporal or frontal lobe.

Similar to patients with acute ischemic stroke, prevention of secondary complications is an essential element of nursing care for patients with ICH. Patients are at risk of aspiration and require careful monitoring of airway clearance, as well as assessment for dysphagia. Additional interventions include meticulous skin care, attention to bowel and bladder management, and strategies to prevent hospital-acquired infections.

SEIZURES

Etiology, Risk Factors, and Pathophysiology

Seizures are rapid, repeated bursts of abnormal electrical activity within the brain that result from an imbalance of excitatory and inhibitory impulses. Signs and symptoms depend on the location of the abnormal activity. A seizure is often a symptom or consequence of an underlying neurologic problem, such as a tumor, hemorrhage, trauma, or infection. Systemic disturbances such as hypoxia, hypoglycemia, drug overdose, and drug or alcohol withdrawal may also cause seizures. Many seizures are considered idiopathic, but treatable causes must be ruled out.

During a seizure, the metabolic demands of the brain for oxygen and glucose increase dramatically. The body tries to keep up with these increased requirements by increasing CBF. If CBF does not keep up with demand, neurons revert to anaerobic metabolism, which leads to secondary ischemia and brain injury.

Clinical Presentation

Clinical presentation varies based on the origin and extent of the brain's abnormal electrical activity. Seizures can be described as focal onset (starting in one area of the cerebral cortex and limited to one hemisphere), generalized onset (rapidly affecting both cerebral hemispheres), or unknown onset.

Focal Seizures

The term focal seizure is preferred over simple partial. If the patient remains aware (with or without the ability to speak) the seizure is termed focal aware. Focal impaired implies that the patient was unaware at some point during the seizure. Focal seizures may present with motor activity such as twitching or jerking in an extremity or one side of the face, sensory symptoms such as an unusual taste or smell, or autonomic sensations such as sweating or vomiting.

Patients with focal seizures may experience an aura (symptoms such as smelling burnt toast) that signal the onset of a seizure. Focal seizures may also present with automatisms (smacking the lips, chewing motions, or fidgeting), purposeless activity such as running or arm jerking, or change in affect such as elation or fear. Focal seizures can progress to a bilateral generalized convulsive seizure.

Generalized Seizures

Generalized seizure replaces the terms *grand mal* and *petit mal*. Generalized seizures are characterized by abnormal electrical discharge that rapidly affects both hemispheres. Motor generalized seizure includes automatism, atonic, clonic, myoclonic, spasm, and hyperkinetic movements (below). Non-motor seizure may include changes in cognitive, emotional, or sensory ability as well as autonomic behaviors.

- *Absence:* Sudden lapse of consciousness and activity that lasts 3 to 30 seconds. Commonly described as a staring spell.
- *Myoclonic:* Sudden, brief muscle jerking of one or more muscle groups. Commonly associated with metabolic, degenerative, and hypoxic causes.
- *Atonic (also called drop attacks):* Sudden loss of muscle tone.
- *Clonic:* Rhythmic muscle jerking.
- *Tonic:* Sustained muscle contraction.
- *Tonic-clonic:* Muscle activity varies between sustained contraction and jerking.

Unknown Onset Seizures

The type of seizure is determined by the first prominent sign or symptom. The term unknown onset seizure is relatively new and used when the practitioner is unable to confidently identify the onset.

Patients are more likely to be injured during a generalized seizure than during a focal seizure and may complain of generalized muscle aches after the seizure stops if convulsions led to sustained muscle activity.

Status Epilepticus

Status epilepticus indicates prolonged or recurring seizures without a return to baseline mental status. The classic definition of *status epilepticus* is a seizure or series of seizures lasting longer than 30 minutes, but treatment is typically instituted much sooner and recent guidelines suggest a definition of seizure activity longer than 5 minutes. Status epilepticus is a medical emergency with a significant mortality rate, higher in the older adults or when the seizure is a symptom of an underlying acute process. There are two primary types of status epilepticus: convulsive status epilepticus and nonconvulsive status epilepticus. In convulsive status epilepticus, seizure activity is readily apparent using clinical observation. In nonconvulsive status epilepticus, no outward clinical seizures may be noted but consciousness is impaired and seizure activity is apparent on EEG.

Diagnostic Testing

Diagnostic testing for patients with seizures may include:

- Laboratory work to identify electrolyte abnormalities, metabolic disorders, or antiepileptic drug levels.
- CT to assess for intracranial processes such as an ICH or tumor.
- MRI to look for structural lesions that may indicate a seizure focus.
- LP when an infectious process (eg, meningitis) is the suspected source of seizure activity.
- EEG to evaluate for seizure activity. One normal EEG does not rule out seizure. Prolonged EEG monitoring may be required.
- Continuous video monitoring in conjunction with continuous EEG recordings correlate clinical phenomena with electrical activity in the brain.
- Intracranial electrodes with continuous EEG monitoring in the evaluation of patients with intractable seizures to identify a focus or foci prior to surgical resection. Intracranial electrodes are inserted via burr holes or a craniotomy.

Principles of Management of Seizures

Management of the patient with seizures focuses on controlling the seizure as quickly as possible, preventing recurrence, maintaining patient safety, and identifying the underlying cause. Observation of seizure type, duration, and any precipitating factors is essential. Following a seizure, patients may experience a period of confusion and altered mental status that slowly resolves. They may complain of a headache or muscle aches. Todd's paralysis describes continued focal symptoms that can persist for up to 36 hours after a seizure. Because of the risk of missing underlying intracranial pathology, patients with focal neurologic deficits following a seizure are diagnosed with Todd's paralysis only after other causes have been ruled out.

Maintaining Patient Safety and Airway Management

From a nursing perspective, the first priority is to protect the patient from injury. Ensure a safe environment during the seizure by clearing objects out of the area. Padded side rails are no longer considered routine care and are indicated only for patients at high risk. During a seizure, attempting to restrain patient movement may result in injury and is avoided.

Airway management assists with maintaining adequate cerebral oxygenation. Maintaining the airway may depend on stopping the seizure. Positioning the patient on his or her side decreases aspiration. Supplemental oxygen is provided. Nothing should be placed in the patient's mouth during a seizure. ECG monitoring, continuous pulse oximetry, and blood pressure monitoring are required in patients with prolonged seizures. Hypoglycemia can induce seizure activity, so a glucose level is checked immediately and treated as appropriate.

Medication Administration for Prolonged Seizures and Status Epilepticus

The average seizure stops within 2 minutes without requiring medication. First-line treatment for patients with prolonged seizures or status epilepticus is administration of a benzodiazepine such as lorazepam. The second medication given is typically levetiracetam, phenytoin, or fosphenytoin. Fosphenytoin is converted to phenytoin in the blood and is preferred because it causes less tissue injury should extravasation occur. Both agents can cause cardiovascular side effects, predominantly treatment-resistant hypotension. The exact mechanism of action for levetiracetam is unknown, but it is generally recognized to stabilize neuronal activity. Cardiac and respiratory status should be closely monitored. If seizure activity continues, the patient will require transfer to the intensive care unit for continuous IV medications. Medications to treat seizures are discussed in more detail in Chapter 7, Pharmacology.

The prolonged muscle activity that occurs with prolonged convulsive seizure activity may cause tissue breakdown and lead to rhabdomyolysis. Serum creatine phosphokinase is elevated and myoglobin may be present in the urine. Hydration is essential to avoid renal dysfunction.

Treatment Options for Patients With Seizures

Many patients require ongoing medication for seizure control. Some common medications include levetiracetam, phenytoin, carbamazepine, oxcarbazepine, valproic acid, lamotrigine, and lacosamide. Approximately two-thirds of patients treated with medication are able to attain good seizure control.

Some patients with seizures uncontrolled by medications may be helped by surgery to remove the seizure focus. These patients most often have seizures originating from the temporal lobe. Selection criteria include intractable seizures that significantly impact quality of life and are uncontrolled by medication, an identifiable unilateral focus of seizure activity, and seizure focus in an area where removal will cause no major neurologic deficit. A craniotomy is used to access and excise the seizure focus. The primary complications are hemorrhage and infection. Patients are kept on their previous seizure medications during the postoperative period. About 50% of patients become seizure free after surgery and an additional 30% experience a significant improvement in seizure control.

For patients with intractable seizures who do not have an identifiable focus, placement of a vagus nerve stimulator (VNS) may be considered. VNS reduces seizure duration, frequency, or intensity by providing intermittent electrical stimulation of the vagus nerve. The exact mechanism of action has not been determined. Roughly one-third of patients with VNS will experience a significant (> 50%) reduction in the number of seizures. Adjunctive therapy with medication is generally indicated.

INFECTIONS OF THE CENTRAL NERVOUS SYSTEM

Meningitis

Meningitis is an acute inflammation of the meninges of the brain and spinal cord. Meningitis can be caused by bacteria, viruses, fungi, or parasites. Risk factors include immunocompromise, trauma, or surgery that disrupts the meninges, and crowded living conditions. Signs and symptoms include fever, headache, neck stiffness, irritability, vomiting, photophobia, altered level of consciousness, seizures, weakness, and cranial nerve deficits. Other signs of meningitis

include Kernig sign (severe pain in the hamstring with knee extension when the hip is flexed 90°) and Brudzinski sign (involuntary flexion of the knees and hips when the neck is flexed). Many patients with meningococcal meningitis have a characteristic rash (petechial rash that progresses to purple blotches). Diagnostic testing includes LP for opening pressure and CSF analysis, blood cultures, and other laboratory tests to look for infection. CT scanning is performed prior to LP in patients with papilledema or focal neurologic findings. Complications of meningitis include hydrocephalus, cerebral edema, and vasculitis. Nursing priorities include management of elevated ICP, implementation of seizure precautions, and prompt administration of antimicrobial therapy. Delays in antimicrobial therapy are associated with worse outcomes. Isolation may be required until the causative organism is identified and treated; notify the infection control practitioner and follow institutional guidelines.

Encephalitis

Encephalitis is inflammation of the brain parenchyma. There are many causes of encephalitis, including arboviruses such as West Nile, but the most common type seen in the United States is encephalitis due to the herpes simplex virus (HSV). HSV encephalitis can result from a new infection, or can represent a reactivation of a preexisting infection. Signs and symptoms include fever, focal or diffuse neurologic changes, headache, and seizures. HSV encephalitis predominately affects the inferior frontal and temporal lobes. Diagnostic testing includes MRI, EEG, and CSF analysis. The diagnosis is often presumed pending specialized testing of the CSF. Empiric therapy is started with an antiviral agent.

Intracranial Abscess

An intracranial abscess is a collection of pus in the brain and can be extradural, subdural, or intracerebral. The infective agent enters the brain through the bloodstream, via an opening in the dura (as may occur with a basilar or open skull fracture or following a neurosurgical procedure), or by direct migration from chronic otitis media, poor dentition, frontal sinusitis, or mastoiditis. Signs and symptoms typically develop over a few weeks and may include headache, seizures, fever, neck pain, focal neurologic signs such as hemiparesis, cranial nerve deficits, and change in level of consciousness. Diagnostic testing includes CT with contrast administration, MRI, EEG, and potentially aspiration of the lesion for culture. Treatment includes prolonged antibiotic therapy (usually 6 weeks) and surgical drainage of the abscess.

NEUROMUSCULAR DISEASES

Although there are a variety of neuromuscular diseases that may result in hospitalization, only a small number of these patients require admission to the progressive care unit. MG,

MS, and GBS often cause respiratory muscle weakness and decreased airway clearance. These patients may be admitted to the progressive care unit for close monitoring of respiratory status. They may also be admitted to ventilator weaning units after initial stabilization in the ICU. In addition, patients with chronic progressive neuromuscular diseases such as amyotrophic lateral sclerosis (ALS) may be admitted to the progressive care unit for management of respiratory failure or other complications.

Myasthenia Gravis

In MG, autoimmune-mediated destruction of acetylcholine receptors results in decreased neuromuscular transmission and muscle weakness. Myasthenia gravis is a chronic disease with periodic exacerbations. Diagnostic testing includes laboratory testing for acetylcholine receptor antibodies, EMG, CT scanning of the chest to evaluate for abnormalities of the thymus, and "Tensilon testing."

Edrophonium chloride (Tensilon) is a short-acting acetylcholinesterase inhibitor that can be administered intravenously. Improvement in symptoms following edrophonium chloride injection is highly suggestive of MG. Adverse effects of edrophonium chloride include bradycardia, asystole, increased oral and bronchial secretions, and bronchoconstriction.

Treatment for acute MG exacerbation includes plasma exchange or IV immunoglobulin in addition to supportive care. Long-term management may include the administration of anticholinesterase medications, thymectomy, or immunosuppression. Priorities of nursing management during an acute exacerbation include close monitoring of respiratory status and prevention of secondary complications.

Multiple Sclerosis

Patients with MS may be admitted to the ICU or progressive care unit with infections, pneumonia, or exacerbation of symptoms (especially neuromuscular respiratory weakness). The typical age of onset is 20 to 50 years and it affects women more than men. One-year mortality rates following an ICU admission are nearly double those for MS patients not admitted to ICU (even after controlling for age and severity of MS).

Guillain-Barré Syndrome

Guillain-Barré syndrome causes progressive muscle weakness, sensory loss, and areflexia due to peripheral nerve demyelination. Symptoms generally start in the lower extremities and ascend. Diagnostic studies include LP and nerve conduction studies. Approximately 25% to 40% of patients require mechanical ventilation. Some patients experience autonomic instability characterized by variations in heart rate and blood pressure. Neuropathic pain related to inflammation and demyelination occurs and requires both pharmacologic and nonpharmacologic treatment. In addition to supportive therapy, patients may receive plasma exchange or IV immunoglobulin. Most patients recover with minimal deficits, but may require weeks to months of hospitalization. Nursing priorities include close monitoring of respiratory status and prevention of complications related to prolonged immobility.

Amyotrophic Lateral Sclerosis

Amyotrophic lateral sclerosis is a progressive disease that affects the motor neurons, causing muscle weakness without affecting sensation or cognition. Patients most commonly present with extremity weakness that is asymmetric and more pronounced distally. Bulbar symptoms such as dysarthria and dysphagia may be present initially, or may develop as the disease progresses. The rapidity of progression varies widely among patients. Eventually, ALS causes respiratory failure due to muscle weakness and decreased airway protection.

Patients with ALS may be admitted to the progressive care unit when airway protection becomes problematic and complications such as pneumonia develop, or if they use assisted ventilation (bilevel positive airway pressure [BiPAP] or mechanical ventilation) at home and require admission for other complications or procedures. Nursing care focuses on decreasing respiratory complications and other complications of immobility, controlling pain, and providing psychological support.

SELECTED BIBLIOGRAPHY

Assessment and Diagnostic Testing

Baumann JJ, Blissitt PA, Stewart-Amidei C. Assessment. In: Bader MK, Littlejohns LR, Olson DM, eds. *AANN Core Curriculum for Neuroscience Nursing*. 6th ed. Glenview, IL: American Association of Neuroscience Nurses; 2016: 63-96.

Bautista C, Cudlip F, Malloy R, Nelson A. Neurodiagnostic tests. In: Bader MK, Littlejohns LR, Olson DM, eds. *AANN Core Curriculum for Neuroscience Nursing*. 6th ed. Glenview, IL: American Association of Neuroscience Nurses; 2016: 97-120.

Chioffi S. Lumbar puncture. In: Wiegand DL, American Association of Critical-Care Nurses, eds. *AACN Procedure for High-acuity, Progressive, and Critical Care*. 7th ed. St. Louis, MO: Elsevier; 2017: 865-872.

D'Andrea A, Conte M, Scarafile R, et al. Transcranial Doppler ultrasound: physical principles and principal applications in neurocritical care unit. *J Cardiovasc Echogr*. 2016;26(2):28-41.

Haymore JB, Patel N. Delirium in the neuro intensive care unit. *Crit Care Nurs Clin North Am*. 2016;28(1):21-35.

McNett M, Amato S, Gianakis A, et al. The FOUR score and GCS as predictors of outcome after traumatic brain injury. *Neurocrit Care*. 2014;21(1):52-57.

Olson DM, Bazil JC. Pupillometer. In: Wiegand DL, American Association of Critical-Care Nurses, eds. *AACN Procedure for High-acuity, Progressive, and Critical Care*. 7th ed. St. Louis, MO: Elsevier; 2017: 880-884.

Sandoval CP. Nonpharmacological interventions for sleep promotion in the intensive care unit. *Crit Care Nurse.* 2017;37(2):100-102.

Schraeder N. Lumbar subarachnoid catheter insertion for cerebrospinal fluid drainage and pressure monitoring. In: Wiegand DL, American Association of Critical-Care Nurses, eds. *AACN Procedure for High-acuity, Progressive, and Critical Care.* 7th ed. St. Louis, MO: Elsevier; 2017: 856-864.

Wijdicks EF. The scope of neurology of critical illness. *Handb Clin Neurol.* 2017;141: 443-447.

Wilson-Pauwels L. *Cranial Nerves: Function and Dysfunction.* 3rd ed. Shelton, CT: People's Medical Pub. House; 2010.

Zhang X, Medow J, Iskandar BJ, et al. Invasive and noninvasive means of measuring intracranial pressure: a review. *Physiol Meas.* 2017;38(8):R143-R182.

Intracranial Pressure

Helbok R, Olson DM, Le Roux PD, Vespa P. Intracranial pressure and cerebral perfusion pressure monitoring in non-TBI patients: special considerations. *Neurocrit Care.* 2014;21(suppl 2):s85-s94.

Lewis LS, Kennedy Madden L, Puccio AM. Intracranial pressure management. In: Bader MK, Littlejohns LR, Olson DM, eds. *AANN Core Curriculum for Neuroscience Nursing.* 6th ed. Glenview, IL: American Association of Neuroscience Nurses; 2016: 185-203.

Olson DM, McNett MM, Lewis LS, Riemen KE, Bautista C. Effects of nursing interventions on intracranial pressure. *Am J Crit Care.* 2013;22(5):431-438.

Olson DM, Parcon C, Santos A, Santos G, Delabar R, Stutzman SE. A novel approach to explore how nursing care affects intracranial pressure. *Am J Crit Care.* 2017;26(2):136-139.

Rogers M, Stutzman SE, Atem FD, Sengupta S, Welch B, Olson DM. Intracranial pressure values are highly variable after cerebral spinal fluid drainage. *J Neurosci Nurs.* 2017;49(2):85-89.

Acute Ischemic Stroke and Hemorrhagic Stroke

Bosel J. Blood pressure control for acute severe ischemic and hemorrhagic stroke. *Curr Opin Crit Care.* 2017;23(2):81-86.

Jauch EC, Saver JL, Adams HP, Jr., et al. Guidelines for the early management of patients with acute ischemic stroke: a guideline for healthcare professionals from the American Heart Association/American Stroke Association. *Stroke.* 2013;44(3):870-947.

Livesay S. *Comprehensive Review for Stroke Nursing.* Chicago, IL: American Association of Neuroscience Nurses; 2014.

Lubitz SA, Parsons OE, Anderson CD, et al. Atrial fibrillation genetic risk and ischemic stroke mechanisms. *Stroke.* 2017;48(6):1451-1456.

Mainali S, Stutzman S, Sengupta S, et al. Feasibility and efficacy of nurse-driven acute stroke care. *J Stroke Cerebrovasc Dis.* 2017;26(5):987-991.

Mehta N, Watkins D. Stent retrieval devices and time prove beneficial in large vessel occlusions: a synopsis of four recent studies for mechanical retrieval and revascularization. *J Neurosci Nurs.* 2015;47(5):296-299.

Seners P, Baron JC. Revisiting 'progressive stroke': incidence, predictors, pathophysiology, and management of unexplained early neurological deterioration following acute ischemic stroke. *J Neurol.* 2018;265(1):216-225.

Supnet C, Crow A, Stutzman S, Olson D. Music as medicine: the therapeutic potential of music for acute stroke patients. *Crit Care Nurse.* 2016;36(2):e1-7.

Seizures

Dawson EA, Gupta PK, Madden CJ, Pacheco J, Olson DM. Arrhythmias in the epilepsy monitoring unit: watching for sudden unexpected death in epilepsy. *J Neurosci Nurs.* 2015;47(3):131-134.

Miller WR. Epilepsy. In: Bader MK, Littlejohns LR, Olson DM, eds. *AANN Core Curriculum for Neuroscience Nursing.* 6th ed. Glenview, IL: American Association of Neuroscience Nurses; 2016: 451-475.

Miller WR, Otte JL, Pleuger M. Perceived changes in sleep in adults with epilepsy. *J Neurosci Nurs.* 2016;48(4):179-184.

Rowe AS, Goodwin H, Brophy GM, et al. Seizure prophylaxis in neurocritical care: a review of evidence-based support. *Pharmacotherapy.* 2014;34(4):396-409.

Infections of the Central Nervous System

Stewart-Amidei C, VanDemark MV, Villnueva NE. Infection and autoimmune conditions. In: Bader MK, Littlejohns LR, Olson DM, eds. *AANN Core Curriculum for Neuroscience Nursing.* 6th ed. Glenview, IL: American Association of Neuroscience Nurses; 2016: 477-510.

Williamson RA, Phillips-Bute BG, McDonagh DL, et al. Predictors of extraventricular drain–associated bacterial ventriculitis. *J Crit Care.* 2014;29(1):77-82.

Neuromuscular Diseases

Brettler S, Merchant K. Movement disorders. In: Bader MK, Littlejohns LR, Olson DM, eds. *AANN Core Curriculum for Neuroscience Nursing.* 6th ed. Glenview, IL: American Association of Neuroscience Nurses; 2016: 527-549.

Marrie RA, Bernstein CN, Peschken CA, et al. Intensive care unit admission in multiple sclerosis: increased incidence and increased mortality. *Neurology.* 2014;82(23):2112-2119.

Evidence-Based Practice

Black AT, Balneaves LG, Garossino C, Puyat JH, Qian H. Promoting evidence-based practice through a research training program for point-of-care clinicians. *J Nurs Adm.* 2015;45(1):14-20.

Carney N, Totten AM, O'Reilly C, et al. Guidelines for the management of severe traumatic brain injury, fourth edition. *Neurosurgery.* 2017;80(1):6-15.

Demaerschalk BM, Kleindorfer DO, Adeoye OM, et al. Scientific rationale for the inclusion and exclusion criteria for intravenous alteplase in acute ischemic stroke: a statement for healthcare professionals From the American Heart Association/American Stroke Association. *Stroke*. 2016;47(2):581-641.

Fried HI, Nathan BR, Rowe AS, et al. The insertion and management of external ventricular drains: an evidence-based consensus statement: a statement for healthcare professionals from the Neurocritical Care Society. *Neurocrit Care*. 2016;24(1):61-81.

Frontera JA, Lewin JJ, 3rd, Rabinstein AA, et al. Guideline for reversal of antithrombotics in intracranial hemorrhage: a statement for healthcare professionals from the Neurocritical Care Society and Society of Critical Care Medicine. *Neurocrit Care*. 2016;24(1):6-46.

Magee WL, Clark I, Tamplin J, Bradt J. Music interventions for acquired brain injury. *Cochrane Database Syst Rev*. 2017;1:Cd006787.

Powers WJ, Derdeyn CP, Biller J, et al. 2015 American Heart Association/American Stroke Association Focused Update of the 2013 guidelines for the early management of patients with acute ischemic stroke regarding endovascular treatment: a guideline for healthcare professionals from the American Heart Association/American Stroke Association. *Stroke*. 2015;46(10):3020-3035.

Torbey MT, Bosel J, Rhoney DH, et al. Evidence-based guidelines for the management of large hemispheric infarction: a statement for health care professionals from the Neurocritical Care Society and the German Society for Neuro-intensive Care and Emergency Medicine. *Neurocrit Care*. 2015;22(1):146-164.

HEMATOLOGIC AND IMMUNE SYSTEMS

Diane K. Dressler

13

KNOWLEDGE COMPETENCIES

1. Analyze laboratory test results used to assess the status of the hematologic and immune systems:
   - Complete blood count (CBC)
   - White blood cell (WBC) differential
   - International normalized ratio (INR)
   - Activated partial thromboplastin time
   - D-dimer

2. Describe the etiology, pathophysiology, clinical manifestations, and interprofessional interventions for common hematological problems in acutely ill patients.

3. Provide comprehensive management for immunosuppressed patients in the acute care setting.

The hematologic and immune systems play a major role in the body's response to illness. Organs and tissues require a continuous supply of oxygen from the red blood cells (RBCs), while the white blood cells (WBCs) provide a first line of defense against infection and mount an immune response. The platelets and other coagulation components are essential for hemostasis. Assessment of these processes and treatment of hematologic and immune problems are an important part of patient management.

SPECIAL ASSESSMENT TECHNIQUES, DIAGNOSTIC TESTS, AND MONITORING SYSTEMS

A complete patient assessment guides the selection of screening tests for hematologic and immune problems. Historical data are particularly important and include family history, occupational exposures, lifestyle behaviors, travel, diet, allergies, past medical problems, surgeries, comorbid conditions, transfusion of blood or blood components, and current medications. Abnormal physical assessment data from each body system collectively assist in the identification of risk factors or acute abnormalities pertinent to hematologic and immune

function. In addition, a variety of laboratory tests including those listed in Table 13-1 assist the clinician to evaluate problems in these systems.

Complete Blood Count

The complete blood count (CBC) is a primary assessment tool for evaluation of the hematologic and immune status. The RBC count and RBC indices, along with the hemoglobin (Hgb) and hematocrit (Hct) levels, provide valuable information regarding the oxygen-carrying capacity of the blood. The total WBC count and the WBC differential reveal the body's ability to fight infection, provide an immune response and to participate in the normal inflammatory process required for tissue restoration. Important information concerning hemostasis is obtained from the platelet count, with additional studies required to fully evaluate the coagulation process.

Red Blood Cell Count

The RBC count is determined by the number of erythrocytes per microliter of blood. Normal values for men are higher than for women. A decrease in the number of RBCs or in

TABLE 13-1. NORMAL VALUES FOR HEMATOLOGIC AND IMMUNE SCREENING TESTS[a]

Laboratory Test	Normal Value
RBC	Males: 4.2-5.4 million/μL
	Females: 3.6-5.0 million/μL
Hgb	Males: 14-17 g/dL
	Females: 12-16 g/dL
Hct	Males: 43%-52%
	Females: 36%-48%
RBC indices	
MCV	84-96 fL
MCH	28-34 pg/cell
MCHC	32-36 g/dL
RDW	11%-14.4%
Reticulocyte count	0.5%-1.5%
WBC	4500-10,500/μL
WBC differential (% of total)	
Neutrophils	50%-70%
Segmented	56%
Bands	0%-3%
Eosinophils	0%-3%
Basophils	0.5%-1.0%
Monocytes	3%-7%
Lymphocytes	25%-40%
T-cells	800-2500 cells/μL
T-helper (CD4) cells	600-1500 cells/μL
Cytotoxic T (CD8) cells	300-1000 cells/μL
Quantitative Immunoglobulins	
IgA	60-400 mg/dL
IgG	700-1500 mg/dL
IgM	60-300 mg/dL
IgE	3-423 IU/mL
Platelet count	150,000-400,000/μL
Bleeding time	3-10 minutes
INR	0.8-1.1
Therapeutic anticoagulation	2.0-3.0
aPTT	30-40 seconds
Therapeutic anticoagulation	1.5-2.5 times normal
ACT	70-120 seconds
Therapeutic anticoagulation	150-210 seconds
Fibrinogen	200-400 mg/dL
D-dimer	< 1.37 nmol/L
Thromboelastogram (TEG)	
Reaction time (R time)	7.5-15 minutes
K time	3-6 minutes
a angle	45 degrees
Maximum amplitude (MA)	5 = 60 mm

Abbreviations: ACT, activated clotting time; aPTT, activated partial thromboplastin time; Hct, hematocrit; Hgb, hemoglobin; Ig, immunoglobulin; INR, international normalized ratio; MCH, mean corpuscular hemoglobin; MCHC, mean corpuscular hemoglobin concentration; MCV, mean corpuscular volume; RBC, red blood cell count; RDW, red blood cell distribution width; WBC, white blood cell count.
[a]Normal values vary between laboratories. Refer to local laboratory standard values when interpreting test results.

the amount of Hgb indicates anemia. Anemia can be due to many factors, including decreased production or increased destruction of RBCs, loss of RBCs by bleeding, vitamin B_{12} deficiency, and/or iron deficiency. An increase in the total number of RBCs occurs as a compensatory mechanism in chronic hypoxia, as an adaptation to high altitude, iron overload, and in some malignant blood disorders. Further assessment of the ability of the bone marrow to produce RBCs is obtained by a reticulocyte count. Reticulocytes are immature red blood cells that are released from the bone marrow. Normally they are present in the blood in small amounts. They mature in 1 to 2 days and prior to their maturation they are not as effective as mature red cells. When there is anemia or blood loss, the bone marrow produces more reticulocytes causing reticulocytosis (an increase in reticulocytes).

Hemoglobin

Hemoglobin is a complex iron-containing protein, which carries oxygen to body tissues and carbon dioxide back to the lungs. As the number of RBCs change, so does the Hgb content. A decline in Hgb to a level as low as 7 g/dL may be well tolerated in some patients, while in others a decline can result in significant symptoms. The rate at which the decline in Hgb level occurs often influences the symptoms and tolerance of the patient. A decline that occurs gradually over time is often tolerated, whereas a rapid decline frequently results in more severe symptoms. Older adults and those with underlying cardiac or pulmonary disorders may become symptomatic with even small changes in the Hgb content of the blood.

Hematocrit

Hematocrit measures the RBC mass in relationship to a volume of blood and is expressed as the percentage of cells per 100 mL of blood. Multiplying the Hgb value by 3 gives an estimate of Hct. The Hct is particularly sensitive to changes in the volume status of the patient. It increases with fluid losses (hemoconcentration) and decreases with increased plasma volume (hemodilution). Interpretation of Hgb and Hct results must take into account the time the values were obtained in relationship to blood volume loss, fluid loss, and/or fluid administration; for example, values obtained immediately after an acute hemorrhage may appear normal, because compensatory mechanisms have not had time to restore plasma volume. Restoration of plasma volume by compensation or crystalloid resuscitation lowers the Hgb and Hct.

Red Blood Cell Indices

The RBC indices (mean corpuscular volume, mean corpuscular hemoglobin, mean corpuscular hemoglobin concentration, and RBC distribution width) are measurements of the size, weight, and Hgb concentration of the individual erythrocytes. These indices are useful in determining the etiology of anemia.

Total White Blood Cell Count

Leukocytes, or WBCs circulating in the blood, are measured as an indicator of the total number of WBCs in the body. Most WBCs are not sampled in a CBC because they are marginated along capillary walls, circulating in the lymphatic system, or residing in lymph nodes and other body tissues.

Increased WBC, or *leukocytosis*, is usually caused by an elevation in one type of WBC. It is most often associated with a normal immune system response to an acute infection, but is also an expected result of other inflammatory processes. Increases in WBCs are known to have both positive and negative effects. Positive effects include phagocytosis of microorganisms in fighting an infection. Potentially destructive effects include the release of reactive oxygen species from neutrophils and excessive amounts of cytokines from macrophages causing damage of healthy tissue and cell death. An abnormal production of leukocytes in the bone marrow occurs in leukemia.

Leukopenia refers to a decrease in the total WBC number. This occurs when bone marrow production is inhibited or when certain infections lead to rapid consumption of WBCs. The life span of a circulating WBC is only hours to days; therefore, a constant replacement process is necessary to prevent leukopenia and immune compromise, which can result in infection and harm to the patient.

White Blood Cell Differential

The differential is a measure of five different categories of leukocytes, with each type reported as a percentage of the total WBC count. The absolute count for each category of white cell (also referred to as a cell line) is calculated by multiplying the percentage of each type of cell by the total WBC count. Increases or decreases in any one cell line help evaluate normal immune response and predict impaired immunity.

Neutrophils, or segmented neutrophils (also called "segs"), are the primary responders to infection and inflammation in the body. They also are an accurate indicator of how the immune system is functioning. With active infections, the bone marrow also releases an immature form of neutrophil called a "band". Bands quickly mature into segmented neutrophils which have greater phagocytic properties to respond to infection. Leukocytosis is usually caused by an increased number of segmented neutrophils and is called neutrophilia. A "left shift" refers to leukocytosis with an increased percentage of bands. Neutropenia, or a decreased number of circulating neutrophils, places the body at increased risk for infection. An absolute neutrophil count (ANC = WBC × [% segmented neutrophils + % segmented bands] × 10) of less than 1000 cells/μL severely compromises immune system response, particularly to bacterial infections.

Monocytes are large phagocytic cells that circulate briefly in the blood before maturing into macrophages which then typically reside in body tissues. These leukocytes are important scavengers of microorganisms and other foreign material. They also activate lymphocytes by presenting antigens to T cells.

Lymphocytes are the WBCs responsible for the body's adaptive (specific) immune responses. Subsets of T and B lymphocytes are assessed by specific cell counts. Lack of properly functioning lymphocytes or inadequate numbers of these cells places the body at risk for bacterial, viral, and fungal infections and certain malignancies. The CD4 cell is a subset of lymphocytes. It is the target of human immunodeficiency virus (HIV) infection leading to the development of acquired immunodeficiency syndrome (AIDS).

Eosinophils increase in numbers and activity during parasitic infections and allergic responses. They attach to parasites and use enzymes to kill them. Increased percentages of these cells are also seen during an allergic response. Basophils are another WBC associated with allergy. They break down during allergic reactions, releasing their intracellular contents such as heparin and histamine, resulting in the allergic symptoms of itching, hives, erythema, swollen mucous membranes, etc.

Platelet Count

The platelet count is determined by the number of platelets per cubic microliter of blood. Platelets are called *thrombocytes* because of their role in the initiation of blood coagulation at the site of damaged blood vessel walls. Two-thirds of the body's platelets are circulating in the blood, with the remaining one-third sequestered within the spleen. Thrombocytopenia (decreased number of platelets) is associated with increased risk of spontaneous bleeding and is caused by decreased production, increased consumption, or excessive destruction of platelets. Hypercoagulability of the blood can result from increased circulating platelets caused by proliferative disorders, malignancies, and inflammation. Qualitative assessment of platelet function is determined by the bleeding time.

Coagulation Studies

International Normalized Ratio

The International Normalized Ratio (INR) evaluates the final coagulation pathway and the time it takes to form a clot. The INR is a calculation developed to standardize interpretation of a previously used test called the prothrombin time (PT). The PT and INR may be reported together, but the INR is the recommended parameter for establishing the therapeutic range for warfarin therapy. The INR is a general test of coagulation, and will be elevated in patients with liver disease, biliary tract disease, and those who are therapeutically anticoagulated with warfarin. It is also elevated in patients with coagulopathies such as disseminated intravascular coagulation (DIC).

Activated Partial Thromboplastin Time

The activated partial thromboplastin time (aPTT) is reported in seconds and is used to evaluate fibrin clot formation stimulated by the pathways of coagulation. This test is used to screen for congenital coagulation disorders and for monitoring anticoagulation with unfractionated (IV) heparin therapy. Prolonged aPTT is also noted in persons with liver disease, vitamin K deficiency, and DIC.

Activated Coagulation Time

The activated coagulation time (ACT) is reported in seconds. The test is used most commonly to monitor effects of unfractionated heparin during and following cardiovascular procedures such as cardiopulmonary bypass and percutaneous coronary interventions. It is generally performed at the point of care.

Fibrinogen

The fibrinogen level is tested during evaluation for bleeding disorders. Fibrinogen is the plasma protein that becomes the fibrin clot. Plasma levels of fibrinogen may be increased during an inflammatory response, pregnancy, or acute infection. Decreased levels are present with liver disease and DIC.

D-Dimer

D-dimer is a very specific indicator of fibrinolysis, the natural process that breaks down fibrin clots. Levels of D-dimer are elevated in thrombotic disorders such as deep venous thrombosis (DVT) and pulmonary emboli (PE). Levels are also elevated during thrombolytic drug therapy and in DIC. It is important to recognize that in addition to pathological conditions, D-dimer is elevated postoperatively and any time a patient has clots that are being broken down by the fibrinolytic process.

Thromboelastogram

Thromboelastography (TEG) testing may be performed to assess clotting activity in patients with coagulopathies such as DIC. This test can be performed at the bedside to evaluate clot formation, clot strength, and breakdown (fibrinolysis).

Additional Tests and Procedures

After obtaining basic laboratory screening tests, additional diagnostic testing is necessary to identify specific disorders in hematologic and immune function. For patients with hematologic disorders, a bone marrow aspiration, or further studies of specific clotting factor assays may be performed. For those with suspected immune disorders, immunoglobulin quantification studies may be indicated.

Blood, sputum, urine, and wound specimens for Gram stain and culture help identify sources of infection. Molecular diagnostic techniques such as polymerase chain reaction (PCR) detect infectious agents not readily cultured, such as viruses. Noninvasive studies such as ultrasound may determine liver, spleen, or lymph node abnormalities. Radiologic procedures (radiographs, CT scans, arteriograms) may be needed to identify malignancy, infection, or hemorrhage.

PATHOLOGIC CONDITIONS

Acutely ill patients often have combined abnormalities involving the hematologic and immune systems. Anemia, immune compromise, and coagulopathy are three distinct problems that may be seen together in acute illness. The patient with chronic immunosuppression and acute infection in the Essential Content Case below typifies this situation. Each of these problems poses major threats to the patient's potential outcome and is evaluated separately.

Anemia

Etiology, Risk Factors, and Pathophysiology

Anemia is defined as a Hgb count less than 12 g/dL and is the most common hematologic disorder. Its etiology may be classified into disorders of RBC production, increased destruction of RBCs, or acute blood loss.

A patient history gives important clues to the etiology of anemia. Decreased production may result from nutritional deficiencies in substrates necessary for RBC production such as iron, folic acid, or vitamin B_{12}. Those at high risk for iron deficiency anemia include children, adolescents, older adults, pregnant women, and patients with malabsorption syndromes. Folic acid deficiency is common in alcoholics. Dietary vitamin B_{12} deficiency may occur in strict vegetarians and also occurs due to a lack of intrinsic factor (postgastrectomy, gastric bypass, or with pernicious anemia) or Crohn disease. Another common cause of anemia is chronic blood loss from the gastrointestinal (GI) tract or from heavy menstruation. Daily blood testing in hospitalized patients may also contribute to anemia, because the patient's bone marrow cannot keep up with the loss.

Anemia may be associated with chronic illnesses, such as renal failure and cancer. Patients with renal failure experience anemia because of reduced production of the hormone erythropoietin. Without adequate erythropoietin, the bone marrow is not stimulated to produce RBCs. Cancer that specifically involves the bone marrow may replace normal bone marrow with malignant cells, disturb the development and maturation process of blood cells, and fill the marrow with immature cells that prevent RBC generation.

Anemia can also occur in cancer patients as a result of treatment-induced bone marrow suppression. Here the bone marrow fails to produce cells, sometimes causing a drop in all three types of blood cells (WBC, RBC, and platelets) known as *pancytopenia*. Medications such as chemotherapeutic agents and some antibiotics suppress the bone marrow and cause anemia. Other causes of anemia include radiation therapy to marrow-producing bones such as the sternum and other long bones in the body. In addition to renal failure and cancer, other chronic disease states may decrease the life span of RBCs leading to anemia when production of new cells by the bone marrow cannot keep up with the losses.

Hemolytic anemia results from excessive destruction of RBCs. This can occur episodically or chronically. Abnormalities intrinsic to the RBC are usually the result of hereditary causes of hemolytic anemia, such as sickle cell disease. Extrinsic sources of hemolysis include immune destruction from an adverse reaction to a medication or a blood transfusion, splenic disorders, damage by artificial heart valves, cardiopulmonary bypass, or use of an intra-aortic balloon pump.

Sickle cell anemia is an inherited Hgb disorder that results in chronic hemolytic anemia and occlusion of blood vessels. The problem is most prevalent in patients who identify as African American and can manifest itself as sickle cell trait, or the more serious sickle cell disease beginning in early childhood. During episodes of low oxygen tension or other stressors such as infection, the RBCs change their shape (to a sickle rather than rounded shape) and adhere to the endothelial lining of blood vessels where they activate coagulation. This results in hemolytic anemia, blood vessel occlusion, and ischemic pain in organs and tissues, a syndrome referred to as *sickle cell crisis*. Management of these crises often includes hospitalization for pain management, hydration, and blood transfusion. Other complications of sickle cell disease include bone disorders, injury to the spleen, and stroke. Specialists in hematology are included in the management of patients with sickle cell anemia. General principles of management include infection prevention, nutrition, and pain management. Hydroxyurea is a cytotoxic drug that can reduce the number of painful crises and hospitalizations and increase survival. Hematopoietic cell transplantation is the only curative option available.

Acute hemorrhage rapidly leads to anemia. Trauma, surgical blood loss, coagulopathy, gastrointestinal bleeding, and bleeding related to anticoagulation are frequently encountered as causes of anemia in critically and acutely ill patient populations. With acute hemorrhage, both cellular components and plasma are lost simultaneously. The remaining cells are normal (normocytic, normochromic) and the main problem is an insufficient number of RBCs. Until volume replacement from fluid resuscitation or mobilization of fluids from extracellular sources occurs, a drop in Hct may not be appreciated. Following an episode of blood loss, the reticulocyte count will generally rise as newly produced immature RBCs are released into the circulation. Rapid loss of blood volume results in hypovolemic shock and cardiovascular instability, further reducing delivery of oxygen to body tissues.

Regardless of the etiology of an anemia, the critical effect of decreased RBCs and Hgb is a decrease in the oxygen-carrying capacity of the blood and a reduction in oxygen content. This may be tolerated if anemia develops slowly and the body can compensate, but may be life threatening if a sudden blood loss occurs resulting in shock or cardiopulmonary collapse.

Clinical Signs and Symptoms

Clinical manifestations are related to the body's compensatory mechanisms that attempt to maintain perfusion of oxygen to vital tissues. Clinical manifestations may not be obvious until the Hgb level is less than 7 g/dL. As compensatory mechanisms are overwhelmed, serious signs and symptoms occur. Patients with pulmonary and cardiovascular disease are less likely to tolerate the effects of anemia and will become symptomatic more quickly.

Cardiovascular

- Tachycardia, palpitations
- Angina
- Decreased capillary refill
- Orthostatic hypotension
- Electrocardiographic (ECG) abnormalities (arrhythmias, ischemic changes)
- Hypovolemic shock (hypotension, tachycardia, decreased cardiac output, increased systemic vascular resistance)

Respiratory

- Increased respiratory rate
- Dyspnea on exertion, progressing to dyspnea at rest

Skin/Musculoskeletal

- Pallor of skin and mucous membranes
- Dusky nail beds
- Decreased skin temperature

Neurologic

- Headache
- Light-headedness
- Ringing in the ears (tinnitus)
- Syncope
- Irritability/agitation
- Restlessness
- Severe fatigue

Abdominal

- Enlarged liver and/or spleen
- Anorexia, nausea, vomiting, pica (craving for inedible or non-nutritional items: ice, clay, soil, paper)

Principles of Management of Anemia

Management of the anemic patient must be guided by the severity of symptoms. Evaluating a change in Hgb and Hct includes assessment of the patient's clinical status and risk of active bleeding. Restoration of adequate blood volume to assure oxygen delivery to the tissues is a priority in critically and acutely ill patients. Identification of the etiology of anemia and resolution of the underlying cause is done simultaneously.

Improving Oxygen Delivery

Oxygen delivery is a product of the amount of Hgb in the blood, the saturation of the Hgb with oxygen, and the cardiac output. Management strategies focus on optimizing each of those components.

1. Administration of supplemental oxygen can increase oxygen saturation. Use of oxygen, particularly during activity, may minimize desaturation and dyspnea.

TABLE 13-2. SUMMARY OF CURRENT GUIDELINE RECOMMENDATIONS ON RED BLOOD CELL TRANSFUSION

1. Decisions regarding the need for transfusion of red blood cells should include assessment of the patient's clinical status, patient preference, and alternative therapy.
2. For hospitalized patients, including the critically ill, who are hemodynamically stable, a restrictive transfusion threshold of 7 g/dL should be used. A threshold of 8 g/dL is recommended for patients with preexisting cardiovascular disease and those undergoing cardiac or orthopedic surgery.
3. Regarding the storage time of blood, patients should receive units of blood selected at any time within the licensed dating period (standard issue).

Data from: Carson JL, Guyatt G, Heddle MN, et al. Clinical practice guidelines from the AABB: Red blood cell transfusion thresholds and storage, JAMA 2016 Nov 15;316(19):2025-2035.

2. Adequate Hgb can be replaced in acute situations only by transfusion of RBCs. Transfusion of packed red blood cells (PRBCs) is considered when blood loss is severe, the patient is actively bleeding, or when the patient is symptomatic. Table 13-2 lists the indications for transfusion.
3. Cardiac output can be optimized with volume replacement, including PRBCs, in situations of bleeding and hypovolemia. Other interventions to improve cardiac output are guided by hemodynamic monitoring and are discussed in Chapter 4.
4. Monitoring vital signs, oxygen saturation, and subjective patient data before, during, and after a change in therapy or activity identifies the patient's ability to tolerate anemia.
5. Limiting strenuous activity and planning periods of rest are important nursing interventions for the anemic patient.

Identifying and Treating Underlying Disease State

Further diagnostic testing may be indicated to determine the etiology of anemia. Radiologic and endoscopic studies to locate sites of bleeding, particularly in the GI tract, may be necessary. Treatment of the underlying cause of anemia may include the following:

1. Administer recombinant human erythropoietin to restore bone marrow production of RBCs in chronic anemia. The response may take several weeks, so it may not be appropriate in situations in which acute correction of anemia is necessary. Chronic kidney disease (CKD) patients and patients receiving chemotherapy may benefit from this treatment.
2. Supplemental oral or parenteral iron replacement may be indicated if iron deficiency anemia is present. Iron depletion is used therapeutically in treating porphyria and iron overload disorders.
3. Vitamin B_{12} and folic acid–related anemia may also require oral or parenteral supplementation.
4. Dietary consultation may be needed prior to discharge to help patients and families plan meals with foods high in iron, folate, or B_{12}.

Minimizing Iatrogenic Blood Loss and Reducing the Need for Transfusion

1. Use small volume collection tubes and microanalysis techniques.
2. Assess the need for routine and additional blood testing to decrease diagnostic blood loss.
3. Use blood salvage systems in surgical patients.
4. Assess the risk of GI bleeding and use prophylactic agents to reduce the risk of GI bleeding if indicated.
5. Screen all patients for anticoagulants and bleeding risk prior to procedures.
6. Accept normovolemic anemia in hemodynamically stable, asymptomatic patients.

Immunocompromise

Etiology, Risk Factors, and Pathophysiology

All acutely ill patients have a high risk for infection because their defense mechanisms are limited by underlying disease, medical therapy, nutritional status, age, and/or physiological stress. The term *immunocompromised* is applied to patients whose immune mechanisms are defective or inadequate. The patient with immunocompromise is more likely to develop an opportunistic infection. Once infection develops, it may quickly progress to sepsis.

Immune system protection from infection is categorized into three levels: natural defenses, innate (general) immunity, and adaptive (specific) immunity. Natural defenses include having intact epithelial surfaces (skin and mucous membranes) with normal chemical barriers (pH, secretions) present and all protective reflexes (blink, swallow, cough, gag, sneeze) intact. The invasive catheters and tubes used in critical and acute care units bypass these protective barriers and allow introduction of pathogens.

When natural defenses are bypassed or overwhelmed, the innate response to infection is activated. Phagocytic WBCs (neutrophils and monocytes) attack the foreign microorganisms, marked by foreign proteins (antigens). The macrophages also play a key role in processing the invading antigen and presenting it to the lymphocytes involved in the adaptive immune response.

Lymphocytes (B cells and T cells) are responsible for the orchestration of an immune response specific to each foreign protein or antigen. B lymphocytes create antigen-specific antibodies or immunoglobulins to aid in the destruction of the invading microorganism and to protect the body from future encounters with the antigen. This is called *humoral immunity*. T lymphocytes have different subsets of cells created to modulate the immune system response (including CD4 helper T cells) and cells that have cytotoxic properties, the CD8 T cells. The immune response of the T lymphocytes is called *cell-mediated immunity*. Both types of lymphocytes work closely together in the specific immune response. However, humoral immunity is the primary protection against bacterial invasion and cell-mediated immunity is effective against infection by viral and fungal organisms, and some malignancies. Additionally, T cells are primarily involved in the rejection of foreign tissue and in delayed hypersensitivity reactions.

Deficiencies in immune system function can be categorized into primary, or congenital, immune system defects and secondary, or acquired, immune system dysfunction. Immune deficiencies may be pinpointed to a specific cell type, a specific antibody, or they may involve abnormalities in multiple components of the immune system. Secondary or acquired immunodeficiencies are the most likely type encountered in critical and acute care patients. Acquired immunodeficiency may be secondary to age, malnutrition, stress, chronic disease states, medications with immunosuppressive effects, cancer and its treatment, HIV infection, and other factors.

Today, an increased number of patients are undergoing organ transplantation and receiving immunosuppressive agents in the transplant setting and for the treatment of autoimmune disorders and certain cancers. Patients who receive organ transplants require lifelong immunosuppressive drug therapy to prevent recognition and rejection of the transplanted tissue by the immune system. Patients typically receive a combination of drugs that affect various components of the immune response. Higher doses are required during the first weeks and months after the transplant. Depending on the type of transplant and the patient's history of rejection episodes, doses are decreased over time to minimize the risk of infection and other complications. Acute cellular rejection may be diagnosed by evidence of failure of the transplanted organ (such as elevated serum creatinine and decreased urine output in a kidney recipient) or by obtaining a biopsy diagnostic of rejection. Rejection is commonly treated by augmented immunosuppression, such as a series of doses of IV methylprednisolone. During and following treatment, these patients are at high risk for infection. Immunosuppressive agents are also used in the management of other disorders such as rheumatoid arthritis, lupus, and other autoimmune diseases.

As new regimens and new chemotherapy agents are used to treat cancer, many of these agents have the potential to produce significant bone marrow suppression and target the body's immune response. More aggressive chemotherapeutic treatment of cancer has led to higher numbers of patients with bone marrow suppression. These patients are at high risk for the development of complications, including pancytopenia, neutropenia, and life-threatening infection.

Neutropenia refers to the state in which the ANC is less than 1000 cells/μL leading to increased susceptibility to infection and sometimes neutropenic fever and sepsis. Many factors contribute to the susceptibility of the neutropenic patient to develop an infection. This includes the cause and duration of neutropenia, functional capability of the existing neutrophils, the patient's defense mechanisms and natural barriers to infection, and endogenous and exogenous flora. The key to preventing severe infection and sepsis is patient education, early detection, and intervention.

Detection of infection in the immunocompromised patient may be difficult since the body's defense mechanisms are suppressed. Lack of neutrophils impairs the patient's ability to mount a vigorous inflammatory response and classic signs and symptoms of infection may be diminished or absent. Redness, febrile response, or even the development of pus may not occur because purulent drainage is largely the result of dying neutrophils at the site of infection. The neutropenic patient can be severely infected and on the verge of becoming septic, and their only complaint may be malaise, somnolence, or pain.

Fever in this patient population is another key sign of infection and warrants aggressive investigation. Since development of fever may not be possible and some patients may even be hypothermic, the nurse must be keenly aware of other signs of sepsis including alterations in mental status, blood pressure, pulse, and respiratory rate that are the result of compensatory mechanisms. The rapid onset of sepsis in a neutropenic patient requires meticulous and frequent assessment to ensure early intervention, as these patients do not present or respond as those with a functional, normal immune system.

HIV is another disorder that leads to immunocompromise. It initially affects helper T cells, decreasing their number and function. This in turn has a profound effect on adaptive immunity. Following diagnosis, the CD4 cells are monitored, and a CD4 count of less than 400/μL is associated with a higher risk of complications. Viral load testing is also performed to measure the amount of viral particles per cubic microliter of blood. As patients receive antiretroviral therapy, the CD4 count may normalize and the viral load decrease. Patients infected with HIV may progress to having AIDS, acquired immune deficiency syndrome, in which they are susceptible to opportunistic infections and certain malignancies. Antiretroviral therapy reduces the progression of HIV infection to AIDS, and increases life expectancy. Patients with HIV may require hospital admission for the management of an opportunistic infection, an adverse reaction to antiretroviral therapy or for a condition or surgery unrelated to their HIV infection.

Clinical Signs and Symptoms[1]
Local Evidence of Inflammation and Infection

- Redness
- Edema
- Warmth
- Pain
- Purulent drainage

General Evidence of Infection

- Fever or hypothermia
- Rigors or shaking chills
- Fatigue and malaise

---

[1] As noted earlier, immune-compromised patients may not show any clinical signs and symptoms of infection The neutropenic patient may have very subtle signs of sepsis; thus heightened vigilance is necessary to expedite treatment.

- Changes in level of consciousness
- Lymphadenopathy
- Tachycardia
- Tachypnea

System-Specific Evidence

Neurologic

- Headache
- Nuchal rigidity
- Changes in mental status, agitation

Respiratory

- Cough
- Change in color, amount of sputum
- Dyspnea, orthopnea
- Pain in chest or pleura

Genitourinary

- Dysuria
- Urgency
- Frequency
- Flank pain
- Abdominal pain
- Cloudy and/or bloody urine

Gastrointestinal

- Nausea
- Vomiting
- Diarrhea
- Cramping abdominal pain
- Enlarged liver or spleen
- Oral or pharyngeal lesions

Principles of Management for Immunocompromised Patients

Patients at high risk for infection must be identified on admission to the unit. Measures to protect and strengthen immune system function are included in the plan of care. All healthcare team members must utilize measures to prevent the development of hospital-associated infections. Close monitoring for signs and symptoms of a local or systemic inflammatory response is especially important to ensure early detection of infection. Identification of the source and likely organisms causing infection allows for initiation of broad-spectrum, empiric antimicrobial coverage. Culture and sensitivity reports guide the choice of antimicrobials specific to the infecting organisms. Care is planned to reduce the risk of exposure to pathogens. Hand hygiene is the main intervention for the prevention of infection. Additionally, the number of lines, tubes, and drains is minimized. Although central lines, indwelling catheters, and other devices are commonplace in critical and acute care settings, the nurse must be vigilant to constantly evaluate the ongoing need for such devices.

Identification of Patients With High Risk of Infection

Risk factors for immunocompromise are as follows:

1. Neonates and older adults
2. Malnutrition

3. Use of medications with known immunosuppressive effects such as glucocorticoids, cancer chemotherapeutic agents, monoclonal antibodies, and transplant immunosuppressive agents
4. Recent radiation therapy to areas of the body that impact bone marrow production
5. Chronic systemic diseases such as renal or hepatic failure or diabetes
6. Diseases involving the immune system such as HIV infection
7. Loss of protective epithelial barriers through:
   - Oral or nasogastric intubation
   - Presence of pressure injuries
   - Burns
   - Surgical wounds
   - Skin and soft tissue trauma
   - Mucositis
   - Altered lymphatics (prior surgery removing lymph nodes)
8. Invasive catheters or prosthetic devices in place such as:
   - Intravascular catheters, including peripheral, central, and arterial lines
   - Indwelling urinary catheters
   - Endotracheal intubation and mechanical ventilation
   - Heart valve replacements
   - Orthopedic hardware such as artificial joints, pins, plates, or screws
   - Dialysis, apheresis catheters, shunts, fistulas, or grafts
   - Cardiovascular devices such as ventricular-assist devices, pacemakers, or implantable defibrillators
   - Ventricular shunts
9. Frequent hospitalizations

Implementing Measures to Protect and Strengthen Immune System Function

1. Take meticulous care of the skin and mucous membranes to prevent loss of barrier protection.
2. Use the enteral route for feeding to maintain caloric intake and normal gut function.
3. Avoid the use of indwelling urinary catheters or remove them as early as possible.
4. Minimize patient stress and the release of endogenous glucocorticoids by relieving pain or using alternative methods such as guided imagery or music for relaxation, and other comfort measures (positioning, massage).
5. Administer colony-stimulating factors (granulocyte colony-stimulating factor [G-CSF] or granulocyte/macrophage colony-stimulating factor [GM-CSF]) to stimulate bone marrow production of neutrophils and monocytes, when appropriate.
6. Administer granulocyte transfusion according to facility protocol.

7. Administer prophylactic antimicrobials as appropriate (such as trimethoprim-sulfamethoxazole for prevention of pneumocystis pneumonia).

Implementing Measures to Prevent Hospital-Associated Infections

1. Educate patients, families, and colleagues about the importance of hand washing, the primary method of preventing hospital-associated infection. All personnel and visitors are to wash their hands before and after contact with the patient.
2. Use private rooms for patients at high risk. Use of protective attire such as masks may be employed according to specific facility protocol.
3. Institute respiratory hygiene/cough etiquette for patients with signs of respiratory infection and appropriate isolation for known or suspected patient infection.
4. Adhere to strict aseptic technique in the care of intravascular catheters and during any invasive procedures.
5. Eliminate environmental sources of infection (eg, leftover fluids used for irrigations). Clean surfaces frequently with recommended disinfectant, including bedside table, equipment, and any surfaces where contamination is likely.
6. Track the date and time fluids, tubing, catheters, and other equipment is initiated and change them according to hospital protocol.
7. Provide healthy food choices and supplements if prescribed to enhance nutrition. Review facility protocol regarding use of filtered water, restriction of fresh fruits and vegetables, and other neutropenic precautions.
8. Encourage use of incentive spirometry, turning, deep breathing, and progressive mobility.
9. Promote recommended immunizations for preventable diseases such as influenza and pneumonia.

Early Detection of Local or System Inflammatory Response and Sepsis

1. Monitor the patient closely for signs and symptoms consistent with infection and sepsis and communicate abnormal findings to the interprofessional team.
2. Initiate the facility's sepsis protocol, when indicated.
3. Collect specimens for culture and sensitivity from potential sources of infection (eg, urine, sputum, blood, stool, wound drainage).
4. Institute antibiotic therapy as directed. See Chapter 11, Multisystem Problems, for more information on the management of sepsis.

Coagulopathies

Etiology, Risk Factors, and Pathophysiology

Patients may develop coagulopathy due to disorders involving platelets, hemostasis, fibrinolysis, thrombosis, or a combination of abnormalities. Acquired disorders of coagulation, as opposed to inherited disorders, are more frequent in critical and progressive care units.

Thrombocytopenia

Platelets initiate the coagulation process at the site of blood vessel injury. Quantitative platelet disorders are associated with bleeding when the platelet count drops to less than 50,000/μL, especially if there is tissue trauma. Spontaneous bleeding can occur at counts of less than 20,000/μL, and counts of 5000 to 10,000/μL create a high risk for hemorrhage. Four general mechanisms are responsible for thrombocytopenia: (1) decreased production of platelets by the bone marrow, (2) shortened survival due to platelet utilization and destruction, (3) sequestration of platelets in the spleen, and (4) intravascular dilution of platelets during transfusion of multiple units of blood and components.

Thrombocytopenia may also be related to immune mechanisms. Drug-induced thrombocytopenia occurs when a drug causes an antigen-antibody reaction. This reaction leads to the formation of immune complexes that destroy platelets by complement-mediated lysis. There are several other types of immune-related thrombocytopenia that are seen in critical and acute care. Heparin-induced thrombocytopenia (HIT) is an immune-mediated reaction to heparin that results in the formation of antiplatelet antibodies that activate platelets and form clots. This then leads to platelet consumption and a precipitous drop in the platelet count. The patient may develop intravascular clotting resulting in clinical thrombosis. Venous thrombosis is most common and may result in limb ischemia and PE. When this syndrome is suspected, all heparin is stopped, and confirmatory testing for HIT antibodies is performed. Treatment options include administration of direct thrombin inhibitors such as argatroban. Patients diagnosed with HIT should not receive heparin again.

Immune thrombocytopenia purpura (ITP) is an acquired disorder that results in the production of IgG antibodies that attack glycoproteins on platelet membranes, destroying the platelets. This disorder was formerly called idiopathic thrombocytopenia, but was renamed when it was identified as an immune process. In adults, ITP may occur as a primary disorder or may be secondary to medications, viral infections, or autoimmune disorders such as systemic lupus erythematosus. For some, the cause may never be determined. Patients may develop petechiae, purpura, and epistaxis. Severe bleeding is possible, especially when the platelet count is less than 20,000/μL. Treatment options include glucocorticoids, intravenous immune globulin (IVIG), administration of rituximab, platelet stimulating agents, platelet transfusion, and, in some cases, splenectomy.

Thrombotic thrombocytopenic purpura (TTP) is a syndrome characterized by thrombocytopenia, hemolytic anemia, renal failure, fever, and neurologic changes. The cause of this disorder is a deficiency of the enzyme ADAMTS13, leading to excessive platelet aggregation and binding to the endothelium of blood vessels. Patients with TTP develop

ESSENTIAL CONTENT CASE

Chronic Immunosuppression

A 35-year-old African American man is admitted to the progressive care unit with dyspnea and altered mental status. The patient's history includes diabetes mellitus and CKD for which he underwent a kidney transplant 3 months ago. Recent kidney function testing suggested possible rejection, and the patient received a course of augmented steroids (ie, increased doses from baseline). Current medications include tacrolimus, mycophenolate mofetil, prednisone, metoprolol, and insulin. Significant findings on admission include the following:

Blood pressure	90/60 mm Hg
Heart rate	116 beats/min
Respiratory rate	28 breaths/min
Temperature	102°F
SpO$_2$	90%
WBC	12,500/µL with 15% bands
Hemoglobin	10.2 g/dL
Hematocrit	30%
Platelets	89,000/µL
Serum glucose	320 mg/dL
Serum creatinine	1.9 mg/dL
Chest x-ray	Infiltrate in the left lower lobe

During the admission interview, the patient is tachypneic, and complains of thirst. He has a dry cough, and crackles are heard over the left lung field. His IV dressing is notably saturated with blood. The physician arrives on the unit and discusses the patient with the progressive care nurse, who knows this patient from previous hospitalizations. Following analysis of the patient's history, physical examination, and diagnostic data, a plan of care is developed.

Case Question 1: What are this patient's risk factors for hematologic and immune problems?

Case Question 2: What should the nursing assessment focus on?

Case Question 3: What therapeutic interventions are the highest priority?

Case Question 4: Analyze the diagnostic test results and outline how the values provide diagnostic information.

Case Question 5: Analyze the assessment data and explain how it will be used to direct patient care.

Case Question 6: What are the most likely working diagnoses?

Case Question 7: What types of consultations should be ordered?

Case Question 8: What are your priority nursing interventions during these first few hours of hospitalization?

Case Question 9: Outline the criteria and considerations for blood transfusion therapy in this patient.

Answers

1. Risk factors for infection include chronic immunosuppression, recently augmented immunosuppression, and diabetes. Risk factors for anemia include CKD and recent surgery. Thrombocytopenia and potential sepsis are risk factors for coagulopathy.
2. Assessment focuses on the evaluation of potential sources of infection and clinical manifestations of infection, anemia and coagulopathy, hyperglycemia, and renal insufficiency.
3. Initial interventions include IV fluids, cultures of sputum, urine, and blood, administration of empiric antibiotics, supplemental oxygen, and respiratory therapy. Implementation of the sepsis protocol is important to consider. Antihypertensives are held, and vital signs frequently monitored.
4. The elevated WBC and high percentage of bands indicate acute infection. The low Hgb and Hct indicate anemia. The low platelet count may be due to sepsis and creates clotting problems. The serum glucose suggests poorly controlled blood sugar possibly due to infection and the recent course of augmented steroids, and frequent testing and management is indicated. The elevated serum creatinine indicates renal insufficiency in the transplanted kidney. The chest x-ray suggests pneumonia.
5. The cough, respiratory distress, and crackles suggest possible pneumonia. The elevated respiratory rate can be indicative of respiratory distress and diabetic ketoacidosis. The thirst may be due to fever and hyperglycemia. The hypotension, tachycardia, tachypnea, fever, low oxygenation, and altered mental status indicate possible sepsis.
6. Working diagnoses include pneumonia with possible sepsis, hyperglycemia, renal insufficiency, anemia, and thrombocytopenia.
7. An infectious disease consultation and if available, a consultation with a diabetic management team are indicated. The renal transplant team needs to be notified of the admission.
8. Nursing priorities include frequent assessment of respiratory status, blood sugar, and kidney function. Collaborative interventions such as fluids, antibiotics, and insulin are administered. Consultants are notified promptly regarding the patient's admission and condition.
9. Red blood cell transfusion is indicated for patients who are hemodynamically unstable and do not respond to administration of IV fluids. Transfusion may also be indicated when there is evidence of active bleeding and inadequate tissue oxygenation.

widespread vascular occlusion in organs, as well as jaundice, purpura, petechiae, and bleeding. Acutely ill individuals may be treated with plasmapheresis.

Hemolytic-uremic syndrome is characterized by thrombocytopenia, hemolytic anemia, and renal failure. It is most often the result of infectious colitis and the toxin released from *Escherichia coli* 0157:H7. Children and older adults are

most seriously affected by this syndrome, and will require hospitalization for supportive care including dialysis.

Patients may have adequate numbers of platelets but still have a bleeding tendency due to qualitative platelet disorders. Drug-induced suppression of platelet function is commonly associated with use of aspirin, clopidogrel, fish oil, vitamin E, and other agents. Renal failure, uremia, and adverse reactions to medications can also contribute to impaired platelet function in acutely ill patients.

Disorders of Hemostasis

Disorders of hemostasis also occur due to inherited abnormalities of coagulation factors. Hemophilia types A and B are congenital deficiencies in factors VIII and IX. Von Willebrand disease represents a deficiency or dysfunction of the plasma protein of the same name. In acute bleeding, replacement of the deficient factor is essential to limit blood loss. Patients with these disorders may require critical or progressive care when undergoing routine surgical procedures or when hospitalized for other medical problems.

Acquired coagulation disorders can be associated with deficient coagulation factor production. This may be caused by a decreased intake of vitamin K, the vitamin essential for the formation of clotting factors II, VII, IX, and X. Intestinal malabsorption, liver disease, use of warfarin, or antibiotic therapy can all contribute to vitamin K deficiency, leading to prolonged INR. Because most coagulation factors are produced in the liver, patients with liver disease have deficiencies of fibrinogen and other factors in addition to deficiencies of the vitamin K–dependent factors.

Many of the medications used routinely in hospitalized patients have anticoagulant and antiplatelet effects (Table 13-3). Therapeutic anticoagulation using heparin, warfarin, and other agents interferes directly with the clotting process. Heparin inhibits the final clotting pathway and its key pro-coagulant thrombin. Decreasing the dose or temporarily stopping a heparin infusion is usually adequate to control minimal bleeding. If bleeding is severe, the antidote to reverse heparin, protamine sulfate, may be administered intravenously. Low-molecular-weight heparin is associated with fewer bleeding and immunological complications. See

Table 13-3 for a list of anticoagulants commonly used in acute care.

Warfarin acts by inhibiting the production of vitamin K–dependent clotting factors. Effects from warfarin take several days to be observed after initiation of the drug, but may persist for many days following administration. The dose of warfarin is titrated to a goal INR, necessitating routine laboratory evaluation for the duration of treatment. Patients who take warfarin are advised to use caution in consuming foods high in vitamin K. If significant bleeding occurs while on warfarin, replacement of vitamin K–dependent factors with transfusion of fresh frozen plasma or prothrombin complex concentrate (PCC) may be necessary. PCC is a lyophilized powder containing pooled factors. It can be quickly reconstituted for emergency administration, and does not require ABO blood typing. Administration of oral or IV vitamin K may also be helpful, but its effectiveness depends on the time needed by the liver to synthesize new clotting factors.

Novel oral anticoagulant (NOAC) agents such as rivaroxaban and dabigatran act by inhibiting factor Xa and thrombin. They do not require laboratory monitoring and do not have dietary restrictions, and thus have a lower treatment burden than warfarin. Evidence to date demonstrates that NOACs are equally effective as warfarin in the prevention of thromboembolism, but carry a similar risk for bleeding. At this time, only dabigatran has a Food and Drug Administration (FDA) approved reversal agent, idarucizumab.

Thrombolytic agents such as alteplase or reteplase are used to dissolve pathologic clots such as venous thrombi, PE, or acute ischemic stroke. They can also cause bleeding from sites where a protective clot previously formed. These agents are used in combination with other anticoagulants, and may precipitate obvious or occult bleeding. Patients who receive these potent thrombolytics and anticoagulants are monitored for any sign of bleeding complications.

DIC is a complex coagulopathy that affects patients who already have another serious illness. See Table 13-4 for a list

TABLE 13-3. ANTICOAGULANTS COMMONLY USED IN ACUTE CARE

Classification	Drug
Factor Xa and thrombin inhibitor	Heparin sodium
Direct thrombin inhibitor	Argatroban
	Bivalirudin (Angiomax)
	Dabigatran (Pradaxa)
Factor Xa inhibitor	Apixaban (Eliquis)
	Fondaparinux (Arixtra)
	Rivaroxaban (Xarelto)
Vitamin K antagonist	Warfarin (Coumadin)
Glycoprotein IIb/IIIa inhibitors	Abciximab (ReoPro)
	Eptifibatide (Integrilin)
	Tirofiban (Aggrastat)
Thrombolytic agents	Alteplase (Activase)
	Reteplase (Retavase)
Antiplatelet agents	Aspirin
	Clopidogrel (Plavix)
	Dipyridamole (Persantine)
	Prasugrel (Effient)
	Ticagrelor (Brilinta)

TABLE 13-4. ETIOLOGIES OF DIC

Infection and Sepsis
- Acute bacterial
- Acute viral, fungal, parasitic

Trauma
- Head injury
- Crushing injury
- Snake venom

Cardiovascular
- Shock
- Extracorporeal circulation

Obstetrical
- Eclampsia and pre-eclampsia
- Amniotic fluid embolism
- Abortion

Immunological
- Blood transfusion reaction

Neoplastic Disease
- Acute leukemia
- Metastatic cancer

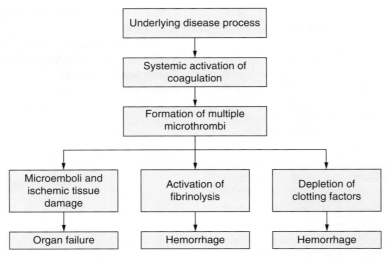

Figure 13-1. Clinical consequences of DIC.

of conditions that can precipitate DIC. The underlying condition triggers the release of proinflammatory cytokines, which activate the coagulation cascade and result in the formation of micro clots. The micro clots obstruct the capillaries of organs and tissues. This initiates a series of events that result in both bleeding and thrombosis. Figure 13-1 outlines the sequence of events that occur in DIC. Acute DIC and hemorrhage can be seen in patients who are seriously ill with sepsis, traumatic injury, and extensive surgery. A chronic form of DIC and associated thrombosis may be seen in patients with cancer.

In DIC, stimulation of the clotting cascade rapidly depletes existing platelets and coagulation factors, consuming them faster than the body can replace them. Depletion of substrates of the coagulation process leaves the body at risk for spontaneous bleeding or hemorrhage from surgical sites, or even minimal trauma.

Simultaneously, multiple tiny clots are formed within the blood and flow to the small vessels where they are trapped. Microcirculatory thrombosis then leads to tissue ischemia, infarction, and organ dysfunction. Single or multisystem organ dysfunction may occur.

Activation of fibrinolysis in DIC releases the enzyme plasmin. Plasmin breaks down some of the fibrin in a physiologic attempt to open the microcirculation, and this produces fibrin degradation products, including D-dimer. Anticoagulant pathways are impaired, further interfering with the balance needed for appropriate hemostasis. Clots are unable to form at new sites of injury, and existing clots are dissolved, leading to bleeding from both old and new sites. Because of the complex pathophysiology, clinical manifestations of DIC are likely to include bleeding from multiple sites and evidence of organ ischemia due to microemboli. Ischemic injury to the skin may cause purpura and color changes in the hands and feet.

Diagnosis of DIC requires careful interpretation of coagulation panel results; there is no single definitive test. Table 13-5 lists the combination of results consistent with

TABLE 13-5. LABORATORY RESULTS SUGGESTING DIC

Test	Abnormality
INR	Elevated
aPTT	Elevated
Platelet count	Decreased
Fibrinogen	Decreased
D-dimer	Increased

DIC. In many cases, absolute certainty regarding a diagnosis of DIC may not be possible, especially in patients with other conditions, such as liver failure, that also cause coagulopathy. With or without a clear diagnosis of DIC, a primary goal of therapy is to treat the underlying condition. In addition, supportive care is provided with volume replacement and support of organ systems, including ventilatory assistance. Significant bleeding is managed with blood and component therapy.

Clinical Signs and Symptoms
Coagulopathy may be a subtle, occult process or a massive, obvious emergency. Assessment must encompass each body system, looking for evidence of abnormality in single or multiple components of the coagulation process.

Abnormal Platelet Numbers or Function
- Petechiae of skin or mucous membranes
- Spontaneous bleeding from gums or nose
- Thrombocytopenia
- Prolonged bleeding time

Abnormal Coagulation Factors
- Hemorrhage into subcutaneous tissue, muscle, or joints
- Ecchymosis, purpura
- Bleeding that is slow to improve with local pressure
- Prolonged INR, aPTT

- Decreased fibrinogen
- Decrease in level of specific coagulation factors

General Assessment for Bleeding or Decreased Organ Perfusion as a Result of Microthrombosis

Skin/Musculoskeletal

- Oozing of blood from multiple sites, including incisions, intravascular catheters
- Petechiae
- Purpura
- Ecchymosis
- Ischemic changes in toes, fingers, nose, lips, ears
- Pain, swelling, and limited joint mobility
- Increased size of body part, increased girth

Neurologic

- Changes in level of consciousness, pupils, movement, or sensation may indicate intracranial bleeding
- Impaired vision with retinal hemorrhage
- Headache

Gastrointestinal

- Blood in gastric aspirate
- Coffee ground emesis or gastric aspirate
- Melena or frank bloody stool
- Abdominal pain
- Enlarged liver or spleen

Genitourinary

- Hematuria
- Decreased urine output
- Vaginal bleeding

Cardiovascular

- Hypotension or labile blood pressure
- Hypovolemia and/or shock (with rapid loss of large volume of blood)

Principles of Management of Coagulopathies

The management of coagulopathy varies with the type and severity of the disorder. The overall goal of therapy is to restore normal hemostasis and prevent/treat hypovolemic shock. Supportive care focuses on the control and prevention of further bleeding and timely provision of therapeutic interventions.

Restoration of Normal Hemostasis

1. Administer blood and components to replace oxygen-carrying capacity, blood volume, and coagulation components. Transfusion is recommended for patients who are actively bleeding or prior to invasive procedures or surgery.
2. Monitor patients for clinical response to transfusion. Positive outcomes include hemodynamic stability, increased oxygenation, and restoration of hemostasis.
3. Monitor for adverse reactions to transfusion. Table 13-6 describes the potential complications of administering blood and blood products. Patients receiving a large number of units of blood and components require additional monitoring for hypothermia, hypocalcemia from citrate stored in blood, and dilution of coagulation components.
4. Transfuse platelets as required to treat quantitative platelet disorders. Platelet dysfunction may improve if the offending agent, such as aspirin, is discontinued. Dialysis improves platelet function in patients with renal failure.
5. Acute replacement of coagulation factors can be accomplished with transfusion of fresh frozen plasma. Cryoprecipitate replaces fibrinogen, factor VIII, and von Willebrand factor. PCC replaces vitamin K–dependent factors. Recombinant factor VIIa may be used for persistent hemorrhage.

TABLE 13-6. **COMPLICATIONS OF BLOOD AND BLOOD COMPONENTS TRANSFUSIONS**

Type of Complication	Key Clinical Signs	Cause	Key Interventions
Acute febrile reaction	Temperature elevation ≥ 1°C or 2°F.	Preexisting antibodies against WBCs or action of cytokines.	Stop the transfusion. Administer antipyretics.
Acute allergic reaction	Urticaria, wheezing, possible anaphylaxis.	Preexisting antibodies.	Stop the transfusion. Administer antihistamine and steroids.
Transfusion-associated circulatory overload (TACO)	Dyspnea, tachypnea, crackles. Cardiogenic pulmonary edema.	Fluid volume overload.	Slow or stop transfusion. Administer diuretic.
Transfusion-related acute lung injury (TRALI)	Acute onset of hypoxemia and non-cardiogenic pulmonary edema within 6 hours of transfusion.	Preexisting antibodies, cytokines, or microparticles within stored blood.	Aggressive respiratory support.
Acute hemolytic reaction	Fever, chills, dyspnea, tachypnea, hypotension, chest and back pain.	Immune destruction of transfused RBCs due to incompatibility of blood.	Stop transfusion. Notify provider and blood bank.
Immune modulation	Acute infections, eg pneumonia.	Depression of immune cells.	Monitor for and recognize signs of infection.
Alloimmunization	Difficulty crossmatching future blood transfusions or donor organs.	Antibodies to RBCs, WBCs, and platelets develop over time.	Monitor previously transfused patients for acute reactions.
Infection transmission	Clinical manifestations are usually delayed, and vary according to the infection.	Transmission of viral diseases such as HIV and CMV. Transmission of bacterial and other organisms.	Bacterial sepsis can lead to an acute reaction with fever, chills, and hypotension.

6. Provide recombinant erythropoietin, iron, and B vitamins to patients with anemia to increase RBC production over time.

Controlling and Preventing Bleeding

1. Modify nursing care measures to minimize trauma and prevent skin and mucous membrane breakdown:
   - Provide gentle oral care.
   - Use electric razor or refrain from shaving.
   - Minimize use of automatic blood pressure cuffs to prevent skin trauma and subcutaneous bleeding; use manual cuffs.
   - Minimize peripheral blood sampling.
   - Avoid IM injections.
   - Use specialty mattress, pad side rails; avoid restraint use.
   - Handle patients gently when turning or moving.
   - Remove adhesive dressings with care.
   - Use low-suction setting to suction endotracheal tube and pharynx.
2. Modify nursing care procedures to control bleeding:
   - Minimize traumatic procedures; apply direct pressure afterward for at least 5 to 10 minutes or until bleeding has stopped.
   - Use ice packs on new hematomas or hemarthroses.
   - Do not dislodge or attempt to remove blood clots from areas of bleeding.
   - Control environment to prevent hypothermia which can worsen coagulopathy.

SELECTED BIBLIOGRAPHY

Anemia

American Association of Blood Banks. *Circular of Information for the Use of Human Blood and Blood Components.* Bethesda, MD: AABB; 2013.

American Society of Anesthesiologists Task Force on Perioperative Blood Management. Practice guidelines for perioperative blood management: an updated report by the American Society of Anesthesiologists Task Force on Perioperative Blood Management. *Anesthesiology.* 2015;122(2):241-275.

Carson JL, Guyatt G, Heddle MN, et al. Clinical practice guidelines from the AABB: red blood cell transfusion thresholds and storage. *JAMA.* 2016. http://jamanetwork.com. Accessed October 27, 2016.

Carlson JL, Stanworth SJ, Roubinian NR, et al. Transfusion thresholds and other strategies for guiding allogeneic red blood cell transfusion. *Cochrane Database Syst Rev.* 2016;10:CD002042.

Clifford L, Jia Q, Yadav H, et al. Characterizing the epidemiology of perioperative transfusion-associated circulatory overload. *Anesthesiology.* 2015;122(1):21-28.

Field JJ, Vichinsky EP, DeBaun MB. Overview of the management and prognosis of sickle cell disease. In: Schrier SL, ed. *Up-To-Date.* www.uptodate.com. Accessed May 10, 2017.

Fischbach F, Dunning MB. *A Manual of Laboratory and Diagnostic Tests.* 9th ed. Philadelphia: Wolters Kluwer Health; 2015.

Gu Y, Estcourt LJ, Doree C, et al. Comparison of a restrictive versus liberal red cell transfusion policy for patients with myelodysplasia, aplastic anaemia, and other congenital bone marrow failure disorders. *Cochrane Database of Syst Rev.* 2015;10:1-4.

National Clinical Guideline Center. *Blood Transfusion.* London: National Institute for Health and Care Excellence (NICE); 2015. http://www.guidelines.gov. Accessed January 30, 2017.

Immunocompromised Patient

American Association of Critical Care Nurses. AANC Practice Alert: Prevention of Aspiration in Adults. 2016. http://www.aacn.org. Accessed May 10, 2017.

American Association of Critical Care Nurses. AACN Practice Alert: Prevention of Catheter-Associated Urinary Tract Infections in Adults. 2017. http://www/aacn.org. Accessed May 10, 2017.

Centers for Disease Control and Prevention. Core infection prevention and control practices for safe healthcare delivery in all settings – recommendations of the Healthcare Infection Control Practices Advisory Committee. 2017. http://www.cdc.gov/hicpac/recommendations/core-practices.html. Accessed March 27, 2017.

Crawford J, Becker PS, Armitage JO, et al. NCCN Clinical Practice Guidelines in Oncology. Myeloid growth factors. *J Natil Compr Canc Netw.* 2014. http//:www.nccn.org/professionalsphysician_gls_guidelines.asp. Accessed May 15, 2017.

Flowers CR, Seidenfeld J, Bow EJ, et al. Antimicrobial prophylaxis and outpatient management of fever and neutropenia in adults treated for malignancy. American Society of Clinical Oncology clinical practice guidelines. *J Clin Oncol.* 2013;31(6):794-819.

Foster M. Reevaluating the neutropenic diet: time to change. *Clin J Oncol Nurs.* 2014;18(2):239-241.

Masur H, Brooks JT, Benson CA, et al. Prevention and treatment of opportunistic infections in HIV-infected adults and adolescents: Updated guidelines from the Centers for Disease Control and Prevention, National Institutes of Health, and HIV Medicine Association of the Infectious Diseases Society of America. *Clin Infec Dis.* 2014;58(9):1308-1311.

Rubin LG, Levin MJ, Ljungman P, et al. 2013 IDSA clinical practice guideline for vaccination of the immunocompromised host. *Clin Infect Dis.* 2014;58(3):e44-e100.

Spruce L, Connor R, Retzlaff KJ. Guideline for prevention of transmissible infections. *2015 Guidelines for Perioperative Practice.* Denver: Association of periOperative Registered Nurses; http//:www.guidelines.gov Accessed May 7, 2017.

Coagulopathy

Agency for Healthcare Research and Quality. Preventing hospital-associated venous thromboembolism: a guide for effective quality improvement. 2015. http://www.ahrq.gov/professionals/quality-patient-safety/patient-safety-resources/resources/vtguide/index.html.

American Association of Critical Care Nurses. AACN Practice Alert: Preventing Venous Thromboembolism in Adults. 2016. http://www.aacn.org. Accessed May 10, 2017.

Coutre S. Clinical presentation and diagnosis of heparin-induced thrombocytopenia. In: Leung LLK, ed. *UpToDate*. www.uptodate.com. Accessed May 24, 2017.

Coutre S. Management of heparin-induced thrombocytopenia. In: Leung LLK, ed. *UpToDate*. www.uptodate.com. Accessed May 24, 2017.

Dirkes S, Wonnacott R. Continuous renal replacement therapy and anticoagulation: what are the options? *Crit Care Nurse*. 2016;36(2):34-40.

Dobesh PP, Fanikos J. New oral anticoagulants for the treatment of venous thromboembolism: understanding differences and similarities. *Drugs*. 2014;74:2015-2032.

Federici AB, Intini D, Lattuada A, et al. Supportive transfusion therapy in cancer patients with acquired defects of hemostasis. *Thromb Res*. 2014;133:S2, S56-S62.

Fontera JA, Lewin JJ, Rabinstein AA, et al. Guideline for reversal of antithrombotics in intracranial hemorrhage: a statement for healthcare professionals from the Neurocritical Care Society and Society of Critical Care Medicine. 2016. http://www.guidelines.gov. Accessed February 22, 2017.

George JN, Arnold DM. Immune thrombocytopenia (ITP) in adults: initial treatment and prognosis.

Goforth CW, Tranberg JW, Boyer P, et al. Fresh whole blood transfusion: military and civilian implications. *Crit Care Nurse*. 2016;36(3):50-57.

Hunt BJ. Bleeding and coagulopathies in critical care. *N Engl J Med*. 2014;370:847-859.

Hurwitz A, Massone R, Lopez BL. Acquired bleeding disorders. *Emerg Med Clin North Am*. 2014;32:691-713.

Jones AR, Frazier SK. Consequences of transfusing blood components in patients with trauma: a conceptual model. *Crit Care Nurse*. 2017;37(2):18-30.

Kahn SR, Lim W, Sunn AS, et al. Prevention of VTE in nonsurgical patients: antithrombotic therapy and prevention of thrombosis, 9th ed. American College of Chest Physicians. *Chest*. 2012;141(2 supp):e195S-e226S.

Katrancha ED, Gonzalez LS. Trauma-induced coagulopathy. *Crit Care Nurse*. 2014;34(4):54-63.

Kearon C, Akl EA, Ornelas J, et al. Antithrombotic therapy for VTE disease: CHEST guideline and expert panel report. *Chest*. 2016;149(2):315-352.

Leung LLK. Clinical features, diagnosis, and treatment of disseminated intravascular coagulation in adults. In: Mannucci, ed. *UpToDate*. www.uptodate.com. Accessed May 10, 2017.

Levi M. Cancer-related coagulopathies. *Thromb Res*. 2014;133:S2, S70-S75.

Levi M. Diagnosis and treatment of disseminated intravascular coagulation. *Int J Lab Hematol*. 2014;36:228-236.

McEvoy MT, Shander A. Anemia, bleeding, and blood transfusion in the intensive care unit: causes, risks, costs, and new strategies. *Am J Crit Care*. 2013;22(6):eS1-eS13.

Menzin J, Sussman M, Nichols C, et al. Use of blood products in patients with anticoagulant-related major bleeding: An analysis of inhospital outcomes. *Am J Health-Syst Pharm*. 2014;71:1635-1645.

National Institute for Health Care Excellence (NICE). Detecting, managing and monitoring haemostasis: viscoelastometric point-of-care testing (ROTEM, TEG and Sonoclot systems). 2014. www.guidelines.gov.

Ozawa S, Nelson T. Clinical applications of prothrombin complex concentrate in blood management in patients. *Crit Care Nurse*. 2017;37(2):49-57.

Paterson TA, Stein DM. Hemorrhage and coagulopathy in the critically ill. *Emerg Med Clin North Am*. 2014;32:797-810.

Squizzato A, Hunt BJ, Kinasewitz GT, et al. Supportive management strategies for disseminated intravascular coagulation. An international consensus. *Thromb Haemost*. 2016;115:896.

GASTROINTESTINAL SYSTEM

14

Beth Quatrara

KNOWLEDGE COMPETENCIES

1. Describe the etiology, pathophysiology, clinical presentation, patient needs, and principles of management for:
   - Acute gastrointestinal bleeding
   - Liver failure
   - Acute pancreatitis
   - Bowel ischemia

- Bowel obstruction
- Bariatric (gastric bypass surgery)

2. Identify nutritional requirements for enterally fed acutely ill patients.

3. List important interventions to decrease the risk for aspiration pneumonia during enteral feeding.

PATHOLOGIC CONDITIONS

Acute Gastrointestinal Bleeding

Upper GI Bleeding

Bleeding from the upper gastrointestinal (GI) tract is a medical emergency associated with morbidity, mortality, and costly care. Prompt and decisive treatment is essential to improve outcomes. Upper GI bleeding is 4 times more common than lower GI bleeding. An acute upper GI bleed is suspected when patients present with syncope, hypotension, or abdominal tenderness, and report melanic stool, hematochezia, and blood or coffee-ground emesis. In addition to anemia, laboratory values typically show an elevation of the blood urea nitrogen (BUN) to creatinine ratio (> 20:1). Although bleeding stops spontaneously in 80% to 90% of cases, patients presenting with sudden blood loss are at risk for hypotension, decreased tissue perfusion, and reduced oxygen-carrying capability. Many organ systems may be adversely affected.

Acute upper GI bleeding has a mortality of 6% to 15% and a high rate of reoccurrence. Many patients with bleeds are rebleeding from a previous upper GI tract lesion. A poor prognosis with upper GI bleeding is associated with age above 65, shock, overall poor health, active bleeding at the time of presentation, elevated creatinine or transaminases, onset of bleeding during hospitalization, and initial low hematocrit. Death is typically not a direct result of blood loss, but is related to age and comorbidities.

Lower GI bleeding

In contrast to upper GI bleeding, lower GI bleeding is defined as bleeding that originates distal to the ligament of Treitz and unlike upper GI bleeding has a lower morbidity and mortality. In fact, the bleeding resolves spontaneously in the vast majority of patients and the mortality rate is less than 5%. Distinguishing upper versus lower GI bleeding by origin is an important consideration because a rapid upper GI bleed may present as the presence of blood in the lower GI tract.

Lower GI bleeding is a common disorder in older adults and may be associated with a host of conditions including infection, hemorrhoids, cancer, diverticulitis, or vascular anomaly. Regardless of the source, lower GI bleeding typically presents as hematochezia. Bleeding sources within the left side of the colon often result in the presence of bright red blood whereas those from the right colon may be mixed with stool and present as a darker shade of red.

TABLE 14-1. COMMON SOURCES OF UPPER GASTROINTESTINAL BLEEDING

Peptic Ulcer Disease
- Gastric ulcer
- Duodenal ulcer

Varices
- Esophageal
- Gastric

Pathologies of the Esophagus
- Tumors
- Mallory-Weiss syndrome
- Inflammation
- Ulcers

Pathologies of the Stomach
- Cancer
- Erosive gastritis
- *Helicobacter pylori* infection
- Tumors

Pathologies of the Small Intestine
- Peptic ulcers
- Angiodysplasia
- Aorto-enteric fistula

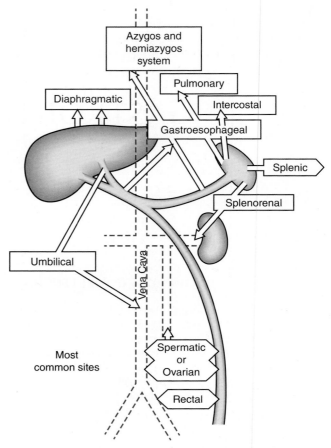

Figure 14-1. The liver with collateral circulation.

Etiology, Risk Factors, and Pathophysiology

A variety of abnormalities within the GI tract can be the source of upper GI bleeding (Table 14-1).

Peptic ulcer disease is the most common cause of upper GI bleeding. Fifty-five percent of patients with gastric ulcers and 39% of patients with duodenal ulcers are hospitalized for acute bleeds. The pathogenesis of peptic ulcer disease is related to hypersecretion of gastric acid, coupled with impaired GI tract mucus secretion. Normally, mucus protects the gastric wall from the erosive effects of acid. Peptic ulcers occur in the stomach and the duodenum and are characterized by a break in the mucosal layer that penetrates the muscularis mucosa (innermost muscular layer), resulting in bleeding. Peptic ulcers are more prevalent in those with a history of alcohol abuse, smoking, chronic renal failure, and nonsteroidal anti-inflammatory drug (NSAID) use. Infection of the mucosa by *Helicobacter pylori,* an organism naturally found in the GI tract, is strongly correlated with 90% to 100% of duodenal ulcers and 60% to 100% of gastric ulcers. However, the increased availability of over-the-counter NSAIDs also contributes to the high prevalence of the condition despite advances in medical management. Of note, many peptic ulcers are asymptomatic and patients can present with a bleeding ulcer without previous GI symptoms.

Gastroesophageal varices develop when there is increased pressure in the portal venous system of the liver. If blood cannot flow easily through the liver because of obstructive disease, it is diverted to collateral channels. These channels are the normally low-pressure vessels found in the distal esophagus (esophageal varices), the veins in the proximal stomach (gastric varices), and in the rectal vault (hemorrhoids) (Figure 14-1). Acute upper GI hemorrhage occurs when esophageal and/or gastric varices rupture from increased portal vein pressure (portal hypertension). Esophagogastric varices do not generally bleed until the portal

pressure exceeds 12 mm Hg. Portal hypertension is most commonly caused by primary liver disease (see next section), liver trauma, or thrombosis of the splenic, mesenteric, or portal veins. Massive upper GI hemorrhage is associated with variceal bleeds.

Mallory-Weiss syndrome is a linear, nonperforating tear of the gastric mucosa near the gastroesophageal junction. The tear is the result of intra-abdominal pressure changes in the stomach that occur with forceful vomiting. Alcohol abuse and inflammatory conditions of the stomach and esophagus are associated with this disorder. Classically, these tears occur in alcoholic patients who experience intense retching and vomiting associated with binge drinking. However, they may also occur in any patient with a history of repeated emesis and other scenarios where the intra-abdominal pressure is suddenly increased.

Angiodysplasia refers to abnormal superficial blood vessels in the GI tract that are prone to bleeding. These abnormal vessels are associated with increased age. The potential for the malformed vessels to bleed is exacerbated with aortic stenosis, chronic renal disease, liver disease, and Von Willebrand disease. This condition is commonly encountered in the outpatient setting and rarely requires admission to the progressive care unit.

ESSENTIAL CONTENT CASE

Upper GI Bleeding

A 52-year-old man is admitted with reports of a 7-hour history of nausea and vomiting with recent emesis of large amounts of "bloody secretions" and frequent "maroon-colored" stools. His mental status is alert but confused. His friend reports that recently he has taken large amounts of NSAIDs due to an acute back injury. A gastric ulcer on the posterior wall of the stomach is diagnosed by upper endoscopy. Significant findings on his admission profile are:

Vital Signs

Blood pressure	84/54 mm Hg lying
Heart rate	132 beats/min; sinus tachycardia
Respiratory rate	28 breaths/min
Temperature	37.3°C (oral)

Respiratory
- Breath sounds clear in all lung fields but diminished

Cardiovascular
- S_1/S_2, no murmurs
- Extremities cool, diaphoretic; pulses present but weak

Abdomen
- Distended with hyperactive bowel sounds (BSs)
- Tender right upper quadrant; no rebound tenderness

Neurologic
- Slightly confused
- Anxious

Genitourinary
- 30 mL of amber cloudy urine following urinary catheter insertion
- Stools liquid maroon, guaiac positive

Arterial Blood Gases
- pH   7.35
- $Paco_2$ 46 mm Hg
- HCO_3 19 mEq/L
- Pao_2 70 mm Hg on room air
- Sao_2 92%

Laboratory
- Hematocrit   24%
- Hemoglobin   6.8 g/dL

- White blood cell count   12,000/mm^3
- Prothrombin time (PT)   11 seconds
- Activated partial thromboplastin time   30 seconds
- Platelet count   110,000/mm^3
- Serum potassium   3.0 mEq/L
- Serum sodium   155 mEq/L
- Serum glucose   207 mg/dL
- Serum BUN   40
- Serum creatinine   1.1
- Liver function testing   Within normal limits

Case Question 1: Initial management of the patient with upper GI bleeding would include:
(A) Volume resuscitation
(B) Hemodynamic stabilization
(C) Identification of the site of bleeding
(D) Initiation of treatment to control bleeding within 24 hours of admission

Case Question 2: After the bleeding site is identified and bleeding is controlled, the drug of choice to treat a nonvariceal bleed is:
(A) Histamine receptor antagonists
(B) Proton pump inhibitors (PPIs)
(C) Antacids
(D) Octreotide/Somatostatin

Answers
1. The correct answer is (A). The fundamental goal for initial management of the patient is volume resuscitation. However, hemodynamic stabilization, identification of the bleeding site, and control of bleeding are all key points for managing the patient with upper GI bleeding. Vital signs are an important indicator of blood loss. If the patient is hemodynamically unstable, resuscitation begins with the administration of 2 to 3 L of crystalloid. Blood products are considered if the response is poor.
2. The correct answer is (B). PPIs are the drug of choice in this patient population as they lead to a more durable and sustained acid suppression. In randomized controlled clinical trials, PPIs are shown to decrease recurrent bleeding.

Erosive gastritis describes gastric lesions that do not penetrate the muscularis mucosa. These are also referred to as stress ulcers. Stress-related ulcers occur frequently in hospitalized patients and those with respiratory failure and coagulopathies have an increased risk of bleeding. Onset of bleeding is sudden and is often the first symptom. However, the bleeding is often minimal and self-limited. The causes of gastritis are multifactorial (Table 14-2), but are most commonly associated with NSAID use, steroid intake, alcohol abuse, and physiologic conditions that cause severe stress (eg, trauma, surgery, burns, radiation therapy, severe medical problems). Alcohol and NSAIDs are known to directly disrupt the mucosal defense mechanisms of the stomach (Figure 14-2). Use of NSAIDs is particularly problematic in older adults and contributes to the increased incidence of symptomatic acute upper GI bleeding in this population. In the progressive and critical care population, particularly patients with neurological or burn injuries, Cushing and Curling stress ulcers may be identified. However, they are rare and only occur in 1.5% of this population.

TABLE 14-2. CAUSES OF GASTRITIS

Alcohol Abuse
NSAID use
Aspirin
Ascriptin
Smoking
Steroids
Severe Physiologic Stress
Burns (Curling ulcer)
CNS disease (Cushing ulcer)
Trauma
Surgery
Medical complications
   Sepsis
   Acute renal failure
   Hepatic failure
Long-term mechanical ventilation

Regardless of the etiology, upper GI bleeding resulting in a significant and sudden loss of blood volume is associated with decreased venous return to the heart, and therefore a decrease in cardiac output (CO). The decrease in CO triggers the release of epinephrine and norepinephrine, causing intense vasoconstriction and tissue ischemia (Figure 14-3). In addition, aldosterone and antidiuretic hormones

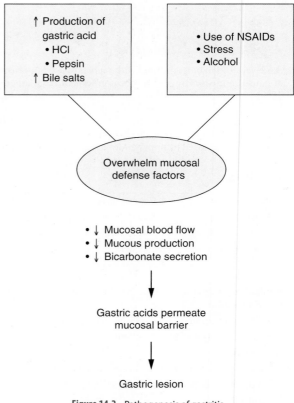

Figure 14-2. Pathogenesis of gastritis.

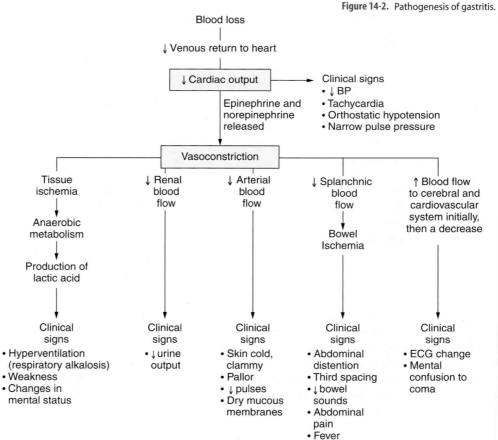

Figure 14-3. Hypovolemic shock.

are released, resulting in sodium and water retention. The clinical signs and symptoms of upper GI hemorrhage are directly related to the effects of the decrease in CO and the vasoconstriction response typically seen in hypovolemic shock.

Clinical Presentation

History

Individuals may have a history of peptic ulcer disease, tobacco abuse, alcohol abuse, liver disease, severe physiologic stress, NSAID use, and anticoagulation or antiplatelet therapy. Older adults are at greater risk for GI bleeding.

Signs and Symptoms

The response to blood loss depends on the rate and amount of blood loss, patient's age, overall health status, and the timing of the initial resuscitation. Specific signs and symptoms may include:

- Hematemesis (bright red blood or coffee ground emesis)
- Melena (black tarry stools)
- Hematochezia (red or maroon stools)
- Nausea and/or early satiety
- Epigastric pain
- Abdominal distention or bloating
- Bowel sounds increased or decreased
- If blood loss is greater than 30% of blood volume, hypotension (orthostatic) and altered functional hemodynamics may indicate a volume deficit.
- Rapid, deep respirations
- Tachycardia
- Fever
- Cold, clammy skin
- Dry mucous membranes
- Decreased pulses
- Weakness
- Decreased urine output
- Anxiety
- Mental status changes
- Restlessness
- Electrocardiographic (ECG) changes consistent with ischemia (eg, ST-segment elevation, arrhythmias)

Diagnostic Tests

- Hematocrit may be normal initially, then decreased with fluid resuscitation and blood loss. The hematocrit may not accurately reflect the actual volume of blood loss because of hemodilution and movement of extravascular fluid. The hematocrit decreases as extravascular fluid enters the vascular space in an attempt to restore volume. This process continues for 24 to 72 hours.
- Hemoglobin may also be normal initially, then decreased with fluid resuscitation and blood loss. It is considered slightly more reliable than hematocrit.

- White blood cell count is elevated due to inflammation.
- Platelet count may be decreased depending on the amount of blood loss.
- Serum sodium is usually elevated initially due to hemoconcentration.
- Serum potassium is usually decreased with vomiting.
- Serum BUN is mildly elevated.
- Serum creatinine is elevated.
- Serum lactate is elevated with severe bleeding.
- PT is usually decreased.
- Activated partial thromboplastin time (aPTT) is usually decreased.
- Arterial blood gases show respiratory alkalosis (early), then later metabolic acidosis with severe shock and hypoxemia.
- Gastric aspirate shows normal or acidotic pH and is guaiac positive.

Principles of Management for GI Bleeding

The fundamental goal of initial treatment is volume resuscitation. The management of the patient with acute GI bleeding focuses on hemodynamic stabilization, identification of the bleeding site, and initiation of definitive medical or surgical therapies to control or stop the bleeding. Measures to decrease anxiety in this patient population are also indicated due to the severity and sudden onset of GI bleeding but sedatives are used sparingly if at all, particularly in patients with liver impairment.

Hemodynamic Stabilization

The initial assessment of the patient with GI bleeding begins with a physical examination in which vital signs and mental status are the most reliable indicators of the amount of blood lost. In the presence of hemodynamic instability, resuscitation begins.

In addition to vital signs and physical assessment, risk stratification tools and laboratory findings help determine the severity of the bleed. The Glasgow Blatchford, Rockall, and AIMS65 scores can be used to predict risk of complications. The Glasgow Blatchford score incorporates measures of BUN, Hgb, systolic BP, pulse, melena, syncope, liver disease, and/or heart failure while the Rockall includes age, shock, and morbidity. The Rockall score does have a secondary set of elements (age, shock, comorbidity, diagnosis, and stigmata of recent bleed) that can be reviewed post-endoscopy to further delineate risk. The AIMS65 score is used preprocedure and consists of five factors including albumin, international normalized ratio (INR), mental status, systolic BP, and age. The use of a risk assessment tool to stratify bleeding and associated mortality is recommended by several consensus groups. Additionally, meta-analyses demonstrate that factors such as active bleeding, hemoglobin less than 10 g/dL, systolic blood pressure less than 100 mm Hg, tachycardia, ulcer size more than 1 to 3 cm, and ulcer location (in the lesser gastric curvature or posterior duodenal bulb) are associated with poor patient outcomes.

1. Monitor and record cardiovascular status (blood pressure, heart rate including orthostatic changes), hemodynamics (central venous pressure [CVP], CO, mean arterial pressure [MAP]), and peripheral pulses. All patients with shock or active bleeding receive resuscitative care in a critical care setting.

2. Insert at least two large-bore intravenous (IV) catheters and begin fluid resuscitation with crystalloid solution (eg, normal saline or lactated ringer solution). Administer fluids to maintain MAP at 65 mm Hg or higher.

3. Administer supplemental oxygen and monitor respiratory function. Airway protection with endotracheal intubation to prevent aspiration is indicated in patients with ongoing hematemesis or altered mental status. Generally, these patients are then transferred to a critical care unit.

4. Obtain blood for measurement of hematocrit, hemoglobin, and clotting studies, as well as for a type and cross-match for packed red blood cells (PRBCs). A Hgb less than 7 to 8 g/dL is considered a marker for transfusion. If the patient also has a history of unstable coronary artery disease or comorbid conditions, a higher threshold is typically used. In patients receiving multiple transfusions, monitoring of ionized calcium levels is required as citrate, contained in the transfused blood, may lower calcium. Estimates for the amount of blood volume lost are most reliably guided by vital sign values and physical assessment (Table 14-3).

5. Administer prescribed IV colloids, crystalloids, or blood products until the patient is stabilized. After the administration of crystalloid fluids, blood products may be considered during the initial resuscitation if the hemodynamic response is poor. PRBCs are used to rapidly increase the hematocrit while providing less volume compared to infusions of whole blood. However, whole blood may be desired with severe hemorrhage as it provides more volume and also includes both plasma and platelets.

Each unit of PRBC increases the hematocrit by 2% to 3% and improves gas exchange. It may take up to 24 hours after blood is administered for changes to be reflected in the hematocrit values, especially if large amounts of crystalloid solutions were administered during the resuscitation period.

6. Monitor coagulation studies (eg, prothrombin time/partial thromboplastin time [PT/PTT], platelet count, and fibrinogen) to determine if the patient requires transfusions of platelets or clotting factors.

7. Monitor fluid balance and renal function (intake and output, daily weight, BUN, creatinine, and hourly urine output). An elevated BUN:creatinine ratio may indicate poor renal perfusion but also occurs when blood is absorbed in duodenum.

8. Insert a nasogastric tube if bleeding is massive (> 40% of blood volume) to assess the rate of bleeding and minimize the risk of aspiration. Placement of a gastric tube in the presence of varices is somewhat controversial and practices vary between institutions. Use of gastric lavage is no longer recommended routinely to minimize bleeding. Some institutions use room temperature saline lavage to clear the stomach prior to endoscopy. Iced saline is no longer used as it lowers core temperature.

9. Position the patient with backrest elevation 30° to 45° to minimize aspiration associated with hematemesis.

10. Monitor temperature and maintain normothermia. Rapid fluid resuscitation, particularly with blood products, can lead to hypothermia which interferes with coagulation. Warming of fluids may be required to prevent hypothermia, if traditional measures are insufficient.

11. Administer medications such as intravenous octreotide and PPIs.

12. Prepare for urgent endoscopic therapy in patients with high risk clinical features such as history of varices, bright red emesis, or Class III or IV hemorrhage. These patients may have improved outcomes when endoscopy is performed within 12 hours. Patients with active bleeding or altered mental status may be transferred to intensive care to undergo

TABLE 14-3. ESTIMATING BLOOD LOSS FROM ACUTE GI BLEEDING (ADVANCED TRAUMA LIFE SUPPORT CLASSIFICATION SYSTEM FOR HYPOVOLEMIC SHOCK)

	Class I	Class II	Class III	Class IV
Blood Loss (mL)	Up to 750	750-1500	1500-2000	> 2000
Blood Loss (% Blood Volume)	Up to 15%	15%-30%	30%-40%	> 40%
Pulse Rate	< 100	> 100	> 120	> 140
Blood Pressure	Normal	Normal	Decreased	Decreased
Pulse Pressure (mmHg)	Normal or increased	Decreased	Decreased	Decreased
Respiratory Rate	14-20	20-30	30-40	> 35
CNS/Mental status	Slightly anxious	Mildly anxious	Anxious, Confused	Confused, lethargy

elective intubation prior to endoscopy. In patients at lower risk, endoscopy is usually performed within 24 hours of admission.

Identify the Bleeding Site

Although the history and physical examination are used to differentiate between upper and lower GI bleeding, endoscopic examination is required to determine the exact site of bleeding and to direct future therapy. Endoscopy allows early direct visualization of the upper GI tract during resuscitation measures.

1. Provide prokinetic agents, if required. The presence of blood in the upper GI tract can impede visualization of the site of bleeding. Prokinetic agents facilitate gastric emptying of retained blood and may be administered prior to endoscopy. Meta-analyses demonstrate that when erythromycin is administered pre-endoscopy, visibility is improved and the need for a repeat procedure is reduced.
2. Administer sedation (eg, midazolam [Versed]) sparingly and institute monitoring protocol.
3. Elevate the head of the bed to a 30° angle (if tolerated) and if intubated, maintain ETT cuff pressure to prevent aspiration.

4. Position the patient in a left lateral decubitus position, which facilitates scope placement, and helps to prevent aspiration of GI contents during endoscopy. Have oral-tracheal suction available at the bedside before the procedure begins.
5. Monitor for cardiac ischemia during the procedure (eg, draw troponin, assess for ST-segment changes [see Chapter 18, Advanced ECG Concepts], arrhythmias).

Institute Therapies to Control or Stop Bleeding

Definitive therapies to treat the bleeding depend on the cause. A general approach for treatment is summarized in Figure 14-4. Administration of PPIs is routine for patients in whom an ulcer is suspected. The PPIs quickly neutralize acids and elevate gastric pH levels, which results in stabilization of the blood clot. An acidic environment will inhibit platelet aggregation and lyse an already formed clot.

In nonvariceal upper GI bleeding, endoscopic treatment is the modality of choice because it is the most effective method to control acute ulcer bleeding, prevent rebleeding, and it is relatively safe procedure. Although individual studies have been too small to show significant advantage for endoscopic therapy in reducing mortality, a meta-analysis indicates that endoscopic therapy is associated with a lower

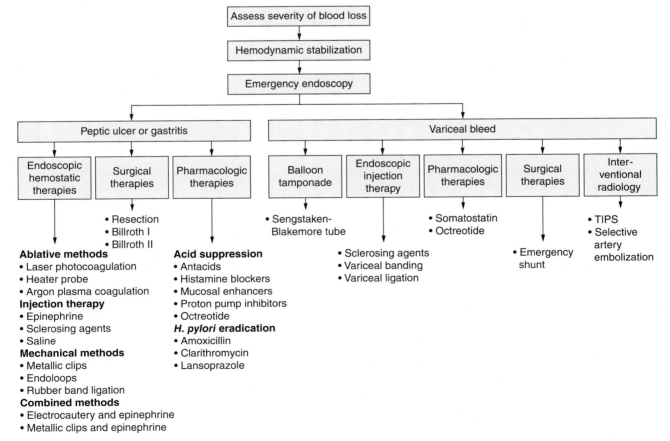

Figure 14-4. Upper GI bleeding treatment guide.

risk of rebleeding and death. While endoscopy carries a risk for complications including GI perforation, precipitation of bleeding, aspiration, cardiac or respiratory compromise, and missed lesions, these rarely occur.

A variety of interventions are used via endoscopy and include ablative or coagulation therapy (laser, monopolar, bipolar, or multipolar electrocoagulation, and heater probe), pharmacologic therapy also known as sclerotherapy, and mechanical and combination therapies. Pharmacologic treatments are easy to use, inexpensive, and available in most settings. The goal is to control bleeding by tamponade, vasoconstriction, and/or an inflammatory reaction after the injection of the selected agent. A saline injection will compress the vessels. Sclerosants such as alcohol, ethanolamine, and polidocanol cause greater vascular thrombosis, but can result in tissue injury and necrosis and are used less frequently. Epinephrine (1:10,000-1:20,000) provides local tamponade, vasoconstriction, and improved platelet aggregation to promote hemostasis. It is the agent of choice in the United States to rapidly control the bleeding site. However, its effects will only last for 20 minutes and therefore is used in combination with an additional more durable thermal or mechanical treatment.

Thermal coagulation methods such as electrocautery and argon plasma coagulation are examples of ablative treatments and are equally effective. Bleeding vessels can also be mechanically compressed using metallic clips, endoloops, or rubber band ligation. Metallic hemo clips are the mechanical treatment of choice and are shown to be as effective as other endoscopic techniques. Combination therapy with epinephrine injection has become the standard treatment for actively bleeding ulcers. Adding a second endoscopic treatment, either an ablative therapy or endoclips, significantly reduces the rate of recurrence, need for surgery, and mortality. It is no longer recommended to use epinephrine alone. If the patient rebleeds, a second attempt with endoscopic control may be considered before surgical intervention or angiography-guided intervention. Rebleeding is more common in patients with variceal bleeds and is highest initially after admission and for the first 24 hours.

The three-stage Forrest classification system is often used at the time of endoscopy to predict rebleeding risk based upon the visual characteristics of the GI lesion/ulcer. Patients with a high-risk for rebleed, as stratified by the Forrest classification system, are often hospitalized for 72 hours of treatment and evaluation. Depending on the risk severity, the patient may remain in the critical or progressive care setting during this time.

Treatment of a Mallory-Weiss tear is supportive therapy. Bleeding episodes are self-limited and the mucosa heals spontaneously within 72 hours in 90% of patients.

Today significant bleeding from stress gastritis is rarely encountered. Patients with a history of gastritis, or those at risk for developing stress-related GI injury, benefit from prophylactic acid-suppressive therapy and from early enteral

TABLE 14-4. PHARMACOLOGIC THERAPIES FOR ULCER DISEASE/GASTRITIS

Agent	Action
Antacids	Acid neutralizers

Histamine blockers
  Cimetidine
  Ranitidine
  Famotidine
  Nizatidine
	Block production of gastric acid (pepsin, HCl) by inhibiting the action of histamine

Cytoprotective agent Sucralfate	Forms protective barrier over ulcer site

Proton pump inhibitors
  Omeprazole (Prilosec)
  Esomeprazole (Nexium)
  Lansoprazole (Prevacid)
  Rabeprazole (Aciphex)
  Pantoprazole (Protonix)-IV
	Suppress secretion of gastric acid

Mucosal barrier enhancers
  Colloidal bismuth
  Prostaglandins
	Protect mucosa from injurious substances

feeding to prevent bleeding. Invasive intervention is rarely required.

In patients with variceal bleeding, pharmacologic treatment to reduce portal hypertension may be considered as preparations are underway for emergent endoscopy. Somatostatin or its analogue octreotide are the vasoactive agents of choice. Continuous intravenous infusion of these agents can temporarily control bleeding so that resuscitation, diagnostic, and therapeutic measures can be completed. Pharmacologic treatments are summarized in Table 14-4. Both sclerotherapy and variceal banding or ligation are used during endoscopy to control variceal bleeding. Currently, balloon tamponade (Sengstaken-Blakemore [S-B] tube) is reserved for patients with massive hemorrhage. Once bleeding is controlled, more definitive therapies can be used.

Treatment of esophageal and gastric varices will also include antibiotic prophylaxis for spontaneous bacterial peritonitis (SBP) in patients with cirrhosis. A third-generation cephalosporin or fluoroquinolone is indicated, as bacteremia is often present in patients with variceal bleeding. Studies demonstrate that administering antibiotics to cirrhotic patients prior to endoscopy decreases infections and mortality.

1. Monitor for complications of endoscopic therapy and/or the sclerosing agents used to treat the ulcer or varix. Complications may include fever and pain due to esophageal spasm, motility disturbances of the esophageal sphincter, and perforation. Systemic complications of endoscopic therapy and/or sclerosing agents also may occur and predominantly affect the cardiovascular and respiratory systems. Cardiovascular effects include heart failure, heart block, mediastinitis, and pericarditis. Respiratory effects include aspiration pneumonia, atelectasis, pneumothorax, embolism, and acute respiratory distress syndrome.

2. Institute pharmacologic therapies as prescribed to treat peptic ulcer disease or gastritis. The most common pharmacologic agents and their actions are reviewed in Table 14-4. PPIs are the drug of choice for the management of patients with non-variceal bleeding. They provide a more durable and sustained acid suppression than histamine receptor antagonists. In randomized clinical trials, treatment with PPIs was correlated to a decrease in recurrent bleeding from ulcer disease, fewer transfusions, less surgery, and shorter length of hospital stay. A typical protocol is to give high dose continuous IV PPIs for 3 days after successful endoscopic treatment for active bleeding (80 mg esomeprazole bolus, 8 mg/h continuous infusion). Yet, newer meta-analyses demonstrate the same benefits with IV BID dosing of 40 mg, until the patient is able to take oral medications. Oral PPIs are commonly recommended for months after an upper GI bleeding episode to allow for healing of the mucosa. Their use is especially beneficial in patients who use chronic NSAIDs or who have had *H. pylori* infection.

3. Administer pharmacologic therapies as prescribed to treat variceal bleeding (Table 14-5). Pharmacologic agents exert their effect by constricting splanchnic blood flow and thereby reducing portal pressure.

4. Consider transfer to the critical care setting if the following therapies are indicated:
   - An intra-aortic balloon pump therapy to achieve temporary vascular control in patients in shock. This therapy optimizes blood pressure, increases aortic diastolic pressure, increases coronary flow, and allows time for rapid resuscitation.
   - A tamponade tube, most commonly the S-B tube (Figure 14-5), to emergently decrease blood flow through the varix and to control bleeding so that endoscopy can be performed. Other tamponade tubes exist but the characteristics are similar to the S-B tube. Endotracheal intubation is performed prior to tube placement to prevent potential aspiration.

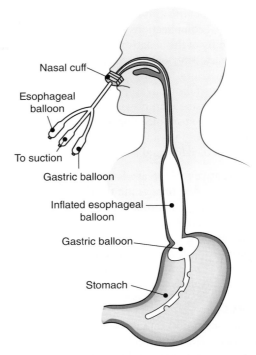

Figure 14-5. Placement of a Sengstaken-Blakemore tube.

Shunt Procedure to Control Bleeding

When severe variceal bleeding cannot be controlled with endoscopic intervention, emergent portal decompression is achieved with the percutaneous transjugular intrahepatic portosystemic shunt (TIPS).

In the TIPS procedure, a stent is used to create a shunt between the hepatic vein and a branch of the portal vein. This decreases the pressure in the portal vein (decreases portal pressure) and subsequently on the varices to prevent rupture and bleeding.

The advantage of the TIPS procedure is that it is less invasive than surgery because the portal circulation is accessed via the right jugular vein. Contraindications to TIPS include severe-progressive liver failure, severe encephalopathy, polycystic liver disease, and severe right heart failure. Complications of the TIPS procedures include puncture of the biliary system, bleeding, infection, and clotting of the stent and stenosis. Postprocedural systemic failure (septic shock, renal failure) and hepatic encephalopathy (see next section) are also associated complications.

Nursing management of the patient undergoing TIPS includes:

1. Monitor blood pressure, ECG, and pulse oximetry throughout the procedure.
2. Administer preprocedure antibiotic coverage for gram-negative organisms as prophylaxis for sepsis.
3. Provide IV sedation.
4. Provide pain medication. Certain parts of the procedure, such as balloon dilation of the intrahepatic tract, can be painful.

TABLE 14-5. PHARMACOLOGIC THERAPIES FOR VARICEAL UPPER GI BLEEDING

Drug	Action	Administration
Somatostatin	Inhibits splanchnic blood flow	250 mcg bolus then continuous IV infusion at 250 mcg/h
Octreotide	Inhibits splanchnic blood flow thus decreasing portal and variceal pressures	50 mcg bolus then IV infusion at 25-50 mcg/h (Off-label use)
Nonselective beta-adrenergic blockers: propranolol, nadolol	Decreases cardiac output and reduces splanchnic flow (decreases portal hypertension)	Administered orally (or IV) to reduce resting pulse by 20% or to 55-60 beats/min

5. Have lidocaine and atropine available to manage potential complications of the procedure. Due to the proximity of the hepatic vein to the right ventricle of the heart, ventricular ectopy can be induced during the procedure.

6. Have crystalloids, vasopressors, PRBCs, and fresh frozen plasma readily available to manage hypotension from sepsis, bleeding, or sedation.

7. Have continuous and intermittent suction ready to manage bleeding and airway patency.

An alternative to TIPS available at some institutions is the balloon-occluded retrograde transvenous obliteration (BRTO) procedure. The procedure involves the occlusion of blood flow to varices by inflating a balloon catheter and instilling a sclerosing agent. The procedure results in a blockage of blood to the varix and the shunting of blood through healthier veins. Further research is needed on the long-term results and effectiveness of BRTO.

Surgical Therapies to Stop Bleeding

Surgery is less common today and is reserved for patients with refractory disease or complications. Patients who experience life-threatening massive bleeding or who continue to bleed despite aggressive medical therapies are candidates for surgery. Surgical therapies include gastric resections such as antrectomy, partial gastrectomy, vagotomy, or combination procedures. An antrectomy or gastrectomy may be performed to decrease the acidity of the duodenum or stomach by removing gastric-acid secreting cells. A vagotomy decreases acid secretion in the stomach by dividing the vagus nerve along the esophagus. Combination procedures are common and one example is the Billroth I, which is a vagotomy and antrectomy with anastomosis of the stomach to the duodenum. A Billroth II consists of a vagotomy, resection of the antrum, and anastomosis of the stomach to the jejunum (Figure 14-6). The latter is preferred over the Billroth I because it does not present the risk for dumping

syndrome. Gastric perforations can be treated by simple closure.

Nursing considerations for patients undergoing surgery to treat GI bleed include:

1. Monitor for fluid and electrolyte imbalances postoperatively due to intraoperative fluid loss and the drains inserted to decompress the stomach or to drain the surgical site.

2. Provide for adequate nutrition to promote wound healing.

3. Monitor the appearance of the incision and surrounding tissue.

4. Document and report all wound drainage (color, amount, odor) and complaints of pain or tenderness.

5. Culture any suspicious drainage.

6. Monitor white blood cell count and temperature trends.

Reducing Anxiety

1. Encourage communication with a calm, interested, and centered approach. If the patient is intubated, consider written communication or use of a communication board.

2. Encourage the patient to identify and apply coping skills used in past difficult situations. These may include family presence, watching TV, listening to music, or relaxation techniques to alleviate anxiety.

3. Offer appropriate reassurance, facts, and information as requested by the patient or family. Explain the progressive care unit routine and procedures to the patient or family. Present information in terms that the patient or family can understand. Repeat and rephrase the information as necessary. Allow time for questions.

4. As appropriate, help the patient to establish a sense of control. Assist the patient to make distinctions among those things he or she can control (eg, bath

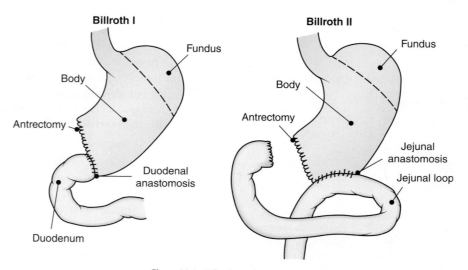

Figure 14-6. Billroth I and II procedures.

time, visitor preferences) and those things that cannot be controlled (eg, need for intravenous fluid and monitoring equipment).

5. Guide the patient to use relaxation exercises and other diversion strategies to decrease anxiety.

Liver Failure

Pathogenesis

The liver, the largest organ in the body, has a central role in regulating the body's metabolism. Metabolic functions include the synthesis of carbohydrates, fats, proteins, and vitamins for nutrition, energy, and key metabolic pathways. Additional processes performed by the liver include the formation of bile, bilirubin metabolism, synthesis of coagulation factors, and detoxification of drugs and toxins. Liver failure may be acute or chronic. Irrespective of the cause of liver injury, inflammation results in damage to hepatocytes, known as "hepatitis." Injured areas are surrounded by scar tissues leading to fibrosis, and after a period of time progressive fibrosis results in cirrhosis or replacement of the normal hepatic tissue with fibrotic tissue. Chronic liver failure is a slow deterioration that evolves over years leading to cirrhosis. Liver dysfunction potentially can be reversed early in the disease as the liver has a regenerative capability; however, fibrotic changes are irreversible resulting in chronic dysfunction and eventual end-stage liver disease.

Acute failure, also known as fulminant hepatic failure, results in a rapid deterioration of liver function in a person without prior liver disease. This cellular insult results in massive cell necrosis leading to a multiorgan dysfunction. Acute liver failure is rare and characterized by a coagulation abnormality (usually an INR ≥ 1.5) and encephalopathy occurring as the result of an insult without previous liver disease. The time between hepatic injury or infection and presentation of either encephalopathy or coagulopathy is usually less than 2 to 6 weeks.

Etiology and Risk Factors

The leading cause of acute liver failure in the United States and Europe is acetaminophen overdose. Other causes include viral hepatitis (A, B, and E), thrombosis, and shock (Table 14-6). Survival in acute liver failure can be categorized into patients in whom intensive care enables recovery of hepatic function and patients who require liver transplantation. Common causes of chronic liver disease include nonalcoholic fatty liver disease (NAFLD), alcoholic liver disease, chronic hepatitis B and C, and hemochromatosis.

NAFLD and a nonalcoholic steatohepatitis (NASH) are the most common causes of chronic liver disease in the Western world, and are becoming more prevalent with increasing rates of obesity. The spectrum of liver disease associated with these syndromes can range from simple steatosis to hepatitis and advanced fibrosis and cirrhosis. They are associated with type 2 diabetes, hyperlipidemia, and metabolic syndrome. In contrast, alcoholic liver injury results from the toxic effects of ethanol on the hepatocytes. Similar to nonalcoholic fatty

TABLE 14-6. COMMON CAUSES OF LIVER FAILURE

Viruses
Hepatitis A, B, C, D, and E
Herpes simplex
Epstein-Barr
Cytomegalovirus
Adenovirus
Parasites
Liver tumors
Toxic ingestion of drugs
Acetaminophen
Halothane
Methyldopa
Toxic ingestion of chemicals and poisons
Chlorinated hydrocarbons
Phosphorus
Nonalcoholic fatty liver disease
Alcohol ingestion
Biliary disease
Cardiac disease
Hepatitis

liver, alcoholic liver conditions may include a spectrum of associated conditions from steatosis to cirrhosis.

Severity Scores

The Child-Pugh classification is a long-standing assessment tool to score hepatic function and estimate cirrhosis severity. This classification is based on two clinical variables and three laboratory values (Table 14-7). Classes define well-compensated disease (Class A) to advanced decompensated disease (Class C).

The Model for End-Stage Liver Disease (MELD) score is another frequently used tool to measure disease severity. The MELD score is a calculation that incorporates age, INR, serum sodium, serum creatinine, and albumin. Additional points are included if the patient undergoes dialysis at least twice in a week. Scores range from 6 to 40 with a higher score associated with higher mortality risk. The MELD score is used by United Network of Organ Sharing (UNOS) to determine hierarchy of transplantation need.

TABLE 14-7. CLINICAL AND LABORATORY PATIENT SCORE FOR INCREASING ABNORMALITY AND SURVIVAL MEASUREMENT

Factor	1 point	2 points	3 points
Total bilirubin (μmol/L)	<34	34-50	>50
Serum albumin (g/L)	>35	28-35	<28
PT INR	<1.7	1.71-2.30	>2.30
Ascites	None	Mild	Moderate to Severe
Hepatic encephalopathy	None	Grade I-II (or suppressed with medication)	Grade III-IV (or refractory)
	Class A	Class B	Class C
Total points	5-6	7-9	10-15
1-year survival	100%	80%	45%

The composite score of these factors is used to provide a severity grade. Grades are: Grade A, 5-6, Grade B 7-8, Grade C 10-15.

TABLE 14-8.　SEQUELAE OF LIVER FAILURE

Sequelae	Outcome	Clinical Manifestations
Impaired splanchnic hemodynamics	Portal hypertension	Varices, acute upper GI bleeding
	Hyperdynamic circulation	Increased CO, decreased SVR, decreased perfusion
Reduced liver metabolic processes	Altered fat, protein, and carbohydrate metabolism	Malnutrition, impaired healing
	Decreased phagocytic function of Kupffer cells	Infection
	Decreased synthesis of blood clotting components	Bleeding
	Decreased removal of activated clotting factors	Emboli
	Decreased metabolism of vitamins and iron	Impaired skin integrity
	Impaired detoxification	Increased ammonia, mental status changes, increased drug levels
Impaired bile formation and flow	Impaired bilirubin metabolism	Jaundice

Clinical Manifestations

Clinical manifestations are directly related to failure of the liver to perform important metabolic processes (Table 14-8). Complications of liver failure include jaundice, ascites, hepatic encephalopathy, hepatopulmonary syndrome, electrolyte imbalance, hepatorenal syndrome, and SBP.

Jaundice

Jaundice is secondary to excessive deposition of bilirubin in tissues including skin, mucous membranes, and sclera, resulting in the characteristic yellow discoloration. This deposition of bilirubin represents failure of the liver to adequately uptake, conjugate, and excrete bilirubin. Jaundice is typically evident when the bilirubin exceeds 2 to 3 mg/dL. The excessive bilirubin in the blood contributes to the urine darkness and pale or clay-colored stools. Pruritus from bile salt accumulation is a commonly associated and uncomfortable symptom.

Ascites

Cirrhosis is the most common cause of ascites, an abnormal collection of fluid in the peritoneal cavity. Liver fibrosis leads to increased pressure in the portal system, obstructing venous flow. This leads to increased nitric oxide, vasodilatation, and renal function compromise with sodium and water retention. Fluid shifts from the intravascular space into the peritoneal space. Decreased intravascular albumin levels and an increase in extravascular protein exacerbate the condition.

Hepatic Encephalopathy

Hepatic encephalopathy defines a spectrum of neuropsychiatric abnormalities that occur with liver failure. This condition most likely results from decreased hepatic clearance of cerebral toxins. Serum ammonia is most often implicated. Ammonia is produced by bacteria in the bowel and converted to urea in the liver for excretion through the kidneys. In liver failure, this function of the liver is impaired, allowing ammonia to directly enter the central nervous system. Because ammonia is neurotoxic, as serum ammonia levels rise, the patient often exhibits signs of impaired cerebral functioning or encephalopathy. These signs can range from minor sensory-perceptual changes such as muscle tremors, slurred speech, or slight mental status changes to marked confusion or profound coma. Asterixis is a common manifestation.

Classifications of deterioration in brain function have been used, from grade I (mild or episodic drowsiness, impaired concentration/intellect, but arousable and coherent); grade II (increased drowsiness, confusion, and disorientation, but able to arouse); grade III (very drowsy, agitated, disoriented, but able to respond to simple verbal commands); and grade IV (unresponsive coma with or without response to painful stimuli). Cerebral edema with elevated intracranial pressure can occur in up to 80% of patients with grade IV encephalopathy and carries a poor prognosis. The cause of cerebral edema is poorly understood. Patients with hepatic encephalopathy need to be carefully assessed for other causes of encephalopathy such as sepsis, uremia, acidosis, alcohol withdrawal, hypoxia, electrolyte abnormalities, and intracerebral bleed.

Hepatopulmonary Syndrome

A critical complication in liver failure, hepatopulmonary syndrome, occurs due to vascular dilation in the lungs leading to impaired gas exchange. Patients with hepatopulmonary syndrome may present with shortness of breath, cyanosis, arterial hypoxemia, and pulmonary edema. Mechanical ventilation may be necessary to provide oxygenation and ventilation. According to studies, hepatopulmonary syndrome has a wide range of prevalence (4%-47%) in cirrhotic patients. However, the critical nature of the condition is clear. Definitive medical treatment is not currently available. Liver transplantation may provide a cure.

Electrolyte Imbalance

A variety of electrolyte imbalances occur in liver failure. Hypoglycemia develops due to massive hepatic cell necrosis, leading to loss of glycogen stores and diminished glucose release. Hypokalemia may occur from inadequate oral intake, increased potassium losses from vomiting, or from medical interventions (eg, nasogastric suction or diuretic therapy). Hypomagnesemia commonly occurs in conjunction with hypokalemia as there is a close relationship between the movement of these electrolytes.

Hypocalcemia is a complication of multiple blood transfusions because the citrate used to anticoagulate stored blood may cause calcium depletion. Hypophosphatemia is also commonly associated with acute liver failure. The exact mechanisms remain unknown. Alkalosis and acidosis may both occur.

Hepatorenal Syndrome

Hepatorenal syndrome, a unique form of renal failure associated with severe liver disease, occurs in up to 40% of patients with advanced cirrhosis. This syndrome represents the most frequent fatal complication of liver failure. The pathogenesis of hepatorenal syndrome is multifactorial and includes portal hypertension resulting in splanchnic vasodilation and eventual sustained renal vasoconstriction and impaired renal perfusion. Precipitating events such as aggressive diuresis and SBP can cause an acute deterioration in renal function. Other than treating contributing conditions, the only definitive treatment for hepatorenal syndrome is liver transplantation. Renal function typically returns to normal after transplant. Without liver transplantation, hepatorenal syndrome is often fatal for the cirrhotic patient. Further research is needed regarding the use of vasoconstricting agents to reverse splanchnic vasodilation and improve outcomes.

Esophageal and Gastric Varices

Esophageal and gastric varices result from portal hypertension and develop in most patients with advanced cirrhosis. Mortality is significant and preventive measures including beta-blockers and endoscopic band ligation are of benefit (see previous section addressing upper GI bleeding). Similarly, prominent veins in the abdominal wall and around the umbilicus (caput medusa) may develop.

Spontaneous Bacterial Peritonitis

Spontaneous bacterial peritonitis is an infected ascitic fluid collection, demonstrated by a polymorphonuclear (PMN) count more than 250 cells/mm³ without an evident intra-abdominal source. SBP occurs in approximately one-quarter of patients admitted with chronic liver failure and ascites. While SBP is a common complication of liver failure, the overall incidence is decreasing due to prophylactic treatment in high-risk populations. A single microbial organism is usually responsible, such as *Escherichia coli*. It is theorized that intestinal translocation of organisms into the ascitic fluid results in infection.

Malnutrition

The liver has multiple nutrition-related functions including metabolism of carbohydrates, fats, and proteins and storage of essential minerals such as iron, copper, and vitamins A, B_{12}, D, and K. In advanced hepatic failure, the impaired ability to synthesize and store glycogen results in rapid muscle loss even during brief periods of decreased nutrient intake. Patients with liver failure frequently require vitamin K supplementation to normalize PT and PTT. Patients with alcohol-related liver disease may require intravenous thiamine to prevent Wernicke encephalopathy and assessment for the risk of withdrawal (see Chapter 11 [Multisystem Problems] for the management of alcohol withdrawal).

Clinical Presentation of Liver Failure

History

- Exposure to contaminated food, water
- Exposure to blood, body fluids
- Alcohol abuse

Signs and Symptoms

Impaired Thought Processes

- Mental status changes (confusion, lethargy)
- Behavioral changes
- Delirium
- Seizures
- Coma

Impaired Gas Exchange

- Hypoxemia
- Pulmonary edema

Fluid Volume Deficit or Excess

- Hypotension
- Skin cool, pale, and dry
- Urine output less than 30 mL/h (< 0.5 mL/kg/h)
- Tachycardia
- Dry mucous membranes

Hyperdynamic Circulation

- Arrhythmias
- Fever
- Palmar erythema (flushed palms)
- Jugular vein distension
- Crackles
- Murmur
- Increased CO
- Decreased systemic vascular resistance

Altered Nutrition

- Decreased appetite
- Muscle wasting
- Nausea and vomiting

Impaired Liver Metabolism

- Jaundice/Icterus
- Dry skin
- Ascites

Diagnostic Tests

- Total bilirubin more than 1.5 mg/dL
- AST more than 40 U/L
- ALT more than 60 U/L
- PT more than 13 seconds
- aPTT more than 45 seconds
- Fibrinogen less than 200 mg/dL
- Albumin less than 3.2 g/dL
- Ammonia more than 45 mg/dL
- Lactate dehydrogenase (LDH) more than 333 U/L

ESSENTIAL CONTENT CASE

Liver Failure

A 47-year-old man is admitted with a 3-day history of shortness of breath, increased confusion, nausea, and weakness. He has a history of upper GI bleeding from esophageal and gastric varices and was recently hospitalized for refractory ascites. He is diagnosed with liver failure due to alcohol abuse and is severely malnourished. Significant findings on his admission profile are:

History
Complaints of decreased appetite for the past 2 months; also complaints of nausea and weakness.

Vital Signs

Blood pressure:	89/52 mm Hg lying
Heart rate:	Sinus tachycardia with frequent PVCs
Respiratory rate:	32 breaths/min; shallow
Temperature:	37°C orally

Cardiopulmonary
- Dyspneic; using accessory muscles
- Rales and coarse rhonchi throughout all lung fields
- S_3/S_4; no murmurs
- Extremities cool, weak pulses
- 4+ pitting edema lower extremities

Neurologic
- Alert, but disoriented to time and place
- Irritable

Abdomen
- Tense ascites, dull to percussion
- Hyperactive BSs in all four quadrants

Genitourinary
- Urine dark, amber, and cloudy (0.3 mL/kg/h via urinary catheter)
- Large hemorrhoid protruding from rectal vault
- Liquid stool; black; guaiac positive

Laboratory Data
Arterial blood gases on 2 L O_2 per nasal cannula

pH	7.46
Paco$_2$	33 mm Hg
Pao$_2$	72 mm Hg
Sao$_2$	87%
HCO$_3^-$	28
Hematocrit	27%

Hemoglobin	8 g/dL
Aspartate transaminase (AST)	80 IU/L
Alanine transaminase (ALT)	84 IU/L
Bilirubin	1.8 mg/dL
PT	18 seconds
aPTT	> 45 seconds
INR	2.0
Fibrinogen	158 mg/dL
Albumin	2.8 g/dL
Potassium	3.0 mEq/L
Sodium	134 mEq/L
Creatinine	2.8 mg/dL
BUN	42 mg/dL
Glucose	80 mg/dL

Urine electrolytes

Sodium	5 mEq/L/day
Potassium	10 mEq/L/day

Case Question 1: Which complication of liver failure is this patient experiencing which contributes to a high risk of mortality?
(A) Hepatorenal syndrome
(B) GI bleeding
(C) Hepatic encephalopathy
(D) Ascites

Case Question 2: Which factor/s contribute/s to malnutrition in the patient with liver failure?
(A) Decreased oral intake
(B) Altered metabolism and storage of nutrients
(C) Altered mental status
(D) All of the above

Answers
1. The correct answer is (A). The most fatal complication of liver failure is hepatorenal syndrome. The risk for hepatorenal syndrome is evident with the low urine output, low BP, low hemoglobin/hematocrit, high BUN/creatinine, electrolyte abnormalities, and ascites.
2. The correct answer is (D). The liver metabolizes carbohydrates, fats, and proteins and also plays a key role in the storage of essential minerals, vitamins, and glycogen. When the liver is not able to synthesize and store glycogen, rapid muscle loss will occur. Altered mental status may lead to a decrease in oral intake which will further compromise nutritional status.

- Ultrasound, endoscopy, endoscopic retrograde cholangiopancreatography (ERCP), liver angiography/biopsy

Principles of Management for Liver Failure
The management of the patient with liver failure is centered on supporting cardiopulmonary status, supporting hematologic and nutritional functions of the liver, and preventing and treating complications.

Support Cardiopulmonary Status

1. Monitor fluid balance. The patient may have a fluid volume deficit related to portal hypertension, ascites, GI bleeding, or coagulation abnormalities. Fluid

overload may be a problem related to sodium excess and hypoalbuminemia. Administer diuretics such as furosemide and spironolactone as prescribed. Weigh patient daily.

2. Monitor abdominal girth when ascites is present and assist with paracentesis if needed. Generally paracentesis is done for patient comfort, to reduce respiratory impingement by the ascites and painful tautness of the abdomen. Large volume paracentesis is defined as removal of more than 5 L of fluid. This requires IV colloid replacement to prevent rapid re-accumulation of ascetic fluid and subsequent dehydration

3. Monitor respiratory status and correlate with arterial blood gas results. Administer oxygen as ordered. Administer sedatives and analgesics cautiously. Assist the patient with maneuvers to improve oxygenation.

Support Hematologic, Nutritional, and Metabolic Functions of the Liver

1. Monitor for signs of bleeding (eg, gastric contents, stools, urine) and test for occult blood. Observe for petechiae and bruising. Monitor hematologic profile.

2. Administer blood and blood products as ordered.

3. Institute measures to prevent variceal bleeding as needed, including beta-blockers.

4. Institute measures to provide for safety and to minimize tissue trauma. Provide for frequent mouth care. Avoid use of rectal tubes.

5. Initiate oral nutrition supplementation or enteral nutrition (EN) as appropriate (see enteral nutrition section of this chapter).

6. Monitor for signs and symptoms of infection. Maintain sterility of invasive lines and tubes. Maintain aseptic technique when performing procedures.

Preventing and Treating Complications

The most common complications of liver failure are hepatic encephalopathy, fluid and electrolyte imbalances, hepatorenal syndrome, and variceal hemorrhage.

1. Institute measures to prevent pressure injury to the skin, particularly in conditions with hypoalbuminemia fluid shifts as well as ascites.

2. Limit the use of medications that are metabolized or detoxified by the liver, especially narcotics and sedatives.

3. Keep the head of bed elevated to prevent aspiration and improve breathing. However, to prevent compression of the lungs by ascites, elevate the patient's head by using the reverse Trendelenburg position when able.

4. Observe for changes in mentation. Institute safety measures if confusion is present. May require endotracheal intubation to protect airway.

5. Perform interventions to reduce ammonia levels. Lactulose is a first-line treatment to decrease gut ammonia production. It can be administered through a nasogastric tube, orally (if alert and without an endotracheal tube), or rectally via a rectal tube (if large friable hemorrhoids are not present). Caution to avoid variceal rupture or tissue trauma is required with any tube insertion. Research demonstrates the efficacy of rifaximin in maintaining remission from hepatic encephalopathy. However, rifaximin is only available as tablets and is not appropriate for acutely ill patients who cannot take medications orally. Perform frequent neurological assessments. Trending serum ammonia levels is not recommended as the levels rarely correlate with degree of encephalopathy.

6. Institute protocols for bleeding risk due to clotting abnormalities and acute upper GI hemorrhage due to variceal rupture (see previous section).

7. Definitive treatment for hepatorenal syndrome is liver transplantation. In acutely ill patients, the use of albumin as an intravascular expander in combination with a vasoconstrictor is recommended and may result in improvement.

Artificial Liver Support Systems

Artificial liver support systems, currently available for investigational use only, may have a role in bridging patients with acute liver failure to transplant or providing support until regeneration of liver function occurs. The basic mechanism of artificial liver support systems is extracorporeal circulation of the patient's blood through filters that remove waste products normally filtered by the liver. These devices have not yet shown a decrease in mortality. Research is underway to optimize the devices.

Liver Transplantation

Liver transplantation has changed the survival of patients with liver failure. The decision to proceed with transplantation requires a detailed assessment and intraprofessional review. The Model for End-Stage Liver Disease, or MELD scoring system, was adopted in 2002 as the index to determine transplant priority. In 2016, UNOS authorized the addition of serum sodium to the MELD calculation when considering transplantation status and established the current MELD score. A higher score is associated with higher mortality risk and subsequent greater priority for transplantation.

Acute Pancreatitis

Acute pancreatitis is inflammation of the pancreas resulting from premature activation of pancreatic exocrine enzymes, such as trypsin, phospholipase A, and elastase within the pancreas. The disease ranges in severity from a mild acute self-limiting form to severe and life threatening. Severe acute pancreatitis occurring in approximately one-fifth of patients with pancreatitis involves autodigestion and necrosis of the pancreas. This pancreatic injury triggers a systemic inflammatory response, which can lead to multisystem organ failure (see Chapter 11, Multisystem Problems). Pancreatitis is categorized into two forms: interstitial edematous pancreatitis, which has a 3% mortality rate, and necrotizing acute pancreatitis, which has a 17% mortality rate. For patients with severe acute pancreatitis with necrosis, the mortality rate is 30%.

The diagnosis of acute pancreatitis is based on at least two of the three following criteria: characteristic abdominal pain or epigastric pain that may radiate to the back; serum amylase or lipase values 2 to 4 times above the normal range; and characteristic findings on imaging, most often ultrasound imaging. In general, serum lipase is more sensitive than serum amylase as a marker of pancreatitis. However, neither is predictive of disease severity or indicative of disease progression. Amylase and lipase are only useful as diagnostic tools. Organ failure and pancreatic necrosis are the two most important markers of severity.

Scoring systems are recommended to accurately identify the severity of acute pancreatitis and determine the appropriate patient care setting. Some of these tools (such as Ranson, Modified Marshall, APACHE IV, and Glasgow-Imrie) have limited to no applicability upon admission and are best applied after full assessment at the 24 to 48-hour mark. Other scoring systems that offer an assessment of disease severity within the first 24 hours have demonstrated clinical usefulness. The Bedside Index of Severity of Acute Pancreatitis (BISAP) is one example. This tool is both accurate and easy to use. The score is calculated on five variables: (1) BUN greater than 25 mg/dL; (2) impaired mental status; (3) presence of two or more criteria of systemic inflammatory response syndrome; (4) age greater than 60; and (5) pleural effusion on imaging. Each variable provides one point and scores of 3, 4, and 5 are associated with higher hospital mortality with a score of 5 associated with ~22% rate of mortality.

Etiologies, Risk Factors, and Pathophysiology

The leading causes of acute pancreatitis are chronic alcohol use and gallstones/biliary tract disease (stones). Drug-induced pancreatitis occurs with less frequency but has been linked to metronidazole, tetracycline, azathioprine, and estrogens as well as others. Less common etiologies are hypertriglyceridemia, hypercalcemia, infectious, autoimmune, vascular, genetic mutations, pancreatic neoplasms, post-ERCP pancreatitis, and idiopathic causes. In fact, 15% to 20% of pancreatitis cases are designated as idiopathic after a complete workup proves inconclusive.

The pathogenesis of acute pancreatitis is not completely understood. The pancreas normally has a protective mechanism, an enzyme called trypsin inhibitor, to prevent activation of enzymes before they reach the duodenum, thereby preventing inflammation of pancreatic cells. Regardless of

TABLE 14-9. COMMON MULTISYSTEM COMPLICATIONS OF ACUTE PANCREATITIS

Pulmonary
Atelectasis
Acute respiratory distress syndrome
Pleural effusions
Cardiovascular
Cardiogenic shock
Neurologic
Pancreatic encephalopathy
Metabolic
Metabolic acidosis
Hypocalcemia
Altered glucose metabolism
Hematologic
Disseminated intravascular coagulation
GI bleeding
Renal
Prerenal failure

the etiology, the process of premature activation of pancreatic enzymes leading to local inflammation and potential necrosis is the defining characteristic of pancreatitis. The activated enzymes can also enter the systemic circulation via the portal vein and lymphatic system, which leads to stimulation of platelet-activating factor and humoral systems (kinin, complement, fibrinolysis). These systems, which normally function to protect against infection, can generate a wide spread inflammatory response which results in damage to multiple organs (Table 14-9; see also Chapter 11, Multisystem Problems). Pancreatic abscess, pseudocyst, peripancreatic fluid collection, and necrosis are localized complications that may occur with fulminant forms of the disease. In severe acute pancreatitis, blood vessels in and around the pancreas may also become disrupted by microthrombi or enzymatic erosion of vasculature, resulting in hemorrhage.

Clinical Presentation
Signs and Symptoms

Pancreatic Inflammation

- *Acute pain:* Severe, relentless, knifelike; midepigastrium or periumbilical
- Abdominal guarding
- Nausea
- Rebound tenderness
- Vomiting
- Abdominal distention
- Hypoactive BS

Fluid Volume Deficit

- Hypotension
- Tachycardia
- Mental status changes
- Cool, clammy skin
- Decreased urine output

Impaired Gas Exchange

- Decreasing PaO_2 (< 60 mm Hg) and SaO_2 (< 90%)

Diagnostic Tests

- Serum amylase more than 140 U/L
- Serum pancreatic isoamylase more than 50% (more sensitive than amylase)
- Serum lipase more than 160 U/dL
- Serum triglycerides more than 1000 mg/dL
- Urine amylase more than 14 U/h (indicative of increased serum amylase)
- Serum calcium less than 8.5 mg/dL
- Serum sodium less than 135 mEq/L
- Serum potassium less than 3.5 mEq/L
- Serum magnesium less than 1.5 mg/dL
- Increased ALT (> 55 U/L), in gallstone pancreatitis
- C-reactive protein (> 3 mg/L)
- Glucose more than 120 mg/dL

Imaging Studies

- Ultrasound abdomen, check for cholelithiasis or choledocholithiasis (but may be obscured by bowel gas)
- Computed tomography (CT), pancreatic protocol CT scan of abdomen
- Endoscopic ultrasound (EUS)
- ERCP
- MRI/magnetic resonance cholangiopancreatography (MRCP)

Principles of Management of Acute Pancreatitis

The management of the patient with acute pancreatitis centers on allaying the release of enzymes and treating complications that can occur with multisystem disease. Interventions within the first 24 hours are essential to improving outcomes including increased survival. These interventions include determining severity with a reliable scoring system, aggressive fluid resuscitation, and other supportive measures such as application of oxygen, intubation, and mechanical ventilations as needed. Patients who demonstrate signs of organ failure (severe acute pancreatitis) are cared for in a critical care unit. Patients who do not demonstrate improvement or in whom there is uncertainty about the diagnosis are considered candidates for CT or MRI/MRCP. Additional principles of management include pain management, reducing pancreatic demands, and supporting other organ systems that may be failing due to the release of inflammatory mediators.

Fluid Resuscitation

Patients with acute pancreatitis experience significant hypovolemia as a result of third space losses, vomiting, and vascular permeability related to inflammatory mediators. Hypovolemia can compromise pancreatic circulation and increase the risk for pancreatic necrosis, so aggressive fluid and electrolyte replacement is essential in the initial management. However, after 48 hours the amount and rate of fluid administration must take into account the risk of fluid overload and consequent compartment syndrome or pulmonary edema.

1. In adults, administer intravenous isotonic crystalloid fluids at a rate of 5 to 10 mL/kg/h or greater if hypotensive with frequent reassessment of fluid needs, particularly within the first 12 to 24 hours. Caution is taken when treating patients with cardiovascular and renal conditions to diminish the risk of fluid overload. Monitor outcomes of fluid replacement therapy, including blood pressure, heart rate, intake and output, preload indicators (central venous pressure [CVP]), skin turgor, capillary refill, mucous membranes, and urine output (goal of greater than 0.5 to 1 mL/kg/h). Studies demonstrate that using the BUN as a marker of effective hydration is helpful in assessing hydration status.

2. Monitor for signs and symptoms of retroperitoneal hemorrhage (low hematocrit and hemoglobin levels). Cullen sign is a bluish discoloration around the periumbilical area, and Grey Turner sign is a bluish discoloration around the flank, indicating blood in the peritoneum. Monitor for increasing abdominal girth.

3. Monitor electrolytes for imbalances related to prolonged vomiting or fluid sequestration. Calcium, sodium, magnesium, and potassium are most commonly affected. Monitor QT intervals on the electrocardiogram and implement seizure precautions with severe hypocalcemia. Hyperglycemia also may be present due to the stress response and impaired secretion of insulin by the islet cells in the inflamed pancreas. Glucose levels need frequent evaluation. If elevated, administer an insulin infusion with hourly glucose assessments and insulin adjustments, then subcutaneous insulin to obtain a normoglycemic state. Hyperglycemia decreases healing and increases infection risk.

Pain Management

Acute pain is a universal sign of acute pancreatitis. It is caused by peritoneal irritation from activated pancreatic exocrine enzymes, edema or distention of the pancreas, or interruption of the blood supply to the pancreas. Treatment of pain is a priority because it increases exocrine enzyme release by the pancreas, extending pancreatic inflammation and worsening hemodynamic instability.

1. Assess the degree of pain using a reliable pain-rating scale.
2. Administer analgesics. In the past, the use of opiate analgesics (eg, morphine, fentanyl) has been discouraged because of the potential for causing increased pressure on the sphincter of Oddi, which in turn may increase pain. Meperidine has been suggested as an alternative to other opioids. However,

no outcome-based studies in patients with acute pancreatitis show that meperidine is superior. In addition, other opioids may provide better pain relief and do not have the seizure risk that occurs with meperidine. No studies or evidence exists to indicate morphine is contraindicated in acute pancreatitis. All analgesics are considered with an understanding of the risks and benefits to the individual patient. Regardless of what analgesic is prescribed, a pain-rating scale is used to evaluate efficacy. In addition, scheduled doses, continuous infusions, and epidural analgesia are important to consider to maintain steady-state analgesia in patients with severe pain.

3. Assess patient anxiety and administer sedatives with analgesics.
4. Assist the patient to a position that promotes comfort. The knee-to-chest position, when possible, may decrease the intensity of the pain. (Refer to Chapter 6 [Pain and Sedation Management] for additional information on pain management.)

Preventing Pancreatic Stimulation
Preventing stimulation of pancreatic exocrine secretion is a priority to interrupt the cycle of pancreatic inflammation.

1. In mild pancreatitis, with decreasing pain, improving labs and no nausea/vomiting or ileus, a low-fat, low-residue diet may be considered within the first 24 to 48 hours.
2. In moderate to severe pancreatitis, EN with jejunal feedings is often preferred to prevent pancreatic stimulation and enzyme secretion and to meet nutritional and caloric needs. With improvement, oral intake may be initiated and advanced as tolerated. New research suggests that early enteral feeding improves outcomes and that oral, gastric, and jejunal feedings may all be feasible.
3. Parenteral nutrition (PN) is not necessary unless enteral feedings are not tolerated.
4. Administer pharmacologic agents as prescribed to block the secretion of pancreatic enzymes or facilitate nutrient absorption.

Treat Local Complications in the Pancreas
Local complications in the pancreas include peripancreatic fluid collections (early peripancreatic fluid collections and pseudocysts) and necrotic collections (acute necrotic collection and walled off necrosis). The Atlanta classification system is used to standardize recognition and definition of these complications. Percutaneous or stent therapies to drain the fluids in and around the pancreas and/or surgical resection or debridement may be required, especially if the pancreas becomes infected. Biliary ERCP and laparoscopic cholecystectomy are indicated for gallstone pancreatitis, once the pancreatic inflammation has abated.

Treat Multisystem Failure
Cardiopulmonary complications due to pancreatic enzyme–induced mediators are the most common multisystem problems. Pancreatic ischemia promotes the release of myocardial depressant factor, causing decreased myocardial contractility and CO. Surgical therapies such as a pancreatic resection may be performed to prevent systemic complications of acute necrotizing pancreatitis by removing necrotic or infected tissue. In some cases, a pancreatectomy may be performed.

1. Administer oxygen therapy to maintain arterial oxygen tension and oxygen saturation. Mechanical ventilation with adjunct therapies to promote maximal alveolar gas exchange is often used to manage acute respiratory distress syndrome (see Chapter 10, Respiratory System).
2. Administer fluids, inotropes, and other vasopressors to support myocardial contractility, CO, and blood pressure (see Chapter 11, Multisystem Problems, for more on sepsis).
3. Institute measures to prevent infection. Monitor for signs and symptoms of sepsis and initiate appropriate treatment, if indicated. Prophylactic antibiotics are not recommended (see Chapter 11, Multisystem Problems).
4. Manage coagulopathies (see Chapter 13, Hematologic and Immune Systems).
5. Treat acute kidney injury if a complicating factor (see Chapter 15, Renal System).

Intestinal Ischemia

Major disorders of the intestine include intestinal ischemia. Vascular occlusion or infarction of the mesenteric vessels is rare but catastrophic and will result in profound illness with a mortality rate of 50%. Intestinal ischemia may present as intestinal angina, ischemic colitis, or intestinal infarction. Ischemic colitis is the most common ischemic injury. Ischemia may be acute or chronic. Acute forms are due to sudden and complete arterial occlusion by emboli, thrombosis of atherosclerotic stenosis, small vessel occlusion, venous thrombosis, or significant vasoconstriction. Gradual occlusion is better tolerated as there is time for collateral circulation to form. Sudden or acute ischemia is poorly tolerated because the bowel is not protected by collateral circulation. There is an extensive mesenteric collateral circulation which protects against ischemic insults. The colon is particularly susceptible to low-flow states, in particular, the splenic flexure, ileocecal junction, and rectosigmoid.

Etiology, Risk Factors, and Pathophysiology
Intestinal ischemia develops from a compromise in blood flow to the intestine, which is inadequate to meet metabolic demands. It is the result of hypoperfusion and reperfusion injury. Both the small intestine and the large bowel can be

affected but ischemic colitis is the most common form of intestinal ischemia. Acute ischemic colitis affects segments of the colon with normal colon on either side of the affected area. The right colon is affected 25% of the time, transverse 10%, left 33%, distal colon 25%, and the entire colon 7%. Disease involving the right side of the colon is usually more severe with the patient at risk for having involvement of the small intestine. Three major arterial trunks—the celiac axis, superior mesenteric artery, and inferior mesenteric artery—comprise the splanchnic (intestinal) circulation. The superior mesenteric artery, the inferior mesenteric artery, and branches of the internal iliac arteries perfuse the colon.

An acute occlusion is usually the result of a cardiogenic embolus with the superior mesenteric artery most frequently affected. The tissue injury that occurs will result in the release of cellular contents and the by-products of anaerobic metabolism into the general circulation. The ischemic bowel loses protein, electrolytes, and fluid into the lumen and wall of the bowel. The third-space extracellular fluid loss decreases the circulating blood volume. Full-thickness necrosis leads to bowel perforation and peritonitis.

The underlying causes of intestinal ischemia are diverse and include decreased CO, hypovolemia, arrhythmias, hypercoagulable states, mechanical obstruction, vascular disease, and trauma. Predisposing drugs include cocaine, cardiac glycosides, and alpha-stimulating sympathomimetic amines (epinephrine, norepinephrine). Older adult patients with systemic atherosclerosis are particularly at risk.

Clinical Presentation
Signs and symptoms will vary depending on the severity of the ischemia and area and length of intestine affected. The most common signs on admission to the hospital are hematochezia due to mucosal sloughing, abdominal pain, and diarrhea.

History
- Obstruction
- Diabetes mellitus
- Dyslipidemia
- Smoking
- Heart failure
- Aortic or coronary artery bypass surgery
- Shock
- Atrial fibrillation
- Atherosclerosis
- Medications: digitalis, diuretics, NSAIDs, catecholamines, and neuroleptics
- Recurrent nonspecific abdominal symptoms

Signs and Symptoms
- Anorexia
- Fever
- Tachycardia
- Leukocytosis
- Metabolic acidosis
- Elevated lactate
- Elevated LDH
- Peritoneal signs (abdominal guarding and rebound tenderness)
- Acute onset, colicky, severe left lower abdominal pain
- Pain out of proportion to abdominal examination findings
- Urgent desire to defecate
- Diarrhea
- Cramping
- Abdominal distention
- Decreased bowel sounds
- Hematochezia (bloody stools)
- Abdominal tenderness
- Ileus
- Nausea and vomiting
- Post-prandial pain
- Muscle rigidity
- Fluid volume deficit

Diagnostic Tests
Diagnosis is based on clinical findings and supported by radiographic corroboration and colonoscopic evaluation. CT or CT arteriography (CTA) scan and magnetic resonance angiography (MRA) or ultrasound are useful in supporting clinical suspicion and for identifying potential complications.

Colonoscopy may also be considered with distinct efforts to avoid overdistending the fragile intestine. The colonoscopy can identify mucosal abnormalities; findings will depend on the stage and severity of the ischemia. The finding of hemorrhagic, dusky mucosa with patches of inflammation is typical. CTA or MRA is indicated if acute mesenteric ischemia involving the small intestine is suspected. Interventional mesenteric arteriography may identify the site of occlusion and in addition can facilitate treatment with transcatheter thrombolysis, stent placement, or vasodilator infusion. A cardiac workup (ECG, Holter monitor, transthoracic echocardiogram) is done to exclude a cardiac source for an embolism.

Principles of Management for Intestinal Ischemia
Patient priorities revolve around treating the intravascular fluid volume deficit and avoiding the use of vasopressors. Generally patients respond to conservative supportive therapy. However in older patients, and in those in whom treatment and surgical intervention is delayed, necrosis and death may ensue. Delayed treatment (> 24 hours from the onset of symptoms) is associated with a mortality rate of more than or equal to 70%.

Medical treatment for intestinal ischemia depends on the presentation and severity of the insult. Supportive care is provided with patients placed on bowel rest, antibiotics, and intravenous fluids. Systemic anticoagulation may also be considered for arterial and venous thrombosis and embolic disease. Hemodynamic status is optimized and vasoconstrictive medications are avoided. The patient is monitored for signs of bowel necrosis such as persistent fever, leukocytosis, peritoneal irritation, or protracted pain or bleeding.

In the case of nonocclusive mesenteric insufficiency, a catheter infusion of a vasodilator, such as papaverine, into the superior mesenteric artery can be given intra-arterially at the time of arteriography. Spasm is considered the primary cause of this type of ischemia.

Exploratory laparotomy with thromboembolectomy or bypass of the occlusion (surgical revascularization) can be performed if the diagnosis is an acute mesenteric occlusion resulting from a clot or an atherosclerotic plaque. Surgery may also be indicated for peritonitis or clinical deterioration suggesting necrotic bowel (increasing abdominal tenderness, guarding, rebound tenderness, rising temperature, and/or paralytic ileus). Twenty percent of patients require surgical intervention for resection of the involved bowel. However, with current advances in endovascular treatments, surgical approaches are less frequent. The options for endovascular approaches such as percutaneous transluminal angioplasty with stent placement avoid the risks associated with an open surgical repair and are more common.

Bowel Obstruction

Bowel obstructions can lead to hospitalization for the management of fluid status, electrolyte abnormalities, and evaluation for surgical treatment. Intestinal transit can be affected by either a mechanical or functional obstruction. Mechanical obstructions can be due to lesions which block the internal lumen (luminal or intrinsic) or by lesions that compress the bowel lumen from the outside of the intestine (extrinsic). Mechanical obstructions can be further classified as either a small-bowel obstruction (SBO) or a large-bowel obstruction (LBO); and complete or partial. Complete obstruction always requires surgical management, whereas a partial obstruction can be managed conservatively with serial examinations and supportive treatment. Ileus and colonic pseudo-obstruction are categorized as functional obstructions.

Etiology, Risk Factors, and Pathophysiology
Small-Bowel Obstruction
Adhesions due to previous surgery are the most common cause of an SBO followed by malignant tumors (peritoneal implants), hernias, and inflammatory bowel disease. Adhesions account for approximately 70% of all SBO. Recent studies reveal that the incidence of SBO is lower in patients who have minimally invasive procedures versus open surgery.

Large-Bowel Obstruction
Colorectal cancer is the most common cause of an LBO in the United States with the descending colon and sigmoid colon being the most common sites of obstruction. Other causes of a mechanical (intraluminal) obstruction include fecal impaction and foreign bodies. Inflammation (diverticulitis or inflammatory bowel disease), ischemia, intussusception, and anastomotic stricture are also intrinsic etiologies. Extrinsic causes include hernias, abscess, volvulus, or tumors in adjacent organs. Adhesions are less likely to lead to obstruction of the large bowel; they are more common in the small bowel.

Early in the course of the obstruction, bowel motility and contractions will increase as the bowel attempts to push contents past the point of obstruction. This can account for diarrhea in the initial presentation. The intestine becomes fatigued, dilates, and contractions are less frequent and intense. Water and electrolytes accumulate in the bowel lumen and lead to dehydration and hypovolemia. Hypochloremia, hypokalemia, and metabolic alkalosis are not uncommon, especially if the patient is vomiting or has high large volume nasogastric tube losses. Abdominal distention can compromise respiratory function. In general, with either an SBO or LBO, a segment of the intestine may be excessively edematous or lumen malrotation may be present. These conditions can result in a blood supply that is compromised or strangulated. The blood supply can also be compromised by the increasing tension related to the abdominal distention. Ischemia may result and, if not treated, can lead to bowel necrosis. The cecum is the most common site of colonic ischemia or perforation, followed by the sigmoid colon.

Ileus
An ileus is intestinal distention and the slowing or absence of the passage of intestinal contents. It is a functional obstruction, so a mechanical cause cannot be identified. Common causes of an ileus are drug induced (anticholinergics, psychotropics, or opioids), metabolic derangements (hyperglycemia, hyperthyroidism), electrolyte abnormalities (such as hypokalemia), neurogenic, and infections. Ileus is most common after abdominal operations and often persists the longest after colon surgery.

Acute Colonic Pseudo-Obstruction
Pseudo-obstruction, also called Ogilvie syndrome, is a chronic condition of recurrent distention of the colon with signs and symptoms of obstruction, in the absence of a physical or mechanical cause. Acute colonic pseudo-obstruction (ACPO) is characterized by the absence of intestinal contractility. The exact cause remains unknown. It is commonly seen in hospitalized or institutionalized patients, older adults, and patients with chronic renal failure, respiratory, cerebral, or cardiovascular disease. It has an unknown prevalence and incidence, and as its name implies, it primarily affects the colon. It is diagnosed only after excluding mechanical LBO.

Clinical Presentation
Signs and symptoms will vary depending on the cause and location of the obstruction.

History
- Prior abdominal surgery
- Ischemia
- Hernia

- Abdominal cancer
- Abdominal radiation
- Inflammatory bowel disease

Signs and Symptoms

- Failure to pass stool or flatus
- Diarrhea
- Crampy or colicky abdominal pain; sometimes localized to periumbilical and epigastric regions, but usually diffuse
- Abdominal distention
- Generalized tenderness
- Nausea and vomiting
- Bowel sounds may be hyperactive or may be absent
- Visible peristalsis
- Tympany
- Tachycardia
- Hypotension
- Fever
- Localized tenderness, rebound, guarding (suggesting peritonitis)

Diagnostic Tests

Plain films of the abdomen will demonstrate whether an obstruction is present. Dilated loops of bowel with air fluid levels are characteristic in the proximal bowel; distal bowel is collapsed. A CT scan of the abdomen and pelvis with oral contrast will show the site of the obstruction, identify the transition zone, and often demonstrates the etiology. It is the diagnostic examination of choice. A small-bowel follow-through or enema study using water-soluble contrast solution may be necessary. Electrolyte disorders are common due to vomiting, diarrhea, lack of oral intake, and inflammatory mediators. The most common electrolyte abnormality is hypokalemia. The patient will exhibit either a metabolic or contraction alkalosis (renal sodium reabsorption in exchange for H^+) or metabolic acidosis (GI bicarbonate loss and hypovolemic tissue hypoperfusion).

Principles of Management for Bowel Obstruction

Treatment options will vary depending on the diagnosis. Initially, a nasogastric tube may be placed to decompress the bowel, the intravascular fluid volume deficit is treated with isotonic fluids, electrolyte abnormalities are corrected, bowel rest is initiated, and antiemetics and antibiotics are administered. Long intestinal tubes are no longer indicated and are associated with longer hospital stays and prolonged ileus. A rectal tube or colonic stent can be used to decompress the distal colon in patients with LBO. These interventions may serve as bridges to surgery or as palliative treatment. Studies demonstrate improved outcomes in bowel obstruction patients who receive prompt surgical consultation for symptoms of pain, nausea, and vomiting.

Treatment of an ileus consists entirely of supportive therapy. The most effective treatment is to address the underlying cause. Metabolic or electrolyte abnormalities are corrected and medications that may be contributing to the ileus are discontinued.

ACPO is treated with the administration of neostigmine, a parasympathomimetic agent. It is important that mechanical causes for the obstruction have been excluded before administering the drug. In the treatment of ACPO, 2.5 mg of neostigmine is given intravenously over 3 minutes. The pseudo-obstruction will resolve within less than 10 minutes with the patient passing stool and flatus. If no response occurs, the dose can be repeated 4 hours later. Bradycardia, bronchospasm, and hypotension are side effects of neostigmine and patients must be monitored with telemetry. Atropine is kept readily available. Patients with cardiac disease are not the candidates for this treatment. Patients who do not respond to neostigmine undergo a colonoscopy for decompression. Surgery is reserved for patients with signs of ischemia, perforation, or whose clinical status deteriorates.

The majority of SBOs will resolve spontaneously with supportive therapy, and therefore are managed nonoperatively. Surgical therapy is required to treat an LBO and may, in some cases, be needed to treat a persistent SBO. However, strangulated obstructions are surgical emergencies and require immediate intervention. Surgical procedures for various types of obstructions may include lysis of adhesions, reduction of hernias, bypass of obstructions, and resection of affected intestine. Self-expandable metallic colon stents may be placed at the time of colonoscopy to decompress the colon and can be a bridge to elective surgery in patients with a malignancy. A permanent or temporary diverting ileostomy or colostomy may be performed. A flexible sigmoidoscopy can be used initially to decompress a sigmoid volvulus; definitive surgery follows.

Both LBO and SBO treatment may include the following components:

1. Administer colloids and crystalloids to treat the fluid volume deficit. Normal saline with potassium supplementation is the replacement fluid of choice. Monitor patient response to fluid resuscitation—hemodynamic parameters (MAP, heart rate), body weight, and intake and output. A urinary catheter may be placed to monitor urine output.
2. Administer antimicrobial therapy to treat intra-abdominal infection. Gram-negative aerobic and anaerobic coverage is appropriate.
3. Elevate the head of bed to promote lung expansion. Use of reverse Trendelenburg, if tolerated, is a preferred position as it minimizes abdominal compression due to flexion at the hips as seen in a sitting position. Assist with deep breathing exercises to promote lung expansion, mobilization of secretions, and relaxation.
4. Administer analgesics for pain as needed. However, avoid excess use of opiates to promote the return of peristalsis.

5. With severe nausea and vomiting, insert a nasogastric tube and apply and maintain suction to drain and decompress the upper GI tract.

6. Monitor and report signs and symptoms of ongoing infection, peritoneal signs, or deterioration in status. Multiple follow-up abdominal radiographs and serial clinical examinations are indicated. Classic symptoms associated with strangulated bowel are leukocytosis, fever, tachycardia, and severe abdominal pain.

7. Provide nutrition as prescribed. Early enteral therapy may be initiated at slow rates as this has been found to promote the return of peristalsis and may assist in maintaining the gut mucosal barrier function. EN is initiated with caution if bowel ischemia is suspected; total parenteral nutrition may be required.

Bariatric (Weight Reduction) Surgery

Bariatric surgery is an option for weight reduction in obese individuals who have not been successful with conservative weight loss strategies such as diet, exercise, and pharmacologic therapy. Candidates for bariatric surgery include those patients with a body mass index (BMI) of 40, or a BMI between 35 and 40 in the presence of obesity-related comorbidities, such as diabetes, hypertension, obstructive sleep apnea, and cardiovascular disease.

Because all patients who have bariatric surgery are obese, and many have comorbid diseases, surgical recovery may be challenging. Diabetes mellitus, nonalcoholic fatty liver disease, coronary artery disease, asthma, obstructive sleep apnea, and other conditions are more common among obese patients and require careful postoperative monitoring.

Surgical Procedure

There are three main types of weight loss surgery: restrictive, malabsorptive, and combined restrictive and malabsorptive. These procedures can be performed via either the laparoscopic or open approach. Laparoscopic is recommended because there is less pain, fewer wound complications, a shorter hospital stay, and quicker recovery. All procedures limit the volume of food eaten and alter gastric emptying. The risk for nutritional deficiencies will vary depending on the surgery performed. The restrictive procedures include the vertical banded gastroplasty (VBG), the laparoscopic adjustable gastric band (LAGB), and the laparoscopic sleeve gastrectomy (LSG). The malabsorptive procedures include the biliopancreatic diversion (BPD), biliopancreatic diversion with duodenal switch (BPD-DS), and duodenal switch (DS). The laparoscopic Roux-en-Y (LRYGB) is categorized as both restrictive and malabsorptive.

The VBG is done infrequently today, but was popular in the 1980s. The upper stomach near the esophagus is stapled vertically to create a small pouch. A band is placed to restrict the outlet from the pouch. With the LAGB, restriction is accomplished by placing an inflatable silicone band around the antrum of the stomach thereby creating a small pouch. The band is connected to an implanted reservoir under the skin, usually just below the rib cage. The pouch opening can be made smaller or larger by inflating or deflating the band via the reservoir.

The LSG, once considered a preliminary step toward LRYGB, has become an acceptable primary bariatric surgery. The procedure reduces the stomach to about 25% of its original size. The majority of the greater curvature of the stomach is removed. The open edges are stapled to form a sleeve or tube with a "banana" shape. The procedure permanently reduces the size of the stomach. Although it is described as a restrictive procedure, recent studies have identified similar metabolic effects as seen with the LRYGB. These effects could potentiate a sense of satiety for patients. Recent studies have shown weight loss after the LSG to be between that seen with the LAGB and LRYGB.

The BPD, BPD-DS, and DS are malabsorptive procedures. These surgeries carry the highest risk for nutritional deficiencies as they significantly alter digestion and absorption of protein, vitamins, and minerals. In general, there are three main components of these surgeries: a partial gastrectomy, the common or nutrient limb, and biliopancreatic limb. The common limb is a 50 to 100 cm portion of distal small bowel where limited digestion and absorption occur, while the biliopancreatic limb is created from the remainder of the proximal small bowel and functions to divert digestive juices to the nutrient or common limb.

The LRYGB results in both restriction and malabsorption and is the gold standard surgery for treating obesity. The stomach is separated with a stapler and a 15-mL pouch is created. The small intestine is divided and the distal stomach, duodenum, and first part of the jejunum are bypassed. The distal end of the jejunum is anastomosed to the pouch (gastrojejunostomy) to allow for emptying while the proximal end is connected side to side to the jejunum (jejunojejunostomy) creating a 75- to 150-cm roux limb. The surgery also has a hormonal effect. Removing the gastric fundus, the primary site of ghrelin production, enhances weight loss by reducing appetite.

Principles of Management for Postoperative Bariatric Surgery

Standard nursing care following bariatric surgery includes assessment of vital signs and incisions, management of pain, pulmonary exercise, and venothromboembolism (VTE) prophylaxis. In addition to standard postoperative care, assessment for, and prevention of, complications inherent to the bariatric surgery procedure and the nuances of the bariatric patient are essential.

Respiratory Insufficiency

Airway obstruction and oxygenation problems are important postoperative concerns following bariatric surgery. Patients with obstructive sleep apnea preoperatively are at higher risk for postoperative respiratory problems. Patients with sleep apnea use their continuous positive airway pressure (CPAP) or bilevel positive airway pressure (BiPAP) machine while in the hospital to help minimize this risk. The increased risk of postoperative oxygenation problems from anesthesia and postoperative analgesics in this vulnerable group requires careful respiratory monitoring for 24 to 48 hours after surgery. Patients with asthma, a common comorbidity with obstructive sleep apnea, need to continue using inhaled medications during the postoperative period.

Assessment for Anastomotic Leaks

Leakage of gastric contents at the site of anastomosis is a potentially life-threatening complication and if not recognized early can lead to overwhelming sepsis. Signs and symptoms of an anastomotic leak include fever, left shoulder pain, tachypnea, and tachycardia. Thirst and hypotension are typically appreciated in progressive sepsis. Abdominal pain may occur, but the absence of it does not preclude the possibility of an anastomotic leak. The only sign of a leak may be unexplained tachycardia.

A leak is diagnosed with either a limited upper GI radiograph or a CT scan. A contained leak can be treated with percutaneous drainage. If the leak is not contained, the patient is returned to the operating room for definitive treatment. A leak could result in an intra-abdominal abscess. The key to treating a leak is to identify it early through watchful monitoring.

Once the upper GI radiograph or CT scan are clear, patients are typically able to begin a gastric bypass diet.

Nausea and Vomiting

Nausea and vomiting are not expected consequences of bariatric surgery. The cause may be mechanical or behavioral. Vomiting is generally very short lived as patients adjust to eating and drinking. Behavioral causes include eating too quickly, overeating, not chewing food well, drinking while eating, or a poor food choice. Dehydration may present as nausea. Anastomotic stricture or another mechanical cause of obstruction must be ruled out. Antiemetics are usually not helpful but may reduce retching that can put strain on the anastomosis and the incision line leading to complications. If the nausea is due to dehydration, the symptoms will resolve with the administration of intravenous fluids. Counseling the patient and addressing anxieties will assist with management of behavioral etiologies.

Prevention of Pulmonary Embolus

Patients having bariatric procedures are at high risk for pulmonary embolus (PE). Early ambulation postoperatively, which can be challenging in this patient population, reduces the risk of DVT and PE. In the immediate postoperative period, DVT and PE prevention requires a combination of subcutaneous weight-based pharmacologic prophylaxis, use of sequential compression devices, and a program of immediate and progressive mobilization. Optimal pain management is important not just for comfort, but to promote mobility. In patients with a prior history of DVT, PE, or a history of a clotting disorder, an inferior vena cava filter may be placed preoperatively.

Skin Care

The bariatric surgery patient is at high risk for pressure injury and poor wound healing. Skin folds harbor moisture, bacteria, and yeast; in addition, the blood supply to adipose tissue is poor. The best skin care is prevention and includes daily inspection of the skin, frequent turning, early ambulation, and special attention to the positioning of catheters and drainage tubes so that they are not hidden within skin folds. Skin care needs to be thorough, paying special attention to the folds under the breasts, back, abdomen, and perineum, as well as the surgical sites or incisions.

Postoperative Medication Alterations

Another important consideration in the care of patients after bariatric surgery is the administration of medications. Because a portion of small bowel has been bypassed, absorption of medications will be impacted. Medications previously given as sustained-released formulations are given in regular-release form to compensate for the changes in absorption. Tolerance of the GI effects of some medications may be altered, and patients are carefully monitored for new or changing side effects.

Many bariatric patients also have hepatic insufficiency from nonalcoholic fatty liver disease. Medication choices take this factor into account and patients are closely monitored for medication effect due to both limited hepatic function as well as decreased absorption.

Resumption of preoperative diabetic medications, both insulin and oral agents, is also carefully monitored. Requirements for glucose control change dramatically immediately after surgery and resuming preoperative doses may lead to hypoglycemia. Postoperatively, diabetic medications such as sulfonylureas and meglitinides are discontinued and insulin doses are adjusted to prevent hypoglycemia. Many patients are able to completely discontinue the use of diabetic medications, including insulin, after surgery.

Patient Education

Recovery from bariatric surgery is a lengthy and involved process, extending beyond surgical healing. Patient education is a critical part of acute nursing care. Patients are taught the signs and symptoms associated with an anastomotic leak before they go home since the leaks can occur weeks following surgery. Nutritional instruction and dietary progression is an important part of the process, and advancing diet properly may reduce nausea, vomiting, and other discomfort following surgery. Patients having malabsorptive procedures remain at long-term risk for vitamin and mineral deficiencies, and are best served by a sure understanding of long-term follow-up and dietary and vitamin/mineral supplementation.

NUTRITIONAL SUPPORT FOR ACUTELY ILL PATIENTS

The negative consequences of malnutrition have been known for centuries, and there is substantial evidence that malnourished hospitalized patients have increased morbidity, compromised surgical outcomes, more ventilator days, and increased mortality rates.

There is accumulating evidence that the route of nutrition support can affect morbidity in the acutely ill patient. Protocols and care bundles for the proper initiation and monitoring of patients on nutrition support may reduce complications.

It is recommended that patients undergo screening for malnutrition upon admission using validated tools. Traditional approaches that incorporate laboratory indicators or other markers (ie, albumin or pre-albumin) are not supported by scientific studies and not recommended. EN is introduced within 24 to 48 hours of admission in acutely ill patients who are unable to maintain sufficient oral intake. Gastric feedings are a reasonable approach if the jejunum is not readily accessible.

Nutritional Requirements

Current recommendations for feeding acutely ill patients suggest approximately 25 total calories/kg/day based on the patient's ideal body weight, or 27.5 total calories/kg/day in the presence of conditions that increase catabolism. A total of 1.2 to 1.5 g/kg/day of protein is also recommended. In severely malnourished patients, reduced calories (15-20 kcal/kg) are initiated to minimize electrolyte shifts from refeeding. When electrolytes are stable, progression to 30 or more calories/kg may be attempted to improve nutrition status. Close monitoring for tolerance is indicated. Controlled trials have demonstrated that overfeeding does not provide increased nutritional benefits, and actually has detrimental effects (Table 14-10).

Nutritional Case: Special Populations

Bariatric Surgery

Nutritional supplementation is standard therapy for all gastric bypass operations. Ongoing monitoring and reinforcement

TABLE 14-10. POTENTIAL CONSEQUENCES OF OVERFEEDING OF MACRONUTRIENTS[a]

Carbohydrate	Fat
Hyperglycemia	Impaired immune response
Synthesis and storage of fat Hepatic steatosis	Fat overload syndrome with neurologic, cardiac, pulmonary, hepatic, and renal dysfunction
Increased carbon dioxide production increasing minute ventilation	Thrombocyte adhesiveness
	Accumulation of lipid in the reticuloendothelial system (RES), leading to RES dysfunction

[a]Remember to look for additional sources of dextrose and fat, such as propofol, intravenous fluids (IVF), continuous venovenous hemodialysis (CVVHD), peritoneal dialysis.
Reproduced with permission from: The University of Virginia Health System from Nutrition Support Traineeship Syllabus, University of Virginia Health System, Charlottesville, VA; Updated June 2013.

of compliance is essential. Medication absorption is also altered in these patients. Ethyl alcohol (ETOH) absorption is enhanced, while sustained release and enteric-coated tablets may pass through undissolved, or unutilized. The efficacy of medications requiring a large volume of food or high-fat meal may be compromised (antifungals, antipsychotics).

Postgastrectomy Syndromes

Gastric resection can predispose patients to both nutritional intolerances and deficiencies. Intolerances include dumping syndrome, fat maldigestion, gastric stasis, and lactose intolerance. Nutrient deficiencies can develop months to years after gastric resections and can result in deleterious clinical consequences. Patients are at higher risk of developing osteoporosis and iron- and vitamin B_{12}–deficiency anemia. Decreased acid production and small bowel bacterial overgrowth most likely play a role in the latter two. Ongoing nutritional monitoring of these patients will prevent deficiencies and identify those in need of intervention.

Parenteral Nutrition

Parenteral nutrition is indicated for malnourished patients and those at risk for becoming malnourished, only if the patient is unable to receive EN (Table 14-11). PN can be lifesaving in some cases, but is not without complications (including bloodstream infections) and is used only when EN is not feasible (Table 14-12). Prospective trials have demonstrated that the metabolic and infectious complications of PN outweigh the benefits in patients without significant malnutrition. Studies have demonstrated that even short-term PN, used to supplement EN in the ICU, does not have benefits and is associated with increased infectious complications and length of stay.

Enteral Nutrition

Current evidence suggests that EN is the preferred method of feeding the acutely ill patient. It is associated with fewer infectious complications, is less expensive, confers some gut immune protection, and diminishes atrophy and attenuation of systemic response (Table 14-13). Patients that do not receive adequate amounts of EN have a greater need for rehabilitation services compared to patients receiving full feedings.

Unfortunately, the delivery of EN is impeded by various situations that occur in progressive care units; for example, EN may be stopped for diagnostic or therapeutic procedures, or in those with clogged or dislodged enteral tubes (Table 14-14).

Successful EN is also thwarted by experiential assumptions and practices, as well as beliefs about how the GI tract functions in acute illness. These unsupported practices are discussed below.

Gastric Residual Volume

Despite the publication of practice guidelines calling for clinicians to avoid measuring gastric residual volumes

TABLE 14-11. INDICATIONS FOR PARENTERAL NUTRITION

Parenteral nutrition is usually indicated in the following situations:
- Documented inability to absorb adequate nutrients via the gastrointestinal tract. This may be due to:
  - Massive small-bowel resection/short-bowel syndrome (at least initially)
  - Radiation enteritis
  - Severe diarrhea
  - Steatorrhea
- Complete bowel obstruction, or intestinal pseudo-obstruction
- Persistent ileus
- Severe catabolism with or without malnutrition when gastrointestinal tract is not usable within 5-7 days
- Inability to obtain enteral access
- Inability to provide sufficient nutrients or fluids enterally
- Pancreatitis accompanied by abdominal pain with jejunal delivery of nutrients
- Persistent GI hemorrhage
- Acute abdomen
- Lengthy GI workup requiring NPO status
- High-output enterocutaneous fistula (> 500 mL) if enteral feeding ports cannot be distally placed
- Trauma requiring repeat surgical procedures

Parenteral nutrition may be indicated in the following situations:
- Enterocutaneous fistula (< 500 mL)
- Inflammatory bowel disease not responding to medical therapy
- Hyperemesis gravidarum when nausea and vomiting persist longer than 5-7 days and enteral nutrition is not possible
- Partial small bowel obstruction
- Intensive chemotherapy/severe mucositis
- Major surgery/stress when enteral nutrition not expected to resume within 7-10 days
- Intractable vomiting when jejunal feeding is not possible
- Chylous ascites or Chylothorax

Reproduced with permission from: The University of Virginia Health System from Nutrition Support Traineeship Syllabus, University of Virginia Health System, Charlottesville, VA; Updated June 2013.

(GRV), the practice continues. However, reliance on isolated high residuals to determine feeding tolerance may be counterproductive.

One of the physiologic functions of the stomach is to act as a reservoir and to control delivery of nutrients into the small bowel. This allows for maximal assimilation with bile salts and pancreatic enzymes. A number of factors contribute to the GRV: endogenous secretions, normal gastric emptying, exogenous fluids, and the cascade effect.

Endogenous Secretions and Exogenous Additions

Two to four liters per day of saliva and gastric secretions are produced above the pylorus. Conservatively, this translates into 3 L of fluid that pass through the pylorus every 24 hours

TABLE 14-12. CONTRAINDICATIONS FOR PARENTERAL NUTRITION

- Functioning gastrointestinal tract
- Treatment anticipated for < 5 days in patients without severe malnutrition
- Inability to obtain venous access
- A prognosis that does not warrant aggressive nutrition support
- When the risks of PN are judged to exceed the potential benefits

Reproduced with permission from: The University of Virginia Health System from Nutrition Support Traineeship Syllabus, University of Virginia Health System, Charlottesville, VA; Updated June, 2013.

TABLE 14-13. BENEFITS OF ENTERAL FEEDING

- Stimulates immune barrier function
- Physiologic presentation of nutrients
- Maintains gut mucosa
- Attenuates hypermetabolic response
- Simplifies fluid/electrolyte management
- More "complete" nutrition than parenteral nutrition
- Less infectious complications (and costs associated with these complications)
- Stimulates return of bowel function
- Less expensive

Reproduced with permission from: The University of Virginia Health System from Nutrition Support Traineeship Syllabus, University of Virginia Health System, Charlottesville, VA; Updated June, 2013.

(an average of 125 mL/h). Once an enteral tube is positioned in the stomach, medications, water flushes, and EN add to this volume. Commonly in acute care, clinicians expect the stomach to be empty or only contain a very small amount of tube feeding or other liquid when checked. However, one study has demonstrated that 40% of healthy volunteers have an average GRV greater than 100 mL.

The Cascade Effect

Patient positioning, either in the supine position or, preferably with backrest elevation 30° or higher, affects GRV measurement. In this position, the stomach partially splits over

TABLE 14-14. COMMON BARRIERS TO OPTIMIZING ENTERAL NUTRITION DELIVERY

- Diagnostic procedures (feedings are stopped)
- Propofol (Diprivan) (calories from the lipid preparation must be calculated as part of the total kcal provided to prevent overfeeding—1.1 cal/mL infused)
- Enteral access issues (clogged/dislodged tubes or obtaining postpyloric access if needed)
- Feedings held due to drug-nutrient interactions
- Hypotensive episodes (patient is often flat in bed necessitating that feedings be turned off)
- Miscalculation of EN requirements
- "NPO" at midnight for tests, surgery, or procedures
- Conditioning regimes and/or therapies that require the feedings to be turned off
- Transportation off the unit
- Hemodialysis (EN is often stopped during hemodialysis if the patient is deemed unstable by the nurse, often after the patient experiences hypotension)
- Perceived or real "GI intolerance or dysfunction"
  - Nausea/vomiting
  - Complaints of fullness
  - Abdominal distention
  - Lack of bowel sounds (see Bowel Sounds)
  - Diarrhea (see Diarrhea Table 14-18)
  - Aspiration risk/no gag (see Aspiration)
  - Gastric residual volume (see Gastric Residual Volume)

A note on checking GRV with jejunal tubes: There is no need to check a GRV with a jejunal tube; there is no "reservoir" to hold EN, hence the flow of EN distally begins immediately.

Reproduced with permission from: The University of Virginia Health System from Nutrition Support Traineeship Syllabus, University of Virginia Health System, Charlottesville, VA; Updated June, 2013.

the spine and is mechanically divided into two parts, the fundus (proximal) and the antrum (distal). Because the fundus is the noncontractile portion of the stomach, contents fill the fundus until they "cascade over" the spine into the antrum and finally exit through the pylorus. Thus, if the patient's feeding port is in the proximal stomach or fundus when the GRV is checked, the aspirated GRV may be erroneous. The GRV in this case may be a function of the patient's supine positioning rather than decreased GI motility.

Checking Gastric Residual Volume

There is no evidence that measuring GRV is a valid assessment of feeding tolerance, elevated GRV is not linked to aspiration, and the practice is not supported by current guidelines. Some of the factors that affect the assessment of GRV are listed below:

1. Type of tube (Salem sump vs Dobhoff-like feeding tube vs a gastrostomy)
2. Location of the gastrostomy on the patient's abdominal wall (fundus, antrum)
3. Position of the patient when GRV is checked (supine, right or left lateral decubitus, prone)
4. Method of aspiration (20-, 35-, 50-, 60-mL syringe vs gravity drainage vs low constant suction)
5. The volume of the aspirate obtained
6. Disposition of the aspirate (eg, reinfused or discarded)
7. The effects of GI stress prophylaxis medications (PPIs) on the production and volume of gastric secretions

For these reasons, measuring GRV is poorly standardized and should not be routinely incorporated into practice. GRV as a valid measure of EN tolerance or whether the amount of GRV is linked to the risk of aspiration pneumonia events has yet to be proven. Until more evidence is available, careful consideration of the need to check GRV is warranted, and the result obtained should never be the only data point used to assess patient tolerance. For clinicians who identify a need to assess GRVs, feedings should not be held for GRVs less than 500 mL unless other signs of intolerance are identifiable.

Aspiration as a complication of Enteral Feeding

Aspiration is the passage of materials into the airway below the level of the vocal cords. The aspirated material may be saliva, nasopharyngeal secretions, bacteria, food, beverage, gastric contents, bile, or any other ingested substance. The incidence of aspiration pneumonia from EN is unclear, because it is difficult to identify an aspiration event and definitions of aspiration vary. Commonly quoted aspiration pneumonia rates in EN patients, however, are between 5% and 36%.

Detection

Several methods of evaluating patients for aspiration risk have been popularized through "conventional wisdom."

These include the routine monitoring of GRVs (discussed above), evaluation of gag reflex, testing tracheal secretions for the presence of glucose, and the addition of blue food color to feeding formulas.

The gag reflex is the least reliable protective reflex in ensuring that aspiration does not occur. More important to airway protection are reliable cough and swallow reflexes.

The presence of glucose in tracheal secretions is not a specific or sensitive method of detecting aspiration of EN. Tracheal glucose can be positive in patients who are not receiving feeding. In addition, some EN formulas have low glucose concentrations and do not result in a positive test when aspirated.

Several studies have demonstrated that adding blue dye to feeding formulas is not a sensitive method for detecting aspiration and is not used to indicate aspiration of gastric contents. In addition, some food dyes are mitochondrial toxins leading the Food and Drug Administration to release a Public Health Advisory Report noting the toxicity associated with the use of FD&C Blue No. 1.

Aspiration Risk
Body Position

The position of the patient is one of the primary factors influencing aspiration risk (Table 14-15). Studies have confirmed that aspiration and pneumonia are significantly more likely when patients are supine with the head of the bed elevated at less than 30°. While the semirecumbent position with head of the bed elevations of greater than or equal to 30° cannot guarantee absolute protection against aspiration, it is a method that is inexpensive and relatively easy to accomplish and monitor. Strict use of semirecumbent position is the most consistent and potent means to reduce the likelihood of aspiration.

Tube Size and Placement Issues

The incidence of aspiration, and subsequently pneumonia, are not affected by the feeding tube size or whether the tube is placed through the nose, mouth, or a gastrostomy stoma. Regardless of the site, confirmation of accurate placement is essential.

TABLE 14-15. PREVENTION OF ASPIRATION

- Maintain backrest elevation of 30°-45° if no contraindication is present to that position.
- Use sedatives as sparingly as possible.
- For tube fed patients, verify appropriate placement of feeding tube every 4 hours.
- For patients receiving gastric feedings, assess for gastrointestinal intolerance every 4 hours.
- For tube fed patients, avoid bolus feedings if high risk for aspiration
- Consult with provider about obtaining a swallow evaluation before oral feedings in recently extubated patients or those intubated for more than 2 days.
- Maintain endotracheal cuff pressures at appropriate level, and ensure that secretions are cleared from above the cuff before it is deflated.

Data from American Association of Critical-Care Nurses. AACN practice alert: Prevention of Aspiration in Adults, Crit Care Nurse. 2016 Feb;36(1):e20-e24.

Moreover, there is evidence that pulmonary injury during bedside placement of feeding tubes occurs more frequently than is generally appreciated. Using a method to provide feedback that the airway has been inadvertently intubated with the feeding tube can decrease the incidence of injury that may occur before the confirmatory radiograph is obtained. Several studies have reported that use of CO_2 detection, electromagnetic guidance, or a preliminary radiograph during placement decreases the incidence of inadvertent pulmonary intubation and injury. It is commonly believed that placing the tip of the feeding tube beyond the pylorus decreases the incidence of aspiration events. However, numerous studies and a meta-analysis on the topic, note that it is unclear if a properly positioned jejunal tube can reduce aspiration risk.

The majority of acutely ill patients in these studies received gastric tube feedings safely and effectively. In studies that used protocols for the prevention of aspiration, very low rates of aspiration pneumonia were demonstrated. From an evidence-based standpoint, the question of jejunal placement of feeding tubes and aspiration risk remains unanswered.

Considering the time and expense associated with jejunal placement of feeding tubes, it is reasonable to use the gastric route unless intolerance is evident. Exceptions to this approach include patients known to be at increased risk for aspiration due to altered anatomy (eg, esophagectomy) or dysmotility (eg, scleroderma, severe gastroparesis). These patients may benefit from jejunally placed tubes.

In congruence with the AACN Practice Alert, techniques to ensure proper placement of enteral tubes are recommended and include: (1) observe for signs of respiratory distress, (2) use capnography to detect inadvertent placement into the lungs, (3) measure pH of aspirates, and (4) observe for visual signs of gastric aspirate (refer to the AACN Practice Alert Initial and Ongoing Verification of Feeding Tube Placement in Adults). Tube placement is verified with radiologic assessment prior to any instillation of feedings, fluids, or medications. Placement is reassessed every 4 hours. The head of bed is raised to 30° to 40° and sedatives are used sparingly. These measures are associated with a reduction in untoward events.

Feeding Rate

The delivery rate of the feeding formula may influence aspiration and pneumonia. Bolus administration of 350 mL reduces lower esophageal sphincter pressure, which may precipitate reflux. Continuous EN (transpyloric feedings) has been associated with more rapidly attained feeding tolerance, but not a significant change in aspiration incidence. In one study, reduced aspiration events were associated with cyclic infusion feedings (16-hour cycle), compared to continuous feedings. The authors postulated that cyclic enteral feedings resulted in a reduction of gastric pH and subsequently prevented colonization of gastric contents. However, randomized trials have failed to demonstrate associations between gastric pH, gastric colonization, or pneumonia incidence between patients fed with cyclic versus continuous feedings.

Pharmacologic Interventions

Prokinetic medications have been evaluated to determine whether they improve EN tolerance. In acutely ill patients, metoclopramide and erythromycin improve gastric emptying, but there are few data on the incidence of aspiration pneumonia associated with the use of the agents.

Bowel Sounds in Enterally Fed Patients

Auscultating the abdomen to determine the presence of BS, and thus GI tract function, is a well-entrenched practice yet has never been validated as a marker of GI tract function. The absence of BS does not preclude the initiation of EN.

Careful initiation of EN in patients without BS may stimulate normal bowel function and the emergence of BS. Research suggests that enteral feeding initiated within the first 24 to 48 hours of ICU admission with or without the presence of BS is safe. Auscultation of BS in the clinical setting varies. Clinician assessment practices differ and include how the quadrants are auscultated, frequency of auscultation, time spent listening for sounds, and interpretation of the sounds. BS are nonspecific markers and hence are best used in conjunction with the overall clinical assessment of the patient if used. Suggested approaches to assessment of GI function when BSs are absent are found in Table 14-16.

Complications of EN: Nausea, Vomiting and Diarrhea

Many factors contribute to nausea and vomiting in the progressive care setting and include medications, the disease process, surgery, procedures, and bedside interventions (eg, placing a nasogastric tube and/or suctioning). After careful assessment and treatment of the underlying cause if possible (Table 14-17), antiemetic medications may allow the continuation of EN while making the patient more comfortable. If antiemetics and/or prokinetics are initiated, they are continued until symptoms abate. Scheduled versus as needed antiemetics may increase efficacy and overall success.

TABLE 14-16. SUGGESTED APPROACHES FOR ASSESSMENT OF GI FUNCTION WHEN BOWEL SOUNDS ARE ABSENT

- Assess need for, and volume of, gastric decompression (ie, compare volume aspirated to normal secretions above the pylorus expected over time frame between aspirations).
- Distinguish significance by differentiating those patients requiring:
  Low constant suction
  Gravity drainage
  An occasional gastric residual check every 4-6 hours (small bowel aspirates should not be checked)
- Abdominal examination—firm, distended, tympanic.
- Presence of nausea, bloating, feeling full, vomiting.
- Evaluate whether patient is passing gas or stool.
- Compare clinical examination with the differential diagnosis, specifically high suspicion for abdominal process.
- Finally, after determining low risk from above, consider a trial of EN at low rate of 10-20 mL/h and clinically observe for any of the symptoms listed above.

Reproduced with permission from: The University of Virginia Health System from Nutrition Support Traineeship Syllabus, University of Virginia Health System, Charlottesville, VA; Updated June, 2013.

TABLE 14-17. SUGGESTED APPROACHES TO REDUCE NAUSEA AND VOMITING IN ENTERALLY FED PATIENTS

1. Review medication profile; change suspected agents to an alternative.
2. Try a prokinetic agent or antiemetic—review orders for PRN vs scheduled doses as well as delivery method.
3. Switch to a more calorically dense product to decrease the total volume infused.
4. Seek transpyloric access of feeding tube.
5. Tighten glucose control to < 200 mg/dL to avoid gastroparesis from hyperglycemia.
6. Consider analgesic alternatives to opiates.
7. If feeding into small bowel, vent gastric port (if available).
8. Consider a proton pump inhibitor in order to decrease sheer volume of endogenous gastric secretions (eg, omeprazole, lansoprazole, esomeprazole, pantoprazole, rabeprazole).
9. If bacterial overgrowth is a possibility, treat with enteral antibiotics.
10. Vent gastric port if available.

Reproduced with permission from: The University of Virginia Health System from Nutrition Support Traineeship Syllabus, University of Virginia Health System, Charlottesville, VA; Updated June, 2013.

Osmolality or Hypertonicity of Formula

Diarrhea in patients on EN is sometimes attributed to the use of hypertonic or hyperosmolar formulas, although no data exist to support this relationship. Diluting formula is thought to reduce this complication by lowering the tonicity and osmolality of the feeding. However, dilution of formula increases nursing time and the risk of contamination, and decreases the nutrient content of the feeding. Therefore, diluting gastric feeding formula is not recommended.

The practice of diluting jejunal feedings is also not scientifically supported. Some believe that full strength tube feeding will not reach isotonicity and therefore should not be delivered straight to the jejunum. However, the GI tract secretes gastric and pancreatobiliary juices (including bicarbonate) to ensure isotonicity. In patients who have received gastrectomies (all the food they eat is delivered directly from the esophagus into the jejunum), normal feedings (albeit smaller portions) are consumed without adverse consequences. Dilution of EN is avoided due to risks of bacterial contamination and confusion with water and feeding volumes.

Diarrhea

Diarrhea occurs in patients in the hospital setting regardless of how they are fed. EN is often implicated as a major cause of diarrhea. However, numerous studies suggest other compelling reasons for diarrhea, such as medications, especially liquid medications most of which contain sorbitol or have a very high osmolality and infectious agents (*Clostridium difficile* in particular). A study on the effects of "Fermentable, Oligo-, Di-, Monosaccharides and Polyols" (FODMAPs) in food suggests that they may adversely affect bowel activity. The study also found that the FODMAPs in many formulas are highly osmotic and fermentable by gut bacteria,

TABLE 14-18. SYSTEMATIC APPROACH TO ASSESSMENT AND MANAGEMENT OF DIARRHEA IN ENTERALLY FED PATIENTS

- Quantify stool volume—determine if it is really diarrhea (> 250 mL/d).
- Review medication list—look for elixirs or suspensions with sorbitol (not always listed on the ingredient list—may need to contact manufacturer).
- Try to correlate timing of diarrhea in relation to start of new medication(s) or change medications to enteral route once enteral access is obtained; common offenders include:
  - Acetaminophen and Guaifenesin elixir
  - Neutra-Phos
  - Lactulose
  - Standing orders for stool softeners/laxatives
- Check for *Clostridium difficile* or other infectious etiologies.
- Try a fiber-containing formula or add a fiber powder (not in poorly perfused or dysmotile gut):
  - Few clinical studies
  - Supports the health of colonocytes
- Added Fructooligosaccharide (FOS) and Fermentable, Oligo-, Di-, Monosaccharides and Polyols (FODMAPs) in some patients may precipitate or aggravate diarrhea.
- Once infectious causes are ruled out:
  - Consider an antidiarrheal agent such as Imodium (may need standing order vs PRN to be effective)
- Check for fecal impaction.
- Check total hang time of EN (should not exceed 8 hours—open systems only).
- Consider providing protein powders by bolus vs adding directly to formulas to decrease contamination risk.
- Check fecal fat as last resort; if negative it does not mean patient is not malabsorbing; if positive, however, there is need to evaluate further.
- Continue to feed.

Reproduced with permission from: The University of Virginia Health System from Nutrition Support Traineeship Syllabus, University of Virginia Health System, Charlottesville, VA; Updated June, 2013.

which then may result in gas, bloating, cramping, and diarrhea. After potential causes for diarrhea have been ruled out (Table 14-18) and addressed, medications to slow GI motility may be warranted.

Flow Rates and Hours of Infusion

Typical infusion rates for the initiation of EN range from 10 to 50 mL/h with increases of 10 to 25 mL every 4 to 24 hours. Little science exists to confirm or refute the efficacy of such regimens. One study has demonstrated that continuous enteral feeding may be started at the final goal rate in acutely ill patients without negative consequences. In the study, feedings started at goal-flow rate did appear to reduce the calorie deficit that frequently accrues in the hospitalized patient. Whether EN runs continuously, nocturnally, during the day, or is given as a bolus, is often institution specific. However, patient-specific factors may also dictate the feeding schedule. For instance, patients on insulin infusions may experience fewer hypoglycemic episodes on continuous infusions of EN.

It is difficult, in fact rare, to achieve goal volumes of EN in acutely ill patients. Frequent interruptions in the delivery of EN are common (see Table 14-14). As a result, it is reasonable to consider "padding" flow rates by basing calculations on less than 24 hours to improve delivery of the desired dose. For example, instead of dividing the goal volume of 1800 mL by 24 hours, to arrive at a flow rate of 75 mL/h, divide by 22 hours to arrive at rate of 80 mL/h, assuming that there will be at least 2 hours during the day when formula infusion is interrupted.

Formula Selection

A vast array of EN formulas are available, including specialty formulas marketed for patients with diabetes, ARDS, hepatic, and renal failure. Other formulas contain nutrients that may modulate immune function, or have nutrients in their most basic (elemental) form for patients with malabsorption syndromes. Medical nutrition products are not required to meet the same level of scientific scrutiny as medications before they are marketed. Adequate outcome data are not available to warrant the use of many of these expensive products. Prospective, randomized trials have demonstrated no advantages of specialized "pulmonary" or "glucose control" feeding formulas. In fact, in a large randomized multicenter trial of a specialized enteral formula with fish oil and antioxidants for patients with acute lung injury, mortality increased with the specialized feeding compared to standard products. The majority of acutely ill patients may be fed with "standard" polymeric tube-feeding formulas. Most formulas provide between 1 and 2 cal/mL.

SELECTED BIBLIOGRAPHY

Upper GI Bleeding

Alhazzani W, Alenezi F, Jaeschke RZ, et al. Proton pump inhibitors versus histamine 2 receptor antagonists for stress ulcer prophylaxis in critically ill patients: a systematic review and meta-analysis. *Crit Care Med.* 2013;41(3):1-13.

Andreyev HJN, Davidson SE, Gillespie C, et al. Practice guidance on the management of acute and chronic gastrointestinal problems arising as a result of treatment for cancer. *Gut.* 2012;61:179-192.

Becq A, Rahmi G, Perrod G, Cellier C., Hemorrhagic angiodysplasia of the digestive tract: pathogenesis, diagnosis, and management. *Gastrointest Endosc.* 2017;86(5):792-806.

Biecker E. Portal hypertension and gastrointestinal bleeding: diagnosis, prevention and management *World J Gastroenterol.* 2013;19(31):5035-5050.

Dworzynski K, Pollit V, Kelsey A, et al. Management of acute upper gastrointestinal bleeding: summary of NICE guidance. *BMJ.* 2012;344:1-5.

El-Tawil AM. Management of non-variceal upper gastrointestinal tract hemorrhage: controversies and areas of uncertainty. *World J Gastroenterol.* 2012;18(11):1159-1165.

Holster I, Kuipers E. Management of acute nonvariceal upper gastrointestinal bleeding: current policies and future perspectives. *World J Gastroenterol.* 2012;18(11):1202-1207.

Hwang J, Fisher D, Ben-Menachem T, et al. The role of endoscopy in the management of acute non-variceal upper GI bleeding. *Gastrointest Endosc.* 2012;75(6):1132-1138.

Hyett B, Abougergi M, Charpentier J, et al. The AIMS65 score compared with the Glasgow-Blatchford in predicting outcomes in upper GI bleeding. *Gastrointest Endosc.* 2013:77:551-557.

Jairath V, Barkun A. Improving outcomes from acute upper gastrointestinal bleeding. *Gut.* 2012;61(9):1246-1249.

Laine L, Jensen D. Management of patients with ulcer bleeding. *Am J Gastroenterol.* 2012;107(3):345-360.

Monteiro S, Cúrdia Gonçalves T, Magalhães J, Cotter J. Upper gastrointestinal bleeding risk scores: who, when and why? *World J Gastrointest Pathophysiol.* 2016;7(1):86-96.

Neumann I, Letelier LM, Rada G, et al. Comparison of different regimens of proton pump inhibitors for acute peptic ulcer bleeding. *Cochrane Database Syst Rev.* 2013;6. doi: 10.1002/14651858. CD007999.pub2.

Sachar H, Vaidya, K, Laine L. Intermittent vs continuous proton pump inhibitor therapy for high-risk bleeding ulcers: a systematic review and meta-analysis. *JAMA Intern Med.* 2014;174(11):1755-1762.

Strate LL, Gralnek IM. American College of Gastroenterology clinical guideline: management of patients with acute lower gastrointestinal bleeding. *Am J Gastroenterol.* 2016;111(4):459-474.

Villanueva C, Colomo A, Bosch A, et al. Transfusion strategies for acute upper gastrointestinal bleeding. *N Engl J Med.* 2013;368:11-21.

Wang B, Zhang JY, Gong JP, et al. Balloon-occluded retrograde transvenous obliteration versus transjugular intrahepatic portosystemic shunt for treatment of gastric varices due to portal hypertension: a meta-analysis. *J Gastro Hepatol.* 2016;31(4):727-733.

Liver Failure

Bachir N, Larson A. Adult liver transplantation in the United States. *Am J Med Sci.* 2012;343(6):462-469.

Baraldi O, Valentini C, Donati G, et al. Hepatorenal syndrome: update on diagnosis and treatment. *World J Nephrol.* 2015;4(5): 511-520.

Bari K, Garcia-Tsao G. Treatment of portal hypertension. *World J Gastroenterol.* 2012;18(11):1166-1175.

Chalasani N, Younossi Z, Lavine J, et al. The diagnosis and management of non-alcoholic fatty liver disease: practice guideline by the American Association for the Study of Liver Diseases, American College of Gastroenterology, and the American Gastroenterological Association. *Hepatol.* 2012;55(6):2005-2023.

Cosarderelioglu C, Coscar A, Gurakar M, Dagher N, Gurakar A. Hepatopulmonary syndrome and liver transplantation: a recent review of the literature. *J Clin Transpl Hepatol.* 2016;4(1):47-53.

Dasher K, Trotter J. Intensive care unit management of liver-related coagulation disorders. *Crit Care Clin.* 2012;28(3):389-398.

Garcia-Tsao G, Abraldes J, Berzigotti A, Bosch J. Portal hypertensive bleeding in cirrhosis: risk stratification, diagnosis, and management: 2016 practice guidance by the American Association for the Study of Liver Diseases. *Hepatol.* 2017;65(1):310-335.

Karvellas C, Subramanian R. Current evidence for extracorporeal liver support systems in acute liver failure and acute-on-chronic liver failure. *Crit Care Clin.* 2016;32(3):439-451.

Lee WM. Recent developments in acute liver failure. *Best Pract Res Clin Gastroenterol*. 2012;26(1):3-16.

Lucey MR, Terrault N, Ojo L, et al. Long-term management of the successful adult liver transplant: 2012 practice guideline by the American Association for the Study of Liver Diseases and the American Society of Transplantation. *Liver Transpl*. 2013;19(1):3-26.

Pericleous M, Sarnowski A, Moore A, Fijten R, Zaman M. The clinical management of abdominal ascites, spontaneous bacterial peritonitis and hepatorenal syndrome: a review of current guidelines and recommendations. *Eur J Gastroenterol Hepatol*. 2015;28(3):10-18.

Rose C. Ammonia-lowering strategies for the treatment of hepatic encephalopathy. *Clin Pharmacol Ther*. 2012;92(3):321-331.

Runyon B. Management of adult patients with ascites due to cirrhosis: update 2012. *Hepatol*. 2013;57(4):1651-1653.

Saad W. Balloon-occluded retrograde transvenous obliteration of gastric varices: concept, basic techniques, and outcomes. *Semin Intervent Radiol*. 2012;29(2):118-128.

Wong F. Recent advances in our understanding of hepatorenal syndrome. *Nat Rev Gastroenterol Hepatol*. 2012;9(7):381-391.

Acute Pancreatitis

Anand N, Park J, Wu B. Modern management of acute pancreatitis. *Gastroenterol Clin North Am*. 2012;41(1):1-8.

Bollen T. Imaging of acute pancreatitis: update of the revised Atlanta classification. *Radiol Clin North Am*. 2012;50:429-445.

Cruz-Santamaria D, Taxonera G, Giner M. Update on pathogenesis and clinical management of acute pancreatitis. *World J Gastrointest Pathophysiol*. 2012;15(3):60-70.

Fischer J, Gardner T. The "golden hours" of management in acute pancreatitis. *Am J Gastroenterol*. 2012;107:1146-1150.

Mirtallo J, Forbes A, McClave S, et al. International consensus guideline for nutrition therapy in pancreatitis. *J Parenter Enteral Nutr*. 2012;36(3):284-289.

Moggia E, Koti R, Belgaumkar AP, et al. Pharmacological interventions for acute pancreatitis. *Cochrane Database Sys Rev*. 2017;4. doi: 10.1002/14651858.CD011384.pub2.

Mounzer R, Langmead CJ, Wu BU, et al. Comparison of existing clinical scoring systems to predict persistent organ failure in patients with acute pancreatitis. *Gastroenterol*. 2012;142(7):1476-1482.

Tenner S, Baillie J, Dewitt J, Vege SS. American College of Gastroenterology guideline: management of acute pancreatitis. *Am J Gastroenterol*. 2013;108(9):1400-1415.

Wu B, Banks P. Clinical management of patients with acute pancreatitis. *Gastroenterol*. 2013;144:1272-1281.

Intestinal Ischemia/Bowel Obstruction

Aliosmanoglu I, Gul M, Kapan M, et al. Risk factors effecting mortality in acute mesenteric ischemia and mortality rates: a single center experience. *Int Surg*. 2013;98(1):76-81.

Brandt L, Feuerstadt P, Longstreth G. Blaszka M. ACG clinical guideline: epidemiology, risk factors, patterns of presentation, diagnosis, and management of colon ischemia (CI). *Am J Gastroenterol*. 2015;110:18-44.

Dayton M, Dempsey D, Larson G, Posner A. New paradigms in the treatment of small bowel obstruction. *Curr Prob Surg*. 2012;49(11):642-717.

De Giorgio R, Cogliandro R, Barbara G, et al. Chronic intestinal pseudo-obstruction: clinical features, diagnosis, and therapy. *Gastroenterol Clin North Am*. 2011;40:787-807.

Maung A, Johnson D, Piper G, et al. Evaluation and management of small-bowel obstruction: an Eastern Association for the Surgery of Trauma practice management guideline. *J Trauma Acute Care Surg*. 2012;73(5 Suppl 4):S362-S369.

Vogel J, Feingold D, Stewart D, et al. Clinical practice guidelines for colon volvulus and acute colonic pseudo-obstruction. *Dis Colon Rectum*. 2016;59:589-600.

Nutrition

American Association of Critical-Care Nurses. AACN Practice Alert: Initial and Ongoing Verification of Feeding Tube Placement in Adults. *Crit Care Nurse*. 2016;36(2):e8-e13.

American Association of Critical-Care Nurses. AACN Practice Alert: Prevention of Aspiration in Adults. 2016. doi: http://dx.doi.org/10.4037/ccn2016831.

Academy of Nutrition and Dietetics. *Critical Illness Evidence-Based Nutrition Practice Guideline*. Chicago, IL: Academy Nutrition Dietetics; 2012.

Burns S, Carpenter R, Blevins C, et al. Detection of inadvertent airway intubation during gastric tube insertion: capnography versus a colorimetric carbon dioxide detector. *Am J Crit Care*. 2006;15(2):188-195.

Davies A, Morrison S, Bailey M, et al. A multicenter, randomized controlled trial comparing early nasojejunal with nasogastric nutrition in critical illness. *Crit Care Med*. 2012;40(8):2342-2348.

McClave S, Taylor B, Martindale R, et al. Guidelines for the provision and assessment of nutrition support therapy in the adult critically ill patient: Society of Critical Care Medicine (SCCM) and American Society for Parenteral and Enteral Nutrition (A.S.P.E.N.). *JPEN J Parenter Enteral Nutr*. 2016;40(2):159-211.

Reignier J, Mercier E, Le Gouge A, et al. Effect of not monitoring residual gastric volume on risk of ventilator-associated pneumonia in adults receiving mechanical ventilation and early enteral feeding: a randomized controlled trial. *JAMA*. 2013;309(3):249-256.

Rice T, Wheeler A, Thompson B, et al. Initial trophic vs. full enteral feeding in patients with acute lung injury: the EDEN randomized trial. *JAMA*. 2012;307(8):795-803.

Online References of Interest

http://www.ginutrition.virginia.edu

Bariatric (Gastric Bypass) Surgery

Boza C, Gamboa C, Salinas J, et al. Laparoscopic roux-en-Y gastric bypass versus laparoscopic sleeve gastrectomy: a case-control study and 3 years of follow-up. *Surg Obes Relat Dis.* 2012;8(3):243-349.

Mechanick J, Youdim A, Jones D, et al. American Association of Clinical Endocrinologists, Obesity Society, American Society for Metabolic & Bariatric Surgery. Clinical practice guidelines for the perioperative nutritional, metabolic, and nonsurgical support of the bariatric surgery patient–2013 update: *Endocr Pract.* 2013;19(2):337-372.

Nguyen N, Nguyen B, Gebhart A, et al. Changes in the makeup of bariatric surgery: a national increase in use of laparoscopic sleeve gastrectomy. *J Am Coll Surg.* 2013;216(2):252-257.

Parikh M, Issa R, McCrillis A, et al. Surgical strategies that may decrease leak after laparoscopic sleeve gastrectomy. A systematic review and meta-analysis of 9991 cases. *Ann Surg.* 2013;257(2):231-237.

Sakran N, Goitein D, Raziel A, et al. Gastric leaks after sleeve gastrectomy: a multicenter experience with 2,834 patients. *Surg Endosc.* 2013;27:240-245.

Saul D, Stephens D, de Cassia Hofstatter R. Preliminary outcomes of laparoscopic sleeve gastrectomy in a Veterans' Affairs medical center. *Am J Surg.* 2012;204(5):e1-e6.

Vidal P, Ramon J, Goday A. Laparoscopic gastric bypass versus laparoscopic sleeve gastrectomy as a definitive surgical procedure for morbid obesity. Midterm results. *Obes Surg.* 2013;23(3):292-299.

von Drygalski A, Andris D, Nuttleman P, Jackson S, Klein J, Wallace J. Anemia after bariatric surgery cannot be explained by iron deficiency alone: results of a large Cohort study. *Surg Obes Relat Dis.* 2011;7:151-156.

15

RENAL SYSTEM

Jie Chen

KNOWLEDGE COMPETENCIES

1. Describe the etiology, pathophysiology, clinical presentation, patient needs, and principles of management of acute kidney injury (AKI).

2. Differentiate between the three types of AKI:
   - Prerenal
   - Intrarenal
   - Postrenal

3. Compare and contrast the pathophysiology, clinical presentation, patient needs, and

management approaches of life-threatening electrolyte imbalances:
   - Sodium (Na$^+$)
   - Potassium (K$^+$)
   - Calcium (Ca^{++})
   - Magnesium (Mg^{++})
   - Phosphorus (PO$_4^-$)

4. Differentiate between the indications for and the efficacy of the different types of renal replacement therapies.

5. Describe the nursing interventions for patients undergoing renal replacement therapy (RRT).

ACUTE KIDNEY INJURY

The most common renal problem seen in acutely ill patients is the development of acute kidney injury (AKI), previously termed as acute renal failure (ARF). AKI is the abrupt decrease in renal function with progressive retention of metabolic waste products (eg, creatinine and urea). Oliguria, urine output of less than 400 mL/day, is a common finding in AKI. The development of AKI in acutely ill patients has an estimated mortality of 40% to 50%, and higher among intensive care unit (ICU) patients (> 50% in most of the studies). Patients who develop AKI due to sepsis have a higher mortality. A history of chronic kidney disease (CKD) complicates the clinical course of any illness.

The RIFLE criteria and Acute Kidney Injury Network (AKIN) criteria are the most commonly used classification systems for AKI (Table 15-1). RIFLE is an acronym for: Risk of renal dysfunction, Injury to the kidney, Failure of kidney function, Loss of kidney function, and End-stage kidney disease.

Etiology, Risk Factors, and Pathophysiology

For the purpose of determining an appropriate plan of care, AKI is often categorized into prerenal, intrarenal, or postrenal. Each category of AKI has different etiologies, pathophysiology, laboratory findings, and clinical presentation. However, the common pathologic pathway for decreased glomerular filtration rate (GFR) is the reduction in renal blood flow. In the acute care setting, the majority of the cases of AKI are caused by the combination of impaired renal perfusion, sepsis, and nephrotoxic agents.

Prerenal Acute Kidney Injury

Physiologic conditions that lead to decreased perfusion of the kidneys, without intrinsic damage to the renal tubules, are identified as prerenal AKI (Figure 15-1). The decrease in renal arterial perfusion causes a decrease in the rate of filtration of blood through the glomerulus. When perfusion pressure falls to less than 80 mm Hg, protective autoregulation is lost, further decreasing glomerular filtration.

TABLE 15-1. RIFLE AND AKIN CRITERIA FOR DIAGNOSIS AND CLASSIFICATION OF AKI

	RIFLE			AKIN	
Class	**SCr[a]**	**Urine Output (common to both)**	**Stage**	**SCr[b]**	
Risk	Increased SCr to > 1.5 × baseline	Urine output < 0.5 mg/kg/h for > 6 h	1	Increase in SCr ≥0.3 mg/dL or increase in SCr to ≥150%-200% of baseline	
Injury	Increased SCr to > 2 × baseline	Urine output < 0.5 mg/kg/h for > 12 h	2	Increase in SCr to >200%-300% of baseline	
Failure	Increased SCr to > 3 × baseline; or an increase of ≥ 0.5 mg/dL to a value of ≥ 4 mg/dL	Urine output < 0.3 mg/kg/h for > 12 h or anuria for > 12 h	3	Increase in SCr to >300% of baseline; or to ≥ 4 mg/dL with an acute increase of ≥ 0.5 mg/dL; or on RRT	
Loss	Need for RRT for > 4 wk				
End Stage	Need for RRT for > 3 mo				

Abbreviations: AKI, acute kidney injury; AKIN, acute kidney injury network; RIFLE, risk, injury, failure, loss, end-stage disease; RRT, renal replacement therapy; SCr, serum creatinine.
[a]For RIFLE, the increase in SCr should be both abrupt (with 1-7 days) and sustained (> 24 hours).
[b]For AKIN, the increase in SCr must occur in less than 48 hours.
Data from Palevsky PM, Liu KD, Brophy PD et al: KDOQI US Commentary on the 2012 KDIGO Clinical Practice Guideline for Acute Kidney Injury, Am J Kidney Dis 2013 May;61(5):649-672.

Renal tubular function, at this point, is still completely normal. As a result of the decreased GFR, the kidneys are unable to adequately filter waste products from the blood. Consequently, more Na⁺ and water are reabsorbed by the kidneys, resulting in oliguria. If the decreased perfusion state persists, irreversible damage to the renal tubules may occur, resulting in intrarenal AKI. Most forms of prerenal AKI are easily reversed by treating the cause and increasing renal perfusion.

Intrarenal Acute Kidney Injury

Physiologic conditions that cause damage to the renal tubule, glomerulus, or renal blood vessels are identified as intrarenal AKI (see Figure 15-1). Following prolonged decreases in renal perfusion, the kidneys gradually suffer damage that is not readily reversed with the restoration of renal perfusion. Acute tubular necrosis is the most common cause of AKI.

When the insult to the kidney is nephrotoxins (medications or other substances that cause direct damage to the

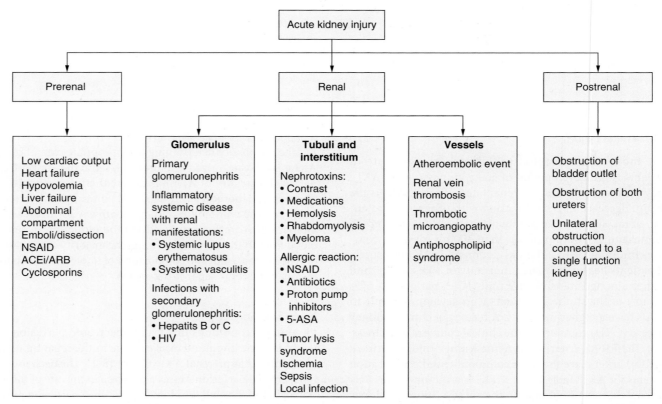

Figure 15-1. Causes of AKI. ACEi, angiotensin-converting enzyme inhibitor; ARB, angiotensin receptor blockers; 5-ASA, 5-aminosalicylic acid; HIV, human immunodeficiency virus; NSAID, nonsteroidal anti-inflammatory drug.

kidney), the nephron damage occurs primarily at the tubular epithelial layer. Because this layer has the ability to regenerate, rapid healing often occurs following nephrotoxic insults. When the insult is ischemic or inflammatory, the nephron's basement membrane is also damaged and regeneration is not possible. Ischemic and inflammatory insults are more likely to cause CKD than nephrotoxic insults.

The underlying pathophysiologic abnormality in intrarenal AKI is renal cellular damage. In healthy kidneys, the glomerulus acts as a filter, preventing the passage of large molecules into the glomerular filtrate. Damage to the glomerulus allows protein and cellular debris to enter the renal tubules, leading to intraluminal obstruction.

Contrast-induced nephropathy (CIN) is seen in about 10% of patients with risk factors receiving contrast media. The risk factors include diabetes, advanced age, CKD, and hypovolemia. Contrast characteristic (osmolality, iconicity, and molecular structure), and high or repetitive doses of intravenous (IV) contrast also impact the risk. CIN is defined as a 25% increase in creatinine or an absolute increase of 0.5 mg/dL from baseline within 48 to 72 hours of intravenous contrast administration. The condition resolves in 7 to 10 days. The patient may be oliguric or may have no decrease in urine output. The pathophysiological changes of CIN are medullary hypoxia that is caused by an initial vasodilation followed by a prolonged renal vasoconstriction, and direct epithelial cell toxicity.

Postrenal Acute Kidney Injury

Physiologic conditions that partially or completely obstruct urine flow from the kidney to the urethral meatus can cause postrenal AKI (see Figure 15-1). Partial obstruction increases renal interstitial pressure, which in turn increases Bowman capsule pressure and opposes glomerular filtration. Complete obstruction leads to urine backup into the kidney, eventually compressing the kidney. With complete obstruction, there is no urine output from the affected kidney. Postrenal failure is an uncommon cause of AKI in acutely ill patients. The treatment for postrenal failure is focused on removing the obstruction.

Clinical Phases

There are three clinical phases of AKI, seen primarily as a result of intrarenal injury. The first, the oliguric phase, begins within 48 hours of the insult to the kidney. In intrarenal AKI, the oliguric phase is accompanied by a significant rise in blood urea nitrogen (BUN) and creatinine. The degree of elevation of these waste products is less pronounced in prerenal AKI. The most common complications seen in this phase are fluid overload and acute hyperkalemia. The oliguric phase may last from a few days to several weeks. The longer the oliguric phase continues, the poorer the patient's prognosis.

The diuretic phase follows the oliguric phase. During this phase, there is a gradual return of renal function. Although the BUN and creatinine continue to rise, there is an increase in urine output. The patient's state of hydration prior to the diuretic phase determines the amount of urine output. A patient who is fluid overloaded may excrete up to 5 L of urine a day and have marked Na^+ wasting. The average time in this phase is 7 to 10 days. Patients must be observed carefully for complications due to fluid and electrolyte deficits. If the patient receives dialysis during the oliguric phase, the diuretic phase may be decreased or absent.

The recovery phase marks the stabilization of laboratory values and can last 3 to 12 months. Some degree of residual renal insufficiency is common following AKI. Some patients never recover renal function and progress to CKD.

Clinical Presentation

The diverse causes of AKI determine the clinical presentation of the patient. AKI can cause multiple organ dysfunction and, therefore, manifests in a variety of ways. Uremia describes the clinical syndrome that accompanies the detrimental effects of renal dysfunction on the other organ systems. The clinical presentation of the patient with uremia reflects the degree of nephron loss and, correspondingly, the loss of renal function.

Signs and Symptoms

- Oliguria (< 400 mL/day) or anuria (< 100 mL/day)
- Tachycardia
- Heart murmur
- Pericardial friction rub
- Hypotension (prerenal)
- Hypertension (intrarenal)
- Jugular vein distension (intrarenal)
- Platelet dysfunction and bleeding
- Dry mucous membranes
- Cool, clammy skin
- Pruritus
- Deep, rapid respirations
- Crackles or rales on lung auscultation
- Vomiting
- Nausea
- Lethargy
- Confusion
- Coma

Diagnostic Tests

Early detection of AKI is critical to prevent further decline in renal function. Laboratory tests are extremely important in diagnosing AKI and evaluating the effectiveness of interventions to treat it. Serum creatinine and BUN are affected by many factors, and in patients with AKI, there is a delay before the rise in serum levels, but these values are still commonly used to evaluate renal function by trending variations of daily levels. A plasma BUN/creatinine ratio greater than 20:1 suggests prerenal AKI as reduced kidney perfusion is associated with an increase in urea reabsorption.

Urinalysis is a useful and inexpensive test to evaluate renal function. Urine sodium values vary as the kidneys attempt to retain or excrete water. Urine volume, specific gravity (SG), and osmolality identify the kidney's ability to excrete and concentrate fluid. Urinalysis findings are normal or almost normal in prerenal AKI. Low urine osmolality is an early finding of AKI as it indicates the loss of kidney concentrating ability. A urine osmolality greater than 500 mOsmol/kg suggests prerenal AKI. Muddy brown granular casts and increased protein in urine are seen in intrarenal AKI. Low urine sodium levels (< 20 mmol/L) are seen in prerenal AKI. In contrast, high urine sodium levels (> 40 mmol/L) are seen in intrarenal AKI.

The fractional excretion of sodium (FeNa) is a valuable indicator of functional renal tubules. FeNa is less than 1% in prerenal injury and more than 1% in intrarenal injury with exceptions, such as in patients with CIN, rhabdomyolysis, and liver diseases. However, calculation of FeNa is not accurate in the setting of diuretic use. In that case, fractional excretion of urea (FeUrea) is used. FeUrea is less than 35% in prerenal injury and more than 35% in intrarenal injury.

There are several novel biomarkers of AKI. Urinary insulin like growth factor-binding protein 7 (IGFBP7) and tissue inhibitor of metalloproteinase-2 (TIMP-2) can be detected at the bedside by using the commercially available and Food and Drug Administration (FDA)-approved NephroCheck Test (a urine test). The increase and decrease of IGFBP7 and TIMP-2 levels from baseline can be used to predict the development of AKI and renal recovery post-AKI events.

Radiologic tests also give important information about the kidneys. A kidney ultrasound may be used to evaluating existing renal disease and exclude postrenal AKI. Both computed tomography (CT) and magnetic resonance imaging (MRI) are able to identify obstruction. Nuclear mercaptoacetyltriglycine-3 (MAG-3) scan can be used to evaluate renal perfusion and tubular function. Doppler ultrasound or arteriogram assesses the patency of the renal vasculature. Contrast use is avoided in all patients with AKI.

Renal biopsy is only considered when prerenal and postrenal AKI have been excluded, and the etiology of the intrarenal AKI is still not clear. In these cases, the findings of renal biopsy are used to guide management.

Physical Assessment

Physical assessment related to the kidneys includes monitoring intake and output, daily weights, and noting a positive or negative fluid balance. Observation of the patient's urine for color, clarity, and odor adds to the assessment. Signs of volume overload may include pulmonary crackles, peripheral edema, jugular venous distention, or an S_3 heart sound. Volume deficit may be denoted by the presence of dry mucus membranes and weak peripheral pulses. Alterations in mental state may indicate uremia. The kidneys help control the internal environment of the body, therefore, when kidney function decreases, the progressive care nurse may see changes in most, if not all, body systems.

Principles of Management of Acute Kidney Injury

The collaborative approach of the healthcare team to the treatment of patients with AKI begins with the recognition of AKI risk. The focus for those at risk is maintenance of adequate renal perfusion and avoidance of renal injury.

Once the patient develops AKI, the goal is to quickly reestablish homeostasis by treating the underlying cause. Management of AKI also includes correction of fluid imbalance, prevention, and correction of life-threatening electrolyte imbalances, treatment of metabolic acidosis, prevention of further renal damage, prevention and treatment of infection, and maintaining adequate nutrition.

Prevention of CIN involves the use of extensive hydration before and after any procedure using contrast media. There is a debate about whether intravenous normal saline or sodium bicarbonate is best for hydration. Patients who are considered to be at risk for CIN may also receive oral acetylcysteine with their hydration but its benefit is uncertain. Diuretics are held during this time. Discontinuing nephrotoxic agents such as aminoglycoside antibiotics, nonsteroidal anti-inflammatory drugs, and chemotherapeutic agents prior to the procedure may also be helpful.

ESSENTIAL CONTENT CASE
Contrast-Induced Nephropathy

A 74-year-old woman was admitted for substernal chest pain, shortness of breath, and weakness. She has a history of type II diabetes mellitus. She underwent diagnostic cardiac catheterization with successful angioplasty and placement of two stents. Postprocedure an infusion of IV fluid was initiated. She is now 4 hours postprocedure and receiving normal saline at 200 mL/h. Vital signs are stable and she has had 50 mL urine output in total so far.

The next morning, serum creatinine has increased from a baseline of 1.2 mg/dL to 1.8 mg/dL. Urine output has remained marginal at 25 to 30 mL/h. Normal saline is continuing at 125 mL/h. The provider decides to keep her one more day to monitor her renal status. On the second postprocedure day, serum creatinine remains at 1.8 mg/dL but urine output has increased to 35 to 40 mL/h. She is discharged to follow up in the office in 3 days.

Case Question 1: What puts this patient at risk of CIN?

Case Question 2: Why is the patient being discharged when the creatinine has not returned to baseline?

Answers
1. The risk factors for developing CIN include a history of diabetes, advanced age, lack of pre-hydration prior to using contrast medium, and the use of increased amounts of contrast media (ie, related to the length of two procedures done at the same time).
2. The patient is discharged to be followed-up as an outpatient because research demonstrates that creatinine returns to baseline within 3 to 5 days in most patients that develop CIN. However, in patients with renal insufficiency, an episode of CIN can lead to CKD.

Correction of Fluid Imbalance

Maintaining fluid balance in the renal failure patient is a challenge. The simultaneous goals of providing enough fluid to ensure adequate renal perfusion and preventing excess fluid and volume overload require close attention. Assessment data that help to determine a patient's fluid status include trending of daily weight, measuring intake and output, especially urine output, and close monitoring of vital signs. Functional hemodynamics described in Chapter 4 (Hemodynamic Monitoring) may provide additional information about the patient's fluid balance. The following interventions are recommended in the management of fluid imbalance:

1. Calculate daily fluid needs. In prerenal disease, fluid replacement must be matched with fluid loss, both in amount and composition. Insensible fluid losses must be considered in this calculation (Table 15-2). Normal saline volume loading before a potential insult in patients at risk for renal dysfunction is a widely accepted practice. Additionally, volume expansion is beneficial in preventing a volume-depleted patient from progressing from prerenal AKI to intrarenal AKI. In contrast, oliguric patients can rarely tolerate more than 1000 mL of fluid per day. It is often necessary to place constraints on other therapies (eg, IV medication administration, nutritional support) during this phase. During the diuretic phase, the patient may require 1 to 4 L of fluid per day to prevent hypovolemia. The patient is frequently allowed to lose more fluid than is replaced in the diuretic phase, to facilitate fluid movement from the interstitial and intracellular spaces into the vascular space.
2. Obtain accurate intake and output measurements, including all insensible losses in the measurements. Fluid therapy decisions are often based on the patient's output.
3. Obtain daily weights. Body weight may decrease by 0.2 to 0.3 kg/day as a result of catabolism. If the patient's weight is stable or increasing, volume overload is suspected. If weight loss exceeds these recommendations, volume depletion or hyper-catabolism may be the cause.
4. Administer diuretics only when the patient is hypervolemic and in consultation with healthcare providers. Increasing dosages may be used in an attempt to determine the optimal dose. Once the diagnosis of AKI is established, diuretics may be used to avoid fluid overload and to potentiate the effects of antihypertensive medications. Potassium-sparing diuretics are typically avoided because K^+ elimination is diminished in AKI. Furosemide, a loop diuretic, is the most common diuretic used in AKI. It works by blocking Na^+ reabsorption in the renal tubules, thereby enhancing excretion of Na^+ and water. It is often used to reduce fluid overload and dialysis frequency in AKI. Furosemide is used cautiously in patients receiving aminoglycoside antibiotics because it potentiates the nephrotoxic effects of these medications, and it increases the risk of ototoxicity.
5. Institute renal replacement therapy (RRT) as needed. There are three types of RRT available. These include intermittent hemodialysis (IHD), peritoneal dialysis (PD), and several forms of continuous renal replacement therapy (CRRT). Each of these is described later in this chapter. Sustained low efficiency dialysis (SLED) is considered one of the continuous therapies. CRRT may be better tolerated in hemodynamically unstable patients who are unable to undergo the abrupt fluid shifts that occur in other forms of dialysis.

Preventing and Treating Life-Threatening Electrolyte Imbalances

There are a number of electrolyte imbalances that can occur in AKI, the most common being hyperkalemia, hypocalcemia, hypermagnesemia, hyperphosphatemia, and bicarbonate deficiency. In AKI, the electrolyte status guides decisions about the type of fluid therapy and the initiation of RRT. The management of these electrolyte disorders is detailed later in this chapter.

Treating Acidosis

Patients with AKI often develop metabolic acidosis, with mild respiratory alkalosis compensation.

1. Administer sodium bicarbonate ($NaHCO_3$) as indicated. Treatment is usually not instituted until the serum bicarbonate level drops to less than 15 to 18 mEq/L. The deficit can be calculated and the serum bicarbonate level or pH reassessed frequently to evaluate the efficacy of treatment. Excessive administration of $NaHCO_3$ can cause metabolic alkalosis, hypocalcemia, and volume overload, especially for patients with lactic acidosis.
2. If a patient is being dialyzed, using a dialysate containing bicarbonate will facilitate buffering of the patient's acidotic state. Dialysates containing bicarbonate are preferred to those with lactate.

Preventing Additional Kidney Damage

In AKI, medications metabolized or excreted by the kidney require adjustment to avoid excessive blood levels and

TABLE 15-2. MINIMAL VOLUMES OF FLUID ASSOCIATED WITH INSENSIBLE FLUID LOSSES

Situation/Condition	Volume
Respiratory losses	500-850 mL/day (dependent on minute ventilation rate)
Fever (loss/°C elevation > 38.0)	200 mL
Diaphoresis	500 mL
Diarrhea	50-200 mL/stool

potential nephrotoxicity. Particular attention must be given to medication scheduling related to RRT schedules. Medications may be eliminated or have their actions potentiated by these therapies. As a result, selected medications, such as antibiotics, are often monitored with peak and trough levels (see Chapter 7 [Pharmacology] for discussion of peak and trough levels). A clinical pharmacist is a helpful resource on appropriate medication selection, dosing, and monitoring during AKI.

1. Modify medication dosing. Because many medications are eliminated by the kidney, dosage and frequency are adjusted in patients with AKI. Medication dosing decisions depend on calculation of the patient's creatinine clearance, which, in turn, is based on the patient's gender, age, height, weight, and serum creatinine level. The phase of AKI and other concomitant treatments help determine the appropriate dose of medication.
2. Administer antihypertensive agents as needed. Hypertension is a frequent problem for many patients with AKI, often requiring concomitant use of several antihypertensive agents. Most antihypertensive agents are not removed by RRT. During hemodialysis, it is important to adjust the dosage schedule of antihypertensive agents to avoid hypotensive episodes. Some antihypertensive agents, however, are eliminated by the kidney. Therefore, dialysis patients receiving these medications may require alterations in their dosages or frequency.

Preventing and Treating Infection

Patients with AKI are at high risk for infection and often require treatment with antimicrobial agents. Selection and dosing of antimicrobial agents is carefully considered to minimize the risk of additional kidney injury. Monitoring of both renal function and drug levels during antimicrobial therapy is necessary to avoid further renal damage. Also, different types of RRT affect drug removal differently and must be considered. Assessment of surgical and line placement sites for signs of infection is imperative.

Maintaining Adequate Nutrition

In patients with AKI, the challenge in the management of nutritional status is to provide a balance between sufficient calories and protein to prevent catabolism, while avoiding problems, such as fluid and electrolyte imbalances that increase the requirement for RRT. The clinical nutritionist is an important resource for the healthcare team. The typical patient with AKI is hypermetabolic, with caloric needs potentially twice normal. Additional stresses, related to the acute illness, can further elevate caloric requirements. Nausea and vomiting, common in uremia, further decrease oral and enteral caloric intake. Adequate nutrition is essential to prevent infection by maintaining the integrity of the immune system and to promote wound healing and tissue repair.

Hyperglycemia is avoided, aiming for a target plasma glucose of 110 to 149 mg/dL.

1. Restrict the patient's fluid, sodium, potassium, and phosphorus intake. Because patients with AKI cannot eliminate wastes, fluid, or electrolytes, their dietary intake of these substances is typically restricted. The degree of restriction depends on the cause and severity of their disease; for example, the level of Na^+ restriction is determined by the cause of AKI and the serum Na^+ level. Some causes lead to Na^+ wasting and others to Na^+ retention. Phosphorus may need to be restricted and Ca^{++} supplemented if the Ca^{++} level is low in conjunction with normal PO_4^- levels.
2. Administer necessary vitamin supplements. Supplementation of folic acid, pyridoxine, and the water-soluble vitamins is most frequently necessary.
3. Consult a dietitian for a diet plan. Dietary requirements change for patients depending on their renal status and the severity of their underlying condition. Although the precise role of nutrition in AKI is controversial, malnutrition is thought to increase morbidity and mortality. Recommendations in the 2016 Guidelines for the Provision and Assessment of Nutrition Support Therapy in the Adult Critically Ill Patient include early initiation of enteral feeding in critically ill patients who are unable to eat.

The usual approach to hypercatabolic states is to provide adequate proteins and carbohydrates for resynthesis of damaged or lost tissue. Protein requirements may range initially from 0.8 to 1 g/kg/day and increase with RRT to 1 to 1.5 g/kg/day to a maximum of 1.7 g/kg/day for patients on CRRT as amino acids are removed. Patients with AKI should not receive more than 30 kcal/kg/day nonprotein calories or 1.3 times the basal energy expenditure, calculated by the Harris-Benedict equation with 30% to 35% of energy coming from lipids. The enteral route is preferred unless contraindicated.

ELECTROLYTE IMBALANCES

The kidneys play a major role in the regulation of fluid and electrolyte balance in the body. Regulation of body fluids and electrolytes helps ensure a stable internal environment, resulting in maximal intracellular function. Any renal dysfunction results in abnormalities in both fluid and electrolyte balance.

For all of the electrolyte disorders, the indications for treatment vary from patient to patient. The signs and symptoms of any electrolyte imbalance are not necessarily determined by the degree of abnormality. Rather, the signs and symptoms are determined by the cause of the condition, as well as the magnitude and rapidity of onset. For many of the electrolyte imbalances, it is difficult to determine at precisely what level signs or symptoms may occur.

Sodium Imbalance: Hyperosmolar Disorders

Etiologies, Risk Factors, and Pathophysiology

Serum osmolality, a measure of the number of particles in a unit of blood volume, is an important indicator of fluid status. Because serum osmolality is determined primarily by the serum Na^+ level, evaluation of Na^+ levels provides valuable information on serum osmolality and potential excesses or deficits of total body water. A quick estimate of serum osmolality can be calculated by simply doubling the serum Na^+ value. Normal serum osmolality values are 285 to 295 mOsm/kg (calculated: 2[Na] mEq/L + serum glucose [mg/dL]/18 + BUN [mg/dL]/2.8). Abnormal serum Na^+ levels are classified as disorders of osmolality, with hyperosmolality referring to high Na^+ levels, which may be indicative of water deficit, or hypo-osmolality referring to low sodium levels, which may be indicative of water excess.

Acutely ill patients often are at risk for disorders of osmolality, with children and older adults at highest risk. As a person ages, the hypothalamus becomes less sensitive to changes in osmolality and is, therefore, less able to alert the body to abnormalities through normal mechanisms. Additionally, the neurologic signs indicative of osmolality disorders are often missed or attributed to age rather than to a physiologic abnormality.

Hyperosmolar disorders are the result of a deficit of water. The causes of hyperosmolality include inadequate intake of water, excessive loss of water, or conditions that cause an inhibition of antidiuretic hormone (ADH). In acutely ill patients, hyperosmolar disorders develop because of inadequate intake, usually related to loss of consciousness or endotracheal intubation, and ADH inhibition, as manifested by diabetes insipidus in a patient with a head injury. The signs and symptoms seen are the results of the ensuing cerebral dehydration. Water is pulled from the intracellular space to enhance intravascular volume, leaving the cells dehydrated.

Clinical Presentation

Signs and Symptoms

- Lethargy
- Restlessness
- Disorientation
- Delusions
- Seizures
- Coma
- Oliguria
- Hypotension
- Tachycardia
- Thirst
- Dry mucous membranes

Diagnostic Tests

- Serum Na^+ more than 145 mEq/L
- Serum osmolality more than 295 mOsm/kg

- In patients who are hypovolemic from extrarenal losses: urine osmolarity more than 600 mOsm/kg with urine Na^+ less than 10 to 20 mEq/L
- In patients who are hypovolemic from renal loss: urine osmolarity 300 mOsm/kg or less with urine Na^+ more than 20 to 30 mEq/L

Sodium Imbalance: Hypo-Osmolar Disorders

Hypo-osmolality disorders are the result of an excess of intravascular water. The causes of hypo-osmolality include excess intake or impaired secretion of water, excess ADH as in the syndrome of inappropriate ADH (SIADH), replacement of volume loss with pure water, and salt-wasting disorders. Hypo-osmolar disorders are extremely common in acutely ill patients, often related to the use of 5% dextrose in water (D_5W) IV solutions. Because these patients have often lost some volume, balanced fluid replacement is extremely important. The neurologic signs and symptoms seen with hypo-osmolar disorders are related to cerebral intracellular swelling, as water moves from the intravascular to the intracellular spaces.

Clinical Presentation

Signs and Symptoms

- Confusion
- Delirium
- Headache
- Seizures
- Muscle twitching
- Coma
- Nausea
- Weight gain
- Anorexia
- Vomiting

Diagnostic Tests

- Serum Na^+ less than 135 mEq/L
- Serum osmolality less than 280 mOsm/kg

Potassium Imbalance: Hyperkalemia

Etiologies, Risk Factors, and Pathophysiology

Hyperkalemia occurs due to increased potassium intake, decreased potassium excretion, and redistribution of K^+ from intracellular to extracellular fluid. Rarely is increased intake a sole cause of hyperkalemia, but in patients with decreased K^+ excretion due to renal impairment it is a contributing factor. The most common causes of hyperkalemia in the acutely ill are AKI, cellular destruction (eg, from crush injuries), and excess supplementation. Because cardiac tissue is sensitive to K^+ levels, hyperkalemia often manifests first as changes in electrical conduction, demonstrated by changes on electrocardiogram (ECG) tracings. Elevated serum K^+ levels alter the conduction of electrical impulses, particularly in cardiac and muscle tissue. These conduction abnormalities can lead to serious cardiac arrhythmias and death.

Clinical Presentation

Because K$^+$ impacts normal neuromuscular and cardiac function, these systems are carefully evaluated when hyperkalemia is suspected. It is important to note that a patient may be experiencing hyperkalemia and may have no symptoms or ECG changes.

Signs and Symptoms

- Vague muscle weakness
- Decreased deep tendon reflexes
- Flaccid paralysis
- Confusion
- Dyspnea
- Palpitations
- Chest pain
- Nausea or vomiting
- Diarrhea
- Cramping
- ECG changes -changes progress and correlate with potassium levels as follows:
  - **5.5-6.5 mEq/L:**
    Tall, peaked T waves
    QT interval may shorten
    ST-segment depression
  - **6.5-8.0 mEq/L:**
    Peaked T waves
    Widened QRS
    Amplified R wave
    Prolonged PR interval
  - **> 8.0 mEq/L:**
    Absence of P wave
    Progressive QRS widening
    Advanced AV block with ventricular escape rhythms, ventricular fibrillation, or asystole

Diagnostic Tests
- Serum K$^+$ > 5.5 mEq/L.

Potassium Imbalance: Hypokalemia
Etiologies, Risk Factors, and Pathophysiology

Hypokalemia occurs with decreased potassium intake, increased potassium excretion or impaired conservation of potassium, excess or abnormal loss, and increased movement of K$^+$ into the cells. In the acutely ill patient, hypokalemia is often related to the use of diuretics and excessive losses through the gastrointestinal tract. Muscle weakness, including cardiac muscle, is the hallmark sign of hypokalemia. Asystole can result from severe hypokalemia. Depressed levels of serum K$^+$ lead to increased irritability of cardiac muscle and neuromuscular cells. Serious cardiac arrhythmias and death may result from hypokalemia.

Clinical Presentation

Signs and Symptoms
- Weakness
- Respiratory muscle weakness, hypoventilation
- Paralytic ileus

- Abdominal distention
- Cramping
- Confusion, irritability
- Lethargy
- ECG Changes
  - Ventricular ectopy and flat, inverted T waves
  - QT interval prolongation
  - U-wave development
  - ST-segment shortening and depression

Diagnostic Tests
- Serum K$^+$ less than 3.5 mEq/L

Calcium Imbalance: Hypercalcemia
Etiologies, Risk Factors, and Pathophysiology

The causes of hypercalcemia are either excess calcium entering the extracellular fluid or insufficient excretion of calcium through the kidneys. Approximately 90% of cases are caused by malignancy or hyperparathyroidism.

Clinical Presentation

Signs and Symptoms
- Weakness
- Lethargy
- Confusion
- Coma
- Nausea or vomiting
- Anorexia
- Constipation
- Pancreatitis
- Dehydration
- Polyuria
- Nocturia
- Renal calculi
- Renal failure
- ECG Changes
  - Arrhythmias
  - Shortened QT interval

Diagnostic Tests
- Serum Ca^{++} more than 10.5 mg/dL

Calcium Imbalance: Hypocalcemia
Etiologies, Risk Factors, and Pathophysiology

True hypocalcemia is rare as it is defined as a decrease in ionized calcium level, which is largely dependent on serum albumin level and serum pH. The causes of hypocalcemia are classified into three categories: decreased absorption of Ca^{++}, increased loss of Ca^{++}, and decreased amounts of physiologically active Ca^{++}. Acutely ill patients may develop hypocalcemia related to either hypoalbuminemia or hypoparathyroidism. The normal level of calcium is critical for normal cell function, neural transmission, membrane stability, bone structure, blood coagulation, and intracellular signaling. Symptomatic patients with classic clinical findings of acute hypocalcemia require immediate medical attention.

Clinical Presentation

Signs and Symptoms

- Positive Chvostek sign (twitching of the facial muscle in response to tapping the skin over the facial nerve)
- Positive Trousseau sign (carpopedal spasm in response to occlusion of circulation to the extremity for 3 minutes)
- Tetany
- Seizures
- Respiratory arrest
- Bronchospasm
- Stridor
- Wheezing
- Paralytic ileus
- Confusion
- Hallucination
- Increased irritability
- ECG Changes
  - Arrhythmias
  - Prolonged QT interval

Diagnostic Tests

- Serum Ca^{++} less than 8.5 mg/dL

Magnesium Imbalance: Hypermagnesemia
Etiologies, Risk Factors, and Pathophysiology

Renal failure is the most common etiology of hypermagnesemia in acutely ill patients and results from an inability to excrete magnesium. Both neuromuscular and cardiac depressions are observed. Hypermagnesemia may also develop when Mg^{++} intake is increased such as when antacids are overused, or in conditions that cause adrenal insufficiency, hypothyroidism, or hyperparathyroidism.

Clinical Presentation

Signs and Symptoms

- Respiratory depression
- Hypotension
- Diminished deep tendon reflexes
- Flaccid paralysis
- Drowsiness
- Lethargy
- ECG Changes
  - Cardiac arrest
  - Prolonged PR and QT intervals
  - Widened QRS
  - Increased T-wave amplitude
  - Bradycardia

Diagnostic Tests

- Serum Mg^{++} more than 2.1 mEq/L; however, patients remain asymptomatic until level more than 3 mEq/L

Magnesium Imbalance: Hypomagnesemia
Etiologies, Risk Factors, and Pathophysiology

Hypomagnesemia frequently occurs in patients with alcoholism and in acutely ill patients and is often associated with hypocalcemia and hypokalemia. Causes of hypomagnesemia include decreased intake, increased excretion, such as with diuretic therapy, and excessive loss of body fluids. The hypomagnesemia seen in the acutely ill is most often the manifestation of compromised nutritional status, secondary to starvation and malabsorption.

Clinical Presentation

Signs and Symptoms

- Muscular weakness
- Positive Chvostek and Trousseau signs
- Nystagmus
- Seizures
- Tetany
- ECG Changes
  - Prolonged PR and QT intervals
  - Broad, flat T waves
  - Ventricular arrhythmias
  - Torsade de pointes

Diagnostic Tests

- Serum Mg^{++} less than 1.6 mEq/L

Phosphate Imbalance: Hyperphosphatemia
Etiologies, Risk Factors, and Pathophysiology

Hyperphosphatemia can result from increased phosphate intake, decreased phosphate excretion, or a disorder that shifts intracellular phosphate to the extracellular space. The most common cause of hyperphosphatemia in all patients, including the acutely ill, is renal injury; the regulation of phosphate in the body depends on the kidneys. Hyperphosphatemia is also seen in milk-alkali syndrome, vitamin D intoxication, hypoparathyroidism, rhabdomyolysis, and tumor lysis. Hyperphosphatemia is often associated with hypocalcemia.

Clinical Presentation

Signs and Symptoms

- Positive Trousseau or Chvostek sign
- Hyperreflexia
- Seizures

Diagnostic Tests

- Serum phosphate more than 4.5 mg/dL

Phosphate Imbalance: Hypophosphatemia
Etiologies, Risk Factors, and Pathophysiology

Hypophosphatemia occurs with hyperparathyroidism, correction of diabetic ketoacidosis, acute respiratory alkalosis, refeeding syndrome, and mesenchymal tumor-induced osteomalacia. Hypophosphatemia is frequently in conjunction with hypercalcemia and is common among renal transplant recipients.

Clinical Presentation

Signs and Symptoms

- Muscle weakness and wasting
- Fatigue
- Confusion
- Bone pain
- Tachycardia
- Anorexia
- Dyspnea
- Seizures

Diagnostic Tests

- Serum phosphate less than 2.5 mg/dL

Principles of Management for Electrolyte Imbalances

Hyperosmolar Disorders

1. Administer free water. Fluid replacement can be given orally, if feasible, or with intravenous administration of D_5W. The goal is to normalize the serum Na^+ level over a 48- to 72-hour period. A gradual return to normal avoids cerebral edema, which may lead to herniation, permanent neurologic deficit, or myelinolysis.
2. During treatment, monitor Na^+ and serum osmolality levels frequently, and perform serial neurologic examinations in order to adjust the rate of correction safely.
3. For patients who are also hypovolemic, intravascular volume is restored with isotonic sodium chloride prior to the correction of water deficit with free water.
4. In the setting of hypervolemia, a loop diuretic may be added to free water administration to increase renal sodium excretion. Those patients with AKI may require RRT for correction.
5. Administer desmopressin (nasally or orally) or vasopressin (IV, IM, subcutaneously) in diabetes insipidus. These medications mimic the action of ADH.

Hypo-Osmolar Disorders

1. Restrict water intake. Mild, asymptomatic hyponatremia often is not treated or is treated only with a water restriction. This is the first-line therapy for patients with SIADH. Demeclocycline, urea, and vasopressin receptor antagonists (Vaptans) may be considered for long-term management.
2. Institute RRT. RRT is indicated for severe fluid overload in the presence of AKI.
3. Administer hypertonic saline. Hypertonic saline may be needed to correct Na^+ levels less than 115 mEq/L when the patient is symptomatic. Careful, slow administration of hypertonic saline is important to avoid sudden shifts in serum osmolality and subsequent osmotic demyelination syndrome. The syndrome consists of neurological symptoms and can be associated with irreversible brain damage.
4. Monitor Na^+ and urine electrolyte levels frequently. The target increase of serum sodium level is 6 mEq/L over 24 hours and an additional mEq/L every 24 hours thereafter until serum sodium level reaches 130 mEq/L.

Hyperkalemia

Of all the potential electrolyte disorders, hyperkalemia is the most life threatening because of potassium's profound impact on the electrophysiology of the heart. Hyperkalemia is also the most common reason for initiation of dialysis in the AKI patients.

1. Initiate cardiac monitoring. Because hyperkalemia affects cardiac tissue, continuous ECG monitoring assists in recognizing cardiac manifestations of altered K^+ levels.
2. Administer calcium salts, such as calcium gluconate in the setting of ECG changes. Calcium elevates the stimulation threshold, protecting the patient from the negative myocardial effects of hyperkalemia. The administration of calcium does not change the serum K^+.
3. Administer hypertonic (50%) glucose and regular insulin intravenously. Insulin acts to drive potassium into the cells on a temporary basis, thereby protecting the heart from the effect of the elevated serum (extracellular) potassium level. Glucose is given to avoid hypoglycemia. All patients, especially patients with AKI, require glucose monitoring because the effects of insulin may be prolonged.
4. Administer medications such as loop or thiazide diuretics to increase renal excretion of extracellular K^+, or cation-exchange resins, such as sodium polystyrene sulfonate (Kayexalate) to increase gastrointestinal excretion of K^+. Patients with impaired renal function have decreased response to diuretic therapy. Kayexalate is administered orally or rectally. It is used in patients who have normal bowel function and are not at risk for constipation or impaction. Repeat dosing without a bowel movement can lead to intestinal necrosis.
5. Institute RRT. Hemodialysis may be necessary to rapidly remove K^+ when the patient's K^+ level cannot be controlled by other methods.
6. Restrict dietary intake of potassium to 40 mEq/day. A dietary restriction is considered conservative management and is usually instituted in conjunction with other therapies aimed at removing potassium from the body.

7. Discontinue medications that inhibit renal potassium excretion, such as potassium-sparing diuretics, sulfamethoxazole-trimethoprim (Bactrim), and angiotensin-converting enzyme (ACE) inhibitors.

Hypokalemia

1. Administer K^+ supplementation. Depending on the severity of the deficit and the patient's status, oral or IV replacements can be given. Ideally, IV supplementation of K^+ is given through a central line due to the irritating nature of K^+ to the tissues. Potassium replacement is given in at least 50 mL of fluid with no more than 20 mEq replaced per hour. It is common for patients to be unable to tolerate more than 10 mEq/h if the supplementation is given through a peripheral intravenous line. Because K^+ is primarily an intracellular cation, allow at least 1 hour after administration for the movement of the K^+ into the cells before evaluating the serum K^+ level. A level obtained too quickly after supplementation is completed may reflect an artificially high serum value. Hemolysis during blood draw may also result in an artificially high level.
2. Evaluate the patient's diuretic therapy. Patients with normal renal function who are on loop diuretics or thiazide diuretics may benefit from changing to potassium-sparing diuretics to prevent hypokalemia.
3. Replace magnesium if low. Correction of hypokalemia may not happen until hypomagnesemia is also corrected as magnesium deficiency exacerbates potassium wasting by increasing distal potassium secretion.

Hypercalcemia

1. Administer normal saline IV and diuretics. In the presence of normal renal function, normal saline infusion followed by loop diuretics reduces Ca^{++} reabsorption and enhances Ca^{++} excretion from the kidneys. Serum sodium, potassium, and magnesium levels are closely monitored, and replaced if needed.
2. Administer corticosteroids. Corticosteroids can be used to decrease absorption of Ca^{++} from the gastrointestinal tract in vitamin D toxicity or external synthesis of 1,25-dihydroxyvitamin D3. Dietary calcium and vitamin D intake are reduced as well.
3. Administer bisphosphonates. Bisphosphonates are the first choice of treatment, especially in cancer-related hypercalcemia. They lower serum calcium by blocking bone resorption and calcitriol synthesis.
4. Administer oral phosphate (PO_4^-) supplementation. PO_4^- binds Ca^{++} so that it is excreted in the stool.
5. Immobility worsens hypercalcemia so ambulation and weight-bearing exercise are encouraged.
6. RRT may be needed to effectively remove Ca^{++}.

Hypocalcemia

1. Administer Ca^{++} supplementation. Calcium-containing antacids may be used. Often Ca^{++} supplementation is done concurrently with the administration of vitamin D. Calcium may be given orally in the form of antacids or intravenously as calcium gluconate or calcium chloride when hypocalcemia is severe. Vitamin D is necessary for Ca^{++} to be absorbed from the gastrointestinal tract.
2. Thiazide diuretics and active forms of vitamin D or calcitriol can be used in patients with hypoparathyroidism.
3. Concurrent hypomagnesemia needs to be corrected before hypocalcemia can be effectively treated.
4. Institute seizure precautions. Patients with hypocalcemia are at risk for developing tetany and seizures.

Hypermagnesemia

1. Discontinue use of Mg^{++}-containing antacids.
2. Administer normal saline and loop diuretics. If the patient has normal renal function, the administration of saline and diuretics promotes excretion of Mg^{++}.
3. Administer calcium gluconate intravenously in order to antagonize neuromuscular and cardiovascular effects of magnesium.
4. Institution of RRT in patients with impaired renal function may be necessary.

Hypomagnesemia

1. Administer Mg^{++} supplementation. Oral administration or Mg^{++} sulfate IV may be used. IV Mg^{++} should not be given faster than 150 mg/min as an abrupt elevation in the serum level will promote magnesium excretion and can result in hypotension. Oral replacement is preferred for asymptomatic patients. However, the oral magnesium salts are not well tolerated as they cause diarrhea.
2. Encourage a magnesium-rich diet, such as green vegetables, beans, nuts, and seeds, etc.

Hyperphosphatemia

1. Limit oral phosphate intake in patients with mild renal impairment.
2. Administer phosphate binders in patients with renal impairment, especially end-stage renal disease (ESRD) patients. They bind with phosphate in the intestine, limiting the absorption. Calcium-containing phosphate binders are preferred.
3. In severe AKI, give normal saline infusion with loop diuretics or begin RRT to lower phosphate levels.

Hypophosphatemia

1. Administer phosphate supplementation. Supplementation can be administered by mouth or IV.
2. Discontinue use of phosphate binders.
3. Encourage a phosphate-rich diet, such as dairy products, meats, and beans, etc.

RENAL REPLACEMENT THERAPY

For many years, IHD and PD were the only modalities of RRT available to manage renal failure with volume overload. Many acutely ill patients cannot tolerate the rapid fluid and electrolyte shifts associated with conventional/intermittent hemodialysis because of hemodynamic instability and cardiac arrhythmias. PD is associated with less abrupt shifts in fluid but cannot be used in patients with recent abdominal surgeries, respiratory distress, bowel diseases, or intra-abdominal infection.

Several alternative modalities to manage acute volume overload and electrolyte disturbances have been introduced since 1977, beginning with continuous arteriovenous hemofiltration (CAVH). The further development of additional CRRTs offers more treatment options for the acutely ill patient with renal injury and hemodynamic instability. These therapies include using a double-lumen venous access and a pump for continuous venovenous hemofiltration (CVVH) and the addition of dialysate for continuous venovenous hemodialysis (CVVHD). Continuous venovenous hemodiafiltration (CVVHDF) combines the principles of CVVH and CVVHD. Using any method of CRRT accomplishes the desirable outcomes of hemodialysis without the complications associated with rapid fluid shifts, such as changes in blood pressure, cardiac arrhythmias, or muscle cramps. Slow

low efficiency dialysis (SLED) involves using hemodialysis at lower flow rates usually over a 12-hour period at night. This therapy also decreases the large fluid shifts problematic for the hemodynamically unstable patient. See Table 15-3 for a summary of CRRT modalities.

The goals of any type of RRT are the removal of excess fluid and toxins and correction of electrolyte imbalances and metabolic acidosis. Each of the RRT modalities is able to accomplish that goal, with varying levels of efficiency. These homeostatic corrections are accomplished through the processes of diffusion (hemodialysis) and/or convection (hemofiltration). Diffusion, the process by which solutes move from an area of high concentration to one of a lesser concentration, provides for movement of fluids and electrolytes between blood and dialysate. Convection occurs as a result of the hydrostatic pressure gradient, which induces the filtration of plasma water across the membrane of the hemofilter. Substitution fluid is usually used to prevent excessive fluid removal. Bicarbonate can be added to the substitution fluid as a buffer.

Access

Before any type of RRT can be performed, access to the bloodstream, for IHD and CRRT or access to the peritoneum, for PD, is necessary. The type of access is determined by the reason for initiation and method of renal replacement. The access can be either temporary or permanent.

Permanent Vascular Access

Permanent access is achieved by placement of either an arteriovenous fistula or graft. A fistula is a surgically created anastomosis between an artery, usually the radial, brachial, or femoral, and an adjacent vein. This anastomosis allows

TABLE 15-3. **SUMMARY OF RENAL REPLACEMENT THERAPIES**

Type	Indications	Contraindications	Complications
Intermittent hemodialysis	Life-threatening fluid/electrolyte imbalances Renal failure Poisoning/drug overdose	Hemodynamic instability Hypovolemia Coagulation disorders	Intradialytic hypotension or hypertension Arrhythmia Muscle cramps Blood loss
Peritoneal dialysis	Fluid/electrolyte imbalances Renal failure	Recent abdominal surgery Abdominal adhesions Peritonitis Respiratory distress Pregnancy	Peritonitis Malnutrition Encapsulating peritoneal sclerosis
Continuous renal replacement therapy SCUF CVVH CVVHD CVVHDF SLED CAVH CAVHD CAVHDF	Fluid/electrolyte imbalances Renal failure Fluid overload	Need for emergent therapy	Filter clotting Worsening uremia for SCUF Hypothermia

Abbreviations: CAVH, continuous arteriovenous hemofiltration; CAVHD, continuous arteriovenous hemodialysis; CAVHDF, continuous arteriovenous hemodiafiltration; CVVH, continuous venovenous hemofiltration; CVVHD, continuous venovenous hemodialysis; CVVHDF, continuous venovenous hemodiafiltration; SCUF, slow continuous ultrafiltration; SLED, slow low efficiency dialysis.

arterial blood to flow through the vein, causing venous enlargement and engorgement. Arteriovenous grafts are placed in patients who do not have adequate vessels to create a fistula. A prosthetic graft is implanted subcutaneously and used to anastomose an artery to a vein.

Permanent access is necessary for patients requiring chronic dialysis. A period of maturation, usually 6 weeks, is necessary before the access can be used. This maturation time allows for the venous side to dilate and the vessel wall to thicken, permitting repeated insertion of dialysis needles.

Temporary Vascular Access

Central venous catheters are used for patients presenting with AKI and for ESRD patients without permanent arteriovenous access or while waiting for the permanent access to mature. Temporary access to the bloodstream is obtained through cannulation of a large-diameter vein, with a large-bore, double- or single-lumen catheter specifically designed for dialysis. These catheters are inserted and maintained similar to other arterial and central venous devices, but are generally larger and reserved for dialysis treatments. A single double-lumen catheter is more commonly used to maximize the filtration and dialysis capabilities of the renal replacement devices.

The catheters can be non-tunneled or tunneled. The tunneled catheter is associated with reduced morbidity and provides better performance. The tunneled catheter can be used for extended periods of time (months to years) with meticulous attention to sterile technique. The location for catheter placement is chosen to maximize blood flow and prevent kinking of the catheter with patient movement. To initiate hemofiltration (CVVH), hemodialysis (CVVHD), or hemodiafiltration (CVVHDF), a single 14- to 16-gauge double-lumen catheter is placed in the subclavian, jugular, or femoral vein. The jugular is the preferred site over the subclavian because use of the subclavian site may lead to central vein stenosis and impede future permanent access. Femoral catheters are used when other accesses are not possible but are less desirable due to increased infection risk and impaired mobility.

Peritoneal Access

Peritoneal catheters are made of Silastic tubing, with side holes along its intraperitoneal portion to allow for fluid exchange, and an attached cuff (or 2 cuffs), soft disk, or balloon to anchor the catheter. When PD needs to be initiated immediately, a rigid stylet, designed for single acute use only, is inserted. Both types of catheters are inserted through small incisions in the abdomen and threaded into the peritoneal space.

Dialyzer/Hemofilters/Dialysate

There are a variety of dialyzers and hemofilters available for use. The type of dialyzer or hemofilter chosen is determined by the patient's condition and the desired outcomes of the RRT. All dialyzers have a blood and dialysate compartment, separated by a semipermeable membrane. The dialyzer has two inlet ports and two outlet ports, one each for blood and dialysate. During dialysis, blood and dialysate are pumped through the dialyzer in opposite directions.

Hemofilters are made of highly permeable hollow fibers or plates. These fibers or plates are surrounded by an ultrafiltrate space and have arterial and venous blood ports. Plasma water and certain solutes are separated from the blood by the hemofilter and drain into a collection device.

Dialysate solution, used in any therapy that has dialysis as a component, is specifically designed to create concentration gradients that optimize the removal of wastes, restoration of acid-base and electrolyte balance, and maintenance of extracellular fluid balance. The specific solution is determined by the patient's condition and desired outcomes. Although standard solutions may initially be used, they can be tailored to meet the individual patient's needs and contain varying concentrations of Na^+, K^+, Mg^+, Ca^{++}, Cl^-, glucose, and buffers.

Procedures

Hemodialysis and Sustained Low Efficiency Dialysis

Initiation of hemodialysis or SLED through a temporary access is accomplished using a procedure called *coupling*. During coupling, the dialysis catheter and the dialysis circuitry are connected, using sterile technique. To initiate dialysis through a permanent access, two 14- or 16-gauge needles are inserted into the dilated vein of the fistula or the graft portion of the synthetic graft. One needle is considered arterial, used for blood outflow, and the other is considered venous, used for blood return.

The basic components of a hemodialysis system are shown in Figure 15-2. Blood, leaving the patient through the arterial needle, is pumped through the circuitry and returned to the patient through the venous needle. A blood pump moves the blood through the dialysis circuitry and dialyzer, allowing for different flow rates. Both arterial and venous pressures are monitored in the circuitry.

Peritoneal Dialysis

Peritoneal dialysis is accomplished through a series of cycles or exchanges. The dialysate, administered into the peritoneal cavity, remains in the cavity for a preset amount of time (dwell time) and then is drained. Each set of these activities is called a cycle or exchange. Dialysate flows into the peritoneal cavity by gravity, taking approximately 10 minutes for 2 L of fluid to infuse. During the dwell time, diffusion and convection occur across the peritoneal membrane. Dwell times are based on patient need. With an optimally functioning catheter, it takes 10 minutes for 2 L of fluid to drain from the abdomen. Other forms of PD include continuous ambulatory peritoneal dialysis (CAPD) and continuous cyclic peritoneal dialysis (CCPD), although these forms are generally

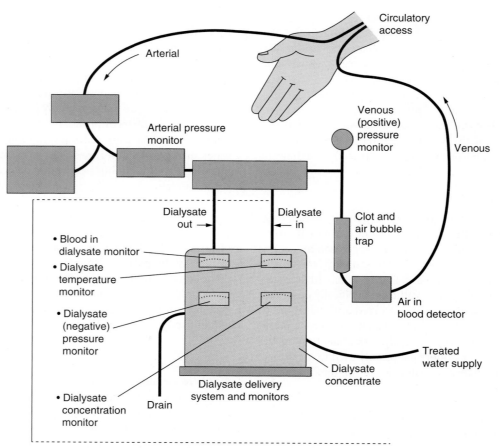

Figure 15-2. Components of a hemodialysis system. (*Reproduced with permission from Thompson JM, McFarland GK, Hirsch JE, et al:* Mosby's Manual of Clinical Nursing. *St Louis, MO: Mosby, 1989.*)

not used in AKI. However, if the patient uses this type of therapy at home for ESRD, it is possible that it will be continued during their hospital admission.

Continuous Renal Replacement Therapy

In CRRT, the blood lines are primed with a saline solution with or without unfractionated heparin as an anticoagulant and then attached to the appropriate vascular access catheter arm (one for outflow and one for inflow). Blood is pumped from the outflow side and passes through the hemofilter. The use of anticoagulation (ie, unfractionated heparin or citrate) assists with blood flow and prolongs the filter life. The blood returns to the body via the inflow tubing after fluid and electrolytes are diffused into the ultrafiltrate. The ultrafiltrate is collected in a bag after removal.

In CVVHD, blood leaves the patient through the outflow catheter and is pumped through a dialyzer rather than a hemofilter. Wastes and fluid are removed and drained into an ultrafiltrate bag. The blood is then returned to the body through the inflow catheter. The dialysate is pumped through the dialyzer countercurrent to blood flow. Figure 15-3 shows the basic setup of CVVHD. In CVVHDF, replacement fluids are given to maintain euvolemia.

Indications for and Efficacy of Renal Replacement Therapy Modes

Each type of RRT is indicated for different clinical situations to achieve identified goals. The goals of therapy are clearly delineated before selection of the type of therapy.

Intermittent Hemodialysis

Intermittent hemodialysis is implemented when urgent therapy is indicated for an acute situation, such as life-threatening hyperkalemia. IHD is contraindicated in patients with hemodynamic instability (although hypotension may be a relative contraindication), hypovolemia, coagulation disorders, or vascular access problems.

Considered the gold standard for the treatment of AKI and ESRD, IHD is the most effective of all of the RRTs. Fluid and uremic wastes can be eliminated from the body during a 4- to 6-hour treatment. Approximately 200 mL of blood is utilized in the circuit, however, and this shift in blood volume can exacerbate hemodynamic instability.

Peritoneal Dialysis

Today, PD is rarely used for acutely ill patients who need dialysis but are unable to tolerate the hemodynamic changes associated with hemodialysis. CRRT is used instead. PD may

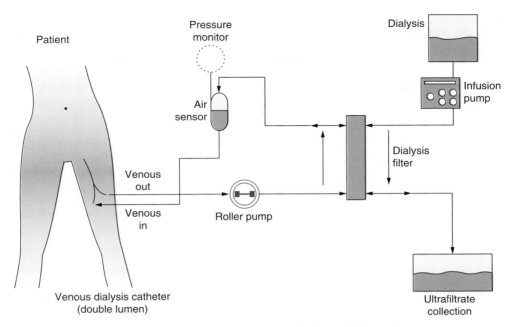

Figure 15-3. Components of a CVVHD system. (*Reproduced with permission from Strohschein BL, Caruso DM, Greene KA. Continuous venovenous hemodialysis. Am J Crit Care. 1994; April 1;3(2):92-99.*)

be performed in a patient who is on chronic PD and hospitalized with an acute illness. Utilizing the peritoneal membrane as the dialyzer, effective elimination of fluid and waste products can be achieved. PD is slower and less effective than hemodialysis.

PD is contraindicated in patients who have had recent or extensive abdominal surgery; who have abdominal adhesions, peritonitis, or respiratory distress; or who are pregnant.

Continuous Renal Replacement Therapy

CRRT is appropriate in patients with hemodynamic instability who require RRT. The specific type of CRRT is selected after considering the patient's fluid and electrolyte status, metabolic needs, and severity of uremia. The most commonly used forms of CRRT are CVVH, CVVHD, or CVVHDF as venous access has more predictable blood flow rate.

Continuous Venovenous Hemofiltration

The main objective of CVVH is fluid removal. Although large changes in blood chemistries are not expected, it is possible for a patient to achieve and maintain a stable volume and composition of electrolytes in the extracellular fluid. The higher the blood flow rate achieved in CVVH, the more solutes that can be removed. Because large volumes of fluid can be removed, the healthcare team has more flexibility in treating patients. Nutrition, a problem in many acutely ill patients, can often be enhanced in these patients because nutrition (even total parenteral nutrition when enteral is contraindicated) can be provided without fear of fluid overload.

CVVH, in some institutions, has become the treatment of choice when patients have contraindications to IHD or PD. Fluid shifts in CVVH are less rapid than with

hemodialysis, making the therapy attractive when persistent hemodynamic instability, especially hypotension, is present. Other patients who may benefit from CVVH are patients with uncontrolled heart failure, pulmonary edema, severe burns, cerebral edema, or hepatorenal syndrome. Patients can be maintained on CVVH for several weeks until either long-term hemodialysis can be initiated or the patient's renal function improves. There are no absolute contraindications for CVVH. Unfortunately, the therapy has to be discontinued for transportation off the unit such as for selected diagnostic tests (eg, computed tomographic scans) and the continuous nature of the therapy limits mobility, particularly if a femoral access is used (eg, out of bed to chair).

Continuous Venovenous Hemodialysis

Continuous venovenous hemodialysis combines the principles of hemofiltration with a slow form of dialysis (see Figure 15-3). The indications for CVVHD are similar to those for hemodialysis. Selection of CVVHD is generally made because a patient is unstable and not able to tolerate the rapid fluid and electrolyte shifts that occur with IHD. CVVHD provides an avenue for hemodynamically unstable patients to achieve a stable fluid and electrolyte balance without further compromise of their status. There are no absolute contraindications for CVVHD. Maintaining patency of the dialyzer is the key to successful CVVHD. Patients with coagulopathies require special monitoring if anticoagulation is used to prevent clotting in the circuit.

Slow Continuous Ultrafiltration

Slow continuous ultrafiltration (SCUF) is primarily for use in patients with a fluid volume excess and some degree of renal function. Because fluid removal is the primary goal, this procedure is performed without simultaneous fluid replacement. There is a minimal impact on the urea and creatinine levels.

General Renal Replacement Therapy Interventions

The frequency of RRT is on the rise. Although each therapy has unique characteristics, all require similar interventions. Careful observations and interventions are essential, as is accurate fluid management. Monitoring includes recording mean arterial pressure, hourly intake and output, daily weights, and state of anticoagulation. Analysis of acid-base and evaluation of serum chemistries for electrolyte balance are also required. The progressive care nurse partners with the dialysis team in assuming responsibility for early recognition and initial interventions for patient and system problems.

Principles of Management

1. Early recognition of the signs and symptoms of AKI is essential in order to correct underlying causes and prevent further decline in renal function.
2. Close monitoring of patients' intake, output, and daily weight during different phases of AKI guides fluid administration, diuretic use, or initiation of RRT. CRRT is frequently utilized for patients who are hemodynamically unstable.
3. Electrolyte imbalance and metabolic acidosis can be life threatening and must be corrected in a timely manner. Frequent laboratory tests are warranted until homeostasis is reestablished.
4. Nephrotoxic agents need to be avoided in all patients with AKI. Medications can be renally adjusted to prevent additional renal damage.
5. Adequate protein and calories are important. Dietician consultation is helpful.

SELECTED BIBLIOGRAPHY

General Renal and Electrolyte

Johnson R, Feehally J, Floege J, eds. *Comprehensive Clinical Nephrology*. 5th ed. Philadelphia, PA: Elsevier Saunders; 2015.

Molzhan A, Butera E, eds. *Contemporary Nephrology Nursing: Principles and Practice*. 2nd ed. Pitman, NJ: American Nephrology Nursing Association; 2007.

Muhsin SA, Mount DB. Diagnosis and treatment of hypernatremia. *Best Pract Res Clin Endocrinol Metab*. 2016;30(2):189-203.

Acute Kidney Injury

Bellomo R, Ronco C, Kellum JA, Mehta RL, Palevsky P. Acute Dialysis Quality Initiative Work Group. Acute renal failure—definition, outcome measures, animal models, fluid therapy and information technology needs: the Second International Consensus Conference of the Acute Dialysis Quality Initiative (ADQI) Group. *Crit Care*. 2004;8:R204-R212.

Fiaccadori E, Maggiore U, Cabassi A, Morabito S, Castellano G, Regolisti G. Nutrition evaluation and manangement of AKI patients. *J Ren Nutr*. 2013;23(3):255-258.

Hertzberg D, Ryden L, Pickering JW, Sartipy U, Holzmann M. Acute kidney injury-an overview of diagnostic methods and clinical management. *Clin Kidney J*. 2017;10(3):323-331.

Isaac S. Contrast-induced nephropathy: nursing implications. *Crit Care Nurse*. 2012;32(3):41-48.

Kidney Disease: Improving Global Outcomes (KDIGO) Acute Kidney Injury Work Group. KDIGO clinical practice guideline for acute kidney injury. *Kidney Int (Suppl)*. 2012;2:1-138.

Palevsky PM, Liu KD, Brophy PD, et al. KDOQI US commentary on the 2012 KDIGO clinical practice guideline for acute kidney injury. *Am J Kidney Dis*. 2013;61(5):649-672.

Subramaniam RM, Suarez-Cuervo C, Wilson RF, et al. Effectiveness of prevention strategies for contrast-induced nephropathy: a systematic review and meta-analysis. *Ann Intern Med*. 2016;164(6):406-416.

Wood S. Contrast-induced nephropathy in critical care. *Crit Care Nurse*. 2012;32(6):15-23.

Renal Replacement Therapy

Golestaneh L, Richter B, Amato-Hayes M. Logistics of renal replacement therapy: relevant issues for critical care nurses. *Am J Crit Care*. 2012;21(2):126-130.

Nissenson AR, Fine RN. *Handbook of Dialysis Therapy*. 5th ed. Philadelphia, PA: Elsevier; 2017.

Tolwani A. Continuous renal-replacement therapy for acute kidney injury. *N Engl J Med*. 2012;367:2505-2514.

Web Resources

Medscape. www.medscape.com. Accessed June 14, 2017.

National Kidney Foundation: guideline and commentaries. www.kidney.org/professionals/guidelines/guidelines_commentaries. Accessed June 14, 2017.

ASPEN/SCCM Guidelines. http://journals.sagepub.com/doi/full/10.1177/0148607115621863. Accessed June 14, 2017.

ENDOCRINE SYSTEM

Mary E. Lough

16

PATHOLOGIC CONDITIONS

Pathologic endocrine conditions are managed in both the critical care and progressive care environments. By far the most common are those associated with hyperglycemic and hypoglycemic states and to that end they are the major focus of this chapter. While not as frequently seen, the chapter also discusses selected pituitary and thyroid disorders.

HYPERGLYCEMIC STATES

Diabetes is a common comorbidity in hospitalized patients. This disease, along with the specter of hyperglycemia, is associated with significant increase in hospital morbidity and mortality. Additionally, many patients, without a history of diabetes, will develop hyperglycemia during their hospitalization.

Hyperglycemia occurs in hospitalized patients due to natural metabolic responses to acute injury and stress. During acute illness, the liver produces and releases glucose in response to glucocorticoids, catecholamines, growth hormone, and various cytokines (interleukin-6 [IL-6], interleukin-1a [IL-1a], and tumor necrosis factor-alpha). As

a result, fat and protein are catabolized and blood glucose surges. Conditions such as myocardial infarction, stroke, surgery, trauma, pain, and sepsis may cause the release of these biological mediators and counterregulatory hormones. In essence, the greater the stress response, the higher the blood glucose will be. To help minimize the adverse outcomes associated with hyperglycemia, rigorous glucose monitoring and effective management of blood glucose are essential. This is usually accomplished in critically ill patients by frequent blood glucose testing paired with a continuous insulin infusion. Infusion protocols, or standing order sets, are often used to standardize treatment and maintain glucose values in the targeted range.

Diabetic Ketoacidosis and Hyperglycemic Hyperosmolar

Diabetic ketoacidosis (DKA) and hyperglycemic hyperosmolar (HHS) are two extremes in the spectrum of decompensated diabetes. The incidence of DKA is defined as acute hyperglycemia with acidosis, and HHS is classified as acute hyperglycemia without acidosis (nonketotic).

Diabetes is a metabolic disease that results in inadequate uptake of glucose by cells, resulting in hyperglycemia. The key disorder in type 1 diabetes mellitus (DM) is minimal or absent insulin secretion by the pancreas. This is often caused by an autoimmune activation where the immune system attacks and destroys the pancreatic beta islet cells that normally produce insulin. Type 2 diabetes usually occurs in older adults, but can occur in youth, and is associated with impaired insulin receptor sensitivity. Insulin production in type 2 DM may initially be normal, and then fall dramatically as the disease progresses. Although hyperglycemia is a shared feature, the etiology, risk factors, pathophysiology, and management priorities vary considerably for each classification of diabetes.

Etiology, Risk Factors, and Pathophysiology

Insulin is normally released from the pancreas by beta islet cells (Islets of Langerhans) in response to an increase in blood glucose. Insulin is necessary for cellular uptake of glucose by most cells in the body. Without insulin, the glucose fails to enter cells and accumulates in the blood, resulting in hyperglycemia and a vascular inflammatory state. Cells deprived of glucose begin to starve, triggering a mobilization of stored glucose via the breakdown of protein and fat (gluconeogenesis) and release of stored glucose from the liver (glycogenolysis). This triggers a complex series of physiologic processes that account for the major signs and symptoms associated with DKA and HHS.

Diabetic Ketoacidosis

The most common precipitating scenarios associated with DKA are underlying or concomitant infection (40%), missed insulin (25%), and newly diagnosed, previously unknown diabetes (15%). Other causes make up about 20% including myocardial infarction, stroke, trauma, and pancreatitis. Although DKA is primarily a complication of type 1 diabetes, it can occur (rarely) in some forms of type 2 diabetes under conditions of extreme stress and extreme hyperglycemia (Table 16-1).

TABLE 16-1. CAUSES OF DKA

Infections
Missed or Inadequate Doses of Insulin (Primarily Type 1 Diabetes)
Initial Presentation of Type 1 Diabetes
Clinical Stressors
- Trauma
- Surgery
- Pregnancy
- Acute illness
- Kidney failure
- Liver failure
- Myocardial infarction/ischemia

Medication-Induced Impairment of Glucose Metabolism
- Thiazide diuretics
- Phenytoin
- Beta-blockers
- Calcium channel blockers
- Steroids
- Epinephrine
- Psychotropics
- Salicylate poisoning

TABLE 16-2. CALCULATION OF ANION GAP (NORMAL < 12 MEQ/L)[a]

$Na^+ - (Cl^- + HCO_3^-)$ = anion gap
Example from DKA case study:
$130 - (94 + 11)$ = 25 mEq/L (anion gap acidosis)
Example from HHS case study:
$152 - (121 + 20)$ = 11 mEq/L (no anion gap)

[a]*Note: Potassium can be added to the sodium but because it is a small number, it is often excluded in the calculation.*

In general, DKA is a biochemical triad of hyperglycemia, ketonemia, and metabolic acidosis with a large anion gap, see Table 16-2. Mild DKA is typically characterized by hyperglycemia (> 300 mg/dL), low bicarbonate level (15-18 mEq/L), and acidosis (pH < 7.30) with ketonemia and ketonuria. While definitions vary, moderate DKA can be categorized by pH of less than 7.2 and serum bicarbonate of 10 to 14 mEq/L, whereas severe DKA has pH of less than 7.1 and bicarbonate below 10 mEq/L. Patients presenting with mild DKA may be alert and responsive. In moderate DKA increasing drowsiness occurs. Severe DKA is associated with a decreased level of consciousness or coma.

DKA can develop in less than 24 hours. The initiating event in DKA is an insufficient or absent level of circulating insulin. This insulin deficiency results in increased fatty acid metabolism, increased liver gluconeogenesis (formation of glucose from amino acids and proteins), and increased secretion of counterregulatory hormones, including glucagon and the stress hormones (catecholamines, cortisol, and growth hormone). Counterregulatory hormones reduce the glucose-lowering effects of insulin, raise blood glucose, and are released in response to stress and other stimuli. The pathogenesis of DKA can be organized into three main components: fluid volume deficit, electrolyte imbalance, and acid-base imbalance (Figure 16-1).

Fluid Volume Deficit With Associated Electrolyte Imbalance in DKA

Because of the insulin deficiency, there is both hyperglycemia and increased amino acid release from cells. The stress response in the body leads to metabolic decompensation, and stress hormones further trigger a rise in plasma glucose and ketones. The hyperglycemia causes an osmotic diuresis and hypotonic losses leading to fluid volume deficits (intracellular and extracellular) and electrolyte losses. As serum glucose exceeds the renal threshold, glycosuria results. In the absence of insulin, protein stores are also broken down by the liver into amino acids and then into glucose for energy. This further increases serum blood glucose, increases urine glucose, and worsens the osmotic diuresis and ketonemia. Urinary losses of water, sodium, magnesium, calcium, and phosphorus cause an increase in serum osmolality and decreased electrolyte levels. Potassium levels may be increased or decreased, depending on the amount of nausea and vomiting, acid-base balance, and fluid status of the patient. This hyperosmolality causes additional fluid shifts from the intracellular to the extracellular space, increasing dehydration. Hypovolemic shock can result from severe fluid

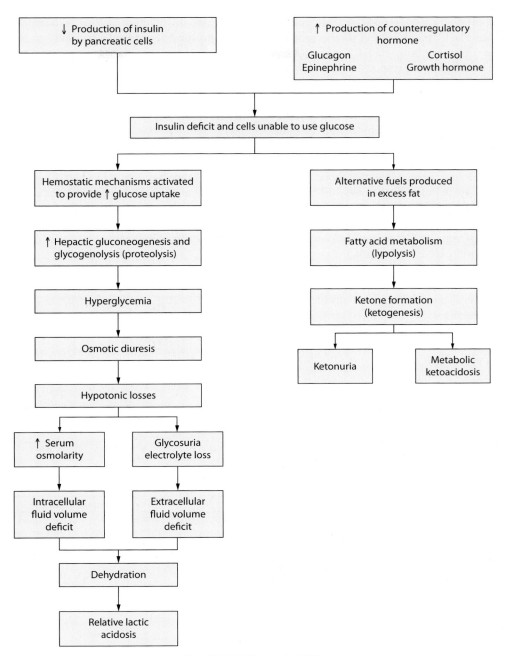

Figure 16-1. Pathogenesis of DKA.

losses in DKA. Volume depletion decreases glomerular filtration of glucose and creates a cycle of progressive hyperglycemia. The increase in serum osmolarity also is thought to further impair insulin secretion and promote insulin resistance. The altered neurologic status frequently seen in these patients is due primarily to brain cell dehydration and serum hyperosmolality.

Acid-Base Imbalance in DKA
Cells without glucose starve and initiate processes to access existing stores of fat and protein to provide energy for body processes (gluconeogenesis). Fats are broken down faster than they can be metabolized in the liver, which results in an accumulation of ketone acids. These ketone acids are usually cleared in peripheral tissues. If the ketogenic pathway is overwhelmed ketone acids accumulate in the blood stream where hydrogen ions (H^+) dissociate, causing a profound metabolic acidosis. Acetone is formed during this process and is responsible for the "fruity breath" found in these patients. Ketones can be quantitatively measured in both blood and urine.

Metabolic acidosis may be worsened with severe fluid volume deficits because hypovolemia results in tissue hypoperfusion and production of lactic acids from anaerobic metabolism. Excess lactic acid results in what is called an *increased anion gap* (increased body acids). Sodium, potassium, chloride, and bicarbonate are responsible for maintaining a normal anion gap in the body, which is normally less than 12 to 14 mEq/L (Table 16-2). The anion gap represents the difference between the cations (Na^{++}, K^{++}), and anions (Cl^-, HCO_3^-). Ketone accumulation, a by-product of gluconeogenesis, causes acidosis and increases the anion gap, often more than 20 mEq/L (see DKA case study).

The normal physiologic response to metabolic acidosis is to produce bicarbonate to buffer the ketones and H^{++} ions. The patient with DKA often has diminished bicarbonate levels because of the osmotic diuresis. The respiratory system attempts to compensate by blowing off carbon dioxide to restore normal blood pH. This explains the deep rapid breathing, called "Kussmaul respirations," often seen in these patients.

Metabolic acidosis also results in potentially life-threatening electrolyte imbalances. Serum potassium is elevated initially in DKA probably due to potassium shifts from the intracellular to the extracellular space because of the acidosis. Later, hypokalemia is common because of insulin-induced transfer of plasma potassium into cells and increased urinary excretion of potassium with the osmotic diuresis.

Correction of Acid-Base Imbalance

In DKA the administration of sufficient intravenous (IV) fluids, insulin, and potassium replacement per hospital protocol is sufficient to reverse acidosis in most cases. Use of IV sodium bicarbonate is not recommended for patients with a pH > 7.0 in DKA. Sodium bicarbonate is not administered to patients with a diagnosis of HHS.

Controversy has existed about use of sodium bicarbonate in DKA with severe acidosis, defined as a pH < 6.9. Guidelines from the American Diabetes Association no longer recommend use of bicarbonate in severe acidosis. A systematic review of randomized controlled trials and case control studies evaluated the use of sodium bicarbonate, versus none, in patients with DKA with a pH between 6.9 and 7.2. There was no difference in normalization of hyperglycemia, and no difference in recovery time in the hospital. Thus, IV fluids, insulin, and potassium replacement per hospital protocol are the recommended strategies to correct acid-base imbalance in DKA.

Hyperosmolar Hyperglycemic States

HHS is classified as hyperglycemia with profound dehydration in the absence of ketosis. The onset of hyperglycemia in HHS is progressive; often with a history of type 2 diabetes, meaning there is some circulating insulin. The extremely severe hyperglycemia in HHS results in profound extracellular fluid volume contraction, marked intracellular dehydration, and excessive loss of electrolytes. In addition, because there is some insulin secretion, lipolysis (fat breakdown) is

suppressed. Therefore, there is no overproduction of ketones and no specific physical signs and symptoms of ketosis (no Kussmaul respirations, no excretion of ketones in the urine, abdominal pain, nausea, vomiting, or anorexia). Without obvious signs and symptoms, patients are unaware their blood glucose is rising and may be unaware of the need for treatment. Sustained osmotic diuresis results, leading to massive volume losses, electrolyte imbalance, and central nervous system (CNS) dysfunction. Mortality rates are higher with HHS, because of the severe volume loss and because it occurs more frequently in older adults. Death results from depression of vital body functions as cardiac and respiratory centers in the brain are depressed, cerebral edema occurs, with cardiovascular decompensation, acute kidney injury, and vascular embolism.

Clinical Presentation: Comparison of DKA and HHS

DKA	HHS
History	
Young adult or adolescent with history of type 1 DM or previously undiagnosed; preexisting infection is common	Older adult with history of type 2 DM, and preexisting chronic illness associated with decreased renal glucose excretion. Concurrent illness frequently precipitates viral infections or pneumonia
Signs and Symptoms	
Nonspecific: Polyuria, polydipsia, weakness, abdominal cramping, stupor, coma	Nonspecific: Polyuria, polydipsia, weakness confusion, coma
Specific: Nausea, vomiting, anorexia, Kussmaul respiration, fruity breath	Specific: None
Diagnostic Tests	
Serum glucose 250-800 mg/dL (usually < 500)	Serum glucose At least 600 mg/dL often > 1000 mg/dL
Serum osmolality < 330 mOsm/kg/H_2O	Serum osmolality > 350 mOsm/kg/H_2O
Ketoacidosis	Ketoacidosis
↓ pH	Not a feature
Mild: < pH 7.20-7.30	pH > 7.30
Moderate: pH 7.10-7.19	
Severe: pH < 7.09	
HCO_3 < 15 mEq/L	HCO_3^- > 15 mEq/L
Serum ketones > 2+	Serum ketones below 2+
Positive urine ketones	Minimal urine ketones
Positive anion gap > 12	Variable anion gap
Dehydration	Dehydration
Volume depletion (decrease intracellular and extracellular)	Severe volume depletion (intracellular and extracellular)
Kidney function	Kidney function
Increased BUN: creatinine ratio	Marked increase in BUN: creatinine ratio
Urine ketones +2	↓ GFR
Electrolyte depletion	Electrolyte depletion
Potassium, magnesium, phosphate, calcium	Potassium, magnesium, phosphate, sodium

Principles of Management for Hyperglycemic Emergencies

The monitoring and management of the patient in acute DKA and HHS revolves around six primary areas:

- fluid replacement
- treatment of hyperglycemia
- electrolyte replacement
- treatment of any underlying disorders
- prevention and management of complications
- patient and family education

Refer to institutional guidelines, protocols, and order-sets for specific glucose monitoring, insulin therapy, and fluid and electrolyte repletion. An overview of these key aspects of care for patients with hyperglycemic conditions follows.

Blood Glucose Monitoring and Point-of-Care Testing

Effective glycemic control is vital for improved morbidity and mortality in critically and acutely ill patients. Frequent assessments of blood glucose levels are commonly performed at the bedside using small quantities of blood obtained from finger sticks, arterial lines, or central venous catheters. At the bedside, a drop of blood is placed onto a chemical reagent strip and inserted into a portable glucometer. This point-of-care (POC) glucometer bedside analysis allows for more rapid interventions to manage critical glycemic disorders than is possible from laboratory glucose analysis. Newer technologies have greatly enhanced both the usability and accuracy of bedside glucometers.

Despite the obvious benefits of POC glucometers and improved technology, inaccuracies of glucose measurements can occur. Studies of critically ill patients have reported significant discrepancies between glucometer POC values and laboratory glucose values. The acceptable discrepancy between glucometer values and laboratory values is ± 15% for blood glucose values according to the United Stated Food and Drug Administration (FDA). Any large discrepancies between laboratory and the bedside glucometers must be investigated. This is particularly urgent in hypoglycemic states. There are many reasons for discrepancies in POC blood glucose values, but one important reason is that these glucometers were not originally developed or intended for use in critically ill and/or unstable patients. The FDA has released stricter industry guidelines for glucometer efficacy and identified acceptable ranges for POC and laboratory glucose value discrepancies.

Errors in blood glucose results may occur due to operator-introduced errors or patient condition. *Operator-introduced issues with POC testing*: A common source of error in glucose measurement is the incorrect operation of the glucometer device. Causes include the use of expired glucose reagent strips or insufficient blood application on the strip. Exogenous glucose contamination of blood samples can occur when venous sampling is obtained at a site above an IV infusion of a glucose-containing solution. All hospitals have written policies and procedures that describe POC standards of care. Generally, if there is an abnormal result with a POC glucometer, a blood sample is sent urgently to the clinical laboratory for verification. Tips for glucometer use are reviewed in Table 16-3.

Patient issues with POC testing: Several clinical conditions may influence POC glucose measurements. The accuracy of glucose measurement is affected by hypotension and vasopressor use that lead to inadequate tissue perfusion in fingers. Confounding factors in critical care that may result in erroneously low blood glucose values include low hemoglobin, high triglycerides, and hypoxemia. Clinical situations that may affect the accuracy of POC glucose monitoring are listed in Table 16-4.

In the future, continuous glucose monitoring (CGM) devices may offer a viable method of glucose monitoring. Subcutaneous CGM devices are used by millions of people with insulin-dependent DM in the outpatient setting. These devices use subcutaneous glucose sensors and have demonstrated that they optimize insulin therapy, metabolic control, and safety in the outpatient setting. Data from the CGM can be downloaded to a computer for a visual display of the patient's continuous glucose levels, as well as daily and weekly glucose trends. These devices also provide safety benefits as they come with hypo- and hyperglycemia alarms. Currently, only the subcutaneous CGM is FDA-approved; in the future, IV glucose sensors are likely to be developed for use in critical care and acute care patients.

Glucose Management With Insulin

A great deal of controversy has existed as to how tightly glucose should be controlled in the hospitalized patient. Earlier studies

TABLE 16-3. TIPS FOR POINT-OF-CARE BLOOD GLUCOMETER USE

- Review the manufacturer's guidelines and hospital procedure before use. User error is the most common reason for inaccurate readings.
- Ensure that the glucometer is calibrated and clean before using.
- For patients with cold hands, warm hand in a warm blanket and let the hand hang down below the level of the heart so that blood can flow to the fingertips.
- Obtain a drop of blood and let it be drawn completely onto the reagent pad. Do not smear the blood.
- Use the side of the finger rather than the underpad as the side has fewer nerve endings (therefore less painful) and more capillaries providing a larger drop of blood.
- Correlate the glucometer device reading with the clinical assessment of the patient.
- Use universal precautions during the entire procedure.

TABLE 16-4. CLINICAL SITUATIONS THAT ALTER ACCURACY OF POINT-OF-CARE BLOOD GLUCOSE MEASUREMENTS

Blood glucose levels > 500 mg/dL or < 75 mg/dL
Inadequate tissue perfusion (hypovolemia and shock)
Vasoactive infusions
Low blood and skin temperature
Hct < 30% (false high reading) or > 55% *(false low reading)*
High blood triglycerides *(false low reading)*
High uric acid *(false low reading)*
High blood oxygen *(false low reading)*
Acetaminophen use *(false low reading)*

reported that tight glucose control using insulin infusions to maintain blood glucose target near 110 mg/dL improved morbidity and mortality in the postsurgical cardiovascular patient population. Unfortunately, "tight glucose control" was associated with an increased risk of severe hypoglycemia and higher mortality in a large randomized controlled trial named NICE-SUGAR. The current recommendations support moderate control, rather than tight glucose control. The American Diabetes Association (ADA) and American Association of Clinical Endocrinologists (AACE) jointly recommend a glucose target between 140 and 180 mg/dL in the critical care setting. The Society of Critical Care Medicine (SCCM) recommends a more conservative blood glucose target of 150 to 180 mg/dL for critically ill patients. In medical surgical units, the ADA/AACE recommends a blood glucose target between 100 and 180 mg/dL.

An insulin infusion is preferable in all hyperglycemic, critically and acutely ill patients, not just those experiencing DKA and hyperosmolar hyperglycemic states (HHSs). Patients at greatest risk are those undergoing major cardiovascular surgery and organ transplants, those with decompensated diabetes (such as DKA and HHS), those in cardiogenic shock or kidney failure, and patients receiving high-steroid doses (Table 16-5). These patients often have increased hepatic glucose production, impaired insulin release and sensitivity, and widely fluctuating blood glucose and insulin needs.

Insulin infusion protocols: In critical illness, IV insulin infusions are preferred over subcutaneous insulin injections due to erratic tissue absorption in the presence of hypotension, generalized edema, and use of vasopressors. An effective insulin infusion protocol incorporates an algorithm that easily adapts to individual patient responses, attains the glucose target quickly with minimal hypoglycemic risk. Infusion rates are increased, decreased, or stopped temporarily based on blood glucose readings and the prescribed algorithm. Whatever protocol is used, it is important to consider the degree of insulin resistance. Patients who are highly insulin resistant may require a much higher hourly infusion rate.

Along with an insulin infusion, hyperglycemic patients will require a tandem infusion of 0.9% normal saline or 5% dextrose and 0.45% normal saline, at a rate commensurate with fluid requirements. A dextrose solution is preferred in patients with diabetes. Most patients also require simultaneous infusion of potassium as insulin is known to drive potassium into cells, especially into liver and muscle cells, which may increase the risk of hypokalemia.

Basal-bolus subcutaneous insulin: When the infusion is discontinued, subcutaneous insulin is often started using basal insulin to mimic normal pancreatic function. Basal insulin is also called long-acting insulin and controls blood glucose throughout the day. Bolus or correctional insulin is fast-acting insulin used to cover food intake and intermittent surges of blood glucose. It is essential that all patients with type 1 DM receive replacement insulin or DKA will ensue. Most hospitals have a protocol for the conversion from the IV insulin infusion to subcutaneous basal insulin with a bolus correction protocol for meals. The subcutaneous long-acting insulin is generally administered 1 to 2 hours before the IV infusion is stopped. This is to prevent hyperglycemia as the IV regular insulin disappears quickly from the bloodstream. Types of insulin are listed in Table 16-6. After discontinuation of the insulin infusion, POC blood glucose testing continues with meals and at bedtime in patients who are eating, or every 4 to 6 hours in patients who cannot take anything by mouth (NPO) or are receiving continuous enteral nutrition.

Hyperglycemia: Management Strategies

In both DKA and HHS, insulin replacement is always needed, although the requirements in DKA are typically lower than HHS.

1. Regular insulin 0.15 U/kg as IV bolus.
2. Initiate low-dose IV insulin at a rate of 0.1 U/kg/h. If serum glucose does not fall by 50 to 70 mg/dL in the first hour, double insulin infusion on an hourly basis until glucose falls by 50 to 70 mg/dL.
3. Monitor serum glucose levels closely and titrate insulin infusion accordingly. Once the serum glucose falls to 250 mg/dL, the insulin infusion is decreased to a rate of 2 to 4 U/h and the IV fluids changed to half normal saline with glucose (D5-1/2NS). This ensures that hypoglycemia does not occur during ongoing treatment of the acute condition. It is essential that insulin infusion continues in the patient with DKA until the serum pH is corrected to avoid intracellular hypokalemia. Additional glucose may be needed to achieve this outcome. A glucose-containing solution is also started in the patient with HHS when serum glucose reaches 250 to 300 mg/dL to protect against cerebral edema.

TABLE 16-5. COMMON INDICATIONS FOR IV INSULIN INFUSIONS

Hyperglycemia in critical illness
Diabetic ketoacidosis (DKA)
Hyperosmolar Hyperglycemic state (HHS)
Total parenteral nutrition

TABLE 16-6. INSULIN ACTION CHART BY TYPE

Type	Onset	Peak	Duration
Rapid Acting (Bolus)			
Humalog (lispro)	< 15 minutes	30-90 minutes	< 5 hours
Novolog (aspart)	10-20 minutes	1-2 hours	3-5 hours
Apidra (glulisine)	10-15 minutes	0.5-1.5 hours	< 3 hours
Humulin R (regular)	40-60 minutes	2-3 hours	4-6 hours
Novolin R (regular)	30 minutes	2-5 hours	8 hours
Intermediate (Basal)			
Humulin N (NPH)	2-4 hours	4-10 hours	14-18 hours
Novolin N (NPH)	90 minutes	4-12 hours	up to 24 hours
Long, "Peakless" (Basal)			
Lantus (glargine)	3-5 hours	minimal	22-26 hours
Levemir (detemir)	2-4 hours	minimal	13-20 + hours

Fluid Replacement: Management Strategies

Replacement of intracellular and extracellular fluid volume deficits is a priority for both DKA and HHS to restore intravascular volume and prevent hemodynamic instability. Fluid replacement is often administered via two peripheral IVs, use of a central venous catheter is uncommon today except in the most critical situations. Initial volume replacement is based on assessment of vascular volume status.

1. Administer normal saline (0.9%). IV fluids are generally infused at rapid rates (1000-2000 mL in the first hour, 1000 mL in the second hour, and then at 500 mL/h) until fluid volume is restored or initially around 15 to 20 mL/kg/h. The blood glucose is expected to fall approximately 75 mg/dL per hour.
2. Some clinicians and clinical laboratories calculate a *corrected serum sodium* value from the measured serum sodium in hyperglycemic states. The corrected value adjusts for the dilution caused by fluid moving from the intracellular to the extracellular space and lowering the serum sodium. If the corrected sodium is normal or high this suggests the patient is dehydrated and requires more fluid volume. The equation is shown in Table 16-7.
3. Titrate the rate of infusion based on blood glucose, urine output, and mean arterial blood pressure. Typically, the patient with HHS has more profound fluid volume deficits, but because the patient may be older and often has other underlying medical problems, the rate of fluid replacement needs to be carefully titrated. Serum glucose falls with initiation of fluids alone. It is critical that insulin therapy not be started without simultaneously correcting the fluid deficit. Otherwise, an acute loss of vascular volume, shock, and increased risk of mortality may occur.
4. When serum glucose reaches 250 mg/dL change IV fluid to 5% dextrose with 0.45 NaCl at 150 to 200 mL/h. Maintain insulin therapy.

Electrolyte Replacement: Management Strategies

Electrolyte deficits are usually present in both DKA and HHS due to the osmotic diuresis. Hypokalemia may be masked by acidosis. Potassium levels rise approximately 0.6 mEq/L for every 0.1 drop in pH.

1. Administer potassium supplements based on serum levels and in accordance with hospital and unit protocols. Replacement of potassium is a priority during the correction of hyperglycemia to avoid hypokalemia during rehydration, when potassium moves into the cell along with glucose and insulin. To avoid

cardiac arrhythmias associated with hypokalemia, delay insulin administration until serum potassium levels are greater than 3.3 mEq/L. The rate of potassium chloride infusion is adjusted according to frequently monitored serum potassium levels and the urine output.
2. Monitor magnesium, calcium, potassium, and phosphate levels every 2 hours during rehydration. Hemodilution will further decrease serum electrolyte levels. Magnesium and calcium replacements are based on serum levels. Total body phosphorous levels are depleted due to osmotic diuresis. This may result in impaired cardiac and respiratory functions. Phosphate deficiencies are usually corrected with volume replacement. If needed, the administration of potassium phosphate 20 mEq/L is one method of phosphate replacement as it replaces both potassium and phosphate simultaneously. Phosphate replacements are not administered in patients with impaired kidney function.

Preventing and Managing Complications

1. Monitor serum glucose, electrolytes (sodium and potassium), and arterial blood gases every 1 to 2 hours until normal levels are attained.
2. Measure serum phosphate and magnesium initially and repeat as necessary.
3. Monitor temperature, blood pressure, heart rate, respiratory rate, pulse oximetry, urinary output, and central venous pressure (CVP; if central line inserted) at frequent intervals.
4. Evaluate neurologic status at frequent intervals. Institute seizure precautions if cerebral edema is suspected.
5. Institute measures to avoid aspiration in patients with altered mental status.
6. Titrate fluid replacement carefully to prevent fluid overload. Auscultate lung sounds and assess urine output.
7. Hyperosmolar patients are at risk for developing thrombosis and some patients may be on anticoagulants.

Patient and Family Education

Teaching patients about self-management of diabetes is essential prior to discharge. Patients requiring ongoing glucose monitoring are evaluated for competency using the glucometer. It is important to first determine the patient's fasting glycemic goal. Underlying patient morbidities, cognitive skills, frailty, and age affect glycemic target goals. In a relatively healthy patient at home, a target fasting glucose between 85 and 140 mg/dL is usually acceptable. Target 2-hour postprandial, blood glucose levels are less than 180 mg/dL whenever possible. These goals are achieved through the use of oral hypoglycemic agents, insulin, and in outpatients, injectable incretins (ie, gastrointestinal

TABLE 16-7. CORRECTION OF SERUM SODIUM LEVELS IN HYPERGLYCEMIA

$$\text{Corrected sodium} = (\text{serum sodium}) + 1.6 \times \left[\frac{\text{glucose (mg/dL)} - 100}{100} \right]$$

hormones that increase the release of insulin from beta cells and enhance glucose metabolism). Accurate glucometer measurements are essential to safely achieve glycemic targets.

Before discharge to home, patients must teach-back how to self-monitor their blood glucose and to test blood levels before each meal and at bedtime, especially if on insulin therapy. Self-monitoring of blood glucose (SMBG) improves safety especially if ongoing insulin dose adjustments are necessary. However, frequent glucose-monitoring schedules may not be feasible, and some patients may struggle with adherence to rigid self-monitoring schedules. Achieving a SMBG strategy that aligns with the patient's needs and goals is important.

The hemoglobin A1C is a blood test that is used to monitor blood glucose over time. The A1C measures the percentage of glucose absorbed by the red blood cells in a 3-month period, a process known as glycation. The American Diabetes Association (ADA) recommends the A1C be measured on all patients with diabetes or hyperglycemia admitted to the hospital, if it has not been measured in the prior 3 months. For ongoing control of blood glucose the A1C target is approximately less than or equal to 6.5% for patients with diabetes. The intent is to achieve a balance between effective blood glucose control while avoiding hypoglycemic episodes.

Table 16-8 outlines required skills for diabetic management. Return demonstrations by the patient or designated caregiver are essential. Instruction regarding the need for routine medical follow-up and the availability of hospital and community resources are important components of the diabetes management plan. The patient is typically discharged on the inpatient insulin doses (via multiple dose insulin or insulin pump). Sometimes a patient who was using preadmission insulin may resume the preadmission regimen unless an adjusted dose is required due to weight loss, decreased kidney function, or marked increase in exercise (typically less insulin is required with these conditions).

Particularly for patients with type 1 DM, education to prevent recurrent DKA is essential. Discuss precipitating factors such as infection and missed insulin doses. If available,

TABLE 16-8. PATIENT EDUCATION: DIABETIC MANAGEMENT SKILLS

Blood glucose monitoring
Insulin administration
Meal planning and counting carbohydrates
Exercise therapy
Urine ketone testing
Sick day management
Recognition of signs and symptoms of hypoglycemia and hyperglycemia
Treatments for hypoglycemia and hyperglycemia
Management of a wearable insulin pump (if used)

Expected Outcomes
1. The patient or caregiver will be able to verbalize essential aspects of diet therapy, meal planning, exercise therapy, sick day management, signs and symptoms of hypoglycemia and hyperglycemia, and treatments for hypoglycemia and hyperglycemia.
2. The patient or caregiver will be able to demonstrate blood glucose monitoring, insulin administration, and urine ketone testing.

contact a diabetes educator to help teach the skills needed to manage diabetes once the patient is stable and ready to receive information.

Patients with type 2 diabetes treated for HHS are usually discharged on oral medications to control blood glucose. Metformin is the principal medication prescribed for type 2 DM due to its insulin sensitizing effects. Other medications may be added, and in some cases a basal insulin is used. All hospitalized patients treated for hyperglycemia require follow-up with their primary care provider and/or an endocrinologist soon after discharge. This is especially true for patients with type 2 DM because of the known association with Metabolic Syndrome. The American Heart Association (AHA) describes Metabolic Syndrome as:

- *Abdominal obesity, defined as a waist circumference of greater than 40 inches in men, and greater than 35 inches in women.*
- *High triglycerides, defined as triglyceride blood level greater than 150 mg/dL.*
- *Low levels of high-density lipoprotein (HDL) cholesterol, defined as a blood level below 40 mg/dL in men or below 50 mg/dL in women.*
- *Hypertension, defined as a systolic blood pressure above 130 mm Hg, or diastolic blood pressure above 85 mm Hg.*
- *Fasting blood glucose above 100 mg/dL.*

Because many of the conditions in Metabolic Syndrome are treatable it is important that patient teaching emphasizes management of the cardiovascular issues as well as diabetes-related health concerns.

Acute Hypoglycemia

Hypoglycemia is a low-blood glucose level and is considered an endocrine emergency. In hospitalized patients an alert level of less than 70 mg/dL is often used. The American Diabetes Association (ADA) now defines clinically significant hypoglycemia as any value less than 54 mg/dL and severe hypoglycemia is defined as any low blood glucose value associated with cognitive impairment. Hypoglycemia results from the imbalance between glucose production and glucose utilization. Of the acute complications, hypoglycemia is most common in insulin-dependent (types 1 and 2) diabetics. Hypoglycemia also can occur with type 2 diabetics who are treated with oral hypoglycemic agents, especially the sulfonylureas: glipizide, glyburide, and glimepiride.

Etiology, Risk Factors, and Pathophysiology
Hypoglycemia can be divided into two categories: fasting hypoglycemia (> 5 hours after a meal) and postprandial hypoglycemia (1-2 hours after a meal) (Table 16-9). *Fasting hypoglycemia* occurs when the normal physiologic response (gluconeogenesis and glycogenolysis) to a falling glucose level is altered and there is an imbalance in glucose production and utilization. Hypoglycemia in a hospitalized patient

ESSENTIAL CONTENT CASE

Diabetic Ketoacidosis

An 18-year-old woman with known type 1 diabetes is in the emergency department (ED) with a diagnosis of DKA. She had run out of her basal insulin (glargine), and was only taking short-acting insulin to cover her meals. During the past 2 days she had been experiencing flu-like symptoms, feeling unwell with abdominal cramping that she attributed to stress over her college examinations. She was brought to the ED by her roommates because she was drowsy and "acting drunk." Significant findings on her admission profile were:

Respiratory rate	38 breaths/min, deep ("fruity" breath)
Blood pressure	98/50 mm Hg
Heart rate	110 beats/min; sinus tachycardia
Temperature	38.7°C
Skin	Warm and flushed
Arterial blood gases	pH 7.09
$PaCO_2$	24 mm Hg
PaO_2	88 mm Hg
HCO_3	11 mEq/L
SaO_2	94%
Serum glucose	440 mg/dL
Serum acetone	4+
Serum ketones	4+
Serum osmolality	310 mOsm/kg
Anion gap	25 mEq/L
Serum potassium	3.2 mEq/L
Serum BUN	28 mg/dL
Serum creatinine	1.5 mg/dL
Serum sodium	130 mEq/L
Serum magnesium	1.0 mg/dL
Serum phosphate	2.2 mg/dL
Serum chloride	94 mEq/L
White blood cell count	14,000/mm³
Urine glucose	2+ (large)
Urine ketone	3+ (large)

Treatment: In the ED, a peripheral IV was started in her right arm and 1 L of 0.9% sodium chloride was infused over 1 hour. When this had infused, a new bag of 0.9% sodium chloride was hung at a rate of 250 mL/h. The low serum potassium level was replaced and potassium rechecked (now 4.0 mEq/L). She was then transferred from the ED to the critical care unit for intensive management of blood glucose, insulin, and assessment of ongoing neurological and metabolic status related to DKA. At this point a second IV was

started in her left arm. An IV insulin bolus was administered, and an insulin infusion started. Hourly blood glucose checks and serum potassium checks were started. Given her elevated white blood cell (WBC) count and elevated temperature urine cultures and blood cultures were obtained.

After 24 hours a total of 6 liters 0.9% sodium chloride was infused, blood glucose was now 298 mg/dL and was managed according to the hospital's DKA insulin protocol. Serum potassium, serum phosphorus, and serum magnesium were replaced per protocol. The anion gap had fallen to 17 indicating that the metabolic acidosis was resolving.

Six hours later the blood glucose reached 250 mg/dL and the IV solution was changed to D5.45% at 150 mL/h. Blood glucose checks continued.

The immediate plan of care is to continue the IV insulin infusion until the anion gap has closed. At that time there will be a transition to a basal-bolus insulin subcutaneous insulin regime with meals.

Case Question 1: Complete the following sentence: Intravenous isotonic 0.9% sodium chloride (normal saline) administered prior to insulin administration will.....
(A) not impact blood glucose levels
(B) dilute blood glucose levels
(C) dangerously raise serum sodium levels
(D) decrease serum potassium levels

Case Question 2: Sodium bicarbonate IV is indicated in DKA in which clinical situation?
(A) High anion gap
(B) pH more than 7.0
(C) pH less than 7.0
(D) Low anion gap

Case Question 3: In type 1 diabetes a person can appear to be "acting drunk" because:
(A) Hyperventilation from Kussmaul ventilation reduces ketone bodies, lowers CO_2 and increases acetone in the bloodstream.
(B) Glucose interacts with glucagon to raise serum alcohol levels.
(C) In DKA the gut microbiome has a fermentation effect that releases powerful peptides into the circulation that cross the blood-brain barrier making a person act inebriated.
(D) Glucose cannot enter the brain cells without insulin.

Answers
1. B
2. C
3. D

with diabetes is most commonly caused by excess insulin, or oral hypoglycemic agents, with insufficient caloric intake.

Glucose is the obligate fuel for the brain and CNS. The brain is unable to synthesize or store glucose and must rely on circulating plasma blood glucose levels for survival. As blood glucose declines rapidly, epinephrine, glucagon, glucocorticoids, and growth hormones are released. Patients

exhibit adrenergic symptoms—tachycardia, anxiety, sweating, trembling, and hunger. These symptoms can occur even if the blood glucose is normal but there is a sudden acute decline (ie, blood glucose level rapidly decreases to 80-90 mg/dL). In moderate to severe hypoglycemic reactions, the CNS is affected, signifying that the brain is being deprived of the glucose it needs.

ESSENTIAL CONTENT CASE

Hyperosmolar Hyperglycemic State

A 72-year-old man was admitted to the MICU with a diagnosis of hyperglycemic crisis. He lives alone with his small dog with family living nearby. His daughter dialed 911 after finding her father confused and barely responsive at his home. She reported that he had experienced a cough for the past week. His history is significant for heart failure and type 2 DM. His daily medications include carvedilol 6.25 mg orally twice a day, Lipitor 40 mg once a day, lisinopril 20 mg orally once a day, furosemide (Lasix) 20 mg orally twice a day, KCl 20 mEq/day orally, and glipizide 10 mg orally twice a day. On arrival in the ED with the paramedics he is barely responsive and unable to answer any questions. He is maintaining an open airway with oxygen supplied via nasal cannula. Significant findings on his admission profile are:

Blood pressure	82/44 mm Hg; MAP 56 mm Hg
Heart rate	121 beats/min
Respiratory rate	14 breaths/min, shallow
Temperature	38.7°C
Skin	Dry, poor turgor; dry mucous membranes
ABG on 2 L/min O_2 per nasal cannula	pH 7.34
$Paco_2$	49 mm Hg
Pao_2	56 mm Hg
HCO_3^-	20 mEq/L
Sao_2	88%
Serum glucose	1467 mg/dL
Serum osmolality	362 mOsm/kg
Anion gap	11 mEq/L
Serum potassium	3.6 mEq/L
Serum BUN	41 mg/dL
Serum creatinine	2.2 mg/dL
Serum sodium	152 mEq/L
Serum phosphate	2.0 mg/dL
Serum chloride	121 mEq/L

Case Question 1: Blood glucose climbs higher in HHS than DKA because:
(A) The pancreas secretes small amounts of insulin in HHS but not in DKA, which raises blood glucose and delays the appearance of symptoms.
(B) Peripheral cellular resistance is protective in DKA but not in HSS which increases blood glucose and symptoms.
(C) Fast acting insulin is contraindicated in DKA but not in HSS making blood glucose rise more quickly.
(D) The hyperosmolar component of HSS forces glucose into the cells delaying symptoms.

Case Question 2: The metabolic acidosis that can occur in HSS is caused by
(A) Ketone acidosis and accumulation of ketone bodies.
(B) Lactic acidosis caused by dehydration and decreased tissue perfusion.
(C) Respiratory acidosis due to decreased respiratory rate and low tidal volume.
(D) Metformin lactic acidosis.

Case Question 3: In hyperglycemic crisis, what is the blood glucose reduction target in the first hour using an insulin infusion?
(A) Decrease blood glucose by 150 to 200 mg/dL
(B) Normalize blood glucose as quickly as possible
(C) Decrease blood glucose by 50 to 70 mg/dL
(D) Maintain blood glucose by until 2 liters of crystalloid have infused

Answers
1. A
2. B
3. C

TABLE 16-9. CAUSES OF HYPOGLYCEMIA (PARTIAL LISTING)

Fasting Hypoglycemia
Excessive insulin dosage
Insulinomas (pancreas tumor)
Decreased need for insulin
  Decreased food intake
  Kidney failure/dialysis
  Liver failure
  Heart failure
Medications
  Oral hypoglycemic agents
  Salicylates
  Beta-adrenergic blockers
Postprandial Hypoglycemia
Excessive insulin effect
Gastric surgery
Other
Alcohol and alcohol binges

Hypoglycemic unawareness is an autonomic neuropathy with potentially serious consequences. Hypoglycemic unawareness is defined as the loss of adrenergic symptoms of hypoglycemia that prompt a patient to act to prevent the progression of severe hypoglycemia and it results from alterations in counterregulation physiology. Both type 1 and 2 diabetics may have deficiencies in counterregulation systems.

Clinical Presentation

Signs and Symptoms

- Mild hypoglycemic symptoms (adrenergic response)
  – Diaphoresis (most common)
  – Tremors
  – Shakiness
  – Tachycardia
  – Paresthesia

- Pallor
- Excessive hunger
- Anxiety
- Moderate to severe hypoglycemic symptoms (CNS or neuroglycopenic symptoms)
  - Headache
  - Inability to concentrate
  - Mood changes
  - Drowsiness
  - Irritability
  - Confusion
  - Impaired judgment
  - Slurred speech
  - Staggering gait
  - Double or blurred vision
  - Morning headaches
  - Nightmares
  - Psychosis (late)
  - Seizures
  - Coma

Diagnostic Tests

- Serum blood glucose (blood test) less than 70 mg/dL
- Fingerstick POC blood glucose less than 70 mg/dL
- Any low blood glucose value with cognitive impairment

Acute Hypoglycemic Management

The management of the patient with acute hypoglycemia depends on the severity of the reaction. Principles of management include normalization of blood glucose concentrations and patient teaching.

Normalization of Blood Glucose

Treatment of the hypoglycemia depends on its severity as described below.

Mild Hypoglycemia

1. Administer 10- to 15-g carbohydrate (Table 16-10). Follow in 10 minutes with another 10 to 15 g if the blood glucose does not improve.
2. Obtain a blood glucose measurement.
3. If the next meal is more than 2 hours away, provide a complex carbohydrate (ie, 4-oz milk).

TABLE 16-10. PATIENT EDUCATION: FOODS WITH 10 TO 15 GRAMS OF CARBOHYDRATE EQUIVALENTS FOR TREATMENT OF MILD HYPOGLYCEMIC REACTIONS

4 oz orange juice
6 oz regular (non-diet) cola
3 glucose tablets
6-8 oz skim milk or milk with 2% fat
3 graham cracker squares
6-8 lifesavers
6 jelly beans
2 tbsp raisins
1 small (2-oz) tube of cake icing

Moderate and Severe Hypoglycemia

1. Administer IV glucose. The initial bolus is 50% dextrose (equivalent of 25-g glucose) followed by a continuous IV infusion until oral replacement is possible.
2. Monitor glucose levels frequently for several hours.

Prevention of Hypoglycemia

1. Teach the early signs and symptoms of hypoglycemia. Instruct the patient to always carry a source of fast-acting carbohydrate (see Table 16-10).
2. Advise the patient not to skip or delay meals and to limit alcohol to no more than 2-oz hard liquor, 8-oz wine, or 24-oz beer per day. It is advisable to never drink on an empty stomach.

Summary: Hyperglycemia and Hypoglycemia

Hypoglycemia and hyperglycemia are frequently encountered in critical and acute care. Hyperglycemia can result from multiple causes including: physiologic stress of critical illness, inadequate insulin in established diabetes, new onset DM, DKA, or HHS. It is important to identify the cause of the hyperglycemia so that the correct treatment plan can be initiated. Most hospitals have protocols that outline treatment goals and procedures for hyperglycemia management. Hyperglycemia predisposes patients to increased infection and to worse cardiovascular outcomes. Achieving glycemic control is a priority intervention in critical care.

Hypoglycemia can be a life-threatening complication of critical illness. It may be precipitated by iatrogenic interventions such as too much insulin or inadequate nutrition. Vigilant monitoring of blood glucose levels is required to prevent neurologic complications or death from low blood glucose.

PITUITARY GLAND FUNCTION AND ASSOCIATED DISORDERS

The pituitary gland is a small gland, about the size of a pea, closely attached to the base of the brain by specialized nerve fibers. The pituitary gland has three lobes: anterior, intermediate, and posterior. The posterior gland is of particular interest in critical and progressive care because dysfunction can result in serious fluid and electrolyte disorders.

Antidiuretic hormone (ADH), also known as arginine vasopressin (AVP), is produced by the hypothalamus and is stored in the posterior pituitary gland. ADH exerts its primary effects in the distal collecting tubules of the kidneys where it acts upon vasopressin-2 (V2) aquaporin receptors to conserve water back to the bloodstream and decreasing serum osmolality. Osmoreceptors in the hypothalamus monitor changes in serum osmolality. An increase of osmolality by 2% leads to ADH release by the posterior pituitary. See Figure 16-2 for an illustration of normal function of the posterior pituitary, and release of ADH in response to dehydration (high serum osmolality) or overhydration (low serum osmolality). Clinical conditions involving the posterior

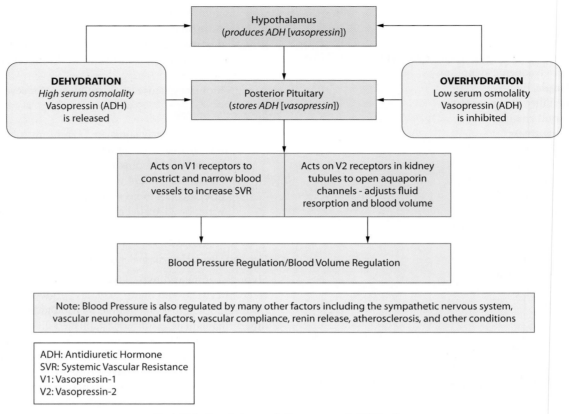

Figure 16-2. Hypothalamus-pituitary-vasopressin (ADH) actions.

pituitary and ADH include the syndrome of inappropriate antidiuretic hormone (SIADH), and diabetes insipidus (DI). Both of these conditions may require admission to a critical care because of serious fluid and electrolyte alterations.

Syndrome of Inappropriate Antidiuretic Hormone Secretion

Etiology, Risk Factors, and Pathophysiology

The syndrome of inappropriate antidiuretic hormone is characterized by excessive release of ADH unrelated to the serum osmolality. Normally, ADH release is controlled by this value (Figure 16-2). The serum osmolality blood test measures the concentration of electrolytes, glucose, and other osmotically active particles in the serum. SIADH is a syndrome of water intoxication and hyponatremia. There are numerous causes of SIADH (Table 16-11).

Exogenous causes of SIADH: Vasopressin (ADH) can be produced by a variety of malignancies, most commonly small-cell carcinoma of the lung. Therefore, patients who develop "idiopathic" SIADH are screened for malignant tumors. SIADH is also commonly associated with pulmonary conditions, metabolic and traumatic neurologic disorders, and medications, particularly chlorpropamide, thiazide diuretics, opiates, and barbiturates.

Clinically, SIADH is distinguished by hyponatremia and water retention that progresses to water intoxication. The seriousness of the signs and symptoms depends on how

TABLE 16-11. ETIOLOGIES OF SYNDROME OF INAPPROPRIATE ANTIDIURETIC HORMONE (SIADH)

Malignancies
Lung
Lymphoma
Gastrointestinal
Pulmonary Disorders
Positive pressure ventilation
Asthma
Pneumonia
Chronic obstructive pulmonary disease (COPD)
Acute respiratory failure
Tuberculosis
Neurological Disorders
Head trauma
Meningitis, encephalitis
Stroke
Brain tumors
Guillain-Barré syndrome
Medications
Vasopressin
Desmopressin
Thiazide diuretics
Opiates
Barbiturates
Nicotine
Antineoplastic drugs
Tricyclic antidepressants
Others
Acquired immunodeficiency syndrome (AIDS)

fast the serum sodium falls. As water intoxication progresses and the serum becomes more hypotonic, brain cells swell, causing neurologic impairment. Without treatment, irreversible brain damage and death can occur.

Clinical Presentation

EARLY

- Urine volume decreased and concentrated
- Nausea
- Vomiting
- Headache
- Impaired taste
- Dulled sensorium
- Muscle weakness and cramps
- Anorexia
- Weight gain
- Crackles
- Dyspnea
- Increased CVP
- Weakness/fatigue

LATE

- Confusion
- Delirium
- Aberrant respirations
- Hypothermia
- Coma
- Seizures

DIAGNOSTIC TESTS

- Serum Na^+ less than 130 mEq/L
- Serum osmolality less than 280 mOsm/kg
- Increased urine osmolality more than 500 mOsm/kg
- Urine sodium more than 20 mEq/L
- Blood urea nitrogen (BUN) and creatinine decreased (hemodilution)
- Urine specific gravity (USG) more than 1.020

Management of SIADH

Principles of management depend on the severity and duration of the hyponatremia. Recognition of early clinical manifestations of SIADH is key to prevent life-threatening complications. Continued assessment of the neuromuscular, cardiac, gastrointestinal, and renal systems is important. Generally, treatment focuses on restricting fluids, replenishing sodium deficits, and in severe cases of hyponatremia using vasopressor-2 (V2) antagonist medications (also called vaptans), a class of diuretics that selectively eliminates water in the urine, and conserves sodium. Treatment of the underlying disorder is also a priority.

Fluid Restriction and Treating Hyponatremia in SIADH

Fluid restriction is the mainstay of treatment and, to be effective, a negative water balance must be achieved.

1. Treatment of mild hyponatremia (sodium level > 125 and < 135 mEq/L) includes fluid restriction of 800 to 1000 mL/day. This allows sodium level to correct over 3 to 10 days.

2. If severe neurologic symptoms of SIADH are present along with severe hyponatremia (< 125 mEq/L), administer hypertonic 3% saline infusion slowly. *To avoid cerebral demyelination, the goal is to only raise the serum sodium by 1 to 2 mEq/H, and no more than 10 to 12 mEq/L in 24 hours.* When the serum sodium has risen above 125 mEq/L, isotonic saline (0.9%) is the usual IV fluid.

3. Frequent mouth care when fluid is restricted. An antiemetic may be necessary to manage nausea.

4. If fluid restriction alone is not effective at raising the serum sodium level, a V2 receptor agonist, also known as vaptans, such as Tolvaptan, may be administered IV. Vaptans are medications that eliminate water while retaining salt and may be used with, or in place of, loop diuretics in dilutional hyponatremia. Oral vaptans are also available. See Chapter 7, Pharmacology.

5. When taking oral diet, add salt to food and consult with a dietician.

6. Assess cardiovascular and respiratory functions closely to evaluate the effects of the excess volume on these systems. Right and left ventricular volumes may increase, causing heart failure. Tachypnea, reports of shortness of breath, and fine crackles are indicators of fluid overload and impending heart failure. Monitor neurologic status closely and protect the patient from self-harm. Institute seizure precautions as necessary.

7. Expected outcomes for the patient with SIADH are listed in Table 16-12.

Diabetes Insipidus

Etiology, Risk Factors, and Pathophysiology

Diabetes insipidus results from a group of disorders in which there is an absolute or relative deficiency of ADH (called *central DI*) or an insensitivity to its effects on the kidney tubules (called *nephrogenic DI*) (Figure 16-3). DI may complicate the course of critically and acutely ill patients and can result in acute fluid and electrolyte disturbances.

There are many causes of DI (Table 16-13). *Central DI* (also called neurogenic DI) results from damage to the hypothalamic/pituitary system. An absolute deficiency of

TABLE 16-12.   EXPECTED OUTCOMES FOR THE PATIENT WITH DIABETES INSIPIDUS (DI) OR SYNDROME OF INAPPROPRIATE ANTIDIURETIC HORMONE (SIADH)

Adequate fluid balance is maintained/restored as evidenced by
- Blood pressure within 10 mm Hg of patient baseline
- Heart rate 60-100 beats/min
- Normal skin turgor
- Peripheral pulses return to baseline
- Serum osmolality 275-295 mOsm/kg
- Serum sodium 135-145 mEq/L
- Urine osmolality appropriate for serum osmolality

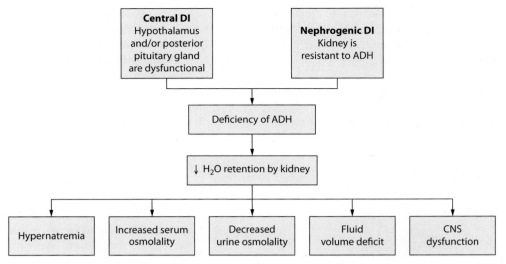

Figure 16-3. Pathogenesis of DI.

ADH results in an impaired ability to concentrate urine, and polyuria of several liters. The result is dehydration. Patients with head trauma or those who have had neurosurgery are at increased risk for up to 7 to 10 days after the injury. DI does not generally present for at least 48 to 72 hours after the initial hypothalamic or pituitary trauma.

Nephrogenic DI is characterized by kidney tubule insensitivity to ADH and develops because of structural or functional changes in the kidney. This results in impaired urine-concentrating ability and free water conservation. Nephrogenic DI is less dramatic than neurogenic DI in its onset and appearance and is usually managed in the outpatient setting.

In *central DI* the ability of the body to increase ADH secretion or respond to ADH is impaired. A high volume of dilute urine and increasing hemoconcentration is evident. Signs and symptoms of dehydration are often present when the thirst mechanism has been impaired or with inadequate fluid replacement. In addition, if a hyperosmolar state exists, intracellular brain volume depletion occurs as water moves from within the brain cells to the plasma. Typically, symptoms of central DI manifest when serum sodium levels exceed 155 mEq/L.

TABLE 16-13. EITOLOGIES OF DIABETES INSIPIDUS (DI)

ADH Insufficiency (Neurogenic DI)
Familial (hereditary)
Trauma
Neoplasms
Infections
    Tuberculosis
    Cryptococcosis
    Syphilis
    Central Nervous System infections
Vascular
    Cerebrovascular hemorrhage
    Cerebrovascular aneurysm
    Cerebral thrombosis
ADH Insensitivity (Nephrogenic DI)
Familial (hereditary)
Medication induced
    Lithium
    Demeclocycline
    Glyburide
    Colchicine
    Amphotericin B
    Gentamicin
    Furosemide
Electrolyte disorders
    Hypokalemia
    Hypercalcemia
Kidney disease
Excessive Water Intake (Secondary DI)
Excessive IV fluid administration
Psychogenic polydipsia (lesion in thirst center)

Clinical Presentation

ADH DEFICIENCY
- Polydipsia (if alert)
- Polyuria (5-20 L in 24 hours)

FLUID VOLUME DEFICIT
- Orthostatic hypotension
- Weight loss
- Tachycardia
- Decreased CVP
- Poor skin turgor
- Dry mucous membranes

INTRACELLULAR BRAIN VOLUME DEPLETION
- Confusion
- Restlessness
- Lethargy
- Irritability
- Seizures
- Coma

Diagnostic Tests

- Water deprivation test (never in critical care)
- Serum sodium more than 155 mEq/L
- Serum osmolality more than 295 mOsm/kg/L
- Urine osmolality inappropriately low with high serum osmolality (< 150 mOsm/kg/L)
- Urine specific gravity decreased
- BUN and creatinine increased (hemoconcentration)

Management of Diabetes Insipidus

The management of the patient in DI is directed at correcting the profound fluid volume deficit and electrolyte imbalances associated with this condition. If fluid losses are not replaced, hypovolemic shock can rapidly develop. Medications that simulate ADH release such as desmopressin acetate (commonly known as DDAVP) is prescribed to treat DI via IV, nasal spray, or oral routes. As with other disorders, identification, diagnosis and treatment of the cause of DI are priorities.

Fluid Volume Replacement

If the patient is alert and the thirst mechanism is not impaired, allow the patient to drink water to maintain normal serum osmolality. In many critically ill patients, this is not possible.

1. Administer hypotonic volume, such as dextrose 5% in water, quarter-strength or half-strength saline, IV as prescribed to restore the hypotonic fluid lost through diuresis. In severe DI, where large amounts of fluid replacement are required, the IV intake is usually titrated to urine output; for example, 400 mL of urine output for 1 hour is replaced with 400 mL IV fluid the next hour. Hypotonic saline solutions are preferred (quarter-strength or half-strength saline). Reduce the serum sodium by approximately 0.5 mEq/L every hour but no more than 12 mEq/L per day.
2. Monitor fluid status: Hourly urine outputs along with measurements of urine specific gravity every 1-2 hours are done along with daily weight and strict intake and output. Monitor for signs of continuing fluid volume deficit. If the serum Na is more than 155 mEq/L, rehydration occurs over 48 hours. A serum sodium more than 170 mEq/L necessitates ICU care due to increased risk of seizures. Expected outcomes for the patient with DI are listed in Table 16-12.
3. Monitor neurologic status continuously. An altered level of consciousness indicates intracellular dehydration of the brain and hypovolemia.
4. Frequent electrolyte monitoring is recommended during the initial phase of treatment.

ADH Administration or Enhancement

In central DI, desmopressin (DDAVP), an ADH analogue, is the drug of choice and is available in subcutaneous, IV, intranasal, and oral preparations. Desmopressin acts on the distal tubules and collecting ducts of the kidney to increase water reabsorption and has very specific actions with little or no ADH-like activity elsewhere in the body. Adjunctive therapies to enhance ADH release include nonhormonal agents such as chlorpropamide, carbamazepine, thiazides, and nonsteroidal anti-inflammatory drugs (NSAIDs).

If the patient is unconscious, injectable DDAVP is given IV or IM 1 to 4 µg every 12 hours until therapeutic goals are achieved, such as a urine output of 2 to 3 mL/kg/h, urine specific gravity 1.010 to 1.020 and serum sodium 140 to 145 mEq/L. In conscious patients, the nasal replacement route is given 10 to 20 µg by spray 2 to 3 times a day. It is important that DDAVP or other ADH analogues not be administered unless serum sodium is at least above 145 mmol/L, as serious hyponatremia may result. Oral formulations of ADH have a slower onset and duration of action and are not useful in acute situations. Major side effects to watch for include headache, abdominal cramps, or allergic reactions such as facial flushing. Monitor for overmedication, which may precipitate hypervolemia. Signs and symptoms of fluid volume excess include dyspnea, hypertension, weight gain, and angina. Hyponatremia is another serious consequence that when it develops rapidly can cause extreme cerebral edema and demyelination syndrome within the CNS. Therefore, close monitoring of serum sodium is necessary.

Summary: Pituitary Gland and DI/SIADH

The pituitary gland is a small pea-size gland that releases ADH to achieve water balance in the body. Alterations in fluid balance impact serum sodium levels. In central DI, the posterior pituitary produces little or no ADH resulting in excess urine output, hypernatremia, and life-threatening dehydration. In SIADH, the posterior pituitary produces excessive quantities of ADH unrelated to physiologic need, causing low urine output, water intoxication, and hyponatremia. Early recognition and prompt treatment are vital for survival.

THYROID GLAND FUNCTION AND ASSOCIATED DISORDERS

The thyroid gland has a shape that resembles a bow tie. The gland wraps around the trachea in the front of the neck. There are two lobes that are connected by a bridge of thyroid tissue called the isthmus. The thyroid gland secretes hormones associated with metabolism that are regulated by a feedback loop as shown in Figure 16-4.

In the normal thyroid feedback loop, the hypothalamus produces thyroid-releasing hormone (TRH), which stimulates the anterior pituitary to release thyroid-stimulating hormone (TSH), and based on the level of circulating hormones, the thyroid gland produces the thyroid hormones thyroxine (T_4) and triiodothyronine (T_3). T_4 is produced in greater quantity but T_3 is more biologically active. When needed, T_4 is converted to T_3 in the peripheral circulation, predominantly by the liver. In the circulation T_4 and T_3 are protein-bound. Ultimately, these hormones are separated from their transport proteins so that metabolically active Free-T_3 and

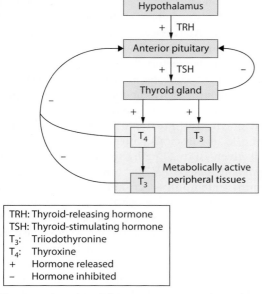

Figure 16-4. Hypothalamus-pituitary-thyroid hormone feedback loop.

Free-T_4 can enter cells. Free-T_3 is the principal thyroid hormone inside cells. Disorders of the thyroid gland are caused by hypersecretion (hyperthyroidism and thyroid storm) and hyposecretion (hypothyroidism and myxedema).

Hyperthyroidism and Thyroid Storm

Hyperthyroidism, also known as thyrotoxicosis, is more common in women than men, occurring in about 2% of the female population (2 in 100), and in approximately 0.002% of the male population (2 in 1000). In this condition, the hyperactive thyroid produces too much thyroid hormone and is not regulated by the normal hypothalamus-pituitary-thyroid feedback loop as described in Figure 16-4.

Hyperthyroidism

The most common cause of hyperthyroidism is *Graves Disease*. This is an autoimmune condition where the immune system produces antibodies that bind to TSH receptors in the thyroid gland causing enlargement of thyroid follicular cells. This causes diffuse thyroid enlargement, with production of excess thyroid hormone, leading to suppression of TSH production from the pituitary gland. In response to the fall in TSH, the thyroid gland increases production of the thyroid hormones T_4 and T_3. On a laboratory blood test, the TSH level is low and circulating thyroid hormone levels are elevated. Hyperthyroidism can also develop after taking the antiarrhythmic medication amiodarone.

Iodine deficiency increases the risk of hyperthyroidism but is rare in wealthy countries, as salt has been supplemented with iodine since the 1920s. Thyroid hormones are involved in all cellular functions, and excess hormone increases metabolism usually leading to increased heart rate, increased temperature, and frequent bowl movements.

Thyroid Storm

Thyroid storm or thyrotoxic crisis is a life-threatening emergency with mortality up to 30%. It is a rare condition in developed countries, typically seen with undiagnosed or under-treated hyperthyroidism. Thyroid storm may be initiated by infection, surgery, or other acute illness. Because thyroid hormones are involved in all metabolic processes, an increase in thyroid hormone availability creates a hypermetabolic state with surges of sympathetic nervous system catecholamine release. This causes dangerously high heart rates, treatment-refractory arrhythmias, increased blood pressure, high temperature, heat intolerance, diarrhea, anxiety, and mental status changes.

Thyroid Storm Management

Emergency management involves immediate administration of beta-blockers (propanol, esmolol) to blunt the sympathetic nervous system receptors, plus medications that block thyroid synthesis and block release of more thyroid hormone (methimazole, propylthiouracil). There are case-reports in the literature that a therapeutic plasma exchange (TPE) via apheresis may remove protein bound T_3 and T_4. Dehydration occurs from fluids lost via the gastrointestinal tract and extreme diaphoresis. Volume resuscitation with monitoring of electrolytes is required. Fever is controlled with acetaminophen and comfort-cooling measures may increase comfort.

Hypothyroidism and Myxedema Coma

Hypothyroidism

As the name suggests, hypothyroidism signals an underactive thyroid with slowed metabolism. The most common cause of hypothyroidism is Hashimoto thyroiditis. This is an autoimmune condition where the immune system makes antibodies against healthy thyroid tissue. Amiodarone (antiarrhythmic medication) can also cause hypothyroidism. Amiodarone has a chemical structure that is similar to thyroxine and it also contains significant amounts of iodine. A high TSH blood level and symptoms of slowed metabolism (weight gain, fatigue, sensitivity to cold) are diagnostic symptoms. Hypothyroidism is more common in women than men. Ongoing critical illness is associated with a downregulation of the hypothalamic-pituitary-thyroid axis with lower levels of circulating thyroid hormones. The specific causes of this change are unknown.

Myxedema Coma

The terms myxedema coma or myxedema crisis are used to describe extreme hypothyroidism. Clinically this is observed as a decreased level of consciousness, respiratory failure, hypothermia, and often heart failure. The onset can be insidious and may only be discovered when a patient is admitted for another cause such as respiratory failure. Mortality can be 25% or higher. Hypothyroidism leads to an extreme hypometabolism that decreases basal metabolic rate, causes bradycardia, hypotension, and low cardiac output. Other clinical signs vary as some patients have periorbital edema, ascites or pericardial effusion, and others may not.

Myxedema Coma Management

Pharmacologic replacement of thyroid hormone is essential. Levothyroxine (synthetic T_4) is administered to replenish hormone stores and increase the metabolic rate. Management involves supportive mechanical ventilation and meticulous nursing care to prevent complications such as hospital-acquired pressure injury (HAPI), ventilator-associated pneumonia (VAP), and sepsis.

Summary: Hyperthyroidism and Thyroid Storm, Hypothyroidism and Myxedema Coma

Severe thyroid dysfunction, whether hyperactive (thyroid storm) or hypoactive (myxedema coma), is rare as a primary diagnosis in critical care. However, it may be helpful to assess for the more common underlying thyroid conditions of hyperthyroidism or hypothyroidism by measuring the TSH level. The TSH value is low in hyperthyroidism, and high in hypothyroidism. This TSH test is useful when a patient who has been admitted for another reason has signs and symptoms not associated with the admitting diagnosis.

ADRENAL GLAND FUNCTION AND ASSOCIATED DISORDERS

The adrenal glands are located on top of the kidney. Although small, they are metabolically important for metabolic and hormonal health. The outer region, called the cortex, is responsible for secretion of glucocorticoids and aldosterone. The inner region, called the medulla, is responsible for secretion of the catecholamine epinephrine. Adrenal gland dysfunction can occur from either hypersecretion or hyposecretion of the hormones in either cortex or medulla (Figure 16-5).

Cushing Syndrome

Cushing syndrome can be primary or secondary. Primary Cushing syndrome is rare. It occurs when the adrenal cortex

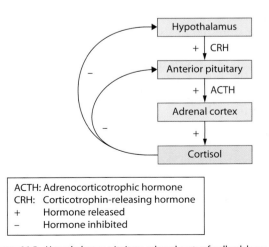

Figure 16-5. Hypothalamus-pituitary-adrenal cortex feedback loop.

produces excessive amounts of the hormone cortisol. The origin may be a pituitary adenoma that produces excessive amounts of adrenocorticotropic hormone (ACTH) that stimulates the adrenal cortex to produce excessive cortisol. ACTH is a component of the hypothalamus-pituitary-adrenal feedback loop that normally regulates cortisol levels. A tumor of the adrenal gland that secretes excess cortisol can also lead to Cushing syndrome.

Secondary Cushing syndrome occurs when a patient is taking long-term glucocorticoids (steroids) for another medical condition. The medical conditions may include corticosteroids to prevent organ transplant rejection, various respiratory conditions, skin conditions, and chronic inflammation. In this circumstance, patients are described as "steroid dependent" because the medications must be tapered off slowly to allow the adrenal glands to recover. If the corticosteroids are stopped abruptly, the patient may be plunged into a life-threatening crisis (see Addisonian crisis discussed later).

Whether Cushing syndrome is primary or secondary, the excess cortisol produces distinct features, including a round face, hirsutism (excess hair growth), fat accumulation on the upper back and abdomen, hyperglycemia, thin skin, bruises, fatigue, weakness, and a compromised immune system with increased vulnerability to infection. It is essential to know if a patient is steroid-dependent as abruptly stopping glucocorticoids leaves the patient without any stress-response protection.

Primary Cushing Syndrome Management

Primary or endogenous Cushing syndrome is rare. It results from a tumor of the pituitary gland that produces excess ATCH and can be removed surgically. Alternatively an adrenal tumor may produce excess cortisol and surgical removal of the affected adrenal gland will resolve the problem.

Steroid-Dependent Patient Management

Secondary or exogenous Cushing syndrome occurs when a patient has been taking corticosteroids for prolonged periods, especially at high dosages. This creates unique challenges in treatment. When a steroid-dependent patient experiences an infection, trauma, surgery, or other medical condition, the adrenal gland cannot increase cortisol output. In this situation, their usual dose of corticosteroids may be inadequate. To compensate, a "stress steroid" regimen may be used to cover the physiologic stress of critical illness and associated procedures. Some hospitals have clinical guidelines/pathways to cover this situation. Addison crisis (discussed later) can be precipitated when glucocorticosteroids are abruptly stopped in a steroid-dependent patient. Corticosteroids are tapered off to avoid complications of cortisol deficiency.

Aldosteronism

The adrenal cortex also produces aldosterone, a mineralo-corticoid hormone important in maintaining salt and water homeostasis. Aldosterone is a component of the renin-angiotensin-aldosterone system (RAAS). In primary aldosteronism, the adrenal cortex secretes excessive amounts of aldosterone unrelated to the RASS feedback loop. An adrenal cortex tumor (aldosteroma) is one of the causes of this rare condition. Patients can present with extreme hypertension, metabolic alkalosis, and life-threatening hypokalemia.

Aldosteronism Management

Emergency management is focused on reducing hypertension and replacing potassium and other electrolytes to within normal limits. If the cause is an aldosteroma, resection of the adrenal tumor will be necessary. There are other causes of aldosteronism and an endocrinology consultation is recommended for a full diagnostic workup.

Addison Disease and Crisis

Adrenal insufficiency, also known as Addison disease, is caused by hyposecretion of glucocorticoids (cortisol) from the adrenal cortex. Simultaneously measuring the serum ACTH and the serum cortisol may confirm the diagnosis in this rare condition. An elevated ACTH with an extremely low cortisol level may be diagnostic. Addison disease can be a difficult diagnosis to make when there are other confounding comorbidities.

If the adrenal gland shuts down completely, this condition is known as an Addisonian crisis. Signature signs and symptoms include critical hypotension, hyperkalemia, hyponatremia, and hypoglycemia. Prompt recognition and intervention are vital to prevent demise.

Addisonian Crisis Management

As soon as the condition is recognized, emergency replacement with IV glucocorticosteroids is vital. Hydration with IV isotonic saline (0.9%) and electrolyte replacement are also priorities. Other supportive treatments will depend on the patient's level of consciousness, respiratory drive, and comorbidities. A thorough assessment by an endocrinologist is recommended once the initial crisis is managed.

Critical Illness-Related Corticosteroid Insufficiency

The physiologic stress associated with critical illness normally stimulates the adrenal gland to produce additional cortisol. However, in critical illness-related corticosteroid insufficiency (CIRCI), the adrenal gland does not respond, so that serum cortisol levels are inadequate to support a therapeutic stress response. Persistent elevation of inflammatory cytokines may be a precipitating and ongoing cause of CIRCI. Patients with CIRCI are vulnerable to infection with hypotensive shock, and to septic shock that is refectory to vasopressor catecholamines.

Diagnosis of CIRCI remains a challenge. Two tests may be helpful: (1) failure of the cortisol level to meaningfully increase ($\leq$ 9 mcg), at a 60-minute time-point following administration of an ACTH-cortisol stimulus (IV cosyntropin 250 mcg), suggests inadequate adrenal function; (2) a random plasma cortisol level below normal (< 10 mcg/dL) suggests inadequate adrenal function.

Guidelines on the use of corticosteroids in critical illness were published by the major critical care medical societies in 2017. The Surviving Sepsis guidelines strongly recommend the use of fluids and antibiotics as first-line therapy to achieve hemodynamic stability (as described in Chapter 11, Multisystem Problems). If hemodynamic stability is not achievable with fluids, antibiotics, and vasopressors, IV hydrocortisone is considered. The 2017 CIRC guidelines also suggest IV hydrocortisone (< 400 mg/day) for 3 days or longer at full dose for refractory septic shock. Corticosteroids are not recommended for sepsis without signs of shock.

The dilemma with pharmacologic glucocorticoids is to balance the known anti-inflammatory properties and potential for shock reversal, against depression of the immune system, and risk of secondary infection. Research on the role of steroids in managing sepsis and shock states is ongoing. For instance, a 2018 report on the ADRENAL trial showed that survivors of septic shock who received infusions of hydrocortisone recovered faster and were less likely to require a blood transfusion than those who received placebo. This same study did not demonstrate a reduced mortality with steroid versus placebo. Readers are referred to the full CIRCI treatment guidelines for more details about the conditions and circumstances under which corticosteroids may be helpful in critical care.

Pheochromocytoma and Catecholamine Crisis

The adrenal medulla normally produces two catecholamines: norepinephrine and epinephrine. In combination with the sympathetic nervous system norepinephrine and epinephrine influence the heart and cardiovascular function. These catecholamines are used as infusions in critical care to mimic normal physiology.

Pheochromocytomas are tumors of the adrenal medulla that produce excessive amounts of norepinephrine and in some cases epinephrine. This can produce a catecholamine crisis manifested by extreme hypertension, tachycardia, hyperglycemia, and increased respiratory rate. Laboratory blood tests to measure the metanephrine level, or a 24-hour urine collection of daily metanephrine level, and imaging studies of the adrenal gland are performed as part of the diagnostic workup.

Pheochromocytoma Management

Definitive treatment requires removal of the tumor usually by minimally invasive laparoscopy. Before and throughout surgery, the blood pressure is aggressively managed with a combination of beta blockade and alpha blockade medications. Usually, hypertension is resolved by removal of the adrenal tumor.

Summary: Adrenal Gland Dysfunction

The adrenal glands are really two endocrine glands in one organ, the outer cortex and inner medulla. Most of the conditions associated with adrenal dysfunction are rare. Commonly seen conditions include Cushing syndrome, which results from excess glucocorticoids, whether endogenous (rare), or from exogenous medications (often seen). Adrenal insufficiency is believed to play a role in acute and chronic critical illness, especially in inflammatory shock states that are unresponsive to vasopressor infusions. Other conditions such as pheochromocytoma, or Addison disease are rarely encountered in critical care.

SELECTED BIBLIOGRAPHY

Blood Glucose Monitoring

American Diabetes Association. Clinical practice recommendations. *Diabetes Care.* 2017;40:S1-S135.

Blood Glucose Monitoring Test. Systems for Prescription. Point-of-Care Use. Guidance for Industry and. Food and Drug Administration. US Department of Health and Human Services. Document issued on October 11th 2016. https://www.fda.gov/downloads/ucm380325.pdf. Accessed June 10, 2017.

Schifman RB, Howanitz PJ, Souers RJ. Point-of-care glucose critical values: a Q-probes study involving 50 health care facilities and 2349 critical results. *Arch Pathol Lab Med.* 2016;140(2):119-124.

Hyperglycemia, DKA, and HHS

American Diabetes Association. Standards of medical care in diabetes-2018. *Diabetes Care.* 2018;41:S1-S159.

Chua HR, Schneider A, Bellomo R. Bicarbonate in diabetic ketoacidosis—a systematic review. *Ann Intensive Care.* 2011; 1(1):23.

Jacobi J, Bircher N, Krinsley J, et al. Guidelines for the use of an insulin infusion for the management of hyperglycemia in critically ill patients. *Crit Care Med.* 2012;40(12):3251-3276.

Moghissi ES, Korytkowski MT, DiNardo M, et al. American Association of Clinical Endocrinologists and American Diabetes Association consensus statement on inpatient glycemic control. *Diabetes Care.* 2009;32(6):1119-1131.

The NICE-SUGAR Study Investigators. Intensive versus conventional glucose control in critically ill patients. *N Engl J Med.* 2009;360:1283-1297.

The NICE-SUGAR Study Investigators. Hypoglycemia and risk of death in critically ill patients. *N Engl J Med.* 2012;367:1108-1118.

Umpierrez G, Korytkowski M. Diabetic emergencies—ketoacidosis, hyperglycaemic hyperosmolar state and hypoglycaemia. *Nat Rev Endocrinol.* 2016;12(4):222-232.

Umpierrez GE, Hellman R, Korytkowski MT, et al. Management of Hyperglycemia in hospitalized patients in non-critical care setting: an endocrine society clinical practice guideline. *J Clin Endocrinol Metab.* 2012;97:16-38.

SIADH and Diabetes Insipidus

Ball S, Barth J, Levy M, Society for Endocrinology Clinical Committee. Society For Endocrinology endocrine emergency guidance: emergency management of severe symptomatic hyponatraemia in adult patients. *Endocr Connect.* 2016;5(5):G4-G6.

Cuesta M, Ortolá A, Garrahy A, Calle Pascual AL, Runkle I, Thompson CJ. Predictors of failure to respond to fluid restriction in SIAD in clinical practice; time to re-evaluate clinical guidelines? *QJM.* 2017;110(8):489-492.

Cuesta M, Thompson CJ. The syndrome of inappropriate antidiuresis (SIAD). *Best Pract Res Clin Endocrinol Metab.* 2016;30(2):175-187.

Hong GK, Payne SC, Jane JA Jr. Anatomy, physiology, and laboratory evaluation of the pituitary gland. *Otolaryngol Clin North Am.* 2016;49(1):21-32.

Robertson GL. Diabetes insipidus: differential diagnosis and management. *Best Pract Res Clin Endocrinol Metab.* 2016;30(2):205-218.

Shepshelovich D, Schechter A, Calvarysky B, et al. Medication-induced SIADH—distribution and characterization according to medication class. *Br J Clin Pharmacol.* 2017;83(8):1801-1807.

Hyperthyroidism and Thyroid Storm

De Leo S, Lee SY, Braverman LE. Hyperthyroidism. *Lancet.* 2016;388(10047):906-918.

McGonigle AM, Tobian AAR, Zink JL, King KE. Perfect storm: therapeutic plasma exchange for a patient with thyroid storm. *J Clin Apher.* June, 2018;33(1):113-116.

Hypothyroidism and Myxedema Coma

Fliers E, Bianco AC, Langouche L, Boelen A. Thyroid function in critically ill patients. *Lancet Diabetes Endocrinol.* 2015;3(10):816-825.

Gish DS, Loynd RT, Melnick S, Nezir S. Myxedema coma: a forgotten presentation of extreme hypothyroidism. *BMJ Case Rep.* 2016; 2016.

Adrenal Gland, Cushing Disease, and Pheochromocytoma

Boonen E, Bornstein SR, Van den Berghe G. New insights into the controversy of adrenal function during critical illness. *Lancet Diabetes Endocrinol.* 2015;3(10):805-815.

Gibbison B, López-López JA, Higgins JP, et al. Corticosteroids in septic shock: a systematic review and network meta-analysis. *Crit Care.* 2017;21(1):78.

Loriaux DL. Diagnosis and differential diagnosis of Cushing's syndrome. *N Engl J Med.* 2017;376(15):1451-1459.

Riester A, Weismann D, Quinkler M, et al. Life-threatening events in patients with pheochromocytoma. *Eur J Endocrinol.* 2015;173(6):757-764.

Rhodes A, Evans LE, Alhazzani W, et al. Surviving Sepsis Campaign: international guidelines for management of sepsis and septic shock: 2016. *Crit Care Med.* 2017;45(3):486-552.

Critical Illness-Related Corticosteroid Insufficiency

Annane D, Pastores SM, Arlt W, et al. Critical illness-related corticosteroid insufficiency (CIRCI): a narrative review from a multispecialty task force of the Society of Critical Care Medicine (SCCM) and the European Society of Intensive Care Medicine (ESICM). *Crit Care Med*. 2017;45(12):2089-2098.

Annene D, Pastores SM, Rochwerg B, et al. Guidelines for the diagnosis and management of critical illness-related corticosteroid insufficiency (CIRCI) in critically ill patients (Part I): Society of Critical Care Medicine (SCCM) and European Society of Intensive Care Medicine (ESICM) 2017. *Crit Care Med*. 2017;45(12):2078-2088.

Pastores S. Annane D, Rochwerg B; and the Corticosteroid Guideline Task Force of SCCM and ESICM. Guidelines for the diagnosis and management of critical illness-related corticosteroid insufficiency (CIRCI) in critically ill patients (Part II): Society of Critical Care Medicine (SCCM) and European Society of Intensive Care Medicine (ESICM) 2017. *Crit Care Med*. 2018;46(1):146-148.

The ADRENAL Trial: Steroids in Septic Shock. 2018. http://rebelem.com/the-adrenal-trial-steroids-in-septic-shock/. Accessed February 16, 2018.

TRAUMA

17

Allen C. Wolfe Jr. and Benjamin W. Hughes

KNOWLEDGE COMPETENCIES

1. Describe the mechanisms of traumatic injury and relate them to accurate assessment of overt and covert injuries.

2. Discuss the common physiologic and psychosocial effects on the patient and family because of major traumatic injury.

3. Identify the unique needs of the trauma patient in critical and progressive care units.

4. Integrate selected management principles to treat trauma patients with thoracic, abdominal, and musculoskeletal injuries.

Trauma is a leading cause of mortality worldwide and an increasing healthcare problem in the United States. In 2016, the World Health Organization (WHO) identified trauma as the leading cause of death in young adults accounting for 10% of all deaths among men and women. Although the death rate is high for this patient population, the disability rate is even greater. In the United States, approximately 30% of all intensive care unit (ICU) admissions are related to traumatic injuries. This chapter focuses on thoracoabdominal, musculoskeletal, and pelvic trauma. Traumatic brain injury (TBI) is the single largest cause of death from injury and is discussed in Chapter 20, Advanced Neurologic Concepts.

SPECIALIZED ASSESSMENT

Trauma patients are unlike other hospitalized patients and require specialized assessment and monitoring. For the trauma victim, admission to the critical care or progressive care setting is sudden and unplanned, without time for psychological preparation or the stabilization of chronic conditions. Trauma patients are often young; however, trauma among older adults is an increasing problem and more complex since they often have additional chronic conditions. Minor injuries can evolve into life-threatening ones if not addressed in initial assessment. Traumatic injuries may be subtle and complications are common. Alcohol or drug use often plays a major role in the cause of the trauma and subsequent treatment. Rehabilitation is frequently needed after injury, and a trauma victim's quality of life may never return to preinjury status. This is especially true for traumatic brain and spinal cord injuries; however, even in lower extremity trauma, it may take a full year for an individual to return to work. Trauma takes a significant emotional and financial toll on the patient, family, and society.

Management of traumatic injury in the initial phases of care occurs in tandem with assessment; for example, the insertion of an advanced airway, establishing intravenous (IV) access and administration of fluids, and pain control may all be provided before the site of hemorrhage is identified and controlled. Internal bleeding is occult and may be missed on the primary survey. External hemorrhage, in contrast, would be obvious in the survey and would be a priority. One of the most important aspects of assessing the traumatically injured patient is to determine the injury based on the mechanism, whether blunt or penetrating trauma. Based on this information, an "index of suspicion" regarding specific injuries is developed during the primary and secondary survey. The goal is to ensure that no occult injuries are overlooked as the plan of care is developed.

Primary, Secondary, and Tertiary Trauma Surveys

The life-threatening nature of trauma often requires that serious physical findings guide immediate management. The primary and secondary surveys reveal immediate life-threatening injuries and direct the trauma team to develop an individualized resuscitation plan.

Initially upon the patient's arrival, a quick visual assessment is completed to determine obvious life threats. These include but are not limited to uncontrolled external injuries, altered mental status, impaled objects, severe respiratory distress, and traumatic amputations. The *primary survey* assesses all life-threatening injuries simultaneously and focuses on ABCDE—Airway, Breathing, Circulation, Disability, and Exposure (Table 17-1). The airway assessment is first and includes examination for obstructions, anatomy distortion,

TABLE 17-1. PRIMARY SURVEY

Airway and C-spine	**Assessment** • Assess patency and airway obstruction **Management** • Basic airway maneuvers—jaw thrust or chin lift accompanied by assessment for foreign bodies in the airway • Insert nasopharyngeal airway or oral pharyngeal airway • Establish a definitive airway if necessary • Maintain C-spine in neutral position with an appropriate device while maintaining airway patency
Breathing	**Assessment** • Assess respiratory rate and depth after exposure of chest and neck area • Assure C-spine immobilization is maintained • Assess for injury to neck to include but not limited to deformity, tracheal deviation, subcutaneous emphysema, etc • Assess for chest wall motion and use of accessory muscle **Management** • Apply high flow oxygen • Maintain airway by definite airway if necessary • Assure CO_2 and pulse oximetry monitoring with intubation • Alleviate tension pneumothorax or seal open pneumothorax

Circulation	**Assessment**
	• Identify source of hemorrhage—internal or external
	• Assess vital signs to include skin color, capillary refill, and pulses
	Management
	• Stop the bleeding
	  • external—direct pressure
	  • internal—locate source and need for operative intervention
	• Establish large bore IV access and obtain blood samples during this process
	• Initiate warmed isotonic (LR or NS) or colloid fluid resuscitation
	• Initiate warming measures to combat hypothermia

Disability	**Assessment** • Assess neurological status to include mental status, pupillary size, and response
Exposure	**Assessment** • Completely disrobe patient but avoid hypothermia

or anything that may block the airway and prevent effective breathing. The breathing assessment includes observation for symmetrical chest movement and depth of respiratory excursion to determine if any part of the airway or lungs has been injured. Circulation is an evaluation of pulse rate and strength, as well as the presence of hemorrhage. Disability includes injuries that affect neurological function. And finally, the E stands for environment/exposure.

Following this rapid survey, the clothing is removed, and a systematic evaluation is completed. This is the *secondary survey* and includes a head to toe systematic review of the patient (Table 17-2). If the patient's status changes at any time during the secondary survey, the practitioner returns to the primary survey to again review the ABCDEs to look for additional or evolving decompensation. Once the patient has awakened and is in acute care setting, a return to the primary survey may be necessary and is called the *tertiary survey*. This methodical approach to trauma assessment is done with any change in the patient's status regardless of where the patient is in the continuum of care.

Diagnostic Studies

Ultrasound, Computed Axial Tomography, and Diagnostic Peritoneal Lavage

Hemorrhage is a major concern and is evaluated during the primary survey. Both external and occult bleeding cases are considered. Secondary survey diagnostic studies may include ultrasound, computed axial tomography (CAT), or/and diagnostic peritoneal lavage (DPL) to diagnose occult thoracoabdominal hemorrhage.

An ultrasound is ideal for an initial screening examination in the trauma patient. This noninvasive procedure can be completed in a few minutes, however, its success in identifying injuries is dependent on the expertise of the person performing the procedure. It is not a replacement for more sensitive imaging studies such as CAT scanning.

A CAT scan, considered the standard for identification of specific injuries in patients with abdominal or thoracic symptoms, is done only if the patient is hemodynamically stable. Unstable patients with an inconclusive ultrasound (bleeding source not identified) may be candidates for a DPL, angiography, or may require an immediate exploratory laparotomy. If a bleeding source is identified by ultrasound, but the patient is hemodynamically unstable, it is considered an acute abdomen and an exploratory laparotomy is required.

Serial physical examinations coupled with ultrasounds are recommended to better evaluate some injuries. This is because the ultrasound examination is limited in identifying retroperitoneal, pancreatic, and pelvic injuries. For example, it is difficult for an ultrasound to conclusively differentiate between fluid (such as urine) and blood in the pelvic area. Refer to Table 17-3 for a comparison of ultrasound, CAT, and DPL.

Cervical Spine Radiograph

A cervical spine (C-spine) radiograph is one of the first diagnostic tests obtained following completion of the primary

TABLE 17-2. SECONDARY SURVEY

Item to Assess	Establishes/Identifies	Assess	Finding	Confirm By
Level of consciousness	• Severity of head injury	• GCS score	• < 8, severe head injury • 9-12, moderate head injury • 13-15, minor head injury	• CT scan • Repeat without paralyzing agents
Pupils	• Type of head injury • Presence of eye injury	• Size • Shape • Reactivity	• Mass effect • Diffuse brain injury • Ophthalmic injury	• CT scan
Head	• Scalp injury • Skull injury	• Inspect for lacerations and skull fractures • Palpable defects	• Scalp laceration • Depressed skull fracture • Basilar skull fracture	• CT scan
Maxillofacial	• Soft tissue injury • Bone injury • Nerve injury • Teeth/mouth injury	• Inspect for visible deformity, malocclusion • Palpation for crepitation	• Facial fracture • Soft tissue injury	• Facial bone x-ray • CT scan of facial bones
Neck	• Laryngeal injury • C-spine injury • Vascular injury • Esophageal injury • Neurologic deficit	• Visual inspection • Palpation • Auscultation	• Laryngeal deformity • Subcutaneous emphysema • Hematoma • Bruit • Platysmal penetration • Pain, tenderness of C-spine	• C-spine x-ray or CT • Angiography/duplex examination • Esophagoscopy • Laryngoscopy
Thorax	• Thoracic wall injury • Subcutaneous emphysema • Pneumo-hemothorax • Bronchial injury • Pulmonary contusion • Thoracic aortic disruption	• Visual inspection • Palpation • Auscultation	• Bruising, deformity, or paradoxical motion • Chest wall tenderness, crepitation • Diminished breath sounds • Muffled heart tones • Mediastinal crepitation • Severe back pain	• Chest x-ray • CT scan • Angiography • Bronchoscopy • Tube thoracostomy • Pericardiocentesis • TE ultrasound
Abdomen/flank	• Abdominal wall injury • Intraperitoneal injury • Retroperitoneal injury	• Visual inspection • Palpation • Auscultation • Determine path of penetration	• Abdominal wall pain/tenderness • Peritoneal irritation • Visceral injury • Retroperitoneal organ injury	• DPL/ultrasound • CT scan • Laparotomy • Contrast GI x-ray studies • Angiography
Pelvis	• Genitourinary (GU) tract injuries • Pelvic fracture(s)	• Palpate symphysis pubis for widening • Palpate bony pelvis for tenderness • Determine pelvic stability only once • Inspect perineum • Rectal/vaginal examination	• GU tract injury (hematuria) • Pelvic fracture • Rectal, vaginal, and/or perineal injury	• Pelvic x-ray • GU contrast studies • Urethrogram • Cystogram • IVP • Contrast-enhanced CT
Spinal cord	• Cranial injury • Cord injury • Peripheral nerve(s) injury	• Motor response • Pain response	• Unilateral cranial mass effect • Quadriplegia • Paraplegia • Nerve root injury	• Plain spine x-rays • CT scan • MRI
Vertebral column	• Column injury • Vertebral instability • Nerve injury	• Verbal response to pain, lateralizing signs • Palpate for tenderness • Deformity	• Fracture vs dislocation	• Plain x-rays • CT scan • MRI
Extremities	• Soft tissue injury • Bony deformities • Joint abnormalities • Neurovascular deficits	• Visual inspection • Palpation	• Swelling, bruising, pallor • Malalignment • Pain, tenderness, crepitation • Absence/diminished pulses • Tense muscular compartments • Neurologic deficits	• Specific x-rays • Doppler examination • Compartment pressures • Angiography

Reproduced with permission from Advanced Trauma Life Support Student Course Manual, 9th ed. American College of Surgeons; 2012.

survey. Trauma patients are presumed to have a C-spine injury until the seven cervical vertebrae have been cleared (ie, determined to be intact) with a radiograph or CAT scan. In most cases of suspected C-spine injury, three plain radiographs are done. These plain radiographs include anterior/posterior view, lateral, and odontoid view. The plain films

identify injuries and are less costly and decrease radiation exposure as compared to CAT scan. However, the CAT scan is the gold standard for assessment of the C-spine. A hard cervical collar is applied to immobilize the neck and is used until the C-spine has been visualized radiographically and no injuries are found. While in the past, all patients with suspected

TABLE 17-3. INDICATIONS, ADVANTAGES, AND DISADVANTAGES OF COMMON DIAGNOSTIC TESTS FOR BLUNT ABDOMINAL TRAUMA

Procedure	Indications	Advantages	Disadvantages
DPL	Decreased BP with suspicion of internal hemorrhage	Easy, rapid, inexpensive	Invasive, unable to pinpoint location of injury, cannot evaluate retroperitoneum
Ultrasound (FAST)	Decreased BP with suspicion of internal hemorrhage	Easy, rapid, inexpensive, noninvasive, can be repeated	Sensitive to operator experience, unable to pinpoint location of injury, cannot evaluate retroperitoneum
CT scan	Normal BP with suspicion of internal hemorrhage	Can pinpoint which organ is damaged, including those in the retroperitoneum	Time consuming, costly, must lie flat

traumatic injury to the C-spine were immobilized until they were transported to the hospital, recent studies suggest that the use of guideline criteria for "selective immobilization in the prehospital setting" may be safely applied to determine the need for immobilization in the field. The use of such guidelines may vary among practice locales.

In hemodynamically unstable trauma patients who are sent to the operating room (OR) without a cleared C-spine, cervical and spinal immobilization is continued until a CT scan is done postoperatively. Because TBI may coexist with a C-spine injury, any patient with an abnormal neurological examination or plain film findings will have CAT scans of the head, C-spine, and other areas of concern such as abdomen, pelvis, and thorax completed at the same time.

Radiographic Studies

Additional radiographic studies to determine the extent of injuries are performed after the primary survey is completed but should not delay resuscitation. Depending on the mechanism of injury, common x-rays may include chest, pelvis, and musculoskeletal studies to name a few.

Serial Examinations

Trauma patients require frequent reexamination to ensure that all injuries are identified, and that the patient's status is not deteriorating. Missed injuries may lead to pain, disability, and death. Repeat assessments by the same provider are recommended, especially in the case of traumatic brain and abdominal injuries as internal bleeding may not be initially evident. Understanding the mechanism of injury and the specific injuries created by destructive blunt or penetrating forces provides the basis of accurate and focused assessments.

Mechanism of Injury

Determining the mechanism of injury provides the trauma team with a means to evaluate for occult injuries. This includes how an injury occurred, the nature of the forces involved, and suspected tissue and organ damage. This knowledge is required when assessing a trauma patient at the scene of the accident, in the emergency department (ED), and in the critical or progressive care unit.

Injuries result when a body is exposed to an uncontrolled outside source of energy that disrupts the body's integrity and/or functional ability. Potential energy sources such as kinetic, penetrating, chemical, thermal, electrical,

or radiating are all considered. The severity of the resultant injury is determined by several factors: the force or speed of impact, the length of the impact or exposure, the total exposed surface area, and related risk factors such as age, gender, preinjury health, and alcohol/drug ingestion.

Mechanisms of injury are typically divided into two major categories: *blunt and penetrating*. *Blunt trauma* is defined as injuries that are not open to the atmosphere and *penetrating* injuries are those in which the body has been pierced. Blunt trauma usually results from motor vehicle or motorcycle collisions, assaults, falls, contact sports injuries, pedestrian/vehicle collisions, or blast injuries. Assessment strategies useful in diagnosing blunt traumatic injuries include physical assessment, ultrasound, DPL, CAT scanning, radiographic studies, angiography, blood count, and blood chemistry analysis. Penetrating trauma is commonly caused by gunshot wounds (GSWs) or knives. Although GSWs are seen less often than stab wounds, mortality is higher due to the velocity and energy displacement of the bullet.

Information related to the mechanism of injury helps determine patterns of injury. Common patterns help clinicians assess trauma patients who are unable to communicate about pain, injury, or other symptoms. Patterns of injury are used to focus the primary and secondary surveys so that diagnostic tests are sequenced appropriately and accomplished efficiently and accurately. For example, in motor vehicle crashes, the common pattern of injury for the unrestrained driver includes the head, pelvis, chest, and musculoskeletal areas (eg, hip, ankle, and foot trauma). Thoracic trauma is often due to impact with a steering wheel. Other patterns of injuries to unrestrained passengers include an increased incidence of craniofacial trauma resulting from hitting the head on the windshield or posterior hip dislocations due to the knee hitting the dashboard at a high rate of speed (Figure 17-1). Fractures of the clavicle and humerus are more frequent among passengers, possibly because of the defensive reflex action of raising the arms prior to impact. The impact of seat belt use and airbags deployment lowers the risk of thoracic injury (Table 17-4). As noted by Rosen in 2013, first-generation airbags deploy with tremendous force at speeds of 140 to 200 mph. Such forces can be lethal, especially to children, in the front passenger seat, particularly when unrestrained by safety belts, or when seated in rear-facing infant seats. A new generation of advanced, less

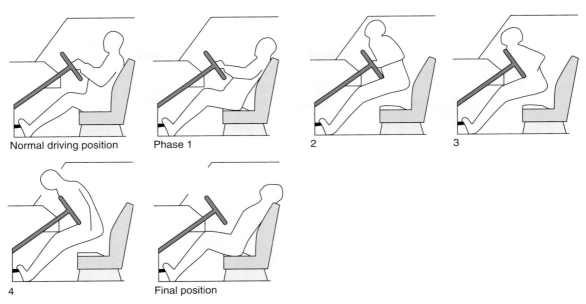

Figure 17-1. Injury mechanism of an unrestrained driver. (*Adapted with permission from Holleran R, Wolfe A, Frakes M. Patient Transport: Principles and Practice. 5th ed. St Louis, MO: Saunders/Elsevier; 2018.*)

Normal driving position — Phase 1 — 2 — 3 — 4 — Final position

forceful air bags has been in use since the late 1990s to reduce air bag–associated injuries.

Patterns of injury have also been identified for victims of falls and pedestrians struck by motor vehicles (Figure 17-2). Knowledge of these patterns of injuries helps prevent further damage or complications during resuscitation. For example, if a patient has sustained a head injury with a high suspicion of basilar skull fracture, an oral gastric tube is preferred over a nasogastric tube. This is because the nasogastric tube may be inadvertently passed through the fracture directly into the brain. A urinary catheter is not inserted if the mechanism of injury suggests bladder rupture or urethral trauma and a more definitive examination such as the retrograde urethrogram or cystogram is warranted.

Physiologic Consequences of Trauma

Traumatic injuries unleash a cascade of vasoactive mediators, such as neurohormones, prostaglandins, and cytokines, which contribute to the body's stress response. However, in severe multisystem trauma, these same mediators that help the trauma patient survive the initial injury may prolong the stress response and contribute to complications and even death. This response is best limited by enhancing the patient's healing ability with supportive physiologic and psychosocial care. Priorities include tissue oxygenation focusing on the three main components of oxygen delivery: cardiac output, hemoglobin level, and oxygen saturation. The trauma patient undergoes continuous vital sign monitoring, including electrocardiogram (ECG), pulse oximetry, and capnography. Pain and anxiety are treated simultaneously.

As previously noted, traumatic injury results in fractures, wounds, and crushed tissues that may not be readily visible. Once the primary trauma survey has been completed and management begins, the head-to-toe, in-depth assessment, *secondary survey,* is initiated and used to create a detailed differential of multiple injuries. From this, definitive care is planned. The nurse assists in stabilizing the patient with IV fluids, ventilatory and circulatory support, while also providing emotional support, especially during diagnostic testing. The nurse has a primary role in addressing pain control and meeting the psychosocial needs of the patient and family.

TABLE 17-4. TRUNCAL AND CERVICAL INJURIES FROM RESTRAINT DEVICES

Restraint Device	Injury
Lap Seat Belt • Compression • Hyperflexion	• Tear or avulsion of mesentery (Bucket Handle) • Rupture of small bowel or colon • Thrombosis of iliac artery or abdominal aorta • Chance fracture of lumbar vertebrae • Pancreatic or duodenal injury
Shoulder Harness • Sliding under the seat belt ("submarining") • Compression	• Intimal tear or thrombosis in innominate, carotid, subclavian, or vertebral arteries • Fracture or dislocation of cervical spine • Rib fractures • Pulmonary contusion • Rupture of upper abdominal viscera
Air Bag • Contact • Contact/deceleration • Flexion (unrestrained) • Hyperextension (unrestrained)	• Corneal abrasions • Abrasions of face, neck, and chest • Cardiac rupture • Cervical spine • Thoracic spine fracture

Courtesy of the National Association of Emergency Medical Technicians (NAEMT).

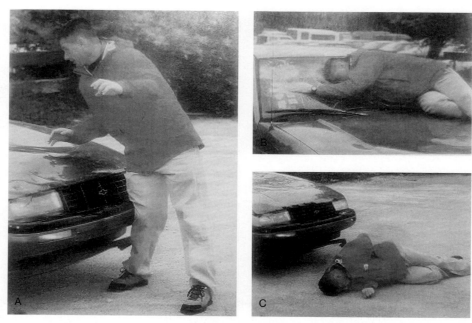

Figure 17-2. Injury mechanism of a pedestrian. (*Courtesy of the National Association of Emergency Medical Technicians (NAEMT).*)

Consequences of traumatic injury include blood loss, tissue destruction, intense pain due to damaged tissues, and altered oxygenation and ventilation. Airway management, fluid balance, aggressive pain control, and wound care are priorities. Stabilization of fractures and surgical repair of injured organs are accomplished in the early post-incident period. Although patients in the ED, critical care unit, or progressive care settings frequently have more than one injured system, a focus on one body system at a time assists in providing an organized management plan.

COMMON INJURIES IN THE TRAUMA PATIENT

Thoracic Trauma

Etiology and Pathophysiology

Thoracic trauma accounts for approximately 25% of all trauma-related deaths and may include injuries created by fractured ribs, blunt cardiac injury, vascular injury, and contused or punctured lung tissue. The most common mechanisms of injury to the chest include blunt trauma (motor vehicle-related injuries) and penetrating trauma from gunshots and stabbings. Common injuries associated with thoracic trauma include tension pneumothorax, open pneumothorax, hemothorax, pulmonary contusion, rib fractures/flail chest, cardiac tamponade, cardiac contusion, blunt cardiac injuries, and aortic disruption. Often a Focused Assessment with Sonography in Trauma (FAST) is initiated early in the evaluative stage to scan for free fluid which suggests bleeding in the peritoneal, pericardial, and pleural cavities. Ultrasound may also be used to evaluate the lungs for pneumothorax. The FAST examination and more

specific diagnostic tools for thoracic and abdominal injuries are described below.

Tension pneumothorax: Accumulation of air within the pleural space due to injury or a laceration of the lung parenchyma may cause a tension pneumothorax. This occurs when the lung parenchyma is no longer intact and air from the lung enters the pleural space but cannot exit. As air accumulates in the pleural space, the positive pressure collapses the lung and shifts the heart and great vessels to the opposite side of the chest. Signs and symptoms are severe respiratory distress, tachypnea, tachycardia, hypotension, hyperresonance and absence of breath sounds on the affected side, chest pain, and distended neck veins (may be flat in severely hypovolemic patients). Tension pneumothorax is a medical emergency. Management includes prompt detection and needle decompression to allow air to escape from the pleural space. A needle decompression consists of insertion of a large bore angiocatheter, preferably a 14G to 16G and length of 4.5 cm in adults. The angiocatheter is inserted into the chest wall on the affected side, at the midclavicular line on the anterior portion of the chest between the second and third intercostal space. An alternate location is the lateral approach on the midaxillary line between the fourth and fifth intercostal space. However, according to recent data, the lateral approach may be less likely to be successful than the anterior approach. Regardless, the goal is to release the life-threatening tension. To that end, provider comfort and experience with the two approaches may guide selection of the location. Once the needle decompression is performed as a lifesaving intervention, a chest tube is required as definitive treatment.

Open pneumothorax: An open pneumothorax is present when there is passage of air in and out of the pleural space from chest wall. This usually occurs when there is a penetrating injury to the chest wall by either a gunshot or stab wound. Definitive treatment for open pneumothorax is a chest tube; however, temporary management until a chest tube can be inserted includes using a three-sided dressing. This results in the closure of the dressing upon inhalation, so ambient air does not flow into the pleural space, and upon exhalation air can escape from the pleural space. If the dressing is completely occlusive, a tension pneumothorax may occur. Should this happen, immediate removal of the dressing generally relieves the increased tension. However, if the tension occurs with the three-sided dressing in place, a needle decompression may be done until a chest tube can be safely placed.

Hemothorax: A hemothorax is defined as blood in the pleural space. Rib fractures are typically the cause. Fracture of the clavicle (first rib) or the second rib is a very serious injury because the subclavian artery and vein are positioned directly under these ribs. A significant force is required to fracture these two ribs, thus potential damage to the underlying vessels is considered dangerous and is carefully assessed. An initial chest x-ray demonstrating a widened mediastinum may be due to a tear in the aorta or one of its major branches. If the hemothorax is large enough and the patient is experiencing respiratory difficulty, a chest tube is placed to drain the hemothorax. If the patient is hemodynamically unstable after chest tube placement, the physician may need to perform an open thoracotomy immediately, or the patient may need to be transported to the OR for exploratory surgery to locate and control the bleeding.

Another option is to attempt a resuscitative endovascular balloon occlusion of the aorta (REBOA). The REBOA procedure is a minimally invasive technique using an intra-aortic balloon occlusion catheter to temporarily occlude the large vessels contributing to bleeding. Once in the aorta, it is directed to the bleeding site to control bleeding and augment afterload in hemorrhagic shock states—a common cause of death after severe injuries. This is similar to an emergency open left thoracotomy to cross clamp the aorta. It can also be used with hemodynamic instability associated with severe pelvic injuries. In this case, the endovascular balloon occludes the lower descending portion of the aorta (called zone 3) versus a higher aortic level.

Pulmonary contusion: A pulmonary contusion is injury to the lung parenchyma, which commonly occurs after blunt injury to the chest. It consists of bleeding into the lung and alveolar capillary membrane disruption. Depending on the severity of the contusion, hypoxemia occurs, which may worsen several days after the injury with progression to respiratory failure and acute respiratory distress syndrome (ARDS). Pulmonary contusions are difficult to identify and diagnose during the initial trauma resuscitation because clinical findings may not become evident for several hours after the injury. Thus knowing the mechanism of injury may help the healthcare team to anticipate such a complication.

Monitoring oxygenation and ventilation with arterial blood gases (ABGs), pulse oximetry, and capnography is necessary to detect subtle changes in pulmonary status. Resuscitative management includes judicious use of IV fluids, support of oxygenation, mechanical ventilation if necessary, and pulmonary toilet.

Fractured ribs: Fractured ribs are common in blunt trauma. Fractured lower ribs can injure the liver or spleen, and upper rib fractures may puncture lung tissue. Pulmonary contusion, hemothoraces, and pneumothoraces are often associated with rib fractures. Also a *flail chest* may occur when several adjacent ribs are fractured in two places, creating a "floating segment" that may puncture the lung and compromise oxygenation and ventilation. Pulmonary contusions are common and anticipated.

Symptoms of flail chest include chest pain and shortness of breath. On observation, a flail chest is indicated by inward movement of the affected side of the chest during inspiration and outward movement during expiration, called "paradoxical breathing." This injury is best assessed when the patient is breathing spontaneously. The paradoxical breathing results in a notable increase in the work of breathing. In addition, the associated pain leads to splinted, shallow respirations, which result in atelectasis, pneumonia, and contribute to fatigue and respiratory failure. Mechanical ventilation may be necessary to stabilize the chest and support oxygenation and ventilation.

Cardiac injuries: Blunt trauma to the thorax may result in damage to the myocardium, coronary arteries, or structures of the heart (septum or valves). These injuries may be subtle and difficult to diagnose but are always suspected. The majority of patients are initially asymptomatic, but some have chest pain, which may be hard to differentiate given the presence of rib fractures and other injuries.

Chest x-ray, ECG, cardiac markers (especially troponin T), transthoracic echocardiography (TTE), and transesophageal echocardiography (TEE) assist in the identification of myocardial injuries both initially and also if the patient is unstable after resuscitative measures. Dysrhythmias also occur in patients with thoracic trauma. Sinus tachycardia, atrial fibrillation, and premature ventricular contractions are most common while ventricular tachycardia and fibrillation are common with extensive myocardial damage.

Cardiac tamponade: A hemopericardium may result in a cardiac tamponade and is a potentially life-threatening complication of both blunt and penetrating chest trauma. The pericardial membrane (sac) is normally stiff and noncompliant. Bleeding into the pericardial sac (effusion) causes compression on the heart, which compromises cardiac function and decreases cardiac output. The rate at which fluid accumulates around the heart in the pericardial sac determines whether the effusion will lead to compression of the heart or compensation (stretching of the sac and accommodation). A rapid accumulation of blood does not allow the pericardial sac to stretch and the tamponade may lead to death unless it is rapidly identified and decompressed.

A chest x-ray may show an enlarged heart, but echocardiography is generally used to confirm diagnosis. Signs such as rapid heart rate (HR), jugular venous distension, low blood pressure (BP), pulsus paradoxus, and finally ventricular fibrillation and cardiac arrest may ensue. Rapid infusion of IV fluids followed by a pericardiocentesis or a cardiac window is the treatment.

Traumatic aortic disruption: An aortic disruption (partial or complete) is a surgical emergency and the most common cause of immediate death in the thoracic trauma patient population. A high index of suspicion and knowledge of mechanism of injury, such as injuries associated with a high-speed motor vehicle collision, may result in an early diagnosis and improved outcomes. A widened mediastinum is typically seen on chest x-ray. Historically, the gold standard for diagnosis was aortography (direct injection of contrast material into the aorta while x-rays are taken). Current technologic enhancements now allow for the confident use of TEE, CAT scan, and MRI without the need for aortagraphy. The survival rate of the patient is directly related to how quickly this injury is diagnosed and the patient is taken to the OR. These patients may require massive transfusions. If so, a Massive Transfusion Protocol (MTP) is initiated as described later in this chapter.

Principles of Management for Thoracic Trauma

Management of the patient with chest trauma is individualized and includes several basic principles:

1. Support of oxygenation, ventilation, and cardiovascular status.
2. Monitoring and care of chest tube drainage and function.
3. Provision of optimal pain control, positioning, and physical care with attention to the promotion of wound healing.
4. Early mobility.
5. Prevention of complications such as infection.
6. Nutrition.

Ventilatory Support

The goals for ventilatory support of the trauma patient are the same as the ventilatory goals for any patient in the critical care or progressive care unit. Management focuses on improving oxygenation and ventilation, maintaining acid-base balance, decreasing the work of breathing, and preventing ventilator-associated conditions (VACs). Mechanical ventilation may be definitive or supportive, depending on the patient's injury and requirements. Definitive care for a flail chest may include the use of the ventilatory support to stabilize the chest wall. Supportive ventilatory care is imperative in the patient with a pulmonary contusion to prevent progression to respiratory failure. The nurse's understanding of both traditional and newer modes and methods of mechanical ventilation is essential to accurately assess patient tolerance of the modes as well as the goals of therapy (see Chapter 5,

Airway and Ventilatory Management, and *Critical Care Essentials* Chapter 20, Advanced Respiratory Concepts: Modes of Ventilation).

Monitoring Chest Tubes

Chest tubes are inserted in patients with chest wall injuries, punctured lung tissue, and those requiring thoracotomy. Care of the patient with chest tubes includes observing for drainage characteristics, signs of a resolving air leak, and prevention of infection. Meticulous sterile technique, insertion site care, and drainage system components and setup are key elements of chest tube management. Trauma patients may have draining wounds and suture lines adjacent to the chest tube site, which can make dressing changes more complicated. Infection surveillance, prevention, and assessments are essential nursing functions for all trauma patients. (See Chapter 10, Respiratory System.)

Pain Control

Appropriate and effective local and systemic pain control are essential for patient comfort and healing. Pain control may also allow for more effective spontaneous breathing and prevent the need for mechanical ventilation in patients with milder degrees of thoracic trauma. Often thoracic injuries result in chest wall splinting, especially with coughing and deep breathing. Both are necessary to avoid atelectasis and pneumonia. Patient-controlled analgesia (PCA), epidural narcotic infusions, or local anesthetics may be used for aggressive pain control in the trauma patient to allow for deep inspiration, the use of incentive spirometers, and effective coughing. These interventions are essential to avoid the need for mechanical ventilation.

Patients report that chest tubes, suctioning, and turning are all extremely painful. Managing a patient's pain aggressively is not only humane, it also allows the patient to focus mental and physical energy on healing. Pain may be controlled with narcotics that act centrally, locally, or regionally, and with medications that act at the periphery to interrupt the painful stimulus. Nonpharmacologic approaches can also operate at the central level through cognitive distraction or relaxation, and peripherally by using positioning or application of heat and cold.

PCA provides for patient control of timing and dosing of pain medication. Epidural PCA is used with success in patients with rib fractures and may decrease the need for mechanical ventilation, an important benefit in older trauma patients. Vigilant nursing care is essential because the epidural catheter may migrate from the pain site and not provide adequate pain relief. A patient's report of pain level and subsequent pain relief are determined at hourly or more frequent intervals as needed. Many critically or acutely ill trauma patients are unable to communicate their needs. Nonverbal pain scales are available (refer to Chapter 6, Pain and Sedation Management).

A variety of nonpharmacologic pain-reducing strategies are useful in patients with trauma, and the nurse may combine these with drug therapy for maximal effect.

Because narcotics have side effects, combining them with non-steroidal anti-inflammatory agents and a cognitive intervention may offer the patient the best pain reduction. Cognitive interventions for pain include relaxation, guided imagery, music therapy, pet therapy, and hypnosis. Clear documentation of the strategies or combinations that work best for the individual is key for continuity of care. This approach requires an established communication system between the patient, family, nurse, and providers. Anxiety and sleeplessness contribute to the pain response and are addressed by asking the patients how they typically try to relax and by eliminating as much environmental noise as possible. Encouraging rest and sleep and limiting patient interruptions enhances pain management approaches. (See Chapter 6, Pain and Sedation Management and Chapter 7, Pharmacology.)

Positioning and Mobility

Early mobilization of the trauma patient promotes oxygenation, ventilation, and prevents other complications of immobility. This includes positioning the patient in and out of bed. Information obtained from a daily chest x-ray may help determine how best to position the patient. Positions to be considered include: sitting, prone, and lateral decubitus. An example of how the concept of therapeutic positioning may be used by the nurse is to position the patient and evaluate for comfort as well as improvement in physical findings such as chest excursion, respiratory rate, pulse oximetry values, ventilator tolerance, and if applicable, hemodynamic data. Continuous lateral rotation and/or prone positioning beds may be helpful for selected injuries or conditions.

ESSENTIAL CONTENT CASE

Cardiac Tamponade

A 17-year-old woman with no past medical history is admitted to the ED after a stabbing × 2 to the upper posterior left side. She is lethargic and in no respiratory distress. Her pulse oximetry reading is 95%, HR 120 beats/min (sinus tachycardia), BP 105/85 mm Hg, and respiratory rate 24 breaths/min non-labored. The team immediately provides supplemental oxygen with a 100% non-rebreather (NRB) and two large bore IV catheters with normal saline (NS) infusions. An emergent FAST examination does not reveal a cardiac tamponade or tension pneumothorax. After the infusion of 1.5 L of NS, the patient's pulse oximetry (Sao_2) reading is 97%, HR 98 beats/min (sinus rhythm), BP 118/80 mm Hg, and respiratory rate (RR) 20 breaths/min non-labored.

The patient is transferred to the surgical intensive care unit (SICU) for 24-hour observation.

In the SICU, the patient continues to be lethargic but has a Glasgow coma scale (GCS) score of 15 and is arousable. She has no pain or distress but her skin is cool. Her tympanic temperature is 98.0°F. Her BP decreases to 75/65 mm Hg, with an HR of 110 beats/min. The NS infusion is increased to wide-open and the physician is called immediately. While the physician is on the way to the SICU, the nurses' reassessment finds clear breath sounds bilaterally and distant heart tones with jugular venous distention. The RR is 24 breaths/min with Sao_2 of 95% on 2 L nasal cannula. The nurse continues the IV boluses until the physician arrives. Upon arrival the physician orders a FAST examination and a change in the oxygen to a 100% NRB.

The team suspects a tamponade but the repeat FAST examination results do not support their suspicion. The patient is unstable so a CT scan cannot be safely completed. Thus, the patient is prepared for emergency exploratory thoracotomy. In the OR, the patient was found to have a large posterior pericardial bloody effusion causing tamponade, which was decompressed. The patient then returns to the SICU postoperatively.

Case Question 1: Which of the following reasons best explains why NS was used versus a vasopressor when the patients BP decreased?
(A) Dextrose solutions are hypotonic and do not expand the vascular bed as well as NS.
(B) The goal is to expand the intravascular volume to offset the pressure caused by the blood in the pericardial sac.
(C) Normal saline is an isotonic fluid.
(D) Vasopressors do not expand the intravascular space.
(E) All of the above.

Case Question 2: Why did two previous FAST examinations fail to show a cardiac tamponade?
(A) The FAST is not 100% predictive in all cases of tamponade.
(B) In cases of penetrating trauma to the chest an exploratory thoracotomy is the standard of care if symptoms of a tamponade persist despite negative FAST findings and if a CT scan cannot be done.
(C) The FAST is user dependent.
(D) All of the above.

Answers
1. Answer is option E: all the above.
    Dextrose solutions may cause an increase in ICP as well as seizures in trauma patients, especially those who are altered mentally. The glucose in the IV fluids may eventually be absorbed and intravascular volume decreases resulting in a decrease in BP. Isotonic fluids (ie, NS, lactated ringers, or colloids) are necessary to expand intravascular volume thus assuring that the volume in the chambers of the heart always exceeds the volume in that surrounds the heart. This prevents further heart compression (cardiac tamponade). Vasopressor use in trauma has been shown to increase mortality in the acute resuscitation phase. This is because vasopressors do not expand the intravascular volume.
2. Answer is D: all the above.
    The FAST is just one tool used to diagnose tamponade and is limited in some cases. It is also user dependent. The CT scan is helpful but if the patient is unstable may not be possible to do. When these two tools do not definitively eliminate the possibility of a tamponade, yet other clinical findings such as vital signs suggest tamponade, an exploratory thoracotomy is necessary.

Abdominal Trauma

Etiology and Pathophysiology

Trauma to the abdomen may occur to organs in three distinct abdominal regions: peritoneal cavity, retroperitoneum, and pelvis. The trauma will be anatomically directly related to the mechanism of injury. The organs most affected by blunt abdominal trauma are the spleen, liver, and kidneys. Most penetrating injuries occur anteriorly thus the intestines are commonly injured. The types of injuries sustained include organ contusions, lacerations, fractures, vascular disruption and hemorrhage, and crush-type tissue damage. Abdominal trauma is frequently not as overt on primary and secondary assessments as other injuries and may be more life threatening.

Evaluation of Abdominal Trauma

Physical examination, the presence of pain, the FAST scan, and the abdominal CAT scan are the main methods used to diagnose potential injuries. These primary diagnostic tools are used to determine if the patient needs to go directly to the OR, angiography, or can be managed more conservatively with close monitoring. Vigilance in nursing assessment for covert changes and observance of trends are the key to identifying abdominal injuries.

Serial physical examinations are labor intensive, but essential to assure detection of bleeding. The FAST examination is used to quickly and efficiently scan the abdomen at the bedside. Repeat FAST examinations may be done as often as necessary (especially during the resuscitation period) to determine a change in intraperitoneal bleeding. While the DPL and angiography may also be used for assessment, the FAST and the abdominal CAT scan are the two diagnostic tools used most often in conventional trauma assessment. Abdominal CAT scanning requires a hemodynamically stable patient, is more expensive, and incurs a higher radiation exposure than FAST examinations.

Historically, if the patient was unable to reliably confirm or deny the presence of abdominal pain, a DPL would be performed. For patient safety during a DPL, a decompressed bladder and stomach is necessary to decrease the likelihood of injury. To perform a DPL, a catheter is inserted just below the umbilicus and NS is infused. The bag is then lowered below the abdomen and the fluid is allowed to drain out. If the fluid comes out bloody or cloudy, there is a high probability of abdominal trauma. A DPL cannot discover a retroperitoneal bleed.

Damage to the spleen is one of the most frequently encountered blunt abdominal trauma injuries. Depending on the severity of splenic injury, interventions range from nonoperative observation, embolization angiography, bed rest for mild lacerations, and finally removal of a massively ruptured spleen. The liver is the second most injured organ in blunt trauma and runs the spectrum from minor injury to severe laceration, requiring operative repair and packing. The bowel, pancreas, and kidneys can be directly injured or sustain secondary injury as a result of poor perfusion and/or inflammation during the trauma, resuscitation, or the critical care phase of recovery.

Typically, presenting signs and symptoms in abdominal trauma include pain and hypovolemia. Complications from abdominal trauma are directly linked to the function of the gastrointestinal tract and include metabolic/nutritional alterations, infections such as peritonitis, and pancreatitis. Patients may require extensive dressing changes if the wound is open or requires multiple surgeries for staged repair of the abdominal organs.

Principles of Abdominal Trauma Management

Selected principles of caring for the patient with abdominal trauma include monitoring for bleeding, infection prevention and management, and initiating early nutritional support (ie, within 24-48 hours) (see Chapter 14, Gastrointestinal System).

Monitoring for Bleeding

Acute hemorrhage is commonly assessed and identified during the primary survey and frequently requires surgery. Occult bleeding may not be initially evident but later discovered during the secondary survey or during care provided by the nurse. Common abdominal injuries that may not initially exhibit early signs and symptoms of bleeding include liver laceration, splenic fractures, and slow retroperitoneal bleeds. In abdominal trauma, understanding the mechanism of injury and performing serial evaluations to detect changes from baseline are key components to assure rapid and effective treatment.

The historical treatment of splenic injuries was splenectomy. However, conventional wisdom is to preserve the spleen, if possible. Currently angiographic embolization repair of the spleen and close observation are more commonly employed. This allows the spleen to heal and preserves its valuable immunoprotective function. If a splenectomy is indicated due to massive injury, patients are given polyvalent pneumococcal vaccine within 72 hours after surgery to prevent infection with pneumococci. Splenectomy patients are immunocompromised for the rest of their lives. Management also includes a minimum of 3 days of bed rest, monitoring for continued bleeding, and interventions to prevent the complications of immobility.

Infection Prevention and Management

Abdominal trauma victims are at high risk for infection, even when surgery has not been performed. For all trauma patients, one of the major nursing care priorities after initial resuscitation is prevention, assessment, and management of infections. Traumatic wounds may be simple lacerations or abrasions from a motor vehicle crash or complex open abdominal surgical wounds that require packing and frequent trips to the OR. Care of the patient with a large abdominal wound is directed by the type of wound (open or closed) and the degree of intracompartment contamination due to the injury and surgery. Careful consideration is also given to the risks and benefits of empiric antimicrobial therapy in patients with contaminated wounds. Dressing changes are frequently performed by the nursing staff thus assessment for signs of infection as well as wound healing is essential. Premedicating and timing of dressing changes around pain medication administration is another important role of the nurse. Trauma patients may have multiple sources of infection, some of which are hospital acquired. The presence of a central line, urinary catheter, endotracheal (ET) tube, nasogastric tube, chest tube, and intravenous lines all increase the risk of infection and potentially sepsis.

Nutritional Support
Nutritional support in the trauma patient is an integral part of care. Management focuses on the route and timing of nutritional support. Other considerations include composition of nutrient formulation, assessment of laboratory tests that are indicators of nutrition, and the selection of enteral versus parenteral feedings. Trauma patients have increased metabolic needs due to a hypermetabolic stress response caused by severe injuries, wound healing, and/or sepsis.

Enteral nutrition is encouraged whenever possible at the earliest time after injury. Even a small amount of nutrition delivered via tube feeding to the gut may be beneficial. A variety of metabolic derangements in the hypermetabolic trauma patient make nutritional support an early imperative. Insertion and maintenance of a feeding tube, percutaneous gastrostomy tube, or jejunostomy tube is often required after injury until the patient can be orally fed. Total parenteral nutrition is recommended only if the gastrointestinal tract can not be used. Accurate nutritional assessment conducted in collaboration with the nutritionist is essential as trauma patients are at risk of complications from overfeeding as well as underfeeding. Diarrhea, inappropriate withholding of tube feedings, and the potential for aspiration are issues that need to be addressed (see Chapter 14, Gastrointestinal System).

Musculoskeletal Trauma

Etiology and Pathophysiology
Approximately 70% to 85% of multisystem traumas involve the musculoskeletal system. Patients in critical or progressive care settings who have extremity or pelvic fractures often have other injuries due to the significant physical impact to the body. Motor vehicle trauma, falls, sports injuries, and industrial trauma are all frequent causes of musculoskeletal trauma. Victims of motorcycle crashes often have severe fractures with extensive soft tissue damage. Massive blood loss, edema of tissues, tissue destruction, and pain accompany musculoskeletal injuries. Major musculoskeletal injuries indicate that the body sustained significant forces. For example, a patient with long bone fractures above and below the diaphragm has an increased likelihood of associated internal torso injuries.

Compartment syndrome is a serious complication of extremity trauma as a result of contused tissue swelling in a specific muscle compartment (Figure 17-3). This may lead to

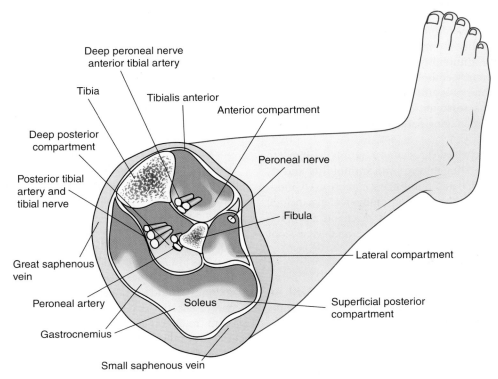

Figure 17-3. Compartments of the lower leg. (*Used with permission from David Hayes, Fulton, MD, 2009.*)

lack of perfusion and nerve compression in the area. Muscle compartments are located in the forearm, leg, hand, foot, thigh, abdomen, and chest. The nurse assesses for signs of compartment syndrome by performing repeated neurovascular checks. However, neurovascular assessment of the five Ps (pain, pallor, pulselessness, paresthesia, paralysis) may not provide accurate early assessment of rising compartment pressures.

Direct assessment of compartment pressures requires the use of a specialized needle that is inserted directly into the tissue compartment. The needle/catheter is attached to the transducer and the compartment pressures are evaluated and monitored. Even open fractures or open abdominal cavities may have significantly increased compartment pressures (normal pressure 0-8 mm Hg). If the compartment pressures are high, a fasciotomy is performed to relieve pressure. A fasciotomy entails surgically opening the skin and fascia to relieve the pressure in a muscle compartment and is the treatment of choice for compartment syndrome. The primary goal of the fasciotomy is to improve perfusion and minimize ischemia and injury to distal tissues.

Additional nursing management consists of immobilization and keeping the extremity level with or below the heart. Elevation of the extremity can worsen the condition. In the event of a severe crush injury, there is a significant release of myoglobin from damaged muscle tissue. Early detection of myoglobin in the urine is treated with generous fluid resuscitation to prevent precipitation in the renal tubules, electrolyte imbalances, and possible acute kidney injury.

Principles of Musculoskeletal Trauma Management
Management of extremity trauma focuses on early stabilization of fractures to prevent further tissue damage, infection, bleeding, and disability. Complications from musculoskeletal trauma include immobility, which can lead to increased incidence of pulmonary emboli, fat emboli, venous thromboemboli (VTE), and pressure injury. Pain control to promote mobility and assessment of neurovascular status are key components to managing patients with musculoskeletal trauma (Table 17-5).

Fractures are repaired early after a traumatic injury to decrease further bleeding and to limit immobility and its complications (eg, VTE and pulmonary embolism). Guidelines for the management of VTE for trauma patients include pharmacologic prophylaxis (if able) and mechanical prophylactic devices, such as sequential compression devices, foot pumps, and vena cava filters (Table 17-6).

Stabilizing Fractures
Improper handling or management of a patient with an injury to the musculoskeletal system may convert a simple problem into a much more serious problem. External fixation is used for pelvic fractures and lower limb fractures. Frequent sensation, movement, and vascular checks on affected extremities are essential. If the presence of pulses is in doubt, Doppler ultrasound is used at the bedside.

Pain Control
Pain control is best achieved with an individualized strategy of medications and nonpharmacologic therapies. Patients respond well when strict attention is paid to pain control and their own unique coping style is encouraged. Patients are expected to move in bed and get out of bed as soon as possible after an injury. Titrated pain medication is generally required to achieve this goal using PCA or a continuous infusion. Nurses are in a unique position to assess patient anxieties regarding the trauma and to promote adequate sleep and rest. Sleep deprivation from a noisy environment, constant worry, and needless pain can exacerbate the patient's discomfort and delay rehabilitation.

COMPLICATIONS OF TRAUMATIC INJURY IN SEVERE MULTISYSTEM TRAUMA
General Concepts
The key to survival for patients with multisystem trauma is to limit the extent of complications and increase the delivery of oxygen to the tissues during the initial phase of resuscitation. Historically, this has been called the "golden hour." The resuscitation goal is to prevent tissue oxygen deprivation due to hypoperfusion and identify and eliminate the cause. Shock, by definition, is hypoperfusion which results in cellular hypoxia, organ dysfunction, and tissue death. When adequate oxygen and blood flow are provided during the resuscitative phase of trauma, the likelihood of complications from shock decreases.

HR and BP are not considered adequate parameters to judge the effectiveness of resuscitation, as they indicate only the body's compensation for the stress of trauma and not real-time tissue oxygenation. Appropriate measures to evaluate resuscitation focus on assessing tissue oxygen delivery, including oxygen transport, delivery, utilization, and end organ function (e.g., mental status, urinary output). Evaluation of base deficit as an indicator of oxygen delivery at the cellular level is invalid. Base deficit is a reasonable prognostic indicator of the effects of the general resuscitation efforts but does not represent tissue oxygenation at the cellular level. Therefore, as the base deficit rises, a serum lactate test may be more helpful to assess perfusion at the cellular level.

To preserve adequate blood flow in the acutely injured trauma patient, permissive hypotension may be used. Permissive hypotension is based on the concept that resuscitation to attain normal BP may increase bleeding from a site that has already "clotted" through the normal clotting cascade process. If permissive hypotension is the goal, large volumes of fluid are not encouraged. Permissive hypotension may be effective in penetrating trauma but generally not with blunt trauma. If a TBI is suspected, permissive hypotension is contraindicated. Perfusion of the brain is a priority (see Chapter 20, Advanced Neurologic Concepts).

Common complications of trauma include infection/sepsis, ARDS, and multiple organ dysfunction. They are

TABLE 17-5. PHYSICAL COMPLICATIONS RELATED TO IMMOBILITY COMMONLY SEEN IN TRAUMA PATIENTS

Body System	Complications	Pathophysiology	Prevention
Neurologic	Potentially affects all body systems from mentation to physical changes.	Caused by decreased level of consciousness; injury to cortex, motor, or sensory systems.	• Neurologic assessment. • Specific focus on the effects seen in other body systems. • Understand neurologic basis of complication.
Respiratory	Fatigue, decreased productivity, infection, pneumonia, respiratory acidosis.	Decreased respiratory movement, unable to mobilize secretions, alterations in blood gases.	• Assessment of respiratory status and changes in level of consciousness. • Mobilization of secretions by turning, coughing, and deep breathing; postural drainage, percussion, vibration, early ambulation, humidification, and hydration.
Cardiovascular	Orthostatic hypotension, fatigue, increased cardiac workload, thrombosis, embolus.	Increased heart rate, CVP, cardiac output, stroke volume in supine position; loss of supporting muscle tone resulting in venous stasis; orthostatic neurovascular receptors cannot adjust to position changes; hypercoagulability and external pressure to vessels.	• Cardiovascular assessment. • Encourage mobilization, exercise, range of motion, positioning. • Antiembolic devices. • Provide adequate hydration. • Avoid Valsalva maneuver.
Gastrointestinal	Anorexia, fatigue, malnutrition, constipation, impaction, bowel obstruction, diarrhea, dehydration.	Negative nitrogen balance and protein deficiency; stress; decreased appetite creates bowel intolerance; muscle weakness; diminished ability to apply abdominal pressure needed for evacuation; psychological factors and position for defecation may increase difficulty.	• Assessment of GI functioning, including baseline history of nutrition, exercise, and bowel habits. • Coordinate bowel plan with nutrition specialist. • Adequate hydration. • Positioning and privacy. • Gastrocolic reflex timing factors; use of digital stimulation. • Stool softeners and suppositories as bowel stimulants. • Adjust tube feedings to avoid constipation or diarrhea. • Small, frequent feedings to increase tolerance and decrease anorexia. • Encourage intake of protein, fluids, bulk forming foods.
Urinary	Urinary reflux, incontinence, urinary stasis, renal calculi, urinary tract infection.	Loss of effect of gravity, urinary stasis in renal pelvis; increased calculi formation from urine sediment in renal pelvis; diminished coordination of sphincters and muscles in supine position; bladder distention, overflow incontinence.	• Assess urinary tract function. • Promote movement and exercise. • Maintain fluid intake. • Decrease calcium intake, increase loss from bones. • Monitor distention and voiding patterns. • Prevent incontinence. • Use upright or sitting position for voiding if possible. • Intermittent catheters preferred to indwelling.
Musculoskeletal	Muscle atrophy, contractures.	Muscles shorten and atrophy; loss of ROM as supporting ligaments, tendons, and capsule lose mobility; loss of ROM becomes permanent; spasticity of antagonistic muscle with weakness of opposing muscle creates contracture.	• Ongoing assessment. • Passive, active, and active-assisted ROM exercises. • Appropriate positioning and body alignment in both bed and chair.
	Osteoporosis, stress fractures, heterotrophic ossification.	Normal bone-building activities depend on weight bearing and movement; increased destruction of bone, release of calcium; bone becomes porous and fragile; abnormal calcification over large joints may also occur.	• Calcium supplement to diet is not recommended. • Promote weight bearing.
Integumentary	Pressure injury; stages I-IV; risk of sepsis with infection due to pressure injury.	Prolonged pressure to skin diminishes capillary blood supply and stops flow of nutrients to cells; necrosis of cells results in skin injury and risk for infection.	• Assessment of skin integrity, nutritional status, and risk factors for breakdown. • Reposition; shift pressure and patient weight frequently. • Check for changes in blanching, sustained redness. • Keep off all red areas. • Massage at-risk areas to promote circulation. • Teach patient to inspect own skin and shift weight. • Increase protein in diet, monitor hydration status. • Take immediate, consistent action on any areas of potential injury.

TABLE 17-6. EVIDENCE-BASED PRACTICE: MANAGEMENT OF VENOUS THROMBOEMBOLISM IN TRAUMA PATIENTS

EVIDENCE-BASED PRACTICE: Venous Thromboembolism (VTE) Prevention	
Prevention (Expected Nursing Practice)	**Levels of Evidence**

1. Assess all patients upon admission to the critical care or progressive care unit for risk factors for VTE. Anticipate orders for (VTE) prophylaxis based on risk assessment (Level D)
2. Risk and treatment for VTE prophylaxis include:
  a. Acute medical patients: low-molecular-weight heparin (LMWH) or low dose unfractionated heparin (LDUH) or fondaparinux (Level B)
  b. General surgery patients: LMWH, LDUH, or mechanical prophylaxis. Examples: antiembolism stockings/graduated compression stockings (GCSs), intermittent pneumatic compression devices (IPCDs), foot impulse devices (FIDs), also known as foot pumps (Level B)
  c. Critical ill patients: LMWH or LDUH (Level A)
  d. High risk for bleeding (trauma): mechanical prophylaxis (Level B)
  e. Use mechanical prophylaxis devices with anticoagulant-based treatment plans (Level D)
3. Discuss current VTE risk factors, the necessity for invasive lines (central venous catheter (CVC) or peripherally inserted central catheter (PICC)), and risk for bleeding. (Level E).
4. Maximize mobility and reduce the time the patient is immobile (Level E)
5. Ambulatory patients are at risk for VTE (Level D)
6. Ensure mechanical prophylaxis devices are properly fitted and in use at all times except for skin assessment and cleaning (Level D)
	1. Level A: Meta-analysis of quantitative studies or meta-synthesis of qualitative studies with results that consistently support a specific action, intervention, or treatment (including systematic review of randomized controlled trials)
	2. Level B: Well-designed, controlled studies with results that consistently support a specific action, intervention, or treatment
	3. Level C: Qualitative studies, descriptive or correlational studies, integrative reviews, systematic reviews, or randomized controlled trials with inconsistent results
	4. Level D: Peer-reviewed professional and organizational standards with the support of clinical study recommendations
	5. Level E: Multiple case reports, theory-based evidence from expert opinions, or peer-reviewed professional organizational standards without clinical studies to support recommendations
	6. Level M: Manufacturer's recommendations only

Data from Hopkins AG. The trauma nurse's role with families in crisis. Crit Care Nurse. 1994;April:14(2):35-43.

discussed below (see also Chapter 10, Respiratory System, and Chapter 11, Multisystem Problems).

Infection, Systemic Inflammatory Response Syndrome, Sepsis/Septic Shock, and Multiple Organ Dysfunction

Trauma patients are at high risk of developing an infection and potentially sepsis. Factors that contribute to this risk include the nature of the injury, the environment in which the injury occurred, the nonsterile conditions in which invasive devices are initially placed, and the multiple invasive procedures, including surgery, that are necessary for resuscitation, stabilization, and management. The procedures performed during resuscitation are at best undertaken under clean conditions.

Infection

The classic signs and symptoms of infection are sometimes difficult to isolate in a recovering trauma patient. Fever, tachycardia, elevated white blood cell count, hyperglycemia, inflammation, pain, and a hyperdynamic state may be indicators of infection and sepsis. These assessment parameters are also common after injury, resuscitation, and during the healing process due to the stress response on immune system. The classic rule in trauma care is that if there is an infection—it needs to be located and treated. When clear identification of an infectious source is elusive, consideration is given to treating the most likely source of infection based on the clinical evidence, particularly if the patient exhibits hemodynamic instability. Meticulous attention to sterile

technique and hand hygiene is essential in this vulnerable patient population.

SIRS and Sepsis

The definitions of systemic inflammatory response syndrome (SIRS) and sepsis are evolving as more distinct entities than previously described. The 2016, Third International Consensus Definitions for Sepsis and Septic Shock (Sepsis-3) define SIRS as an *appropriate* inflammatory response to a clinical insult, such as an infection, inflammation, or injury. In contrast to previous definitions, SIRS is not defined as a precursor to sepsis and septic shock. Sepsis is defined by a dysregulated response, which results in the release of many mediators, leading to end organ damage. Current guidelines suggest that assessment of mortality potential secondary to sepsis and septic shock is best done using the Sequential (Sepsis-related) Organ Failure Assessment (SOFA) score and the Quick SOFA (qSOFA) tools. The reader is referred to an in-depth discussion of sepsis, septic shock, SOFA, and qSOFA scores in Chapter 11, Multisystem Problems.

MODS

Multiple organ dysfunction syndrome (MODS) refers to progressive damage to two or more organs that may result in a permanent change in organ function. In the trauma patient, MODS may be due to infection and sepsis but also may occur as a result of excessive blood loss. Regardless of the etiology, unless hypoperfusion and shock are rapidly or adequately reversed, the organs sustain ischemia, inflammation, injury, and possibly infarction. The clinical presentation of organ dysfunction may have a rapid onset or take several days. Organ dysfunction is identified by signs and symptoms associated with organ failure such as ARDS, pancreatitis, acute kidney injury, and hepatic insufficiency. Delivering oxygen to the tissues by maintaining increased blood flow during resuscitation and early acute care phases can decrease the duration of hypoperfusion, limit anaerobic metabolism and avoid lethal complications.

Achieving adequate oxygen delivery to the tissues requires oxygen, hemoglobin, and sufficient cardiac output to meet cellular requirements. This is often accomplished with large volume fluid resuscitation or multiple blood transfusions in the trauma patient. MTPs are used to guide the use of large volumes of blood products (eg, the administration of more than 10 units of packed red blood cells within 24 hours). In such cases, multiple types of blood components (whole blood, packed red blood cells, fresh frozen plasma, cryoprecipitate, and platelets) are used. The different blood products address the restoration of blood volume, tissue oxygenation, and the correction of coagulation and acid-base abnormalities.

It is recommended that when a trauma patient needs either a massive transfusion of blood products or fluids, the nurse administers these fluids via a fluid warmer to prevent hypothermia. Trauma patients suffering from hypothermia do not respond normally to the administration of blood and fluid resuscitation, and coagulopathy may develop or worsen. The concurrent presence of hypothermia, acidosis, and coagulopathy is known as the trauma triad or triangle of death. Mortality may be increased to over 90%, if this combination of disorders is not reversed.

Trauma patients are at risk of experiencing significant complications after massive fluid/blood administration. Hypothermia, coagulopathy, acidosis, electrolyte imbalances, transfusion-related acute lung injury (TRALI), transfusion-associated circulatory overload (TACO), transfusion-associated immunomodulation (TRIM) (a down regulation of immune function or immunosuppression), and posttransfusion infections have all been attributed to massive fluid or blood replacement. Monitoring for and treating these complications are essential aspects of trauma care.

Acute Respiratory Distress Syndrome

Patients with trauma have an increased incidence of ARDS (see Chapter 10, Respiratory System). Precipitating factors for ARDS in the trauma patient include direct or indirect injury to the lungs. Examples of direct injury include smoke inhalation, rib fractures, aspiration, and large pulmonary contusions. Indirect injury may be due to sepsis, massive fluid and/or blood resuscitation, and prolonged hypoperfusion states (shock), which can lead to an inflammatory insult and alveolar infiltration.

Standard treatment for ARDS is supportive and includes mechanical ventilation, oxygen titrated to maintain Pao_2 more than or equal to 60 mm Hg, positive-end expiratory pressure (PEEP), and ventilatory modes and methods to recruit closed alveoli and decrease lung injury (see *Critical Care Essentials* Chapter 20, Advanced Respiratory Concepts: Modes of Ventilation). In addition to mechanical ventilation, another method to improve oxygenation is positioning for optimal ventilation and perfusion. This is a unique challenge for the critically or acutely ill trauma patient because their traumatic injuries may preclude many positions; for example, the patient with an unstable pelvic fracture, a spinal cord injury, or lower extremity fractures may be difficult or impossible to turn. Meticulous nursing care to prevent VACs is a priority for all trauma patients receiving mechanical ventilation.

PSYCHOLOGICAL CONSEQUENCES OF TRAUMA

Any illness places stresses on patients and families, and this is often magnified in critically or acutely ill trauma patients. Trauma injury is by nature unexpected. It typically affects young, healthy individuals and can launch both the patient and the family into a cycle of chaos and crisis. Common responses to trauma include anxiety, anger, fear, grief, loss, guilt, depression, denial, sleeplessness, and hopelessness.

Fear begins immediately as the awake trauma patient is transported from the scene. Fear is related to the unknown, the specifics of the injuries, and impact on the patient's future, including body image, family, and career. Loss typifies the experience of trauma and can be characterized as loss of physical functioning, loss of quality of life, or even loss of significant others due to the traumatic event. Guilt may ensue as the patient may perceive responsibility for the event (directly or indirectly), and this may be overwhelming. Depression and denial are common coping mechanisms during personal crises and may be exhibited in a variety of ways by trauma victims. It is noted that although the injuries are sustained by the patient, the family members and friends are also frequently traumatized.

Monitoring the patient's response to injury is as much the responsibility of the nurse as monitoring the patient's BP. Just as there are long-term physiologic effects of a low BP (shock), so there are long-term psychological effects of unmet or unidentified emotional needs. There are also psychoneuroimmunology responses that may impact the physical recovery. Assessing the emotional response to injury is an important part of comprehensive care. Talk to the patient and listen to responses and perceptions. Help them identify and articulate concerns and fears.

Fear creates anxiety in the trauma patient, and unrelieved pain may worsen anxiety. With the intense monitoring and frequent care interruptions commonly present in the critical or progressive care environment, sleep may be minimal and fragmented. A vicious cycle is thus initiated whereby sleeplessness leads to an increased perception of pain, which in turn creates needless anxiety and inhibits sleep.

Viewing these responses as cyclical emphasizes that the nurse may intervene anywhere in the cycle of responses and make a major impact on all three; for example, providing pain-relieving strategies that permit sleep automatically decreases anxiety. A focus on information sharing may ease the patient's mind so that sleep can occur, and pain perception decreases. The nurse has a significant role in intervening to stop this vicious cycle through a variety of holistic strategies.

All families of trauma patients experience a crisis. Families may have no idea of how to act or what the healthcare team expects of them. Clinicians have a key role in providing support and information to meet family needs and in identifying family coping mechanisms. Knowing the phases of family emotional response and suggested interventions is useful. Early assessment of family system structure, relationship process, and family functioning are keys to effective management of the psychosocial needs of the patient and family. Getting to know and working with family members in trauma care is essential and can be best facilitated with flexible visiting policies, and family presence during rounds, procedures, and codes when appropriate. Inviting family members to participate in decisions about the plan of care is also essential. Shared decision making is a key component of patient and family-centered health care. The healthcare team, the family, and the patient together can make decisions that are based on risk, clinical evidence, and outcomes as they relate to the patient's preferences and values.

SELECTED BIBLIOGRAPHY

General Trauma

American Association of Critical-Care Nurses. AACN Practice Alert: Family Presence During Resuscitation and Invasive Procedures. https://www.aacn.org/clinical-resources/practice-alerts.

American Association of Critical-Care Nurses. AACN Practice Alert: Preventing Venous Thromboembolism in Adults. https://www.aacn.org/clinical-resources/practice-alerts.

American Association of Critical-Care Nurses. AACN Practice Alert: Family Presence: Visitation in the Adult ICU. https://www.aacn.org/clinical-resources/practice-alerts.

American Institute of Ultrasound in Medicine, American College of Emergency Physicians. AIUM practice guideline for the performance of the focused assessment with sonography for trauma (FAST) examination. *J Ultrasound Med.* 2014;33:2047.

Aresco C. Trauma. In: Morton P, Fontaine D, eds. *Critical Care Nursing: A Holistic Approach.* 10th ed. New York, NY: Philadelphia Wolters Kluwer Health/Lippincott Williams & Wilkins; 2013.

ATLS Subcommittee, American College of Surgeons' Committee on Trauma, International ATLS Working Group. *Advanced Trauma Life Support Student Course Manual.* 9th ed. Chicago, IL: ACS; 2012.

Catherine JK, Gena SS. Metabolic and nutritional management in the trauma patient. In: McQuillan K, Makic M, Whalen E, eds. *Trauma Nursing: From Resuscitation Through Rehabilitation.* 4th ed. St Louis, MO: Saunders Elsevier; 2009.

Davis JS, Satahoo SS, Butler FK. An analysis of prehospital deaths: Who can we save? *J Trauma Acute Car Surg.* 2014;77(2): 213-218.

Feliciano DV, Mattox KL, Moore, EE. Trauma. *Nursing Core Course Provider Manual.* 7th ed. New York, NY: McGraw Hill; 2014.

Frawley P. Thoracic trauma. In: McQuillan K, Makic M, Whalen E, eds. *Trauma Nursing: From Resuscitation Through Rehabilitation.* 4th ed. St Louis, MO: Saunders Elsevier; 2009.

Gomez D, Berube M. Identifying targets for potential interventions to reduce rural trauma deaths: a population-based analysis. *J Trauma.* 2010;69:633-639.

Holleran R, Wolfe A, Frakes, M. *Patient Transport: Principles and Practice.* 5th ed. St Louis, MO: Saunders Elsevier; 2018.

Jones K. Abdominal injuries. In: McQuillan K, Makic M, Whalen E, eds. *Trauma Nursing: From Resuscitation Through Rehabilitation.* 4th ed. St Louis, MO: Saunders Elsevier; 2009.

Kleber C, Giesecke MT, Tsokos M. Trauma-related preventable deaths in Berlin 2010: need to change prehospital management strategies and trauma management education. *World J Surg.* 2013;37:1154-1161.

Lawrence G, Grim R, Bell T, Camey D, Ahuja V. The impact of seatbelt use and air bag deployment on blunt thoracic aortic injury. *Am J Surg.* 2013;79(11):E335-E336.

National Association of Emergency Technicians (U.S.), Pre-Hospital Trauma Life Support Committee, American College of Surgeons, Committee on Trauma. Kinematics of trauma. *Prehospital Trauma Life Support (PHTLS).* 8th ed. Burlington, MA: Jones and Bartlett Learning; 2016: chap 5.

Rushton C, Reina M, Reina D. Building trustworthy relationships with critically ill patients and families. *AACN Adv Crit Care.* 2007;18:19-30.

Sanchez LD, Straszewski S, Saghir A. Anterior versus lateral needle decompression of tension pneumothorax: comparison by computed tomography chest wall measurement. *Acad Emerg Med.* 2011;18:1022-1026.

Singer M, Deutschman CS, Seymour CW, et al. The Third International Consensus Definitions for Sepsis and Septic Shock (Sepsis-3). *JAMA.* 2016;315:801-810. doi:10.1001/jama.2016.0287.

Snyder KA, Veronese VR. Genitourinary injuries and renal management. In: McQuillan K, Makic M, Whalen E, eds. *Trauma Nursing: From Resuscitation Through Rehabilitation.* 4th ed. St Louis, MO: Saunders Elsevier; 2009.

Stannard A, Eliason JL, Rasmussen TE. Resuscitative endovascular balloon occlusion of the aorta (REBOA) as an adjunct for hemorrhagic shock. *J Trauma.* 2011;71:1869-1872.

WHO. World Health Organization. 2016. Health statistics and information systems. 2016. www.who.int/healthinfo/global_burden_disease/en/. Accessed May 16, 2017.

ADVANCED CONCEPTS

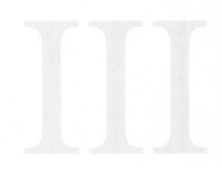

ADVANCED ECG CONCEPTS

Carol Jacobson

18

KNOWLEDGE COMPETENCIES

1. Identify electrocardiogram (ECG) characteristics and treatment approaches for each of the following advanced dysrhythmias:
   - Supraventricular tachycardias (SVTs)
   - Wide QRS beats and rhythms
2. Using the 12-lead ECG, determine the following:
   - Bundle branch blocks
   - QRS axis

- Patterns of myocardial ischemia, injury, and infarct
3. Identify ECG characteristics of single- and dual-chamber pacemakers during normal and abnormal functioning.
4. Identify ECG characteristics of Brugada syndrome (BrS) and long QT syndromes.

THE 12-LEAD ELECTROCARDIOGRAM

The 12-lead electrocardiogram (ECG) records electrical activity as it spreads through the heart from 12 different leads, which are in turn recorded by electrodes placed on the arms and legs, and in specific spots on the chest. Each lead represents a different "view" of the heart and consists of two electrodes. A bipolar lead has two poles—one positive and one negative. A unipolar lead has one positive pole and a reference pole that is a point in the center of the chest that is mathematically determined by the ECG machine. The standard 12-lead ECG consists of six frontal plane limb leads that record electrical activity traveling up/down and right/left in the heart, and six precordial leads that record electrical activity in the horizontal plane traveling anterior/posterior and right/left. Limb leads are recorded by electrodes placed on the arms and legs, and precordial leads are recorded by electrodes placed on the chest (Figure 18-1).

A camera analogy makes the 12-lead ECG easier to understand. Each lead of the ECG represents a picture of the electrical activity in the heart taken by the camera. In any lead, the positive electrode is the recording electrode or the camera lens. The negative electrode tells the camera which way to "shoot" its picture and determines the direction in which the positive electrode records. When the positive electrode sees electrical activity traveling toward it, it records an upright deflection on the ECG. When the positive electrode sees electrical activity traveling away from it, it records a negative deflection (Figure 18-2). If the electrical activity travels perpendicular to a positive electrode, no activity is recorded. The standard 12-ECG records three bipolar frontal plane leads (leads I, II, and III) and three unipolar frontal plane leads (aVR, aVL, and aVF). In addition, there are six unipolar precordial leads: V_1, V_2, V_3, V_4, V_5, and V_6.

The three bipolar frontal plane leads are illustrated in Figure 18-3A. In each lead, the camera represents the positive pole of the lead. In lead I, the positive electrode is on the left arm and the negative electrode is on the right arm. Any electrical activity in the heart that travels toward the positive electrode (camera lens) on the left arm is recorded as an upright deflection and any activity traveling away from it is recorded as a negative deflection. In lead II, the positive electrode is on the left leg and the negative electrode is on the right arm. Any electrical activity traveling toward the left leg electrode (camera lens) is recorded as an upright deflection and any activity traveling away from it toward the right arm electrode is recorded as a negative deflection. In lead III, the

425

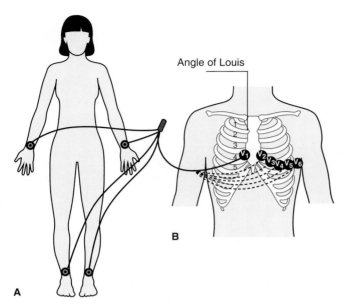

Angle of Louis

B

A

Figure 18-1. **(A)** Limb electrodes can be placed anywhere on arms and legs. Standard placement is shown here on wrists and ankles. **(B)** Chest electrode placement. V_1 = fourth intercostal space to right of sternum; V_2 = fourth intercostal space to left of sternum; V_3 = halfway between V_2 and V_4 in a straight line; V_4 = fifth intercostal space at mid clavicular line; V_5 = same level as V_4 at anterior axillary line; V_6 = same level as V_4 at midaxillary line.

positive electrode is on the left leg and the negative electrode is on the left arm. Any electrical activity coming toward the left leg electrode (camera lens) is recorded upright and any traveling away from it toward the left arm is recorded negative. The view of the heart by the bipolar leads can be compared to a wide-angle camera lens.

The three unipolar frontal plane leads, aVR, aVL, and aVF, are illustrated in Figure 18-3B. The camera represents the location of the positive electrode: on the right shoulder for aVR, on the left shoulder for aVL, and at the foot (left leg) for aVF. The "negative end" of the unipolar lead is a reference spot in the center of the chest that is mathematically determined by the ECG machine. The same principles apply to unipolar leads: any electrical activity traveling toward the

positive electrode is recorded as an upright deflection and any traveling away from it is recorded as a negative deflection. The six unipolar precordial leads are recorded from their locations on the chest as shown in Figure 18-3C. The view of the heart by unipolar leads can be compared to a telephoto lens on the camera, "zooming in" on the electrical activity in the heart.

The hexaxial reference system (or axis wheel) is formed when the six frontal plane leads are moved together in such a way that they bisect each other in the center (Figure 18-4A). Each lead is labeled at its positive end to make it easy to remember where the positive electrode is. In Figure 18-4B, the hexaxial reference system is superimposed over a drawing of the heart to illustrate how each lead views the heart.

The normal sequence of depolarization through the heart begins with an electrical impulse originating in the sinus node, high in the right atrium, and spreading leftward through the left atrium and downward toward the atrioventricular (AV) node, low in the right atrium (Figure 18-5A). Leads I and aVL, with their positive electrodes (camera lens) on the left side of the body, record this leftward electrical activity as an upright P wave, and leads II, III, and aVF, with their positive electrodes at the bottom of the heart, record the downward spread of activity as upright P waves. Lead aVR, with its positive electrode on the right shoulder, sees the electrical activity moving away from it and records a negative P wave.

As the impulse spreads through the AV node, no electrical activity is recorded because the AV node is too small to be recorded by surface leads. As the impulse exits the AV node, it moves through the bundle of His and enters the right and left bundle branches. The left bundle branch sprouts some Purkinje fibers high on the left side of the septum that carry the impulse into the septum and cause it to depolarize first in a left-to-right direction. The electrical impulse then enters the Purkinje system of both ventricular free walls simultaneously and depolarizes them from endocardium to epicardium, as shown by the small arrows through the ventricular wall in Figure 18-5A. The millions of electrical forces travel through the heart in three dimensions simultaneously, but if averaged together they move downward, leftward, and

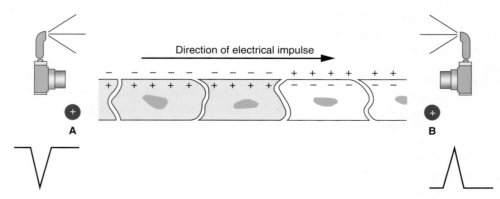

Direction of electrical impulse

A   **B**

Figure 18-2. A strip of cardiac muscle depolarizing in the direction of the arrow. A positive electrode at **(B)** sees depolarization coming toward it and records an upright deflection. A positive electrode at **(A)** sees depolarization going away from it and records a negative deflection.

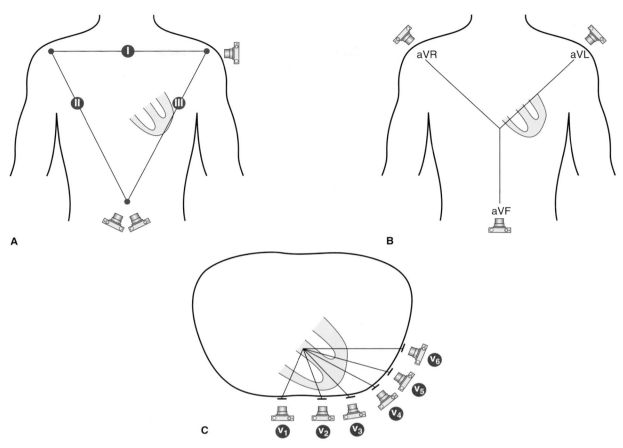

Figure 18-3. The 12 leads of the ECG. The camera represents the location of the positive, or recording, electrode in each lead. **(A)** Bipolar frontal plane leads I, II, and III. **(B)** Unipolar frontal plane leads aVR, aVL, and aVF. **(C)** Unipolar precordial leads V_1 to V_6.

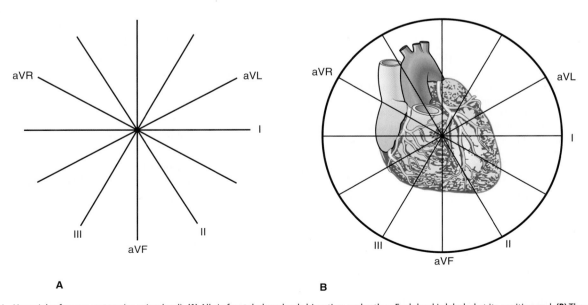

Figure 18-4. Hexaxial reference system (or axis wheel). **(A)** All six frontal plane leads bisecting each other. Each lead is labeled at its positive end. **(B)** The axis wheel superimposed on the heart to demonstrate each lead's view of the heart. Leads I and aVL face the left lateral wall; leads II, III, and aVF face the inferior wall.

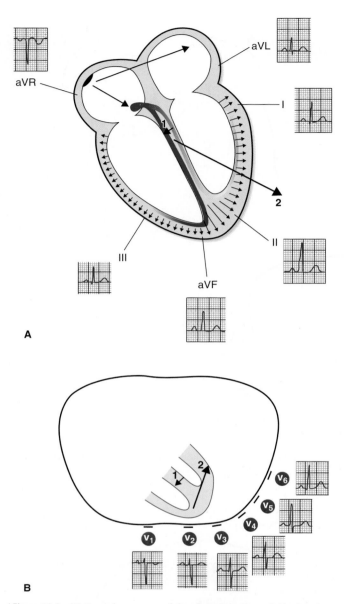

Figure 18-5. (A) Normal sequence of depolarization through the heart as recorded by each of the frontal plane leads. **(B)** Cross-section of the thorax illustrating how the six precordial leads record normal electrical activity in the ventricles. The small arrow (1) shows the initial direction of depolarization through the septum, followed by the direction of ventricular depolarization, indicated by the larger arrow (2).

posteriorly toward the large left ventricle, as indicated by the large arrow in the same figure. This large arrow represents the mean axis, which is the net direction of electrical depolarization through the ventricles when all the smaller arrows are averaged together.

The QRS complex is recorded as the ventricles depolarize. Leads I and aVL, with their positive electrodes on the left side of the body, see the septum depolarizing away from them and record a small negative deflection (Q wave). These leads then see the large left ventricular free wall depolarizing toward them and record an upright deflection

(R wave). Leads II, III, and aVF, with their positive electrodes at the bottom of the heart, may not see septal activity at all and record no deflections. However, if these leads see septal electrical activity coming slightly toward them, they record a positive deflection. As the forces continue moving downward toward leads II, III, and aVF, an upright deflection (R wave) is recorded. Lead aVR, positive on the right shoulder, sees all activity moving away from it and records a negative deflection (QS complex). Figure 18-5A illustrates how the six frontal plane leads record normal electrical activity as it spreads through the atria and ventricles.

The six precordial leads record electrical activity traveling in the horizontal plane. Figure 18-5B illustrates the position of the precordial leads and how they record electrical activity as it spreads through the ventricles. Lead V_1 is located on the front of the chest and records a small R wave as the septum depolarizes toward it from left to right. It then records a deep S wave as depolarization spreads away from it through the thick left ventricle. As the positive electrode is moved across the precordium from the V_1 to the V_6 position, it records progressively more left ventricular forces and the R wave gets progressively larger. Lead V_6 is located on the left side of the chest and may record a small Q wave as the septum depolarizes from left to right away from the positive electrode, and it records a large R wave as electrical activity spreads toward the positive electrode through the thick left ventricle. Normal R wave progression means that the R wave becomes progressively larger from V_1 to V_6, or that the R wave in V_1 is a minimal part of the QRS complex and the R wave in V_6 is the dominant part of the QRS complex.

In addition to P waves and QRS complexes, the ECG records T waves as the ventricles repolarize. Normal T waves are slightly asymmetrical with an ascending limb that is more gradual than the descending limb. T waves are usually upright in leads I, II, and V_{3-6}, and negative in lead aVR. T waves can vary in other leads. A normal T wave is not taller than 5 mm in a limb lead or 10 mm in a chest lead. Tall T waves can indicate hyperkalemia or myocardial ischemia or infarction.

The ST segment begins at the end of the QRS complex (the J point) and ends at the beginning of the T wave. It is normally at the baseline (the isoelectric segment between the T wave and the next P wave) and should not stay on the baseline for longer than 0.12 second (Figure 18-6). The ST segment should gently curve upward into the T wave without forming a sharp angle. Normal ST-segment elevation and depression is discussed under "ST-Segment Monitoring" later in this chapter.

The U wave is sometimes seen following the T wave, and when present it should be smaller than the T wave and point in the same direction as the T wave. U waves are thought to represent repolarization of the midmyocardial cells (M-cells) in the ventricles. Large U waves can be seen in hypokalemia and with certain drugs, like quinidine. Inverted U waves can indicate myocardial ischemia.

Lead II

Lead V₁

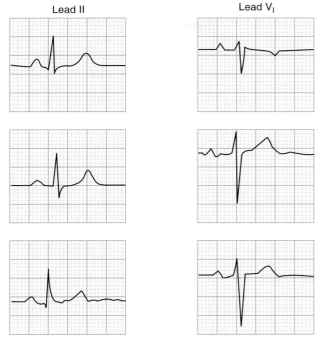

Figure 18-6. Normal ST segment and T waves.

Figure 18-7 shows a normal 12-lead ECG. Normal sinus rhythm is present, and the QRS axis is +45°. P waves are normal (they are flat in V_2, but this is not necessarily abnormal), and T waves are normal. The QRS complex is normal (0.08-second wide), there are no abnormal Q waves, and R-wave progression is normal across the precordium. The ST segment is at baseline in all leads. This ECG is used for comparison as abnormalities are discussed throughout this chapter.

Axis Determination

The *hexaxial reference system* (axis wheel) forms a 360° circle surrounding the heart that by convention is divided into 180 positive degrees (+180°) and 180 negative degrees (−180°) (Figure 18-8). The normal QRS axis is defined as −30° to +90° because most of the electrical forces in a normal heart are directed downward and leftward toward the large left ventricle. Left axis deviation is defined as an axis of −31° to −90° and occurs when most of the forces move in a leftward and superior direction, as can happen in a variety of conditions, such as left ventricular hypertrophy, left anterior fascicular block, inferior myocardial infarction (MI), or left bundle branch block (LBBB) (Table 18-1). Right axis deviation is

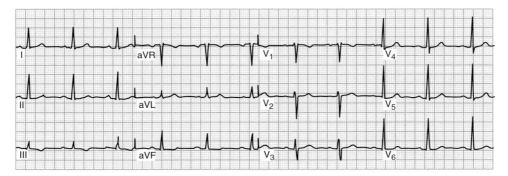

Figure 18-7. Normal 12-lead ECG.

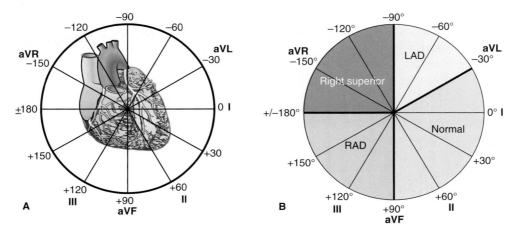

Figure 18-8. **(A)** Degrees of the axis wheel. **(B)** Normal axis = −30° to + 90°; left axis deviation = −31° to −90°; right axis deviation = +91° to +180°; right superior axis = −90° to −180°.

TABLE 18-1. SUMMARY OF CAUSES OF AXIS DEVIATIONS

Axis: −30° to +90°
• Normal

Left Axis Deviation: −31° to −90°
• Left ventricular hypertrophy
• Left anterior fascicular block
• Inferior myocardial infarction
• Left bundle branch block
• Congenital defects
• Ventricular tachycardia
• Wolff-Parkinson-White syndrome

Right Axis Deviation: +91° to +180°
• Right ventricular hypertrophy
• Left posterior fascicular block
• Right bundle branch block
• Dextrocardia
• Ventricular tachycardia
• Wolff-Parkinson-White syndrome

Right Superior Axis: −90° to −180°
• Ventricular tachycardia
• Bifascicular block

defined as +91° to +180° and occurs when most of the forces move rightward, as can happen in conditions such as right ventricular hypertrophy, left posterior fascicular block, and right bundle branch block (RBBB) (see Table 18-1). When most of the forces are directed superior and rightward between −90° and −180°, the term *right superior axis* is used. This axis can occur with ventricular tachycardia and occasionally with bifascicular block.

The mean frontal plane QRS axis can be determined in a number of ways. The most accurate method is to average the forces moving right and left with those moving up and down because this represents the frontal plane, lead I is the "pure" right/left lead, and lead aVF is the "pure" up/down lead; it is easiest to use these two perpendicular leads to calculate the mean axis. Figure 18-9A shows the frontal plane leads of a 12-lead ECG. Leads I and aVF are shown enlarged along with the axis wheel with small dash marks along the axes of lead I and lead aVF (Figure 18-9B). These dash marks

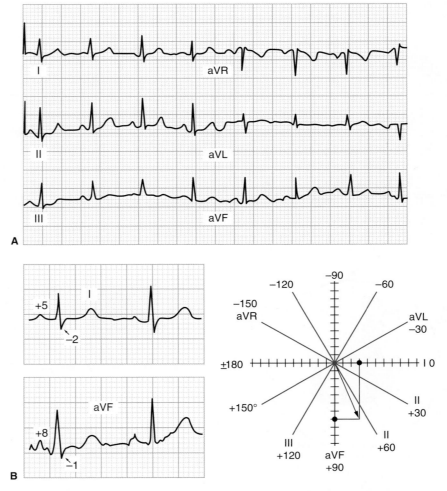

Figure 18-9. Calculating the mean QRS axis. **(A)** The six frontal plane leads of an ECG. **(B)** Leads I and aVF enlarged. See the text for instructions on calculating the axis using leads I and aVF on the axis wheel.

represent the small, 1-mV boxes on the ECG paper. To determine the mean QRS axis, follow these steps:

1. Look at the QRS complex in lead I and count the number of positive and negative boxes. Mark the net vector along the appropriate end of lead I on the axis wheel. In Figure 18-9B, the QRS complex in lead I is five boxes positive and two boxes negative, resulting in a net three boxes positive, or + 3. Count three dash marks toward the positive end of lead I and put a mark on the axis wheel at that spot.
2. Look at the QRS complex in aVF and follow the same procedure as above. In this example, the QRS complex in aVF is eight boxes positive and has two very small negative deflections that equal approximately one box when combined, resulting in a net +7. Count seven dash marks along the positive end of aVF's axis and place a mark at that spot.
3. Draw a perpendicular line down from the mark on lead I's axis and a perpendicular line across from the mark on aVF's axis.
4. Draw a line from the center of the axis wheel to the spot where the two perpendicular lines meet. This line represents the mean QRS axis. In the example in Figure 18-9B, the axis is about +65°.

A quick but less precise method of axis determination is to place the axis in its proper quadrant of the axis wheel by looking at leads I and aVF, because these leads divide the wheel into four quadrants. As illustrated in Figure 18-10, if both of these leads are positive, the axis falls in the normal quadrant, 0° to +90°. If lead I is positive and aVF is negative, the axis falls in the left quadrant, 0° to −90°. If lead I is negative and aVF is positive, the axis falls in the right quadrant, +90° to +180°. If both leads are negative, the axis falls in the right superior quadrant or "no-man's-land" −90° to −180°. Locating the correct quadrant is sometimes adequate, but because 30° of the left quadrant is considered normal, it is necessary to be more precise in describing the axis when it falls in the left quadrant. To "fine-tune" the axis when it is in the left quadrant, look at lead II. If lead II has a positive QRS, the axis is in the normal part of the left quadrant (0 to −30°); if it has a negative QRS, the axis is left deviated (−31° to −90°).

Using the ECG in Figure 18-11A, first place the axis in the appropriate quadrant by using leads I and aVF. Lead I is upright and aVF is negative, placing the axis in the left quadrant. However, because 30° of the left quadrant is considered normal, we need to fine-tune the axis to determine where within the left quadrant it actually falls. Since lead II is mostly negative, the axis is deviated to the left. The axis wheel shows how to count boxes in this example. The axis is −60°.

Using the ECG in Figure 18-11B, place the axis in the appropriate quadrant. Because lead I is negative and aVF is positive, the axis is in the right quadrant. The axis wheel shows how boxes are counted in this example. The axis is +130°.

Bundle Branch Block

When one of the bundle branches is blocked, the ventricles depolarize asynchronously. Bundle branch block is characterized by a delay of excitation to one ventricle and an abnormal spread of electrical activity through the ventricle whose

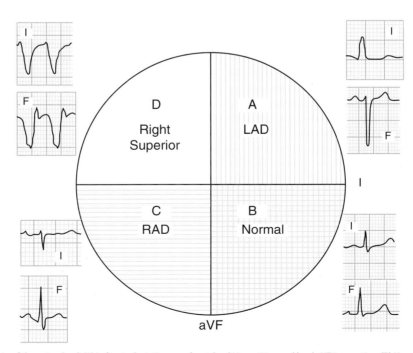

Figure 18-10. The four quadrants of the axis wheel. **(A)** Left axis deviation quadrant; lead I is positive and lead aVF is negative. **(B)** Normal axis quadrant; leads I and aVF are both positive. **(C)** Right axis deviation quadrant; lead I is negative and lead aVF is positive. **(D)** Right superior quadrant; leads I and aVF are both negative. (*Reproduced with permission from Marriott HJL. Practical Electrocardiography, 8th ed. Baltimore, MD: Williams & Wilkins; 1988.*)

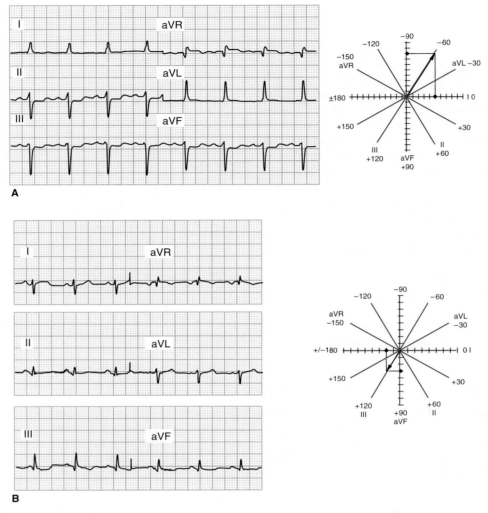

A

B

Figure 18-11. **(A)** Frontal plane leads demonstrating left axis deviation. Lead I is five boxes positive; aVF is two boxes positive and ten boxes negative for a net of −8. The axis is −60°. **(B)** Frontal plane leads demonstrating right axis deviation. Lead I is two boxes positive and four boxes negative for a net of −2; lead aVF is one box negative and four boxes positive for a net of +3. The axis is +120°.

bundle is blocked. This delayed conduction results in widening of the QRS complex to 0.12 second or more and a characteristic pattern best recognized in precordial leads V_1 and V_6 and limb leads I and aVL.

Normal ventricular depolarization as recorded by leads V_1 and V_6 is illustrated in Figure 18-12. The positive electrode for V_1 is located on the front of the chest at the fourth intercostal space to the right of the sternum, close to the right ventricle. The positive electrode for V_6 is located in the left midaxillary line at the fifth intercostal space, close to the left ventricle. Lead V_1 records a small R wave as the septum depolarizes from left to right toward the positive electrode. It then records a negative deflection (S wave) as the main forces travel away from the positive electrode toward the left ventricle, resulting in the normal rS complex in V_1. Lead V_6 may record a small Q wave as the septum depolarizes left to right away from the positive electrode. It then records a tall R wave as the main forces travel toward the left ventricle, resulting in

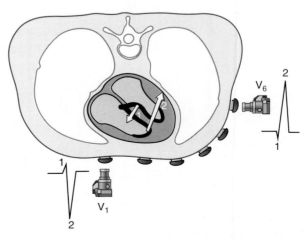

Figure 18-12. Normal ventricular depolarization as recorded by leads V_1 and V_6.

the normal qR complex in V₆. When both ventricles depolarize together, the QRS width is less than 0.12 second.

Right Bundle Branch Block

The presence of a block in the right bundle branch causes a different spread of electrical forces in the ventricles and thus a different pattern to the QRS complex. Three separate forces occur, as seen in Figure 18-13A.

1. Septal activation occurs first from left to right (*arrow 1*), resulting in the normal small R wave in V_1 and small Q wave in V_6.
2. The left ventricle is activated next through the normally functioning left bundle branch. Depolarization spreads normally through the Purkinje fibers in the left ventricle (*arrow 2*), causing an S wave in V_1 as the impulse travels away from its positive electrode and an R wave in V_6 as the impulse travels toward the positive electrode in V_6.
3. The right ventricle depolarizes late and abnormally as the impulse spreads via cell-to-cell conduction through the right ventricle (*arrow 3*). This abnormal activation causes a wide second R wave (called R prime [R′]) in V_1 as it travels toward the positive electrode in V_1. It also results in a wide S wave in V_6 as it travels away from the positive electrode in V_6. Because muscle cell-to-cell conduction is much slower than conduction through the Purkinje system, the QRS complex widens to 0.12 second or greater.

RBBB can be recognized by a wide rSR′ pattern in V_1 and a wide qRs pattern in V_6, I, and aVL, because the positive electrode in these two limb leads is located on the left side of the body. The ECG in Figure 18-13B illustrates RBBB.

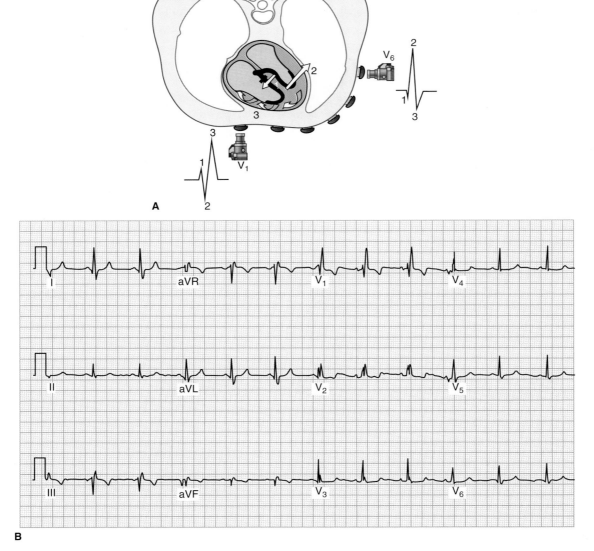

Figure 18-13. **(A)** Ventricular depolarization with RBBB as recorded by leads V_1 and V_6. **(B)** 12-lead ECG illustrating RBBB.

Left Bundle Branch Block

Figure 18-14 illustrates the spread of electrical forces through the ventricles when the left bundle branch is blocked. In LBBB, the septum does not depolarize in its normal left-to-right direction because the block occurs above the Purkinje fibers that normally activate the left side of the septum. This results in the loss of the normal small R wave in V_1 and loss of the Q wave in V_6, I, and aVL. Two main forces occur in LBBB:

1. The right ventricle is activated first through the Purkinje fibers (*arrow 1*). Because the right ventricular free wall is so much thinner than that of the left ventricle, forces traveling through it are often not recorded in V_1. Sometimes a small, narrow R wave is recorded in V_1 during LBBB, and this wave is most likely the result of forces traveling through the right ventricular free wall.
2. The left ventricle depolarizes late and abnormally as the impulse spreads via cell-to-cell conduction through the thick left ventricle (*arrow 2*). This causes V_1 to record a wide negative QS complex as the impulse travels away from its positive electrode. The lateral leads V_6, I, and aVL record a wide R wave as the impulse travels through the large left ventricle toward their positive electrodes. The QRS widens to 0.12 second or greater due to the slow cell-to-cell conduction in the left ventricle.

LBBB can be recognized by a wide QS complex in V_1 and wide R waves with no Q waves in V_6, I, and aVL. The ECG in Figure 18-14B illustrates LBBB.

Acute Coronary Syndrome

The term *acute coronary syndrome* (ACS) is used to refer to the pathophysiologic continuum that begins with plaque rupture in a coronary artery and ultimately results in cell necrosis (infarction), if the process is not arrested. ACS encompasses three distinct phases of this continuum: (1) unstable angina (UA), (2) non–ST-elevation MI (NSTEMI), and (3) ST-elevation MI (STEMI). The terms STEMI and

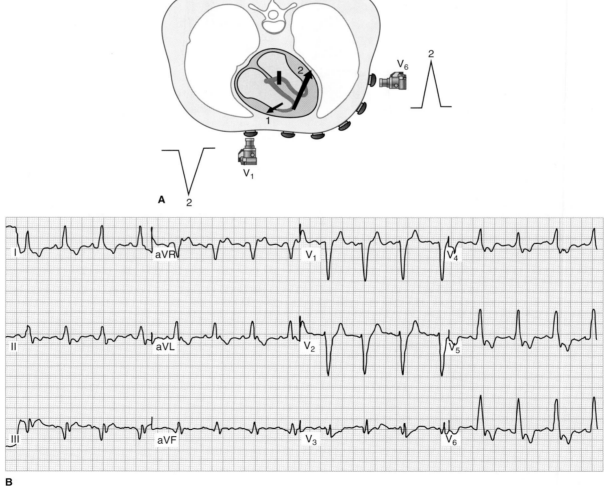

Figure 18-14. **(A)** Ventricular depolarization with LBBB as recorded by leads V_1 and V_6. **(B)** 12-lead ECG illustrating LBBB.

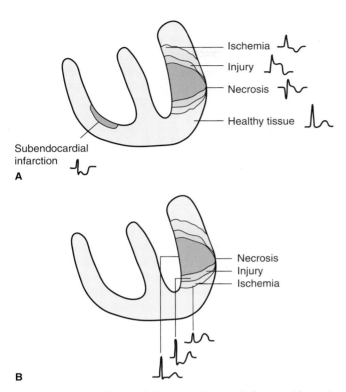

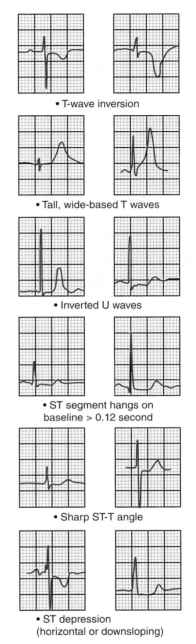

Figure 18-15. Zones of myocardial ischemia, injury, and infarction with associated ECG changes. **(A)** Indicative changes of ischemia, injury, and necrosis seen in leads facing the injured area. **(B)** Reciprocal changes often seen in leads not directly facing the involved area.

Figure 18-16. ECG patterns associated with myocardial ischemia.

NSTEMI refer to the presence or absence of ST elevation on the admission ECG in a patient who is having an MI as diagnosed by elevated biochemical markers in the blood. Once an infarction has occurred, the terms Q-wave or non–Q-wave MI indicate the ultimate presence or absence of Q waves on the ECG.

MI can occur because of blockage of a coronary artery with thrombus or from severe and prolonged ischemia due to coronary artery spasm or unrelieved obstruction of a coronary artery. When infarction does occur, there are three "zones" of tissue damage, each of which produces characteristic changes on the ECG (Figure 18-15).

Myocardial ischemia can result in several changes on the ECG (Figure 18-16). The most familiar patterns of ischemia are horizontal or downsloping ST-segment depression of 0.5 mm or more, and T-wave inversion. Other indicators of ischemia include an ST segment that remains on the baseline longer than 0.12 second; an ST segment that forms a sharp angle with the upright T wave; tall, wide-based T waves; and inverted U waves.

Myocardial injury is most often indicated by ST-segment elevation of 1 mm or more above the baseline in leads facing the infarcted area (Figure 18-17). Other signs of acute injury include a straightening of the ST segment that slopes up to the peak of the T wave without spending any time on the baseline; tall, peaked T waves; and symmetric T-wave inversion.

Necrosis or death of myocardial tissue is indicated on the ECG by development of Q waves that are greater than 0.03 second wide or 25% of the ensuing R-wave amplitude (see Figures 18-5A and 18-9 for normal Q waves and Figures 18-18 and 18-19 for abnormal Q waves). Q waves can develop transiently with severe ischemia and with non–Q wave MI, although Q waves are more commonly seen with necrosis that extends through the full thickness of the myocardial wall (transmural infarction). Necrosis that involves just the endocardial layer of the myocardium typically does not result in Q waves on the ECG and is referred to as a non–Q wave MI. In any case, the presence of abnormal

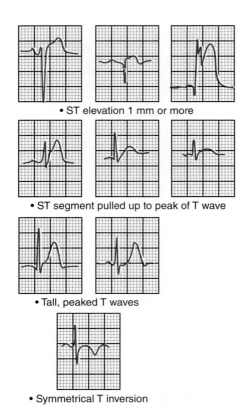

- ST elevation 1 mm or more

- ST segment pulled up to peak of T wave

- Tall, peaked T waves

- Symmetrical T inversion

Figure 18-17. ECG patterns associated with acute myocardial injury.

Q waves is still considered to be ECG evidence of myocardial necrosis.

The ECG reflects the evolution of the infarction from the acute stage through the fully evolved stage. Very early MI often causes peaking and widening of the T waves followed within minutes by ST-segment elevation. ST-segment elevation can persist for hours to several days but resolves more quickly with successful reperfusion. Once the ST segment has returned to baseline, ECG evidence of the acute infarction stage is lost. Q waves appear within hours of pain onset and usually remain forever, although sometimes Q waves disappear with very early reperfusion. T-wave inversion occurs within hours after infarction and can last for months. T waves often return to their previous upright position within a few months after acute MI. Thus, an *evolving infarct* is one in which serial ECGs show ST segments returning toward baseline, the development of Q waves, and T-wave inversion. The term *old infarction* or *infarct of undetermined age* is used when the first ECG recorded shows Q waves, ST segment at baseline, and T waves either inverted or upright, indicating that an MI occurred at some point in the past.

Locating the Infarction From the ECG

ST-segment elevation, Q waves, and T-wave inversion are recorded in leads facing the damaged myocardium and are called the *indicative changes of infarction*. Leads not facing the involved tissue often show changes related to the loss of electrical forces (depolarization and repolarization) in the damaged tissue. These leads record mirror-image changes that are called *reciprocal changes*. Figure 18-15 illustrates indicative and reciprocal changes associated with MI, and Table 18-2 lists leads in which indicative and reciprocal changes are found in each of the major types of MI.

Anterior wall MI is recognized by indicative changes in leads facing the anterior wall precordial leads V_1 to V_4 (see Figure 18-18). Reciprocal changes are often recorded in the

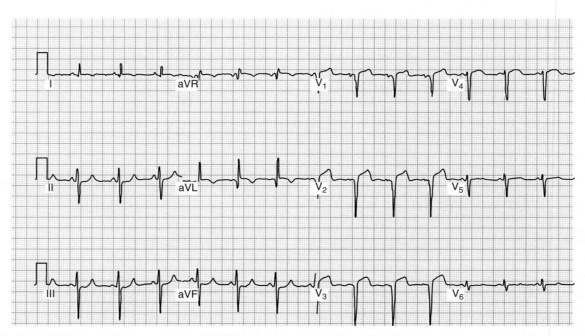

Figure 18-18. 12-lead ECG demonstrating acute anterior wall MI. Q waves are present in V_1 to V_3 and ST-segment elevation is present in V_1 to V_4. An abnormal Q wave is also present in aVL.

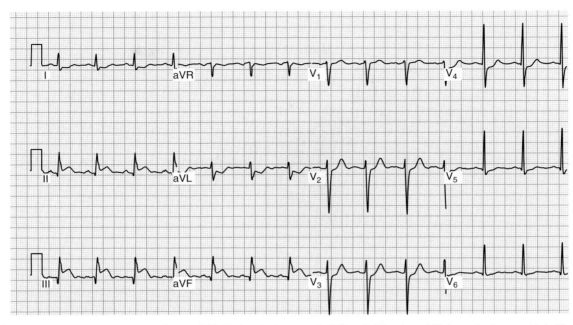

Figure 18-19. 12-lead ECG demonstrating acute inferior wall MI. ST elevation is present in II, III, and aVF; reciprocal ST depression is present in I, aVL, and V_2 to V_4. Q waves can be seen in III and aVF.

TABLE 18-2. ECG CHANGES ASSOCIATED WITH MYOCARDIAL INFARCTION

Location of MI	Indicative Changes (ST Elevation)	Reciprocal Changes (ST Depression)
Anterior	V_1-V_4 (not necessarily all of these leads) aVR with proximal LAD occlusion	II, III, aVF, V5 with proximal LAD occlusion
Septal	V_1, V_2	V_5 with proximal LAD occlusion
Anterolateral	V_1-V_6, I, aVL	II, III, aVF
Inferior	II, III, aVF	I, aVL
Posterior	Posterior leads V_8, V_9	V_1-V_3
Lateral	I, aVL, V_5, V_6	II, III, aVF
Right ventricle	Right side leads V_3R-V_6R	

inferior leads II, III, and aVF, and sometimes in V_5 with proximal left anterior descending (LAD) artery stenosis. Inferior wall MI is diagnosed by indicative changes in leads II, III, and aVF (see Figure 18-19), and reciprocal changes are often seen in leads I and aVL. Lateral wall MI presents with indicative changes in leads I, aVL, and/or V_5 and V_6, with reciprocal changes in leads II, III, and aVF (Figure 18-20). Posterior wall MI is less obvious because in the standard 12-lead ECG there are no leads that face the posterior wall, and therefore there are no indicative changes recorded (Figure 18-21). The diagnosis is suspected when ST segment depression is present in the anterior leads, especially V_1 and V_2 but often all the way to V_4. Reciprocal changes seen in these leads include a taller R wave than normal (mirror image of the Q wave

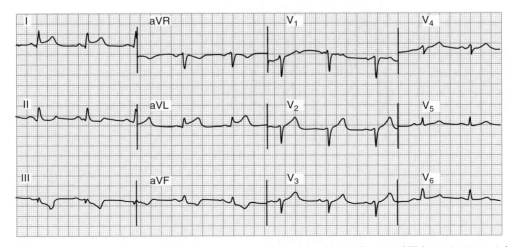

Figure 18-20. 12-lead ECG demonstrating acute lateral wall MI. ST elevation is present in leads I and aVL, and reciprocal ST depression is seen in leads II, III, and aVF.

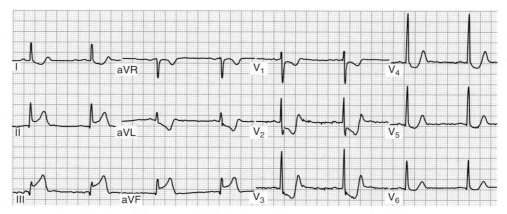

Figure 18-21. 12-lead ECG demonstrating acute inferior and posterior MI. ST elevation is present in leads II, III, and aVF (inferior leads), and ST depression is present in all of the V leads. ST depression in V_1 to V_3 is indicative of posterior MI. The ST depression in V_4 to V_6 is reciprocal to the inferior MI.

that would be recorded over the posterior wall), ST-segment depression (mirror image of the ST elevation from the posterior wall), and upright, tall T waves (mirror image of the T-wave inversion from the posterior wall). Posterior leads V_7, V_8, and V_9 should be recorded whenever posterior wall MI is suspected (Figure 18-23B).

Right ventricular MI occurs in up to 45% of inferior MIs; therefore, it usually is associated with indicative changes in the inferior leads II, III, and aVF (Figure 18-22). In addition, it is not uncommon to see ST elevation in V_1 as well, because V_1 is the chest lead that is closest to the right ventricle. ST elevation in V_1, together with ST elevation in the inferior leads, is suspicious for right ventricular MI. Another clue is discordance between the ST segment in V_1 and the ST segment in V_2.

Normally, when the ST segment in V_1 is elevated, it is related to anterior or septal MI, in which case the ST in V_2 is also elevated. *Discordance* means that the ST segments do not point in the same direction—V_1 shows ST elevation while V_2 is either normal or shows ST depression. This finding is suspicious for right ventricular MI. The American Heart Association (AHA) and the American College of Cardiology (ACC) have recommended that right-sided chest leads V_3R and V_4R be recorded in all patients presenting with ECG evidence of acute inferior wall infarction. Leads V_3R through V_6R develop ST elevation when acute right ventricular MI is present. Lead V_4R is the most sensitive and specific lead for recognition of right ventricular MI. Figure 18-23A shows location of right-sided chest leads and Figure 18-23B shows location of posterior leads.

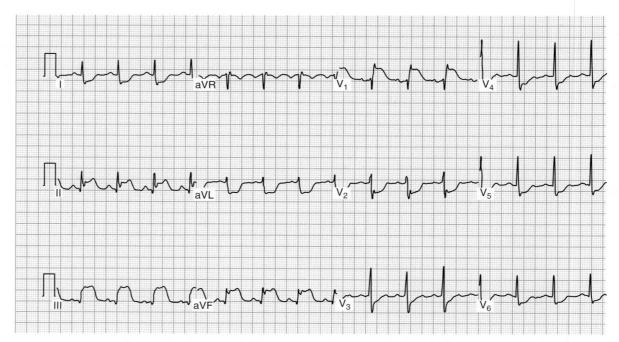

Figure 18-22. 12-lead ECG demonstrating acute right ventricular MI. ST elevation is present in II, III, aVF, and V_1; reciprocal ST depression is present in all other leads. Note the discordant ST elevation in V_1 and ST depression in V_2.

ESSENTIAL CONTENT CASE

Acute MI

You are caring for a patient who is admitted with acute chest pain. His VS are stable but he is complaining of 8/10 chest pain, which began 2 hours ago and has steadily increased. This is his initial ECG (A):

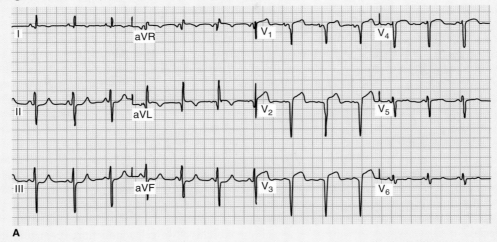

A

The cath lab is not yet ready for this patient, so while waiting to transport him you initiate ST segment monitoring. The ST segment alarm rings and when you check the patient you see higher ST elevation on the monitor. You get another ECG (B):

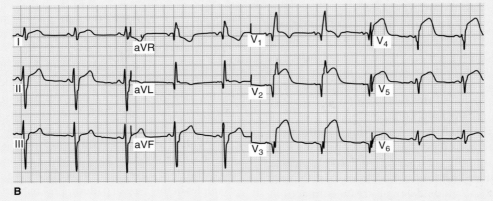

B

Case Question 1: What is your interpretation of the initial ECG (A), rhythm, QRS axis, bundle branch block, and ST segments?

Case Question 2: What would be a good lead for ST segment monitoring in this patient? Describe how to initiate ST segment monitoring.

Case Question 3: What is your interpretation of the second ECG (B), rhythm, QRS axis, bundle branch block, and ST segments?

Case Question 4: What is the significance of these changes and what complications can result?

Answers
1. The rhythm is sinus rhythm in the 80s. The QRS axis is about −45°. There is no bundle branch block present. There is ST segment elevation in leads V_2 to V_4 and slight ST depression in leads II, III, and aVF. The interpretation is anterior wall STEMI.
2. Since this is an anterior wall MI, lead V_3 is the best lead for ST segment monitoring. If you only have one V lead available, then you will lose your best dysrhythmia monitoring lead (V_1), but V_3 would be a good choice for ST segment monitoring. The ST baseline reference point should be the patient's current ST segment levels (not the isoelectric line) so that if there is any change from the current ST position, the monitor will alarm. The ST measuring point is 0.06 second (60 msec) after the J point (the point where the QRS ends and the ST segment begins).
3. The rhythm is sinus rhythm. The QRS axis has shifted even more leftward and is now about −70°. There is now RBBB. The combination of significant left axis deviation and RBBB indicates probable bifascicular block: RBBB and left anterior hemiblock. The ST segments are even higher now and ST elevation extends all the way from V_2 to V_6.
4. The higher ST segment elevation indicates extension of the MI. Bifascicular block means that two of the three pathways of conduction into the ventricle are blocked, creating a high potential for third degree AV block. This patient needs to get to the cath lab and get his artery opened!

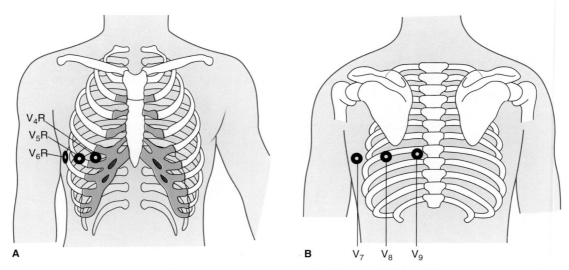

Figure 18-23. **(A)** Right side chest leads. V$_4$R at right fifth intercostal space, mid clavicular line; V$_5$R at right fifth intercostal space, anterior axillary line; V$_6$R at right fifth intercostal space, midaxillary line. **(B)** Posterior leads: V$_7$ at posterior axillary line; V$_8$ at tip of scapula; V$_9$ next to spine.

Preexcitation Syndromes

Preexcitation means early activation of the ventricle by supraventricular impulses that reach the ventricle through an accessory conduction pathway faster than they travel through the AV node. Many people have tracts of tissue, often referred to as "bypass tracts" or "accessory pathways," that can carry electrical impulses directly from atria to ventricles, bypassing the delay in the AV node and causing early and abnormal depolarization of the ventricles. These accessory pathways can be found anywhere around the tricuspid or mitral valve rings. The most common type of preexcitation syndrome is the Wolff-Parkinson-White syndrome, in which the impulse travels down the accessory pathway from the atria directly into the ventricles, completely bypassing AV node delay. Other anatomic connections exist that can bypass the normal AV node delay or create connections between different parts of the conduction system and the ventricles and cause variations of the preexcitation pattern. Fibers originating in the atria and inserting into the bundle of His have been demonstrated anatomically and can result in a short PR interval and normal QRS complex (formerly called Lown-Ganong-Levine syndrome).

Wolff-Parkinson-White Syndrome

In Wolff-Parkinson-White syndrome, the ventricle is stimulated prematurely by an electrical impulse traveling through the accessory pathway while the impulse simultaneously descends normally through the AV node (Figure 18-24A). Impulses travel faster through the accessory pathway because they bypass the normal AV node delay. Part of the ventricle receives the impulse early via the accessory pathway and begins to depolarize before the rest of the ventricle is activated through the His-Purkinje system. Early stimulation of the ventricle results in a short PR interval and a widened QRS complex as the impulse begins to depolarize the ventricle via

muscle cell-to-cell conduction. Premature stimulation of the ventricle causes a characteristic slurring of the initial part of the QRS complex, called a delta wave. The remainder of the QRS complex is normal because the rest of the ventricle is depolarized normally through the Purkinje system. This preexcitation results in ventricular fusion beats as the ventricles are depolarized simultaneously by the impulse coming through the accessory pathway and through the normal AV node. The degree of preexcitation varies, depending on the relative rates of conduction down the accessory pathway and through the AV node, and it determines the length of the PR interval and size of the delta wave (Figure 18-24).

Wolff-Parkinson-White syndrome is recognized on the ECG by the presence of a short PR interval (< 0.12 second) and delta waves in many leads. Figure 18-25 shows two examples of this type of pattern. Preexcitation syndromes are clinically significant because the presence of two pathways into the ventricle is a setup for reentrant tachycardias, which occur frequently in people with accessory pathways and are a part of the "syndrome" of Wolff-Parkinson-White. See the section Supraventricular Tachycardias later in this chapter for more information on dysrhythmias associated with accessory pathways.

Treatment

Wolff-Parkinson-White syndrome does not require treatment unless it is associated with symptomatic tachycardias. Specific therapy depends on the mechanism of the tachyarrhythmia, the effect of drugs on conduction through the AV node and the accessory pathway, and on the patient's tolerance of the dysrhythmia. The section on supraventricular tachycardias later in this chapter discusses drug treatment of tachycardias associated with accessory pathways.

Radiofrequency (RF) catheter ablation of the bypass tract provides a cure for the tachyarrhythmias associated

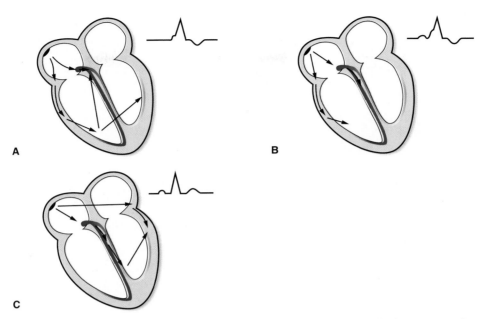

Figure 18-24. Varying degrees of preexcitation. **(A)** Maximal preexcitation when the ventricles are activated totally by the accessory pathway. **(B)** Less-than-maximal preexcitation when the ventricles are activated by the impulse traveling through both the accessory pathway and the normal AV conduction system. **(C)** Concealed accessory pathway. The ventricles are activated through the normal AV conduction system with no participation of the accessory pathway, resulting in a normal PR interval and normal QRS complex.

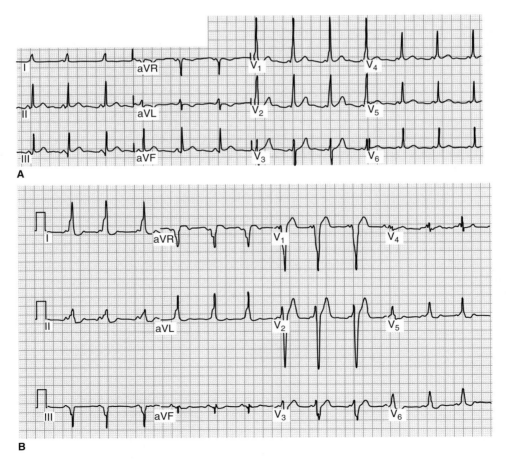

Figure 18-25. (A) 12-lead ECG demonstrating Wolff-Parkinson-White syndrome with short PR interval and delta waves. Lead V_1 is positive, indicating a posterior accessory pathway. **(B)** Wolff-Parkinson-White syndrome with short PR and delta waves with a negative V_1, indicating an anterior or right-sided accessory pathway.

Type 1   Type 2

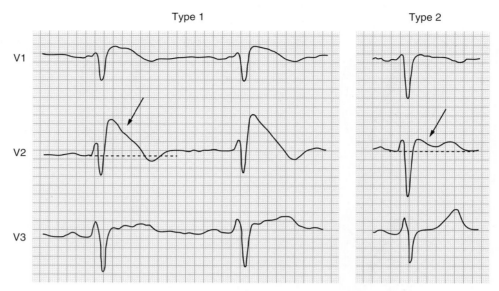

Figure 18-26. Two ECG patterns of Brugada syndrome. Type I shows the coved ST segment elevation and T-wave inversion and is considered the diagnostic pattern. Type 2 shows the saddle-back type ST elevation with an inverted T wave in V_1 and upright T wave in V_2.

with accessory pathways in many patients. RF ablation is an invasive procedure that requires the introduction of several catheters into the heart through the venous and sometimes arterial systems. An electrophysiology study is done first to record intracardiac signals and determine the mechanism of the tachycardia. The electrophysiology study confirms the presence and location of the accessory pathway, participation of the pathway in maintaining the tachycardia, and conduction characteristics of the accessory pathway. A special ablation catheter is then positioned next to the bypass tract and RF energy is delivered through the catheter to the tract, destroying the tissue and preventing it from being able to conduct. Permanent tissue damage in the accessory pathway is the goal of RF ablation, and when successful, it prevents further episodes of tachycardia.

Brugada Syndrome

Brugada syndrome is an inherited channelopathy involving mutations of the SCN5A gene that participates in regulation of cardiac sodium channels. It is associated with a high incidence of VT/VF and sudden cardiac death (SCD) in people with structurally normal hearts. BrS is estimated

to be responsible for at least 4% of all sudden deaths and at least 20% of sudden deaths in patients with structurally normal hearts. It is seen worldwide but is most prevalent in Southeast Asia, occurs most often in men (8:1 male to female ratio), and typically manifests in the third or fourth decade of life.

BrS is characterized by ST-segment elevation and an RBBB-type QRS pattern in leads V_1 to V_3, typically without the dominant S waves in the lateral leads that is seen with true RBBB. Three patterns of ST elevation were initially described, but current consensus is that there are two patterns typical of BrS (Figure 18-26): (1) type 1 ECG pattern with a coved ST segment elevation more than or equal to 2 mm, descending with an upward convexity into a negative T wave; (2) type 2 ECG pattern with a saddle-back shaped ST elevation of more than or equal to 0.5 mm followed by an upright or biphasic T wave. Only the type 1 pattern is considered diagnostic (Figure 18-27). BrS is diagnosed by the presence of a type 1 or coved-type ST-segment elevation in more than one right precordial lead (V_1-V_3) plus one of the following conditions: documented VF or polymorphic VT, a family history of SCD at a young age (< 45 years), a

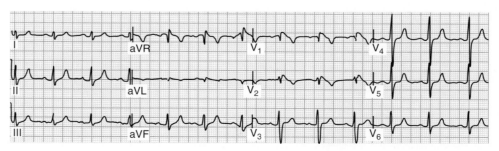

Figure 18-27. 12-lead ECG showing type I Brugada pattern in a young man with syncope.

type 1 ECG in family members, otherwise unexplained syncope, nocturnal agonal respiration, or inducibility of VT/VF with programmed electrical stimulation. The diagnosis is also considered positive when a type 2 ECG pattern present at baseline converts to the diagnostic type 1 pattern after sodium channel blocker administration, along with one or more of the above clinical criteria. These characteristic ECG changes are transient or variable in some patients, thus the ECG can be non-diagnostic even when BrS is present.

The mainstay of therapy for BrS is an implantable cardioverter defibrillator (ICD). ICD implantation is a class I recommendation for survivors of cardiac arrest due to VF or hemodynamically unstable sustained VT not because of a reversible cause, and a class IIa recommendation for patients with BrS who have had syncope or documented VT. Quinidine is the only drug that has been shown to be effective in preventing ventricular dysrhythmias in patients with BrS. The best way to manage asymptomatic BrS patients is still debated.

The QT Interval and Long-QT Syndromes

The QT interval is measured from the beginning of the QRS complex to the end of the T wave and is used clinically as a reflection of ventricular repolarization time. The QT interval is heart rate dependent; it shortens at faster heart rates and lengthens at slower heart rates, therefore, the measured QT interval must be corrected for heart rate (QTc = QT corrected for heart rate). A normal QTc is less than 0.46 second (460 msec) in women and less than 0.45 second (450 msec) in men. A prolonged QTc indicates abnormally prolonged ventricular repolarization and is associated with torsades de pointes (TdP) and SCD. The most commonly used method of correcting the measured QT interval for heart rate is the Bazett formula:

QTc = measured QT interval divided by the square root of the preceding R-R interval (all measurements in seconds).

Figure 18-28 illustrates how to use the Bazett formula. A QTc more than 500 msec increases the risk of developing TdP.

Long-QT syndrome (LQTS) can be acquired or congenital. The acquired type is usually due to medications that prolong ventricular repolarization or to electrolyte abnormalities, especially hypokalemia or hypomagnesemia. The congenital type is owing to gene mutations that affect ion channels on the cardiac cell membrane and is hereditary. Both types of QT-interval prolongation increase the risk of TdP and can be a cause of SCD.

The AHA's practice standards for ECG monitoring in hospital settings lists the following indications for QT-interval monitoring:

1. Initiation of a medication known to cause TdP
2. Overdose from potentially proarrhythmic agents
3. New-onset bradyarrhythmias
4. Severe hypokalemia or hypomagnesemia

Each facility should develop a protocol that defines a single consistent method of QT-interval monitoring that is used by all practitioners responsible for cardiac monitoring.

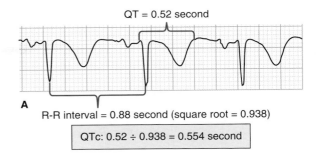

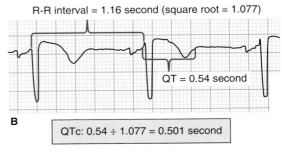

Figure 18-28. Two examples showing Bazett correction for measured QT intervals.

The protocol should define the equipment used (manual or electronic), the method for determining the end of the T wave, the formula for heart-rate correction, criteria for lead selection, and require that whichever lead is chosen should be used for serial measurements in the same patient.

The American Association of Critical-Care Nurses (AACN) practice alert on dysrhythmia monitoring in adults lists the following guidelines for QT interval monitoring:

1. Measure QT interval and calculate QTc (rate-adjusted QT interval) by using the same lead where there is a T-wave amplitude of at least 2 mm and a clearly identified T-wave end.
2. Do not include a distinctly separate U wave in the measurement of the QT interval.
3. Assess and document QTc at least once per shift in patients who meet criteria for QT interval monitoring as identified in the American Heart Association Scientific Statement: Practice Standards for Electrocardiographic Monitoring in Hospital Settings. Also consider QTc monitoring as a routine practice in patients with one or more risk factors for TdP.
4. Assess QTc more frequently in patients with baseline QTc prolongation, the initiation or dosage increase of a drug that prolongs QTc, or in patients with other warning signs for TdP observed on the monitor.
5. Assess QTc before and after administration of a medication that prolongs the QTc by using the same lead, the same device, and the same formula for heart-rate correction.
6. Use QTc to differentiate TdP from polymorphic ventricular tachycardia (PVT) with normal QT interval.

7. Report a QTc greater than 0.50 second (500 msec) or any increase in the QTc of more than 0.06 second (60 msec) after administration of a QTc-prolonging medication. Report any new finding of a QTc greater than 0.50 second (500 msec).

8. Review the patient's medication list for actual or potential QT-prolonging medications whenever QT prolongation is a concern. Consider collaboration with a clinical pharmacist when reviewing the medication profile.

Acquired Long-QT Syndrome

The most common cause of acquired LQTS is pharmacologic therapy. Many medications prolong the QT interval by inhibiting potassium channels that are responsible for repolarization of cardiac cells. The most common classes of drugs that prolong the QT interval and cause TdP include antiarrhythmics, antibiotics, antipsychotic and antidepressant drugs, antihistamines, and gastric motility agents. A list of drugs commonly associated with Tdp is available at www.crediblemeds.com but also may be found in selected drug references and/or hospital pharmacies. Episodes of TdP in the acquired form of LQTS are most commonly precipitated by short-long RR intervals, such as those caused by a ventricular premature beat (short cycle) followed by a compensatory pause (long cycle). Episodes of TdP are also associated with bradycardia or frequent pauses in the rhythm, thus, the acquired type is commonly referred to as pause-dependent LQTS.

The risk of developing TdP from medications increases in the presence of hypokalemia or hypomagnesemia, high doses or rapid intravenous (IV) infusion of QT prolonging agents, or combined use of multiple medications that also prolong the QT interval or slow medication metabolism. Other risk factors for TdP include heart failure (HF) or myocardial ischemia, liquid protein weight-loss diets or starvation, bradycardia or sudden pauses in rhythm, acute neurological events (eg, subarachnoid hemorrhage), older age, female sex, and genetic predisposition to QT prolongation. Significant changes in QTc after initiation of a medication associated with TdP include an increase in QTc of more than 60 msec from the baseline QTc, or a QTc more than 500 msec. Other warning signs of TdP during medication administration include widening or distortion of the T wave, development of enlarged U waves or T-U waves, exaggerated T-U wave distortion on beats terminating pauses, T-wave alternans (alternating T-wave amplitude from beat to beat), and premature ventricular contraction (PVC) couplets or short runs of polymorphic VT occurring on the T wave of the beat terminating a pause.

Treatment of TdP includes identifying and managing the cause, discontinuing any causative agents, and correcting electrolyte imbalances. IV magnesium can be administered to control episodes of TdP until the cause is corrected. Overdrive atrial or ventricular pacing at a rate of 80 beats/min or faster can prevent the pauses that may precipitate episodes of TdP and cause the QT interval to shorten as the heart rate is increased. Pacing and magnesium are temporary management strategies until the cause is eliminated. If TdP becomes sustained or degenerates into VF, defibrillation with an unsynchronized shock is required to terminate the episode.

Congenital Long-QT Syndromes

Congenital LQTS involves mutations in several genes that control potassium or sodium channels on cardiac cells. Thirteen different types of congenital LQTS have been identified and are named LQT1 through LQT13. The three most common are LQT1, LQT2, and LQT3, which are responsible for up to 90% of genotyped cases of LQTS. LQT1 and LQT2 are due to mutations of genes that affect potassium channel function (KCNQ1 and KCNH2), and LQT3 is because of mutations of the SCN5A gene that affects sodium channel function. The three main types of mutations all present with long QT intervals but differ from each other in several ways. The ECG in LQT1 often has wide, broad-based T waves that cause the prolonged QT interval, and dysrhythmia events often occur during physical activity, especially swimming or diving. In LQT2, the ECG often shows notched T waves in multiple leads, and dysrhythmia events are typically triggered by emotional upset or loud noises, such as alarm clocks or telephones. LQT3 usually shows long-ST segments, which are responsible for the long-QT interval, and dysrhythmia events commonly occur at rest or during sleep. T wave abnormalities are often present in all three types. There is overlap between these types in terms of ECG and clinical presentation. Figure 18-29 illustrates the three main types of congenital LQTS.

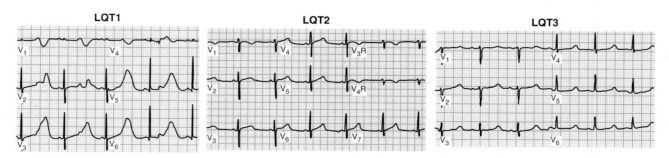

Figure 18-29. Representative V leads from the three major types of LQTS. The LQT1 patient is a 2-year-old girl who is in second-degree AV block with 2:1 conduction. The LQT2 patient is a 13-year-old girl who had a cardiac arrest at a slumber party. The LQT3 patient is a 17-year-old boy who had a "seizure."

Patients with congenital LQTS often present in childhood or in their teens. They may be asymptomatic and their LQTS is incidentally discovered when they are screened after a syncopal episode or when a family member is diagnosed with LQTS. Symptoms can range from palpitations and dizziness to seizures to cardiac arrest. The diagnosis is made by family history and a careful review of symptoms, triggering events if they can be identified, and the ECG. Genetic testing can identify the genotype and help direct therapy.

Treatment depends on severity of symptoms and risk stratification. Lifestyle modifications include avoiding competitive sports and extreme exertion, especially swimming in LQT1 patients. Patients with LQT2 should avoid startling loud noises such as alarm clocks or telephones. Hypokalemia and hypomagnesemia must be avoided, and electrolyte loss due to vomiting, sweating, etc, should be replaced. All LQTS patients should avoid medications known to prolong the QT interval. Beta-blockers are the mainstay of medical therapy for all patients with LQTS and are especially effective in decreasing the incidence of exercise-induced events and SCD in LQT1 and LQT2 patients. They are less effective in LQT3. ICD implantation is a class I recommendation for any patient who has had a cardiac arrest owing to VT or VF in which no reversible cause is identified. ICD is a class IIa recommendation for patients with long-QT syndrome who have syncope and/or VT while receiving beta-blockers.

ADVANCED DYSRHYTHMIA INTERPRETATION

The study of cardiac rhythms provides a never-ending challenge to those interested in learning about dysrhythmias. In most basic ECG classes, the content presented is limited to basic rhythms originating in the sinus node, atria, AV junction, and ventricles, and to basic AV conduction abnormalities, all of which are described in Chapter 3 of this text. Rarely does time permit the inclusion of more advanced concepts. This section discusses some of these more advanced concepts of dysrhythmia interpretation and provides clues to aid in recognition of selected dysrhythmias not usually covered in a basic course.

Supraventricular Tachycardias

Supraventricular tachycardia (SVT) describes a rapid rhythm that arises above the level of the ventricles (atria or AV junction) or utilizes the atria or AV node as part of the circuit that maintains the tachycardia but whose exact origin is not known. Usually, SVT is used to describe a narrow QRS tachycardia where atrial activity (P waves) cannot be identified, and therefore the origin of the tachycardia cannot be determined from the surface ECG. The presence of the narrow QRS indicates the supraventricular origin of the rhythm and conduction through the normal His-Purkinje system into the ventricles.

Sometimes SVT conducts with bundle branch block, which results in a wide QRS but does not change the fact that the rhythm is supraventricular in origin. Thus, *SVT* can be used for narrow QRS tachycardias whose mechanism is uncertain or for wide QRS tachycardias that are known to be coming from above the ventricles.

SVTs can be classified into those that are AV nodal passive and those that are AV nodal active. *AV nodal passive SVTs* are those in which the AV node is not required for the maintenance of the tachycardia but serves only to passively conduct supraventricular impulses into the ventricles. Examples of AV nodal passive dysrhythmias include atrial tachycardia, atrial flutter, and atrial fibrillation, all of which originate within the atria and do not need the AV node to sustain the atrial dysrhythmia. In these rhythms, the AV node passively conducts the atrial impulses into the ventricles but does not participate in the maintenance of the dysrhythmia itself. *AV nodal active tachycardias* require participation of the AV node in the maintenance of the tachycardia. The two most common causes of a regular, narrow QRS tachycardia are AV nodal reentry tachycardia (AVNRT) and circus movement tachycardia (CMT) using an accessory pathway, both of which require the active participation of the AV node in maintaining the tachycardia.

Atrial fibrillation is a supraventricular rhythm that is usually easily recognized because of its irregularity, but atrial tachycardia, atrial flutter, junctional tachycardia, AVNRT, and CMT can all present as regular, narrow QRS tachycardias whose mechanism often cannot be determined from the ECG. Because AVNRT and CMT are the most common causes of a regular, narrow QRS tachycardia, they are discussed in detail here.

Atrioventricular Nodal Reentry Tachycardia

In people with AVNRT, the AV node has two pathways that are capable of conducting the impulse into the ventricles. One pathway conducts more rapidly and has a longer refractory period than the other pathway (Figure 18-30A). In AVNRT, a reentry circuit is set, usually using a slowly conducting pathway just outside the body of the AV node as the antegrade limb into the ventricle and the faster conducting pathway in the AV node as the retrograde limb back into the atria (Figure 18-30C).

The sinus impulse normally conducts down the fast pathway into the ventricles, resulting in a normal PR interval of 0.12 to 0.20 second. If a PAC occurs and enters the AV node before the fast pathway with its longer refractory period has recovered its ability to conduct, the impulse conducts down the slow pathway into the ventricle because of its shorter refractory period (Figure 18-30B). This slow conduction causes the PR interval of the PAC to be longer than the PR interval of sinus beats. The long conduction time through the slow pathway allows the fast pathway time to recover, making it possible for the impulse to conduct backward through the fast pathway into the atria. This returning impulse may then reenter the slow pathway, which is again ready to conduct antegrade because of its short refractory period, thus setting up a reentry circuit within the AV

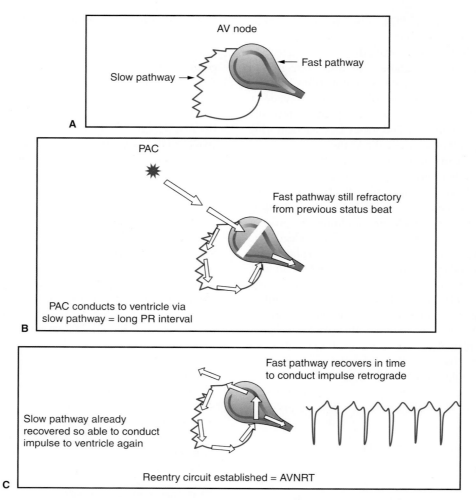

Figure 18-30. Mechanism of AVNRT. **(A)** Illustrates the dual AV nodal pathways responsible for AVNRT. The normal AV node is the fast-conducting pathway with a long refractory period; the slow-conducting pathway lies outside the AV node and has a shorter refractory period. **(B)** A PAC finds the fast pathway still refractory but is able to conduct through the slow pathway. **(C)** When the impulse arrives at the end of the slow pathway, it finds the AV node recovered and ready to conduct retrograde to the atria. The slow pathway has already recovered due to its short refractory period and is able to conduct the same impulse back into the ventricle. This sets up the reentry circuit and causes AVNRT.

node and resulting in AVNRT. Figure 18-30C illustrates the mechanism of the most common type of AVNRT in which antegrade conduction occurs over the slow pathway and retrograde conduction over the fast pathway. The resulting rhythm is usually a narrow QRS tachycardia because the ventricles are activated through the normal His-Purkinje system. P waves are either not seen at all or are barely visible peeking out at the tail end of the QRS complex because the atria and ventricles depolarize almost simultaneously (Figure 18-31A and B). In the presence of preexisting bundle branch block or rate-dependent bundle branch block, the QRS in AVNRT is wide.

In about 4% of cases of AVNRT, the impulse conducts antegrade into the ventricle through the fast pathway and retrograde into the atria through the slow pathway, reversing the circuit within the AV node. This reversal of the circuit in the AV node results in P waves that appear immediately in front of the QRS because atrial activation is delayed because

of slow conduction backward through the slow pathway. These P waves are inverted in inferior leads because the atria depolarize in a retrograde direction.

Treatment

AVNRT is an AV nodal active SVT because the AV node is required for the maintenance of the tachycardia. Therefore, anything that causes block in the AV node, such as vagal stimulation or drugs like adenosine, beta-blockers, or calcium channel blockers, can terminate the rhythm. AVNRT is usually well tolerated unless the rate is extremely rapid. Episodes can become frequent and, if not controlled with drugs, can interfere with lifestyle. Many people learn to stop the rhythm by coughing or breath holding, which stimulates the vagus nerve. Acute medical treatment involves administering any drug that blocks AV node conduction, but adenosine is usually used first because of its rapid effect, short duration of action, and lack of significant side effects. RF ablation can

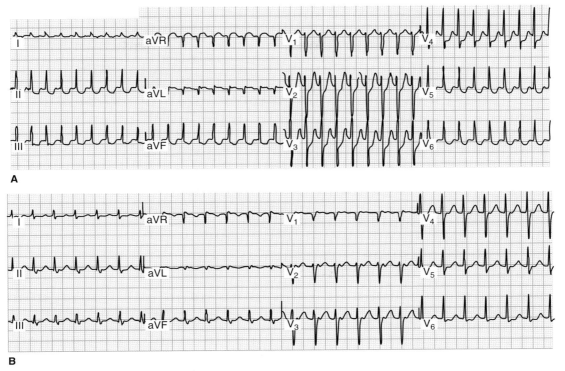

Figure 18-31. **(A)** AVNRT, rate 214. No P waves are visible. **(B)** AVNRT, rate 150. P waves distort the end of the QRS complex in leads II, III, aVF, and V_1 to V_3. (*Reproduced with permission from Woods SL, Froelicher ES, Motzer SA, et al. Cardiac Nursing, 3rd ed. Philadelphia, PA: JB Lippincott; 1995.*)

destroy the slow pathway and prevent recurrence of the dysrhythmia. Refer to Table 3-4 in Chapter 3 for recommendations on management of AVNRT.

Circus Movement Tachycardia

Circus movement tachycardia (CMT) is an SVT that occurs in people who have accessory pathways (see the section Preexcitation Syndromes earlier). *AV reentrant tachycardia (AVRT)* is also used to describe this dysrhythmia, but to avoid confusion between AVRT and AVNRT, *circus movement tachycardia* is used here.

In CMT, an impulse travels a reentry circuit that involves the atria, AV node, ventricles, and accessory pathway. *Orthodromic* is used to describe the most common type of CMT, in which the impulse travels antegrade through the AV node into the ventricles and retrograde back into the atria through the accessory pathway (Figure 18-32A). The result is a regular, narrow QRS tachycardia because the ventricles are activated through the normal His-Purkinje system. In the presence of bundle branch block, a wide QRS pattern is present. Because the atria and ventricles depolarize separately, P waves, if visible at all, are seen following the QRS complex in the ST segment or between two QRS complexes, usually closest to the first QRS.

Antidromic describes the rare form of CMT in which the accessory pathway conducts the impulse from atria to ventricles and the AV node conducts it retrograde back to the atria (Figure 18-32B). Antidromic CMT is a regular wide QRS tachycardia because the ventricles depolarize abnormally through the accessory pathway. This form of SVT is often indistinguishable from ventricular tachycardia on the ECG.

Treatment

CMT is an AV nodal active tachycardia because the AV node is necessary for maintenance of the dysrhythmia. Vagal maneuvers and drugs that block AV conduction can be used to terminate an episode of tachycardia. Acute treatment is aimed at slowing conduction through the AV node with a vagal maneuver or medications such as adenosine, beta-blockers, or calcium channel blockers, or at slowing accessory pathway conduction with antiarrhythmics such as procainamide or ibutilide. See Table 3-4 in Chapter 3 for recommendations for management of CMT.

Atrial Fibrillation in Wolff-Parkinson-White Syndrome

Atrial fibrillation occurs more frequently in people with accessory pathways than in the general population and can be life threatening. Atrial flutter and fibrillation are especially dangerous in the presence of an accessory pathway because the pathway can conduct impulses rapidly and without delay into the ventricles, resulting in dangerously fast ventricular rates (Figure 18-33). These rapid ventricular rates can degenerate into ventricular fibrillation and result in sudden death. When atrial fibrillation is the mechanism of the tachycardia in Wolff-Parkinson-White syndrome, the QRS complex is

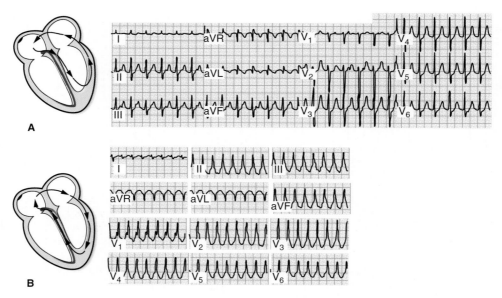

Figure 18-32. (A) Orthodromic circus movement tachycardia. P waves are visible on the upstroke of the T wave in leads II, III, aVF, and V₁ to V₃. (*Reproduced with permission from Woods SL, Froelicher ES, Motzer SA, et al. Cardiac Nursing, 3rd ed. Philadelphia, PA: JB Lippincott; 1995.*) **(B)** Antidromic circus movement tachycardia.

wide and bizarre due to conduction of the impulses into the ventricle through the bypass tract. The ventricular response to the atrial fibrillation is irregular and very rapid, often approaching rates of 300 beats/min or more because of lack of delay in conduction through the accessory pathway. Atrial fibrillation with accessory pathway conduction must be recognized and differentiated from atrial fibrillation conducting through the AV node because treatment is different for the two situations. When accessory pathway conduction is known or suspected, flecainide, ibutilide, or procainamide are recommended because they prolong the refractory period of the accessory pathway and slow ventricular rate, and they may convert the atrial fibrillation to sinus rhythm.

Verapamil often is used to slow AV conduction in atrial fibrillation conducting into the ventricles through the AV node, but it can be very dangerous and even lethal when used in the presence of an accessory pathway. Digitalis, verapamil,

diltiazem, and IV amiodarone are contraindicated in preexcited atrial fibrillation because they can result in ventricular fibrillation. See Table 3-4 in Chapter 3 for management of preexcited atrial fibrillation.

Polymorphic Ventricular Tachycardias

Polymorphic ventricular tachycardia refers to VT with unstable, continuously varying QRS morphology often occurring at rates of approximately 200 beats/min. It can occur in short repetitive runs, longer sustained runs, or can degenerate into VF and cause SCD. PVT can be classified based on whether it is associated with a normal or prolonged QT interval.

Polymorphic VT with a normal QT interval can occur in the presence of ventricular ischemia during ACS or following MI, although it is not a common dysrhythmia. Figure 18-34 shows PVT in a patient during acute anterior-wall MI. Therapy of PVT associated with ischemia should be

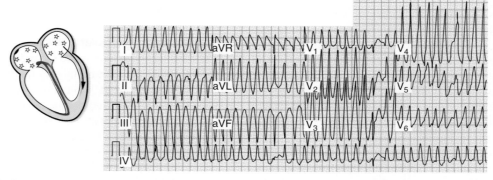

Figure 18-33. Atrial fibrillation conducting into the ventricle through an accessory pathway. Note the extremely short RR intervals in the V leads. QRS is fast, wide, and irregular.

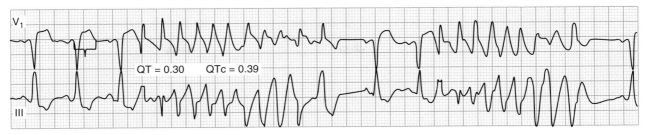

Figure 18-34. Polymorphic VT with a normal QT interval. This patient was having an acute MI (note ST elevation in lead V₁).

directed toward relieving the ischemia by either surgery or percutaneous coronary intervention (PCI). Beta-blockers are recommended for PVT if ischemia is suspected. For recurrent PVT in the absence of a long-QT interval, IV amiodarone is useful and lidocaine may be helpful. If PVT becomes sustained or degenerates to VF, defibrillation with an unsynchronized shock is necessary. Table 3-6 in Chapter 3 summarizes recommendations for managing PVT.

Torsades de pointes means "twisting of the points" and describes polymorphic VT that occurs with abnormal ventricular repolarization. This abnormal repolarization presents on the ECG as an abnormally prolonged QT or QTU interval. See the section on long-QT syndromes in this chapter for more information on long-QT syndromes.

Characteristic ECG findings of TdP include: (1) markedly prolonged QT intervals with wide TU waves; (2) initiation of the dysrhythmia by an R-on-T PVC with a long coupling interval; and (3) wide, bizarre, multiform QRS complexes that change direction frequently, appearing to twist around the isoelectric line (Figure 18-35). Ventricular rate during TdP is commonly 200 to 250 beats/min. TdP is usually self-terminating and occurs in repeated episodes, but it can deteriorate into ventricular fibrillation.

Differentiating Wide QRS Beats and Rhythms

Determining the origin of a wide QRS beat or a wide QRS tachycardia is one of the most common problems encountered when caring for monitored patients. A supraventricular beat with abnormal, or aberrant, conduction through the ventricles, can look almost identical to a beat that originates in the ventricle. The problem with aberration is that it can mimic ventricular dysrhythmias, which require different therapy and carry a different prognosis than aberrancy. Aberrancy is always secondary to some other primary disturbance and does not itself require treatment. Nurses must be able to identify accurately which mechanism is responsible for the wide QRS rhythm being observed whenever possible, initiate appropriate treatment when needed, and avoid inappropriate treatment.

Mechanisms of Aberration

Aberrancy is the temporary abnormal intraventricular conduction of supraventricular impulses. Aberration occurs whenever the His-Purkinje system or ventricle is still partly refractory when a supraventricular impulse attempts to travel through it. The refractory period of the conduction system is directly proportional to preceding cycle length. Long cycles are followed by long refractory periods, and short cycles are followed by short refractory periods. An early supraventricular beat, such as a PAC, may enter the conduction system during a portion of its refractory period, forcing conduction through the ventricles to occur in an abnormal manner. Beats that follow a sudden lengthening of the cycle may conduct aberrantly because of the increased length of the refractory period that occurs when the cycle lengthens (Figure 18-36). The right bundle branch has a longer refractory period than the left; therefore, aberrant beats tend to conduct most often with an RBBB pattern, although LBBB aberration is common in people with cardiac disease.

Electrocardiographic Clues to the Origin of Wide QRS Beats and Rhythms

P Waves

If P waves can be seen during a wide QRS tachycardia, they are very helpful in making the differential diagnosis of aberration versus ventricular ectopy. Atrial activity, represented by the P wave on the ECG and preceding a wide QRS beat or run of tachycardia, strongly favors a supraventricular origin of the dysrhythmia. Figure 18-37 shows three wide QRS beats that could easily be mistaken for PVCs if not for the obvious presence of the early P wave initiating the run.

An exception to the preceding P-wave rule occurs with end-diastolic PVCs. *End-diastolic PVCs* occur at the end of diastole, after the sinus P wave has been recorded but before it has a chance to conduct through the AV node into the ventricle. Figure 18-38 shows sinus rhythm with an end-diastolic PVC occurring immediately after the sinus P wave. Here, the P wave preceding the wide QRS is merely a coincidence and does not indicate aberrant conduction. The PR interval is much too short to have conducted that QRS complex. In addition, the P wave preceding the wide QRS is not early; it is the regularly scheduled sinus beat coming on time. Thus, early P waves that precede early wide QRS complexes are usually "married to" those QRSs and indicate aberrant conduction, while "on-time" P waves in front of end-diastolic PVCs are not early and do not cause the wide QRS.

P waves seen during a wide QRS tachycardia also can be very helpful in making the differential diagnosis between SVTs with aberration and ventricular tachycardia. If P waves

ESSENTIAL CONTENT CASE

Patient With Syncope

A 20-year-old patient was admitted with a head laceration after an episode of syncope with seizure. He had one previous episode of "fainting" about a month ago but did not seek medical care. His BP is 126/72 mm Hg, heart rate 50 beats/min, and complains of pain at the laceration site but is awake, oriented, and cooperative. This is the 12-lead ECG obtained as part of his workup for syncope:

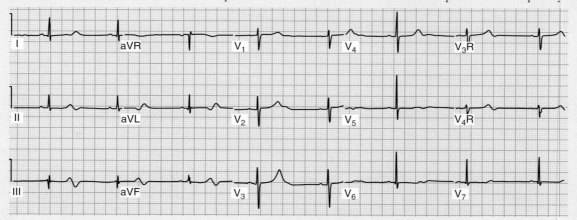

Case Question 1: What is your interpretation of this ECG, rhythm, QRS axis, and bundle branch block?

Case Question 2: Is there anything on the ECG that might indicate a cause of his "seizure?"

You put him on the bedside monitor and set the alarms. He remains stable for the next few hours, then you hear his monitor alarm. When you enter the room, he is complaining of extreme dizziness and says he feels like he might pass out. This is his rhythm on the monitor:

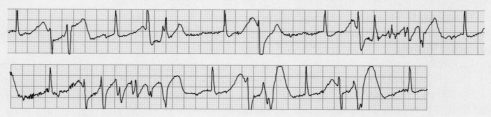

Case Question 3: What is this rhythm?

Case Question 4: What treatment is indicated for this rhythm acutely and long term?

In the next minute, the following rhythm appears:

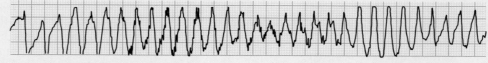

Case Question 5: What is the treatment now?

Answers

1. The rhythm is sinus bradycardia. The QRS axis is normal. There is no bundle branch block.
2. The QT interval is long, about 0.58 second (580 ms) in lead II and 0.60 second (600 ms) in lead V_2. The T waves are biphasic or notched. This is a form of congenital long-QT syndrome, which increases the risk of TdP and SCD. Patients often present with syncope, or seizures that are due to episodes of TdP that last long enough to result in loss of consciousness.
3. The basic rhythm appears to be sinus (narrow QRS beats) with PVC couplets and short runs of TdP.
4. Treatment of short runs of TdP includes IV magnesium or overdrive pacing to shorten the QT interval. Any drugs that might contribute to QT interval prolongation should be discontinued, and any electrolyte imbalances need to be corrected. Beta-blockers are the mainstay of long-term treatment of congenital long-QT syndrome. Patients who continue to have significant ventricular dysrhythmias on beta-blockers or who experience an SCD event should receive an ICD implant.
5. This strip represents a sustained run of TdP. Long runs that do not terminate spontaneously cause loss of consciousness and usually degenerate into VF. Defibrillation is the treatment for sustained TdP.

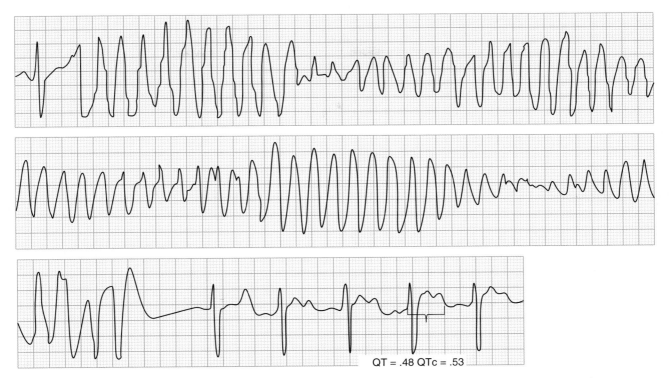

Figure 18-35. Torsades de pointes. Note characteristic "twisting" appearance during VT and the long-QT interval during sinus rhythm.

QT = .48 QTc = .53

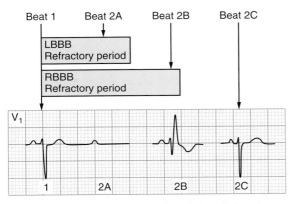

Figure 18-36. Diagram of refractory periods in the bundle branches and the effect of cycle length on conduction. The right bundle has a longer refractory period than the left. Beat 2A occurs so early that it cannot conduct through either bundle branch. Beat 2B encounters a refractory right bundle and conducts with RBBB. Beat 2C falls outside the refractory period of both bundles and is able to conduct normally.

are seen associated with every QRS, the rhythm is supraventricular in origin (Figure 18-39A). P waves that occur independently of the QRS and have no consistent relationship to QRS complexes indicate the presence of AV dissociation, which means that the atria and the ventricles are under the control of separate pacemakers and strongly favors ventricular tachycardia (Figure 18-39B).

QRS Morphology

The shape of the QRS complex is very helpful in determining the origin of a wide QRS rhythm. When using QRS morphology clues, it is extremely important to examine the correct leads and apply the criteria only to leads that have been proven helpful. Many practitioners prefer to monitor with lead II because usually it shows an upright QRS complex and clear P wave. Lead II, however, has no value in determining

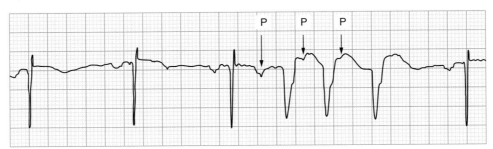

Figure 18-37. Sinus rhythm with PACs and three wide QRS beats that could be mistaken for ventricular tachycardia. Note the P waves preceding the wide QRS complexes, indicating aberrant conduction. (*Reproduced with permission from Woods SL, Froelicher ES, Motzer SA, et al. Cardiac Nursing, 3rd ed. Philadelphia, PA: JB Lippincott; 1995.*)

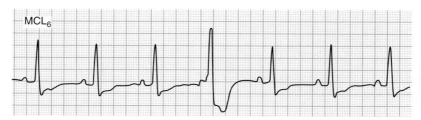

Figure 18-38. Sinus rhythm with an end-diastolic PVC. The P wave preceding the PVC is the sinus P wave that coincidentally occurs just before the PVC. (*Reproduced with permission from Woods SL, Froelicher ES, Motzer SA, et al. Cardiac Nursing, 3rd ed. Philadelphia, PA: JB Lippincott; 1995.*)

the origin of a wide QRS rhythm. The single best dysrhythmia monitoring lead is V_1, followed by V_6 and V_2 in certain situations.

When applying QRS morphology criteria for wide QRS rhythms, it is helpful to first decide whether the QRS complexes have an RBBB morphology or an LBBB morphology. RBBB morphology rhythms have an upright QRS in lead V_1, while LBBB morphology rhythms have a negative QRS complex in V_1.

When dealing with a wide QRS rhythm of RBBB morphology (upright in V_1), follow these steps to evaluate QRS morphology (Figures 18-40 and 18-41A):

1. Look at V_1 and determine if the upright QRS complex is monophasic (R wave), diphasic (qR), or triphasic (rsR'). Monophasic and diphasic complexes favor a ventricular origin, if the left peak ("rabbit ear") is taller. A taller right rabbit ear does not favor either diagnosis. A triphasic rsR' is typical of RBBB aberration in V_1.
2. Look at V_6 and determine whether the QRS is monophasic (all negative QS), diphasic (rS), or triphasic (qRs). A monophasic or diphasic complex in V_6 favors a ventricular origin, and the triphasic qRs complex is typical of RBBB aberration in V_6.

If the QRS has an LBBB morphology (negative in V_1), follow these steps to evaluate morphology (Figures 18-40 and 18-41B):

1. Look at V_1 or V_2 (both are helpful in this case) and determine if the R wave (if present) is wide or narrow. A wide R wave of more than 0.03 second favors a ventricular rhythm, and a narrow R wave favors a supraventricular origin with LBBB aberration.
2. Next look at the downstroke of the S wave in V_1 or V_2. Slurring or notching on the downstroke favors a ventricular origin. LBBB aberration typically slurs on the upstroke if it slurs at all.
3. Measure from the onset of the QRS complex to the deepest part of the S wave in V_1 or V_2. A measurement of more than 0.06 second favors a ventricular rhythm and a narrower measurement favors LBBB aberration. Note that this measurement can be prolonged due to either a wide R wave or slurring on the downstroke of the S wave, either one of which favors the ventricular origin of the rhythm.
4. Look at V_6 and determine whether a Q wave is present. Any Q wave (either a QS or qR complex) favors a ventricular origin.

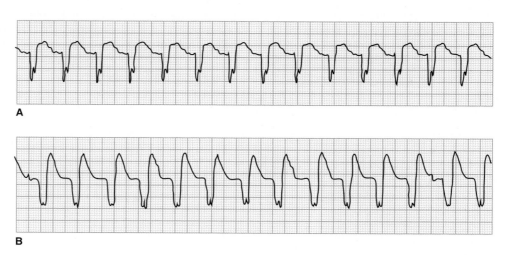

Figure 18-39. Two very similar, wide QRS tachycardias. **(A)** Sinus tachycardia, rate 115. P waves can be seen on the downslope of the T wave preceding each QRS, indicating a supraventricular origin of the tachycardia. **(B)** P waves are independent of QRS complexes, indicating AV dissociation, which favors ventricular tachycardia. (*Reproduced with permission from Woods SL, Froelicher ES, Motzer SA, et al. Cardiac Nursing, 3rd ed. Philadelphia, PA: JB Lippincott; 1995.*)

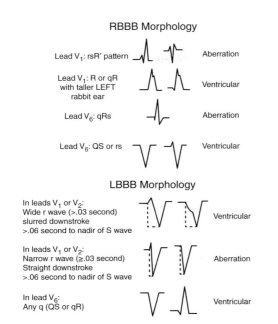

RBBB Morphology

Lead V₁: rsR′ pattern   Aberration

Lead V₁: R or qR
with taller LEFT   Ventricular
rabbit ear

Lead V₆: qRs   Aberration

Lead V₆: QS or rs   Ventricular

LBBB Morphology

In leads V₁ or V₂:
Wide r wave (>.03 second)   Ventricular
slurred downstroke
>.06 second to nadir of S wave

In leads V₁ or V₂:
Narrow r wave (≥.03 second)   Aberration
Straight downstroke
>.06 second to nadir of S wave

In lead V₆:
Any q (QS or qR)   Ventricular

Figure 18-40. Morphology clues for wide QRS beats and rhythms with RBBB and LBBB patterns.

Concordance

Concordance means that all the QRS complexes across the precordium from V₁ through V₆ point in the same direction; positive concordance means they are all upright, and negative concordance means they are all negative (Figure 18-42A).

Negative concordance favors a diagnosis of ventricular tachycardia when it occurs in a wide QRS tachycardia, and positive concordance favors ventricular tachycardia as long as Wolff-Parkinson-White syndrome can be ruled out.

FUSION AND CAPTURE BEATS

Ventricular fusion beats occur when the ventricles are depolarized by two different wavefronts of electrical activity at the same time. Fusion often results when a supraventricular impulse travels through the AV node and begins to depolarize the ventricles at the same time that an impulse from a ventricular focus depolarizes the ventricles. When two different impulses contribute to ventricular depolarization, the resulting QRS shape and width are determined by the relative contributions of both the supraventricular and the ventricular impulses. In the presence of a wide QRS tachycardia, the presence of fusion beats indicates AV dissociation, which means that the atria and ventricles are under the control of separate pacemakers. Capture beats occur when the supraventricular impulse manages to conduct all the way into and through the ventricle, depolarizing ("capturing") the ventricle and resulting in a normal QRS in the midst of the wide QRS tachycardia. The presence of fusion and capture beats in a wide QRS tachycardia is strong evidence supporting the diagnosis of ventricular tachycardia, but they occur rarely and cannot be counted on to make the diagnosis. Figure 18-42B shows fusion beats in a wide QRS tachycardia. Helpful ECG clues for differentiating aberrancy from ventricular ectopy are summarized in Table 18-3.

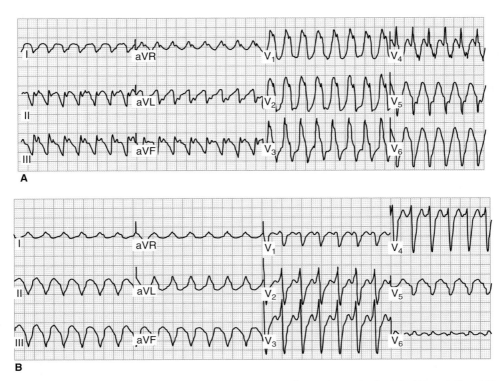

Figure 18-41. 12-lead ECG of ventricular tachycardia. **(A)** With RBBB morphology. Note monophasic R wave with taller left rabbit ear in V₁ and QS complex in V₆. **(B)** With LBBB morphology. Note wide R wave in V₁ and V₂, and qR pattern in V₆.

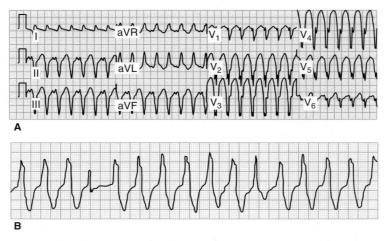

Figure 18-42. **(A)** 12-lead ECG of ventricular tachycardia with negative concordance. **(B)** Rhythm strip of ventricular tachycardia with fusion beats.

ST-SEGMENT MONITORING

Many bedside monitors have software programs that allow for continuous monitoring of the ST segment in addition to routine dysrhythmia monitoring. In patients who have undergone thrombolytic therapy or a PCI procedure to treat acute MI, continuous ST-segment monitoring can detect ischemia related to reocclusion of the involved artery. ST-segment monitoring is also useful in detecting silent ischemia (ischemic episodes that occur in the absence of chest pain or other symptoms) that would otherwise go unnoticed with symptom and dysrhythmia monitoring alone. Early detection of ischemic changes is critical in identifying patients who need interventions to reestablish blood flow to myocardium before permanent damage occurs.

ST elevation in leads facing damaged myocardium is the ECG sign of myocardial injury. ST depression is often recorded as a reciprocal change in leads that do not directly face the involved myocardium (see Table 18-2). In addition, ST depression can be recorded in leads facing ischemic tissue. Therefore, either ST elevation or ST depression indicates myocardium at risk for infarction. The sooner the artery is opened and blood flow reestablished to ischemic or injured

tissue, the more myocardium is salvaged and the fewer complications and deaths occur.

Measuring the ST Segment

Clinically significant ST-segment deviation is defined as ST elevation or depression 1 mm or more from the baseline, or isoelectric line, measured 60 msec (0.06 second) after the J point. The J point is the point at which the QRS ends and the ST segment begins. Figure 18-43A illustrates a normal ST segment, and Figure 18-43B illustrates ST-segment elevation and depression.

ST-segment monitoring software in newer bedside monitors defines the baseline and the ST-segment measuring point. It also sets default alarm parameters so the equipment can audibly notify the nurse when the patient's ST segment falls outside the defined parameters. Most monitors allow the user to redefine the baseline, reset the J point, choose where the ST segment is measured, and change the alarm parameters to account for individual patient variations. The monitor then displays the ST-segment measurement in millimeters on the screen, and most monitors also allow for trending of the ST segment over specified time intervals.

TABLE 18-3. ECG CLUES FOR DIFFERENTIATING ABERRATION FROM VENTRICULAR ECTOPY

	Aberrancy	Ventricular Ectopy
P waves	Precede QRS complexes	Dissociated from QRS or occur at rate slower than QRS; if 1:1 V-A conduction is present, retrograde P waves follow every QRS
Precordial QRS concordance	Positive concordance may occur with WPW	Negative concordance favors VT; positive concordance favors VT if WPW ruled out
Fusion or capture beats		Strong evidence in favor of VT
QRS axis	Often normal; may be deviated to right or left	Right superior axis favors VT; often deviated to left or right
RBBB QRS morphology	Triphasic rsR′ in V_1; triphasic qRs in V_6	Monophasic R wave or diphasic qR complex in V_1; left "rabbit ear" taller in V_1; monophasic QS or diphasic rS in V_6
LBBB QRS morphology	Narrow R wave (< 0.04 second) in V_1; straight downstroke of S wave in V_1 (often slurs or notches on upstroke); usually no Q wave in V_6	Wide R wave (> 0.03 second) in V_1 or V_2; slurring or notching on downstroke of S wave in V_1; delay of greater than 0.06 second to nadir of S wave in V_1 or V_2; any Q wave in V_6

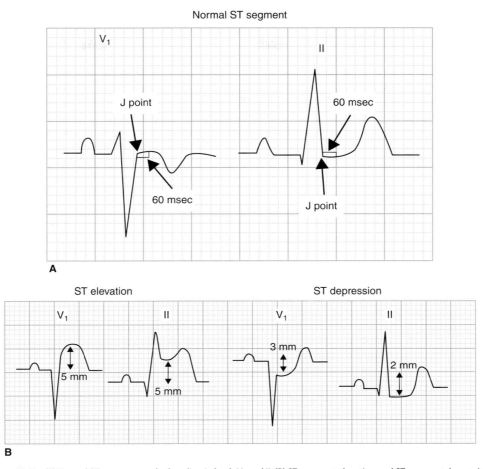

Figure 18-43. **(A)** Normal ST segment on the baseline in leads V₁ and II. **(B)** ST-segment elevation and ST-segment depression.

Choosing the Best Leads for ST-Segment Monitoring

Some monitoring systems offer continuous 12-lead ECG monitoring, which eliminates the need to select the "best" leads to monitor for a given clinical situation. Most younger generation bedside monitors offer at least two leads for simultaneous ECG monitoring and some offer three leads. The best single lead for dysrhythmia monitoring is V₁, with V₆ being next best. Using two or three leads for ST-segment monitoring is optimal because a single lead may miss significant ST-segment deviations. Since most current bedside monitors allow for the use of only one V lead at a time, using V₁ as the dysrhythmia monitoring lead (or V₆ if V₁ is not available because of dressings, etc) means that limb leads must be used for ST-segment monitoring. The best limb leads are discussed below.

The best way to choose leads for ST-segment monitoring is to know the patient's "ischemic fingerprint." To determine the patient's ischemic fingerprint, obtain a 12-lead ECG during a pain episode or with inflation of the balloon during PCI and note which leads show the most ST-segment displacement (either elevation or depression) during the acute ischemic event. Choose the lead or leads with the most ST-segment displacement as the bedside ST-segment monitoring leads.

If no ischemic fingerprint is available, use a lead or leads that have been determined through research to be best for the artery involved (Table 18-4). The limb leads that have been shown to best detect ischemia related to all three major coronary arteries (right coronary, left anterior descending, and circumflex) are leads III and aVF. In the case of the right coronary artery (RCA), leads III and aVF directly face the inferior wall supplied by this artery and record ST elevation with inferior wall injury. The left anterior descending and circumflex artery supply the anterior and lateral walls, respectively. Because these walls are not directly faced by leads III and aVF, ST-segment depression is recorded as a reciprocal

TABLE 18-4. RECOMMENDED LEADS FOR CONTINUOUS ECG MONITORING

Purpose	Best Leads
Dysrhythmia detection	V₁ (V₆ next best)
RCA ischemia, inferior MI	III, aVF
LAD ischemia, anterior MI	V₃ (or V₂; III, or aVF if V lead not available)
Circumflex ischemia, lateral MI	V₆, (I or aVL if V lead not available; III, aVF good reciprocal leads)
RV infarction	V₄R
Axis shifts	I and aVF together

TABLE 18-5. EVIDENCE-BASED PRACTICE: ST-SEGMENT MONITORING

Patient Selection

Class I: ST-segment monitoring recommended for the following types of patients:

- Patients in the early phase of acute coronary syndromes (unstable angina, "rule-out MI, ST elevation MI, non–ST-elevation MI").[a]
- Patients presenting to emergency department with chest pain or anginal equivalent symptoms.[a]
- Patients who have undergone nonurgent percutaneous coronary intervention and who have suboptimal angiographic results.[a]
- Patients with possible variant angina due to coronary vasospasm.[a]

Class II: ST-segment monitoring may be of benefit in some patients but is not considered essential for all:

- Patients with post-acute MI (after 24-48 hours).[a]
- Patients who have undergone nonurgent, uncomplicated percutaneous coronary intervention.[a]
- Patients at high risk for ischemia after cardiac or noncardiac surgery.[a]
- Pediatric patients at risk of ischemia or infarction due to congenital or acquired conditions.[a]

Electrode Application

- Make sure skin is clean and dry before applying monitoring electrodes.[a,b]
- Place electrodes according to manufacturer recommendations when using a derived 12-lead ECG system.[a,b]
- When using a 3- or 5-wire-monitoring system, place electrodes as follows:
  - Place arm electrodes in infraclavicular fossa close to shoulder[a,b] or on top or back of shoulder as close to where arm joins torso as possible.
  - Place leg electrodes at lowest point on rib cage or on hips.[a,b]
  - Place V_1 electrode at the fourth intercostal space at right sternal border.[a,b]
  - Place V_6 electrode in a straight line from V_4 at left midaxillary line.
- Mark electrode placement with indelible ink.[a,b]
- Change electrodes daily.[b]

Lead Selection

- Monitor all 12 leads continuously if ST segment mapping is available.[b]
- Use V_1 (or V_6 if V_1 is not possible due to dressings, etc) for arrhythmia monitoring in all multilead combinations.
- Choose the ST-segment monitoring lead according to the patient's "ischemic fingerprint" obtained during an ischemic event whenever possible.[b] Use the lead with the largest ST-segment deviation (elevation or depression).[b]
- If no ischemic fingerprint is available, use either lead III[a,b] or aVF (whichever has tallest QRS complex) for ST-segment monitoring.
- Lead V_3 is the best lead for detecting anterior wall ST-segment deviation,[b] but it can only be used if the chest lead is not being used for arrhythmia monitoring in lead V_1.

Alarm Limits

- Establish baseline ST level with patient in the supine position.[a,b]
- Set ST alarm parameters at 1 mm above and below the patient's baseline ST level in patients at high risk for ischemia.[a,b]
- Set ST alarm parameters at 2 mm above and below the patient's baseline ST level in more stable patients.[a]

Data compiled from:
[a]*Drew BJ, Califf RM, Funk M. Practice standards for electrocardiographic monitoring in hospital settings.* Circulation. 2004;110:2721-2746.
[b]*AACN Practice Alert: Ensuring Accurate ST Segment Monitoring. American Association of Critical Care Nurses.* Crit Care Nurse. 2016;36:e18-e25.

change when anterior or lateral wall injury occurs. Table 18-5 summarizes critical elements of ST-segment monitoring.

CARDIAC PACEMAKERS

Chapter 3, Interpretation and Management of Basic Cardiac Rhythms, describes the components of a temporary pacing system and basic pacemaker operation. This section discusses single-chamber and dual-chamber pacemaker function and evaluation of pacemaker rhythm strips for appropriate capture and sensing.

Cardiac pacemakers are classified by a standardized five-letter pacemaker code that describes the location of the pacing wire(s) and the expected function of the pacemaker. Table 18-6 illustrates the five-letter code. The first letter in the pacemaker code describes the chamber that is paced (A = atrium, V = ventricle, D = dual [atrium and ventricle], 0 = none). The letter in the second position describes the chamber where intrinsic electrical activity is sensed (A = atrium, V = ventricle, D = dual, 0 = none). The letter in the third position describes the pacemaker's response to sensing of intrinsic electrical activity (I = inhibited, T = triggered, D = dual [inhibited or triggered], 0 = none). The fourth letter indicates the presence or absence of rate modulation, and the fifth letter describes multisite pacing functions. To know how a pacemaker should function, it is necessary to know at a minimum the first three letters of the code, which describe where the pacemaker is supposed to pace, where it is supposed to sense, and what it should do when it senses. The last two letters representing advanced pacemaker function are not covered in this text; see the recommended references at the end of the chapter.

Three types of temporary pacing are commonly used in critical care or telemetry settings. The first is transvenous pacing through a wire introduced into the apex of the right ventricle via a peripheral or central vein and set in the demand mode (sensitive to intrinsic ventricular activity). Ventricular pacing is always done in the demand mode to avoid the delivery of pacing stimuli into the vulnerable period of the cardiac cycle, which could induce ventricular tachycardia or fibrillation (see Chapter 3, Interpretation and Management of Basic Cardiac Rhythms). This type of pacing is described by the pacemaker code as a VVI pacemaker— it paces the ventricle, senses intrinsic ventricular electrical activity, and inhibits its output when sensing occurs.

The second type of pacing done in critical care or telemetry is temporary epicardial pacing (either atrial, ventricular,

TABLE 18-6. PACEMAKER CODES

First Letter: Chamber Paced	Second Letter: Chamber Sensed	Third Letter: Response to Sensing	Fourth Letter: Rate Modulation	Fifth Letter: Multisite Pacing[a]
0 = None	0 = None	0 = None	0 = None	0 = None
A = Atrium	A = Atrium	I = Inhibited	R = Rate modulation	A = Atrial
V = Ventricle	V = Ventricle	T = Triggered		V = Ventricular
D = Dual (A&V)	D = Dual (A&V)	D = Dual (I&T)		D = Dual

[a] *Multisite indicates either pacing in both atria or both ventricles or pacing multiple sites within a chamber.*

TABLE 18-7. **DUAL-CHAMBER PACING MODES**

Mode	Chamber(s) Paced	Chamber(s) Sensed	Response to Sensing
DVI	Atrium and ventricle	Ventricle	Inhibited
VDD	Ventricle	Atrium and ventricle	Atrial sensing triggers ventricular pacing Ventricular sensing inhibits ventricular pacing
DDI	Atrium and ventricle	Atrium and ventricle	Inhibited
DDD	Atrium and ventricle	Atrium and ventricle	Atrial sensing inhibits atrial pacing, triggers ventricular pacing Ventricular sensing inhibits atrial and ventricular pacing

or dual chamber) via pacing wires attached to the atria and/or ventricles during cardiac surgery. If atrial pacing is done with no sensing of atrial electrical activity, also called asynchronous mode, the pacemaker operates as an A00 pacemaker—it paces the atria, does not sense, and therefore does not respond to intrinsic atrial activity. If atrial pacing is done with sensing of atrial electrical activity, also called the demand mode, the pacemaker operates as an AAI pacemaker—it paces the atria, senses atrial activity, and inhibits its output when it senses. Dual-chamber pacing can be done in several modes involving pacing and sensing functions in one or both chambers and described by the pacemaker code according to the mode chosen. The two most common dual-chamber modes used with temporary epicardial pacing (and occasionally with temporary transvenous pacing) are DVI (paces atria and ventricles, senses only in the ventricle, and inhibits pacing output when sensing occurs) and DDD (paces both chambers, senses both chambers, and either triggers or inhibits pacing output in response to sensing). The common dual-chamber pacing modes are listed in Table 18-7.

The third type of temporary pacing is external (transcutaneous) pacing. External pacing is done in emergency situations requiring immediate pacing when placement of a temporary transvenous pacing wire is not feasible. External pacing is not as reliable as transvenous or epicardial pacing and is used as a temporary measure until transvenous pacing can be instituted. External pacing is briefly described in Chapter 3, Interpretation and Management of Basic Cardiac Rhythms.

Evaluating Pacemaker Function

Evaluating pacemaker function requires knowledge of the mode of pacing expected (VVI, AAI, etc); the minimum rate of the pacemaker, or pacing interval; and any other programmed parameters in the pacemaker. The basic functions of a pacemaker include stimulus release, capture, and sensing. *Stimulus release* refers to pacemaker output, or the ability of the pacemaker to generate and release a pacing impulse. *Capture* is the ability of the pacing stimulus to result in depolarization of the chamber being paced. *Sensing* is the ability of the pacemaker to recognize and respond to intrinsic electrical activity in the heart. Pacemaker operation is evaluated according to these three functions. Single-chamber pacemaker evaluation is much less complicated than dual-chamber evaluation. Because single-chamber ventricular pacing is a

very common type of temporary pacing in critical care and telemetry units, VVI pacemaker evaluation is discussed here.

VVI Pacemaker Evaluation

Stimulus release, capture, and sensing must all be assessed when evaluating VVI pacemakers. A VVI pacemaker is expected to pace the ventricle at the set rate unless spontaneous ventricular activity occurs to inhibit pacing. The set rate of the pacemaker, or *pacing interval,* is measured from one pacing stimulus to the next consecutive stimulus. Pacemakers have a *refractory period,* which is a period following either pacing or sensing in the chamber, during which the pacemaker is unable to respond to intrinsic activity. During the refractory period, the pacemaker in effect has its eyes closed and is not able to see spontaneous activity. In a normally functioning VVI pacemaker, pacing spikes occur at the set pacing interval and each spike results in a ventricular depolarization (capture). If spontaneous ventricular activity occurs (either a normally conducted QRS or a PVC), that activity is sensed and the next pacing stimulus is inhibited. Figure 18-44A and B shows normal VVI pacemaker function.

Stimulus Release

Stimulus release depends on a pacemaker with enough battery power to generate the electrical impulse, and on an intact pacemaker lead system to deliver the electrical stimulus to the heart. The presence of a pacer spike on the rhythm strip or monitor indicates that the stimulus was released from the generator and entered the body. The presence of the spike does not indicate where the stimulus was delivered (eg, atria or ventricles), only that it entered the body somewhere. Total absence of pacing stimuli, when they should be present, can indicate a faulty pulse generator or battery, or a break or disconnection in the lead system. Pacing stimuli also can be absent when pacing is inhibited by the sensing of intrinsic electrical activity. Figure 18-45 illustrates total loss of stimulus release in a patient whose pacemaker battery was depleted.

Capture

Capture is indicated by a wide QRS complex immediately following the pacemaker spike and represents the ability of the pacing stimulus to depolarize the ventricle. Loss of capture is recognized by the presence of pacer spikes that are

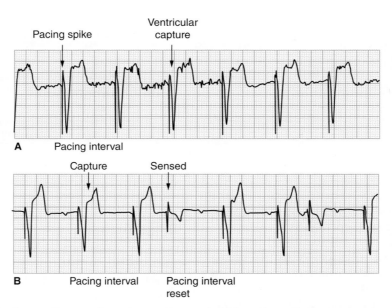

Figure 18-44. Normal VVI pacemaker function. **(A)** Pacing electrical activity ("pacer spike") followed by a wide QRS complex indicating ventricular capture. Pacemaker sensing cannot be evaluated because no intrinsic QRS complexes are present. **(B)** Pacemaker capture and sensing both normal. Intrinsic QRS complexes are sensed, inhibiting ventricular pacing output, and resetting the pacing interval. Absence of intrinsic ventricular electrical activity causes pacing to occur with capture.

not followed by paced ventricular complexes (Figure 18-46). Causes of loss of capture include:

- Inadequate stimulus strength, which can be corrected by increasing the electrical output of the pacemaker (turning up the milliampere level).
- Pacing wire out of position and not in contact with myocardium, which can be corrected by repositioning the wire and sometimes the patient.
- Pacing lead positioned in infarcted tissue, which can be corrected by repositioning the wire to a place where the myocardium is not injured and is capable of responding to the stimulus.
- Electrolyte imbalances or medications that alter the heart's response to the pacing stimulus
- Delivery of a pacing stimulus during the ventricle's refractory period when the heart is physiologically unable to respond to the stimulus. This problem occurs with loss of sensing (undersensing) and can be corrected by correcting the sensing problem (Figure 18-47A).

Sensing
Sensing of intrinsic ventricular electrical activity inhibits the next pacing stimulus and resets the pacing interval. Sensing cannot occur unless the pacemaker is given the opportunity

to sense. It must be in the demand mode and there must be intrinsic ventricular activity that occurs for the pacemaker to have an opportunity to sense. In Figure 18-44A, sensing cannot be evaluated because there is no intrinsic ventricular activity that occurs, and therefore the pacemaker is not given an opportunity to sense. In Figure 18-44B, the occurrence of two spontaneous QRS complexes provides the pacemaker with an opportunity to sense. In this example, sensing occurred normally, as indicated by the absence of the next expected pacing stimulus and resetting of the pacing interval by the intrinsic QRS complex.

Two sensing problems can occur: undersensing (Figures 18-47A and 18-48A) and oversensing (Figure 18-48B). Undersensing, also called "failure to sense" or "loss of sensing," can be caused by:

- Asynchronous (fixed rate) mode in which the sensing circuit is off. This problem can be corrected by turning the sensitivity control to the demand mode.
- Pacing catheter out of position or lying in infarcted tissue, which can be corrected by repositioning the wire. Pacing wire repositioning must be done by a physician; however, turning the patient onto his or her side sometimes temporarily works when the pacing wire loses contact with the ventricle.

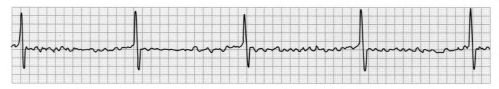

Figure 18-45. Absence of stimulus release in a patient with a permanent pacemaker. Underlying rhythm is atrial fibrillation with complete AV block and a very slow ventricular rate. The battery in the pacemaker generator was depleted.

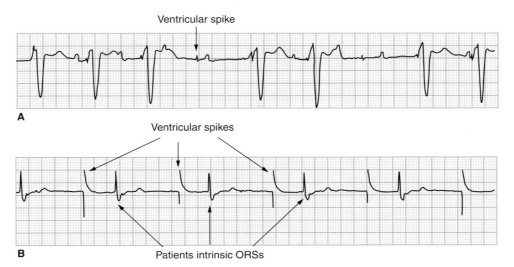

Figure 18-46. (A) VVI pacemaker with intermittent loss of capture. **(B)** VVI pacemaker with total loss of capture.

- Intrinsic QRS voltage too low to be sensed by the pacemaker. Turning the sensitivity control clockwise or decreasing the sensitivity number increases the sensitivity of the pacemaker and makes it able to "see" smaller intrinsic electrical signals. Repositioning the wire sometimes helps.
- Break in connections, battery failure, or faulty pulse generator. Check and tighten all connections along

the pacing system, and replace the battery if it is low. A chest x-ray may detect wire fracture. Change the pulse generator if problems cannot be corrected any other way.
- Intrinsic ventricular activity falling in the pacemaker's refractory period. If a spontaneous QRS complex occurs during the time the pacemaker has its eyes closed, the pacemaker cannot see it. This event occurs

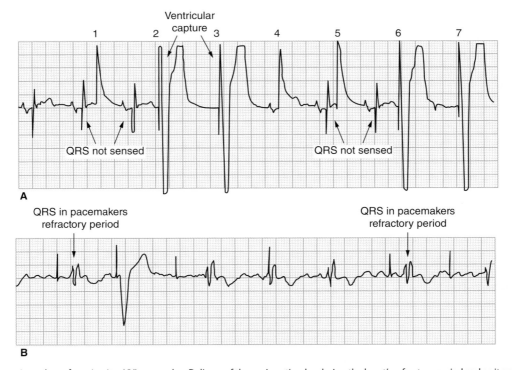

Figure 18-47. (A) Intermittent loss of sensing in a VVI pacemaker. Delivery of the pacing stimulus during the heart's refractory period makes it appear that capture is lost as well. Because the heart is physiologically unable to respond to the pacing stimulus when it falls in the refractory period, this is not a capture problem. Pacer spikes 1, 2, 5, and 6 should not have occurred; their presence is due to loss of sensing. Pacer spike 4 occurred coincident with the normal QRS complex, resulting in a "pseudofusion" beat, and does not represent loss of sensing. **(B)** Loss of capture in a VVI pacemaker. Only one pacer spike captures the ventricle. Two QRS complexes occur during the pacemaker's refractory period and thus are not sensed. This does not represent loss of sensing because the pacemaker has its "eyes closed" during the time intrinsic ventricular activity occurred.

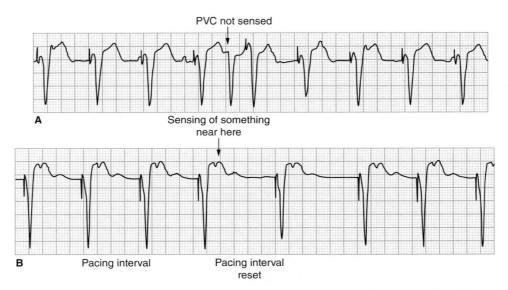

Figure 18-48. **(A)** Undersensing in a VVI pacemaker. The PVC is not sensed and pacing occurs at the programmed pacing interval, resulting in a pacemaker spike on the T wave of the PVC. **(B)** Oversensing in a VVI pacemaker. The pacing rate slows for two intervals, presumably due to sensing of something near the T wave, which resets the pacing interval from the point where sensing occurred.

when the pacemaker fails to capture, which can allow an intrinsic QRS to occur during the pacemaker's refractory period. This problem is due to loss of capture and does not reflect a sensing malfunction (see Figure 18-47B).

Oversensing means that the pacemaker is so sensitive that it inappropriately senses internal or outside signals as QRS complexes and inhibits its output. Common sources of outside signals that can interfere with pacemaker function include electromagnetic or RF signals, or electronic equipment in use near the pacemaker. Internal sources of interference can include large P waves, large T-wave voltage, local myopotentials in the heart, or skeletal muscle potentials (see Figure 18-48B). Because a VVI pacemaker is programmed to inhibit its output when it senses, oversensing can be a dangerous situation in a pacemaker-dependent patient, resulting in ventricular asystole. Oversensing is usually due to the sensitivity control being set too high, which can be corrected by turning the sensitivity dial counterclockwise and reducing the pacemaker's sensitivity. It is recommended that the sensitivity control be set between the 1 and 3 o'clock positions on the dial (about 2 mV) rather than all the way to the right, unless a higher sensitivity is required to make the pacemaker sense QRS complexes.

Stimulation Threshold Testing

The stimulation threshold is the minimum output of the pacemaker necessary to capture the heart consistently. The stimulation threshold changes over time. When the pacing lead is first placed, the stimulation threshold is usually very low. Over time, the threshold increases and it takes more output to result in capture. When caring for a patient with a temporary pacemaker, stimulation threshold testing

should be done every shift until a stable threshold is reached. Once the threshold has been determined, set the output 2 to 3 times higher than threshold to ensure an adequate safety margin for capture. To determine the stimulation threshold, follow these steps:

- Verify that the patient is in a paced rhythm. The pacing rate may need to be temporarily increased to override an intrinsic rhythm.
- Watch the monitor continuously while slowly decreasing output by turning the output control counterclockwise.
- Note when the pacing stimulus no longer captures the heart (a pacing spike not followed by a paced beat).
- Slowly increase the output until 1:1 capture resumes. This is the stimulation threshold.
- Set the output 2 to 3 times higher than threshold (ie, if threshold is 2 mA, set output between 4 and 6 mA).

DDD Pacemaker Evaluation

Dual-chamber pacemakers have become very complicated, with multiple programmable parameters and varying functions depending on the manufacturer. It is impossible to present dual-chamber pacemaker function in detail in a single chapter. To understand dual-chamber pacemaker function, it is necessary to understand the timing cycles involved in dual-chamber pacing. More detailed information on dual-chamber pacemaker function is available in the references at the end of this chapter. In this section, the major timing cycles are defined and basic DDD pacemaker evaluation is covered in a very generic manner, because each pacemaker is different depending on the manufacturer. Dual-chamber pacemakers can function in a variety of modes (see Table 18-7).

Because the DDD mode is most commonly used, basic DDD function is described here.

According to the pacemaker code, DDD means both chambers (atria and ventricles) are paced, both chambers are sensed, and the mode of response to sensed events is either inhibited or triggered, depending on which chamber is sensed. When atrial activity is sensed, pacing is triggered in the ventricle after the programmed AV delay unless intrinsic conduction to the ventricle occurs. When ventricular activity is sensed, all pacemaker output is inhibited.

The following timing cycles determine dual-chamber pacemaker function:

- *Pacing interval* (or lower rate limit): The base rate of the pacemaker is measured between two consecutive atrial pacing stimuli. The pacing interval is a programmed parameter.
- *AV delay* (or AV interval): The amount of time between atrial and ventricular pacing, or the "electronic PR interval." This is measured from the atrial pacing spike to the ventricular pacing spike and is a programmed parameter.
- *Atrial escape interval* (or VA interval): The interval from a sensed or paced ventricular event to the next atrial pacing output. The VA interval represents the amount of time the pacemaker waits after it paces in the ventricle or senses ventricular activity before pacing the atrium. The atrial escape interval is not a programmed parameter but is derived by subtracting the AV delay from the pacing interval. Its length can be estimated by measuring from a ventricular spike to the next atrial pacing spike.
- *Total atrial refractory period* (TARP): The period of time following a sensed P wave or a paced atrial event during which the atrial channel will not respond to sensed events (ie, "has its eyes closed"). The TARP consists of the AV delay and the PVARP (see later).
- *Post ventricular atrial refractory period* (PVARP): The period of time following an intrinsic QRS or a paced ventricular beat during which the atrial channel is refractory and will not respond to sensed atrial activity. PVARP is a programmable parameter but is not evident on a rhythm strip.
- *Blanking period*: The very short ventricular refractory period (VRP) that occurs with every atrial pacemaker output. The ventricular channel "blinks its eyes" so it does not sense the atrial output and inappropriately inhibits ventricular pacing. The blanking period is a programmable parameter but is not evident on a rhythm strip.
- *Ventricular refractory period*: The period of time following a paced ventricular beat or a sensed QRS during which the ventricular channel ignores intrinsic ventricular activity (ie, "has its eyes closed"). VRP is a programmable parameter but is not evident on a rhythm strip.

- *Maximum tracking interval* (or upper rate limit): The maximum rate at which the ventricular channel will track atrial activity. The upper rate limit prevents rapid ventricular pacing in response to very rapid atrial activity, such as atrial tachycardia or atrial flutter. The maximum tracking interval is a programmable parameter and usually is set according to how active a patient is expected to be and how fast a ventricular rate is likely to be tolerated.

Because a dual-chamber pacemaker has both atrial and ventricular pacing and sensing functions, evaluation includes assessing atrial capture, atrial sensing, ventricular capture, and ventricular sensing. To evaluate dual-chamber pacemaker function accurately, it is necessary to know the following information: mode of function (DDD, DVI, etc), minimum rate, upper rate limit, AV delay, PVARP, and VRPs. In the real world of bedside nursing, this information is not always available, so we do the best we can with what we have. The following sections briefly discuss the issues of assessing atrial and ventricular capture and sensing in a dual-chamber pacing system.

Atrial Capture

Atrial capture, unlike ventricular capture, is not always easy to see. Often, the atrial response to pacing is so small that it cannot be seen in many monitoring leads, so we cannot rely on the presence of a P wave following every atrial pacer spike as evidence of atrial capture. If a clear P wave is present after every atrial pacemaker spike, atrial capture can be assumed. In the absence of a clear P wave, atrial capture can only be assumed when a normally conducted QRS complex follows an atrial pacer spike within the programmed AV delay. If the atrial spike captures the atrium and there is intact AV conduction, the presence of the normal QRS indicates that the atrium must have been captured for conduction to occur into the ventricles before the ventricular pacing stimulus was delivered. Because a DDD pacemaker paces the ventricle at a preset AV interval following atrial pacing, the presence of a ventricular paced beat following an atrial paced beat does not verify capture, because the ventricle paces at the end of the AV delay whether atrial capture occurs or not. Therefore, atrial capture can only be assumed when there is an obvious P wave after every atrial pacing spike or when an atrial pacing spike is followed by a normal QRS within the programmed AV delay.

Atrial Sensing

Atrial sensing is verified by the presence of a spontaneous P wave that is followed by a paced ventricular beat at the end of the programmed AV delay. If a P wave is sensed, it starts the AV delay and ventricular pacing is triggered at the end of the AV delay unless AV conduction is intact and results in a normal QRS. The presence of a normal P wave followed by a normal QRS only proves that AV conduction is intact, not that the pacemaker is sensing electrical activity in the atria.

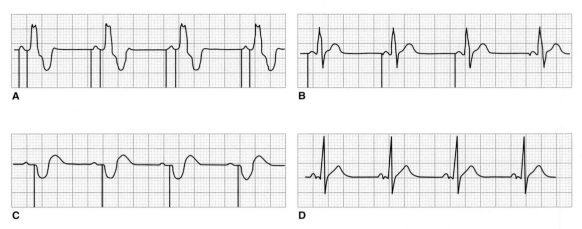

Figure 18-49. Four states of DDD pacing. **(A)** Atrial and ventricular pacing (AV sequential pacing state). **(B)** Atrial pacing, ventricular sensing. **(C)** Atrial sensing, ventricular pacing (atrial tracking state). **(D)** Atrial and ventricular sensing (inhibited pacing state).

Therefore, atrial sensing is verified by a spontaneous P wave followed by a paced QRS.

Ventricular Capture

Ventricular capture is recognized by a wide QRS immediately following a ventricular pacing spike. Ventricular capture is much easier to recognize than atrial capture and is no different than with single-chamber ventricular pacing.

Ventricular Sensing

Ventricular sensing can only be verified if there is spontaneous ventricular activity present for the pacemaker to sense. Ventricular sensing is verified when an atrial pacer spike followed by a normal QRS inhibits the ventricular pacing spike, which is the same event that proves atrial capture. If a QRS is sensed before the next atrial pacing spike is due, both the atrial and ventricular pacing stimuli are inhibited and the VA interval (atrial escape interval) is reset.

Dual-chamber pacemakers are capable of operating in four states of pacing: atrial and ventricular pacing (AV sequential pacing state), atrial pacing with ventricular sensing, atrial sensing with ventricular pacing (atrial tracking state), and atrial and ventricular sensing. All four states of pacing can occur within a short period of time, and the timing cycles determine which state of pacing is done. Figure 18-49 shows the four states of dual-chamber pacing, and Figure 18-50 illustrates the basic principles of dual-chamber pacemaker evaluation.

Cardiac Resynchronization Therapy With Biventricular Pacing

Patients with chronic HF often have intraventricular conduction delays (especially LBBB) that result in ventricular dyssynchrony and impair cardiac function. This intraventricular conduction delay causes electrical and mechanical abnormalities in ventricular function that interfere with ventricular filling, impair cardiac output, worsen mitral regurgitation, and contribute to mortality in patients with HF. LBBB causes both electrical and mechanical abnormalities that result in ventricular dyssynchrony. Interventricular dyssynchrony refers to the time delay between right and left ventricular contraction, where the right ventricle (RV) depolarizes and contracts before the left ventricle (LV). Intraventricular dyssynchrony refers to the abnormal segmental contraction within the LV as it depolarizes late and abnormally in LBBB.

When the RV contracts before the LV, the septum depolarizes and contracts with the RV instead of with the LV. Since the septum normally contributes to LV ejection by contracting with the LV, normal septal function is lost in LBBB. Since the septum contracts with the RV, it is relaxed by the time the LV begins contracting, and increasing pressure in the LV causes paradoxical septal motion by pushing the septum into the RV. In LBBB, the papillary muscles that are responsible for holding the mitral valve leaflets tight depolarize late and fail to keep valve leaflets from everting into the atria during LV systole, resulting in mitral regurgitation. The combination of paradoxical septal wall motion and mitral regurgitation contribute to the already reduced LV stroke volume

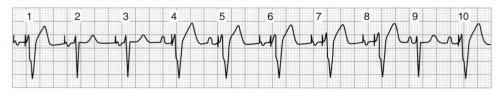

Figure 18-50. DDD pacemaker operating in all four states of pacing. Beats 1, 6, 7, and 8 illustrate AV sequential pacing (A pace and V pace); beats 2 and 3 illustrate atrial pacing and ventricular sensing; beats 4, 5, and 10 illustrate atrial sensing and ventricular pacing; beat 9 is an intrinsic beat with normal P wave and normal conduction to the ventricle. Atrial capture is proven evident in beats 1, 2, 3, 6, 7, and 8; atrial sensing is verified by beats 4, 5, and 10; ventricular capture is evident in beats 1, 4, 5, 6, 7, 8, and 10; ventricular sensing is verified by beats 2, 3, and 9.

that occurs in HF. Portions of the LV that are activated first contract before those portions that are activated late, creating mechanical dyssynchrony that reduces systolic function by about 20%, reduces stroke volume, increases wall stress, and delays relaxation.

Cardiac resynchronization therapy (CRT) is biventricular pacing aimed at improving electromechanical activity in the failing heart. The goals of CRT are to improve hemodynamics by restoring ventricular synchrony, and improve quality of life via symptom relief. CRT devices can be stand-alone pacemakers or combination ICD and biventricular pacemakers (CRT-D). Class I recommendations for CRT include patients with the following characteristics: HF with New York Heart Association (NYHA) class II, III, or ambulatory IV symptoms; left ventricular ejection fraction less than 35%; presence of significant intraventricular conduction delay (QRS duration > 150 msec); sinus rhythm; and symptoms in spite of optimal guideline directed medical therapy for HF. Class IIa indications include patients with LVEF less than 35% and NYHA class II, III, or ambulatory IV symptoms with QRS duration between 120 and 149 msec; those with non-LBBB pattern wide QRS of more than 150 msec; those with atrial fibrillation who are likely to be near 100% ventricular paced; and those undergoing new or replacement device implantation with anticipated requirement for more than 40% ventricular pacing.

CRT is accomplished by placing standard pacing leads in the right atrium and into the right ventricular apex as is done for normal dual-chamber pacing. A third lead is advanced through the coronary sinus and into a lateral or posterior left ventricular vein for pacing of the LV (Figure 18-51).

The goal in biventricular pacing is to cause both ventricles to depolarize and contract simultaneously, thus eliminating the interventricular and intraventricular dyssynchrony that occurs during LBBB. The AV interval is often programmed shorter than intrinsic AV conduction in order to force the ventricles to pace rather than allowing intrinsic conduction to occur. Biventricular pacing causes both ventricles to contract simultaneously and allows the septum to contract with the LV. Controlling the AV delay restores the normal timing between left atrial and left ventricular contraction, allowing the LV papillary muscles to contract earlier and put tension on the mitral valve leaflets to reduce or prevent mitral regurgitation. Biventricular pacing allows the LV to complete contraction and begin relaxation earlier, which increases filling time and improves "atrial kick."

Electrocardiographic evaluation of biventricular pacemaker function is more complicated than single ventricle pacing from the right ventricular apex. Pacing from the RV apex creates an LBBB pattern with a wide negative QRS complex in lead V_1. Left ventricular pacing is more complicated due to the fact that the LV lead can be placed in either a lateral or posterior LV vein and can be located in an apical or a basal site within the vein. The resulting QRS varies in morphology, depending on the location of the LV lead, but, in general, LV pacing produces an RBBB pattern with a wide upright QRS complex in lead V_1. It makes logical sense that pacing both ventricles simultaneously would result in a narrow QRS complex preceded by a pacemaker spike, but this narrowing is not always obvious with biventricular pacing. Loss of capture in one or the other ventricle should cause a change in the morphology of the paced QRS that would

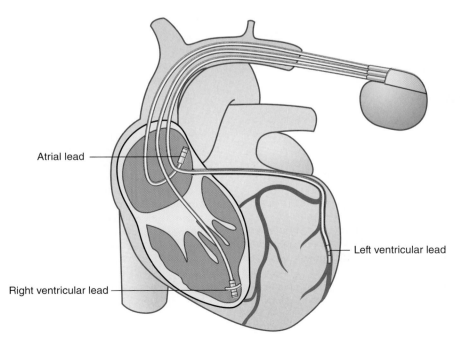

Figure 18-51. Lead placement for biventricular pacing.

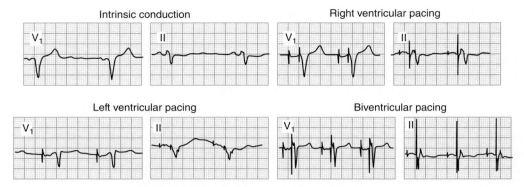

Figure 18-52. ECG in biventricular pacing.

indicate single-chamber pacing from the ventricle that is still being captured. A shift in the frontal plane axis may also occur with loss of capture in one ventricle.

Some experts recommend recording four 12-lead ECGs at the time of implant: during intrinsic conduction, in the course of RV pacing with capture, in LV pacing with capture, and during biventricular pacing with capture in both ventricles. These ECGs should be examined to determine which lead best demonstrates an obvious difference between the four pacing states recorded, then the best lead should be used as the monitoring lead for pacemaker evaluation. Figure 18-52 shows leads V_1 and II recorded during intrinsic conduction, RV pacing, LV pacing, and bi-ventricular pacing. Note the similarity between the intrinsic QRS with LBBB and the RV paced QRS, which produces an "iatrogenic" LBBB pattern. The ventricular pacing spike is not visible in lead V_1 in LV pacing, and the QRS is negative during LV pacing in this patient as opposed to the more common upright QRS during LV pacing. The QRS during biventricular pacing is narrower than the intrinsic beats and the single-chamber paced beats. Lead V_1 would be a good monitoring lead for this patient due to the differences in QRS morphology among these four examples.

SELECTED BIBLIOGRAPHY

Electrocardiography

Bayes de Luna A, Goldwasser D, Fiol M, Bayes-Genis A. Surface electrocardiography. In: Fuster V, Harrington RA, Narula J, Eapen ZJ, eds. *Hurst's the Heart*. 14th ed. New York, NY: McGraw Hill; 2017.

Elizari M, Acunzo RS, Ferreiro M. Hemiblocks revisited. *Circulation*. 2006;115:1154-1163.

Jacobson C, Marzlin K, Webner C. *Cardiovascular Nursing Practice: a Comprehensive Resource Manual and Study Guide for Clinical Nurses*. 2nd ed. Burien, WA: Cardiovascular Nursing Education Associates; 2014.

Mirvis DM, Goldberger AL. Electrocardiography. In: Mann DL, Zipes DP, Libby P, Bonow RO, Braunwald E, eds. *Braunwald's Heart Disease: A Textbook of Cardiovascular Medicine*. 10th ed. Philadelphia, PA: Elsevier; 2015: 114-154.

Sgarbossa EB, Pinski SL, Barbagelata A, et al. Electrocardiographic diagnosis of evolving acute myocardial infarction in the presence of left bundle-branch block. *N Engl J Med*. 1996;334:481-487.

Acute Coronary Syndrome

Moliterno DJ, Januzzi JL. Evaluation and management of non-ST-segment elevation myocardial infarction. In: Fuster V, Harrington RA, Narula J, Eapen ZJ, eds. *Hurst's the Heart*. 14th ed. New York, NY: McGraw Hill; 2017.

Patel MR, Singh M, Gersh BJ, O'Neill W. ST-segment elevation myocardial infarction. In: Fuster V, Harrington RA, Narula J, Eapen ZJ, eds. *Hurst's the Heart*. 14th ed. New York, NY: McGraw Hill; 2017.

Long QT Syndrome and Brugada Syndrome

Antzelevitch C, Brugada P, Borggrefe M. Brugada syndrome: recent advances and controversies. *Circulation*. 2008;10(5):376-383.

Bayes de Luna A, Brugada J, Baranchuk A, et al. Current electrocardiographic criteria for diagnosis of Brugada pattern: a consensus report. *J Electrocardiol*. 2012;45:433-442.

Priori SG, Napolitano C. Genetics of channelopathies and clinical implications. In: Fuster V, Harrington RA, Narula J, Eapen ZJ, eds. *Hurst's the Heart*. 14th ed. New York, NY: McGraw Hill; 2017.

Priori SG, Wilde AM, Horie M, et al. HRS/EHRA/APHRS expert consensus statement on the diagnosis and management of patients with inherited primary arrhythmia syndromes. *Heart Rhythm*. 2013;10(12):1932-1963.

Dysrhythmias

Bradfield JS, Boyle NG, Shivkumar K. Ventricular arrhythmias. In: Fuster V, Harrington RA, Narula J, Eapen ZJ, eds. *Hurst's the Heart*. 14th ed. New York, NY: McGraw Hill; 2017.

Calkins H. Supraventricular tachycardia: atrial tachycardia, atrioventricular nodal reentry, and Wolff-Parkinson-White syndrome. In: Fuster V, Harrington RA, Narula J, Eapen ZJ, eds. *Hurst's the Heart*. 14th ed. New York, NY: McGraw Hill; 2017.

Miller JM, Zipes DP. Diagnosis of cardiac arrhythmias. In: Mann DL, Zipes DP, Libby P, Bonow RO, Braunwald E, eds. *Braunwald's Heart Disease*. 10th ed. Philadelphia, PA: Elsevier; 2015: 662-684.

Pacemakers

Barold SS, Herweg B, Giudici M. Electrocardiographic follow-up of biventricular pacemakers. *Ann Noninvasive Electrocardiol.* 2005;10(2):231-255.

Kenny T. *The Nuts and Bolts of Cardiac Pacing.* Malden, MA: Blackwell Futura; 2005.

Swerdlow CD, Wang PJ, Zipes DP. Pacemakers and implantable cardioverter-defibrillators. In: Mann DL, Zipes DP, Libby P, Bonow RO, Braunwald E, eds. *Braunwald's Heart Disease: A Textbook of Cardiovascular Medicine.* 10th ed. Philadelphia, PA: Elsevier; 2015: 721-747.

Upadhyay GA, Singh JP. Pacemakers and defibrillators. In: Fuster V, Harrington RA, Narula J, Eapen ZJ, eds. *Hurst's the Heart.* 14th ed. New York, NY: McGraw Hill; 2017.

Evidence Based Practice

Drew BJ, Ackerman MJ, Funk M. Prevention of Torsade de Pointes in hospital settings. *J Am Coll Cardiol.* 2010;55:934-947.

Drew BJ, Califf RM, Funk M. Practice standards for electrocardiographic monitoring in hospital settings. *Circulation.* 2004;110:2721-2746.

Epstein AE, DiMarco JP, Ellenbogen KA. ACC/AHA/HRS 2008 guidelines for device-based therapy of cardiac rhythm abnormalities: a report of the American College of Cardiology/American Heart Association Task Force on Practice Guidelines. *Circulation.* 2008;117:e350-e408.

Hancock EW, Deal BJ, Mirvis DM. AHA/ACCF/HRS recommendations for the standardization and interpretation of the electrocardiogram part V: electrocardiogram changes associated with cardiac chamber hypertrophy. A scientific statement from the American Heart Association Electrocardiography and Arrhythmias Committee, Council on Clinical Cardiology; the American College of Cardiology Foundation; and the Heart Rhythm Society. *Circulation.* 2009;119:e251-e261.

Page RL, Joglar JA, Caldwell MA, et al. ACC/AHA/HRS Guideline for the management of adult patients with supraventricular tachycardia: a report of the American College of Cardiology/American Heart Association Task Force on Practice Guidelines and the Heart Rhythm Society. *Circulation.* 2016;133:e506-e574.

Priori SG, Blomstrom-Lundqvist C, Mazzanti A, et al. 2015 ESC guidelines for the management of patients with ventricular arrhythmias and the prevention of sudden cardiac death. *Eur Heart J.* 2015;36:2793-2867.

Rautaharju PM, Surawicz B, Gettes LS. AHA/ACCF/HRS recommendations for the standardization and interpretation of the electrocardiogram part IV: the ST segment, T and U waves, and the QT interval. A scientific statement from the American Heart Association Electrocardiography and Arrhythmias Committee, Council on Clinical Cardiology; the American College of Cardiology Foundation; and the Heart Rhythm Society. *Circulation.* 2009;119:e241-e250.

Surawicz B, Childers R, Deal BJ, Gettes LS. AHA/ACCF/HRS recommendations for the standardization and interpretation of the electrocardiogram part III: intraventricular conduction disturbances: a scientific statement from the American Heart Association Electrocardiography and Arrhythmias Committee, Council on Clinical Cardiology; the American College of Cardiology Foundation; and the Heart Rhythm Society. *Circulation.* 2009;119:e235-e240.

Tracy CM, Epstein AE, Darbar D. 2012 ACCF/AHA/HRS focused update of the 2008 guidelines for device-based therapy of cardiac rhythm abnormalities: a report of the American College of Cardiology Foundation/American Heart Association Task Force on Practice Guidelines. *Circulation.* 2012;126:1784-1800.

Wagner GS, Macfarlane P, Wellens H, et al. AHA/ACCF/HRS recommendations for the standardization and interpretation of the electrocardiogram: part VI: acute ischemia/infarction: a scientific statement from the American Heart Association Electrocardiography and Arrhythmias Committee, Council on Clinical Cardiology; the American College of Cardiology Foundation; and the Heart Rhythm Society. *Circulation.* 2009;119:e262-e270.

Webner C, Marzlin K. AACN practice alert: accurate dysrhythmia monitoring in adults. *Crit Care Nurse.* 2016;36(6):e26-e34.

ADVANCED CARDIOVASCULAR CONCEPTS

19

Barbara Leeper

KNOWLEDGE COMPETENCIES

1. Describe the etiology, pathophysiology, clinical presentation, patient needs, and principles of management of:
   - Cardiomyopathy
   - Valvular disease
   - Pericarditis
   - Aortic aneurysm
   - Cardiac transplantation

2. Compare and contrast the principles of management of:
   - Cardiomyopathy
   - Valvular disease
   - Pericarditis
   - Aortic aneurysm
   - Cardiac transplantation

3. Identify indications for, complications of, and nursing management of patients receiving ventricular assist device (VAD) therapy.

PATHOLOGIC CONDITIONS

Cardiomyopathy

Cardiomyopathy is a disease involving destruction of the cardiac muscle fibers, causing impairment of myocardial function and decreased cardiac output (CO). The body responds to this with initiation of several neuroendocrine responses including activation of the sympathetic nervous system and renin-angiotensin-aldosterone chain. The prevailing result is marked vasoconstriction, retention of sodium and water, and further myocyte injury. This process contributes to remodeling of ventricular myocytes and the downward spiral of cardiomyopathy. The cause of cardiomyopathy is often unknown. Cardiomyopathies are commonly classified into three types: dilated, hypertrophic, and restrictive (Figure 19-1).

Dilated cardiomyopathy, the most common type of cardiomyopathy, is commonly caused by coronary artery disease and is associated with impaired myocardial contractility and increased ventricular filling pressures. Coronary artery disease contributes to ventricular remodeling thereby reducing ejection fraction. The two case studies presented later in this chapter involve patients with dilated cardiomyopathy.

Hypertrophic cardiomyopathy may occur in both the young and the older adults. Hypertrophic cardiomyopathy is often categorized as obstructive or nonobstructive. Ventricular hypertrophy occurs in both types. The diagnosis of obstructive hypertrophic cardiomyopathy is made if hypertrophy of the intraventricular septum is also present. This is the congenital form and is often referred to as hypertrophic obstructive cardiomyopathy (HOCM). In the past, other terms used to describe this type of cardiomyopathy were idiopathic hypertrophic subaortic stenosis (IHSS) and asymmetric septal hypertrophy (ASH). The hypertrophied septum obstructs left ventricular outflow tract just below the aortic valve, thereby limiting ejection. Blood volume is "trapped" within the left ventricular chamber.

Restrictive cardiomyopathy is the least common of the three types. A classic finding for this type of cardiomyopathy is ventricular fibrosis caused by infiltration of the cardiac myocytes with abnormal cells such as sarcoid or amyloid

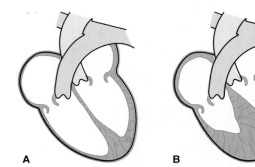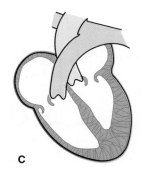

Figure 19-1.   Types of cardiomyopathies. **(A)** Dilated (cardiac dilation and impaired contractility). **(B)** Hypertrophic (decreased size of ventricular chambers and increased ventricular muscle mass). **(C)** Restrictive (decreased ventricular compliance).

disease. The fibrotic muscle tissue becomes very rigid with decreased compliance, thus limiting distention during diastole.

Etiology and Pathophysiology

A variety of conditions may cause or contribute to the development of cardiomyopathy (Table 19-1). As noted previously, coronary artery disease is the most common cause of dilated cardiomyopathy in the United States.

Pathophysiology of Dilated Cardiomyopathy

Dilated cardiomyopathy begins with gradual destruction of the myocardial fibers impairing myocardial contraction. As the disease progresses, left ventricular dilation occurs with increased blood volume in the left ventricle at the end of diastole. Additionally, ventricular compliance is reduced, which contributes to an increase in filling pressures (ie, left ventricular end-diastolic pressure [LVEDP]) and a decrease

in CO. Left atrial volume and pressure eventually increase as the atrium struggles to overcome the higher LVEDP and eject blood into the left ventricle. The increased left atrial pressure often leads to an increased pulmonary capillary pressure as the higher filling pressures are reflected back into the pulmonary vascular bed leading to the development of pulmonary hypertension. Right ventricular failure will eventually occur as the right ventricle has a limited capacity to increase its force of contraction against the higher pressures in the pulmonary vascular bed. Eventually, the right ventricle will dilate along with the left ventricle. In addition, the atrioventricular valves (mitral and tricuspid) may develop insufficiency due to the dilated chambers stretching the papillary muscle and interfering with the closure of the valves.

Pathophysiology of Hypertrophic Cardiomyopathy

Patients with hypertrophic cardiomyopathy have a greatly thickened ventricular wall (see Figure 19-1). It is not uncommon for the ventricular chamber size to be dramatically reduced due to hypertrophy. In obstructive cardiomyopathy, the intraventricular septum is also involved in the hypertrophic process, whereas in nonobstructive cardiomyopathy the septum is relatively normal. Common causes of the nonobstructive form include aortic stenosis and hypertension. The hypertrophied ventricle becomes rigid, reducing ventricular compliance and distension. Myocardial contractility becomes impaired, resulting in a decreased stroke volume and CO.

If HOCM is present, left ventricular systolic ejection will be further compromised by obstruction of the outflow tract as the anterior leaflet of the mitral valve presses against an enlarged intraventricular septum.

Stress is placed on the left atrium as it attempts to propel blood forward into the stiff left ventricle. It is not uncommon for left atrial enlargement to develop as the left atrium is forced to contract against high left ventricular resistance.

Pathophysiology of Restrictive Cardiomyopathy

The ventricles of patients with restrictive cardiomyopathy become rigid as fibrotic tissue infiltrates the myocardium. The stiffness of the ventricles decreases the compliance, or distensibility, of the ventricles, thus limiting ventricular filling and increasing end-diastolic pressures. Myocardial

TABLE 19-1.   ETIOLOGY OF CARDIOMYOPATHY

Dilated Cardiomyopathy
- Idiopathic
- Coronary artery disease
- Toxins, such as lead, alcohol, cocaine
- Chemotherapeutic agents
- Viral, bacterial, or fungal infections
- Chagas disease (parasitic)
- Peripartum or postpartum status
- Hemochromatosis
- Scleroderma
- Hypertension
- Microvascular spasm

Hypertrophic Cardiomyopathy
- Idiopathic
- Congenital
- Aortic stenosis

Restrictive Cardiomyopathy
- Idiopathic
- Myocardial fibrosis
- Hypertrophy
- Amyloidosis
- Hemochromatosis
- Scleroderma

ESSENTIAL CONTENT CASE
Cardiomyopathy Case 1

A 56-year-old man was admitted to the emergency room with shortness of breath. His chest x-ray revealed an enlarged heart and pulmonary congestion. His 12-lead electrocardiogram (ECG) was consistent with left ventricular hypertrophy and his rhythm was atrial fibrillation (AF) with a ventricular rate of 102. Clinical findings included bilateral crackles auscultated one-third up from the bases, +4 pitting edema of the bilateral lower extremities to the mid-calf, jugular venous distension (JVD), an S_3, and a systolic murmur heard best at the apex. An emergency echocardiogram showed impaired contractility of a dilated left ventricle.

Case Question 1: After the patient is admitted and his diagnosis is confirmed, the initial priority for his medical management is:
(A) Initiate inotropic support
(B) Obtain electrophysiology consult for a biventricular pacemaker workup
(C) Administer a diuretic to reduce fluid overload
(D) Administer carvedilol to control the ventricular rate

Case Question 2: The most likely cause of a systolic murmur in this patient is:
(A) Aortic stenosis
(B) Mitral insufficiency
(C) Tricuspid stenosis
(D) Pulmonic insufficiency

Answers
1. C is the correct answer. A diuretic is indicated to reduce his signs and symptoms of significant fluid overload.
2. B is the correct answer. Mitral insufficiency produces a systolic murmur (valve is leaking when it should be closed) that is heard best at the apex. Murmurs of the aortic and pulmonary valves are heard best at the second intercostal spaced on the right sternal border (aortic) and left sternal border (pulmonic). Murmurs from the tricuspid valve are heard at the fourth intercostal space at the left sternal border.

contractility is impaired, leading to decreases in CO. As with the other types of cardiomyopathy, atrial workload is increased as the atria attempt to propel blood forward into stiff ventricles. Often, the atrioventricular valves become insufficient and the pressures in the pulmonary vascular bed and peripheral venous bed increase, leading to edema.

Clinical Presentation
Patients may be asymptomatic for lengthy periods of time (months to years) prior to being diagnosed with a cardiomyopathy. By the time patients develop symptoms, myocardial contractility may be significantly impaired. The heart rate (HR) increases initially as the heart attempts to maintain an adequate CO. As the disease progresses and/or during physical exertion, the impaired myocardium is no longer able to maintain an adequate CO to meet the metabolic demands of the tissues in spite of the increased HR.

ESSENTIAL CONTENT CASE
Cardiomyopathy Case 2

A 32-year-old woman was admitted to the progressive care unit at 31 weeks' gestation with dyspnea and fatigue. She had bilateral basilar crackles, and her oxygen saturation via pulse oximetry was 88%. Her neck veins were markedly distended with head of bed up at 45°. Her vital signs were blood pressure (BP) 88/62 mm Hg, HR 112 beats/min, and respiratory rate (RR) 28 breaths/min. An echocardiogram showed a markedly dilated left ventricle with diffuse hypokinesis and an ejection fraction of 20% to 25%. A central line was placed in her right subclavian vein.

A dobutamine infusion was initiated at 5 mcg/kg/min and oxygen was applied at 6 L/min via nasal cannula.

Case Question 1: The most likely medical diagnosis for this patient is:
(A) HOCM
(B) Restrictive cardiomyopathy
(C) Peripartum cardiomyopathy
(D) Idiopathic cardiomyopathy

Case Question 2: Her clinical presentation indicates possible volume overload as evidenced by:
(A) HR 112/minute
(B) Distended neck veins
(C) EF 20%-25%
(D) SpO_2 88%

Case Question 3: Your plan of care for this patient includes which of the following:
(A) Improve oxygen delivery to the tissues
(B) Increase myocardial contractility
(C) Careful management of preload as blood volume is normally 1.5 times higher during pregnancy
(D) Education about self-management of heart failure and coping strategies
(E) All of the above

Answers
1. C is the correct answer. Her symptoms presented at 31 weeks gestation.
2. B is the correct answer given her clinical presentation of dyspnea and the presence of bibasilar crackles confirming the cause of the elevated central venous pressure (CVP) and pulmonary artery occlusion pressure (PAOP).
3. E is the correct answer. All of the strategies are important for the management of this patient.

Dilated Cardiomyopathy

1. Inability to maintain adequate CO:
   - Fatigue
   - Weakness
   - Sinus tachycardia
   - Pulsus alternans
   - Narrowed pulse pressure
   - Decreased CO
2. Increased left ventricular filling pressures (LVEDP)
   - Dyspnea
   - Orthopnea
   - Paroxysmal nocturnal dyspnea

- Crackles
- S_3/S_4
- Dysrhythmias (AF, ventricular tachycardia or fibrillation)
- Systolic murmur associated with mitral valve insufficiency
- Abnormal hemodynamic profile:
  - Increased pulmonary artery systolic (PAS) and pulmonary artery diastolic (PAD) pressures
  - Elevated PAOP
  - Increased systemic vascular resistance (SVR)
  - Elevated V wave on PAOP waveform with mitral valve insufficiency
3. Increased right ventricular filling pressures:
  - Peripheral edema
  - Jugular vein distention (JVD)
  - Hepatomegaly
  - Elevated V wave on the right atrial (RA) waveform and systolic murmur associated with tricuspid valve insufficiency
4. Increased atrial pressures:
  - Palpitations
  - S_4 may develop as the atria attempt to eject blood into stiff ventricles.
  - Atrial dysrhythmias may occur, such as premature atrial complexes (PACs) or AF, due to increased atrial pressure
  - Elevated A wave on PAOP waveform
  - Elevated RA pressures
  - Elevated A wave on the RA waveform

Hypertrophic Cardiomyopathy

1. Inability to maintain adequate CO:
  - Angina
  - Syncope
  - Fatigue
  - Sinus tachycardia
  - Ventricular fibrillation
  - CO is initially normal, then decreases
2. Increased ventricular filling pressures:
  - Dyspnea
  - Orthopnea
  - Dysrhythmias, such as premature ventricular contractions or ventricular tachycardia
  - Abnormal hemodynamic profile:
    – Elevated PAS and PAD pressures
    – Elevated PAOP pressure
    – Increased SVR
3. Increased atrial pressure:
  - S_4 may develop as the atria attempt to eject blood into rigid ventricles
  - Atrial dysrhythmias may occur (eg, PAC, AF) due to the increased atrial pressure
  - Palpitations
  - Elevated A wave on PAOP waveform
  - Elevated RA pressure

4. Left ventricular outflow tract obstruction:
  - Systolic murmur as blood flows through a narrowed outflow tract due to septal hypertrophy; heard at apex

Restrictive Cardiomyopathy

Signs and symptoms of restrictive cardiomyopathy and pericarditis are similar. Diagnosis can usually be made after an echocardiogram.

1. Inability to maintain adequate CO:
  - Activity intolerance
  - Weakness
  - Sinus tachycardia
  - Dysrhythmias
  - Decreased CO/cardiac index (CI)
2. Increased left ventricular filling pressures:
  - Dyspnea
  - JVD
  - S_3
  - Narrowed pulse pressure
  - Systolic murmur with mitral valve insufficiency
3. Abnormal hemodynamic profile:
  - Elevated PAS, PAD, and PAOP pressures
  - Elevated SVR
  - Elevated V wave on PAOP waveform with mitral valve insufficiency
4. Increased right ventricular pressures:
  - Peripheral edema
  - Hepatomegaly
  - Jaundice
  - JVD
  - Systolic murmur with tricuspid valve insufficiency
  - Kussmaul sign (increased neck vein distention with inspiration)
  - Elevated V wave on the RA waveform if tricuspid valve insufficient
5. Increased atrial pressures:
  - Palpitations
  - S_4 may develop as the atria attempt to eject blood into rigid ventricles
  - Atrial dysrhythmias may occur (eg, PACs, AF) due to the increase in atrial pressure
  - Elevated A wave on PAOP waveform
  - Elevated RA pressure
  - Elevated A wave on the RA waveform

Diagnostic Tests

Dilated Cardiomyopathy

- *Chest x-ray:* Left ventricular dilation with potential enlargement and dilation of all four cardiac chambers
- *12-lead ECG:* ST-segment and T-wave changes; left axis deviation; left ventricular hypertrophy and bundle branch block (left bundle branch block most common)
- *Echocardiography:* Dilated left ventricle with an increase in chamber size (other chambers may be

enlarged also); diminished ventricular contractility; decreased septal wall movement; elevated ventricular volumes and decreased ejection fraction

Hypertrophic Cardiomyopathy

- *Chest x-ray:* Normal or left atrial and ventricular hypertrophy
- *12-lead ECG:* ST-segment and T-wave changes; septal Q waves due to septal hypertrophy; left ventricular hypertrophy
- *Echocardiography:* Thickened ventricular walls with a decrease in chamber size; left ventricular outflow obstruction created by thickened ventricular septum and motion of mitral valve leaflet

Restrictive Cardiomyopathy

- *Chest x-ray:* Normal or slight enlargement of left atria and ventricle
- *12-lead ECG:* ST-segment and T-wave changes; low QRS amplitude
- *Echocardiography:* Thickened ventricular walls; enlarged atria; diminished ventricular contractility; decreased ventricular volumes; elevated ventricular end-diastolic pressures

Principles of Management of Cardiomyopathy

The primary objectives in the management of cardiomyopathy are to treat the underlying cause (if known); maximize cardiac function; assist the patient and family members to cope with a debilitating, chronic disease; and prevent complications associated with cardiomyopathy.

Improvement of Cardiac Function

Dilated Cardiomyopathy

1. *Improve myocardial oxygenation:* As ventricular dilation occurs, ventricular wall tension increases, increasing the myocardial workload and oxygen consumption. Oxygen therapy is initiated as necessary to increase oxygenation delivery. Pulse oximetry, mixed venous oxygenation saturation (Svo_2) or central venous oxygen saturation ($Scvo_2$), and arterial blood gases are helpful in guiding sufficient oxygen therapy. If the patient has an Svo_2 catheter or PA catheter, monitoring the Svo_2 is also an accurate means of assessing oxygenation status.
2. *Increase myocardial contractility:* Inotropic agents including β1 receptor stimulating agents (eg, dobutamine) and phosphodiesterase inhibitors (eg, milrinone) produce a positive inotropic effect (eg, strengthen myocardial contractility) and cause mild vasodilation, thereby reducing the workload of the failing ventricle.
3. *Decrease preload and afterload:* Diuretics decrease excess fluid and lower ventricular end-diastolic volumes; fluid and sodium restrictions also may be necessary. Vasodilators (eg, isosorbide dinitrate, hydralazine) dilate arterial and venous vessels,

decreasing venous return and resistance to ventricular systolic ejection (afterload).
4. *Administer beta-blockers* (eg, metoprolol, carvedilol, bisoprolol) to reduce the risk of sudden cardiac death (VF, VT), as well as prevent further deterioration of the myocytes.
5. *Administer angiotensin-converting enzyme (ACE) inhibitors, angiotensin II receptor blockers (ARBs), or angiotensin receptor neprilysin inhibitors (ARNIs)* to block the negative effects of angiotensin II on the cardiac cells, as well as reduce ventricular afterload. ARNIs are never given conjunction with ARB or ACE inhibitor and are started only after a minimum of 36 hours has passed since the last ACE inhibitor or ARB dose.
6. *Mechanical cardiac assist devices* (eg, intra-aortic balloon therapy, VAD therapy), and in some critical situations extracorporeal membrane oxygenation (ECMO), may be instituted to assist with improving CO/CI and oxygen delivery to the tissues.
7. *Dual-chamber biventricular pacemaker/implantable cardioverter defibrillator:* Refer to Chapter 9, Cardiovascular System (section Improvement of Left Ventricular Function).
8. *Ventricular reconstruction procedure:* This is a surgical procedure focusing on removal of a ventricular aneurysm and scar tissue on the left ventricle, usually a result of a myocardial infarction (MI). The left ventricle is returned to its normal shape and is able to contract more efficiently.
9. *Cardiac transplantation* may be necessary if medical therapy does not relieve patient symptoms.

Hypertrophic Cardiomyopathy

The management of the patient with hypertrophic cardiomyopathy focuses on promoting myocardial relaxation and decreasing left ventricular obstruction.

1. *Decrease myocardial contractility:* Use beta-blockers to decrease HR, contractility, and myocardial oxygen consumption.
2. *The following medications are usually contraindicated in patients with hypertrophic cardiomyopathy:*
   - Diuretics, because a decrease in fluid volume decreases ventricle filling pressures and CO.
   - Inotropes (eg, dobutamine, milrinone), because an increase in contractility contributes to an increase in the left ventricular outflow obstruction.
   - Vasodilators (eg, nitroglycerin, nitroprusside), because they decrease end-diastolic volume, leading to an increase in left ventricular outflow obstruction.
3. *Reduce physical and psychological stress:* Patients with hypertrophic cardiomyopathy are at an increased risk for sudden cardiac death, which may occur during stressful periods. Strenuous physical activity and psychological stress are avoided. In addition, sudden

changes in position are avoided, because the heart cannot respond to fluid shifts created by sudden position changes. Valsalva maneuver is also avoided. Teach patients strategies to enhance self-relaxation. Relaxation therapy may include rhythmic breathing, biofeedback, and imagery.

4. *Cardiac surgery:* Myectomy may be indicated for individuals who do not respond to medical management and have severe left ventricular outflow obstruction. Myectomy involves removal of a portion of the enlarged intraventricular septum in an attempt to decrease left ventricular outflow obstruction and improve myocardial functioning.

5. *Ethanol septal ablation:* Ethanol septal ablation involves instilling absolute alcohol (98% ethanol) into selected septal perforator branches of the left anterior descending coronary artery, resulting in a therapeutic MI. The result is reduced left ventricular outflow obstruction and improved CO. The procedure is performed in the cardiac catheterization laboratory by the interventional cardiologists. This procedure is less risky than myectomy because it is less invasive.

Restrictive Cardiomyopathy

Decrease preload: Diuretics, sodium and fluid restrictions, and vasodilators decrease ventricular end-diastolic volumes. The rigid ventricle is very sensitive to small fluid changes, significantly increasing ventricular end-diastolic pressure.

Facilitate Coping

For most patients, cardiomyopathy is a chronic, potentially life-threatening disease. Patients and their families often face an uncertain long-term prognosis. Emotions may vacillate as the family struggles to cope with the implications of the disease and its effect on lifestyle. Emphasis is placed on assisting the patient to remain active and to cope with a progressive disease. Involvement of the family unit in symptom management is also important. Relaxation therapy can benefit not only the patient, but also the family. Goals of care discussions that include options for palliative and hospice care are essential components of patient management when the prognosis is poor or treatment options are limited.

Preventing and Managing Complications

1. *Dysrhythmias:* Continuous electrocardiogram (ECG) monitoring; observe for potential side effects of cardiac medications; encourage family to learn cardiopulmonary resuscitation (CPR).

2. *Hemodynamic instability* may require that the patient be managed in an ICU for invasive monitoring with insertion of a pulmonary artery catheter. The patient will be managed based on trends in hemodynamic parameters (ie, RA, PAS, PAD, and PAOP pressures; CO; CI; SVR; and PVR).

3. *Thromboembolic event:* Anticoagulation is necessary for patients with severely compromised left ventricular function and for patients with AF. In both circumstances, thrombi may develop due to increased fluid volume and stasis.

4. *Endocarditis:* Antibiotic prophylaxis is recommended for patients with valve involvement. Prophylaxis is provided prior to dental work, surgery, or other invasive procedures.

Valvular Heart Disease

Heart valve disorders result from both congenital and acquired causes. Valves on the left side of the heart are more commonly affected because they are constantly exposed to higher pressures. Normally, when a valve opens, there are no pressure gradients between the chambers or vessels above and below the valve. As the heart valve disease progresses, pressure gradients between the two structures develop.

Heart valve disorders are commonly classified as valve stenosis or valve insufficiency. A stenotic valve has a narrowed opening, that is, it does not open fully thereby reducing the amount of blood flowing through it. An insufficient valve does not close properly, thus permitting some blood to flow backward instead of forward. Heart valve insufficiency is also referred to as valvular regurgitation. Valvular dysfunction may affect one or more valves.

The development of valvular heart disease is usually a gradual process. As the case study illustrates below, the patient's valve problems began with a bacterial endocarditis 15 years prior to the onset of her symptoms of mitral valve insufficiency.

Etiology and Pathophysiology

Both congenital and acquired diseases can cause heart valve disorders (Table 19-2). Congenital valve disorders may affect any of the four valves causing stenosis or insufficiency. An example of a congenital valve disorder is an aortic valve with only two, instead of three, cusps. The bicuspid valve is associated with an increase in turbulence as blood flows through the narrowed orifice. The individual may become symptomatic later in life when fibrotic tissue and calcium deposits form on the abnormal valve, leading to stenosis. This is often referred to as "senile aortic stenosis."

There are three types of acquired valve disorders: degenerative disease, rheumatic disease, or infective endocarditis. Degenerative disease may occur as the valve is damaged over time due to constant mechanical stress. This may occur with aging, or may be aggravated by conditions such as hypertension. Hypertension places significant pressure on the aortic valve, often causing insufficiency.

Individuals who develop rheumatic fever often experience valvular disease years later. Rheumatic disease contributes to gradual fibrotic changes of the valve, in addition to calcification of the valve cusps. Shortening of the chordae tendineae also may occur. Rheumatic fever commonly affects the mitral valve.

TABLE 19-2. ETIOLOGY OF VALVULAR DISORDERS

Mitral Stenosis
- Rheumatic disease
- Endocarditis
- Degenerative process

Mitral Insufficiency
- Dilated cardiomyopathy
- Rheumatic disease
- Congenital
- Endocarditis
- Mitral valve prolapse
- Papillary muscle dysfunction
- Chordae tendineae dysfunction

Aortic Stenosis
- Rheumatic disease
- Congenital (bicuspid valve)
- Degenerative process

Aortic Insufficiency
- Rheumatic disease
- Congenital
- Hypertension
- Endocarditis
- Marfan syndrome

Tricuspid Stenosis
- Rheumatic disease
- Congenital
- Endocarditis

Tricuspid Insufficiency
- Rheumatic disease
- Dilated cardiomyopathy
- Marfan syndrome
- Endocarditis
- Ebstein anomaly
- Congenital
- Secondary to left-sided valve disease
- IV drug use

Pulmonic Stenosis
- Rheumatic disease
- Congenital
- Endocarditis

Pulmonic Insufficiency
- Primary pulmonary artery hypertension
- Secondary to left-sided valve disease
- Marfan syndrome
- Endocarditis

Infective endocarditis may occur as a primary or secondary infection. The infectious organism destroys the value tissue. Table 19-2 lists other conditions that cause valvular heart disease.

Pathophysiology of Mitral Stenosis

Several processes occur that together cause stenosis or narrowing of the mitral valve orifice (Figure 19-2). Gradual fusion of the commissures (the valve leaflet edges) and fibrosis of the valve leaflets are common. In addition, calcium deposits may invade the valve leaflets, further impeding their movement. As the mitral valve becomes increasingly stenotic, the left atrium has to generate significant amounts of pressure to propel blood forward through the mitral valve and into the left ventricle. Left atrial pressures are commonly increased,

ESSENTIAL CONTENT CASE
Heart Valve Disorder

A 48-year-old woman was admitted to the progressive care unit with increasing shortness of breath and fatigue. She had bacterial endocarditis 15 years ago, which resulted in mitral valve insufficiency. On admission, she was in normal sinus rhythm with frequent premature atrial contractions, and her vital signs were BP of 150/94 mm Hg, HR 110 beats/min, and RR 26 breaths/min. Chest auscultation revealed crackles in the left lower lung field. The patient reported minimal urine output in the last 24-48 hours.

Case Question: The initial priority for medical management of this patient will be to:
(A) Improve oxygen delivery to the tissues
(B) Consider initiation of an inotrope
(C) Initiate a sodium nitroprusside infusion to reduce the BP
(D) Consider a diuretic to decrease preload

Answer
1. D is the correct answer. Her increased RR with crackles in her lungs and diminished urine out indicate she is retaining fluid. A diuretic will address this.

with left atrial dilation occurring as the stenosis worsens. Increased left atrial pressures may lead to increased pulmonary vascular pressures (pulmonary hypertension) contributing to the development of right-sided ventricular failure.

Pathophysiology of Mitral Insufficiency

Adequate closure of the mitral valve is important so that blood is ejected forward into the aorta, not backward into the left atrium, during ventricular systole. Damage to the mitral valve can affect the valve's ability to close properly (Figure 19-3). During ventricular systole, as blood is ejected forward into the aorta, blood is also ejected backward through the insufficient mitral valve. This abnormal blood flow contributes to an increase in left atrial volume, pressure, and eventually dilation. Increased left atrial pressures may lead to increased pulmonary vascular pressures and right-sided heart failure. The left ventricle usually dilates and hypertrophies over time as end-diastolic volumes increase and CO decreases.

Mitral insufficiency is often associated with dilated cardiomyopathy. As the left ventricle dilates, the papillary muscles are stretched and no longer able to maintain closure of the mitral valve during ventricular systole. Acute mitral insufficiency may occur due to dysfunction or rupture of the papillary muscles. Papillary muscle contraction contributes to preventing the valve leaflets from everting back into the left atrium during ventricular systole. Papillary muscles may rupture during an acute MI if blood supply to the tissue is diminished or absent during the infarct. Loss of a papillary muscle causes sudden, severe insufficiency of the mitral valve, resulting in rapid increase in both left ventricular and atrial volumes and pressures. The high left-sided pressures

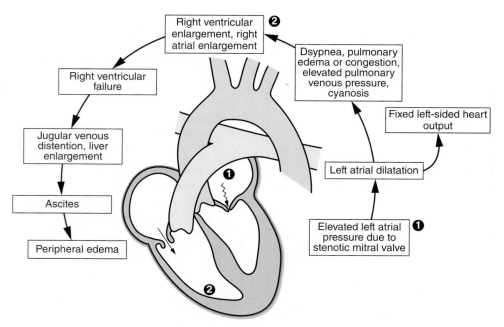

Figure 19-2. Cardiovascular effects of mitral stenosis.

affect the pulmonary vascular system leading to acute pulmonary edema. Unlike chronic mitral insufficiency, in acute mitral insufficiency, there is no time for the heart to compensate for the sudden increases in volume and pressure.

Pathophysiology of Aortic Stenosis
A similar process occurs in aortic stenosis as in mitral stenosis (Figure 19-4). Fusion of the commissures, fibrosis of the valve leaflets, and calcium deposits may occur on the aortic valve leaflets, impeding their movement. When aortic stenosis occurs, the left ventricle has to generate a significant amount of pressure to propel blood forward through the aortic valve into the aorta. Increased left ventricular pressure contributes to left ventricular dilation and hypertrophy, as well as decreases in CO. Left atrial volume and pressure increase as the left atrium must generate more pressure to

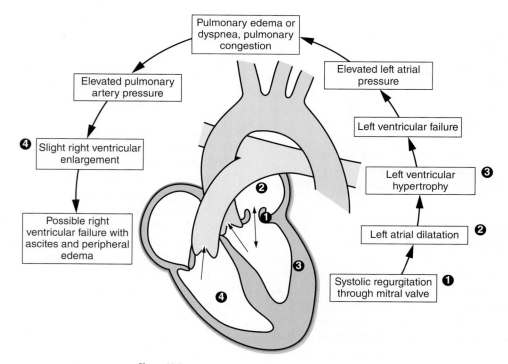

Figure 19-3. Cardiovascular effects of mitral insufficiency.

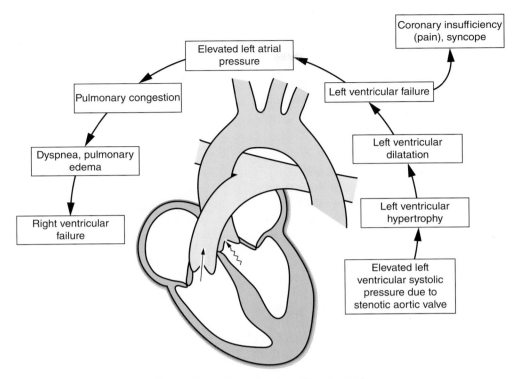

Figure 19-4. Cardiovascular effects of aortic stenosis.

eject blood into the left ventricle. Left atrial dilation may eventually occur. The elevated left-sided pressures are reflected back into the pulmonary vascular system and to the right side of the heart, eventually causing right heart failure.

Pathophysiology of Aortic Insufficiency

A similar process occurs in aortic insufficiency as in mitral insufficiency (Figure 19-5). Adequate closure of the aortic valve is even more important than adequate closure of the mitral

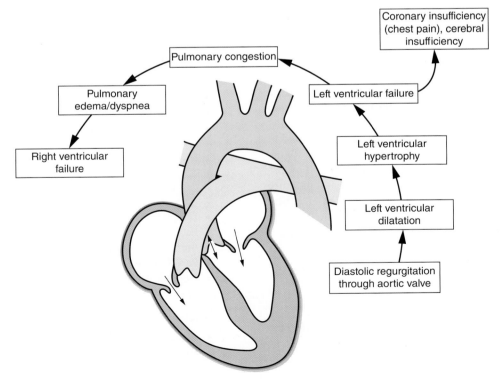

Figure 19-5. Cardiovascular effects of aortic insufficiency.

valve. If the aortic valve does not close properly, blood flows backward from the aorta into the left ventricle during diastole. This can seriously affect forward blood flow into the aorta, and thus CO. This causes significant increases in the volume and pressure of the left ventricle contributing to the gradual development of left ventricular dilation and hypertrophy. As with other left-sided valvular disease, pulmonary vascular pressures increase contributing to the development of right heart failure.

Pathophysiology of Tricuspid Stenosis

Fused commissures or fibrosis of the valve leaflets may also narrow the tricuspid valve orifice. RA pressures increase as the right atrium attempts to propel blood forward into the right ventricle. Eventually, RA dilation occurs and the increased right atrial pressure is reflected back into the venous system.

Pathophysiology of Tricuspid Insufficiency

Damage to the tricuspid valve that prevents complete closure during ventricular systole causes the abnormal ejection of blood through the tricuspid valve into the right atrium. Right atrial volumes and pressures increase, eventually leading to dilation and possible decreases in CO. In recent years, tricuspid insufficiency commonly occurs with dilated cardiomyopathy. As the right ventricle dilates, the papillary muscles are stretched and are unable to maintain closure of the valve during ventricular systole. This frequently accompanies mitral insufficiency.

Pathophysiology of Pulmonic Stenosis

Pulmonic stenosis develops as the pulmonic valve orifice becomes narrowed. Right ventricular pressures increase as the right ventricle attempts to eject blood forward into the pulmonary artery. Over the time, right ventricular dilation may occur, with decreases in right-sided CO. The increased pressure may back up into the right atrium, causing an increase in volume and pressure, and eventually leading to dilation. This can lead to volume and pressure increases in the venous system.

Pathophysiology of Pulmonic Insufficiency

Closure of the pulmonic valve prevents blood from backing up from the pulmonary artery into the right ventricle during diastole. An insufficient pulmonic valve permits blood to flow backward into the right ventricle during diastole. Right-sided CO decreases as blood flows backward instead of forward. An increase in right ventricular volume and pressure occurs, which may eventually lead to dilation. The increased pressures may be reflected back into the right atrium and the venous system. Pulmonic stenosis and insufficiency are rarely seen in adults and are much more common in children. They are usually caused by a congenital defect.

Clinical Presentation

Mitral and Aortic Disease

The following signs and symptoms are found in all of the valvular disorders of the left side of the heart:

- Dyspnea
- Fatigue

- Increased pulmonary artery pressures (PASs, PAD, PAOP)
- Decreased CO

Mitral Stenosis

- Palpitations
- Hemoptysis
- Hoarseness
- Dysphagia
- JVD
- Orthopnea
- Cough
- Diastolic murmur
- Atrial dysrhythmias (PACs, AF)
- Elevated A wave on PAOP pressure waveform

Mitral Insufficiency

- Paroxysmal nocturnal dyspnea
- Orthopnea
- Palpitations
- S_3 and/or S_4
- Crackles
- Systolic murmur
- Atrial dysrhythmias
- Elevated V wave on PAOP pressure waveform

Aortic Stenosis

- Angina
- Syncope
- Decreased SVR
- S_3 and/or S_4
- Systolic murmur
- Narrowed pulse pressure

Aortic Insufficiency

- Angina
- S_3
- Diastolic murmur
- Widened pulse pressure
- de Musset sign (nodding of the head)

Tricuspid and Pulmonic Valve Disease

The following signs and symptoms are found in all of the valvular disorders of the right side of the heart:

- Dyspnea
- Fatigue
- Increased RA pressures
- Peripheral edema
- Hepatomegaly
- JVD

Tricuspid Stenosis

- Atrial dysrhythmias
- Diastolic murmur
- Decreased CO
- Elevated A wave on RA pressure waveform

Tricuspid Insufficiency
- Conduction delays
- Supraventricular tachycardia (SVT)
- Systolic murmur
- Elevated V wave on RA pressure waveform

Pulmonic Stenosis
- Cyanosis
- Systolic murmur
- Elevated A wave on RA pressure waveform

Pulmonic Insufficiency
- Diastolic murmur
- Elevated A wave on RA pressure waveform

Diagnostic Tests
- *Chest x-ray:* Shows specific cardiac chamber enlargement, pulmonary congestion, presence of valve calcification
- *12-lead ECG:* Useful in the diagnosis of right ventricular, left ventricular, and left atrial hypertrophy
- *Echocardiogram:* Demonstrates the size of the four cardiac chambers, presence of hypertrophy, specific valve dysfunction, ejection fraction, and amount of regurgitant flow, if present
- *Radionuclide studies:* Identify abnormal ejection fraction during inactivity and activity
- *Cardiac catheterization:* Determines cardiac chamber pressures, ejection fraction, regurgitation, and pressure gradients, if present

Principles for Management of Valvular Disorders
The primary objectives in the management of valvular disorders are to maximize cardiac function, reduce anxiety, and prevent complications.

Maximize Cardiac Function
1. *Improve oxygenation delivery:* As ventricular dilation occurs, there is an increase in ventricular wall tension, myocardial workload, and oxygen consumption. Oxygen therapy is initiated, as necessary, to increase oxygen saturation. Pulse oximetry, arterial blood gases, and mixed venous oxygenation saturation (Svo_2) monitoring in the ICU are helpful in guiding supplemental oxygen therapy.
2. *Decrease preload:* Diuretics decrease excess fluid and ventricular end-diastolic volumes. Fluid and sodium restrictions also may be necessary. (*Exception:* Preload reduction is not part of the management plan for patients with aortic insufficiency, because decreased left ventricular end-diastolic volumes may adversely affect CO by increasing backward flow.)
3. *Decrease afterload:* Afterload reduction may be indicated for patients with increased SVR and impaired left ventricular function (eg, aortic stenosis or mitral insufficiency).

4. *Improve contractility:* Inotropic agents (eg, dobutamine, milrinone) increase myocardial contractility and improve CO.
5. *Modify activity:* Activity limitation helps reduce myocardial oxygen consumption. Teach patients the importance of alternating periods of activity with periods of rest.
6. *Balloon valvuloplasty may be an option for stenotic mitral or aortic valves:* A percutaneous catheter is inserted via the femoral artery under fluoroscopy and the balloon is inflated at the stenotic lesion in an effort to force open the fused commissures and improve valve leaflet mobility.

Surgical Management
Cardiac surgery is indicated when medical management does not alleviate patient symptoms. Patients may have better surgical outcomes if surgery is done prior to left ventricular dysfunction.

1. *Valve repair:* An increasing trend is to have dysfunctional valves repaired instead of replaced. The hemodynamic function of the inherent valve is superior to any prosthetic valve. In addition, the risks associated with valve replacement are avoided. An open commissurotomy may be performed to relieve stenosis of any of the four heart valves. During open commissurotomy, the fused commissures are incised, thus mobilizing the valve leaflets. Valve leaflet reconstruction also may be done using pericardial patches to repair tears in valve leaflets. Chordae tendineae reconstruction may be performed to elongate fibrotic tendineae or to shorten excessively stretched tendineae. An annuloplasty ring may also be inserted to correct dilation of the valve annulus.
2. *Prosthetic valve replacement:* Replacement of the native valve with a prosthetic, or artificial, valve is done for severely damaged valves or when repair is not possible. The entire native valve is removed and replaced with a mechanical or biological (porcine, bovine, or allograft [homograft or autograft]) prosthetic valve.
3. *Postoperative management* after cardiac surgery is similar to coronary artery bypass surgery management (see Chapter 9, Cardiovascular System). Special considerations for patients having valve repair or replacement include the following:
   - *Maintain adequate preload:* Patients with valvular heart disease, particularly aortic insufficiency and mitral insufficiency, are usually accustomed to increased end-diastolic volumes. Although the valve is repaired, the heart needs time to adjust to the hemodynamic changes. Generally, fluids are adjusted based on patient weight postoperatively as well as pulmonary symptoms, chest x-ray, and vital signs.

- *Monitor for conduction disturbances:* The mitral, tricuspid, and aortic valves lie in close proximity to conduction pathways. Temporary or permanent cardiac pacing may be needed to manage postoperative conduction disorders.
- *Initiate anticoagulation therapy:* Anticoagulation therapy is usually initiated for patients having valve replacement after the epicardial pacing wires are removed. This may be as early as the first postoperative day.

4. *Maze Procedure:* If the patient had AF or flutter preoperatively, the surgeon may perform a Maze procedure, ablating the area around the pulmonary veins in an effort to prevent return of the atrial dysrhythmia postoperatively.

5. *Transcatheter aortic valve replacement (TAVR):* Technological advances have allowed for the development of a minimally invasive approach to aortic valve replacement. In this approach, a prosthetic tissue valve is placed via a stent-like introducer catheter. The valve may be inserted through the femoral artery and placed across the native aortic valve. Another approach is transapical where a small incision is made in the anterior chest wall and the device is deployed through the left ventricular apex into the aortic valve position. Both approaches avoid the use of cardiopulmonary bypass (CPB). Currently, this procedure is limited to patients who are older (eighth or ninth decade) and who are too debilitated to tolerate the traditional surgical approaches to aortic valve replacement. The patient often experiences near immediate relief of symptoms and is discharged home within a couple of days.

6. *Transaortic approach:* In this approach, a ministernotomy is performed and the valve is accessed via the aorta. The benefit of this approach may include a decreased risk of postoperative bleeding compared to the transapical approach. A valve-in-valve procedure is another recently developed approach. This involves introducing a prosthetic tissue valve, using the transcatheter approach, into a previously implanted prosthetic tissue valve. The valve-in-valve TAVR approach was trialed in the Partner 2 study and found to have positive outcomes in those individuals who had a surgically implanted valve earlier that required replacement but the patient was no longer a surgical candidate. This is gaining increasing popularity—but still early in its use. Clinical trials are underway using the transcatheter approach for mitral valve and tricuspid valve replacement. Expect this to take a longer time to perfect due to the complexity of the mitral valve anatomy.

Reducing Anxiety
Teach the patient relaxation techniques. Deep breathing or imagery may help alleviate anxiety, especially when symptoms of valve dysfunction occur.

Preventing and Managing Complications

1. *Dysrhythmias:* Maintaining continuous ECG monitoring and performing daily 12-lead ECGs promote early recognition of cardiac dysrhythmias. Many cardiac medications can affect cardiac rhythm and these side effects can be observed with ECG monitoring

2. *Hemodynamic instability:* Hemodynamic monitoring may be invasive using a pulmonary artery catheter, minimally invasive using a central venous catheter and/or arterial pressure monitoring, or completely noninvasive. Generally, the patient is managed based on trends in hemodynamic monitoring.

3. *Thromboembolic event:* Anticoagulation is necessary for patients with severely compromised left ventricular function or AF, and after valve surgery. Lifelong anticoagulation therapy is indicated for patients after mechanical valve replacement. Short-term anticoagulation therapy is usually initiated for patients having a biological valve replacement.

4. *Endocarditis:* Antibiotic prophylaxis is recommended for patients with valve disorders and for patients with prosthetic valves. Prophylaxis is provided prior to dental work, surgery, or other invasive procedures. Prior to discharge, teach the patient and family the importance of prophylaxis.

5. *Prosthetic valve dysfunction:* Biological valve dysfunction usually develops slowly with gradual signs and symptoms (eg, presence of a new murmur, dyspnea, syncope). Mechanical valve dysfunction may occur slowly or suddenly. Rapid valve dysfunction requires an emergency intervention as the patient presents with signs and symptoms of acute cardiac failure (hypotension, tachycardia, low CO/CI, heart failure, cardiac arrest).

Pericarditis

Pericarditis is a chronic or acute inflammation of the pericardial lining of the heart. Acute pericarditis usually occurs secondary to another disease process and usually resolves within 6 weeks. Chronic pericarditis, however, may last for months.

Pericarditis may lead to pericardial effusion or cardiac tamponade. Pericardial effusion occurs as fluid builds up within the pericardial sac. Cardiac tamponade can occur as the pericardial fluid compresses the heart, restricts ventricular end-diastolic filling, and compromises cardiac function.

The case study is an example of the importance of accurate diagnosis of patients with chest pain. The pain of pericarditis may be similar to anginal pain, but the treatment is very different.

Etiology and Pathophysiology
A number of different conditions and situations can cause pericarditis (Table 19-3). Common causes include MI, infections, neoplasm, radiation therapy, and uremia.

TABLE 19-3. ETIOLOGY OF PERICARDITIS

Idiopathic
Infections (viral/bacterial)
Myocardial infarction
Cardiac surgery
Neoplasm
Radiation therapy
Rheumatic disease
Lupus erythematosus
Scleroderma
Uremia
Medication induced

Normally, the pericardial sac contains a small amount of clear serous fluid, typically less than 50 mL. This fluid lies between the visceral and the parietal pericardium and lubricates the surface of the heart as it expands and contracts. An inflammation of the pericardium causes friction between the visceral and the parietal pericardial layers.

Inflammation of the pericardium causes an increase in pericardial fluid production, with increases of up to 1 liter or more. A gradual buildup of fluid may have little compromising effect on the heart as the pericardium expands and normal hemodynamics is not altered. A sudden increase in pericardial fluid, however, dramatically impairs the hemodynamic status.

Chronic pericarditis causes fibrotic changes within the pericardial lining. The visceral and parietal pleura eventually adhere to each other, restricting the filling of the heart. This condition may be referred to as constrictive pericarditis. The pressure created by the constricted pericardium affects the heart's ability to distend properly, causing decreases in end-diastolic volume and CO. These changes may contribute to increases in ventricular end-diastolic atrial pressures, leading to increases in pulmonary vascular and venous system pressures

Clinical Presentation
Acute Pericarditis

- Sharp, stabbing, burning, dull, or aching pain in the substernal or precordial area, which increases with movement, inspiration, or coughing, or when the patient is in a recumbent position
- Pericardial friction rub
- Fever
- Sinus tachycardia
- Dyspnea, orthopnea
- Cough
- Fatigue
- Narrowed pulse pressure
- Hypotension
- Dysrhythmias
- Elevated cardiac pressures (PA, PAOP, RA)
- Decreased CO
- Peripheral edema
- JVD

ESSENTIAL CONTENT CASE
Pericarditis

A woman had an acute anterior MI 7 days ago. She was readmitted to the progressive care unit with sharp, substernal chest pain worsening with inspiration, shortness of breath, and ST-segment elevation in the precordial leads and in leads I and II. The chest pain was unrelieved with nitroglycerin. Her pain did improve after receiving 4 mg of morphine IV. The pain went away completely when she sat up and leaned forward so that her nurse could auscultate posterior breath sounds.

Case Question 1: A classic sign of pericarditis is:
(A) Sharp pain on inspiration relieved by leaning forward
(B) Distended neck veins
(C) Narrow pulse pressure
(D) Cough

Case Question 2: An important nursing action for this patient is to:
(A) Continue to administer morphine for pain
(B) Encourage patient to ambulate as much as possible
(C) Alleviate anxiety by informing patient this is not another heart attack
(D) Encourage deep breathing exercises to expand the lung

Answers
1. A is the correct answer. A sharp pain on inspiration relieved by leaning forward is a classic sign of pericarditis. Neck vein distention may accompany pericarditis but is not always present.
2. C is the correct answer. Many patients believe the onset of chest pain indicates they are having another MI. It is important to inform the patient that it is not.

Chronic Pericarditis

- Dyspnea
- Anorexia
- Fatigue
- Abdominal discomfort
- Weight gain
- Activity intolerance
- JVD
- Peripheral edema
- Hepatomegaly
- Kussmaul sign (increase in RA pressure during inspiration)

Diagnostic Tests

- *Chest x-ray:* Normal or enlarged heart; chronic pericarditis may reveal a decrease in heart size.
- *ECG:* ST-segment elevation in precordial leads (V leads) and leads I, II, or III; T-wave inversion after ST-segment returns to isoelectric line; decrease in QRS voltage.
- *Echocardiogram:* Presence of increased fluid in pericardial sac; chronic, constrictive pericarditis may

demonstrate a thickened pericardium and diminished ventricular contractility.

- *Laboratory:* Elevated sedimentation rate and elevated white blood cell (WBC); causative organisms may be identified from blood cultures.
- *CT/MRI scan:* Detects a thickened pericardium for patients with chronic pericarditis.

Principles of Management of Pericarditis

The primary principles of management of pericarditis are to correct the underlying cause, relieve pain and promote comfort, relieve pericardial effusion, and prevent and manage complications associated with pericarditis.

Promoting Comfort and Relieving Pain

1. *Decrease pain:* Teach the patient that chest pain may be decreased or relieved by sitting up and/or leaning forward. Analgesics such as, colchicine, and nonsteroidal anti-inflammatory agents administered around the clock assist in pain relief.
2. *Promote relaxation:* Teach the patient relaxation techniques such as progressive muscle relaxation and visualization. This may assist the patient to cope. Relaxation techniques that include deep breathing are avoided because pericardial pain usually increases with deep inspiration.
3. *Limit activity:* This is especially important during the acute period of inflammation. Activity can be gradually increased as fever and chest pain decrease. Assist patients to find a position of comfort. Patients often are more comfortable sitting up and leaning slightly forward.

Correcting the Underlying Cause

1. *Decrease pericardial inflammation:* Nonsteroidal anti-inflammatory agents (eg, indomethacin, ibuprofen) assist to decrease inflammation of the pericardium and the associated pain. Chronic, recurrent pericarditis may require corticosteroid therapy.
2. *Eliminate infection:* If the cause of the pericarditis is an infectious process, appropriate medications, including antibiotic therapy, are necessary.

Relieving Pericardial Effusion

1. *Pericardiocentesis:* A needle or small catheter is introduced subxiphoid into the pericardial sac and fluid is withdrawn via the needle or is attached to a catheter and drained into a vacuum bottle. This procedure is performed to remove fluid from the pericardium and improve myocardial function. Culture specimens of the drained fluid are obtained and sent to the laboratory for analysis. The drain may be left in for several days until the volume of drainage is minimal.
2. *Pericardiotomy/pericardial window:* This is a surgical procedure in which a section of the pericardium is removed in an effort to decrease pericardial pressure

on the heart and to allow pericardial fluid to drain more readily. A drain may be inserted into the pericardium and tunneled down across the diaphragm into the peritoneal cavity. This permits the excess fluid to drain continuously into the peritoneal space where it is eventually absorbed into the lymph system. It may be performed for recurrent pericardial effusions.
3. *Pericardiectomy:* This involves surgically removing the entire pericardium. This may be necessary for chronic pericarditis that is refractory to other interventions.

Preventing and Managing Complications

1. *Monitor for signs and symptoms of acute heart failure:* These include hypotension, tachycardia, increased RR, extreme dyspnea, decreased oxygen saturation, decreased peripheral pulses, and decreased urinary output. Oxygen therapy and inotropic agents assist in improvement of myocardial contractility. Assessment of the need for surgical intervention for pericarditis may be indicated.
2. *Cardiac tamponade:* Monitor for signs and symptoms of cardiac tamponade. These include hypotension, tachycardia, tachypnea, dyspnea, pulsus paradoxus, narrowed pulse pressure, muffled heart sounds, and distended neck veins. Another sign of tamponade is equalization of pressures, when hemodynamic assessment reveals PAS, PAD, PAOP, and CVP that fall within a close range. Emergency pericardiocentesis is necessary to prevent further hemodynamic compromise.

Aortic Aneurysm

An aortic aneurysm is an area of aortic wall dilation. Aneurysms are most prevalent in men, commonly occurring during their early 50s to late 60s. Without treatment, mortality associated with aortic aneurysms is high.

Aneurysms frequently are classified by types (Figure 19-6). A fusiform aneurysm is characterized by distention of the entire circumference of the affected portion of the aorta. A saccular aneurysm is characterized by distention of one side of the aorta. The distention of a saccular aneurysm resembles a bulging sac. Aneurysms may also be classified according to their location (Figure 19-7):

- *Ascending:* Between the aortic valve and the innominate artery
- *Transverse:* Between the innominate artery and the left subclavian artery
- *Descending:* From the left subclavian artery to the diaphragm
- *Thoracoabdominal:* From above the diaphragm to the aortic bifurcation

Aneurysms have the potential to dissect or rupture. Dissection occurs when the intimal aortic wall is disrupted and

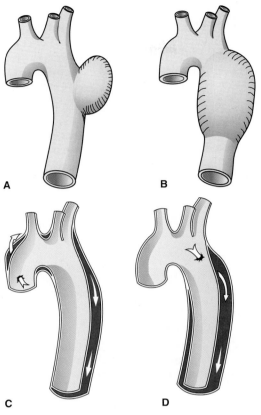

Figure 19-6. Diagram of different types of aortic aneurysms. **(A)** Saccular aneurysm. **(B)** Fusiform aneurysm. **(C, D)** Two aortic dissections. (*Reproduced with permission from Underhill SL, Woods SL, Sivarajan ES, et al:* Cardiac Nursing. *Philadelphia, PA. JB Lippincott; 1982.*)

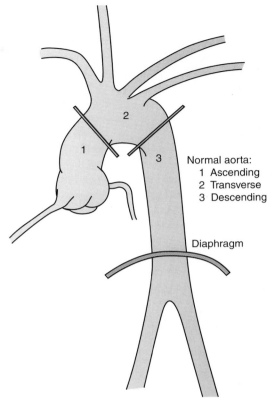

Normal aorta:
1 Ascending
2 Transverse
3 Descending

Diaphragm

Figure 19-7. Classification of aortic aneurysms according to location. (*Reproduced with permission from Seifert PC.* Cardiac Surgery. *St Louis, MO: Mosby Yearbook; 1994.*)

blood extends into the aortic vessel layers (see Figures 19-6C and 19-6D). Rupture occurs when all three layers of the aorta are disrupted and massive hemorrhage occurs. Both dissection and rupture are life-threatening events. The case study demonstrates the sudden onset of signs and symptoms associated with aortic rupture and the emergent need for life-saving interventions.

Etiology and Pathophysiology

Aortic aneurysms are caused by a variety of conditions, including atherosclerosis, genetic link, congenital abnormality, hypertension, Marfan syndrome, and trauma to the chest.

The aorta is composed of three layers: the intima, media, and tunica adventitia. Aneurysm development is initiated by degeneration of smooth muscle cells and elastic tissue in the medial layer of the aorta. This weakens the vessel wall, potentially leading to dilation of all layers of the aorta. The aortic wall may be further weakened with age, as well as from hypertension.

As the aortic aneurysm gradually expands, there is an increase in the risk for aortic dissection. Dissection begins with a tear in the intima. Blood leaves the central aorta via the intimal tear and flows through the medial layer of the aorta (see Figures 19-6C and 19-6D). This creates a false lumen. As

the amount of blood increases in the medial layer, the pressure in the false lumen increases, compressing the central aorta (see Figure 19-6D). This compression may decrease or totally obstruct blood flow through the aorta and/or its arterial branches. Dissections are classified as acute if they have occurred less than 2 weeks since the onset of symptoms. They are classified as chronic if they occurred more than 2 weeks since the onset of symptoms.

Two additional classifications exist for identifying the location of aortic dissections (Figure 19-8). The first (Stanford classification) classifies the dissection as type A, involving the ascending aorta, or type B, involving the descending aorta (distal to the left subclavian artery). Type A requires immediate surgical intervention whereas type B is managed medically until surgery is deemed necessary. Another classification system for aortic dissection has three categories for the dissection: type I, the original intimal tear begins in the ascending aorta and the dissection extends to the descending aorta; type II, the original intimal tear begins and is contained in the ascending aorta; and type III, the original intimal tear begins and is contained in the descending aorta.

Clinical Presentation

Patients rarely demonstrate early signs of an aortic aneurysm. Diagnosis is commonly made during a routine physical examination or chest x-ray. Signs and symptoms

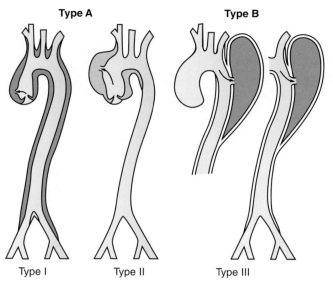

Figure 19-8. Classification for the location of aortic dissections. The Stanford system classifies aortic dissections based on involvement (type A) of the ascending aorta or noninvolvement (type B). The DeBakey system classifies dissections into types I, II, or III. (*Reproduced with permission from DeBakey ME. Surgical management of dissecting aneurysms of the aorta. J Thorac Cardiovasc Surg. 1965;49:131; adapted with permission from Seifert PC. Cardiac Surgery. St Louis, MO: Mosby Yearbook; 1994.*)

of an aortic aneurysm occur as the aneurysm enlarges and compresses adjacent organs, structures, and/or nerve pathways.

Thoracic Aneurysm

Often times thoracic aneurysm is asymptomatic until the growing aneurysm puts pressure on surrounding nerves and organs

- Chest pain
- Back pain
- Dysphagia
- Hoarseness, cough
- Dyspnea
- Different BPs when comparing right and left arms
- Different pulses when comparing right and left peripheral pulses

Abdominal Aneurysm

- Dull, constant abdominal, side, low back, lumbar pain or groin pain
- Abdominal mass
- Pulsations in the abdomen
- Reduced lower extremity pulses
- Nausea and/or vomiting

Aortic Dissection

- Ripping, tearing, or splitting pain, located at the anterior chest or posterior chest between the scapula, of an intense or excruciating nature
- Dyspnea
- Syncope

ESSENTIAL CONTENT CASE

Aortic Aneurysm

A 62-year-old man was admitted to the progressive care unit with substernal chest pain. The chest pain was unrelieved by nitroglycerin. The pain decreased in intensity after 8 mg of morphine sulfate. His admitting ECG was normal. His chest x-ray revealed a widened mediastinum, and an aortogram demonstrated a thoracic aneurysm. He has nitroprusside infusing at 1.0 mcg/kg/min to maintain his systolic BP below 100 mm Hg. Suddenly, the patient yells out, "The pain, the pain . . . it's back . . . it's even worse than before." A rapid assessment reveals the following:

BP	190/100 mm Hg
HR	110 beats/min
RR	30 breaths/min
Color	Gray
Skin	Moist and cool
Pain	Rated 10 on a 0 to 10 scale, described as tearing in the middle of his chest and between his shoulder blades

Case Question 1: Following relief of the patient's pain with morphine and notification of the physician, the nurse anticipates the patient will need:
(A) STAT chest x-ray
(B) STAT CT scan of the chest
(C) Cardiac catheterization
(D) STAT MRI

Case Question 2: Based on the description of the location of the pain, the nurse suspects the dissection is located in the:
(A) Ascending thoracic aorta
(B) Transverse thoracic aorta
(C) Descending thoracic aorta
(D) Abdominal aorta

Case Question 3: Medical management of a thoracic aortic aneurysm is focused on:
(A) Maintaining the systolic BP less than 120 mm Hg
(B) Maintaining the diastolic BP less than 40 mm Hg
(C) Maintaining the HR less than 100 beats/min
(D) Reducing the CO to less than 2.0 L/min

Answers
1. B is the correct answer. The CT will reveal the location and extent of the aneurysm.
2. C is the correct answer. Chest pain is a common symptom associated with a dissection of the descending thoracic aorta.
3. A is the correct answer. It is important to maintain the systolic pressure at 120 or below to prevent further dissection or rupture of the aneurysm.

- Abdominal discomfort or bloating
- Extremity weakness
- Oliguria or hematuria
- Hemiparesis, hemiplegia, or paraplegia

- Speech or visual disturbances
- Decreased hemoglobin and hematocrit
- Loss of consciousness

Aortic Rupture

- Sudden cessation of pain
- Recurrence of pain
- Signs and symptoms of shock, with the exception of BP (high in rupture), including tachycardia, increased RR, pallor, moist skin, and restlessness

Diagnostic Tests

- *Chest x-ray:* Shows the dilated aorta, widening of the mediastinum, and mediastinal mass.
- *CT/MRI scan:* Determines the size of the aorta, size of the aneurysm, extent of a dissection, involvement of additional arterial branches, lumen diameter, and wall thickness.
- *Echocardiogram:* Can sometimes visualize the location and size of an aneurysm. Transesophageal echo (TEE) may be more helpful, particularly in visualizing thoracic aneurysms and when dissection is suspected.
- *Aortography:* Determines the origin, size, and location of the aneurysm and involvement of additional arterial branches

Principles for Management of Aortic Aneurysm

The primary objectives in the management of aortic aneurysm are relieving pain and anxiety, lowering BP and thereby decreasing stress on the aneurysm, surgical repair if necessary, patient teaching, and prevention of complications.

Relieving Pain and Anxiety

Administer narcotics (eg, morphine) as necessary. Unrelieved pain is likely to increase anxiety, tachycardia, and hypertension, all of which may aggravate the condition. Relaxation therapy, with deep breathing exercises or imagery, may be extremely helpful.

Decreasing Stress on Aneurysm Wall

1. *Decrease afterload:* Vasodilators (eg, nitroprusside, nicardipine, esmolol) may be prescribed to lower BP and thus pressure on the aneurysm. BPs are maintained as low as possible (systolic blood pressure 90-120 mm Hg), without compromising perfusion to vital organs.
2. *Decrease preload:* Limit oral and IV fluids, decrease sodium intake, and administer diuretics as indicated. A decrease in preload decreases the circulating blood volume, thus decreasing pressure on the site of the aneurysm.
3. *Decrease myocardial contractility* with beta-blockers (eg, esmolol, labetalol). A decrease in the strength of each cardiac contraction decreases the pulsatile pressure on the aneurysm.

Patient and Family Teaching

1. *Follow-up:* If the patient is to be medically managed, follow-up chest x-rays, CT scans, MRI scans, and/or ultrasounds will be needed at 6-month intervals to assess the status of the aneurysm. The importance of these studies is stressed.
2. *Diet modification:* Teach the patient and family the importance of following a low-sodium diet. Consult a nutritionist for recipes and tips for food preparation.
3. *Smoking cessation:* Connect patient with programs available to assist with smoking cessation.
4. *Physical/psychological stress modification:* Teach the patient and family the hazardous effects of stress and the importance for modification. Discuss activity limitations and relaxation therapy.
5. *Medications:* Teach the patient and family the importance of adherence with the medication regimen. Stress that the medications are essential even though the patient may be asymptomatic.

Surgical Management

Surgery is indicated for acute aneurysm rupture, aortic dissection in the ascending aorta, aortic dissection refractory to medical therapy, and asymptomatic patients with a fusiform aneurysm 6 cm or more in diameter (normal diameter is 2.5-3 cm).

1. During surgery the aortic aneurysm is resected and a prosthetic graft is sutured in place. The original aortic wall may be wrapped around the prosthetic graft for additional support.
2. If an acute dissection or rupture occurs and the patient is waiting for the operating room team to arrive:
   - Administer narcotics for pain.
   - Titrate vasodilators to maintain the patient's BP as low as possible (90-120 mm Hg if tolerated). This decreases the pressure on the aneurysm.
   - Administer fluids to prevent hypovolemia.
   - Administer blood replacement products to maintain adequate hemoglobin and hematocrit levels. If rupture occurs, the chest and abdomen will be opened emergently. The patient has a high risk of mortality or complications, including cerebral anoxia, severe hypovolemic shock, and multiorgan dysfunction syndrome (MODS).
3. Postoperative management:
   - Same interventions as described to relieve pain and anxiety and decrease stress on the aorta wall. It is important to decrease pressure on the repaired aorta so that suture lines can heal and bleeding is kept to a minimum.
   - Continuous ECG and hemodynamic monitoring.
   - Complete assessment (including a focused neurologic assessment) once per shift after the patient

leaves the ICU. These patients are at risk to develop hemiparesis of the lower extremities following surgical repair of the aneurysm.

- Gradual rewarming to prevent postoperative shivering, which increases BP and places additional stress on suture lines.
- Maintain adequate oxygenation with ventilator management or supplemental oxygen.
- Progressive mobility according to institution standards and surgeon preference.
- Monitor renal function (urine output, blood urea nitrogen [BUN]), and creatinine, especially if the aorta was cross-clamped above the renal arteries.

Preventing and Managing Complications

1. *Hemorrhage:* Hourly assessment of vital signs and hemodynamic parameters. Daily assessment of hemoglobin and hematocrit.
2. *Dysrhythmia:* Continuous ECG monitoring; daily 12-lead ECGs; monitoring electrolytes and replacing as indicated.
3. *Hemodynamic instability:* Arterial and PAP monitoring; manage hemodynamic parameters based on trends.
4. *Altered perfusion:* Arteries originating from the aorta may be compromised, leading to MI, cerebral insufficiency/cerebrovascular accident, bowel necrosis, renal failure, paraplegia, and limb ischemia. Assess and monitor the patient for these conditions.
5. *Aortic insufficiency:* Aortic insufficiency may develop if the aneurysm is located in the ascending aorta. Enlargement or dissection of the aneurysm may dilate or damage the aortic valve, causing signs of acute heart failure and pulmonary edema.

Cardiac Transplantation

From the early work of Dr. Christian Barnard in 1967, cardiac transplantation has evolved over four decades to a standard modality for the treatment of end-stage cardiac disease. When medical, surgical, or pharmacologic interventions have failed to improve quality of life and functional capacity, cardiac transplantation offers patients improved survival. The international survival rate is 80% to 90%, 75% at 1 year, and 56% at 10 years. The primary indications for cardiac transplantation include cardiomyopathies or ischemic heart disease. Other indications include heart valve disease, congenital heart disease, and myocarditis.

Candidate Selection

Candidates for cardiac transplant usually have a poor prognosis without transplant and are in New York Heart Association (NYHA) functional class III or IV or American Heart Association (AHA) Stage D. Some patients require a cardiac

TABLE 19-4. GENERAL INDICATIONS FOR CARDIAC TRANSPLANTATION

Criteria for Consideration of Heart Transplantation in Advanced Heart Failure

General Indications:
- Dilated cardiomyopathy
- Ischemic cardiomyopathy
- Congenital heart disease for which no conventional therapy exists or for which conventional therapy has failed
- Ejection fraction less than 20%
- Pulmonary vascular resistance of less than 2 Wood units
- Age younger than 70 years
- Ability to comply with medical follow-up care
- Absence of tobacco use

Updated Criteria:[a]
- An estimated 1 year survival of less than 80%, as calculated by the Seattle Heart Failure Model or Heart Failure Survival Score in high/medium risk range
- Right heart catheterization should be performed on all adult candidates in preparation for listing and periodically until transplanted
- After LVAD, reevaluation of hemodynamics should be done after 3 to 6 months to ascertain reversibility of pulmonary hypertension
- Recommend weight loss to achieve body mass index less than or equal to 35 kg/m^2
- Severe symptomatic cerebrovascular disease
- Assessment of frailty (three of five possible symptoms: unintentional weight loss ≥ 10 lb within the past years, muscle loss, fatigue, slow walking speed, and low levels of physical activity
- Retransplantation is indicated for those patients who develop significant cardiac allograft vasculopathy with refractory cardiac allograft dysfunction, without evidence of ongoing rejection

[a]Data from Mehra MR, Hannan MM, Semigran MJ, et al. The 2016 International Society for Heart Lung Transplantation listing criteria for heart transplant: A 10 year update, J Heart Lung Transplant 2016 Jan;35(1):1-23.

assist device such as the IABP, VAD, or ECMO to maintain adequate hemodynamic stability while awaiting transplantation. Because of the shortage of available organs and the complexity of post-transplant care, the patient must pass an extensive screening process to ascertain that he or she is appropriate for the candidate list (Table 19-4). Patients must be emotionally stable and free of alcohol, drug addictions, and tobacco use. They must demonstrate a commitment to the rigors of being a candidate and eventual recipient through adherence to their medical regimens.

The period of waiting for an available donor can be extremely stressful for patients and their families. It is important to explore their perceptions of the transplant process, what outcomes they are anticipating, and what methods they have utilized to cope in the past. Support group participation or meetings with a psychiatric clinical nurse specialist or nurse practitioner may be beneficial. Fear of death and acute illness may heighten the patient's anxiety. Family members may need proximity to the patient, and this may assist in alleviating anxiety. Incorporating their involvement in direct patient care may enhance their coping abilities.

Pretransplant Process

The greatest delay for cardiac transplantation occurs because of the shortage of donors. When a brain-dead donor is identified, he or she must be carefully managed to maintain cardiovascular stability and avoid electrolyte and renal complications. The United Network for Organ Sharing (UNOS) coordinates the allocation of organs based on a nationwide waiting list. The donor must be of a compatible ABO blood type to the recipient and of similar body size and weight. The recipient is tested for relative immunologic compatibility with the donor to avoid hyperacute rejection. Panel-reactive antibody screening is performed using the recipient's serum with a random pool of lymphocytes. If no lymphocyte destruction occurs, the cross-match is negative and the transplant may proceed. The donor's cardiac function must be normal as assessed by an echocardiogram, nuclear studies, or cardiac catheterization. The donor should have stable hemodynamic profiles on minimal inotropic support.

This process may take several hours, and it is imperative that the patient and family be frequently updated and made aware of the clinical plan of care. Pretransplant teaching is reviewed to clarify misconceptions and correct knowledge deficits. If CO is compromised, decreased cerebral perfusion may compromise the attention span. During this time, the recipient needs close monitoring to maintain cardiovascular stability. The recipient may require antiarrhythmic therapy, inotropes, diuretics, or after-load reduction agents to achieve major organ perfusion adequate for cellular function. Anticoagulation therapy may be instituted to decrease risk of embolization secondary to AF, reduced left ventricular function, or peripheral venous stasis.

Unstable patients may be maintained on cardiac assist devices such as the IABP, VAD, or ECMO to promote stabilization or to "bridge" to transplantation.

Transplant Surgical Techniques

In the past, there were two surgical options for cardiac transplantation. Today, almost all are orthotopic transplants in which the recipient's heart is removed and replaced by the donor's heart in the normal anatomic position (Figure 19-9). The surgical approach is a median sternotomy; the recipient's heart is incised at the superior and inferior vena cavae, pulmonary artery, and aorta. The donor's and recipient's vena cavae, aortas, and pulmonary arteries are aligned and anastomosed. This technique is called the bicaval technique.

Another technique, which is less common, is the biatrial technique. This method involves removing the native heart but leaving the superior/posterior aspects of both atria. This will leave the native SA node intact and may result in double P waves on the ECG tracing (see Figure 19-9). In both techniques, the donor's heart is denervated and therefore receives no sympathetic or parasympathetic influence from the recipient's nervous system. Changes in CO after heart transplant depend on noncardiac mediators.

The other surgical option was a heterotopic approach, which is interesting from a historical perspective. It was used in about 5% of cardiac transplants at one point and was also known as a piggyback approach. The donor's heart was placed to the right side of the pleural cavity and performed as an auxiliary pump for the native heart (Figure 19-10). This was used as an option in a size mismatch between donor and recipient or for severe pulmonary hypertension. This approach is rarely performed any more.

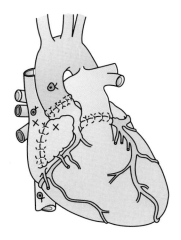

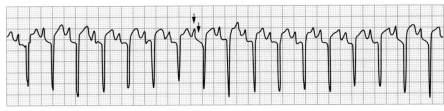

Figure 19-9. Orthotopic method of transplantation using a biatrial approach. Both the donor and the recipient SA nodes are intact (X). This results in an ECG tracing as shown. Arrows in the ECG strip show the double P wave at independent rates. (*Reproduced with permission from Morton PG, Fontaine DK. Critical Care Nursing: A Holistic Approach, 9th ed. Philadelphia: Lippincott Williams & Wilkins; 2009.*)

ESSENTIAL CONTENT CASE

Cardiac Transplant

A 54-year-old, white, married, unemployed man is admitted to the progressive care unit for idiopathic cardiomyopathy after an orthotopic heart transplant (OHT) 2 days ago. He has a mediastinal chest tube draining 60 mL of sanguineous fluid per hour, atrial and ventricular epicardial wires, and a left radial arterial line. CO, cardiac index, and SVR are being monitored using a minimally invasive device connected to the arterial catheter.

Temperature	35.88°C
BP	140/82 mm Hg
HR	90 beats/min NSR without ectopy; remnant P wave present
RR	18 breaths/min
CO	3.80 L/min
Urine	60 mL/h
CI	2.0 L/min/m²
Mediastinal tube	60 mL/h
SVR	1800 dyne/s/cm⁵
SvO_2	58%
SpO_2	96%
Neurologic	Moves all extremities on command; neurologically intact

Case Question 1: Which of the following hemodynamic measurements would contribute to the CI of 2.0 l/min/m²?
(A) HR 90 beats/min
(B) SVR 1800 dynes/s/cm⁵
(C) SvO_2 58%
(D) RR 18 breaths/min

Case Question 2: Which of the following treatments would be appropriate to increase the CO/CI?
(A) Dobutamine to improve ventricular contractility
(B) Dopamine to improve renal perfusion
(C) Sodium nitroprusside to reduce afterload
(D) Esmolol to control the HR

Answers
1. B is the correct answer. The increased SVR reflects an increased afterload on the left ventricle causing an increased cardiac workload.
2. C is the correct answer. Sodium nitroprusside is an arterial vasodilator and will reduce the SVR thereby reducing myocardial work.

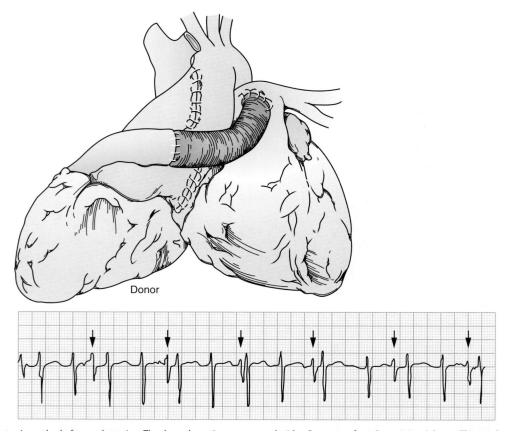

Donor

Figure 19-10. Heterotopic method of transplantation. The donor heart is anastomosed with a Dacron graft to the recipient's heart. This results in an ECG tracing as shown. Arrows point to the "extra" QRS at an independent rate. (*Reproduced with permission from Smeltzer SC, Bare BG.* Brunner & Suddarth's Textbook of Medical-Surgical Nursing, *10th ed. Philadelphia: Lippincott Williams & Wilkins; 2004.*)

Principles of Management of Cardiac Transplantation

The postsurgical care is similar to care following conventional open heart surgery (see Chapter 9, Cardiovascular System). The primary objectives in the early postoperative period include stabilizing cardiovascular function, monitoring altered immune response and graft protection, and providing post-transplant psychological adjustment.

Stabilizing Cardiovascular Function

1. *Cardiac denervation:* Postoperatively there is loss of vagal influence, and the patient usually has a higher resting HR than normal.
   - The post-transplant patient requires more stabilization prior to exercise or position changes to avoid orthostasis due to these effects from denervation. With loss of vagal tone, and if the sinus rate decreases, there is a stronger potential for junctional rhythms to result.
   - Surgical manipulation and postoperative edema may decrease donor SA node automaticity, and therefore the patient may require temporary pacing or isoproterenol (Isuprel) to increase the HR.
   - If dysrhythmias such as SVT occur, beta-blockers or calcium channel blockers are used to decrease HR in these circumstances. It is important to assess the patient for response to isoproterenol, because the medication can increase myocardial oxygen consumption.
   - Denervation also creates a more long-term concern in these patients because the patient no longer experiences angina if the myocardium becomes ischemic. Pain impulses are not transmitted to the brain, so patients must be taught to report other signs of declining cardiac function (ie, decreased exercise tolerance). This is seen in chronic rejection where even with diffuse coronary artery disease, the patient does not experience angina. The patient transplanted for ischemic cardiac disease may find this difficult to comprehend.
2. *Ventricular failure:* Any element of pulmonary hypertension can result in right ventricular dysfunction and eventually compromise left ventricular function also. Inotropic and vasodilating agents may be required to enhance cardiac function. It is essential to rule out any cardiac injury during harvesting and implantation that may have an impact on cardiac function. Review of the operative procedure can help rule out reperfusion injuries or post-bypass problems.
3. *Bleeding:* Risk factors include CPB, altered coagulation factors if right ventricular failure compromised hepatic function, and preoperative anticoagulation therapy. The recipient's pericardium may be enlarged from pretransplant cardiomegaly. With a smaller donor heart, there is more room for blood accumulation without early detection. If there is greater than 100 to 200 mL/h of bleeding for 2 hours, the patient may need to return to the OR. All medications are reviewed for potential effect on platelet function and coagulation factors.

Monitoring Altered Immune Response and Graft Protection

After cardiac transplantation, the patient is pharmacologically managed with immunosuppressive treatment for graft protection, titrating for the best graft function with the least adverse effects. By virtue of these agents, patient survival has been tremendously enhanced, with a decrease in the need for retransplantation.

1. *Immunosuppression:* Most patients are maintained on triple-therapy immunosuppression, such as tacrolimus (Prograf®), mycophenolate mofetil (CellCept®), and corticosteroids.
   - Tacrolimus (Prograf®), is indicated for both prevention of and management of organ rejection. It is classified as a calcineurin inhibitor, which inhibits the phosphate required for IL2 production. The effect is limiting T-lymphocyte activation. Tacrolimus is used in combination with mycophenolate mofetil and is generally preferred over cyclosporine. Adverse effects include prolonging QTc intervals and producing hyperkalemia. Potassium levels are monitored closely. A daily trough level is measured to assess therapeutic dosage and avoid toxicity.
   - Cyclosporine inhibits certain T-cells, creating a selective immunosuppression. T-cells dependent on humoral immunity continue intact and no bone marrow suppression occurs. T-cell lymphocytes become unresponsive to interleukin (IL)-1, ultimately preventing maturation of helper and cytotoxic T-cells. Adverse effects include hypertension, nephrotoxicity, hepatotoxicity, hirsutism, tremors, and gum hyperplasia. When the first intravenous (IV) dose is administered, it is important to assess the patient closely for potential histamine-type reactions with cardiovascular collapse. This is related to the IV solution preparation and is not seen with the oral preparation. A daily trough level is measured to assess therapeutic dosage and avoid toxicity.
   - Basiliximab (Simulect) is an immunosuppressive agent that is an IL-2 antagonist. It is indicated for patients with renal insufficiency related to their chronic low CO because it is renal sparing. This medication is given preoperatively and then 2 to 4 days postoperatively.
   - Mycophenolate mofetil has potent cytotoxic effects on lymphocytes. It inhibits the proliferative responses of T and B lymphocytes to both mitogenic and allospecific stimulation. It also suppresses antibody formation against B lymphocytes.

It is given in 1.5-g dose twice a day. The side effects include gastrointestinal tract ulceration, nausea, vomiting, and diarrhea. It has severe neutropenic effects and can cause anemia, leukopenia, and thrombocytopenia.

- Corticosteroids are administered to both prevent and treat rejection. They are able to decrease antibody production and inhibit antigen-antibody production, as well as interfere with production of mediators IL-1 and IL-2. Both their anti-inflammatory and immunosuppressive properties offer the patient benefits. Immediately postoperatively, they are administered in high doses, and then tapered over the next 6 months. However, if the patient experiences two or more episodes of acute rejection, he/she remains on a maintenance dose. In situations of acute or chronic rejection, the patient may be "pulsed" with steroids. These doses are 500 to 1000 mg IV every day for 3 days, during which other steroids are discontinued. The patient then resumes the maintenance dose of steroids. Complications from steroid treatment are numerous and include infection, hyperlipidemia, diabetes, hypertension, osteoporosis, sodium and water retention, metabolic alkalosis, peptic ulceration, pancreatitis, increased appetite, adrenopituitary suppression, lymphocytopenia, opportunistic infections, and aseptic necrosis of femoral and humoral heads. The patient often receives ulcer prophylaxis with a histamine blocker or antacids. Strict fluid and electrolyte balance must be maintained, and close assessment must be maintained for glucose intolerance. The anti-inflammatory response may mask an infection; therefore, identification of malaise, anorexia, myalgias, change in wound appearance, cough, or sore throat must be reported. With all these immunosuppressive agents, the patient has an intrinsic risk for malignancies and needs comprehensive teaching regarding this and all preventive therapies.
- Newer therapies offer further improvement in transplant outcomes. Muromonab-CD3 (Orthoclone OKT3), a monoclonal antibody, may be given to reverse acute rejection, although it is rarely used. Antibodies that react with T3 cells' surface antigens are produced, interfering with T-cell antigen recognition and making it more difficult for active T-cells to recognize the target organ. Muromonab-CD3 is administered for a 10- to 14-day course of therapy as a daily bolus dose of 5 to 10 mg IV. There is a danger of flash pulmonary edema, so patients receiving this medication are closely monitored, with emergency intubation equipment on hand, and often premedicated with steroids, acetaminophen, and diphenhydramine. Cyclosporine is usually held during the period of Muronab-CD3

administration, and then titrated back up during the last 3 days of treatment. CD3 levels are monitored in the laboratory on the fourth and tenth days of therapy to assess effectiveness. Some centers utilize a monoclonal or polyclonal antibody for induction therapy in the immediate postoperative period. Others reserve medications such as Muromonab-CD3 for rescue therapy.

2. *Infection risk:* The immunosuppressive medications decrease the normal immune response, increasing the risk for nosocomial or suprainfections. Transplant patients are more susceptible to infection with common bacterial pathogens such as *Escherichia coli*, enterococci, staphylococcus and streptococcus organisms. In addition, opportunistic infections such as CMV and pneumocystis pose a threat to patients who are immunocompromised. In the immediate post-transplant period, when steroid doses are highest, the patient is more vulnerable to these infections. Infections are a major cause of morbidity and mortality, and prevention and early detection are crucial.

- The most challenging aspect of determining an infection is the clinical presentation, which is often masked by immunosuppressive therapy. The patient may not mount a fever or develop a high WBC as rapidly because of this therapy. It is imperative to assess the individual trend in each patient and have a strong suspicion for infection if patients appear more fatigued, complain of sore throats, develop a new cough, or run low-grade temperatures. Bacterial, fungal, viral, and protozoal infections may compromise the post-transplant recipient.
- Meticulous skin care to decrease dermal injuries, adequate nutrition and hydration, removing all invasive devices as soon as possible, and limiting unnecessary procedures may assist in reducing the risk for sepsis. Patients and families receive thorough education regarding the risk of infection transmission. Antimicrobial therapy is instituted postoperatively while invasive devices are in place but their use is limited to avoid growth of antibiotic-resistant organisms. Thorough skin and oral assessments as part of the routine examination of the patient can help identify viral or fungal infections.

3. *Assessing for rejection:* Following transplant, patients undergo routine endomyocardial biopsy to rule out rejection (Figure 19-11). Under fluoroscopy, utilizing a cardiac bioptome via the right internal jugular vein into the right ventricle, multiple (three to five) samples are taken of the myocardium to rule out rejection. If one or more of these samples demonstrates rejection, the patient is treated with the appropriate protocol (pulsed steroids or monoclonal antibodies). These biopsies are performed serially post-transplant

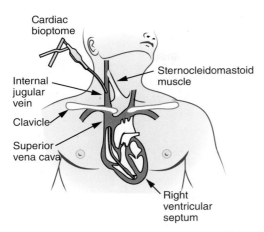

Figure 19-11. Endomyocardial biopsy technique. (*Reproduced with permission from Smith SL: Tissue and Organ Transplantation: Implications for Professional Nursing Practice. St Louis, MO: Mosby-Year Book, 1990.*)

during clinic visits to monitor for rejection. Other diagnostic procedures such as transesophageal echocardiogram and chest x-ray are often performed on a routine basis as well. Cyclosporine or tacrilimus levels are measured monthly. These data provide further guidance for earlier detection of rejection.

Providing Post-Transplant Psychological Adjustment

Many emotions impact the post-transplant patient. Often the patient and family have altered their roles and responsibilities during the illness. The post-transplant goal is to encourage role readjustment and resumption of pre-illness activities of daily living. The return to independence may frighten patients after the security of the hospital environment.

1. Involvement in a transplant support group may benefit the patient and family, reduce anxieties, and clarify misconceptions. Meeting other recipients may validate their feelings and enhance the patient's adjustments.
2. Some recipients experience body image concerns related to hirsutism and increased weight. Reviewing safe methods for dealing with these changes may decrease their concerns.
3. Weight loss may be enhanced through dietary counseling and participation in cardiac rehabilitation activities.
4. Discussions about quality-of-life issues can heighten the positive side of transplantation.
5. Steroids may cause periods of mood swings from episodes of depression to euphoria. Counseling with the patient and family may reduce confusion over the cause of personality changes. During pulsed steroid therapy, it is very important to assess for steroid psychosis. Closer monitoring and reassurance during this therapy may assist in diminishing this side effect.

Ventricular Assist Devices

Patients with cardiogenic shock following an MI, coming off CPB, or with cardiomyopathies may require additional assistance when CO remains low despite maximal medical therapy. When maximal medical therapy is inadequate, a VAD may be appropriate. The goals of utilizing a VAD are to reduce myocardial ischemia and workload, limit permanent cardiac damage, and restore adequate organ perfusion.

Indications

Patients with end-stage cardiac disease, patients who have recently come off CPB, and patients with cardiogenic shock following acute MI are candidates for VAD therapy. In some cases, insertion of a VAD is as a "bridge" until cardiac transplant takes place. The patient's status on the transplant list may or may not change once the VAD is in place. In other cases, such as post-MI, a patient may undergo VAD placement in the hope of myocardial recovery and eventual weaning from the device. This is often referred to as "bridge to recovery or decision". Once the VAD is inserted and the patient recovers, the patient is discharged home. Some patients experience myocardial recovery after VAD placement and can then undergo surgical removal. The VAD is removed when the myocardium has recovered to the point of consistently ejecting an adequate CO. After VAD removal, the patient is monitored closely for reoccurrence of heart failure symptoms. VAD is also used as "destination therapy" in which a nonsurgical/non-transplant candidate undergoes VAD placement with the expectation of ongoing dependence on the device. In those cases, the VAD remains in place until the patient dies or a decision is made to remove the device.

The appropriate selection of a candidate for these devices is based on hemodynamic criteria. If cardiovascular compromise persists despite increasing preload, reducing afterload, and instituting maximal medication doses, a VAD may be critical to achieve survival. Appropriate parameters to consider for VAD placement are:

- CI less than 2 L/min/m^2
- SVR more than 2100 dyne/s/cm^5
- Mean arterial pressure more than 60 mm Hg
- Left or right atrial pressure more than 20 mm Hg
- Urine output more than 30 mL/h
- PAOP more than 15 to 20 mm Hg

The exclusion criteria for use of a VAD include the following:

- Acute cerebral vascular damage
- Cancer with metastasis
- Renal failure (unrelated to cardiac failure)
- Severe hepatic disease
- Coagulopathy
- Sepsis, resistant to therapy
- Severe pulmonary disease
- Severe peripheral vascular disease

- Psychological instability
- Alcohol, drug addiction, or tobacco use

General Description of Ventricular Assist Device Principles

The VAD unloads the native ventricle or ventricles by way of artificial ventricles or a blood pump. CO is enhanced by blood circulating at a physiologic rate and by augmenting systemic and coronary circulation.

VAD support is predominately utilized for the left ventricle. However, if the right ventricle is compromised, support can be provided to both ventricles. This would necessitate separate VADs, yet the systems would function in tandem.

VADs can be used for postcardiotomy support as a bridge to recovery, a bridge to transplant, or as destination therapy. VADs can be nonpulsatile pumps (roller, centrifugal, or axial flow) or pulsatile pumps (pneumatically or electromagnetically driven). Previously, most VADs were inserted in the operating room but percutaneous placement is also an option, depending on the patient's condition and the indication for VAD therapy. There are several approaches for cannula insertion depending on the type of device being used and whether support is needed for one or both ventricles.

Examples of VADs that are used as a bridge to recovery following cardiac surgery include the Bio-medicus system and the Abiomed 5000 BVS system. The Bio-medicus is a continuous-flow centrifugal pump and usually requires a perfusionist at the bedside for monitoring and troubleshooting. The bedside nurse can often manage the Abiomed 5000 BVS system. There are smaller VADs that can be inserted in the cardiac catheterization laboratory using a percutaneous approach via the femoral vein and/or femoral artery. These include the Tandem Heart® and the Abiomed Impella® devices. The Tandem Heart involves inserting a cannula into the right atrium via the femoral vein. The cannula is introduced across the fossa ovalis into the left atrium. Arterialized blood is removed from the left atrium, circulated through an axial flow device, and reintroduced into the arterial circulation via a cannula that has been inserted into the aorta via the femoral artery. The Abiomed Impella is inserted percutaneously through the femoral artery, up the aorta, and introduced across the aortic valve. The device is designed to augment the patient's CO. Blood is removed from the left ventricle and delivered into the ascending aorta.

VADs commonly used as a bridge to transplant include the HeartMate II (Figure 19-12), HeartMate III, and HeartWare VAD. The HeartMate II and III and HeartWare VAD are axial flow devices. The axial flow devices are usually not associated with a palpable pulse initially. Often, as the heart regains contractility over a period of several weeks, the pulse will return.

The HeartMate II and the HeartWare HVAD system have both been Food and Drug Administration (FDA) approved for destination therapy. Destination therapy implies that the patient is not a candidate for transplant and will not be placed on the waiting list for a transplant.

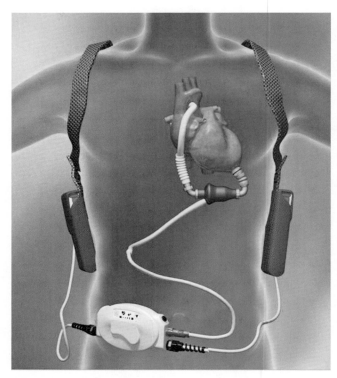

Figure 19-12. HeartMate II left ventricular assist system. (*Used with permission from Thoratec Corporation Pleasanton, CA.*)

The devices used as a bridge to transplant or for destination therapy are all LVADs. They all require an incision from the sternal notch to the umbilicus. A large cannula is inserted into the apex of the left ventricle and connected to the inflow port of LVAD with an outflow cannula inserted into the aorta. The LVAD is implanted outside the peritoneum just below the diaphragm. The driveline (power cord) is brought through the skin and connected to a power source. The driveline exit site requires meticulous care to prevent infection.

The LVAD has a monitor that provides the flow rate (similar to CO) and other information pertinent to the device. These devices can achieve flow rates that support adequate oxygen delivery to the tissues while reducing cardiac workload.

Weaning and Recovery

The plan for weaning depends on hemodynamic stability and the recovery of the patient's other organ systems following the period of poor perfusion. A thorough evaluation of the patient helps identify evidence of continued organ damage and guides the decision for weaning. Pharmacologic support is maintained at a stable level with good major organ perfusion.

The arterial line waveform is assessed for the dicrotic notch appearance, indicating that there is adequate left ventricular pressure for aortic opening. The VAD is turned down at small increments to assess tolerance throughout the weaning process. Heparin must be initiated before weaning and the device never set at less than 2 L/min flow to avoid clot formation. At completion of weaning, the patient returns to the operating room for surgical removal.

Principles of Management of Ventricular Assist Devices

The primary objectives in managing the patient with a VAD are to optimize CO, maximize coping, and prevent complications.

Optimizing Cardiac Output

1. In the initial period after insertion, the risk of biventricular failure still is paramount and the patient must be closely evaluated. Cardiovascular profiles are measured every 2 to 4 hours and changes in CO and CI or the device flow rates are reported to the physician. Pharmacologic support is titrated to achieve the most stable mean arterial pressure, adequate flow rates and adequate SvO_2.
2. Assessing the VAD for proper function is essential to achieving an improved cardiovascular profile. As myocardial recovery occurs, more support occurs from the heart and less from the VAD. The patient can then support CO without as much mechanical support.

Maximizing Coping

The patient and family may be overwhelmed by the suddenness of the disease, the progressive care unit environment, the equipment related to the VAD, and the threat of loss of life. Transplantation, if discussed, may significantly increase their stress. They may require intense information sharing and clarification of misconceptions.

1. Promote emotional and psychological adaptation, assess for nonverbal clues of fear or anxiety and give frequent updates regarding goals for the day and the present plan of care. The advanced practice nurse and the patient's primary nurse may coordinate this communication.
2. Provide realistic information related to prognosis. Twenty to forty percent of patients on VAD die awaiting a donor heart, and families need support to cope with this possibility. Early involvement with social work and chaplains also may assist patients and families. Closely assess for other situational stressors and review prior coping strategies the patient or family found helpful.
3. If the device has been implanted as destination therapy, the patient and family need to be taught the following:
   - How to perform dressing changes
   - How to change from the battery-powered unit to the base power unit and the reverse
   - How to hand pump the device if there is a total loss of power if appropriate for the type of device
   - What equipment the patient should always have when leaving home or the base power unit

The patient and family education process begins in the ICU as soon as the patient is awake and alert. The nursing staff on the progressive care unit continues the education and assist with a skills check off as the patient and family develop competence. Prior to discharge home, the emergency medical services (EMS) system in the patient's home community is notified about the patient returning to his community.

Preventing Complications

1. *Thromboembolism:* Anticoagulation therapy may include heparin, dextran, or aspirin to reduce the risk for thromboembolism. Peripheral vascular impairment may occur secondary to vascular catheters. Frequent neurovascular checks are performed and any change reported immediately. Assess for the five Ps of vascular complications:
   - Pallor
   - Pain
   - Paresthesia
   - Paralysis
   - Pulselessness
2. *Bleeding:* Monitor hemoglobin, hematocrit, and coagulation factors frequently. Assess all catheter sites and wounds for oozing. For patients awaiting transplant, maintaining a narrow therapeutic range with anticoagulation is essential so that reversal of therapy can be achieved if a donor heart is available. Ideally the partial thromboplastin time (PTT) is 1.5 times normal or activated clotting levels are appropriate for the device. The anticoagulation therapy may increase the propensity for cardiac tamponade to occur. This is a surgical emergency and may require reoperation for stabilization. Clues to this complication include the following:
   - Elevated atrial pressures/neck vein distention
   - Reduced CO as pump cannot fill properly
   - Elevated pulmonary pressures
   - Diastolic equalization
   - Reduced mean arterial pressure
   - Declining MvO_2
3. *Right ventricular failure:* Observe for development of elevated central venous pressure/neck vein distention combined with low to normal PAOP.
4. *Dysrhythmias:* Monitor ECG continuously. Patients may require antiarrhythmic medication or electrical cardioversion. Biventricular support may maintain nearly normal hemodynamics during dysrhythmias. Assess the effect of dysrhythmias on CO and augment the VAD accordingly. Treat all electrolyte abnormalities aggressively to enhance contractility. Validate with physicians whether CPR may be performed for asystole, depending on the specific VAD.
5. *Decreased renal function:* Monitor renal function including BUN and creatinine daily, and urine output. Use nephrotoxic medications with caution and

ensure that doses are based on creatinine clearance. Use vasopressor to enhance renal perfusion, if appropriate. Maintain adequate fluid balance so preload is within normal limits. Monitor urinalysis for potential abnormalities, and avoid any period of hypotension as that will cause further injury to the kidneys.

6. *Infection:* Monitor closely for signs of infection as patients on VADs have large cannulas exiting the skin, which can be portals of entry for pathologic organisms. Patients on VAD support are also more prone to infections because of their underlying fragility. Patients awaiting transplant may be become ineligible for the surgery if they become septic. The best plan of action is prevention and includes:
   - Perform hand hygiene before and after all patient care activities
   - Use strict aseptic technique
   - Pan-culture for temperature more than 101°F (38.33°C)
   - Monitor wounds for erythema, exudate, or edema
   - Assess for leukocytosis or increase in bands on differential count

7. *Immobility:* Provide meticulous skin care and frequent position changes to reduce the risk of dermal injury during the patient's critical illness. Reduce the risk of catabolism by giving nutritional support. Collaborate with physical therapy to provide bedside exercise that prevents muscle mass loss and negative nitrogen balance. Apply foot splints to diminish the risk of foot drop.

8. *Poor device performance:* Evaluate the VAD performance routinely and with any change in the patient's clinical status. Dangers related to VAD mechanical problems include thrombus formation, inflow obstructions, or device failures. Device failure may result in inadequate or no systemic perfusion, so emergency measures must be implemented rapidly (Table 19-5).

TABLE 19-5. EMERGENCY MEASURES FOR VAD FAILURE OR CARDIAC ARREST

- Backup VAD in place and ready for operation if mechanical failure occurs.
- CPR is usually not recommended. Should refer to manufacturer's guidelines.
- Assess availability of blood products should emergency transfusions be necessary.
- Have vascular clamps available for cannula disconnections.
- Educate all team members regarding emergency measures if problem with VAD occurs.
- Patients can be safely cardioverted and defibrillated with VAD in place.
- Connect to emergency power outlets in case of an electrical outage.

ESSENTIAL CONTENT CASE
Thinking Critically

A patient was transferred yesterday to the progressive care unit from cardiac surgery. He was admitted to the hospital with mitral insufficiency and 2 days ago had a St. Jude mechanical valve inserted into the mitral position. He has a central line in place via the right subclavian vein. The initial assessment shows:

Temperature	37.6°C
HR	Temporarily atrial paced at 80 beats/min
BP	86/60 mm Hg
RR	16 breaths/min
RA	3 mm Hg
SpO$_2$	95%

Case Question 1: What is the probable reason for his hypotension?
(A) Hypervolemia
(B) Impaired myocardial contractility
(C) Hypovolemia
(D) Increased afterload

Case Question 2: What interventions should be immediately initiated to improve his cardiac status?
(A) Dobutamine to improve ventricular contractility
(B) Sodium nitroprusside to reduce afterload
(C) Increase HR to 90 beats/min
(D) Administer volume to increase preload

Answers
1. C is the correct answer. Hypovolemia is the most likely answer based on his low CVP and pulmonary artery pressures. The SVR is increased in response to the low CO/CI as a compensatory mechanism.
2. D is the correct answer. Administration of volume will normalize the pressures and improve the CO/CI.

SELECTED BIBLIOGRAPHY

General Cardiovascular

Fuster V, Harrington RA, Narula J, Eapan ZJ. *Hurst's The Heart.* 14th ed. New York, NY: McGraw Hill Companies; 2017.

Good VS, Kirkwood PL. *Advanced Critical Care Nursing.* 2nd ed. St Louis, MO: Elsevier; 2018.

Hardin S, Kaplow R. *Cardiac Surgery Essentials for Critical Care Nursing.* 2nd ed. Sudbury, MA: Jones & Bartlett Publishing; 2010.

Mann DL, Zipes DP, Libby P, eds. *Braunwald's Heart Disease: A Textbook of Cardiovascular Medicine.* 10th ed. Philadelphia, PA: Saunders Elsevier; 2015.

Moser DK, Riegel B. *Cardiac Nursing: A Companion to Braunwald's Heart Disease.* Canada: Saunders; 2008.

Woods SL, Froelicher ESS, Motzer SA, Bridges EJ. *Cardiac Nursing.* 6th ed. Philadelphia, PA: Lippincott, Williams & Wilkins; 2010.

Cardiomyopathy

Albert NM. Fluid management strategies in heart failure. *Crit Care Nurse*. 2012;32(2):20-31.

Bloom MW, Cole RT, Butler J. Evaluation and management of acute heart failure. In: Fuster V, Harrington RA, Narula J, Eapan ZJ. *Hurst's The Heart*. 14th ed. New York, NY: McGraw Hill Companies; 2017: chap 71.

Felker GM, Teerlink, JR. Diagnosis and management of acute heart failure. In: Mann DL, Zipes DP, Libby P, eds. *Braunwald's Heart Disease: A Textbook of Cardiovascular Medicine*. 10th ed. Philadelphia, PA: Saunders Elsevier; 2015: 484-511.

Lee CS, Tkacs NC. Current concepts of neurohormonal activation in heart failure. *AACN Adv Crit Care*. 2008;19(4):364-385.

Leeper B, Legge D. Resynchronization therapy for management of heart failure. *Crit Care Nurs Clin North Am*. 2003;15(4):467-476.

Lewis PS, Boyd CM, Hubert NE, Steele MC. Ethanol-induced therapeutic myocardial infarction to treat hypertrophic obstructive cardiomyopathy. *Crit Care Nurse*. 2001;21(2):20-34.

Hasenfuss G, Mann DL. Pathophysiology of heart failure. In: Mann DL, Zipes DP, Libby P, eds. *Braunwald's Heart Disease: A Textbook of Cardiovascular Medicine*. 10th ed. Philadelphia, PA: Saunders Elsevier; 2015: 454-472.

Mann DL, Felker GM, eds. *Heart Failure: A Companion to Braunwald's Heat Disease*. 3rd ed. ST Louis, MO: Elsevier; 2016.

Paul S. Diastolic dysfunction. *Crit Care Nurs Clin North Am*. 2003;15(4):495-500.

Paul S. Ventricular remodeling. *Crit Care Nurs Clin North Am*. 2003;15(4):407-412.

Piano MR, Prasun M. Neurohormone activation. *Crit Care Nurs Clin North Am*. 2003;15(4):413-422.

Quinn B. Pharmacologic treatment of heart failure. *Crit Care Nurs Q*. 2007;30(4):299-306.

Heart Transplantation

Freeman R, Koerner E, Clark C, Halabicky K. The path from heart failure to cardiac transplant. *Crit Care Nurs Q*. 2016;39(3):207-215.

Freeman R, Koerner E, Clark C, Halabicky K. Cardiac transplant: postoperative management. *Crit Care Nurs Q*. 2016;39(3):214-226.

Jasiak NM, Park JM. Immunosuppression tips in solid organ transplantation: essentials and practical tips. *Crit Care Nurs Q*. 2016;39(3):227-240.

Kittleson MM, Patel JK, Kobashigawa JA. History and overview of cardiac transplantation. In: Fuster V, Harrington RA, Narula J, Eapan ZJ. *Hurst's The Heart*. 14th ed. New York, NY: McGraw Hill Companies; 2017.

Mehra MR, Canter CE, Hannan MM, et al. The 2016 International Society for Heart Lung Transplantation listing criteria for heart transplantation: a 10 year update. *J Heart Lung Transplant*. 2016;35(1):A1-A10.

Schonder KS. Pharmacology of immunosuppressive medications in solid organ transplantation. *Crit Care Nurs Clin North Am*. 2011;23(3):405-423.

Valvular Disorders

Blaisdell MW, Good L, Gentzler RD. Percutaneous transluminal valvuloplasty. *Crit Care Nurse*. 1989;9(3):62-68.

Hill KM. Surgical repair of cardiac valves. *Crit Care Nurs Clin North Am*. 2007;19(4):353-360.

Holloway S, Feldman T. An alternative to valvular surgery in the treatment of mitral stenosis: balloon mitral valvotomy. *Crit Care Nurse*. 1997;17(3):27-36.

Leeper B. Valvular disease and surgery. In: Good VS, Kirkwood PL, eds. *Advanced Critical Care Nursing*. 2nd ed. St Louis, MO: Elsevier, 2018.

Nauer KA, Schouchoff B, Demitras K. Minimally invasive aortic valve surgery. *Crit Care Q*. 2000;23(1):66-71.

Otto CM, Bonow RO, eds. *Valvular Heart Disease. A Companion to Braunwald's Heart Disease*. 4th ed. Philadelphia, PA: Saunders Elsevier; 2013.

Piaschyk M, Cyr AM, Wetzel A, et al. A journey through heart valve surgery. *Crit Care Nurs Clin North Am*. 2011;23(4):587-605.

Pericarditis

Dziadulewicz L, Shannon-Stone M. Postpericardiotomy syndrome: a complication of cardiac surgery. *AACN Clin Issues Crit Care Nurs*. 1998;9(2):464-470.

Hamel W. Care of patients with an indwelling pericardial catheter. *Crit Care Nurse*. 1998;18(5):40-45.

Kloos JA. Characteristics, complications and treatment of acute pericarditis. *Crit Care Nurs Clin North Am*, 2015;27(4):483-497.

LeWinter MM, Hopkins WE. Pericardial diseases. In: Mann DL, Zipes DP, Libby P, eds. *Braunwald's Heart Disease: A Textbook of Cardiovascular Medicine*. 10th ed. Philadelphia, PA: Saunders Elsevier; 2015: 454-472.

Thoraco-Abdominal Aneurysms

Anderson LA. Abdominal aortic aneurysm. *J Cardiovasc Nurs*. 2001;15(4):1-14.

Dolinger C, Strider DV. Endovascular interventions for descending thoracic aortic aneurysms: the pivotal role of the clinical nurse in post-operative care. *Vasc Nurs*. 2010;28:147-153.

Fairman RM, Wang GJ. Thoracic and thoracoabdominal aortic aneurysms: endovascular treatment. In: Cronenwett JL, Johnston W, eds. *Rutherford's Vascular Surgery*. Philadelphia, PA: Saunders Elsevier; 2014: 2046-2061.

Lam CH, Vatakencherry G. Spinal cord protection with a cerebrospinal fluid drain in a patient undergoing thoracic endovascular aortic repair. *J Vasc Radio*. 2010;21:1343-1346.

Leeper B, Lovasik D. Cerebrospinal drainage systems: external ventricular and lumbar drains. In: Littlejohns LR, Bader MK, eds. *AACN-AANN Protocols for Practice: Monitoring Technologies in Critically Ill Neuroscience Patients*. Sudbury, MA: Jones & Bartlett Publishers; 2009: 71-102.

Upchurch GR. Thoracic and thoracoabdominal aortic aneurysms: evaluation and decision making. In: Cronenwett JL, Johnston W, eds. *Rutherford's Vascular Surgery*. Philadelphia, PA: Saunders Elsevier; 2014: 2084-2101.

Woo EY, Damrauer SM. Thoracic and thoracoabdominal aortic aneurysms: open surgical treatment. In: Cronenwett JL, Johnston W, eds. *Rutherford's Vascular Surgery*. Philadelphia, PA: Saunders Elsevier; 2014: 2024-2045.

Ventricular Assist Devices

Aaronson KS, Pagani FD. Mechanical circulatory support. In: Mann DL, Zipes DP, Libby P, eds. *Braunwald's Heart Disease: A Textbook of Cardiovascular Medicine*. 10th ed. Philadelphia, PA: Saunders Elsevier; 2015: 590-599.

Christensen DM. Physiology of continuous-flow pumps. *AACN Adv Crit Care.* 2012;22(1):46-54.

Doty D. Ventricular assist device and destination therapy candidates from preoperative selection through end of hospitalization. *Crit Care Nurs Clin North Am.* 2015;27(4):551-564.

Hagan K, Casanova-Ghosh E. Postcardiotomy cardiogenic shock: the role of ventricular assist devices. *Crit Care Nurs Clin North Am.* 2007;19(4):427-444.

Kurien S, Hughes KA. Anticoagulation and bleeding in patients with ventricular assist devices. *AACN Adv Crit Care.* 2012;23(1):91-98.

Litton KA. Demystifying ventricular assist devices. *Crit Care Nurs Q.* 2011;34(3):200-207.

Myers TJ. Temporary ventricular assist devices in the intensive care unit as a bridge to decision. *AACN Adv Crit Care.* 2012;23(1):55-68.

O'Shea G. Ventricular assist devices: what intensive care unit nurses need to know about post-operative management. *AACN Adv Crit Care.* 2012;23(1):69-83.

Puhlman M. Continuous-flow left ventricular assist device and the right ventricle. *AACN Adv Crit Care.* 2012;23(1):86-90.

Puhlman M, Bingham A. Ventricular assist devices. In: Wiegand DL, ed. *AACN Procedure Manual for High Acuity, Progressive, and Critical Care.* 7th ed. St Louis, MO: Elsevier; 2017.

Rose EA, Moskowitz AJ, Packer M, et al. The REMATCH trial: rationale, design and end points. *Ann Thorac Surg.* 1999;67:723-730.

Savage L. Quality of life among patients with a left ventricular assist device: what is new? *AACN Clin Issues.* 2003;14:64-72.

Intraaortic Balloon Pump

Castellucci D. Intraaortic balloon pump management. In: Weigand D, ed. *AACN Procedure Manual.* 6th ed. Philadelphia, PA: Saunders Elsevier; 2011: 443-463.

Murks C, Juricek C. Balloon pumps inserted via the subclavian artery: bridging the way to heart transplant. *AACN Adv Crit Care.* 2016;27(3):301-315.

Quall SJ. *Comprehensive Intraaortic Balloon Pumping.* St Louis, MO: CV Mosby; 1984.

Evidence-Based Practice/Guidelines

Baddour LM, Wilson WR, Bayer AS, et al. Infective endocarditis in adults: diagnosis, antimicrobial therapy, and management of complications: a scientific statement for healthcare professionals from the American Heart Association. *Circulation*, 2015. doi.org/10.1161/CIR.0000000000000296.

Bonow RO, Nishimura RA, Otto CM, et al. 2014 ACC/AHA guideline for management of patients with valvular heart disease. *Circulation.* 2014:129:e521-e643.

Peura JL, Colvin-Adams M, Francis GS, et al. Recommendations for the use of mechanical circulatory support: device strategies and patient selection. A scientific statement from the American Heart Association. *Circulation.* 2012;126:2648-2667.

Yancy CW, Jessup M, Bozkurt B et al. 2017 ACC/AHA/HFSA focused update on the 2013 ACCF/AHA/guideline for the management of heart failure: a report of the American College of Cardiology/American Heart Association Task Force on Clinical Practice Guidelines and the Heart Failure Society of America. *Circulation.* 2017; doi:10.1161/CIR.0000000000000509.

ADVANCED NEUROLOGIC CONCEPTS

20

DaiWai M. Olson and Kathrina Siaron

KNOWLEDGE COMPETENCIES

1. Compare and contrast the pathophysiology, clinical presentation, patient needs, and management approaches for the following conditions:
   - Subarachnoid hemorrhage (SAH)
   - Traumatic brain injury

   - Acute spinal cord injury (SCI)
   - Brain tumor
2. Describe intracranial monitoring technology and implications for nursing care.
3. Describe the use of lumbar drainage of cerebrospinal fluid (CSF) and implications for nursing care.

SUBARACHNOID HEMORRHAGE

Etiology, Risk Factors, and Pathophysiology

Subarachnoid hemorrhage (SAH) can result from trauma, aneurysm, or other vascular malformations. This chapter focuses on SAH due to the rupture of an intracranial aneurysm (aneurysmal subarachnoid hemorrhage [aSAH]). Intracranial aneurysms usually occur in the circle of Willis at arterial bifurcations or trifurcations (Figure 20-1). Aneurysms vary in size and shape; *saccular* (also called *"berry"*) aneurysms are the most common and most amenable to treatment. When an intracranial aneurysm ruptures, blood is expelled from within the vessel into vulnerable brain tissue. The blood takes the path of least resistance, which is most often into the subarachnoid space. Subsequently, a clot may form in the ventricular system or in the brain parenchyma. In some patients, blood in the subarachnoid space causes hydrocephalus by obstructing cerebrospinal fluid (CSF) flow through the ventricles or by clogging the arachnoid granulations that reabsorb CSF. Although the mechanism is not well-understood, arterial narrowing (commonly referred to as *"vasospasm"* or *"cerebral artery vasospasm"*) occurs in a significant number of patients in the days following aneurysm rupture and can cause delayed cerebral ischemia (DCI) or delayed ischemic neurological deficit (DIND). There are several scales used to grade the severity of aSAH. The Hunt and Hess scale and the World Federation of Neurological Surgeons (WFNS) scale (Table 20-1) are the commonly used.

Risk factors for intracranial aneurysm formation include: smoking, hypertension, family history of intracranial aneurysms, and certain genetic disorders (autosomal dominant polycystic kidney disease, Ehlers-Danlos syndrome). Roughly 10% to 15% of patients have multiple aneurysms. Risk factors associated with aneurysm rupture include: size of the aneurysm, hypertension, smoking, age (risk increases with age, peaking at age 50-60), and the use of stimulants (cocaine, amphetamines). Aneurysmal SAH is more common in men until the age of 50 and more common in women after the age of 50.

Mortality and morbidity associated with aSAH is substantial but improving. Approximately 40% of individuals with aSAH will die either at the time of rupture or during hospitalization. Two-thirds of aSAH survivors are left with some type of neurological deficit. Predictors of outcome after aSAH include neurologic condition on admission, age, comorbidities, and the amount of blood noted on the initial computed tomography (CT) scan.

Clinical Presentation

Most patients are asymptomatic until the time of aneurysm rupture, but some have prodromal signs such as headaches

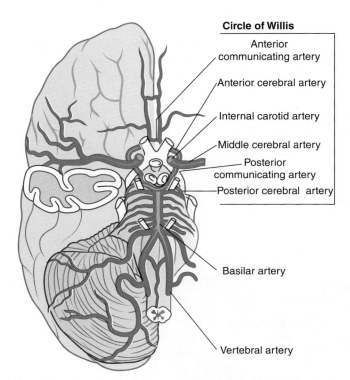

Circle of Willis

Anterior communicating artery

Anterior cerebral artery

Internal carotid artery

Middle cerebral artery

Posterior communicating artery

Posterior cerebral artery

Basilar artery

Vertebral artery

Figure 20-1. The circle of Willis as seen from below the brain. (*Reproduced with permission from Phipps WJ, Marek JF, Monahan FD, et al: Medical-Surgical Nursing: Health and Illness Perspectives. St Louis, MO: Mosby; 2003.*)

or visual changes. Upon aneurysm rupture, many patients experience a sudden, severe headache, sometimes described as "thunderclap," "explosive," or "the worst headache of my life." Transient or prolonged loss of consciousness may occur. Episodes of acute hypertension or intense physical activity may increase the pressure on an aneurysm and cause rupture. Bystanders may describe seizure-like activity; it is unclear whether this is an actual seizure or abnormal posturing related to a sudden increase in intracranial pressure (ICP). Other common signs and symptoms include nausea and vomiting, stiff neck, vision changes, mental status

changes, and photophobia. Focal deficits such as hemiparesis, hemiplegia, or aphasia may also occur.

Diagnostic Tests

Computerized Tomography Scan

A CT scan is used to determine whether a SAH has occurred and to assess for hydrocephalus. CT scan will detect subarachnoid blood in almost all patients if performed within the first 3 days of symptom onset. As the blood in the subarachnoid space starts to break down, the sensitivity of the CT scan decreases. CT angiography (see Chapter 12, Neurological System) can be performed quickly at the time of the initial scan and may reveal the aneurysm location. The amount of blood present on the initial CT scan is predictive of vasospasm risk.

Magnetic Resonance Imaging and Magnetic Resonance Angiogram

Magnetic resonance imaging (MRI) and magnetic resonance angiogram (MRA) are used to identify aneurysm location and look for other vascular abnormalities. These studies are especially useful in patients with a negative CT or CT angiogram.

Lumbar Puncture

A lumbar puncture (LP) is performed when the CT fails to demonstrate SAH in a patient with a history highly suspicious for SAH. LP is avoided in patients with signs or symptoms of increased ICP due to the risk of cerebellar tonsillar herniation. LP is performed at least 6 to 12 hours after the onset of symptoms to allow red blood cells (RBCs) in the CSF to start to break down. This breakdown in RBCs gives a yellow tinge to the CSF after centrifugation. This pigmentation is called xanthochromia and will not be present if blood in the CSF is only due to a traumatic LP.

Cerebral Angiography

Although computed tomography angiography (CTA) done at the time of the initial CT scan detects many aneurysms, cerebral angiography (catheter angiography) remains the gold

TABLE 20-1. SEVERITY OF SUBARACHNOID HEMORRHAGE CLASSIFICATION SCALES

Grade	Hunt and Hess	World Federation of Neurological Surgeons	Fisher
	Based on Symptoms	**Based on Assessment**	**Based on Diagnostic Imaging**
0	Unruptured		
I	Asymptomatic or minimal headache, nuchal rigidity	Glasgow Coma Score = 15 Motor deficit = Absent	No blood detected on brain CT
II	Moderate to severe headache, nuchal rigidity, no neurological deficit other than cranial nerve palsy	Glasgow Coma Score = 13-14 Motor deficit = Absent	Diffuse thin layer of subarachnoid blood (vertical layers < 1 mm thick)
III	Drowsiness, confusion, mild focal deficit	Glasgow Coma Score = 13-14 Motor deficit = Present	Localized clot or thick layer of subarachnoid blood (vertical layers ≥ 1 mm thick)
IV	Stupor, moderate to severe hemiparesis, possible early decerebrate rigidity and vegetative disturbances	Glasgow Coma Score = 7-12 Motor deficit = Present or absent	Intracerebral or intraventricular blood with diffuse or no subarachnoid blood
V	Deep coma, decerebrate rigidity, moribund appearance	Glasgow Coma Score = 3-6 Motor deficit = Present or absent	

ESSENTIAL CONTENT CASE

Subarachnoid Hemorrhage

A 54-year-old loan officer experienced a sudden onset of a severe headache while at work. She was taken to the emergency department of a local hospital where she described her headache as the "worst headache of my life." CT scan confirmed the diagnosis of SAH. Angiography revealed an aneurysm of the left anterior communicating artery at the junction of the left anterior cerebral artery. The aneurysm was successfully coiled and she returned to the intensive care unit (ICU) following the procedure. The next day, the patient was transferred to the progressive care unit (PCU).

Case Question 1: Describe nursing priorities of care for this patient.

On the fifth day post-bleed, the nurse noted that this previously neurologically intact patient was difficult to arouse. Once awake, the patient also had right upper extremity weakness and difficulty in speaking.

Case Question 2: What actions should the nurse anticipate?

The patient was taken to radiology where a CT and CTA revealed normal postoperative changes and arterial narrowing, especially of the left middle cerebral artery. Her symptoms improved transiently with induced hypertension, but then recurred. Catheter angiography confirmed severe narrowing of the left middle cerebral artery. Intra-arterial verapamil was infused with radiologic improvement. Postprocedure, the patient was able to speak (although confused) and move her right arm with 4 out of 5 strength (ie, against resistance). Following several days in the ICU, she was transferred to the PCU. Her neurologic examination continued to improve and she was discharged home on post-bleed day 14 with outpatient speech therapy to address occasional word-finding difficulty and subtle cognitive deficits.

Answers

1. Nursing priorities of care include close monitoring of neurologic status and volume status. Maintenance of euvolemia is important to decrease the risk of DCI due to vasospasm, and close monitoring of neurologic status allows prompt intervention if complications develop. Other priorities of care include pain management, encouraging mobility, and prevention of hospital-acquired infections.
2. The nurse prepares the patient for a stat CT scan and potentially an angiogram. Fluid balance is checked and fluid administration may be ordered. The cause of neurological decline is likely cerebral ischemia due to vasospasm, which will be treated with induced hypertension and endovascular measures.

standard to identify the location, size, and shape of the aneurysm or other vascular anomalies. The initial angiogram may fail to reveal an aneurysm in approximately 10% to 20% of patients with SAH. If no aneurysm is seen on the first angiogram, a repeat angiogram after approximately a week will reveal an aneurysm in a small number of these patients. A

negative angiogram with a distinct pattern of bleeding on CT scan may indicate a nonaneurysmal perimesencephalic SAH; patients with this diagnosis have an excellent prognosis.

Angiogram is also often used to guide endovascular treatment (described later) for many patients who are found to have aneurysms without a bleed. Additionally, it can also be used to detect arterial narrowing in patients with neurological decline in the days following aneurysm rupture. Angioplasty may be used to treat the arterial narrowing.

Principles of Management of Aneurysmal Subarachnoid Hemorrhage

Patients who survive the initial rupture of a cerebral aneurysm are at risk for complications that increase their chances for morbidity and death. Primary central nervous system (CNS) complications include rebleeding, hydrocephalus, and DCI due to arterial narrowing. Arterial narrowing correlates temporally with the breakdown of subarachnoid blood and is due to a combination of arterial spasm and inflammatory changes that thicken the vessel wall. This phenomenon is commonly referred to as "vasospasm," although the current understanding of the pathophysiology behind it and how it leads to DCI is incomplete. Despite this, the terminology is commonly used in practice and will be used in this text to reflect arterial narrowing after aSAH.

Rebleeding

Prior to the aneurysm being secured with surgical clipping or intravascular coiling, the biggest risk to the patient is aneurysmal re-rupture (or "rebleed"). This risk is highest within the first 24 hours, with a significantly higher probability of death. Signs and symptoms of rebleeding include a sudden reappearance or increase in headache, nausea and vomiting, decreased level of consciousness, and new focal neurologic deficits. Neurologic assessments should be performed hourly (or more frequently if indicated) to promptly identify changes related to rebleeding or hydrocephalus. If an external ventricular drain (EVD) is present, careful management is essential to prevent overdrainage of CSF, which can result in rebleeding due to a change in transmural pressure. The most definitive method to prevent rebleeding is to secure the aneurysm using surgical clipping or endovascular embolization. Both methods are discussed below.

In the interim between admission and definitive treatment, strategies such as blood pressure and ICP management may be used to decrease bleeding risk. Avoidance of activities that raise the patient's blood pressure and/or ICP, as well as the administration of medications to control pain, nausea, and other sources of discomfort are effective strategies. The goal of blood pressure management is to treat hypertension without dropping the blood pressure to a level that decreases cerebral perfusion. Systolic BP goals with an upper range of 150 to 160 mm Hg are common. The use of agents that can be titrated is recommended, and calcium channel blockers are often preferred. Vasodilating agents are avoided. Bed rest is typically ordered prior to securing the aneurysm. Prophylaxis for venous thromboembolism (VTE), including sequential compression stockings and pneumatic compression devices, is implemented. Stool softeners are used to prevent straining due to constipation. Pain is treated with analgesics, usually short-acting narcotics so that accurate neurological assessment is possible. Anxiety is reduced through explanations of care and psychological support.

Two management options exist to secure the aneurysm and prevent re-rupture: surgical clipping of the aneurysm via craniotomy and endovascular embolization of the aneurysm via catheter angiography. Management at a facility that offers both treatment modalities and frequently treats patients with aSAH is recommended to optimize outcomes. The decision to secure the aneurysm via open craniotomy versus an endovascular procedure is made on the basis of aneurysm location and morphology, comorbidities, and the severity of neurologic deficits on admission. When the aneurysm is amenable to treatment by either modality, endovascular management is generally performed. The aneurysm is secured as soon as possible prior to the period of time when patients are most at risk for vasospasm. With the aneurysm secured, standard management strategies for vasospasm can be implemented without the risk of causing additional hemorrhage.

Aneurysm clipping is performed via a craniotomy incision. The surgeon carefully dissects tissue away from the aneurysm and places a titanium or titanium alloy clip across the base (Figure 20-2). Different sizes and shapes of clips are available. Following surgery, the patient is initially admitted to the ICU for management. Follow-up radiologic studies may be done, including CT scanning to look for bleeding at the operative site and angiography to evaluate clip position.

Endovascular embolization decreases rebleeding risk by preventing blood flow into the aneurysm. Using cerebral angiography, the interventional radiologist threads a wire with a helical platinum coil at the tip into the cerebral vasculature. The coil is manipulated into the body of the aneurysm and detached from the wire using a small electrical current. The neck of the aneurysm must be narrow enough for the coils to be retained inside the aneurysm instead of floating back out into the vessel lumen. Figure 20-3 depicts endovascular coil embolization of an aneurysm with a narrow neck (berry or saccular aneurysm). If the neck is wide, special stents may be used to assist with coiling or to span the aneurysm (*stent-assisted clipping*). Multiple coils may be needed to completely fill the aneurysm. The coils cause the aneurysm to clot, preventing blood flow into the aneurysm and decreasing the likelihood of rebleed. The primary risks associated with coil embolization are aneurysmal rupture during the procedure and ischemia related to clot formation in the vessel lumen.

Patients with aSAH return to the ICU after aneurysm clipping or endovascular treatment. At some institutions, neurologically stable patients without other ICU needs may be transferred to a progressive care unit (PSU) after 24 to 48 hours to be monitored for vasospasm and other complications.

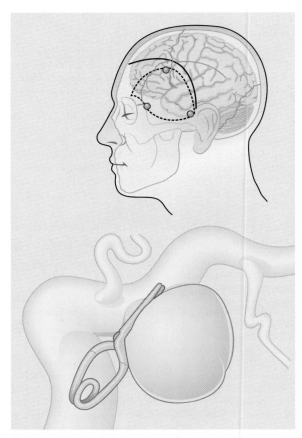

Figure 20-2. Clipping of a posterior communicating artery aneurysm. The clip is placed across the base of the aneurysm so that it can no longer fill with blood, but blood flow can continue through the parent artery.

Hydrocephalus

An SAH disrupts normal CSF flow through two mechanisms: (1) intraventricular blood may create a blockage in the ventricular drainage system and cause CSF to build

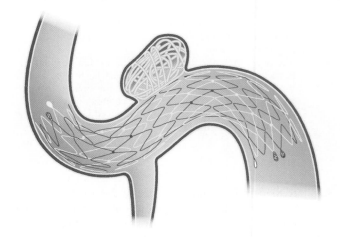

Figure 20-3. Stent-assisted coiling of a wide neck aneurysm. After the coils are placed and detached during an endovascular procedure, a stent is placed to keep the coils within the aneurysm sac.

up (*obstructive* or *noncommunicating hydrocephalus*), or (2) the arachnoid granulations that absorb CSF may become blocked with cellular debris, resulting in decreased reabsorption of CSF (*communicating hydrocephalus*). Signs and symptoms of acute hydrocephalus relate to increased ICP. Acute obstructive hydrocephalus after SAH may be managed by the placement of an EVD (see section on ICP monitoring and management at the end of this chapter). Patients with sustained obstructive hydrocephalus or ventriculomegaly will require a ventriculoperitoneal (VP) shunt.

Late or chronic hydrocephalus can develop weeks after SAH. These patients present with a headache, gait instability, incontinence, and cognitive decline. Treatment is placement of a VP shunt.

Delayed Cerebral Ischemia Due to Arterial Narrowing (Vasospasm)

Arterial narrowing occurs in many patients after aSAH and may cause decreased perfusion, potentially leading to DCI and infarction of cerebral tissue. As previously noted, several mechanisms contribute to arterial narrowing, commonly referred to as "vasospasm." Vasospasm typically develops 3 to 14 days after initial hemorrhage, with peak incidence around day 7, and is the biggest contributor to morbidity and mortality rates in patients with SAH who survive to hospital admission. Approximately one-third of patients with aneurysmal SAH will develop delayed ischemic neurologic deficits (DIND) due to vasospasm, and another third will have angiographic evidence of arterial narrowing without neurologic decline. The amount of blood on the initial CT scan is a good predictor of the risk of vasospasm and DCI.

At many institutions, transcranial Doppler studies (TCDs, see Chapter 12, Neurological System) are used to monitor for the development of vasospasm. TCDs assess blood flow velocity in select arteries; the velocity increases as the vessels become narrower. TCDs are noninvasive and can be performed at the bedside, but accuracy varies based on patient and operator characteristics. CT angiography can also be used to look for vasospasm but, as with aneurysm diagnosis, catheter angiography remains a standard. Vasospasm is suspected in any patient who develops sudden neurologic deficits, especially a decrease in level of consciousness, paresis, paralysis of a limb or one side of the body, or aphasia. If any neurologic change is detected, the physician is notified immediately. Early identification of neurologic deficits allows rapid intervention to improve perfusion and prevent infarction.

Maintenance of euvolemia is essential to decrease the risk of DCI. Careful attention to fluid balance is important and must include recognition of insensible fluid loss. Dehydration increases blood viscosity and decreases cerebral perfusion. SAH patients are at risk for dehydration because of cerebral salt wasting, in which too much sodium is excreted, leading to increased water loss and hypovolemia. If serum sodium falls, volume restriction is contraindicated because of an increased risk of DIND. Infusion of hypertonic saline (usually 1.8% NaCl - 3% NaCl) is often used for treatment of hyponatremia.

Nimodipine, a calcium channel blocker, does not significantly decrease angiographic vasospasm, but a clinical trial of nimodipine demonstrated improved outcomes at 3 months after aSAH. Vasospasm can also be treated using an endovascular approach with transluminal balloon angioplasty or direct infusion of a calcium channel antagonist (such as verapamil) or a phosphodiesterase-3 inhibitor (milrinone) into the artery in spasm.

"Triple-H" therapy (hypertension, hypervolemia, and hemodilution) is no longer recommended. Recent guidelines support the maintenance of euvolemia by matching fluid output with an equal volume of intravenous fluid, thereby maintaining the patient's overall volume at a steady state. Accurate output measurement is crucial when matching fluids, therefore these patients may require an indwelling urinary catheter.

Blood pressure goals for vasospasm vary based on the patient's response but are typically in the range of 160 to 200 mm Hg. If previously transferred to the PCU, patients requiring treatment for vasospasm may be readmitted to the ICU for additional management.

Clinical management of aSAH is still an evolving field; there are many ongoing clinical trials related to the monitoring and treatment of this condition.

Additional Management Strategies and Prevention of Complications

Prophylactic anticonvulsants may be given to patients with SAH for a short period (approximately 3-7 days) immediately following presentation. Patients who demonstrate clinical or electrographic seizures are treated according to standard seizure management (see Chapter 12, Neurological System) and remain on anticonvulsants throughout hospitalization. Systemic complications of SAH include myocardial dysfunction, cardiac arrhythmias, and neurogenic pulmonary edema. These complications typically occur within hours of the initial hemorrhage. Patients are also at risk for complications of immobility such as infections and deep venous thrombosis (DVT).

TRAUMATIC BRAIN INJURY

Etiology, Risk Factors, and Pathophysiology

The major causes of traumatic brain injury (TBI) are falls, motor vehicle accidents (MVAs), "struck by/against" events (such as injury from falling debris), and assault. Together, these make up over 80% of all TBI-related admissions. While TBI from falls are more commonly the cause of TBI in the very young and elderly, MVA is more likely the cause for persons aged 15 to 44 years. The incidence of TBI is higher in males than females and higher in children aged 0 to 4 years compared to all other age groups. Despite an increase in the rate of TBI admissions, the rate of TBI-related deaths has been steadily declining. Rates of hospitalization and death are highest in those older than 75 years. TBI ranges from mild (causing a brief change in consciousness) to very severe (causing prolonged unresponsiveness or even death).

TBI severity can be classified using the Glasgow Coma Scale (GCS) score (see Chapter 12, Neurological System). Mild brain injury refers to patients with a GCS score of 13 to 15, moderate indicates a GCS score of 9 to 12, and patients with a score of 8 or less are categorized as having severe brain injury. Although a higher GCS is associated with better outcomes, TBI does not have to be severe to cause long-term impact. Even mild TBI can cause significant functional deficits that become apparent in the weeks and months following the injury. Patients with mild TBI and an abnormal CT scan may be admitted to the PCU; likewise, patients currently admitted to the PCU for other injuries may also be diagnosed with mild TBI. Patients with moderate TBI and a stable or improving neurologic examination may be admitted directly to the PCU at some institutions. However, most of these patients are initially admitted to the ICU and later transferred to the PCU for continued care. Patients with severe TBI will be directly admitted to the ICU.

Mechanism of Injury

TBI occurs as the result of blunt trauma (a direct blow to the head), penetrating trauma (missile or impaled object), or blast injury.

Blunt injury occurs as a consequence of:

- *Deceleration:* The head is moving and strikes a stationary object (eg, pavement).
- *Acceleration:* A moving object (eg, baseball bat) strikes the head.
- *Acceleration-deceleration:* The brain moves rapidly within the skull, resulting in a combination of two injury-causing forces. This is common with MVAs.
- *Rotation:* Twisting motion of the brain occurs within the skull, usually due to side impact.
- *Deformation/compression:* Direct injury to the head changes the shape of the skull, resulting in compression of brain tissue.

In the United States, gunshot wound (GSW) is the most common type of penetrating brain trauma. The degree of injury caused by a GSW varies based on the type of firearm, bullet type, and trajectory of the bullet. The bullet destroys tissue, after which shock waves and cavity formation occur along the bullet's path. Some bullets will ricochet once inside the skull, creating more tissue destruction. Other causes of penetrating brain injury include nail guns and stab wounds. Surgical management of penetrating trauma to the brain differs from the management of closed injury, but many of the issues relevant to progressive care nurses remain the same.

Awareness of TBI due to blast injury caused by an explosion has increased in recent years. The individual may be hit by flying debris or may be thrown by the force of the blast, causing blunt or penetrating trauma. The brain is also thought to be sensitive to the initial over pressurization wave, with damage occurring as the result of the diffuse impact of intense pressure on brain structures.

Skull Fractures

Skull fractures can result in injury to the underlying brain tissue or may occur in isolation. Skull fractures are classified as linear, depressed, or basilar.

- *Linear skull fractures* resemble a line or single crack in the skull. Generally, they are not displaced and require no treatment.
- *Depressed skull fractures* are characterized by an inward depression of bone fragments. Surgery to elevate the depressed bone may be required. In the case of an open fracture, the wound is also washed out in the operating room to decontaminate the area and decrease the risk of infection.
- *Basilar skull fractures* involve the base of the skull, including the anterior, middle, or posterior fossa. Clinical manifestations of a basilar skull fracture include periorbital ecchymosis (raccoon's eyes), mastoid ecchymosis (Battle's sign), rhinorrhea (CSF or blood leaking from the nose), otorrhea (CSF or blood leaking from the ears), hemotympanum (blood behind the tympanic membrane), conjunctival hemorrhage, and cranial nerve dysfunction. The presence of otorrhea or rhinorrhea indicates a dural tear with an increased risk of meningitis. Although most CSF leaks stop spontaneously, those that persist may require surgical repair. Management of a CSF leak includes elevating the head of bed, antibiotics, and occasionally a lumbar drainage of CSF to decrease pressure on the healing dura.

Primary Brain Injury

The damage that results from TBI is due to both the primary insult and the secondary injury produced by ongoing intracranial and systemic complications. Primary injury can be described as *focal* (resulting in local damage at the site of injury) or *diffuse* (affecting the whole brain). *Focal injuries* take up space and can cause tissue compression, increased ICP, brain shift, and herniation. Examples of focal injury include cerebral contusions and hematomas. *Diffuse brain injuries* involve microscopic damage to cells deep in the white matter. They occur as lateral head motion produces angular movement of the brain within the skull, causing shearing or stretching of axonal nerve fibers. Damage is variable and dependent on the amount of accelerative force transmitted to the brain. Focal and diffuse brain injuries do not typically occur in isolation; for example, a patient with a focal cerebral contusion is also likely to have some component of diffuse brain injury.

Examples of primary injury:

- *Contusion:* Contusions are cortical bruises caused by the brain impacting the inside of the skull. They may be described as *coup* (occurring at the site of impact) or *contrecoup* (occurring opposite the site of impact). The frontal and temporal lobes are common sites of contusions. Clinical presentation depends on the site

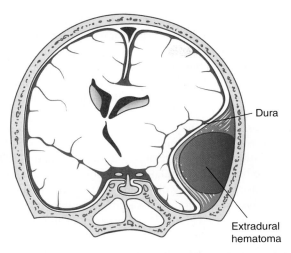

Figure 20-4. Schematic illustration of an epidural hemorrhage. (*Reproduced with permission from Waxman SG:* Clinical Neuroanatomy. *New York, NY: Lange Medical Books/McGraw-Hill; 2003.*)

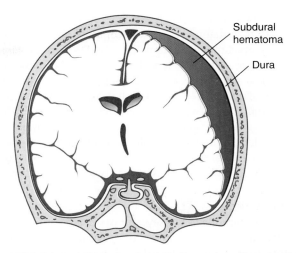

Figure 20-5. Schematic illustration of a subdural hemorrhage. (*Reproduced with permission from Waxman SG:* Clinical Neuroanatomy. *New York, NY: Lange Medical Books/McGraw-Hill; 2003.*)

and extent of brain injury. Progressive focal edema and mass effect may result in neurologic deterioration. The severity of injury may not be apparent on the initial CT scan, because bleeding into the contused or lacerated tissue often occurs later and results in intracerebral hematoma. Repeat CT scanning may be performed to evaluate for injury progression.

- *Epidural hematoma:* (EDH, Figure 20-4). An EDH is a bleeding located above the dura (between the dura and the skull). EDH is often associated with skull fractures that lacerate an underlying artery, and is most common in the temporal region due to tearing of the middle meningeal artery. Patients may have a lucid interval, especially if the injury is very focal (ie, struck by a baseball or other solid object) and then deteriorate rapidly as bleeding displaces brain structures and causes increased ICP. While a lucid interval suggests EDH, not all patients follow this course. Symptoms of EDH include a decrease in consciousness, headache, seizures, vomiting, hemiparesis, and pupillary dilation. Management includes emergency surgery to evacuate the hematoma.

- *Subdural hematoma:* (SDH, Figure 20-5.) SDH is blood that accumulates below the dura (within the subdural space, between the dura and the arachnoid layers). This creates direct pressure on the brain. SDH results from rupture of the bridging veins between the brain and the dura, bleeding from contused or lacerated brain tissue, or extension from an intracerebral hematoma. SDH is described as acute if symptoms begin within the first 48 hours after injury. Many patients experience significant symptoms immediately following the injury or much sooner than 48 hours. Patients with acute SDH present with progressive decline in level of consciousness, headache, agitation, and confusion. Motor deficits, pupillary

changes, and cranial nerve dysfunction may be seen reflecting the primary brain injury and compressive effects. Treatment of acute SDH consists of evacuation of the hematoma by craniotomy.

- Blood may also collect in the subdural space more slowly, over days to weeks (subacute SDH) or weeks to months (chronic SDH). Symptom onset is insidious because the brain can better compensate for this slow increase in mass. Symptoms include an increasingly severe headache, confusion, drowsiness, and, possibly, seizures, pupillary abnormalities, or motor dysfunction. Predisposing conditions include advanced age, alcoholism, and disorders or treatments that result in prolonged coagulation times (ie, if the patient routinely takes anticoagulants for a separate disease process). Treatment of subacute or chronic SDH includes evacuation via burr holes or a craniotomy.

- *Traumatic subarachnoid hemorrhage:* Traumatic SAH can occur alone or in combination with other types of primary brain injury and may be present in up to one-third of severe TBI cases. The risk of symptomatic vasospasm is thought to be less than that associated with aneurysmal SAH, perhaps because the amount of blood seen in the subarachnoid space is typically less with traumatic SAH than in aneurysmal SAH. In patients who present with traumatic SAH, the possibility that the patient experienced an aneurysmal SAH (which then caused the traumatic event) should be investigated, especially if the events preceding the trauma are unclear.

- *Diffuse injury:* Diffuse TBI exists on a continuum from cerebral concussion to severe diffuse axonal injury (DAI). Cerebral concussion is a transient neurologic dysfunction caused by rapid acceleration-deceleration or by a sudden blow to the head. Symptoms of concussion include headache, confusion, disorientation, and amnesia; most symptoms resolve without intervention. Patients with severe DAI typically experience an immediate and prolonged loss of consciousness and display abnormal posturing. The initial CT scan may appear normal, show signs of diffuse cerebral edema (decreased ventricle size, loss of differentiation between gray and white matter, and loss of sulci), or show very small areas of hemorrhage (punctate hemorrhage). The clinical course and outcome are dependent upon the severity of axonal injury.

Secondary Brain Injury

Patients with moderate to severe TBI are at significant risk for secondary brain injury. Secondary injury refers to the complications that result from pathophysiologic changes caused by the primary injury. Care is directed at minimizing secondary injury by improving the supply of oxygenated blood to the brain and decreasing cerebral metabolic demands. Major contributors to secondary injury include the following:

- *Hypoxemia:* The brain needs a constant supply of oxygen to function. It is very sensitive to any insult that creates hypoxemia. Examples include pneumonia, atelectasis, chest trauma, neurogenic pulmonary edema, airway obstruction, and pulmonary embolus. Hypoxemia results in cerebral tissue hypoxia and anaerobic metabolism. Anaerobic metabolism produces less energy (ATP) than aerobic metabolism—thereby increasing metabolic demand—and results in a number of metabolic byproducts, including lactic acid. These metabolic byproducts cause further cell damage and apoptosis.
- *Hypotension:* Hypotension resulting in decreased cerebral perfusion (SBP < 90 mm Hg) is associated with increased risk of mortality after TBI. Hypotension decreases cerebral blood flow, resulting in tissue ischemia and buildup of waste products. Mortality risk increases with multiple episodes of hypotension.
- *Anemia:* Anemia causes secondary injury by decreasing oxygen delivery to the brain. The optimal hematocrit in patients with cerebral insults is still under investigation.
- *Hypo- or hyperglycemia:* The brain cannot store glucose and is dependent on a constant supply of nutrients to maintain metabolic function. Hypoglycemia must be avoided because it disrupts this supply and leads to cellular dysfunction. Significant hypoglycemia is uncommon following TBI. Hyperglycemia is more common and is associated with increased mortality; it is unclear if elevated blood glucose is a marker of injury severity or if it contributes to pathologic changes that increase mortality.
- *Increased intracranial pressure:* Increased ICP (> 20-25 mm Hg) may negatively affect cerebral perfusion and the viability of neurons. The major sources of increased ICP after brain injury are cerebral edema and expanding lesions such as hematomas. Compression of blood vessels can result in ischemia and infarction of specific areas. Edema may be diffuse or localized at the site of the injury, with edema occurring 2 to 5 days after injury.
- *Loss of autoregulatory mechanisms:* Autoregulatory mechanisms maintain constant cerebral blood flow within a wide range of blood pressures and ICP. The ability to autoregulate blood flow may be compromised or entirely disabled in an injured brain. This increases the brain's susceptibility to ischemia caused by decreased blood flow. The extent of autoregulatory damage varies from patient to patient.
- *Hypo- or hypercapnia:* Hypocapnia decreases cerebral blood flow by increasing pH and causing cerebral vasoconstriction. Decreased cerebral blood flow lowers the ICP but creates a potentially ischemic state. Hypercapnia results in cerebral vasodilation and increases ICP, which may contribute to secondary injury; careful management is therefore warranted in order to achieve an optimal balance.
- *Biochemical changes:* A number of biochemical changes occur following TBI, including the release of excitatory amino acids, free radical production, inflammation, and abnormal calcium shifts. A complete explanation of these underlying processes is beyond the scope of this text. Multiple factors contribute to changes in cellular function and can cause cell death. Much research has been completed in an attempt to stop these biochemical changes and confer neuroprotection; to date, none of these trials have demonstrated significant improvement in outcomes.
- *Increased metabolic demands:* Fever, agitation, and seizures increase metabolic demand. Fever has been shown to significantly increase the ICP and can be due to an infectious process or injury to the hypothalamus. A seizure places extreme stress on the body and significantly increases systemic metabolic demand, which may worsen or cause an anoxic injury.

Clinical Presentation

Patients with TBI often present with external signs of trauma to the head, such as ecchymosis, lacerations, and abrasions. Level of consciousness is the most important indicator of severity of injury and is assessed using the GCS. A decreasing GCS or a change in pupil size/reactivity both indicate neurologic decline and warrant immediate provider notification. The type, location, and severity of TBI determine specific neurologic assessment findings. Patients may display hemiparesis, hemiplegia, language deficits, cognitive changes, or behavioral changes. If the injury is severe, the patient may display flexor or extensor posturing, as well as autonomic instability (eg, fever, tachycardia, or hypertension).

Patients with mild TBI may not display focal deficits such as hemiplegia or hemiparesis, but instead report a variety of physical, cognitive, and emotional symptoms. Signs and symptoms of mild TBI include headache, nausea/vomiting, dizziness, balance disturbance, visual problems, fatigue, photophobia, and sensitivity to sound. Patients often report difficulty concentrating, decreased short-term memory, slowed thought processes, irritability, anxiety, sadness, and increased emotion. Sleep disturbances are also common following mild TBI and include both drowsiness/increased need for sleep and difficulty sleeping.

Diagnostic Tests

Brain CT is used to rapidly identify intracranial hematomas. Other bleeding (such as into the subarachnoid space), contusions, skull fractures, and cerebral edema can be detected on CT as well. MRI is useful in the detection of DAI, brain stem injury, and vascular injury but is not typically included in the initial evaluation. The diagnostic workup of the TBI patient includes a search for other injuries as appropriate to the mechanism of injury.

Principles of Management of Traumatic Brain Injury

Management priorities for patients with TBI vary based on the severity of injury.

Mild Traumatic Brain Injury (GCS 13-15)

Patients with mild TBI and an abnormal CT scan may be admitted to the PCU for serial neurologic examination or for monitoring and management of other injuries. These patients require education regarding the possible sequelae of mild TBI, including headaches, difficulty concentrating, dizziness, fatigue, irritability, decreased processing speed, and sleep disturbances. Resources for follow-up are provided to the patient and family. In most cases, the symptoms will resolve, but future reevaluation by a neuropsychologist or rehabilitation professional is recommended if symptoms persist.

Moderate Traumatic Brain Injury (GCS 9-12)

Moderate TBI poses a significant challenge to the healthcare team. A number of these patients will decline and require aggressive management similar to patients with severe TBI. Others will improve without intervention. Patients with moderate TBI who are admitted to the PCU should be monitored very closely, with neurological assessments performed at least hourly. Changes in these exams warrant immediate action by the healthcare team.

Severe Traumatic Brain Injury (GCS Less Than or Equal to 8)

The initial management of patients with severe TBI takes place in the ICU and is focused on optimizing functional recovery by minimizing secondary brain injury. In addition, other injuries must be identified and treated. An understanding of the early management of these patients gives the progressive care nurse insight into the patient's overall hospital course, which is often helpful in supporting families. In addition, these general principles can be applied to any patient with TBI who is experiencing neurologic worsening.

General principles of management for the patient with severe TBI include:

- *Airway management:* Patients with a GCS of 8 or less require intubation and mechanical ventilation. Patients with TBI are treated with spine precautions until injury to the spinal column can be ruled out, so manual in-line stabilization of the cervical spine is used during intubation. Once the patient's condition has stabilized, a tracheostomy is often performed to allow for faster ventilator weaning and facilitate rehabilitation.

- *Oxygenation:* Hypoxemia is avoided because it worsens secondary brain injury. Patients with severe TBI may vomit and aspirate prior to airway placement, or may have thoracic injuries which may complicate pulmonary management. The need for ventilator support and meticulous pulmonary care often continues following transfer from the ICU.

- *Ventilation:* In general, the goal of management is to maintain a normal $Paco_2$. Hypoventilation causes cerebral vasodilation, which may increase ICP. Prolonged or prophylactic hyperventilation is not recommended because it causes cerebral vasoconstriction, which lowers ICP but may cause cerebral ischemia.

- *Fluid and volume management:* The goal of fluid management is to maintain euvolemia. Hypotonic solutions are avoided because they increase cerebral edema. Patients with TBI, especially those with autonomic instability due to DAI, often have large insensible losses due to diaphoresis and fever and are at risk for dehydration. Patients with injury to the hypothalamus or pituitary gland are at risk for diabetes insipidus (DI) or syndrome of inappropriate antidiuretic hormone (SIADH), further complicating fluid management. For more information on DI and SIADH, refer to Chapter 16, Endocrine.

- *Managing increased ICP:* Initially, an ICP monitor is placed in patients with severe TBI to help guide management. Treatment is initiated when ICP is sustained above 20 mm Hg (see Special procedures: Invasive Monitoring of Intracranial Pressure and Management of a Patient with a Lumbar Drain at the end of this chapter). These patients are often managed in the ICU, but increased ICP can also occur in patients with moderate TBI who are admitted to the PCU. It can also occur in response to late complications of severe TBI, such as hydrocephalus. Nursing measures to prevent and manage elevations in ICP are discussed in Chapter 12, Neurological System. Of note, steroids worsen outcomes following TBI and should therefore be avoided.

- *Supporting cerebral perfusion:* Hypotension (SBP < 90 mm Hg) is associated with a poor outcome in TBI patients. Cerebral perfusion pressure (CPP, calculated by subtracting ICP from MAP) is an indirect indicator of cerebral blood flow. Goal CPP may vary based on the clinical scenario and other monitors of cerebral perfusion, but a CPP of less than 50 mm Hg is avoided because of the high likelihood of resulting cerebral ischemia.

- *Preventing increased cerebral oxygen demand:* Seizures, fever, and agitation increase cerebral oxygen demand and are avoided. An anticonvulsant is used to prevent posttraumatic seizures during the first 7 days after injury. Beyond the first week, continued seizure prophylaxis does not impact the development of posttraumatic seizures and is not recommended. Fever is known to be detrimental to the injured brain. For every 1°C increase in temperature, cerebral metabolism increases by approximately 6%. To prevent additional demands on the injured brain, fevers are aggressively controlled. However, it is important to manage shivering when treating fevers because shivering markedly increases cerebral metabolic demand. Agitation also increases demand. Strategies to avoid agitation include maintaining a calm, quiet environment and if severe, it may warrant the use of sedatives or anxiolytics. Pain management is very important; short-acting medications are preferred to allow ongoing accurate evaluations of mental status.

Preventing Secondary Complications

Common secondary complications include pneumonia and other infections, VTE including pulmonary embolism (PE), gastric ulcers and bleeding, and pressure injury to the skin. Nutrition may be started within the first 3 days after injury. VTE prophylaxis is initiated on admission with pneumatic compression devices. Pharmacologic prophylaxis varies by practitioner and type of TBI. To decrease the risk of PE,

inferior vena cava (IVC) filters are indicated in patients who develop DVTs but cannot receive anticoagulation.

Complications of immobility are common in patients with TBI. Progression of activity is optimized with early spine clearance. Institutional protocols vary, but typically include a series of spine x-rays, CT scanning, and MRIs to rule out injury to the bones and ligaments of the spine.

Promoting Recovery After Traumatic Brain Injury

Most patients progress through a series of recovery stages, during which they become more alert, then agitated, then purposeful and more appropriate. The Rancho Los Amigos scale (Table 20-2) is useful in tracking patient recovery, planning interventions, and educating family members. Managing agitation is frequently challenging in patients with TBI. Environmental strategies are very important; a calm demeanor maintained by staff and family members is essential to minimizing agitation. One person speaks at a time and the patient is allowed extra time to respond to questions. Consistent staff members are assigned to care for the patient to promote continuity of care whenever possible. All lines and tubes, such as indwelling bladder catheters and IVs, are removed as soon as possible. Medications are often prescribed as part of managing agitation in patients with TBI but should be used in the smallest doses possible for the shortest time possible because they may slow recovery and confuse neurological assessments. Restraints are avoided unless patient or staff safety is compromised.

The best care for patients with TBI includes input from multiple disciplines. Physical therapy, occupational therapy, nutrition, and social work are consulted early in the patient's hospital course. The speech therapist provides expert assistance with swallowing issues, language, and cognition. Consultation with the rehabilitation provider and a neuropsychologist may also be helpful.

TABLE 20-2. RANCHO LOS AMIGOS LEVELS OF COGNITIVE FUNCTIONING SCALE AFTER HEAD TRAUMA

Level	Response	Description
1	None	Completely unresponsive to any stimulus
2	Generalized	Reacts inconsistently and nonpurposefully to stimuli; may respond with physiologic changes, gross body movements, or utterances
3	Localized	Reacts specifically but inconsistently to stimuli; responds directly to a stimulus; shows vague awareness of self and body; may pull at tubes and react to discomfort
4	Confused, agitated	Heightened state of activity but unable to process information correctly; reacts to internal confusion; nonpurposeful behavior with confabulation present; cries, screams, and manifests aggressive behavior; cannot discriminate among people; performs gross motor activities but not self-care activities
5	Confused, inappropriate	Follows simple commands; may show agitated behavior from inability to cope with external demands; gross inattention to environment, easily distracted; impaired memory and inappropriate verbalization; cannot initiate tasks; often uses things incorrectly
6	Confused, appropriate	Displays goal-directed behavior but requires direction from others; follows simple commands; shows carryover of information from previously learned tasks; memory problems persist; inconsistently oriented to time and place; increased awareness of self and others
7	Automatic, appropriate	Oriented in hospital and home settings; performs tasks in robotlike manner; superficial awareness of own condition but lacks good problem-solving abilities; carryover for new learning; independent in self-care activities; needs structure but can initiate tasks of interest
8	Purposeful, appropriate	Alert and oriented; few memory problems; can begin vocational rehabilitation; carryover for new learning; social, emotional, and intellectual capacities may be decreased from pretrauma level

Data from Malkmus D, Booth, B, Kodimer C. Rehabilitation of the Head Injured Adult—Comprehensive Cognitive Management. Downey, CA: Professional Staff Association of the Rancho Los Amigos Hospital; 1980.

Family Education and Support

TBI alters the life of the injured individual and their family forever. The unpredictable nature of their recovery from brain injury can be difficult to comprehend. Family members may feel that information provided by different caregivers is inconsistent or that insufficient information is being provided. They express the need to be involved in care—to be "part of the team."

Nurses can best support patients and families by providing direct, honest communication (including acknowledging the difficulty of providing a definitive prognosis) and by recognizing their need to be present and involved in care. The transition from the ICU to the PCU is often a stressful time for family members. While there is less uncertainty about whether or not the patient will live, the extent of the patient's recovery remains unknown. Intensive and progressive care nurses can decrease family members' anxiety by collaborating to provide continuity of care and consistent education about the stages of recovery.

TRAUMATIC SPINAL CORD INJURY

Etiology, Risk Factors, and Pathophysiology

Common causes of SCI include MVAs, falls, acts of violence, accounting for over 80% of all SCIs. Sports-related injuries account for approximately 9% of SCI and medical or surgical procedures account for approximately 5% of SCI. Nearly 60% of SCIs involve the cervical cord and result in partial or complete tetraplegia (loss of function in all four limbs). The average age at time of injury has increased and is now at 42 years old. Over 80% of individuals with SCI are male. SCI results in varying degrees of paralysis and loss of sensation below the level of injury, which can impact physical, emotional, and social function. Similar to brain injury, deficits are due to both the initial impact (primary injury) and the ongoing physiologic changes (secondary injury).

The spinal column consists of stacked vertebrae joined by bony facet joints and intervertebral disks. Ligaments provide structure and support to prevent the vertebrae from moving. The ring-like structure of the stacked vertebrae creates a hollow canal through which the spinal cord runs. SCI occurs when something (ie, bone, disk material, or foreign object) enters the spinal canal and disrupts the spinal cord or its blood supply. Mechanisms of injury include hyperflexion, hyperextension, axial loading/vertical compression, rotation, and penetrating trauma (Figure 20-6). Damage to the spinal cord can be characterized as concussion, contusion, laceration, transection, hemorrhage, or damage to the blood vessels that supply the spinal cord. *Concussion* causes temporary loss of function. *Contusion* is bruising of the spinal cord that includes bleeding into the spinal cord, subsequent edema, and possible neuronal death from compression by the edema or damage to the tissue; the extent of neurologic deficit depends on the severity of the contusion. *Laceration* is an actual tear in the spinal cord that results in permanent injury. *Transection* is a severing of the spinal cord resulting in complete loss of function below the level of the injury. The

most obvious example of cord laceration or transection is a penetrating injury that disrupts the cord. Damage to the blood vessels that supply the spinal cord can result in ischemia and infarction, or hemorrhage due to vessel tearing.

Regardless of the type of primary injury, secondary insults occur from cellular damage to the spinal cord, vascular damage, structural changes in the gray and white matter, and subsequent biochemical responses. Blood flow to the spinal cord is decreased during the acute phase of injury, resulting in changes in metabolic function, destruction of cell membranes, and the release of free radicals. Patients may develop neurogenic shock following cervical and upper thoracic cord injury. Neurogenic shock occurs due to loss of sympathetic nervous system input from the T1 to L2 area of the spinal cord, which normally increases heart rate and constricts the blood vessel walls. Loss of sympathetic outflow results in bradycardia and decreased vascular resistance. Blood pools in the peripheral vasculature, resulting in hypotension and decreased cardiac output. Neurogenic shock contributes to hypoperfusion and secondary injury.

Clinical Presentation

Assessment of the patient with SCI begins with evaluation of circulation, airway, and breathing, with attention to the immobilization of the spine to prevent further injury during the assessment and any subsequent interventions. The focus then shifts to obtaining a baseline assessment of motor and sensory function. Assessment of motor function and sensory level is performed at least every 4 hours during the acute postinjury period. Decreased motor function may be seen with swelling at the injury site, loss of vertebral alignment, or intrathecal hematoma formation. Changes in function warrant immediate provider notification.

The degree of injury (complete or incomplete) and the level of the affected spinal cord determine the severity of the deficits displayed by the patient. Acute SCI can result in the temporary suppression of reflexes controlled by segments below the level of injury, a phenomenon referred to as "*spinal shock*." Formal determination of complete versus incomplete SCI cannot be made until spinal shock is resolved. *Complete SCI* results in total loss of sensory and motor function below the level of injury due to complete interruption of motor and sensory pathways. *Incomplete SCI* results in mixed loss of motor and sensory function because some spinal tracts remain intact. Syndromes associated with incomplete SCI are described in Table 20-3.

Deficits caused by SCI relate to the level at which the injury occurs (cervical, thoracic, or lumbar). Cervical and lumbar injuries are more common because these areas have the greatest flexibility and movement. A cervical injury can result in paralysis of all four extremities or tetraplegia (previously called quadriplegia). Injuries to the thoracic and lumbar areas can result in paraplegia. The American Spinal Injury Association (ASIA) scale may be used to assess and document motor and sensory function. Specific functional losses from SCI are summarized in Figure 20-7.

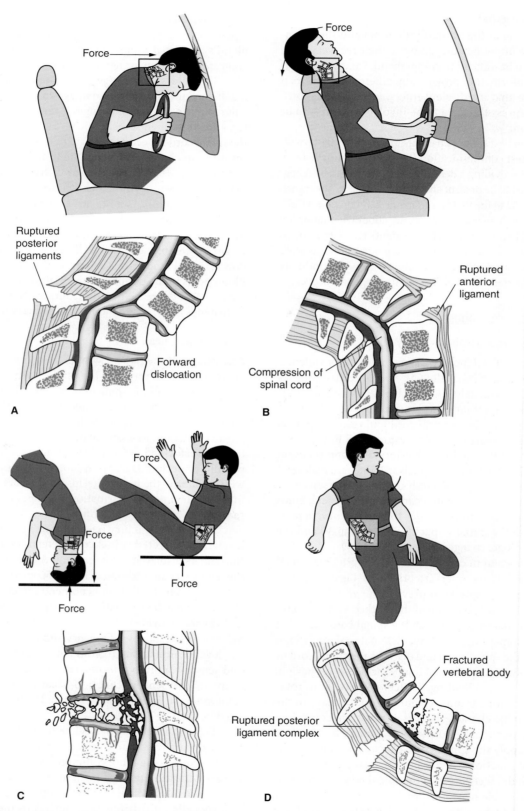

Figure 20-6. Mechanisms of spinal cord injury. **(A)** Hyperflexion. **(B)** Hyperextension. **(C)** Axial loading/vertical compression. **(D)** Rotation. (*Reproduced with permission from Phipps WJ, Marek JF, Monahan FD, et al:* Medical-Surgical Nursing: Health and Illness Perspectives. *St Louis, MO: Mosby; 2003.*)

TABLE 20-3. INCOMPLETE SCI SYNDROMES

Syndrome	Pathophysiology	Motor Function Below Level of Injury	Sensory Function Below Level of Injury
Central cord syndrome	Injury to central gray matter with preservation of outer white matter	Weakness/paralysis of upper extremities greater than lower extremities	Sensory loss greater in upper extremities than lower extremities
Anterior cord syndrome	Injury to anterior portion of spinal cord, disruption of blood flow through anterior spinal artery	Paralysis	Loss of pain and temperature with preservation of vibration and position sense
Posterior cord syndrome	Injury to posterior column	None	Loss of vibration and position sense with preservation of pain and temperature sensation
Brown-Séquard syndrome	Lateral injury to one side of the cord	Ipsilateral motor paralysis	Ipsilateral loss of vibration and position sense with contralateral loss of pain and temperature sensation

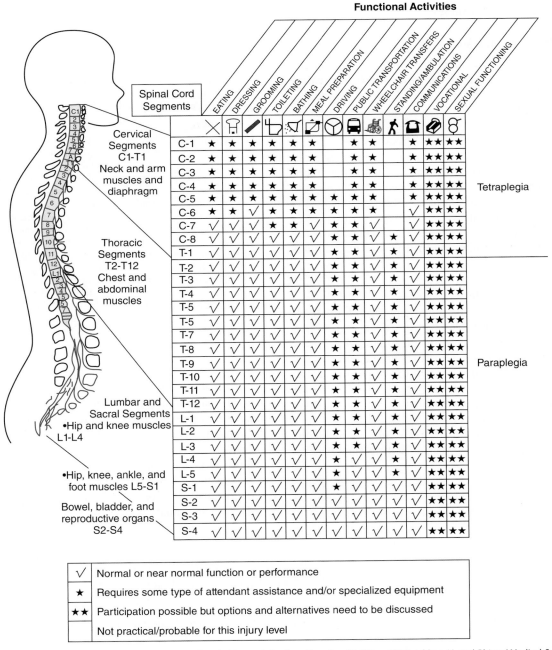

Figure 20-7. Spinal cord injury functional activity chart. (*Reproduced with permission from Monahan FD, Phipps WJ, Neighbors M, et al.* Phipps' Medical-Surgical Nursing: Health and Illness Perspectives, *8th ed. Philadelphia, PA: Mosby Elsevier; 2006.*)

Diagnostic Tests

Immobilization of the spinal column is maintained through-out the trauma evaluation to prevent additional injury. Cervical, thoracic, and lumbar spine x-rays identify the presence of injury to the vertebral column, although these tests are increasingly being replaced with specially constructed CT images. In addition to injury to the vertebral column, CT reveals many injuries to the spinal cord itself, such as bleeding or significant compression. Most patients with suspected SCI undergo an MRI to reveal more subtle signs of injury to the cord and soft tissue, like injury to the supporting ligaments. Injury to the ligaments and spinal cord is possible even without bony abnormalities.

Principles of Management of Acute Spinal Cord Injury

As with brain injury, education focuses on prevention of primary injury and initial management focuses on decreasing secondary injury and preventing complications. Priorities of management include:

Immobilization and Prevention of Further Injury

Patients with potential SCI are immobilized with a rigid cervical collar and a backboard in the prehospital environment, followed by a rigid cervical collar and bed rest in the hospital until an injury is ruled out or confirmed clinically and by radiograph. Some mattresses (such as air mattresses) do not provide adequate stability to the spinal column; special care to follow manufacturer and institutional guidelines is necessary.

Supporting Oxygenation and Ventilation

Altered respiratory function is a major problem for patients with high thoracic or cervical SCI. Impaired oxygenation contributes to secondary injury. The mnemonic "3, 4, 5, keep the lungs alive" helps to recall that the phrenic nerve, which supplies motor and sensory input to the diaphragm, arises from the C3-C5. Patients with complete injuries at or above the C2 level require mechanical ventilation due to the loss of diaphragmatic innervation.

Patients with cervical or thoracic injuries below the level of diaphragmatic innervation will initiate breaths but still experience respiratory compromise due to the paralysis of the intercostal and abdominal muscles. Paralysis of the intercostal muscles causes the chest wall to be flaccid. Contraction of the diaphragm creates a negative pressure in the thoracic cavity and the intercostal muscles retract, decreasing lung capacity. Upright positioning creates further downward displacement of the diaphragm and increases intercostal retraction; therefore, flat positioning can improve respiratory function in patients with cervical or thoracic SCI. Abdominal binders can also be useful, especially during physical activity (rehabilitation). With time, the intercostal muscles become spastic and the chest wall no longer collapses with inspiration, allowing for improved ventilation.

Pulmonary function is closely monitored in patients with cervical and thoracic SCI. Ongoing assessment of maximal inspiratory pressure (MIP) and forced vital capacity (FVC) allow early identification of impending respiratory failure. In general, a patient who is unable to generate an MIP of at least -20 cm H_2O or a vital capacity of greater than 10 to 15 mL/kg requires intubation and mechanical ventilation. Noninvasive ventilation may be considered but does not address problems related to inadequate clearance of secretions.

Hemodynamic Support

Neurogenic shock occurs in patients with cervical or thoracic injury and causes significant hemodynamic alterations, including bradycardia and hypotension. Management focuses on the following:

- *Differentiating neurogenic shock from other types of shock.* SCI can mask the signs and symptoms of other trauma, including hemorrhage in the abdomen or pelvis.

- *Administration of intravenous fluids and vasopressors.* Hypotension due solely to neurogenic shock reflects fluid displacement into the vasodilated periphery; it is not a true lack of fluid volume. As with all trauma patients, adequate fluid resuscitation is important, but continued fluid administration will not correct hypotension and can lead to pulmonary edema or heart failure, especially in patients with comorbidities. Norepinephrine is frequently used to counter the loss of sympathetic tone and to provide inotropic and chronotropic support. Research suggests that maintaining MAP more than 85 mm Hg in the week following injury may improve neurologic outcomes. Pending definitive evidence, target blood pressure varies by practitioner. At most institutions, patients requiring vasopressor support due to neurogenic shock or for blood pressure augmentation will be managed in the ICU.
- *Monitoring for bradycardia.* Patients with SCI above T6 may experience bradycardia. This can be profound in patients with cervical injury, even progressing to asystole. Bradycardia occurs more frequently during suctioning; the risk can be lessened but not eliminated by maintaining adequate oxygenation and ventilation. Symptomatic bradycardia is treated with atropine, although some patients may require pacemaker placement.

Neuroprotection

There are no currently approved neuroprotective agents that improve outcomes after SCI. Neuroprotection is an area of ongoing research, and includes both pharmacologic and nonpharmacologic strategies.

Decompression and Stabilization

Early management of SCI includes decompression of the spinal canal and stabilization of the spinal column. In patients with cervical injury, traction may be used to realign the spinal column and relieve pressure on the spinal cord. Traction devices include bed-based (ie, Gardner-Wells tongs) and personalized thoracolumbar sacral orthosis (TLSO) equipment. Nursing responsibilities during traction placement include patient monitoring, pain management, and administration of sedating agents. Decompression of the spinal cord can also be accomplished surgically. Rapid surgical intervention is indicated for patients with worsening neurologic examination and ongoing spinal cord compression.

Stabilization of the spinal column does not improve neurologic function but enables the patient to be mobilized without causing additional damage to the spinal cord. In patients who require operative decompression of the spinal canal, the spinal column is stabilized at the time of surgery using rods, screws, or other hardware. For other patients, the timing of surgical stabilization may vary. Surgery is commonly performed within 24 hours of injury if the patient's cardiorespiratory status is stable because early surgery decreases secondary complications and length of stay. Some fractures can be managed without surgery by immobilizing the spinal column and allowing the bones to heal. Immobilization is achieved using a cervical collar, halo vest, or other orthotic device. Skin care is a primary concern for these patients because pressure injury can occur at contact points with the brace, especially in patients with decreased sensation.

Bladder and Bowel Management

Areflexia caused by spinal shock leads to urinary retention. An indwelling catheter may be placed on admission and maintained until a program of scheduled intermittent catheterization is implemented.

A bowel program is initiated soon after admission and typically includes daily stool softeners, glycerin or bisacodyl suppositories, and digital stimulation. For patients with injuries at or above T6, an anesthetic jelly is used to decrease the risk of autonomic dysreflexia (see Prevention and Management of Complications later in section). The goal of the bowel program is for the patient to have a bowel movement at planned intervals without incontinence between scheduled evacuations. An effective bowel program decreases constipation, limits incontinence, decreases the risk for pressure injury, and increases the patient's sense of control.

Managing Pain

Pain following SCI impacts functional recovery and can be challenging to treat. During the immediate postinjury period, many patients experience musculoskeletal pain and neuropathic pain (described as a burning sensation, paresthesia, or hypersensitivity). Medications for management include opiates and muscle relaxants as well as neuropathic agents such as gabapentin and pregabalin. Antidepressants and anticonvulsants are also useful in the treatment of neuropathic pain. Some patients benefit from nonpharmacologic methods such as massage, visual imagery, and distraction.

Managing Anxiety

Fear, uncertainty, and anxiety are common emotions following SCI. The psychological and emotional trauma of SCI can be overwhelming. Sudden paralysis does not allow patients or family members to prepare for this major insult. Anxiety results from the hospital environment, feelings of total dependence, sensory deprivation, powerlessness, and an unknown future.

A trusting relationship must be established between the patient and the healthcare team. Use of eye contact, patience, honesty, and consistency are reassuring to the patient. Encouraging self-care within the patient's abilities decreases feelings of complete dependence. Whenever possible, the patient is allowed choices within the daily care routine. Contracting with the patient may be helpful in setting limits for some patients. The family and significant others are also incorporated into the plan of care.

Prevention and Management of Complications

The prevention and effective management of complications maximizes rehabilitation potential. Common complications include:

- *Respiratory complications:* Respiratory complications are common and contribute to morbidity and mortality. Chest physiotherapy and assisted coughing ("quad" coughing) are used in both ventilated and nonventilated patients. In addition, a mechanical cough assist device (in-exsufflator) can be used to clear secretions. This device imitates a physiologic cough by providing a deep breath via positive pressure followed by negative pressure. Standard measures to prevent hospital-acquired pneumonia, such as head of bed elevation and oral care, are implemented.
- *Gastrointestinal problems:* Paralytic ileus is common immediately following injury. Initially, an orogastric or nasogastric tube may be placed for decompression, especially in patients with cervical or thoracic injuries. The current recommendation is for enteral nutrition to be started within 48 hours of injury. Patients with acute SCI may also have an increased risk for stress ulcers and require prophylactic medications.
- *Pressure injury:* The patient with SCI is at high risk for pressure injury due to decreased blood flow to the skin and decreased cutaneous response to focal pressure. Meticulous skin care is essential. Skin inspection is performed at least twice daily and pressure reduction strategies are implemented. Early in the hospitalization, the patient who requires assistance with repositioning is encouraged to request that assistance at scheduled intervals. This increases the patient's sense of control and self-care responsibility, which is associated with improved long-term outcomes.
- *Orthostatic hypotension:* Blood pools in the lower extremities due to loss of sympathetic vascular tone. Nursing strategies to decrease orthostatic hypotension include application of gradient compression stockings and elastic wraps to the legs, hydration, and gradual progression to an upright position. If these measures are ineffective, medication to raise blood pressure may be ordered.
- *Altered thermoregulation:* Individuals with SCI at or above the T6 level are unable to conserve heat by vasoconstriction or shivering. Heat loss is compromised by the inability to sweat below the level of injury.
- *Venothromboembolism:* Recommended strategies for prevention during acute hospitalization include mechanical prophylaxis for all patients starting at the time of admission, followed by low-molecular-weight heparin or the combination of low-dose unfractionated heparin and intermittent pneumatic compression. To prevent pulmonary embolus, IVC filters can be placed in patients who cannot receive pharmacologic prophylaxis.

- *Spasticity:* During spinal shock, there is a total loss of motor function below the level of injury. Flaccid paralysis progresses to spastic paralysis as spinal shock resolves. Measures to decrease spasticity in the acute postinjury phase include frequent range-of-motion exercises and medications. Occupational and physical therapy are consulted early in the course of hospitalization.
- *Autonomic dysreflexia:* Autonomic dysreflexia (also called autonomic hyperreflexia) is a life-threatening complication that occurs in individuals with SCI at or above T6 due to unopposed sympathetic response below the level of injury. It can occur any time after spinal shock has resolved. Autonomic dysreflexia results from a variety of stimuli, including an overdistended bladder (most common), a full rectum, infections, skin stimulation, pressure injuries, and pain. The stimulus causes massive vasoconstriction that clinically presents with elevation of blood pressure (relative to the patient's baseline). Other signs and symptoms include headache, nasal congestion, nausea, blurred vision, flushing and diaphoresis above the level of injury, and feelings of apprehension or anxiety. In some individuals, the only sign of autonomic dysreflexia is elevated blood pressure. Autonomic dysreflexia is a medical emergency and the provider is promptly notified. Treatment includes moving the patient into a sitting position, and promptly identifying and treating the underlying cause (eg, bladder distention, bowel impaction).

Monitor blood pressure and pulse closely and administer short-acting antihypertensive agents as ordered. The timing of pharmacologic intervention varies based on patient characteristics, suspected cause of the event, and institutional guidelines. Careful attention to bowel and bladder management aids in the prevention of autonomic dysreflexia.

Future Spinal Cord Injury Treatment

Currently, much research is focused on SCI. The major areas of investigation include limiting the neuronal damage caused by secondary injury (neuroprotection), enhancing regrowth of neurons (nerve regeneration), and encouraging increased activity of functioning neurons (synaptic plasticity). One resource for patients and families who request information about clinical trials is a website sponsored by the National Institutes of Health (www.clinicaltrials.gov).

BRAIN TUMORS

Etiology, Risk Factors, and Pathophysiology

The epidemiology of brain tumors varies widely based on tumor type. When all primary CNS tumors are grouped together, the incidence is higher in women than men. This overall gender difference is attributable to increased incidence of meningiomas in women. Prognosis varies based on age (younger patients have a better prognosis), tumor type, degree of tumor differentiation, functional status at diagnosis, and anatomic tumor location. The most common brain tumors are meningiomas, gliomas, and metastatic lesions. Intracranial tumors are classified by distinguishing criteria.

Primary Versus Secondary

Primary intracranial tumors originate from the cells and structures in the brain. Secondary or metastatic intracranial tumors originate from structures outside the brain, such as primary tumors of the lung or breast.

Histologic Origins

During the early stage of embryonic development, there are two types of undifferentiated cells—the neuroblasts and the glioblasts. The neuroblasts become neurons, while the glioblasts form a variety of cells that support, insulate, and metabolically assist the neurons. The glioblasts are collectively referred to as glial cells and are subdivided into astrocytes, oligodendrocytes, and ependymal cells. This is the basis of a broad category of intracranial tumors called gliomas. Gliomas are subdivided into astrocytomas, oligodendrogliomas, oligoastrocytomas (also called mixed gliomas), and ependymomas. Gliomas are graded based on histologic criteria related to the degree of differentiation from the parent cell. Higher-grade tumors are more malignant. Glioblastoma multiforme (GBM) is a rapidly growing, poorly differentiated tumor. GBM is the most aggressive brain tumor and carries the worst prognosis.

A meningioma is a tumor that arises from the meninges. Meningiomas tend to grow slowly and compress rather than invade the brain. Prognosis is excellent if the tumor is in a surgically accessible location. Neuromas (also called schwannomas) are noninvasive, slow-growing tumors that arise from the Schwann cells, which produce myelin. Pituitary adenomas, located in the pituitary gland, can be secretory or nonsecretory. Secretory tumors increase the production of hormones such as prolactin, growth hormone, adrenocorticotropic hormone, thyrotropin, or gonadotropin. Nonsecretory pituitary tumors cause symptoms through mass effect; patients commonly present with visual changes due to the compression of the optic chiasm. Pituitary tumors are treated with pharmacologic agents, surgery, radiation therapy, or a combination of these modalities. The tumors described here are the ones most likely to be encountered in practice; other less common types of brain tumors are beyond the scope of this text.

Anatomic Location

This refers to the actual site of the tumor, such as the frontal lobe, temporal lobe, pons, or cerebellum. Knowing the location of the tumor helps predicting deficits based on the normal functions of that anatomic area. Anatomic location also can refer to the location of the tumor in reference to the tentorium. Supratentorial refers to tumors located above the tentorium (cerebral hemispheres), and infratentorial refers to tumors located below the tentorium (brain stem and cerebellum).

Benign Versus Malignant

The distinction between benign and malignant intracranial tumors is based on histologic examination. Tumors made up of well-differentiated cells are "benign" and the prognosis is generally better than if cells are poorly differentiated (ie, GBM). However, a histologically benign tumor can be surgically inaccessible. This benign tumor continues to grow and ultimately contributes to a decline in neurologic function and even death. Benign tumors may convert to more histologically malignant types as they develop.

Clinical Presentation

Brain tumors occupy space, causing compression of brain structures, infiltration of tissue that controls functions, and displacement of normal tissue. Brain tumors disrupt the blood-brain barrier and cause cerebral edema. CSF flow may be obstructed by the tumor itself or the edema, leading to hydrocephalus. Tumors are often vascular and bleed, causing additional neurologic deficits.

The most common initial signs and symptoms of intracranial tumors are headache, seizures, papilledema, and vomiting. Headache is usually progressive in severity and worse after lying flat, for example upon awakening from sleep. Clinical presentation may also include decreased level of consciousness, pupillary changes, visual abnormalities, and personality changes. Additional signs and symptoms depend upon the area of the brain that is being compressed or infiltrated (Table 20-4).

Diagnostic Tests

CT and MRI are used to differentiate tumors from abscesses and to identify tumor location and characteristics. Functional MRI detects physiologic changes using MRI scanning during physical and cognitive activity and is helpful in mapping language, sensory, and motor function affected by the lesion. Magnetic resonance spectroscopy (MRS) and positive emission tomography (PET) scans evaluate cerebral metabolism and are used to provide information about how aggressive a tumor is (a more aggressive tumor will display higher metabolic activity), and to differentiate necrosis or scarring from tumors. Additional testing includes cerebral angiography, visual field and funduscopic examination, audiometric studies, and endocrine studies. If the lesion is suspected to be metastatic, further diagnostic tests are needed to identify the primary tumor site, if not already known. A biopsy of the lesion determines tumor type and degree of differentiation. Biopsy may be performed via a burr hole using stereotactic guidance or may be done as part of a craniotomy for tumor resection.

TABLE 20-4. CLINICAL PRESENTATION OF BRAIN TUMORS RELATED TO LOCATION

Location	Clinical Presentation
Frontal lobe	Inappropriate behavior Inattentiveness Inability to concentrate Emotional lability Quiet but flat affect Expressive aphasia Seizures Headache Impaired memory
Parietal lobe	Hyperesthesia Paresthesia Astereognosis (inability to recognize an object by feeling it) Autotopagnosia (inability to locate or recognize parts of the body) Loss of left-right discrimination Agraphia (inability to write) Acalculia (difficulty in calculating numbers)
Temporal lobe	Psychomotor seizures Receptive aphasia
Occipital lobe	Visual loss in half of the visual field seizures
Pituitary and hypothalamus region	Visual deficits Headache Hormonal dysfunction of the pituitary gland Water imbalance and sleep alterations in tumors of the hypothalamus
Ventricles	Symptoms of increased ICP associated with obstruction of CSF flow
Cerebellum	Ataxia Incoordination Symptoms of increased ICP associated with obstruction of CSF flow

Principles of Management of Intracranial Tumors

Treatment modalities are used alone or in any combination. Variables considered in selecting appropriate treatment include the type of tumor, its location and size, related symptoms, and the general condition of the patient.

Corticosteroids

A corticosteroid, typically dexamethasone, is administered to decrease vasogenic cerebral edema. Steroids are started in patients with brain tumors when the presence of cerebral edema is noted. Significant improvements in neurologic status can be seen soon after initiation of therapy. Side effects of steroid therapy include gastric irritation, mood swings, fluid retention, hyperglycemia, myopathy, insomnia, and increased risk of infection.

Surgery

The goal of surgery is to resect as much of the tumor as possible with minimal harm to normal tissue. In most cases, a craniotomy is done to provide access for resection. Total resection is curative for some tumor types. Some tumors cannot be completely removed because of location or histologic type. A partial resection of the tumor mass temporarily relieves the symptoms of compression, and increased ICP

may be relieved. If CSF flow is obstructed, treatment includes surgical placement of a shunt to reroute CSF from the ventricular system to another part of the body (usually the peritoneal space) where it can be reabsorbed.

Several strategies are available to decrease the morbidity associated with surgery. Intraoperative MRI is available at some centers and is most often used when the lesion is in or near the motor strip, difficult to access, or small and potentially hard to locate. Intraoperative MRI can be used alone or in conjunction with cortical mapping techniques. With cortical mapping, the patient is anesthetized for the initial part of the surgery, then awakened and asked to perform certain tasks, allowing the surgeon to avoid areas of the brain that control speech or motor function. Stereotactic techniques allow targeted biopsy or resection based on previously obtained images.

Most patients undergo elective operations for intracranial tumors and may be admitted to the PCU postoperatively. Postoperative management includes monitoring neurologic status, controlling pain, and preventing and managing complications. Potential complications in the immediate postoperative period include:

- *Hematoma formation:* Clinical signs include increasing headache, decreasing level of consciousness, and the development of new focal neurologic signs. If an intracranial bleed is suspected, a brain CT scan is obtained immediately. If significant bleeding is found, the patient is returned to the operating room for surgical removal of the hematoma and management of bleeding points.
- *Cerebral edema:* Postoperative cerebral edema may occur due to the long surgical procedure and/or the retraction of brain tissue to expose the operative area. Cerebral edema is suspected if the patient presents postoperatively with greater neurologic deficits than were present preoperatively. A CT scan is obtained and treatment is initiated with mannitol or hypertonic saline to decrease edema. As noted previously, dexamethasone is useful in the management of tumor-related edema.
- *Infection:* Infection can occur following surgery because of contamination in the operating room or a defect in the dura, which allows communication of the cerebral spinal fluid with the atmosphere.
- *Venous thromboembolism:* Neurosurgical patients are at increased risk for VTE. Preventive measures to decrease this risk include the use of intermittent pneumatic compression devices, early progression of activity, and low doses of subcutaneous unfractionated heparin.
- *Diabetes insipidus:* DI is caused by a disturbance in the posterior lobe of the pituitary gland, which secretes antidiuretic hormone (ADH). If ADH is not secreted in sufficient amounts, the patient will produce large volumes of dilute urine with a low specific

gravity. Significant fluid and electrolyte imbalances with dehydration can result. Management includes IV therapy that correlates with urine output (or allowing the patient to drink fluids as needed to quench thirst and administration of aqueous vasopressin or desmopressin acetate (DDAVP). The patient's hydration status, electrolytes (especially sodium), and serum osmolarity are monitored closely. DI is common following surgery for pituitary tumors.

Radiation Therapy

Radiation therapy preferentially destroys tumor cells because they are rapidly dividing, but affects normal cells also. The treatment dose depends on the histologic type, radioresponsiveness, location of the tumor, and patient tolerance. Increased edema is a common complication of radiation therapy. Patients typically remain on dexamethasone throughout treatment. Special techniques, such as stereotactic radiosurgery or gamma knife radiation, focus concentrated radiation from many directions on the tumor site and reduce radiation to normal tissue.

Chemotherapy

Chemotherapy is used to slow or stop the proliferation of abnormal cells. One commonly used agent in the treatment of high-grade gliomas is temozolomide (Temodar). Temozolomide is administered orally and is generally well-tolerated by patients.

Prevention and Management of Seizures

The incidence of seizures in patients with brain tumors ranges from 20% to 50% in high-grade gliomas. Antiepileptic drugs are often given prophylactically to patients with supratentorial tumors. When seizures do occur, they are managed according to the guidelines described in Chapter 12, Neurological System. Any seizure in the immediate postoperative period prompts an emergent CT scan to look for hematoma formation.

Special Considerations: Transsphenoidal Resection of Pituitary Tumors

The surgical management of patients with pituitary tumors differs because a transsphenoidal approach may be used (Figure 20-8). Transsphenoidal resection uses a special technique to reach pituitary tumors by going through the sphenoid sinus. An incision may be made under the patient's upper lip or an endonasal approach may be used. Because the pituitary gland secretes a number of hormones, endocrine disturbances are common both before and after surgery. Care in the postoperative period is similar to that described for patients undergoing a craniotomy, but certain assessments are emphasized. Because the pituitary gland is located near the optic chiasm, visual acuity and visual field testing is essential. The patient is closely monitored for CSF leak and is instructed not to blow his or her nose or lean over (these

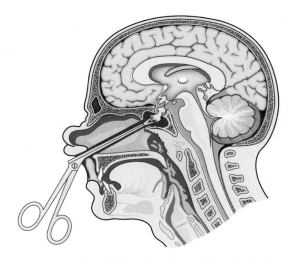

Figure 20-8. Transsphenoidal hypophysectomy. (*Reproduced with permission from Urden LD, Stacy KM, Lough ME: Thelan's Critical Care Nursing, 4th ed. St Louis, MO: Mosby; 2002.*)

actions increase the likelihood of nasal CSF leaks). Nasal packing, if present, is typically removed by the physician on the first or second postoperative day. Serum cortisol is monitored because the patient will no longer secrete adrenocorticotropic hormone if the anterior pituitary was resected. Close monitoring of fluid balance and electrolytes is required because of the risk of DI. DI is caused by insufficient amounts of ADH, which is produced by the posterior lobe of the pituitary gland. If ADH is not secreted in sufficient amounts, the patient will produce large volumes of dilute urine. Significant fluid and electrolyte imbalances with dehydration can result. Intake and output are measured frequently (initially every hour in the ICU). Electrolytes (especially sodium) and urine specific gravity are monitored frequently, typically every 4 to 6 hours. Serum and urine osmolality may also be monitored. Management of DI includes allowing the patient to drink fluids as needed to quench thirst. Management may also include matching the output with intravenous fluid therapy and the administration of aqueous vasopressin or desmopressin acetate (DDAVP).

SPECIAL PROCEDURES: INVASIVE MONITORING OF INTRACRANIAL PRESSURE

Intracranial pressure is most often measured via a catheter inserted into the ventricles or a probe inserted into the brain parenchyma (Figure 20-9). Several systems exist, but the basic setup for EVD ICP monitoring includes a catheter, transducer (either external or integrated into the catheter), and collection device for CSF. The catheter is placed via a burr hole into the anterior horn of the lateral ventricle. The zero point of the drainage system is leveled at the external landmark of the foramen of Monro and the setup is zeroed to atmospheric pressure using manufacturer's specifications. Different external landmarks for the foramen

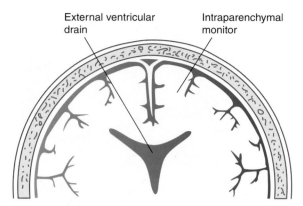

Figure 20-9. Primary sites for ICP monitoring: external ventricular drain placement and intraparenchymal bolt placement.

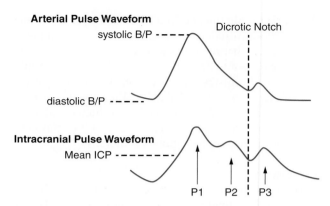

Figure 20-10. Components of a normal ICP waveform.

of Monro are reported in the literature (tragus, halfway between the outer canthus of the eye and the tragus, external auditory meatus); follow institutional protocols to maintain consistency among caregivers. The transducer senses the pressure exerted by the CSF in the ventricles and translates it into a waveform on the monitor. The advantage of using an intraventricular catheter for monitoring is that CSF can be drained, providing a treatment modality for increased ICP. CSF drainage is controlled by adjusting the height of the system relative to the foramen of Monro. If the drainage system is raised, CSF drainage decreases; when the drainage system is lowered, CSF drainage increases. Continuous CSF drainage is associated with higher risk of complications. Rapid drainage of CSF can result in ventricular collapse, which is why CSF is drained in a controlled manner based on a predetermined ICP. This is accomplished by opening the system to allow CSF drainage only when the ICP exceeds a specified value. CSF drainage is monitored for amount (trended hourly), color, and clarity. An occlusive dressing is maintained over the catheter site. Risks associated with intraventricular catheter placement include infection and hemorrhage caused by catheter placement. Sterile technique is essential when the catheter is placed and whenever the system is manipulated (ie, when sampling for CSF or changing drainage bags).

Intracranial pressure is also commonly monitored using a transducer inserted into the brain parenchyma. These monitors are easier to insert and have a lower rate of infection than intraventricular catheters. Leveling to the foramen of Monro is not required. Fiberoptic and strain gauge transducers are connected directly to an independent monitor, which provides an ICP reading. Other technology is available to monitor ICP, including some devices that allow re-zeroing after monitor insertion, but these are less commonly used in practice. Normal ICP is 0 to 15 mm Hg in adults.

Intracranial Pressure Waveforms

With continuous ICP monitoring, there are fluctuations in waveforms that correlate with specific physiologic events.

Examination of these waveforms can be helpful in evaluating changes in the patient's condition.

The ICP pulse waveform is a continuous, real-time pressure display that corresponds to each heartbeat. The normal pulse wave has three or more defined peaks representing blood and CSF flow within the cranium: P1 (percussion wave), P2 (tidal wave), and P3 (dicrotic wave).

The pulse waveform at low pressures is a descending saw-toothed pattern with a distinct P1 (Figure 20-10). As mean ICP rises, a progressive elevation of P2 occurs, causing the pulse waveform to appear more rounded. When P2 is equal to or higher than P1, decreased compliance exists (Figure 20-11).

Trend recordings compress continuous ICP recording data to reflect general trends in ICP over longer time periods (minutes to hours). Three distinct pressure waves have been identified (see Figure 20-10). A waves (plateau waves) are sudden increases in pressure lasting 5 to 20 minutes. They begin from a baseline of an already elevated ICP (> 20 mm Hg) and reflect cerebral ischemia. B waves are sharp, rhythmic oscillations of pressure (up to 50 mm Hg) occurring every 0.5 to 2 minutes. They are not clinically significant, but may progress to A waves. C waves are small rhythmic waves with pressures up to 20 mm Hg occurring 4 to 8 times per minute. They relate to normal changes in systemic arterial pressure, and their clinical significance is unknown.

CPP is a measurement of the pressure at which blood reaches the brain. CPP is an indirect reflection of CBF. It is calculated by subtracting ICP from mean arterial pressure (CPP = MAP − ICP). Decreased CPP occurs as the result of an increase in ICP, a decrease in mean arterial pressure, or both. A CPP of at least 50 to 60 mm Hg is necessary for adequate cerebral perfusion. CPP below 30 mm Hg results in irreversible neuronal hypoxia.

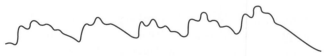

Figure 20-11. ICP waveform demonstrating decreased compliance.

SPECIAL PROCEDURES: MANAGEMENT OF A PATIENT WITH A LUMBAR DRAIN

Lumbar drains are used in the PCU to manage communicating hydrocephalus, and in patients with CSF leakage following neurosurgery or trauma to decrease pressure against the dura and allow it to heal (Figure 20-12). Lumbar drains are also used to improve spinal cord perfusion in the immediate postoperative period following thoracoabdominal aneurysm repair. The process for placing a lumbar drain is similar to performing a LP (see Chapter 12, Neurological System). The physician threads the catheter into the subarachnoid space of the lumbar spine. Nursing responsibilities during placement include assistance with patient positioning and the administration of pain medications and sometimes sedation. Once the lumbar catheter has been placed, it is connected to an external drainage system. The amount of CSF drainage is determined by the height of the system, which corresponds to the amount of pressure within the spinal subarachnoid space. The lumbar drain may be left open so that CSF flows into the collection chamber whenever the pressure in the spinal subarachnoid space exceeds the pressure created by the height of the column of fluid in the drainage system or a certain amount of CSF may be drained every hour. Alternatively, an external transducer can be connected to the system to measure pressure within the spinal subarachnoid space, with orders to allow drainage only when the pressure exceeds a predetermined limit. Based on the reason for CSF drainage and individual provider preference, the system may be kept open to drain continuously or allowed to drain only when the pressure exceeds a certain value.

The zero reference for leveling the drip chamber and transducer vary based on reason for drainage, provider preference, and institutional protocol. Common sites for leveling include the shoulder, the external auditory meatus, and the level of insertion. Nursing priorities when caring for a patient with a lumbar drain include maintaining the system at the ordered height (eg, 10 cm H_2O above the external auditory meatus). If the system is placed below the ordered height, overdrainage of CSF may result and can lead to the development of subdural hemorrhage or even herniation. If the lumbar drainage system is placed too high, CSF drainage may be inadequate for the desired purpose. Other potential complications include infection, bleeding, and sensory deficits related to nerve root injury or irritation. An occlusive sterile dressing is maintained at the insertion site. Practices related to mobilizing the patient with a lumbar drain vary; follow institutional standards and provider order.

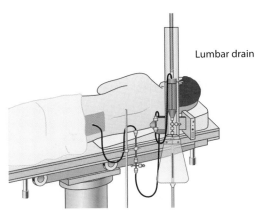

Figure 20-12. Lumbar drain.

SELECTED BIBLIOGRAPHY

Subarachnoid Hemorrhage

Censullo JL, Harris C, Keigher KM, Livesay SL. Hemorrhagic stroke. In: Bader MK, Littlejohns LR, Olson DM, eds. *AANN Core Curriculum for Neuroscience Nursing*. 6th ed. Glenview, IL: American Association of Neuroscience Nurses; 2016: 247-266.

Glisic EK, Gardiner L, Josti L, et al. Inadequacy of headache management after subarachnoid hemorrhage. *Am J Crit Care*. 2016;25(2):136-143. doi:10.4037/ajcc2016486.

Lantigua H, Ortega-Gutierrez S, Schmidt JM, et al. Subarachnoid hemorrhage: who dies, and why? *Crit Care*. 2015;19:309. doi:10.1186/s13054-015-1036-0.

Olson DM, Zomorodi M, Britz GW, Zomorodi AR, Amato A, Graffagnino C. Continuous cerebral spinal fluid drainage associated with complications in patients admitted with subarachnoid hemorrhage. *J Neurosurg*. 2013;119(4):974-980. doi:10.3171/2013.6.JNS12240.3.

Rockett H, Thompson HJ, Blissitt PA. Fever management practices of neuroscience nurses: what has changed? *J Neurosci Nurs*. 2015;47(2):66-75. doi:10.1097/jcn.0000000000000118.

Safavi-Abbasi S, Wilson CD, Ghafil C, Spetzler RF. Meta-analysis comparing continuous and intermittent cerebrospinal fluid drainage in aneurysmal subarachnoid hemorrhage. *J Neurol Surg B*. 2016;77:A083. doi:10.1055/s-0036-1579871.

Yousef KM, Balzer JR, Bender CM, et al. Cerebral perfusion pressure and delayed cerebral ischemia after aneurysmal subarachnoid hemorrhage. *Am J Crit Care*. 2015;24(4):e65-71. doi:10.4037/ajcc2015913.

Traumatic Brain Injury

Bader MK, Stutzman SE, Palmer S, et al. The Adam Williams initiative: collaborating with community resources to improve care for traumatic brain injury. *Crit Care Nurse*. 2014;34(6):39-47. doi:10.4037/ccn2014112.

Bengualid V, Talari G, Rubin D, Albaeni A, Ciubotaru RL, Berger J. Fever in trauma patients: evaluation of risk factors, including traumatic brain injury. *Am J Crit Care*. 2015;24(2):e1-5. doi:10.4037/ajcc2015856.

Mahdavi Z, Pierre-Louis N, Ho TT, Figueroa SA, Olson DM. Advances in cerebral monitoring for the patient with traumatic brain injury. *Crit Care Nurs Clin North Am*. 2015;27(2):213-223. doi:10.1016/j.cnc.2015.02.002.

McNett M, Amato S, Gianakis A, et al. The FOUR score and GCS as predictors of outcome after traumatic brain injury. *Neurocrit Care*. 2014;21(1):52-57. doi:10.1007/s12028-013-9947-6.

Menon DK, Ercole A. Critical care management of traumatic brain injury. *Handb Clin Neurol*. 2017;140:239-274. doi:10.1016/b978-0-444-63600-3.00014-3.

Wijayatilake DS, Talati C, Panchatsharam S. The monitoring and management of severe traumatic brain injury in the United Kingdom: is there a consensus? A national survey. *J Neurosurg Anesthesiol*. 2015;27(3):241-245. doi:10.1097/ana.0000000000000143.

Spinal Cord Injury

Catapano JS, Hawryluk GW, Whetstone W, et al. Higher mean arterial pressure values correlate with neurologic improvement in patients with initially complete spinal cord injuries. *World Neurosurg*. 2016;96:72-79. doi:10.1016/j.wneu.2016.08.053.

Hawryluk G, Whetstone W, Saigal R, et al. Mean arterial blood pressure correlates with neurological recovery after human spinal cord injury: analysis of high frequency physiologic data. *J Neurotrauma*. 2015;32:1958-1967.

Mahanes D, McNett M, Miller Niklash D, Thompson R. Traumatic spine injuries. In: Bader MK, Littlejohns LR, Olson DM, eds. *AANN Core Curriculum for Neuroscience Nursing*. 6th ed. Glenview, IL: American Association of Neuroscience Nurses; 2016: 359-412.

Reintam Blaser A, Starkopf J, Alhazzani W, et al. Early enteral nutrition in critically ill patients: ESICM clinical practice guidelines. *Intensive Care Med*. 2017;43(3):380-398. doi:10.1007/s00134-016-4665-0.

Shank CD, Walters BC, Hadley MN. Management of acute traumatic spinal cord injuries. *Handb Clin Neurol*. 2017;140:275-298. doi:10.1016/b978-0-444-63600-3.00015-5.

Waring WP, Biering-Sorensen F, Burns S, et al. 2009 review and revisions of the international standards for the neurological classification of spinal cord injury. *J Spinal Cord Med*. 2010;33(4):346-352.

Brain Tumors

Batich KA, Reap EA, Archer GE, et al. Long-term survival in glioblastoma with cytomegalovirus pp65-targeted vaccination. *Clin Cancer Res*. 2017;23(8):1898-1909. doi:10.1158/1078-0432.ccr-16-2057.

Lally-Goss D, Strayer A, Sullivan C. Nervous system tumors. In: Bader MK, Littlejohns LR, Olson DM, eds. *AANN Core Curriculum for Neuroscience Nursing*. 6th ed. Glenview, IL: American Association of Neuroscience Nurses; 2016: 431-449.

Ryu JA, Bang OY, Suh GY, et al. Ischemic stroke in critically ill patients with malignancy. *PLoS One*. 2016;11(1):e0146836. doi:10.1371/journal.pone.0146836.

Schiff D, Lee EQ, Nayak L, Norden AD, Reardon DA, Wen PY. Medical management of brain tumors and the sequelae of treatment. *Neuro Oncol*. 2015;17(4):488-504. doi:10.1093/neuonc/nou304.

Intracranial Pressure Monitoring

Lewis LS, Kennedy Madden L, Puccio AM. Intracranial pressure management. In: Bader MK, Littlejohns LR, Olson DM, eds. *AANN Core Curriculum for Neuroscience Nursing*. 6th ed. Glenview, IL: American Association of Neuroscience Nurses; 2016: 185-203.

Mahdavi ZK, Olson DM, Figueroa SA. Association patterns of simultaneous intraventricular and intraparenchymal intracranial pressure measurements. *Neurosurgery*. 2016;79(4):561-567.

Olson DM, Parcon C, Santos A, Santos G, Delabar R, Stutzman SE. A novel approach to explore how nursing care affects intracranial pressure. *Am J Crit Care*, 2017;26(2):136-139. doi:10.4037/ajcc2017410.

Roh D, Park S. Brain multimodality monitoring: updated perspectives. *Curr Neurol Neurosci Rep*. 2016;16(6):56. doi:10.1007/s11910-016-0659-0.

Tackla R, Hinzman JM, Foreman B, Magner M, Andaluz N, Hartings JA. Assessment of cerebrovascular autoregulation using regional cerebral blood flow in surgically managed brain trauma patients. *Neurocrit Care*. 2015;23(3):339-346. doi:10.1007/s12028-015-0146-5.

Evidence-Based Guidelines

Al-Mufti F, Mayer SA. Neurocritical care of acute subdural hemorrhage. *Neurosurg Clin N Am*. 2017;28(2):267-278. doi:10.1016/j.nec.2016.11.009.

Bushnell C, McCullough LD, Awad IA, et al. Guidelines for the prevention of stroke in women: a statement for healthcare professionals from the American Heart Association/American Stroke Association. *Stroke*. 2014;45(5):1545-1588. doi:10.1161/01.str.0000442009.06663.48.

Carney N, Totten AM, O'Reilly C, et al. Guidelines for the management of severe traumatic brain injury, Fourth Edition. *Neurosurgery*. 2016. doi:10.1227/neu.0000000000001432.

Connolly ES, Rabinstein AA, Carhuapoma JR, et al. Guidelines for the management of aneurysmal subarachnoid hemorrhage: a guideline for healthcare professionals from the American Heart Association/American Stroke Association. *Stroke*. 2012;43(6):1711-1737. doi:10.1161/STR.0b013e3182587839.

Fried HI, Nathan BR, Rowe AS, et al. The insertion and management of external ventricular drains: an evidence-based consensus statement: a statement for healthcare professionals from the neurocritical care society. *Neurocrit Care*. 2016;24(1):61-81. doi:10.1007/s12028-015-0224-8.

Helbok R, Olson DM, Le Roux PD, Vespa P. Intracranial pressure and cerebral perfusion pressure monitoring in non-TBI patients: special considerations. *Neurocrit Care*. 2014;21(suppl 2):s85-s94. doi:10.1007/s12028-014-0040-6.

Kernan WN, Ovbiagele B, Black HR, et al. Guidelines for the prevention of stroke in patients with stroke and transient ischemic attack: a guideline for healthcare professionals from the American Heart Association/American Stroke Association. *Stroke*. 2014;45(7):2160-2236. doi:10.1161/str.0000000000000024.

Sandsmark DK, MacKenzie L, Kofke WA. How should traumatic brain injury be managed. In: Deutschman CS, Neligan PJ, eds. *Evidence-Based Practice of Critical Care*. 2nd ed. 2016: 441-449.

KEY REFERENCE INFORMATION

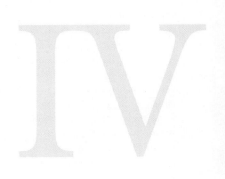

NORMAL LABORATORY REFERENCE VALUES

21

Suzanne M. Burns and Sarah A. Delgado

Category	Abbreviation	Definition	Normal Value	Formula
Acid Base				
	pH		7.35-7.45	
	$PaCO_2$	Partial pressure of arterial carbon dioxide	35-45 mm Hg	
	PaO_2	Partial pressure of arterial oxygen	75-100 mm Hg	
	Bicarbonate		18-22 mmol/L	
	Base deficit/ base excess		(−3)−(+3)	
	Lactate		0.5-1 mmol/L	
Cardiac and Hemodynamic				
	BSA	Body surface area	Meters squared (m^2)	Value obtained from a nomogram based on height and weight
	CI	Cardiac index	2.5-4.3 L/min/m^2	$CI\left(L/min/m^2\right) = \dfrac{\text{cardiac output (L/min)}}{\text{body surface area } (m^2)}$
	CK	Creatinine kinase	< 120 mcg/L	
	CK-MB	Creatinine kinase MB band	< 3 ng/mL	
	CO	Cardiac output	4-8 L/min	CO = stroke volume × heart rate
	CVP	Central venous pressure	2-8 mm Hg	
	EF	Ejection fraction	Greater than 60%	$\text{Ejection fraction} = \dfrac{SV}{EDV}$
	HR	Heart rate	60-100 beats/min	
	LVSW	Left ventricular stroke work	8-10 g/m/m^2	LVSW = SI × MAP × 0.0144
	MAP	Mean arterial pressure	> 70 mm Hg	$\text{MAP estimate} = \dfrac{(\text{Systolic} + 2\,\text{Diastolic})}{3}$
	PAD	Pulmonary artery diastolic	8-15 mm Hg	
	PAS	Pulmonary artery systolic pressure	16-24 mm Hg	
	PAOP	Pulmonary artery occlusion pressure	8-12 mm Hg	PAOP obtained via swan-ganz catheter.
	PVR	Pulmonary vascular resistance	100-250 dynes/s/cm^{-5}	$PVR = (dynes/s/cm^5) = \dfrac{PAM\,(mm\,Hg) - PAOP\,(mm\,Hg) \times 80}{\text{cardiac output (L/min)}}$
	RVEDV	Right ventricular end-diastolic volume	100-160 mL	SV/EF
	RVSW	Right ventricular stroke work	51-61 g/m/m^2	RVSW = SI × MAP × 0.0144
	SV	Stroke volume	60-100 mL/beat	CO/HR × 1000

(continued)

Category	Abbreviation	Definition	Normal Value	Formula
	SVI	Stroke volume index	33-47 mL/m²/beat	$SI\ (mL/min/m^2) = \dfrac{stroke\ volume}{body\ surface\ area}$
	SVR	Systemic vascular resistance	800-1200 dynes-s/cm^{-5}	$SVR = 80 \times (MAP-RAP)/CO$
	SVRI	Systemic vascular resistance index	1970-2390 dynes-sec/cm^{-5}/m²	$80 \times (MAP - RAP)/CI$
	Myoglobin	Female	10-65 ng/mL	
	Myoglobin	Male	10-95 ng/mL	
	Troponin I	Troponin I	< 0.4 ng/mL	
	Troponin T	Troponin T	< 0.1 ng/mL	
Functional Hemodynamics				
	SPV	Systolic pressure variation	> 10 mm Hg	$SBP_{max} - SBP_{min}$
		SPV%	> 10%	$[(SBP_{max} - SBP_{min})/(SBP_{max}+SBP_{min}/2)] \times 100$
	PPV	Pulse pressure variation	> 12.5%	$[(PP_{max} - PP_{min})/PP_{max}+PP_{min}/2)] \times 100$
	SVV	Stroke volume variation	> 12%	$[(SV_{max} - SV_{min})/SV_{max}+SV_{min}/2)] \times 100$
Endocrine				
	ACTH	Adrenocorticotropic hormone	10-50 pg/mL Levels are usually less than 20 pg/mL in afternoon Less than 5-10 pg/mL at midnight	
	ADH	Antidiuretic hormone	1-5 pg/mL	
	Cortisol	Cortisol	10-20 ug/dL in the early morning 3-10 ug/dL afternoon < 5 ug/dL after usual bedtime Great deal of variation	
	T3	Serum triiodothyronine	80-180 ng/dL	
	T4	Serum thyroxine	4.6-12 ug/dL	
	TSH	Serum thyrotropin (thyroid-stimulating hormone)	0.5-6 mIU/L	
Hematology				
	RBC	Red blood count	Males: 4.2-5.4 million/μL Females: 3.6-5.0 million/μL	
	Retic count	Reticulocyte count	0.5%-1.5%	
	WBC	White blood cell count	4500-10500/μL	
	WBC differential (% of total)	As below		
		Neutrophils *Segmented Bands*	50%-70% 56% 0%-3%	
		Eosinophils	0%-3%	
		Basophils	0.5%-1.0%	
		Monocytes	3%-7%	
		Lymphocytes	25%-40%	
		Platelet count	150,000-400,000/μL	
		Bleeding time	3-10 minutes	
	INR	International Normalized Ratio *Therapeutic anticoagulation*	0.8-1.1 2.0-3.0	
	aPTT	Activated partial thromboplastin time *Therapeutic anticoagulation*	30-40 sec 1.5-2.5 times the mean normal value	
	ACT	Activated clotting time Therapeutic anticoagulation	70-120 sec 150-210 sec	
	Fibrinogen	Fibrinogen	200-400 mg/dL	
	D-dimer	D-dimer	< 1.37 nmol/L	

(continued)

Category	Abbreviation	Definition	Normal Value	Formula
Immunology				
	IgA	Immunoglobulin A	60-400 mg/dL	
	IgG	Immunoglobulin G	700-1500 mg/dL	
	IgM	Immunoglobulin M	60-300 mg/dL	
	IgE	Immunoglobulin E	3-423 IU/mL	
Liver Function				
	Albumin		35-50 g/L	
	Total protein		6-8.3 g/dL	
	Bilirubin	Total	2-20 μmol/L	
		Direct	0-6 μmol/L	
	ALP	Alkaline phosphatase	50-100 U/L	
	AST	Aspartate aminotransferase	5-30 U/L	
	ALT	Alanine aminotransferase	5-30 U/L	
Pulmonary				
	A-a gradient	Alveolar-arterial oxygen gradient	When on 100% Fio_2 A-a gradient ~75 mm Hg, on 21% Fio_2 A-a gradient ~10-15 mm Hg	A-a = gradient. See formula for calculation of Alveolar O_2. Arterial (pao_2) obtained via arterial blood gas.
	$C(a-v)O_2$	Arteriovenous oxygen content difference	4-6 mL/100 mL	$C(a-v)O_2$ (mL/100 mL or vol%) = $Cao_2 - Cvo_2$ (calculation for Cao_2 and Cvo_2 are below)
	Cao_2	Arterial oxygen content	~20 vol%	Cao_2 (mL O_2/100 mL blood or vol%) = (Hb × 1.39) Sao_2 + (Pao_2 × 0.0031)
	Cvo_2	Mixed venous oxygen content	~15 vol%	Cvo_2 (ml O_2/100 mL blood or vol%) = (Hb × 1.39) Svo_2 + (Pvo_2 × 0.0031)
	Cdyn	Dynamic compliance	~30-40 mL/cm H_2O	Cdyn = Vt/PIP−PEEP
	Cstat	Static compliance	~50 mL/cm H_2O	Cstat = VT/Plat−PEEP
	FRC	Functional residual capacity	2400 mL (dependent on height)	Measured in a pulmonary function laboratory
	NIP	Negative inspiratory pressure (also called NIF or negative inspiratory force)	−75 to 100 cm H_2O (the more negative the number, the stronger the force of the inspiration)	Measured at bedside or in a pulmonary function laboratory
	O_2 extraction ratio	Oxygen extraction ratio	0.25	$O_2 \text{ extraction ratio} = \dfrac{C(a-v)O_2}{CaO_2}$
	Pao_2	Mean partial pressure of oxygen in alveolus	104 mm Hg	$Pao_2 = Fio_2$ (Pbar−PH_2O)−$Paco_2$/RQ
	$Paco_2$	Partial pressure of carbon dioxide in arterial blood	35-45 mm Hg	$Paco_2$ obtained via arterial blood gas.
	Pao_2	Partial pressure of oxygen in arterial blood	Will vary with patient's age and the Fio_2. Pao_2 on room air: 80-100 mm Hg, on 100% Pao_2: ≥ 500 mm Hg	Pao_2 obtained via arterial blood gas.
	$Pvco_2$	Partial pressure of carbon dioxide in mixed venous blood	38-55 mm Hg	$Pvco_2$ obtained from the distal port of the PA catheter
	Pvo_2	Partial pressure of oxygen in mixed venous blood	35-45 mm Hg -will vary with the Fio_2, cardiac output, and oxygen consumption	Pvo_2 obtained from the distal port of the PA catheter
	QS/QT	Right-to-left shunt (percentage of cardiac output flowing past nonventilated alveoli or the equivalent)	5%-8%	$Qs/QT(\%) = \dfrac{0.0031 \times P(A-a)O_2}{C(a-v)O_2 + (0.0031 \times P[A-a]O_2)} \times 100$
	RQ	Respiratory quotient	0.8	$RQ = \dfrac{Vco_2}{VO_2}$
	Sao_2	Percentage of oxyhemoglobin saturation of arterial blood	96%-100% (on room air)	
	VO_2	Oxygen consumption	~250 mL/min	
	Svo_2	Percentage of oxyhemoglobin saturation of mixed venous blood	60%-80% (on room air)	

(continued)

Category	Abbreviation	Definition	Normal Value	Formula
	VO_2	Oxygen consumption	~ 250 mL/min	
	VC	Vital capacity	65-75 mL/kg	
	VCO_2	Carbon dioxide production	~ 200 mL/min	
	VC	Vital capacity	65-75 mL/kg	
	V_D/V_T	Dead space to tidal volume ratio	0.25-0.40	$VD/VT = \dfrac{Paco_2 - PEco_2}{Paco_2}$
	V_T	Tidal volume	6-8 mL/kg	
Renal	ACR	Albumin to creatinine ratio	More than 30 mg per gram	
	BUN	Blood urea nitrogen	7-20 mg/dL	
	Creatinine (serum)		Women: 0.6-1.1 mg/dL Men: 0.7-1.3 mg/dL	
	CrCl	Creatinine clearance	88-128 mL/min for women and 97-137 mL/min for men	
	FENa	Fractional excretion of sodium	< 1% in prerenal injury > 1% in intrarenal injury	FENa = [Na (urine) × creatinine (serum)] / [(Na (serum) × creatinine (urine)] × 100
	FEUrea	Fractional excretion of urea	< 35% indicates prerenal injury > 35% indicates intrarenal injury	[Cr (serum) × Urea (urine)] / Urea (serum) × Cr (urine)] × 100
	GFR	Glomerular filtration rate	> 90 mL/min/1.73 m^2	
	Microalbumin (urine)		> 30 mg	Microalbumin (urine)
	Sosm	Osmolality (serum)	285-295 mOsm/kg	Sosm = (2 × serum Na, in mmol/L) + [glucose, in mg/dL]/18 + [blood urea nitrogen, in mg/dL]/2.8

PHARMACOLOGY TABLES

Earnest Alexander

TABLE 22-1. INTRAVENOUS MEDICATION ADMINISTRATION GUIDELINES

Drug	Usual IV Dose Range[a]	Standard Dilution	Infusion Times/Comments/Drug Interactions
Abciximab			
Bolus dose	0.25 mg/kg	In 250 mL	Bolus infused over 1-65 minutes
Infusion dose	0.125 mcg/kg/min for 12 hours		Maximum infusion rate = 10 mcg/min
Acetaminophen	1 g q6h		Maximum dose of 4 g in 24 hours
Acetazolamide	5-10 mg/kg/24 h or 250 mg qd-qid	Undiluted	Infuse over 1-3 minutes with maximum infusion rate of 500 mg/min
Acyclovir	5-15 mg/kg q8h	In 100 mL	Infuse over at least 60 minutes
Adenosine	6 mg initially, then 12 mg × 2 doses PRN	Undiluted	Inject over 1-2 seconds
			Drug interactions: theophylline (1); persantine (2); caffeine; carbamazepine
Alteplase			
Acute MI	100 mg over 3 hours	100 mg in 200 mL	In acute MI, infuse 10 mg over 2 minutes, then 50 mg over 1 hour, and then 40 mg over 2 hours.
PE	100 mg over 2 hours		
Ischemic stroke	0.9 mg/kg (not to exceed 90 mg)		10% of total dose as IV bolus over 1 minute, then remaining 90% as IV infusion over 60 minutes
Amikacin			
Standard dose	5-7.5 mg/kg q12h	In 50 mL	Infuse over 30 minutes
Single daily dose	15-20 mg/kg q24h	In 50 mL	Drug interactions: neuromuscular blocking agents (3)

			Therapeutic levels:
			  Peak: 20-40 mg/L; trough: < 8 mg/L
			  Single daily dose: trough level at 24 hours = 0 mg/L; peak levels unnecessary

Amiodarone	150-300 mg, which may be followed by 150 mg IV × 1 PRN		Infuse continuously at 1 mg/min for 6 hours then reduce to 0.5 mg/min for 18 hours
Ammonium chloride	mEq Cl = Cl deficit (in mEq/L) × 0.2 × wt (kg)	100 mEq in 500 mL	Maximum infusion rate is 5 mL/min of a 0.2-mEq/mL solution; correct 1/3 to 1/2 of Cl deficit while monitoring pH and Cl; administer remainder as needed
Amphotericin B colloidal dispersion (ABCD)	3-5 mg/kg q24h	In 500 mL; final concentration range 0.16-0.83 mg/mL	Infuse at 1 mg/kg/h
Amphotericin B deoxycholate	0.5-1.5 mg/kg q24h	In 250 mL	Infuse over 2-6 hours
			Do not mix in electrolyte solutions (eg, saline, lactated Ringer solution)

(continued)

TABLE 22-1. INTRAVENOUS MEDICATION ADMINISTRATION GUIDELINES (continued)

Drug	Usual IV Dose Range[a]	Standard Dilution	Infusion Times/Comments/Drug Interactions
Amphotericin B lipid complex (ABLC)	3-5 mg/kg q24h	In 250 mL	Infuse over 2 hours; maximum rate of 2.5 mg/kg/h
Amphotericin B liposomal	3-7 mg/kg q24h	In 250 mL	Infuse over 1-2 hours
Ampicillin	0.5-3 g q4-6h	In 100 mL	Infuse over 15-30 minutes
Ampicillin/sulbactam	1.5-3 g q6h	In 100 mL	Infuse over 15-30 minutes
Argatroban			
Percutaneous coronary intervention	350 mcg/kg bolus, followed by 25 mcg/kg/min infusion	250 mg in 250 mL	Infuse bolus over 3-5 minutes; titrate to aPTT or ACT
Heparin-induced thrombocytopenia with thrombosis	0.5-1 mcg/kg/min in critically ill	250 mg in 250 mL	Titrate to aPTT; initial dose increased to 2 mcg/kg/min in non-critically ill
Aztreonam	0.5-2 g q6-12h	In 100 mL	Infuse over 15-30 minutes
Bivalirudin			
Percutaneous coronary intervention	1 mg/kg bolus, followed by 2.5 mg/kg/h × 4 hours; if necessary 0.2 mg/kg/h for up to 20 hours	250 mg in 500 mL	Infuse bolus over 2 minutes; titrate to aPTT or ACT
Percutaneous coronary intervention with heparin-induced thrombocytopenia with thrombosis	0.75 mg/kg bolus, followed by 1.75 mg/kg/h × 4 hours; if necessary 0.2 mg/kg/h for up to 20 hours	250 mg in D5W 500 mL	Infuse bolus over 2 minutes; titrate to aPTT or ACT
Bumetanide			
Bolus dose	0.5-1 mg	Undiluted	Maximum injection rate: 1 mg/min
Infusion dose	0.5-2 mg/h	2.4 mg in 100 mL	Continuous infusion
Calcium (elemental)	Ca chloride 1-2 g	In 50-100 mL	Ca chloride 1 g = 272 mg (13.6 mEq) of elemental calcium
	Ca gluconate 1-2g	In 50-100 mL	Ca gluconate 1 g = 90 mg (4.65 mEq) of elemental calcium
Cefazolin	0.5-2 g q6-8h	In 50 mL	Infuse over 15-30 minutes
Cefepime	1-2 g q8-12h	In 100 mL	Infuse over 15 minutes
Cefotaxime	1-2 g q4-6h	In 50 mL	Infuse over 15-30 minutes
Cefotetan	1-2 g q12h	In 50 mL	Infuse over 15-30 minutes
Cefoxitin	1-2 g q4-6h	In 50 mL	Infuse over 15-30 minutes
Ceftazidime	0.5-2 g q8-12h	In 50 mL	Infuse over 15-30 minutes
Ceftriaxone	0.5-2 g q12-24h	In 50 mL	Infuse over 15-30 minutes
Cefuroxime	0.75-1.5 g q8h	In 50 mL	Infuse over 15-30 minutes
Chlorothiazide	0.5-1 g qd-bid	In 18 mL	Inject over 3-5 minutes
Chlorpromazine	10-50 mg q4-6h	Dilute to final concentration of 1 mg/mL	Inject at 1 mg/min
Ciprofloxacin	200-400 mg q8-12h	Premix solution 2 mg/mL	Infuse over 60 minutes
			Drug interactions: theophylline, warfarin (7)
Cisatracurium			
Bolus dose	0.15-0.2 mg/kg	Undiluted	Monitor TOF
Infusion dose	1-3 mcg/kg/min	200 mg in 200 mL	
Clevidipine	1-32 mg/h	Undiluted	Continuous infusion; average infusion rate is 21 mg/h
Clindamycin	150-900 mg q8h	In 50 mL	Infuse over 30-60 minutes
Conivaptan			
Bolus dose	20 mg	In 100 mL	Infuse over 30 minutes
Infusion dose	20 mg	In 250 mL	Infuse over 24 hours
Conjugated Estrogens	0.6 mg/kg/d × 5 days	In 50 mL	Infuse over 15-30 minutes
Cosyntropin	0.25 mg IV	Undiluted	Inject over 60 seconds
Cyclosporine	5-6 mg/kg q24h	In 100 mL	Infuse over 2-6 hours
			Drug interactions: digoxin (8); erythromycin (9); amphotericin, NSAID (10)
			IV dose = 1/3 PO dose
			Therapeutic levels: trough: 50-400 ng/mL (whole blood—HPLC)

TABLE 22-1. INTRAVENOUS MEDICATION ADMINISTRATION GUIDELINES (continued)

Drug	Usual IV Dose Range[a]	Standard Dilution	Infusion Times/Comments/Drug Interactions
Dantrolene			
Bolus dose	1-2 mg/kg	Revonto 20 mg in 60 mL Ryanodex 250 mg in 5 mL	Administer as rapidly as possible
Maximum dose	10 mg/kg/24h		Do not dilute in dextrose or electrolyte-containing solutions
Maintenance dose	2.5 mg/kg q4h × 24h	Revonto 20 mg in 60 mL Ryanodex 250 mg in 5 mL	Infuse Revonto solution over 60 minutes Inject Ryanodex suspension IV push for malignant hyperthermia treatment or over at least 1 minute for prevention
Daptomycin	4-6 mg/kg q24h	250 or 500 mg in 50 mL	Infuse over 30 minutes
Desmopressin	0.3 mcg/kg	In 50 mL	Infuse over 15-30 minutes
Dexamethasone	0.5-20 mg	In 50 mL	May give doses ≤ 10 mg undiluted IVP over 60 seconds
Dexmedetomidine			
Bolus dose	1 mcg/kg	200 mcg in 50 mL or 400 mcg in 100 mL	Infuse bolus over 10 minutes
Infusion dose	0.2-1.5 mcg/kg/h		
Diazepam	2.5-5 mg q2-4h	Undiluted	Inject 2-5 mg/min Active metabolites contribute to activity
Digoxin			
Digitalizing dose	8-12 mcg/kg total loading dose divided into 3 doses	Undiluted	Inject over 3-5 minutes; first dose equaling one-half the total, then remaining half in 2 equally divided doses at 6- to 8-hour intervals. Use ideal body weight for dosing. Reduce dosing in renal insufficiency.
Maintenance dose	0.125-0.25 mg q24h		Drug interactions: amiodarone, cyclosporine, quinidine, verapamil (8) Therapeutic levels: 0.5-2.0 ng/mL
Diltiazem			
Bolus dose	0.25-0.35 mg/kg	Undiluted	Inject over 2 minutes
Infusion dose	5-15 mg/h	125 mg in 125 mL	Continuous infusion (final conc = 1 mg/mL)
Diphenhydramine	25-100 mg IV q 2-4h	Undiluted	Inject over 3-5 minutes Competitive histamine antagonist, doses > 1000 mg/24 h may be required in some instances
Dobutamine	2.5-20 mcg/kg/min	500 mg in 250 mL standard concentration; 1000 mg in 250 mL double concentration	Continuous infusion
Dopamine			
Renal dose	< 5 mcg/kg/min	400 mg in 250 mL	Continuous infusion
Inotrope	5-10 mcg/kg/min	400 mg in 250 mL	Continuous infusion
Pressor	> 10 mcg/kg/min	400 mg in 250 mL	Continuous infusion
Doripenem	500 mg q8h	In 100 mL	Infuse over 60 minutes
Doxycycline	100-200 mg q12-24h	In 250 mL	Infuse over 60 minutes
Droperidol	0.625-10 mg q1-4h	Undiluted	Inject over 3-5 minutes
Enalaprilat	0.625-1.25 mg q6h	Undiluted	Inject over 5 minutes Initial dose for patients on diuretics is 0.625 mg
Epinephrine	1-30 mcg/min	1 mg in 250 mL	Continuous infusion
Eptifibatide			
Bolus dose	180 mcg/kg	Undiluted	Maximum infusion duration of 72 hours; maximum bolus dose is 22.6 mg
Infusion dose	2 mcg/kg/min until discharge or CABG		Maximum infusion rate is 15 mg/h
Ertapenem	1 g q24h	1 g in 50 mL	Infuse over 30 minutes
Erythromycin	0.5-1 g q6h	In 250 mL	Infuse over 60 minutes Drug interactions: theophylline (4); cyclosporine (9)
Erythropoietin	12.5-600 U/kg 1-3 × per week	Undiluted	Inject over 3-5 minutes

(continued)

TABLE 22-1. INTRAVENOUS MEDICATION ADMINISTRATION GUIDELINES (continued)

Drug	Usual IV Dose Range[a]	Standard Dilution	Infusion Times/Comments/Drug Interactions
Esmolol			
Bolus dose	500 mcg/kg	Undiluted	Inject over 60 seconds
Infusion dose	50-400 mcg/kg/min	5 g in 500 mL	Continuous infusion
Ethacrynic acid	50 mg	In 50 mL	Inject over 3-5 minutes
			Maximum single dose 100 mg
Famotidine	20 mg q12h	In 100 mL	Infuse over 15-30 minutes
Fenoldopam			
Infusion dose	0.1-1.6 mcg/kg/min	20 mg in 250 mL	Titrate to BP
Fentanyl			
Bolus dose	25-100 mcg q1-2h	Undiluted	Inject over 5-10 seconds
Infusion dose	50-300 mcg/h	Undiluted	Continuous infusion
Filgrastim	1-20 mcg/kg × 2-4 weeks	In 50 mL	Preferred route of administration is subcutaneous
Fluconazole	100-800 mg q24h	Premix solution 2 mg/mL	Maximum infusion rate 200 mg/h
Flumazenil			
Reversal of conscious sedation	0.2 mg initially, then 0.2 mg q60s to a total of 1 mg	Undiluted	Inject over 15 seconds
			Maximum dose of 3 mg in any 1-hour period
Benzodiazepine overdose	0.2 mg initially, then 0.3 mg × 1 dose, then 0.5 mg q30s up to a total of 3 mg	Undiluted	Inject over 30 seconds
			Maximum dose of 3 mg in any 1-hour period
Continuous infusion	0.1-0.5 mg/h	5 mg in 1000 mL	Continuous infusion
Foscarnet			
Induction dose	60 mg/kg q8h	Undiluted or diluted to less than or equal to 12 mg/mL	Infuse over 1 hour; undiluted requires central line and diluted can be administered peripherally
Maintenance dose	90-120 mg/kg q24h	Undiluted or diluted to less than or equal to 12 mg/mL	Infuse over 2 hours; undiluted requires central line and diluted can be administered peripherally
Fosphenytoin		In 250 mL	Infuse no faster than 150 mg/min
Status epilepticus			
Loading dose	15-20 mg PE/kg		Maximum infusion rate 150 mg PE/min
Nonemergency			
Loading dose	10-20 mg PE/kg		Maximum infusion rate 150 mg PE/min
Maintenance dose	4-6 mg PE/kg/d		Maximum infusion rate 150 mg PE/min
Furosemide			
Bolus dose	10-100 mg q1-6h	Undiluted	Maximum injection rate 40 mg/min
Infusion dose	10-40 mg/h	100 mg in 100 mL	Continuous infusion
Ganciclovir	2.5-5 mg/kg q12h	In 100 mL	Infuse over 1 hour
Gentamicin			
Loading dose	2-3 mg/kg	In 50 mL	Infuse over 30 minutes
Maintenance dose	1-2.5 mg/kg q8-24h	In 50 mL	Infuse over 30 minutes
Extended interval dose	5-7 mg/kg q24h	In 50 mL	Infuse over 30 minutes
			Critically ill patients have an increased volume of distribution requiring increased doses
			Drug interactions: neuromuscular blocking agents
			Therapeutic levels: Peak: 3-12 mg/L, varies based on indication Trough: < 2 mg/L
			Extended interval dose: trough level at 24 hours = 0 mg/L; peak levels unnecessary
Glycopyrrolate	5-15 mcg/kg	Undiluted	Inject over 60 seconds
Granisetron	10 mcg/kg	In 50 mL	Infuse over 15 minutes
Haloperidol (lactate)			
Bolus dose	1-10 mg q2-4h	Undiluted	Inject over 3-5 minutes
Infusion dose	10 mg/h	100 mg in 100 mL	Continuous infusion is not generally recommended
			In urgent situations the dose may be doubled every 15-20 minutes until an effect is obtained
			Decanoate salt is only for IM administration

(continued)

TABLE 22-1. INTRAVENOUS MEDICATION ADMINISTRATION GUIDELINES (continued)

Drug	Usual IV Dose Range[a]	Standard Dilution	Infusion Times/Comments/Drug Interactions
Heparin			
Treatment of DVT, PE, arterial thromboembolism, or mural thrombosis			
Bolus dose	80 Units/kg	Undiluted	Titrate to PTT or antifactor Xa; drug interactions: nitroglycerin (11)
Maintenance dose	18 Units/kg/h	25,000 Units in 500 mL	Titrate to PTT or antifactor Xa; drug interactions: nitroglycerin (11)
ST-elevation myocardial infarction (STEMI), non-ST-elevation myocardial infarction (NSTEMI)			
Bolus dose	50-100 Units/kg	Undiluted	Titrate to ACT, PTT or antifactor Xa; drug interactions: nitroglycerin (11)
Maintenance dose	12 Units/kg/h	25,000 Units in 500 mL	Titrate to ACT, PTT or antifactor Xa; drug interactions: nitroglycerin (11)
Hydralazine	10-25 mg q2-4h	Undiluted	
Hydrochloric acid	mEq = $(0.5 \times BW \times (103 - \text{serum Cl}))$	100 mEq in 1000 mL	Maximum infusion rate 0.2 mEq/kg/h
Hydrocortisone	12.5-100 mg q6-12h	Undiluted	Inject over 60 seconds
Hydromorphone	0.5-2 mg q4-6h	Undiluted	Inject over 60 seconds
			Dilaudid-HP available as 10 mg/mL
Ibutilide			Infuse over 10 minutes
Patient 60 kg or more	1 mg	In 50 mL	Repeat dose possible 10 minutes after completion of initial bolus
Patient less than 60 kg	0.01 mg/kg		
Imipenem	0.5-1 g q6-8h	In 100 mL	Infuse over 30-60 minutes
Isoproterenol	1-10 mcg/min	2 mg in 500 mL	Continuous infusion
Labetalol			
Bolus dose	10-20 mg, then double q10 min (maximum total dose of 300 mg)	Undiluted	Inject over 2 minutes
Infusion dose	1-4 mg/min	200 mg in 160 mL	Continuous infusion
Levetiracetam	200-1500 mg q12h		Usual maximum of 3000 mg daily
Levofloxacin	250-750 mg q24-48h	In 50-150 mL	Infuse over 60 minutes (250 mg, 500 mg)
			Infuse over 90 minutes (750 mg)
Levothyroxine	25-200 mg q24h	Undiluted	Inject over 5-10 seconds
			IV dose = 75% of PO dose
Lidocaine			
Bolus dose	1 mg/kg	Undiluted	Inject over 60 seconds
Infusion dose	1-4 mg/min	2 g in 500 mL	Continuous infusion
			Drug interactions: cimetidine (6)
			Therapeutic levels: 1.5-5.0 mg/L
Linezolid	600 mg q12h	600 mg in 300 mL	Infuse over 30-120 minutes
			Linezolid may exhibit a yellow color that can intensify over time without adversely affecting potency
Lorazepam			
Bolus dose	0.5-2 mg q1-4h	Dilute 1:1 before administration	Inject 2 mg/min
Infusion dose	0.06 mg/kg/h	20 mg in 250 mL	Monitor for lorazepam precipitate in solution
			Use in-line filter during continuous infusion to avoid infusing precipitate into patient
Magnesium (elemental)			Magnesium 1 g = 8 mEq
Magnesium deficiency	25 mEq over 24 hours followed by 6 mEq over the next 12 hours	25 mEq in 1000 mL	Continuous infusion
Acute myocardial infarction	15-45 mEq over 24-48 hours followed by 12.5 mEq/day for 3 days	25 mEq in 1000 mL	Continuous infusion

(continued)

TABLE 22-1. **INTRAVENOUS MEDICATION ADMINISTRATION GUIDELINES (continued)**

Drug	Usual IV Dose Range[a]	Standard Dilution	Infusion Times/Comments/Drug Interactions
Ventricular arrhythmias	16 mEq over 1 hour followed by 40 mEq over 6 hours	40 mEq in 1000 mL	16 mEq (2 g) may be diluted in 100 mL D_5W and infused over 1 hour
Mannitol			
Diuretic		Undiluted	Inject over 30-60 minutes
Bolus dose	0.25-0.5 g/kg		
Maintenance dose	0.25-0.5 g/kg q4h		
Cerebral edema	1-2 g/kg over 30-60 minutes		
Meperidine	25-100 mg q2-4h	Undiluted	Inject over 60 seconds
			Avoid in renal failure
Meropenem	0.5-2 g q8-24h	In 50 mL or undiluted	Infuse over 15-30 minutes or bolus dose over 3-5 minutes
Methadone	5-20 mg qd	Undiluted	Inject over 3-5 minutes
			Accumulation with repetitive dosing
Methyldopate	0.25-1 g q6h	In 100 mL	Infuse over 30-60 minutes
Methylprednisolone	10-500 mg q6h	Undiluted	Inject over 60 seconds
Metoclopramide			
Small intestine intubation	10 mg × 1	Undiluted	Inject over 3-5 minutes
Antiemetic	2 mg/kg before chemotherapy, then 2 mg/kg q2h × 2, then q3h × 3	In 50 mL	Infuse over 15-30 minutes
Metoprolol	5 mg q2min × 3 for MI; 1.25-10 mg q6-12h for HTN	Undiluted	Inject over 3-5 minutes
Metronidazole	500 mg q6-8h	Premix solution 5 mg/mL	Infuse over 30 minutes
Midazolam			
Bolus dose	0.025-0.35 mg/kg q1-2h	Undiluted	Inject 0.5 mg/min
Infusion dose	0.5-5 mcg/kg/min	50 mg in 100 mL	Continuous infusion
			Unpredictable clearance in critically ill patients
			Drug interactions: cimetidine (6)
Morphine			
Bolus dose	2-10 mg	Undiluted	Inject over 60 seconds
Infusion dose	2-30 mg/h	100 mg in 100 mL	Continuous infusion
Moxifloxacin	400 mg q24h	400 mg in 250 mL	Infuse over 60 minutes
Nafcillin	0.5-2 g q4-6h	In 100 mL	Infuse over 30-60 minutes
Naloxone			
Postoperative opiate depression			
Loading dose	0.1-0.2 mg q2-3min	Undiluted	Infuse over 60 minutes
Infusion dose	3-5 mcg/kg/h	2 mg in 250 mL	Continuous infusion
Opiate overdose			
Loading dose	0.4-2 mg q2-3min	Undiluted	Infuse over 60 seconds
Infusion dose	2.5-5 mcg/kg/h	2 mg in 250 mL	Continuous infusion
Neostigmine	25-75 mcg/kg	Undiluted	Inject over 60 seconds
Nesiritide			
Bolus dose	2 mcg/kg		Monitor for hypotension
Infusion dose	0.01 mcg/kg/min	1.5 mg in 250 mL	
Nitroglycerin	10-300 mcg/min	50 mg in 250 mL	Continuous infusion
			Drug interactions: heparin (11)
Norepinephrine	4-30 mcg/min	4 mg in 250 mL	Continuous infusion
Ondansetron			
Chemotherapy-induced nausea and vomiting	32 mg 30 minutes before chemotherapy	In 50 mL	Infuse over 15-30 minutes
Postoperative nausea and vomiting	4 mg × 1 dose	Undiluted	Inject over 2-5 minutes
Oxacillin	0.5-2 g q4-6h	In 100 mL	Infuse over 30 minutes

(continued)

TABLE 22-1. INTRAVENOUS MEDICATION ADMINISTRATION GUIDELINES (continued)

Drug	Usual IV Dose Range[a]	Standard Dilution	Infusion Times/Comments/Drug Interactions
Pamidronate	60-90 mg × 1 dose	In 1000 mL	Infuse over 24 hours
			Metabolite contributes to activity
			Drug interactions: aminoglycosides (3); anticonvulsants (5)
Penicillin G	8-24 MU divided q4h or as continuous infusion	In 100 mL IVPB; higher volumes feasible for continuous infusion	Infuse over 15-30 minutes for IVPB, or administered as continuous infusion
Pentamidine	4 mg/kg q24h	In 50 mL	Infuse over 60 minutes
Phentolamine			
Bolus dose	2.5-10 mg prn q5-15 min	Undiluted	Inject over 3-5 minutes
Continuous infusion	1-10 mg/min	50 mg in 100 mL	Continuous infusion
Phenylephrine	20-200 mcg/min	15 mg in 250 mL	Continuous infusion; 0.5 mg over 20-30 seconds
Phenytoin			
Status epilepticus		Undiluted	Drug interactions: cimetidine; neuromuscular blocking agents
Bolus dose	15-20 mg/kg		Therapeutic total levels: 10-20 mg/L
			Therapeutic free levels: 1-2 mg/L
			Maximum infusion rate is 50 mg/min
Infusion dose	5 mg/kg/day (divided into 2 or 3 doses)		Maximum infusion rate is 50 mg/min
Phosphate (potassium)	0.08-0.64 mmol/kg	Function of K^+ concentration	Infuse over 6-8 hours
			1 mmol of PO_4 = P 31 mg
			Solution should be made no more concentrated than 0.4 mEq/mL K^+
Piperacillin/tazobactam	2.25-4.5 g IV q6-8h	In 100 mL	Infuse over 30 minutes
			Each 2.25-g vial contains 2 g piperacillin and 0.25 g tazobactam
Potassium chloride	5-40 mEq/h	10-40 mEq in 100-1000 mL	Cardiac monitoring should be used with infusion rates > 20 mEq/h
Propranolol			
Bolus dose	0.5-1 mg q5-15 min	Undiluted	Infuse over 60 seconds
Infusion dose	1-4 mg/h	50 mg in 500 mL	Continuous infusion
Protamine	< 30 min: 1-1.5 mg/100 Units; 30-60 minutes: 0.5-0.75 mg/ 100 Units; > 120 min: 0.25-0.375 mg/100 Units	50 mg in 5 mL	Inject over 3-5 minutes; do not exceed 50 mg in 10 minutes
Pyridostigmine	100-300 mcg/kg	Undiluted	Use to reverse long-acting neuromuscular blocking agents
			Inject over 60 seconds
Quinidine gluconate	600 mg initially, then 400 mg q2h, maintenance 200-300 mg q6h	800 mg in 50 mL	Infusion rate 1 mg/min; use cardiac monitor
			Therapeutic levels: 1.5-5 mg/L
Quinupristin/dalfopristin	7.5 mg/kg q8-12h	In 250 mL	Infuse over 60 minutes
			Central line preferred
			Flush with D_5W after peripheral infusion to minimize venous irritation
Ranitidine			
IVPB	50 mg q6-8h	In 50 mL	Infuse over 15-30 minutes
			IVP dose should be injected over at least 5 minutes
Infusion dose	6.25 mg/h	150 mg in 150 mL	Continuous infusion
Succinylcholine	0.6-2 mg/kg	Undiluted	Inject over 60 seconds
Tacrolimus	50-100 mcg/kg/day	5 mg in 250 mL	Continuous infusion, with targeted dose administered over 24 hours
Tenecteplase	30-50 mg	In 10 mL	Inject over 5 seconds; incompatible with dextrose solutions. Lines must be flushed prior to administration
Thiamine	100 mg qd, or 200-500 mg q8h for 5-7 days for treatment of Wernicke/Korsakoff syndrome	In 50 mL	Infuse over 15-30 minutes

(continued)

TABLE 22-1. INTRAVENOUS MEDICATION ADMINISTRATION GUIDELINES (continued)

Drug	Usual IV Dose Range[a]	Standard Dilution	Infusion Times/Comments/Drug Interactions
Tirofiban			
Bolus dose	25 mcg/kg	25 mg in 500 mL	Bolus infused over less than 5 minutes
Infusion dose	0.1 mcg/kg/min for 12-24 hours after angioplasty or atherectomy		
Tobramycin			
Loading dose	2-3 mg/kg	In 50 mL	Infuse over 30 minutes
Maintenance dose	1.5-2.5 mg/kg q8-24h	In 50 mL	Infuse over 30 minutes
Extended internal dose	5-7 mg/kg q24h		Critically ill patients have an increased volume of distribution requiring increased doses
			Drug interactions: neuromuscular blocking agents (3)
			Therapeutic levels
			Peak: 4-10 mg/L
			Trough: < 2 mg/L
Trimethoprim-sulfamethoxazole			
Common infections	4-5 mg/kg q12h	TMP 16 mg-SMX 80 mg per 25 mL	Infuse over 60 minutes
PCP	5 mg/kg q6h	TMP 16 mg-SMX 80 mg per 25 mL	Infuse over 60 minutes
			Therapeutic levels: 100-150 mg/L
Vancomycin	15 mg/kg q12h	In 250-500 mL	Infuse over at least 1 hour to avoid "red-man" syndrome
			Therapeutic levels
			Trough: < 20 mg/L
Vasopressin			
GI hemorrhage	0.2-0.3 U/min	50 Units in 50 mL	Maximum infusion rate 0.9 U/min
Septic shock	0.01-0.04 U/min		
Vecuronium			
Intubating dose	0.1-0.28 mg/kg	Undiluted	Inject over 60 seconds
Maintenance dose	0.01-0.015 mg/kg	Undiluted	Inject over 60 seconds
Infusion dose	1 mcg/kg/min	20 mg in 100 mL	Continuous infusion
			Metabolite contributes to activity
			Drug interactions: aminoglycosides (3); anticonvulsants (5)
Verapamil			
Bolus dose	0.075-0.15 mg/kg	Undiluted	Inject over 1-2 minutes
			Continuous infusion
			Drug interactions: digoxin (8)

[a]Usual dose ranges are listed; refer to appropriate disease state for specific dose.

Abbreviations: ACT, activated clotting time; aPTT, activated partial thromboplastin time; bid, twice a day; HF, heart failure; conc, concentration; D₅W, destrose-5%-water; DVT, deep venous thrombosis; HPLC, high-performance liquid chromatography; IM, intramuscular; IV, intravenous; IVP, IV push; IVPB, IV piggyback; MI, myocardial infarction; NS, normal saline; NSAID, nonsteroidal anti-inflammatory drug; PCP, pneumocystis carinii pneumonia; PE, pulmonary embolism; PO, orally; prn, as needed; PTT, partial thromboplastin time; qd, daily; SW, sterile water; TOF, train-of-four.

Drug interactions: (1) antagonizes adenosine effect; (2) potentiates adenosine effect; (3) potentiates effect of neuromuscular blocking agents; (4) inhibits theophylline metabolism; (5) antagonizes effect of neuromuscular blocking agents; (6) metabolism inhibited by cimetidine; (7) metabolism inhibited by ciprofloxacin; (8) increased digoxin concentrations; (9) metabolism inhibited by erythromycin; (10) increased nephrotoxicity; (11) increased heparin requirements.

TABLE 22-2. ORAL MEDICATION ADMINISTRATION GUIDELINES

Drug	Usual Oral Dose Range	Comments
Acetazolamide	250-500 mg qd-tid	May take with food to decrease GI upset
Acyclovir	400 mg bid or 200 mg tid-5 times/day	May take with or without food
Ampicillin	250-500 mg q6h	Take on empty stomach
Atenolol	25-100 mg qd	May take with or without food
Bumetanide	0.5-5 mg qd-bid (maximum of 10 mg)	
Calcium (elemental)	500-2000 mg divided 2-4 times/day	Take with meals to increase absorption
Cephalexin	250-1000 mg q6h	May take with food to decrease GI upset
Chlorothiazide	500-1000 mg qd-bid	
Chlorpromazine	10-25 mg q4-6h	
Cimetidine	300 mg qid or 800 mg qhs, or 400 mg bid	
Ciprofloxacin	250-750 mg qd-bid	Do not take with dairy products, calcium-fortified juices, oral multivitamins, or mineral supplements because of a decrease in ciprofloxacin absorption
Clindamycin	150-450 mg q6-8h	May take with or without food
Cyclosporine	1-15 mg/kg/day divided twice daily	Administer consistently with relation to time of day and meals for consistent levels
Dantrolene	25-100 mg bid-qid	
Desmopressin	0.1-1.2 mg daily divided 2-3 times/day	
Dexamethasone	4-10 mg qd-bid	May take with food to decrease GI upset
Diazepam	2-10 mg bid-qid	
Diazoxide	3-8 mg/kg/day divided 2-3 times/day	
Digoxin	0.125-0.5 mg qd	
Diltiazem	120-540 mg daily divided 1-2 times/day	Do not crush long-acting dosage forms. Capsules may be opened and pellets swallowed (without chewing pellets)
Diphenhydramine	25-150 mg daily divided 1-4 times/day	
Doxycycline	100 mg bid	Take with food to decrease GI upset. Do not take with dairy products or iron/calcium supplements due to decreased doxycycline absorption
Enalapril	2.5-40 mg daily divided 1-2 times/day	
Erythromycin	250-800 mg q6-12h	Do not crush enteric-coated dosage forms. GI upset, including diarrhea, is common. May take with food to decrease GI upset
Ethacrynic acid	50-400 mg daily divided 1-2 times/day	
Famotidine	20-40 mg daily divided 1-2 times/day	
Fluconazole	100-800 mg qd	
Furosemide	20-600 mg daily divided 1-4 times/day	Should be given on an empty stomach, however may take with food to decrease GI upset
Granisetron	1 mg bid or 2 mg qd	
Haloperidol	0.5-10 mg bid-tid	
Hydralazine	10-125 mg bid-qid	Take with food
Labetalol	100-400 mg bid	
Levofloxacin	250-750 mg qd	Do not take with dairy products, calcium-fortified juices, oral multivitamins, or mineral supplements because of a decrease in levofloxacin absorption
Levothyroxine	12.5-50 mcg qd	Take on empty stomach
Linezolid	400-600 mg q12h	
Lorazepam	1-10 mg daily divided 2-3 times/day	
Metoclopramide	5-10 mg tid	
Metoprolol	25-450 mg daily divided 2-3 times/day	Do not crush or chew extended release tablets
Metronidazole	250-750 mg daily divided 1-4 times/day	Take on empty stomach, however may take with food to decrease GI upset
Morphine	10-30 mg q3-4h prn	May take with food to decrease GI upset
Moxifloxacin	400 mg qd	Do not take with dairy products, calcium-fortified juices, oral multivitamins, or mineral supplements because of a decrease in moxifloxacin absorption
Nitroglycerin	2.5-9 mg bid-qid	
Ofloxacin	200-400 mg bid	Do not take with dairy products, calcium-fortified juices, oral multivitamins, or mineral supplements because of a decrease in ofloxacin absorption
Ondansetron	8-24 mg daily divided 1-3 times/day	
Phenytoin	5 mg/kg/day divided 1-3 times/day	Tube feedings decrease phenytoin absorption
Prednisolone	5-60 mg qd	May take with food to decrease GI upset

(continued)

TABLE 22-2. ORAL MEDICATION ADMINISTRATION GUIDELINES (continued)

Drug	Usual Oral Dose Range	Comments
Propranolol	30-320 mg daily divided 2-4 times/day	May take with or without food, however must be taken consistently (with or without food)
Ranitidine	300-600 mg daily divided 1-2 times/day	
Theophylline	400-900 mg daily divided 1-4 times/day	Long-acting preparations should be taken with a full glass of water, swallowed whole, or cut in half if scored. Do not crush. Extended release capsules may be opened and the contents swallowed (do not chew pellets)
Torsemide	2.5-20 mg qd	
Trimethoprim-sulfamethoxazole	6-20 mg/kg/day divided 2-4 times/day	Take with 8 oz. of water on empty stomach
Verapamil	120-480 mg daily divided 1-4 times/day	

TABLE 22-3. VASOACTIVE AGENTS

Agent and Dose	α	β_1	β_2	DM	SM	VD	VC	INT	CHT	Comments
Inotropes										
Dobutamine										Useful for acute management of low cardiac output states
2-10 mcg/kg/min	1+	3+	2+	—	—	1+	1+	3+	1+	
> 10-20 mcg/kg/min	2+	4+	3+	—	—	2+	1+	4+	2+	
Isoproterenol	—	4+	3+	—	—	3+	—	4+	4+	Used primarily for temporizing treatment of life-threatening bradycardia
2-10 mcg/kg/min										
Milrinone										Useful for acute management of low cardiac output states; can be combined with dobutamine
Loading dose: 50 mcg/kg over 10 min										
Maintenance dose: 0.375-0.75 mcg/kg/min	—	—	—	—	2+	2+	—	3+	3+	
Mixed										
Dopamine										Doses > 20-30 mcg/kg/min usually produce no added response
2-5 mcg/kg/min	—	3+	—	4+	—	—	—	2+	1+	
5-10 mcg/kg/min	—	4+	2+	4+	—	—	—	4+	2+	
10-20 mcg/kg/min	3+	4+	1+	—	—	—	3+	3+	3+	
Epinephrine										Mixed vasoconstrictor/inotrope; stronger inotrope than norepinephrine; does not constrict coronary or cerebral vessels; give as needed to maintain BP
0.01-0.05 mcg/kg/min	1+	4+	2+	—	—	1+	1+	4+	2+	
0.05 mcg/kg/min	4+	3+	1+	—	—	—	3+	3+	3+	
Vasopressors[a]										
Norepinephrine										Mixed vasoconstrictor/inotrope; give as needed to maintain BP (usually ≤ 20 mcg/min)
2-20 mcg/min titrate to effect	4+	2+	—	—	—	—	4+	1+	2+	
Phenylephrine										Pure vasoconstrictor without direct cardiac effect; may cause reflex bradycardia; useful when other pressors cause tachyarrhythmias; give as much as needed to maintain BP
Start at 30 mcg/min IV and titrate	4+	—	—	—	—	—	4+	—	—	
Vasopressin										Pure vasoconstrictor without direct cardiac effect; may cause gut ischemia if dose is increased > 0.04 U/min
0.01-0.04 U/min	—	—	—	—	—	—	4+	—	—	
Vasodilators										
Nitroglycerin										Tachyphylaxis, headache
20-100 mcg/min	—	—	—	—	4+	4+ A < V	—	—	1+	
Nitroprusside										Monitor thiocyanate levels if infusion duration > 48 hours; maintain thiocyanate level < 10 mg/dL
0.5-10 mcg/kg/min	—	—	—	—	4+	4+ A = V	—	—	1+	

[a]*Vasopressors usually are given by central vein and should be used only in conjunction with adequate volume repletion. All can precipitate myocardial ischemia. All except phenylephrine can cause tachyarrhythmias.*

Abbreviations: α_1, α_1-adrenergic; β_1, β_1-adrenergic; β_2, β_2-adrenergic; A, arterial; CHT, chronotropic; A, DM, dopaminergic; INT, inotropic; SM, smooth muscle; VC, vasoconstrictor; VD, vasodilator; V, venous.

Modified with permission from Oronato JC: Clinics in Emergency Medicine: Cardiovascular Emergencies. New York, NY: Churchill Livingstone; 1986.

TABLE 22-4. ANTIARRHYTHMIC AGENTS

Agents	Indications	Dosage	Comments
Class IA			
Quinidine	Ventricular ectopy; conversion of atrial fibrillation and atrial flutter; WPW	Quinidine sulfate: 200-300 mg PO q6h Quinidine gluconate: 324-648 mg PO q8h	Diarrhea, nausea, headache, dizziness; hypersensitivity reactions including thrombocytopenia; hemolysis; fever hepatitis; rash QT prolongation; increased digoxin level
			Dosage adjustment should be made when switching from one salt to another: Quinidine sulfate (83% quinidine), gluconate (62% quinidine), polygalacturonate (60% quinidine)
			Therapeutic range: 1.5-5 mg/L
Procainamide	Ventricular ectopy; conversion of atrial fibrillation and atrial flutter; WPW	15-17 mg/kg bolus, infused at 20-30 mg/min, followed by continuous infusion at 1-4 mg/min	Usual initial maintenance dose is about 50 mg/kg/day Therapeutic range procainamide : 4-10 mcg/mL Therapeutic range NAPA: 10-20 mcg/mL
Disopyramide	Ventricular ectopy; conversion of atrial fibrillation and atrial flutter; WPW	100-300 mg PO q6h; SR: 100-300 mg PO q12h	Anticholinergic effects; negative inotropy; QT prolongation Therapeutic range: 2-4 mg/L
Class IB			
Lidocaine	Malignant ventricular ectopy; WPW	1.5 mg/kg IV over 2 minutes, then 1-4 mg/min	No benefit in atrial arrhythmias Seizures; paresthesias; delirium; levels increased by cimetidine; minimal hemodynamic effects
			Therapeutic range: 1.5-5 mg/L
Mexiletine	Malignant ventricular ectopy	150-300 mg PO q6-8h with food	No benefit in atrial arrhythmias
			Less effective than IA and IC agents
			Nausea; tremor; dizziness; delirium; levels increased by cimetidine
			Therapeutic range: 0.5-2 mg/L
Class IC			
Flecainide	Life-threatening ventricular arrhythmias refractory to other agents	100-200 mg PO q12h	Proarrhythmic effects; moderate negative inotropy; dizziness; conduction abnormalities
	Prevention of symptomatic, disabling, paroxysmal supraventricular arrhythmias, including atrial fibrillation or flutter and WPW in patients without structural heart disease		Therapeutic range: 0.2-1 mg/L
Propafenone	Life-threatening ventricular arrhythmias refractory to other agents	150-300 mg PO q8h	Proarrhythmic effects; negative inotropy; dizziness; nausea; conduction abnormalities
	SVT, WPW, and paroxysmal atrial fibrillation or flutter in patients without structural heart disease		
Class II (beta-blocking agents)			
Propranolol	Slowing ventricular rate in atrial fibrillation, atrial flutter, and SVT; suppression of PVCs	Up to 0.5-1 mg IV, then 1-4 mg/h (or 10-100 mg PO q6h)	Not cardioselective; hypotension; bronchospasm; negative inotropy
Esmolol	Slowing ventricular rate in atrial fibrillation, atrial flutter, SVT, and MAT	Loading dose: 500 mcg/over 1 minute; Maintenance dose: 50 mcg/kg/min; rebolus and increase q5min by 50 mcg/kg/min to maximum of 400 mcg/kg/min	Cardioselective at low doses; hypotension; negative inotropy; very short half-life
Metoprolol	Slowing ventricular rate in atrial fibrillation, atrial flutter, SVT, and MAT	Initial IV dose: 5 mg q5min up to 15 mg, then 25-100 mg PO q8-12h	Cardioselective at low doses; hypotension; negative inotropy
Class III			
Amiodarone	Life-threatening ventricular arrhythmias, supraventricular arrhythmias, including WPW refractory to other agents	800-1600 mg PO qd for 1-3 weeks, then 600-800 mg PO qd for 4 weeks, then 100-400 mg PO qd	Half-life > 50 days; pulmonary fibrosis; corneal microdeposits; hypo/hyperthyroidism; bluish skin; hepatitis; photosensitivity; conduction abnormalities; mild negative inotropy; increased effect of coumadin; increased digoxin level
			Therapeutic range: 1-2.5 mg/L
Sotalol	Life-threatening ventricular arrhythmia	80-160 mg PO q12h; may increase up to 160 mg PO q8h	Beta-blocker with class III properties; proarrhythmic effects; QT prolongation
Dofetilide	Conversion of atrial fibrillation	250-500 mcg orally twice a day	Dose adjusted based on QTc interval and creatinine clearance

(continued)

TABLE 22-4. ANTIARRHYTHMIC AGENTS (continued)

Agents	Indications	Dosage	Comments
Class IV (calcium channel antagonists)			
Verapamil	Conversion of SVT; slowing ventricular rate in atrial fibrillation, atrial flutter, and MAT	IV bolus: 5-10 mg over 2-3 minutes (repeat in 30 min prn) Continuous infusion: 2.5-5 mcg/kg/min PO: 40-160 mg PO q8h	Hypotension; negative inotropy; conduction disturbances; increased digoxin level; generally contraindicated in WPW
Diltiazem	Conversion of SVT; slowing ventricular rate in atrial fibrillation, atrial flutter, and MAT	IV bolus: 0.25 mg/kg over 2 minutes (repeat in 15 minutes prn with 0.35 mg/kg IV) Maintenance infusion: 5-15 mg/h PO: 30-90 mg PO q6h	Hypotension; less negative inotropy than verapamil; conduction disturbances; rare hepatic injury; generally contraindicated in WPW
Miscellaneous agents			
Adenosine	Conversion of SVT, including WPW	6-mg rapid IV bolus; if ineffective, 12-mg rapid IV bolus 2 minutes later; follow bolus with fast flush; use smaller doses if giving through central venous line	Flushing; dyspnea; nodal blocking effect increased by dipyridamole and decreased by theophylline and caffeine; very short half-life ($\approx$ 10 seconds)
Atropine	Initial therapy for symptomatic bradycardia	0.5-mg IV bolus; repeat q5min prn to total of 2 mg IV	May induce tachycardia and ischemia
Digoxin	Slowing AV conduction in atrial fibrillation and atrial flutter	Loading dose: 0.5 mg IV, then 0.25 mg IV q4-6h up to 1 mg; maintenance dose: 0.125-0.375 mg PO/IV qd	Heart block; arrhythmias; nausea; yellow vision; numerous drug interactions; generally contraindicated in WPW Therapeutic range: 0.5-2.0 mg/mL

Abbreviations: AV, atrioventricular; IV, intraventricular; MAT, multifocal atrial tachycardia; NAPA, N-acetylprocainamide; PO, per oral; PVC, premature ventricular complex; SR, sustained release; SVT, supraventricular tachycardia; WPW, Wolff-Parkinson-White.

TABLE 22-5. THERAPEUTIC DRUG MONITORING

Drug	Usual Therapeutic Range	Usual Sampling Time
Antibiotics		
Amikacin	Peak: 20-40 mg/L	Peak: 30-60 minutes after a 30-minute infusion
	Trough: < 10 mg/L	Trough: Just before next dose
Chloramphenicol	Peak: 10-25 mg/L	Peak: 30-90 minutes after a 30-minute infusion
	Trough: 5-10 mg/L	Trough: Just before the next dose
Flucytosine	Peak: 50-100 mg/L	Peak: 1-2 hours after an oral dose
	Trough: < 25 mg/L	Trough: Just before the next dose
Gentamicin	Peak: 4-10 mg/L	Peak: 30-60 minutes after a 30-minute infusion
	Trough: < 2 mg/L	Trough: Just before the next dose
Tobramycin	Peak: 4-10 mg/L	Peak: 30-60 minutes after a 30-minute infusion
	Trough: < 2 mg/L	Trough: Just before the next dose
Vancomycin	Trough: < 20 mg/L	Trough: Just before the next dose
Sulfonamides (sulfamethoxazole, sulfadiazine, cotrimoxazole)	Peak: 100-150 mg/L	Peak: 2 hours after 1-hour infusion Trough: Not applicable
Antiarrhythmics		
Digoxin	0.5-2 mcg/L	Peak: 8-12 hours after administered dose Trough: Just before next dose
Lidocaine	1.5-5 mg/L	Anytime during a continuous infusion
Procainamide/NAPA	Procainamide: 4-10 mg/L NAPA: 10-20 mg/L	
Quinidine	1.5-5 mg/L	Trough: Just before next dose
Anticonvulsants		
Carbamazepine	4-12 mg/L	Trough: Just before next dose
Pentobarbital	20-50 mcg/L	IV: Immediately after IV loading dose: anytime during continuous infusion
Phenobarbital	15-40 mg/L	Trough: Just before next dose
Phenytoin	10-20 mg/L	IV: 2-4 hours after dose Trough: PO/IV: Just before next dose Free phenytoin level: 1-2 mg/L
Valproic acid	50-100 mg/L	Trough: Just before next dose
Miscellaneous		
Cyclosporine	50-150 ng/mL (whole blood, HPLC)	Trough: IV, PO: Just before next dose

CARDIAC RHYTHMS, ECG CHARACTERISTICS, AND TREATMENT GUIDE

Carol Jacobson

23

Rhythm	ECG Characteristics	ECG Sample	Treatment
Normal sinus rhythm (NSR)	• Rate: 60-100 beats/min. • Rhythm: Regular. • P waves: Precede every QRS; consistent shape. • PR interval: 0.12-0.20 second. • QRS complex: 0.04-0.10 second.		• None.
Sinus bradycardia	• Rate: < 60 beats/min. • Rhythm: Regular. • P waves: Precede every QRS; consistent shape. • PR interval: Usually normal (0.12-0.20 second). • QRS complex: Usually normal (0.04-0.10 second). • Conduction: Normal through atria, AV node, bundle branches, and ventricles.		• Treat only if symptomatic. • Atropine 0.5 mg IV. • Temporary pacing may be necessary until cause is corrected.
Sinus tachycardia	• Rate: > 100 beats/min. • Rhythm: Regular. • P waves: Precede every QRS; consistent shape. • PR interval: Usually normal (0.12-0.20 second); may be difficult to measure if P waves are buried in T waves. • QRS complex: Usually normal (0.04-0.10 second). • Conduction: Normal through atria, AV node, bundle branches, and ventricles.		• Treat underlying cause.
Sinus arrhythmia	• Rate: 60-100 beats/min. • Rhythm: Irregular; phasic increase and decrease in rate, which may or may not be related to respiration. • P waves: Precede every QRS; consistent shape. • PR interval: Usually normal. • QRS complex: Usually normal. • Conduction: Normal through atria, AV node, bundle branches, and ventricles.		• Treatment is usually not required.
Sinus arrest	• Rate: Usually within normal range, but may be in the bradycardia range. • Rhythm: Irregular due to absence of sinus node discharge. • P waves: Present when sinus node is firing and absent during periods of sinus arrest. When present, they precede every QRS complex and are consistent in shape. • PR interval: Usually normal when P waves are present. • QRS complex: Usually normal when sinus node is functioning and absent during periods of sinus arrest, unless escape beats occur. • Conduction: Normal through atria, AV node, bundle branches, and ventricles when sinus node is firing. When the sinus node fails to form impulses, there is no conduction through the atria.		• Treat underlying cause. • Discontinue drugs that may be causative. • Minimize vagal stimulation. • For frequent sinus arrest causing hemodynamic compromise, atropine 0.5 mg IV may increase heart rate. • Pacemaker may be necessary for refractory cases.

Premature atrial contraction

- Rate: Usually within normal range.
- Rhythm: Usually regular except when PACs occur, resulting in early beats. PACs usually have a noncompensatory pause.
- P waves: Precede every QRS. The configuration of the premature P wave differs from that of the sinus P waves.
- PR interval: May be normal or long depending on the prematurity of the beat. Very early PACs may find the AV junction still partially refractory and unable to conduct at a normal rate, resulting in a prolonged PR interval.
- QRS complex: May be normal, aberrant (wide), or absent, depending on the prematurity of the beat.
- Conduction: PACs travel through the atria differently from sinus impulses because they originate from a different spot. Conduction through the AV node, bundle branches, and ventricles is usually normal unless the PAC is very early.

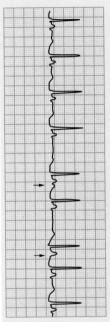

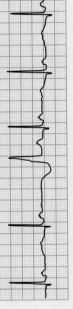

PACs conducted normally in the ventricle.

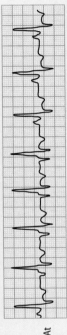

PAC conducted abnormally in the ventricle.

- Treatment is usually not necessary.
- Treat underlying cause.
- Drugs (eg, beta-blockers, disopyramide, flecainide, propafenone) can be used if necessary.

Wandering atrial pacemaker

- Rate: 60-100 beats/min.
- Rhythm: May be slightly irregular.
- P waves: Varying shapes (upright, flat, inverted, notched) as impulses originate in different parts of the atria or junction. At least three different P-wave shapes should be seen.
- PR interval: May vary depending on proximity of the pacemaker to the AV node.
- QRS complex: Usually normal.
- Conduction: Conduction through the atria varies as they are depolarized from different spots. Conduction through the bundle branches and ventricles is usually normal.

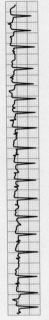

- Treatment is usually not necessary.
- Treat underlying cause.
- For symptoms from slow rate, use atropine.

Multifocal atrial tachycardia

- Rate: Faster than 100.
- Rhythm: Irregular.
- P waves: Varying shapes (upright, flat, inverted, notched) as impulses originate in different parts of the atria or junction. At least three different P-wave shapes should be seen. Often misdiagnosed as atrial fibrillation.
- PR interval: May vary depending on proximity of the pacemaker to the AV node.
- QRS complex: Usually normal.
- Conduction: Conduction through the atria varies as they are depolarized from different spots. Conduction through the bundle branches and ventricles is usually normal.

- Treat underlying cause.
- Acute rate control: IV beta-blockers, IV verapamil.
- Oral beta-blockers, verapamil, diltiazem.
- Maintain normal Mg^{++} and K^{+} levels.

(continued)

Rhythm	ECG Characteristics	ECG Sample	Treatment
Atrial tachycardia	• Rate: Atrial rate is 120-250 beats/min. • Rhythm: Regular unless there is variable block at the AV node. • P waves: Differ in shape from sinus P waves because they are ectopic. Precede each QRS complex but may be hidden in preceding T wave. When block is present, more than one P wave appears before each QRS complex. • PR interval: May be shorter than normal but often difficult to measure because of hidden P waves. • QRS complex: Usually normal but may be wide if aberrant conduction is present. • Conduction: Usually normal through the AV node and into the ventricles. In atrial tachycardia with block, some atrial impulses do not conduct into the ventricles. Aberrant ventricular conduction may occur if atrial impulses are conducted into the ventricles while the ventricles are still partially refractory.		• Eliminate underlying cause and decrease ventricular rate. • Adenosine may be effective in some ATs. • IV beta-blockers, verapamil, or diltiazem can slow ventricular rate. • Flecainide, propafenone, amiodarone, sotalol, and dofetilide may be effective for ongoing management. • Cardioversion may be successful for reentry AT but not for automatic AT. • Radiofrequency ablation is often successful.
Atrial flutter	• Rate: Atrial rate varies between 250 and 350 beats/min, most commonly 300. Ventricular rate varies depending on the amount of block at the AV node. • Rhythm: Atrial rhythm is regular. Ventricular rhythm may be regular or irregular due to varying AV block. • P waves: Flutter waves (F waves) are seen, characterized by a very regular, "sawtooth" pattern. One F wave is usually hidden in the QRS complex, and when 2:1 conduction occurs, F waves may not be readily apparent. • FR interval (flutter wave to the beginning of the QRS complex): May be consistent or may vary. • QRS complex: Usually normal; aberration can occur. • Conduction: Usually normal through the AV node and ventricles.	 	• Cardioversion is preferred for markedly reduced cardiac output. • Beta-blockers, verapamil, or diltiazem for ventricular rate control. IV amiodarone can be used for rate control if systolic heart failure. • Oral dofetilide or IV ibutilide for pharmacological conversion. • Amiodarone, dofetilide, or sotalol to maintain sinus rhythm. • Radiofrequency ablation is usually successful.
Atrial fibrillation	• Rate: Atrial rate is 400-600 beats/min or faster. Ventricular rate varies depending on the amount of block at the AV node. In new atrial fibrillation, the ventricular response is usually quite rapid, 160-200 beats/min; in treated atrial fibrillation, the ventricular rate is controlled in the normal range of 60-100 beats/min. • Rhythm: Irregular. One of the distinguishing features of atrial fibrillation is the marked irregularity of the ventricular response. • P waves: Not present. Atrial activity is chaotic with no formed atrial impulses visible. Irregular F waves are often seen and vary in size from coarse to very fine. • PR interval: Not measurable; there are no P waves. • QRS complex: Usually normal; aberration is common. • Conduction: Conduction within the atria is disorganized and follows a very irregular pattern. Most of the atrial impulses are blocked within the AV junction. Those impulses that are conducted through the AV junction are usually conducted normally through the ventricles. If an atrial impulse reaches the bundle branch system during its refractory period, aberrant intraventricular conduction can occur.	 	• Eliminate underlying cause. • Cardiovert, if hemodynamically unstable. • Calcium channel blockers and beta-blockers are used to slow ventricular rate. • Flecainide, dofetilide, propafenone, ibutilide, and amiodarone are used to convert to sinus. • Amiodarone, dofetilide, dronedarone, flecainide, propafenone, or sotalol are used for maintenance of sinus rhythm. • Radiofrequency ablation often successful.

		Characteristics	Treatment
Premature junctional complexes	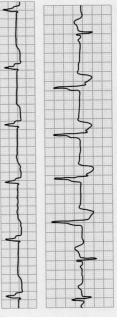 ↑ PJC	• Rate: 60-100 beats/min or whatever the rate of the basic rhythm. • Rhythm: Regular except for occurrence of premature beats. • P waves: May occur before, during, or after the QRS complex of the premature beat and are usually inverted. • PR interval: Short, usually 0.10 second or less, when P waves precede the QRS. • QRS complex: Usually normal but may be aberrant if the PJC occurs very early and conducts into the ventricles during the refractory period of a bundle branch. • Conduction: Retrograde through the atria; usually normal through the ventricles.	• Treatment is usually not necessary.
Junctional rhythm		• Rate: Junctional rhythm, 40-60 beats/min; accelerated junctional rhythm, 60-100 beats/min; junctional tachycardia, 100-250 beats/min. • Rhythm: Regular. • P waves: May precede or follow QRS. • PR interval: Short, 0.10 second or less if P waves precede QRS. • QRS complex: Usually normal. • Conduction: Retrograde through the atria; normal through the ventricles.	• Treatment is rarely needed unless rate is too slow or too fast to maintain adequate CO. • Atropine is used to increase rate. • Verapamil, propranolol, or beta-blockers are used to decrease rate. • Withhold digitalis, if digitalis toxicity is suspected.
Premature ventricular complexes		• Rate: 60-100 beats/min or the rate of the basic rhythm. • Rhythm: Irregular because of the early beats. • P waves: Not related to the PVCs. Sinus rhythm is usually not interrupted by the premature beats, so sinus P waves can often be seen occurring regularly throughout the rhythm. • PR interval: Not present before most PVCs. If a P wave happens, by coincidence, to precede a PVC, the PR interval is short. • QRS complex: Wide and bizarre; > 0.10 second in duration. May vary in morphology (size, shape) if they originate from more than one focus in the ventricles. • Conduction: Wide QRS complexes. Some PVCs may conduct retrograde into the atria, resulting in inverted P waves following the PVC.	• Eliminate underlying cause. • Drug therapy is not usually used, but, if desired, lidocaine, amiodarone, procainamide, beta-blockers may be effective.
Ventricular rhythm		• Rate: < 50 beats/min for ventricular rhythm and 50-100 beats/min for accelerated ventricular rhythm. • Rhythm: Usually regular. • P waves: May be seen but at a slower rate than the ventricular focus, with dissociation from the QRS. • PR interval: Not measured. • QRS complex: Wide and bizarre. • Conduction: If sinus rhythm is the basic rhythm, atrial conduction is normal. Impulses originating in the ventricles conduct via muscle cell-to-cell conduction, resulting in the wide QRS complex.	• For ventricular escape rhythms, use atropine to increase sinus rate and overdrive ventricular rhythm. • Use ventricular pacing to increase ventricular rate if escape rhythm is too slow.

(continued)

Rhythm	ECG Characteristics	ECG Sample	Treatment
Monomorphic ventricular tachycardia	• Rate: Ventricular rate is faster than 100 beats/min. • Rhythm: Usually regular but may be slightly irregular. • P waves may be seen but will not be related to QRS complexes (dissociated from QRS complexes). If sinus rhythm is the underlying basic rhythm, regular P waves are often buried within QRS complexes. • PR interval: Not measurable because of dissociation of P waves from QRS complexes. • QRS complex: Wide and bizarre; > 0.10 second in duration. • Conduction: Impulse originates in one ventricle and spreads via muscle cell-to-cell conduction through both ventricles. There may be retrograde conduction through the atria, but more often the sinus node continues to fire regularly and depolarize the atria normally.		• Treatment depends on how rhythm is tolerated. • Lidocaine, amiodarone, or procainamide should be given if patient is stable. • Cardioversion is preferred for hemodynamic instability. • Defibrillation should be performed if VT is pulseless. • Radiofrequency ablation is successful for some monomorphic VTs.
Ventricular tachycardia (polymorphic)	• Regularity: irregular. • Rate: > 100 beats/min, often very fast. • P waves: none associated with VT. • PR interval: none. • QRS width: > 0.12 second, multiple shapes. • QT interval is normal (< 0.47 sec)	V1 QT interval is normal (QTc = 0.39 sec)	• Treat ischemia with beta-blockers, angioplasty/stent, or CABG. • IV magnesium or overdrive pacing can be used until the cause is corrected. • Defibrillate if it becomes sustained with loss of consciousness.
Torsades de pointes (Polymorphic VT associated with prolonged QT interval)	• Regularity: irregular. • Rate: > 100 beats/min, often very fast. • P waves: none associated with VT. • PR interval: none. • QRS width: > 0.12 seconds, multiple shapes, often appears to twist around the baseline. • QT interval is prolonged; QTc > 0.50 seconds increases risk.	QT interval is very long (0.76 sec)	• Discontinue causative drugs. • Correct electrolyte imbalances. • IV amiodarone or lidocaine may be used. • Defibrillate if it becomes sustained with loss of consciousness.
Ventricular fibrillation	• Rate: Rapid, uncoordinated, ineffective. • Rhythm: Chaotic, irregular. • P waves: None seen. • PR interval: None. • QRS complex: No formed QRS complexes seen; rapid, irregular undulations without any specific pattern. • Conduction: Multiple ectopic foci firing simultaneously in ventricles and depolarizing them irregularly and without any organized pattern. Ventricles are not contracting.		• Immediate defibrillation. • CPR required until defibrillator is available. • Amiodarone, lidocaine, magnesium are commonly used. • After conversion, use IV antiarrhythmic that facilitates conversion to prevent recurrence.
Ventricular asystole	• Rate: None. • Rhythm: None. • P waves: May be present if the sinus node is functioning. • PR interval: None. • QRS complex: None. • Conduction: Atrial conduction may be normal if the sinus node is functioning. There is no conduction into the ventricles.		• Provide immediate CPR. • Give IV epinephrine. • Identify and treat cause.

Type	ECG	Description	Treatment
First-degree AV block		• Rate: Can occur at any sinus rate, usually 60-100 beats/min. • Rhythm: Regular. • P waves: Normal; precede every QRS. • PR interval: Prolonged above 0.20 second. • QRS complex: Usually normal. • Conduction: Normal through the atria, delayed through the AV node. Ventricular conduction is normal.	• Treatment is usually not necessary.
Second-degree AV block type I (Wenckebach; Mobitz I)		• Rate: Can occur at any sinus or atrial rate. • Rhythm: Irregular. Overall appearance of the rhythm demonstrates "group beating." • P waves: Normal. Some P waves are not conducted to the ventricles, but only one at a time fails to conduct to the ventricle. • PR interval: Gradually lengthens in consecutive beats. The PR interval preceding the pause is longer than that following the pause. • QRS complex: Usually normal unless there is associated bundle branch block. • Conduction: Normal through the atria, progressively delayed through the AV node until an impulse fails to conduct. Conduction ratios can vary, with ratios as low as 2:1 (every other P wave is blocked), up to high ratios such as 15:14 (every 15th P wave blocked).	• Treatment depends on conduction ratio, ventricular rate, and symptoms. • Atropine is used for slow ventricular rate. • No treatment is given with normal ventricular rate. • Hold digitalis, beta-blockers, and calcium channel blockers. • Temporary pacemaker may be needed for slow ventricular rate.
Second-degree AV block type II (Mobitz II)		• Rate: Can occur at any basic rate. • Rhythm: Irregular because of blocked beats. • P waves: Usually regular and precede each QRS. Periodically a P wave is not followed by a QRS complex. • PR interval: Constant before conducted beats. The PR interval preceding the pause is the same as that following the pause. • QRS complex: Usually wide due to associated bundle branch block. • Conduction: Normal through the atria and through the AV node but intermittently blocked in the bundle branch system and fails to reach the ventricles. Conduction through the ventricles is abnormally slow owing to associated bundle branch block. Conduction ratios can vary from 2:1 to only occasional blocked beats.	• Pacemaker is often needed. • Atropine is not recommended.

(continued)

Rhythm	ECG Characteristics	ECG Sample	Treatment
High-grade (advanced) AV block	• Rate: Atrial rate < 135 beats/min. • Rhythm: Regular or irregular, depending on conduction pattern. • P waves: Normal; present before every conducted QRS, but two or more consecutive P waves are not followed by QRS complexes. • PR interval: Constant before conducted beats; may be normal or prolonged. • QRS complex: Usually normal in type I and wide in type II advanced blocks. • Conduction: Normal through the atria. Two or more consecutive atrial impulses fail to conduct to the ventricles. Ventricular conduction is normal in type I and abnormally slow in type II advanced blocks.		• Treatment is necessary if patient is symptomatic. • Atropine may increase ventricular rate. • Pacemaker is often required.
Third-degree AV block (complete)	• Rate: Atrial rate is usually normal; ventricular rate is < 45 beats/min. • Rhythm: Regular. • P waves: Normal but dissociated from QRS complexes. • PR interval: No consistent PR intervals because there is no relationship between P waves and QRS complexes. • QRS complex: Normal if ventricles controlled by a junctional rhythm; wide if controlled by a ventricular rhythm. • Conduction: Normal through the atria. All impulses are blocked at the AV node or in the bundle branches, so there is no conduction to the ventricles. Conduction through the ventricles is normal if a junctional escape rhythm occurs, and abnormally slow if a ventricular escape rhythm occurs.		• Pacemaker. • Atropine is usually not effective. • With severely decreased cardiac output, perform CPR until pacemaker available.
Ventricular paced rhythm with capture	• Rate: Depends on programmed pacing rate. • Rhythm: Regular. • P waves: Absent or present but dissociated from QRS complexes. • PR interval: None. • QRS complex: Pacemaker spike followed immediately by wide, bizarre QRS complex. • Rate: Depends on programmed pacing rate.		• None.
Ventricular paced rhythm without capture	• Conduction: Abnormal. • ECG characteristics depend on nature of intrinsic rhythm. • Pacemaker spike has no fixed relationship to QRS complexes.		• Increase mA. • Reposition patient to reestablish contact of pacing lead with myocardium. • If hemodynamically unstable, treat as third-degree AV block or asystole as necessary.

INDEX